Optum

ICD-10-PCS

The complete official code set

Codes valid from October 1, 2022
through September 30, 2023

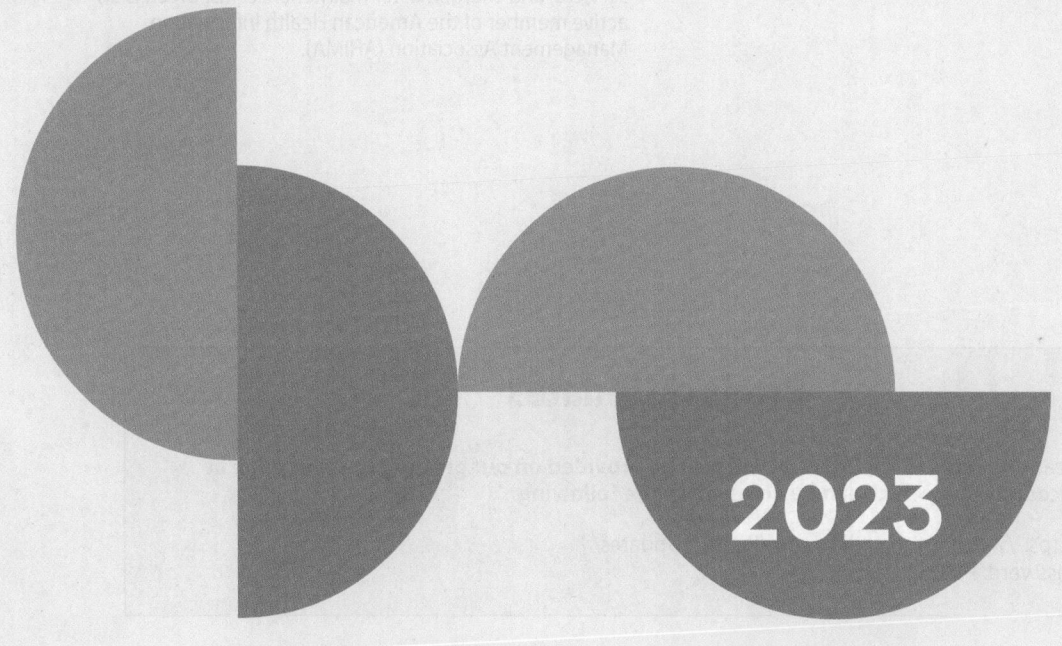

2023

optumcoding.com

Notice

ICD-10-PCS: The Complete Official Code Set is designed to be an accurate and authoritative source regarding coding and every reasonable effort has been made to ensure accuracy and completeness of the content. However, Optum makes no guarantee, warranty, or representation that this publication is accurate, complete, or without errors. It is understood that Optum is not rendering any legal or other professional services or advice in this publication and that Optum bears no liability for any results or consequences that may arise from the use of this book. Please address all correspondence to:

Optum
2525 Lake Park Blvd
Salt Lake City, UT 84120

Our Commitment to Accuracy

Optum is committed to producing accurate and reliable materials.

To report corrections, please email customerassistance@optum.com. You can also reach customer service by calling 1.800.464.3649, option 1.

Copyright

Property of Optum, Inc. Optum and the Optum logo are trademarks of Optum, Inc. All other brand or product names are trademarks or registered trademarks of their respective owner.

© 2022 Optum, Inc. All rights reserved.

Made in the USA
ISBN 978-1-62254-838-5 (Spiral)
ISBN 978-1-62254-839-2 (Softbound)

Acknowledgments

Marianne Randall, CPC, *Product Manager*

Anita Schmidt, BS, RHIA, AHIMA-approved ICD-10-CM/PCS Trainer, *Subject Matter Expert*

LaJuana Green, RHIA, CCS, *Subject Matter Expert*

Stacy Perry, *Manager, Desktop Publishing*

Tracy Betzler, *Senior Desktop Publishing Specialist*

Hope M. Dunn, *Senior Desktop Publishing Specialist*

Katie Russell, *Desktop Publishing Specialist*

Kate Holden, *Editor*

Anita Schmidt, BS, RHIA, AHIMA-approved ICD-10-CM/PCS Trainer

Ms. Schmidt has expertise in ICD-10-CM/PCS, DRG, and CPT with more than 15 years' experience in coding in multiple settings, including inpatient, observation, and same-day surgery. Her experience includes analysis of medical record documentation, assignment of ICD-10-CM and PCS codes, and DRG validation. She has conducted training for ICD-10-CM/PCS and electronic health record. She has also collaborated with clinical documentation specialists to identify documentation needs and potential areas for physician education. Most recently she has been developing content for resource and educational products related to ICD-10-CM, ICD-10-PCS, DRG, and CPT. Ms. Schmidt is an AHIMA-approved ICD-10-CM/PCS trainer and is an active member of the American Health Information Management Association (AHIMA) and the Minnesota Health Information Management Association (MHIMA).

LaJuana Green, RHIA, CCS

Ms. Green is a registered health information administrator with over 35 years of experience in multiple areas of information management. She has proven expertise in the analysis of medical record documentation, assignment of ICD-10-CM and PCS codes, DRG validation, and CPT code assignment in ambulatory surgery units and the hospital outpatient setting. Her experience includes serving as a director of a health information management department, clinical technical editing, new technology research and writing, medical record management, utilization review activities, quality assurance, tumor registry, medical library services, and chargemaster maintenance. Ms. Green is an active member of the American Health Information Management Association (AHIMA).

Product Updates

Significant updates to this manual will also be provided on our product updates page at Optumcoding.com, which can be accessed at the following:

https://www.optumcoding.com/ProductUpdates/
Password: PCS23

Procedure	Code
231. Sacrococcygeal fusion with bone graft from same operative site, open	
232. Interphalangeal fusion of left great toe, percutaneous pin fixation	
233. Suture repair of left radial nerve laceration	
234. Laparotomy with suture repair of blunt force duodenal laceration	
235. Perineoplasty with repair of old obstetric laceration, open	
236. Suture repair of right biceps tendon (upper arm) laceration, open	
237. Closure of abdominal wall stab wound	
238. Cosmetic face lift, open, no other information available	
239. Bilateral breast augmentation with silicone implants, open	
240. Cosmetic rhinoplasty with septal reduction and tip elevation using local tissue graft, open	
241. Abdominoplasty (tummy tuck), open	
242. Liposuction of bilateral thighs	
243. Creation of penis in female patient using tissue bank donor graft	
244. Creation of vagina in male patient using synthetic material	
245. Laparoscopic vertical (sleeve) gastrectomy	
246. Left uterine artery embolization with intraluminal biosphere injection	

Obstetrics

Procedure	Code
1. Abortion by dilation and evacuation following laminaria insertion	
2. Manually assisted spontaneous abortion	
3. Abortion by abortifacient insertion	
4. Bimanual pregnancy examination	
5. Extraperitoneal C-section, low transverse incision	
6. Fetal spinal tap, percutaneous	
7. Fetal kidney transplant, laparoscopic	
8. Open in utero repair of congenital diaphragmatic hernia	
9. Laparoscopy with total excision of tubal pregnancy	
10. Transvaginal removal of fetal monitoring electrode	

Placement

Procedure	Code
1. Placement of packing material, right ear	
2. Mechanical traction of entire left leg	
3. Removal of splint, right shoulder	
4. Placement of neck brace	
5. Change of vaginal packing	
6. Packing of wound, chest wall	
7. Sterile dressing placement to left groin region	
8. Removal of packing material from pharynx	
9. Placement of intermittent pneumatic compression device, covering entire right arm	
10. Exchange of pressure dressing to left thigh	

Administration

Procedure	Code
1. Peritoneal dialysis via indwelling catheter	
2. Transvaginal artificial insemination	
3. Infusion of total parenteral nutrition via central venous catheter	
4. Esophagogastroscopy with Botox injection into esophageal sphincter	
5. Percutaneous irrigation of knee joint	
6. Systemic infusion of recombinant tissue plasminogen activator (r-tPA) via peripheral venous catheter	
7. Transabdominal in vitro fertilization, implantation of donor ovum	
8. Autologous bone marrow transplant via central venous line	
9. Implantation of anti-microbial envelope with cardiac defibrillator placement, open	
10. Sclerotherapy of brachial plexus lesion, alcohol injection	
11. Percutaneous peripheral vein injection, glucarpidase	
12. Introduction of anti-infective envelope into subcutaneous tissue, open	

Measurement and Monitoring

Procedure	Code
1. Cardiac stress test, single measurement	
2. EGD with biliary flow measurement	
3. Right and left heart cardiac catheterization with bilateral sampling and pressure measurements	
4. Temperature monitoring, rectal	
5. Peripheral venous pulse, external, single measurement	
6. Holter monitoring	
7. Respiratory rate, external, single measurement	
8. Fetal heart rate monitoring, transvaginal	
9. Visual mobility test, single measurement	
10. Left ventricular cardiac output monitoring from pulmonary artery wedge (Swan-Ganz) catheter	
11. Olfactory acuity test, single measurement	

Extracorporeal or Systemic Assistance and Performance

Procedure	Code
1. Intermittent mechanical ventilation, 16 hours	
2. Liver dialysis, single encounter	
3. Cardiac countershock with successful conversion to sinus rhythm	
4. IPPB (intermittent positive pressure breathing) for mobilization of secretions, 22 hours	
5. Renal dialysis, 12 hours	
6. IABP (intra-aortic balloon pump) continuous	
7. Intraoperative cardiac pacing, continuous	
8. Intraoperative ECMO (extracorporeal membrane oxygenation), central	
9. Controlled mechanical ventilation (CMV), 45 hours	
10. Pulsatile compression boot with intermittent inflation	

Extracorporeal or Systemic Therapies

Procedure	Code
1. Donor thrombocytapheresis, single encounter	
2. Bili-lite phototherapy, series treatment	
3. Whole body hypothermia, single treatment	
4. Circulatory phototherapy, single encounter	
5. Shock wave therapy of plantar fascia, single treatment	
6. Antigen-free air conditioning, series treatment	
7. TMS (transcranial magnetic stimulation), series treatment	
8. Therapeutic ultrasound of peripheral vessels, single treatment	
9. Plasmapheresis, series treatment	
10. Extracorporeal electromagnetic stimulation (EMS) for urinary incontinence, single treatment	

Osteopathic

Procedure	Code
1. Isotonic muscle energy treatment of right leg	
2. Low velocity-high amplitude osteopathic treatment of head	
3. Lymphatic pump osteopathic treatment of left axilla	
4. Indirect osteopathic treatment of sacrum	
5. Articulatory osteopathic treatment of cervical region	

Other Procedures

Procedure	Code
1. Near infrared spectroscopy of leg vessels	
2. CT computer assisted sinus surgery	
3. Suture removal, abdominal wall	
4. Isolation after infectious disease exposure	
5. Robotic assisted open prostatectomy	
6. In vitro fertilization	

Chiropractic

Procedure	Code
1. Chiropractic treatment of lumbar region using long lever specific contact	
2. Chiropractic manipulation of abdominal region, indirect visceral	
3. Chiropractic extra-articular treatment of hip region	
4. Chiropractic treatment of sacrum using long and short lever specific contact	
5. Mechanically-assisted chiropractic manipulation of head	

Imaging

Procedure	Code
1. Noncontrast CT of abdomen and pelvis	
2. Intravascular ultrasound, left subclavian artery	
3. Fluoroscopic guidance for insertion of central venous catheter in SVC, low osmolar contrast	
4. Chest x-ray, AP/PA and lateral views	
5. Endoluminal ultrasound of gallbladder and bile ducts	
6. MRI of thyroid gland, contrast unspecified	
7. Esophageal videofluoroscopy study with oral barium contrast	

Procedure	Code
8. Portable x-ray study of right radius/ulna shaft, standard series	
9. Routine fetal ultrasound, second trimester twin gestation	
10. CT scan of bilateral lungs, high osmolar contrast with densitometry	
11. Fluoroscopic guidance for percutaneous transluminal angioplasty (PTA) of left common femoral artery, low osmolar contrast	

Nuclear Medicine

Procedure	Code
1. Tomo scan of right and left heart, unspecified radiopharmaceutical, qualitative gated rest	
2. Technetium pentetate assay of kidneys, ureters, and bladder	
3. Uniplanar scan of spine using technetium oxidronate, with first-pass study	
4. Thallous chloride tomographic scan of bilateral breasts	
5. PET scan of myocardium using rubidium	
6. Gallium citrate scan of head and neck, single plane imaging	
7. Xenon gas nonimaging probe of brain	
8. Upper GI scan, radiopharmaceutical unspecified, for gastric emptying	
9. Carbon 11 PET scan of brain with quantification	
10. Iodinated albumin nuclear medicine assay, blood plasma volume study	

Radiation Therapy

Procedure	Code
1. Plaque radiation of left eye, single port	
2. 8 MeV photon beam radiation to brain	
3. IORT of colon, 3 ports	
4. HDR brachytherapy of prostate using low dose palladium-103, unidirectional source	
5. Electron radiation treatment of right breast, with custom device	
6. Hyperthermia oncology treatment of pelvic region	
7. Contact radiation of tongue	
8. Heavy particle radiation treatment of pancreas, four risk sites	
9. LDR brachytherapy to spinal cord using iodine	
10. Whole body Phosphorus 32 administration with risk to hematopoietic system	

Physical Rehabilitation and Diagnostic Audiology

Procedure	Code
1. Bekesy assessment using audiometer	
2. Individual fitting of left eye prosthesis	
3. Physical therapy for range of motion and mobility, patient right hip, no special equipment	
4. Bedside swallow assessment using assessment kit	
5. Caregiver training in airway clearance techniques	
6. Application of short arm cast in rehabilitation setting	
7. Verbal assessment of patient's pain level	
8. Caregiver training in communication skills using manual communication board	

Procedure	Code
9. Group musculoskeletal balance training exercises, whole body, no special equipment	
10. Individual therapy for auditory processing using tape recorder	

Mental Health

Procedure	Code
1. Cognitive-behavioral psychotherapy, individual	
2. Narcosynthesis	
3. Light therapy	
4. ECT (electroconvulsive therapy), unilateral, multiple seizure	
5. Crisis intervention	
6. Neuropsychological testing	
7. Hypnosis	
8. Developmental testing	
9. Vocational counseling	
10. Family psychotherapy	

Substance Abuse Treatment

Procedure	Code
1. Naltrexone treatment for drug dependency	
2. Substance abuse treatment family counseling	
3. Medication monitoring of patient on methadone maintenance	
4. Individual interpersonal psychotherapy for drug abuse	
5. Patient in for alcohol detoxification treatment	
6. Group motivational counseling	
7. Individual 12-step psychotherapy for substance abuse	
8. Post-test infectious disease counseling for IV drug abuser	
9. Psychodynamic psychotherapy for drug dependent patient	
10. Group cognitive-behavioral counseling for substance abuse	

New Technology

Procedure	Code
1. Infusion of terlipressin via peripheral venous catheter	
2. Transcatheter dilation of left peroneal artery with 2 SAVAL stents	

Answers to Coding Exercises

Medical Surgical Section

Procedure	Code
1. Excision of malignant melanoma from skin of right ear	0HB2XZZ
2. Laparoscopy with excision of endometrial implant from left ovary	0UB14ZZ
3. Percutaneous needle core biopsy of right kidney	0TB03ZX
4. EGD with excisional gastric biopsy	0DB68ZX
5. Open endarterectomy of left common carotid artery	03CJ0ZZ
6. Excision of basal cell carcinoma of lower lip	0CB1XZZ
7. Open excision of tail of pancreas	0FBG0ZZ
8. Percutaneous biopsy of right gastrocnemius muscle	0KBS3ZX
9. Sigmoidoscopy with sigmoid polypectomy	0DBN8ZZ
10. Open excision of lesion from right Achilles tendon	0LBN0ZZ
11. Open resection of cecum	0DTH0ZZ
12. Total excision of pituitary gland, open	0GT00ZZ
13. Explantation of left failed kidney, open	0TT10ZZ
14. Open left axillary total lymphadenectomy	07T60ZZ (RESECTION is coded for cutting out a chain of lymph nodes.)
15. Laparoscopic-assisted vaginal hysterectomy	0UT9FZZ
16. Right total mastectomy, open	0HTT0ZZ
17. Open resection of papillary muscle	02TD0ZZ (The papillary muscle refers to the heart and is found in the *Heart and Great Vessels* body system.)
18. Total retropubic prostatectomy, open	0VT00ZZ
19. Laparoscopic cholecystectomy	0FT44ZZ
20. Endoscopic bilateral total maxillary sinusectomy	09TQ8ZZ, 09TR8ZZ
21. Amputation at right elbow level	0X6B0ZZ
22. Right below-knee amputation, proximal tibia/fibula	0Y6H0Z1 (The qualifier *High* here means the portion of the tib/fib closest to the knee.)
23. Fifth ray carpometacarpal joint amputation, left hand	0X6K0Z8 (A *complete* ray amputation is through the carpometacarpal joint.)
24. Right leg and hip amputation through ischium	0Y620ZZ (The *Hindquarter* body part includes amputation along any part of the hip bone.)
25. DIP joint amputation of right thumb	0X6L0Z3 (The qualifier *low* here means through the distal interphalangeal joint.)
26. Right wrist joint amputation	0X6J0Z0 (Amputation at the wrist joint is actually complete amputation of the hand.)
27. Trans-metatarsal amputation of foot at left big toe	0Y6N0Z9 (A *partial* amputation is through the shaft of the metatarsal bone.)
28. Mid-shaft amputation, right humerus	0X680Z2
29. Left fourth toe amputation, mid-proximal phalanx	0Y6W0Z1 (The qualifier *High* here means anywhere along the proximal phalanx.)
30. Right above-knee amputation, distal femur	0Y6C0Z3

Procedure	Code
31. Cryotherapy of wart on left hand	0H5GXZZ
32. Percutaneous radiofrequency ablation of right vocal cord lesion	0C5T3ZZ
33. Left heart catheterization with laser destruction of arrhythmogenic focus, A-V node	02583ZZ
34. Cautery of nosebleed	093K7ZZ
35. Transurethral endoscopic laser ablation of prostate	0V508ZZ
36. Percutaneous cautery of oozing varicose vein, left calf	0Y3J3ZZ
37. Laparoscopy with destruction of endometriosis, bilateral ovaries	0U524ZZ
38. Laser coagulation of right retinal vessel, percutaneous	085G3ZZ (The *Retinal Vessel* body-part values are in the *Eye* body system.)
39. Thoracoscopic pleurodesis, left side	0B5P4ZZ
40. Percutaneous insertion of Greenfield IVC filter	06H03DZ
41. Forceps total mouth extraction, upper and lower teeth	0CDWXZ2, 0CDXXZ2
42. Removal of left thumbnail	0HDQXZZ (No separate body-part value is given for thumbnail, so this is coded to *Fingernail*.)
43. Extraction of right intraocular lens without replacement, percutaneous	08DJ3ZZ
44. Laparoscopy with needle aspiration of ova for in vitro fertilization	0UDN4ZZ
45. Nonexcisional debridement of skin ulcer, right foot	0HDMXZZ
46. Open stripping of abdominal fascia, right side	0JD80ZZ
47. Hysteroscopy with D&C, diagnostic	0UDB8ZX
48. Liposuction for medical purposes, left upper arm	0JDF3ZZ (The *Percutaneous* approach is inherent in the liposuction technique.)
49. Removal of tattered right ear drum fragments with tweezers	09D77ZZ
50. Microincisional phlebectomy of spider veins, right lower leg	06DY3ZZ
51. Routine Foley catheter placement	0T9B70Z
52. Incision and drainage of external anal abscess	0D9QXZZ
53. Percutaneous drainage of ascites	0W9G3ZZ (This is drainage of the cavity and not the peritoneal membrane itself.)
54. Laparoscopy with left ovarian cystotomy and drainage	0U914ZZ
55. Laparotomy and drain placement for liver abscess, right lobe	0F9100Z
56. Right knee arthrotomy with drain placement	0S9C00Z
57. Thoracentesis of left pleural effusion	0W9B3ZZ (This is drainage of the pleural cavity)
58. Phlebotomy of left median cubital vein for polycythemia vera	059C3ZZ (The median cubital vein is a branch of the basilic vein)
59. Percutaneous chest tube placement for right pneumothorax	0W9930Z
60. Endoscopic drainage of left ethmoid sinus	099V4ZZ
61. External ventricular CSF drainage catheter placement via burr hole	009630Z
62. Removal of foreign body, right cornea	08C8XZZ

Procedure	Code
63. Percutaneous mechanical thrombectomy, left brachial artery	03C83ZZ
64. Esophagogastroscopy with removal of bezoar from stomach	0DC68ZZ
65. Foreign body removal, skin of left thumb	0HCGXZZ (There is no specific value for thumb skin, so the procedure is coded to *Hand*.)
66. Transurethral cystoscopy with removal of bladder stone	0TCB8ZZ
67. Forceps removal of foreign body in right nostril	09CKXZZ (Nostril is coded to the *Nasal mucosa and soft tissue* body-part value.)
68. Laparoscopy with excision of old suture from mesentery	0DCV4ZZ
69. Incision and removal of right lacrimal duct stone	08CX0ZZ
70. Nonincisional removal of intraluminal foreign body from vagina	0UCG7ZZ (The approach *External* is also a possibility. It is assumed here that since the patient went to the doctor to have the object removed, that it was not in the vaginal orifice.)
71. Right common carotid endarterectomy, open	03CH0ZZ
72. Open excision of retained sliver, subcutaneous tissue of left foot	0JCR0ZZ
73. Extracorporeal shockwave lithotripsy (ESWL), bilateral ureters	0TF6XZZ, 0TF7XZZ (The *Bilateral Ureter* body-part value is not available for the root operation FRAGMENTATION, so the procedures are coded separately.)
74. Endoscopic retrograde cholangiopancreatography (ERCP) with lithotripsy of common bile duct stone	0FF98ZZ (ERCP is performed through the mouth to the biliary system via the duodenum, so the approach value is *Via Natural or Artificial Opening Endoscopic*.)
75. Thoracotomy with crushing of pericardial calcifications	02FN0ZZ
76. Transurethral cystoscopy with fragmentation of bladder calculus	0TFB8ZZ
77. Hysteroscopy with intraluminal lithotripsy of left fallopian tube calcification	0UF68ZZ
78. Division of right foot tendon, percutaneous	0L8V3ZZ
79. Left heart catheterization with division of bundle of HIS	02883ZZ
80. Open osteotomy of capitate, left hand	0P8N0ZZ (The capitate is one of the carpal bones of the hand.)
81. EGD with esophagotomy of esophagogastric junction	0D948ZZ
82. Sacral rhizotomy for pain control, percutaneous	018R3ZZ
83. Laparotomy with exploration and adhesiolysis of right ureter	0TN60ZZ
84. Incision of scar contracture, right elbow	0HNDXZZ (The skin of the elbow region is coded to *Lower Arm*.)
85. Frenulotomy for treatment of tongue-tie syndrome	0CN7XZZ (The frenulum is coded to the body-part value *Tongue*.)
86. Right shoulder arthroscopy with coracoacromial ligament release	0MN14ZZ

Procedure	Code
87. Mitral valvulotomy for release of fused leaflets, open approach	02NG0ZZ
88. Percutaneous left Achilles tendon release	0LNP3ZZ
89. Laparoscopy with lysis of peritoneal adhesions	0DNW4ZZ
90. Manual rupture of right shoulder joint adhesions under general anesthesia	0RNJXZZ
91. Open posterior tarsal tunnel release	01NG0ZZ (The nerve released in the posterior tarsal tunnel is the tibial nerve.)
92. Laparoscopy with freeing of left ovary and fallopian tube	0UN14ZZ, 0UN64ZZ
93. Liver transplant with donor matched liver	0FY00Z0
94. Orthotopic heart transplant using porcine heart	02YA0Z2 (The donor heart comes from an animal [pig], so the qualifier value is *Zooplastic*.)
95. Right lung transplant, open, using organ donor match	0BYK0Z0
96. Transplant of large intestine, organ donor match	0DYE0Z0
97. Left kidney/pancreas organ bank transplant	0FYG0Z0, 0TY10Z0
98. Replantation of avulsed scalp	0HM0XZZ
99. Reattachment of severed right ear	09M0XZZ
100. Reattachment of traumatic left gastrocnemius avulsion, open	0KMT0ZZ
101. Closed replantation of three avulsed teeth, lower jaw	0CMXXZ1
102. Reattachment of severed left hand	0XMK0ZZ
103. Right open palmaris longus tendon transfer	0LX50ZZ
104. Endoscopic radial to median nerve transfer	01X64Z5
105. Fasciocutaneous flap closure of left thigh, open	0JXM0ZC (The qualifier identifies the body layers in addition to fascia included in the procedure.)
106. Transfer left index finger to left thumb position, open	0XXP0ZM
107. Percutaneous fascia transfer to fill defect, right neck	0JX43ZZ
108. Trigeminal to facial nerve transfer, percutaneous endoscopic	00XK4ZM
109. Endoscopic left leg flexor hallucis longus tendon transfer	0LXP4ZZ
110. Right scalp advancement flap to right temple	0HX0XZZ
111. Resection right breast with TRAM flap reconstruction, open	0HTT0ZZ, 0HRT076 (Code both the resection and the replacement per guideline B3.18)
112. Skin transfer flap closure of complex open wound, left lower back	0HX6XZZ
113. Open fracture reduction, right tibia	0QSG0ZZ
114. Laparoscopy with gastropexy for malrotation	0DS64ZZ
115. Left knee arthroscopy with reposition of anterior cruciate ligament	0MSP4ZZ
116. Open transposition of ulnar nerve	01S40ZZ
117. Closed reduction with percutaneous internal fixation of right femoral neck fracture	0QS634Z
118. Trans-vaginal intraluminal cervical cerclage	0UVC7DZ
119. Cervical cerclage using Shirodkar technique	0UVC7ZZ
120. Thoracotomy with banding of left pulmonary artery using extraluminal device	02VR0CZ
121. Restriction of thoracic duct with intraluminal stent, percutaneous	07VK3DZ

Procedure	Code
122. Craniotomy with clipping of cerebral aneurysm	03VG0CZ (The clip is placed lengthwise on the outside wall of the widened portion of the vessel.)
123. Nonincisional, transnasal placement of restrictive stent in right lacrimal duct	08VX7DZ
124. Catheter-based temporary restriction of blood flow in abdominal aorta for treatment of cerebral ischemia	04V03DJ
125. Percutaneous ligation of esophageal vein	06L33ZZ
126. Percutaneous embolization of left internal carotid-cavernous fistula	03LL3DZ
127. Laparoscopy with bilateral occlusion of fallopian tubes using Hulka extraluminal clips	0UL74CZ
128. Open suture ligation of failed AV graft, left brachial artery	03L80ZZ
129. Percutaneous embolization of vascular supply, intracranial meningioma	03LG3DZ
130. Percutaneous embolization of right uterine artery, using coils	04LE3DT
131. Open occlusion of left atrial appendage, using extraluminal pressure clips	02L70CK
132. Percutaneous suture exclusion of left atrial appendage, via femoral artery access	02L73ZK
133. ERCP with balloon dilation of common bile duct	0F798ZZ
134. PTCA of two coronary arteries, LAD with stent placement, RCA with no stent	02703DZ, 02703ZZ (A separate procedure is coded for each artery dilated, since the device value differs for each artery.)
135. Cystoscopy with intraluminal dilation of bladder neck stricture	0T7C8ZZ
136. Open dilation of old anastomosis, left femoral artery	047L0ZZ
137. Dilation of upper esophageal stricture, direct visualization, with Bougie sound	0D717ZZ
138. PTA of right brachial artery stenosis	03773ZZ
139. Transnasal dilation and stent placement in right lacrimal duct	087X7DZ
140. Hysteroscopy with balloon dilation of bilateral fallopian tubes	0U778ZZ
141. Tracheoscopy with intraluminal dilation of tracheal stenosis	0B718ZZ
142. Cystoscopy with dilation of left ureteral stricture, with stent placement	0T778DZ
143. Open gastric bypass with Roux-en-Y limb to jejunum	0D160ZA
144. Right temporal artery to intracranial artery bypass using Gore-Tex graft, open	031S0JG
145. Tracheostomy formation with tracheostomy tube placement, percutaneous	0B113F4
146. PICVA (percutaneous in situ coronary venous arterialization) of single coronary artery	02103D4
147. Open left femoral-popliteal artery bypass using cadaver vein graft	041L0KL
148. Shunting of intrathecal cerebrospinal fluid to peritoneal cavity using synthetic shunt	00160J6
149. Colostomy formation, open, transverse colon to abdominal wall	0D1L0Z4
150. Open urinary diversion, left ureter, using ileal conduit to skin	0T170ZC
151. CABG of LAD using pedicled left internal mammary artery, open off-bypass	02100Z9

Procedure	Code
152. Open pleuroperitoneal shunt, right pleural cavity, using synthetic device	0W190JG
153. Percutaneous placement of ventriculoperitoneal shunt for treatment of hydrocephalus	00163J6
154. End-of-life replacement of spinal neurostimulator generator, multiple array, in lower abdomen	0JH80DZ (Taking out of the old generator is coded separately to the root operation Removal)
155. Percutaneous insertion of spinal neurostimulator lead, lumbar spinal cord	00HV3MZ
156. Percutaneous replacement of broken pacemaker lead in left atrium	02H73JZ (Taking out the broken pacemaker lead is coded separately to the root operation Removal.)
157. Open placement of dual chamber pacemaker generator in chest wall	0JH606Z
158. Percutaneous placement of venous central line in right internal jugular, with tip in superior vena cava	02HV33Z
159. Open insertion of multiple channel cochlear implant, left ear	09HE06Z
160. Percutaneous placement of Swan-Ganz catheter in pulmonary trunk	02HP32Z (The Swan-Ganz catheter is coded to the device value Monitoring Device because it monitors pulmonary artery output.)
161. Bronchoscopy with insertion of Low Dose Pd-103 brachytherapy seeds, right lung	0BHK81Z, DB11BBZ
162. Open insertion of interspinous process device into lumbar vertebral joint	0SH00BZ
163. Open placement of bone growth stimulator, left femoral shaft	0QHY0MZ
164. Cystoscopy with placement of brachytherapy seeds in prostate gland	0VH081Z
165. Percutaneous insertion of Greenfield IVC filter	06H03DZ
166. Full-thickness skin graft to right lower arm, autograft (do not code graft harvest for this exercise)	0HRDX73
167. Excision of necrosed left femoral head with bone bank bone graft to fill the defect, open	0QR70KZ
168. Penetrating keratoplasty of right cornea with donor matched cornea, percutaneous approach	08R83KZ
169. Excision of abdominal aorta with Gore-Tex graft replacement, open	04R00JZ
170. Total right knee arthroplasty with insertion of total knee prosthesis	0SRC0JZ
171. Tenonectomy with graft to right ankle using cadaver graft, open	0LRS0KZ
172. Mitral valve replacement using porcine valve, open	02RG08Z
173. Percutaneous phacoemulsification of right eye cataract with prosthetic lens insertion	08RJ3JZ
174. Transcatheter replacement of pulmonary valve using of bovine jugular vein valve	02RH38Z
175. Total left hip replacement using ceramic on ceramic prosthesis, without bone cement	0SRB03A
176. Aortic valve annuloplasty using ring, open	02UF0JZ
177. Laparoscopic repair of left inguinal hernia with marlex plug	0YU64JZ
178. Autograft nerve graft to right median nerve, percutaneous endoscopic (do not code graft harvest for this exercise)	01U547Z
179. Exchange of liner in femoral component of previous left hip replacement, open approach	0SUS09Z (Taking out of the old liner is coded separately to the root operation Removal)

Procedure	Code
180. Anterior colporrhaphy with polypropylene mesh reinforcement, open approach	0JUC0JZ
181. Implantation of CorCap cardiac support device, open approach	02UA0JZ
182. Abdominal wall herniorrhaphy, open, using synthetic mesh	0WUF0JZ
183. Tendon graft to strengthen injured left shoulder using autograft, open (do not code graft harvest for this exercise)	0LU207Z
184. Onlay lamellar keratoplasty of left cornea using autograft, external approach	08U9X7Z
185. Resurfacing procedure on right femoral head, open approach	0SUR0BZ
186. Exchange of drainage tube from right hip joint	0S2YX0Z
187. Tracheostomy tube exchange	0B21XFZ
188. Change chest tube for left pneumothorax	0W2BX0Z
189. Exchange of cerebral ventriculostomy drainage tube	0020X0Z
190. Foley urinary catheter exchange	0T2BX0Z (This is coded to *Drainage Device* because urine is being drained.)
191. Open removal of lumbar sympathetic neurostimulator lead	01PY0MZ
192. Nonincisional removal of Swan-Ganz catheter from right pulmonary artery	02PYX2Z
193. Laparotomy with removal of pancreatic drain	0FPG00Z
194. Extubation, endotracheal tube	0BP1XDZ
195. Nonincisional PEG tube removal	0DP6XUZ
196. Transvaginal removal of brachytherapy seeds	0UPH71Z
197. Transvaginal removal of extraluminal cervical cerclage	0UPD7CZ
198. Incision with removal of K-wire fixation, right first metatarsal	0QPN04Z
199. Cystoscopy with retrieval of left ureteral stent	0TP98DZ
200. Removal of nasogastric drainage tube for decompression	0DP6X0Z
201. Removal of external fixator, left radial fracture	0PPJX5Z
202. Trimming and reanastomosis of stenosed femorofemoral synthetic bypass graft, open	04WY0JZ
203. Open revision of right hip replacement, with readjustment of prosthesis	0SW90JZ
204. Adjustment of position, pacemaker lead in left ventricle, percutaneous	02WA3MZ
205. External repositioning of Foley catheter to bladder	0TWBX0Z
206. Taking out loose screw and putting larger screw in fracture repair plate, left tibia	0QWH04Z
207. Revision of totally implantable VAD port placement in chest wall, causing patient discomfort, open	0JWT0WZ
208. Thoracotomy with exploration of right pleural cavity	0WJ90ZZ
209. Diagnostic laryngoscopy	0CJS8ZZ
210. Exploratory arthrotomy of left knee	0SJD0ZZ
211. Colposcopy with diagnostic hysteroscopy	0UJD8ZZ
212. Digital rectal exam	0DJD7ZZ
213. Diagnostic arthroscopy of right shoulder	0RJJ4ZZ
214. Endoscopy of maxillary sinus	09JY4ZZ
215. Laparotomy with palpation of liver	0FJ00ZZ
216. Transurethral diagnostic cystoscopy	0TJB8ZZ
217. Colonoscopy, discontinued at sigmoid colon	0DJD8ZZ
218. Percutaneous mapping of basal ganglia	00K83ZZ
219. Heart catheterization with cardiac mapping	02K83ZZ
220. Intraoperative whole brain mapping via craniotomy	00K00ZZ

Procedure	Code
221. Mapping of left cerebral hemisphere, percutaneous endoscopic	00K74ZZ
222. Intraoperative cardiac mapping during open heart surgery	02K80ZZ
223. Hysteroscopy with cautery of post-hysterectomy oozing and evacuation of clot	0W3R8ZZ
224. Open exploration and ligation of post-op arterial bleeder, left forearm	0X3F0ZZ
225. Control of post-operative retroperitoneal bleeding via laparotomy	0W3H0ZZ
226. Reopening of thoracotomy site with drainage and control of post-op hemopericardium	0W3D0ZZ
227. Arthroscopy with drainage of hemarthrosis at previous operative site, right knee	0Y3F4ZZ
228. Radiocarpal fusion of left hand with internal fixation, open	0RGP04Z
229. Posterior approach spinal fusion at L1-L3 level with BAK cage interbody fusion device, open	0SG10AJ
230. Intercarpal fusion of right hand with bone bank bone graft, open	0RGQ0KZ
231. Sacrococcygeal fusion with bone graft from same operative site, open	0SG507Z
232. Interphalangeal fusion of left great toe, percutaneous pin fixation	0SGQ34Z
233. Suture repair of left radial nerve laceration	01Q60ZZ (The approach value is *Open*, though the surgical exposure may have been created by the wound itself.)
234. Laparotomy with suture repair of blunt force duodenal laceration	0DQ90ZZ
235. Perineoplasty with repair of old obstetric laceration, open	0WQN0ZZ
236. Suture repair of right biceps tendon (upper arm) laceration, open	0LQ30ZZ
237. Closure of abdominal wall stab wound	0WQF0ZZ
238. Cosmetic face lift, open, no other information available	0W020ZZ
239. Bilateral breast augmentation with silicone implants, open	0H0V0JZ
240. Cosmetic rhinoplasty with septal reduction and tip elevation using local tissue graft, open	090K07Z
241. Abdominoplasty (tummy tuck), open	0W0F0ZZ
242. Liposuction of bilateral thighs	0J0L3ZZ, 0J0M3ZZ
243. Creation of penis in female patient using tissue bank donor graft	0W4N0K1
244. Creation of vagina in male patient using synthetic material	0W4M0J0
245. Laparoscopic vertical (sleeve) gastrectomy	0DB64Z3
246. Left uterine artery embolization with intraluminal biosphere injection	04LF3DU

Obstetrics

Procedure	Code
1. Abortion by dilation and evacuation following laminaria insertion	10A07ZW
2. Manually assisted spontaneous abortion	10E0XZZ (Since the pregnancy was not artificially terminated, this is coded to *Delivery* because it captures the procedure objective. The fact that it was an abortion will be identified in the diagnosis code.)
3. Abortion by abortifacient insertion	10A07ZX
4. Bimanual pregnancy examination	10J07ZZ
5. Extraperitoneal C-section, low transverse incision	10D00Z1
6. Fetal spinal tap, percutaneous	10903ZA
7. Fetal kidney transplant, laparoscopic	10Y04ZS
8. Open in utero repair of congenital diaphragmatic hernia	10Q00ZK (Diaphragm is classified to the *Respiratory* body system in the *Medical and Surgical* section.)
9. Laparoscopy with total excision of tubal pregnancy	10T24ZZ
10. Transvaginal removal of fetal monitoring electrode	10P073Z

Placement

Procedure	Code
1. Placement of packing material, right ear	2Y42X5Z
2. Mechanical traction of entire left leg	2W6MX0Z
3. Removal of splint, right shoulder	2W5AX1Z
4. Placement of neck brace	2W32X3Z
5. Change of vaginal packing	2Y04X5Z
6. Packing of wound, chest wall	2W44X5Z
7. Sterile dressing placement to left groin region	2W27X4Z
8. Removal of packing material from pharynx	2Y50X5Z
9. Placement of intermittent pneumatic compression device, covering entire right arm	2W18X7Z
10. Exchange of pressure dressing to left thigh	2W0PX6Z

Administration

Procedure	Code
1. Peritoneal dialysis via indwelling catheter	3E1M39Z
2. Transvaginal artificial insemination	3E0P7LZ
3. Infusion of total parenteral nutrition via central venous catheter	3E0436Z
4. Esophagogastroscopy with Botox injection into esophageal sphincter	3E0G8GC (Botulinum toxin is a paralyzing agent with temporary effects; it does not sclerose or destroy the nerve.)
5. Percutaneous irrigation of knee joint	3E1U38Z
6. Systemic infusion of recombinant tissue plasminogen activator (r-tPA) via peripheral venous catheter	3E03317
7. Transabdominal in vitro fertilization, implantation of donor ovum	3E0P3Q1
8. Autologous bone marrow transplant via central venous line	30243G0
9. Implantation of anti-microbial envelope with cardiac defibrillator placement, open	3E0102A
10. Sclerotherapy of brachial plexus lesion, alcohol injection	3E0T3TZ

Procedure	Code
11. Percutaneous peripheral vein injection, glucarpidase	3E033GQ
12. Introduction of anti-infective envelope into subcutaneous tissue, open	3E0102A

Measurement and Monitoring

Procedure	Code
1. Cardiac stress test, single measurement	4A02XM4
2. EGD with biliary flow measurement	4A0C85Z
3. Right and left heart cardiac catheterization with bilateral sampling and pressure measurements	4A023N8
4. Temperature monitoring, rectal	4A1Z7KZ
5. Peripheral venous pulse, external, single measurement	4A04XJ1
6. Holter monitoring	4A12X45
7. Respiratory rate, external, single measurement	4A09XCZ
8. Fetal heart rate monitoring, transvaginal	4A1H7CZ
9. Visual mobility test, single measurement	4A07X7Z
10. Left ventricular cardiac output monitoring from pulmonary artery wedge (Swan-Ganz) catheter	4A1239Z
11. Olfactory acuity test, single measurement	4A08X0Z

Extracorporeal or Systemic Assistance and Performance

Procedure	Code
1. Intermittent mechanical ventilation, 16 hours	5A1935Z
2. Liver dialysis, single encounter	5A1C00Z
3. Cardiac countershock with successful conversion to sinus rhythm	5A2204Z
4. IPPB (intermittent positive pressure breathing) for mobilization of secretions, 22 hours	5A09358
5. Renal dialysis, 12 hours	5A1D80Z
6. IABP (intra-aortic balloon pump) continuous	5A02210
7. Intra-operative cardiac pacing, continuous	5A1223Z
8. Intraoperative ECMO (extracorporeal membrane oxygenation), central	5A15A2F
9. Controlled mechanical ventilation (CMV), 45 hours	5A1945Z
10. Pulsatile compression boot with intermittent inflation	5A02115 (This is coded to the function value *Cardiac Output*, because the purpose of such compression devices is to return blood to the heart faster.)

Extracorporeal or Systemic Therapies

Procedure	Code
1. Donor thrombocytapheresis, single encounter	6A550Z2
2. Bili-lite phototherapy, series treatment	6A601ZZ
3. Whole body hypothermia, single treatment	6A4Z0ZZ
4. Circulatory phototherapy, single encounter	6A650ZZ
5. Shock wave therapy of plantar fascia, single treatment	6A930ZZ
6. Antigen-free air conditioning, series treatment	6A0Z1ZZ
7. TMS (transcranial magnetic stimulation), series treatment	6A221ZZ

Procedure	Code
8. Therapeutic ultrasound of peripheral vessels, single treatment	6A750Z6
9. Plasmapheresis, series treatment	6A551Z3
10. Extracorporeal electromagnetic stimulation (EMS) for urinary incontinence, single treatment	6A210ZZ

Osteopathic

Procedure	Code
1. Isotonic muscle energy treatment of right leg	7W06X8Z
2. Low velocity-high amplitude osteopathic treatment of head	7W00X5Z
3. Lymphatic pump osteopathic treatment of left axilla	7W07X6Z
4. Indirect osteopathic treatment of sacrum	7W04X4Z
5. Articulatory osteopathic treatment of cervical region	7W01X0Z

Other Procedures

Procedure	Code
1. Near infrared spectroscopy of leg vessels	8E023DZ
2. CT computer assisted sinus surgery	8E09XBG (The primary procedure is coded separately.)
3. Suture removal, abdominal wall	8E0WXY8
4. Isolation after infectious disease exposure	8E0ZXY6
5. Robotic assisted open prostatectomy	8E0W0CZ (The primary procedure is coded separately.)
6. In vitro fertilization	8E0ZXY1

Chiropractic

Procedure	Code
1. Chiropractic treatment of lumbar region using long lever specific contact	9WB3XGZ
2. Chiropractic manipulation of abdominal region, indirect visceral	9WB9XCZ
3. Chiropractic extra-articular treatment of hip region	9WB6XDZ
4. Chiropractic treatment of sacrum using long and short lever specific contact	9WB4XJZ
5. Mechanically-assisted chiropractic manipulation of head	9WB0XKZ

Imaging

Procedure	Code
1. Noncontrast CT of abdomen and pelvis	BW21ZZZ
2. Intravascular ultrasound, left subclavian artery	B342ZZ3
3. Fluoroscopic guidance for insertion of central venous catheter in SVC, low osmolar contrast	B5181ZA
4. Chest x-ray, AP/PA and lateral views	BW03ZZZ
5. Endoluminal ultrasound of gallbladder and bile ducts	BF43ZZZ
6. MRI of thyroid gland, contrast unspecified	BG34YZZ
7. Esophageal videofluoroscopy study with oral barium contrast	BD11YZZ
8. Portable x-ray study of right radius/ulna shaft, standard series	BP0JZZZ
9. Routine fetal ultrasound, second trimester twin gestation	BY4DZZZ

Procedure	Code
10. CT scan of bilateral lungs, high osmolar contrast with densitometry	BB240ZZ
11. Fluoroscopic guidance for percutaneous transluminal angioplasty (PTA) of left common femoral artery, low osmolar contrast	B41G1ZZ

Nuclear Medicine

Procedure	Code
1. Tomo scan of right and left heart, unspecified radiopharmaceutical, qualitative gated rest	C226YZZ
2. Technetium pentetate assay of kidneys, ureters, and bladder	CT631ZZ
3. Uniplanar scan of spine using technetium oxidronate, with first-pass study	CP151ZZ
4. Thallous chloride tomographic scan of bilateral breasts	CH22SZZ
5. PET scan of myocardium using rubidium	C23GQZZ
6. Gallium citrate scan of head and neck, single plane imaging	CW1BLZZ
7. Xenon gas nonimaging probe of brain	C050VZZ
8. Upper GI scan, radiopharmaceutical unspecified, for gastric emptying	CD15YZZ
9. Carbon 11 PET scan of brain with quantification	C030BZZ
10. Iodinated albumin nuclear medicine assay, blood plasma volume study	C763HZZ

Radiation Therapy

Procedure	Code
1. Plaque radiation of left eye, single port	D8Y0FZZ
2. 8 MeV photon beam radiation to brain	D0011ZZ
3. IORT of colon, 3 ports	DDY5CZZ
4. HDR brachytherapy of prostate using low dose palladium-103, unidirectional source	DV10BB1
5. Electron radiation treatment of right breast, with custom device	DM013ZZ
6. Hyperthermia oncology treatment of pelvic region	DWY68ZZ
7. Contact radiation of tongue	D9Y57ZZ
8. Heavy particle radiation treatment of pancreas, four risk sites	DF034ZZ
9. LDR brachytherapy to spinal cord using iodine	D016B9Z
10. Whole body Phosphorus 32 administration with risk to hematopoietic system	DWY5GFZ

Physical Rehabilitation and Diagnostic Audiology

Procedure	Code
1. Bekesy assessment using audiometer	F13Z31Z
2. Individual fitting of left eye prosthesis	F0DZ8UZ
3. Physical therapy for range of motion and mobility, patient right hip, no special equipment	F07L0ZZ
4. Bedside swallow assessment using assessment kit	F00ZHYZ
5. Caregiver training in airway clearance techniques	F0FZ8ZZ
6. Application of short arm cast in rehabilitation setting	F0DZ7EZ (Inhibitory cast is listed in the equipment reference table under E, *Orthosis*.)
7. Verbal assessment of patient's pain level	F02ZFZZ

Procedure	Code
8. Caregiver training in communication skills using manual communication board	F0FZJMZ (Manual communication board is listed in the equipment reference table under M, *Augmentative/ Alternative Communication*.)
9. Group musculoskeletal balance training exercises, whole body, no special equipment	F07M6ZZ (Balance training is included in the motor treatment reference table under *Therapeutic Exercise*.)
10. Individual therapy for auditory processing using tape recorder	F09Z2KZ (Tape recorder is listed in the equipment reference table under *Audiovisual Equipment*.)

Mental Health

Procedure	Code
1. Cognitive-behavioral psychotherapy, individual	GZ58ZZZ
2. Narcosynthesis	GZGZZZZ
3. Light therapy	GZJZZZZ
4. ECT (electroconvulsive therapy), unilateral, multiple seizure	GZB1ZZZ
5. Crisis intervention	GZ2ZZZZ
6. Neuropsychological testing	GZ13ZZZ
7. Hypnosis	GZFZZZZ
8. Developmental testing	GZ10ZZZ
9. Vocational counseling	GZ61ZZZ
10. Family psychotherapy	GZ72ZZZ

Substance Abuse Treatment

Procedure	Code
1. Naltrexone treatment for drug dependency	HZ94ZZZ
2. Substance abuse treatment family counseling	HZ63ZZZ
3. Medication monitoring of patient on methadone maintenance	HZ81ZZZ
4. Individual interpersonal psychotherapy for drug abuse	HZ54ZZZ
5. Patient in for alcohol detoxification treatment	HZ2ZZZZ
6. Group motivational counseling	HZ47ZZZ
7. Individual 12-step psychotherapy for substance abuse	HZ53ZZZ
8. Post-test infectious disease counseling for IV drug abuser	HZ3CZZZ
9. Psychodynamic psychotherapy for drug dependent patient	HZ5CZZZ
10. Group cognitive-behavioral counseling for substance abuse	HZ42ZZZ

New Technology

Procedure	Code
1. Infusion of terlipressin via peripheral venous catheter	XW03367
2. Transcatheter dilation of left peroneal artery with 2 SAVAL stents	X27U395

Contents

What's New for 2023 iii

Introduction 1
   ICD-10-PCS Manual 1
   Medical and Surgical Section (Ø) 4
   Obstetrics Section (1) 7
   Placement Section (2) 7
   Administration Section (3) 8
   Measurement and Monitoring
      Section (4) 8
   Extracorporeal or Systemic Assistance and Performance
      Section (5) 9
   Extracorporeal or Systemic Therapies Section (6) 10
   Osteopathic Section (7) 10
   Other Procedures Section (8) 11
   Chiropractic Section (9) 11
   Imaging Section (B) 11
   Nuclear Medicine Section (C) 12
   Radiation Therapy Section (D) 13
   Physical Rehabilitation and Diagnostic Audiology Section (F) 13
   Mental Health Section (G) 14
   Substance Abuse Treatment Section (H) 15
   New Technology Section (X) 15

ICD-10-PCS Index and Tabular Format 17
   Index 17
   Code Tables 17

ICD-10-PCS Additional Features 19
   Use of Official Sources 19
   Table Notations 19
   Appendixes 20

**ICD-10-PCS Official Guidelines for Coding
and Reporting 2023** 23
   Conventions 23
   Medical and Surgical Section Guidelines (section Ø) 24
   Obstetric Section Guidelines (section 1) 29
   Radiation Therapy Section Guidelines (section D) 29
   New Technology Section Guidelines (section X) 30

Index 31

ICD-10-PCS Tables 131
   Central Nervous System and Cranial Nerves 131
   Peripheral Nervous System 153
   Heart and Great Vessels 171
   Upper Arteries 193
   Lower Arteries 219
   Upper Veins 243
   Lower Veins 263
   Lymphatic and Hemic Systems 283
   Eye 301
   Ear, Nose, Sinus 319
   Respiratory System 339

   Mouth and Throat 355
   Gastrointestinal System 373
   Hepatobiliary System and Pancreas 401
   Endocrine System 415
   Skin and Breast 425
   Subcutaneous Tissue and Fascia 443
   Muscles 463
   Tendons 485
   Bursae and Ligaments 499
   Head and Facial Bones 521
   Upper Bones 541
   Lower Bones 561
   Upper Joints 579
   Lower Joints 599
   Urinary System 623
   Female Reproductive System 639
   Male Reproductive System 659
   Anatomical Regions, General 675
   Anatomical Regions, Upper Extremities 687
   Anatomical Regions, Lower Extremities 697
   Obstetrics 707
   Placement 711
   Administration 717
   Measurement and Monitoring 729
   Extracorporeal or Systemic Assistance and Performance 733
   Extracorporeal or Systemic Therapies 735
   Osteopathic 737
   Other Procedures 739
   Chiropractic 741
   Imaging 743
   Nuclear Medicine 773
   Radiation Therapy 783
   Physical Rehabilitation and Diagnostic Audiology 801
   Mental Health 813
   Substance Abuse Treatment 815
   New Technology 817

Appendixes 827
   Appendix A: Components of the Medical and Surgical
      Approach Definitions 827
   Appendix B: Root Operation Definitions 830
   Appendix C: Comparison of Medical and Surgical
      Root Operations 835
   Appendix D: Body Part Key 837
   Appendix E: Body Part Definitions 853
   Appendix F: Device Classification 865
   Appendix G: Device Key and Aggregation Table 867
   Appendix H: Device Definitions 876
   Appendix I: Substance Key/Substance Definitions 882
   Appendix J: Sections B–H Character Definitions 887
   Appendix K: Hospital Acquired Conditions 896
   Appendix L: Procedure Combination Tables 915
   Appendix M: Coding Exercises and Answers 932

What's New for 2023

The Centers for Medicare and Medicaid Services is the agency charged with maintaining and updating ICD-10-PCS. CMS released the most current revisions, a summary of which may be found on the CMS website at https://www.cms.gov/medicare/icd-10/2023-icd-10-pcs.

Due to the unique structure of ICD-10-PCS, a change in a character value may affect individual codes and several code tables.

Change Summary Table

2022 Total	New Codes	Revised Titles	Deleted Codes	2023 Total
78,229	331	0	64	78,496

ICD-10-PCS Code Totals, By Section

Medical and Surgical	68,024
Obstetrics	304
Placement	861
Administration	1,257
Measurement and Monitoring	422
Extracorporeal or Systemic Assistance and Performance	51
Extracorporeal or Systemic Therapies	46
Osteopathic	100
Other Procedures	78
Chiropractic	90
Imaging	2,978
Nuclear Medicine	463
Radiation Therapy	2,056
Physical Rehabilitation and Diagnostic Audiology	1,380
Mental Health	30
Substance Abuse Treatment	59
New Technology	297
Total	78,496

ICD-10-PCS Table Changes Highlights

- New qualifier Laser Interstitial Thermal Therapy (LITT) added to the root operation table, Destruction, in the following body systems:
  - Central Nervous System and Cranial Nerves
  - Respiratory System
  - Gastrointestinal System
  - Hepatobiliary System and Pancreas
  - Endocrine System
  - Skin and Breast
  - Male Reproductive System
- New qualifier Rapid Deployment Technique added to root operation table Replacement in the Heart and Great Vessels body system for the body part Aortic Valve and device value Zooplastic Tissue
- New qualifier values Prostatic Artery, Right and Prostatic Artery, Left, added to root operation table Occlusion in the Lower Arteries body system for body parts Internal Iliac Artery, Right, and Internal Iliac Artery, Left, respectively

- New qualifier values Bladder; Ureter, Right; Ureter, Left; and Ureters, Bilateral, added for body part Small Intestine and new qualifier value Bladder added for body part Large Intestine in the root operation table Transfer in the Gastrointestinal System body system
- New device value Infusion Device added for body part Skull in the root operation tables Removal and Revision in the Head and Facial Bones body system
- Approach values Via Natural or Artificial Opening and Via Natural or Artificial Opening Endoscopic added to body part Neck in the root operation table Drainage in the Anatomical Regions, General, body system
- New row added to root operation table Assistance, Physiological Systems, in the Extracorporeal or Systemic Assistance and Performance section to capture continuous supersaturated oxygenation of the Cardiac body system
- Qualifier value Supersaturated removed from Circulatory body system in the root operation table Assistance, Physiological Systems, in the Extracorporeal or Systemic Assistance and Performance section
- New row added to the root operation MRI, Respiratory System, in the Imaging section to capture the use of Hyperpolarized Xenon 129 (Xe-129) for the body part Lungs, Bilateral
- Modality qualifier value of Laser Interstitial Thermal Therapy removed from all root operation tables, Other Radiation, in the Radiation Therapy section
- Seven new tables added to the New Technology section:
  - X0H Nervous System, Insertion
  - X0Z Nervous System, Other Procedures
  - XF5 Hepatobiliary System and Pancreas, Destruction
  - XKU Muscles, Tendons, Bursae and Ligaments, Supplement
  - XNH Bones, Insertion
  - XRH Joints, Insertion
  - XRR Joints, Replacement
- One table deleted from the New Technology section:
  - XK0 Muscles, Tendons, Bursae and Ligaments, Introduction

New Definitions Addenda

Section 0 – Medical and Surgical
Body Part Definitions

ICD-10-PCS Value	Definition	
Internal Iliac Artery, Left	Add	Prostatic artery
	Add	Superior vesical artery
Internal Iliac Artery, Right	Add	Prostatic artery
	Add	Superior vesical artery
Add Peritoneal Cavity	Add	Abdominal cavity
Add Skin, Perineum	Add	Perianal skin
Superior Vena Cava	Add	Cavoatrial junction

Section 0 – Medical and Surgical Device Definitions

ICD-10-PCS Value	Definition	
Interbody Fusion Device in Lower Joints	Add Add Add Add	COALESCE® radiolucent interbody fusion device COHERE® radiolucent interbody fusion device nanoLOCK™ interbody fusion device Titan Endoskeleton™
Interbody Fusion Device in Upper Joints	Add Add Add Add	COALESCE® radiolucent interbody fusion device COHERE® radiolucent interbody fusion device nanoLOCK™ interbody fusion device Titan Endoskeleton™
Internal Fixation Device, Sustained Compression for Fusion in Lower Joints	Delete Delete Add Add	DynaNail Mini® DynaNail® DynaClip® (Forte) DynaNail® (Hybrid)(Mini)
Internal Fixation Device, Sustained Compression for Fusion in Upper Joints	Delete Delete Add Add	DynaNail Mini® DynaNail® DynaClip® (Forte) DynaNail® (Hybrid)(Mini)
Nonautologous Tissue Substitute	Add	MIRODERM™ Biologic Wound Matrix
Spinal Stabilization Device, Interspinous Process for Insertion in Lower Joints	Add	X-Spine Axle Cage
Spinal Stabilization Device, Interspinous Process for Insertion in Upper Joints	Add	X-Spine Axle Cage

Section 3 – Administration Substance Definitions

ICD-10-PCS Value	Definition	
Hematopoietic Stem/Progenitor Cells, Genetically Modified	Delete Delete	OTL-103 OTL-200
Add Other Substance	Add Add Add	CBMA (Concentrated Bone Marrow Aspirate) Defitelio MarrowStim™ PAD Kit for CBMA (concentrated bone marrow aspirate)

Section X – New Technology Root Operation Definitions

ICD-10-PCS Value	Definition	
Fusion	Delete Delete	Explanation: The body part is joined together by fixation device, bone graft, or other means. Includes/Examples: Spinal fusion, ankle arthrodesis
Add Other Procedures	Add	Definition: Methodologies which attempt to remediate or cure a disorder or disease.
Replacement	Delete Delete	Explanation: The body part may have been taken out or replaced, or may be taken out, physically eradicated, or rendered nonfunctional during the Replacement procedure. A Removal procedure is coded for taking out the device used in a previous replacement procedure. Includes/Examples: Total hip replacement, bone graft, free skin graft

Section X – New Technology Device/Substance/Technology Definitions

ICD-10-PCS Value	Definition	
Delete Bezlotoxumab Monoclonal Antibody	Delete	ZINPLAVA™
Add Afamitresgene Autoleucel Immunotherapy	Add	afami-cel
Add Betibeglogene Autotemcel	Add	beti-cel
Add Broad Consortium Microbiota-based Live Biotherapeutic Suspension	Add	REBYOTA®
Ciltacabtagene Autoleucel	Add	CARVYKTI™
Delete Concentrated Bone Marrow Aspirate	Delete	CBMA (concentrated bone marrow aspirate)
Delete Defibrotide Sodium Anticoagulant	Delete	Defitelio
Delete Interbody Fusion Device, Nanotextured Surface in New Technology	Delete	nanoLOCK™ interbody fusion device
Delete Interbody Fusion Device, Radiolucent Porous in New Technology	Delete	COALESCE® radiolucent interbody fusion device
	Delete	COHERE® radiolucent interbody fusion device
Delete Skin Substitute, Porcine Liver Derived in New Technology	Delete	MIRODERM™ Biologic Wound Matrix
Delete Zooplastic Tissue, Rapid Deployment Technique in New Technology	Delete Delete Delete Delete	EDWARDS INTUITY Elite valve system INTUITY Elite valve system, EDWARDS Perceval sutureless valve Sutureless valve, Perceval
Add Daratumumab and Hyaluronidase-fihj	Add	Darzalex Faspro®
Add Engineered Allogeneic Thymus Tissue	Add	RETHYMIC®

ICD-10-PCS Value		Definition	
Add	Inebilizumab-cdon	Add	UPLIZNA®
Add	Internal Fixation Device with Tulip Connector in New Technology	Add	iFuse Bedrock™ Granite Implant System
Add	Maribavir Anti-infective	Add	LIVTENCITY™
Add	Neurostimulator Lead in New Technology	Add	Ischemic Stroke System (ISS500)
		Add	ISS500 (Ischemic Stroke System)
Add	Neurostimulator Lead with Paired Stimulation System in New Technology	Add	Vivistim® Paired VNS System Lead
Add	Posterior Spinal Motion Preservation Device in New Technology	Add	TOPS™ System
Add	Posterior Vertebral Tether in New Technology	Add	LigaPASS 2.0™ PJK Prevention System
Add	Synthetic Substitute, Lateral Meniscus in New Technology	Add	NUsurface® Meniscus Implant
Add	Synthetic Substitute, Medial Meniscus in New Technology	Add	NUsurface® Meniscus Implant
Add	Tabelecleucel Immunotherapy	Add	tab-cel®
Add	Taurolidine Anti-infective and Heparin Anticoagulant	Add	DefenCath™

List of Updated Files

2023 Official ICD-10-PCS Coding Guidelines

- New guideline B3.19 added and guidelines B4.1c and B6.1a revised in response to public comment and internal review.
- Downloadable PDF

2023 ICD-10-PCS Code Tables and Index (Zip file)

- Code tables for use beginning October 1, 2022.
- Downloadable PDF, file name is pcs_2023.pdf
- Downloadable xml files for developers, file names are icd10pcs_tables_2023.xml, icd10pcs_index_2023.xml, icd10pcs_definitions_2023.xml
- Accompanying schema for developers, file names are icd10pcs_tables.xsd, icd10pcs_index.xsd, icd10pcs_definitions.xsd

2023 ICD-10-PCS Codes File (Zip file)

- ICD-10-PCS Codes file is a simple format for nontechnical uses, containing the valid FY2023 ICD-10-PCS codes and their long titles.
- File is in text file format, file name is icd10pcs_codes_2023.txt
- Accompanying documentation for codes file, file name is icd10pcsCodesFile.pdf
- Codes file addenda in text format, file name is codes_addenda_2023.txt

2023 ICD-10-PCS Order File (Long and Abbreviated Titles) (Zip file)

- ICD-10-PCS order file is for developers, provides a unique five-digit "order number" for each ICD-10-PCS table and code, as well as a long and abbreviated code title.
- ICD-10-PCS order file name is icd10pcs_order_2023.txt
- Accompanying documentation for tabular order file, file name is icd10pcsOrderFile.pdf
- Tabular order file addenda in text format, file name is order_addenda_2023.txt

2023 ICD-10-PCS Final Addenda (Zip file)

- Addenda files in downloadable PDF, file names are tables_addenda_2023.pdf, index_addenda_2023.pdf, definitions_addenda_2023.pdf
- Addenda files also in machine readable text format for developers, file names are tables_addenda_2023.txt, index_addenda_2023.txt, definitions_addenda_2023.txt

2023 ICD-10-PCS Conversion Table (Zip file)

- ICD-10-PCS code conversion table is provided to assist users in data retrieval, in downloadable Excel spreadsheet, file name is icd10pcs_conversion_table_2023.xlsx
- Conversion table also in machine readable text format for developers, file name is icd10pcs_conversion_table_2023.txt
- Accompanying documentation for code conversion table, file name is icd10pcsConversionTable.pdf

Introduction

ICD-10-PCS: The Complete Official Code Set is your definitive coding resource for procedure coding in acute inpatient hospitals. In addition to the official ICD-10-PCS Coding System Files, revised and distributed by the Centers for Medicare and Medicaid Services (CMS), Optum's coding experts have incorporated Medicare-related coding edits and proprietary features, such as coding tools and appendixes, into a comprehensive and easy-to-use reference.

This manual provides the most current information that was available at the time of publication. For updates to official source documents that may have occurred after this manual was published, please refer to the following:

- **CMS International Classification of Disease, 10th Revision, Procedural Coding System (ICD-10-PCS):**

  https://www.cms.gov/medicare/icd-10/2023-icd-10-pcs

- **CMS Inpatient Prospective Payment System Proposed Rule, FY2023**

  https://www.cms.gov/medicare/acute-inpatient-pps/fy-2023-ipps-proposed-rule-home-page

- **CMS Inpatient Prospective Payment System Proposed Rule, FY 2023 - Proposed, version 40, MS-DRG Grouper software, Definitions Manual files and Medicare Code Editor (MCE) files**

  https://www.cms.gov/Medicare/Medicare-Fee-for-Service-Payment/AcuteInpatientPPS/MS-DRG-Classifications-and-Software

- **American Hospital Association (AHA) Coding Clinics**

  https://www.codingclinicadvisor.com/

ICD-10-PCS Code Structure

All codes in ICD-10-PCS are seven characters long. Each character in the seven-character code represents an aspect of the procedure, as shown in the following diagram of characters from the main section of ICD-10-PCS, called the Medical and Surgical section.

	Section	Body System	Root Operation	Body Part	Approach	Device	Qualifier
Characters:	1	2	3	4	5	6	7

One of 34 possible alphanumeric values—using the digits Ø–9 and letters A–H, J–N, and P–Z—can be assigned to each character in a code. The letters O and I are not used so as to avoid confusion with the digits Ø and 1. A code is derived by choosing a specific value for each of the seven characters, based on details about the procedure performed. Because the definition of each character is a function of its physical position in the code, the same value placed in a different position means something different; the value Ø as the first character means something different from Ø as the second character or as the third character, and so on.

The first character always determines the broad procedure category, or section. The second through seventh characters have the same meaning within a specific section, but these meanings can change in a different section. For example, the sixth character means "device" in the Medical and Surgical section but "qualifier" in the Imaging section.

ICD-10-PCS Manual

Index

Codes may be found in the index based on the general type of procedure (e.g., resection, transfusion, fluoroscopy), or a more commonly used term (e.g., appendectomy). For example, the code for percutaneous intraluminal dilation of the coronary arteries with an intraluminal device can be found in the Index under *Dilation*, or a synonym of *Dilation* (e.g., angioplasty). The Index then specifies the first three or four values of the code or directs the user to see another term.

Example:

> **Dilation**
>   Artery
>   Coronary
>   One Artery Ø27Ø

Based on the first three values of the code provided in the Index, the corresponding table can be located. In the example above, the first three values indicate table Ø27 is to be referenced for code completion.

The tables and characters are arranged first by number and then by letter for each character (tables for ØØ-, Ø1-, Ø2-, etc., are followed by those for ØB-, ØC-, ØD-, etc., followed by ØB1, ØB2, etc., followed by ØBB, ØBC, ØBD, etc.).

Note: The Tables section must be used to construct a complete and valid code by specifying the last three or four values.

Tables

The tables in ICD-10-PCS provide the valid combination of character values needed to build a unique procedure code. Each table is preceded by the first three characters of the code, along with their descriptions. In the Medical and Surgical section, for example, the first three characters contain the name of the section (character 1), the body system (character 2), and the root operation performed (character 3).

Listed underneath the first three characters is a table comprising four columns and one or more rows. The four columns in the table specify the last four characters needed to complete the ICD-10-PCS code. Depending on the section, the labels for each column may be different. In the Medical and Surgical section, they are labeled body part (character 4), approach (character 5), device (character 6), and qualifier (character 7). Each row in the table specifies the valid combination of values for characters 4 through 7.

Table 1: Row from table Ø27

Ø Medical and Surgical
2 Heart and Great Vessels
7 Dilation   Definition: Expanding an orifice or the lumen of a tubular body part

Explanation: The orifice can be a natural orifice or an artificially created orifice. Accomplished by stretching a tubular body part using intraluminal pressure or by cutting part of the orifice or wall of the tubular body part.

Body Part Character 4	Approach Character 5	Device Character 6	Qualifier Character 7
Ø Coronary Artery, One Artery 1 Coronary Artery, Two Arteries 2 Coronary Artery, Three Arteries 3 Coronary Artery, Four or More Arteries	Ø Open 3 Percutaneous 4 Percutaneous Endoscopic	4 Intraluminal Device, Drug-eluting 5 Intraluminal Device, Drug-eluting, Two 6 Intraluminal Device, Drug-eluting, Three 7 Intraluminal Device, Drug-eluting, Four or More D Intraluminal Device E Intraluminal Device, Two F Intraluminal Device, Three G Intraluminal Device, Four or More T Intraluminal Device, Radioactive Z No Device	6 Bifurcation Z No Qualifier

For instance, table 1 above shows the first row from table Ø27 in ICD-10-PCS. The values Ø27 specify the section *Medical and Surgical (Ø)*, the body system *Heart and Great Vessels (2)*, and the root operation *Dilation (7)*. As shown, the root operation (Dilation) is also accompanied by its corresponding definition and explanation. Note, a definition of the root operation is provided for every table in ICD-10-PCS; however, an explanation may not always be applicable.

In total, this single row can be used to construct 240 unique procedure codes. The valid codes shown in table 2 (below) are constructed using the body part (character 4) value of Ø, Coronary artery, one artery, combined with all valid approach (character 5) values, device (character 6) values, and a qualifier (character 7) value of Z, No Qualifier.

Table 2: Code titles for dilation of one coronary artery (Ø27Ø)

Ø27004Z	Dilation of Coronary Artery, One Artery with Drug-eluting Intraluminal Device, Open Approach
Ø27005Z	Dilation of Coronary Artery, One Artery with Two Drug-eluting Intraluminal Devices, Open Approach
Ø27006Z	Dilation of Coronary Artery, One Artery with Three Drug-eluting Intraluminal Devices, Open Approach
Ø27007Z	Dilation of Coronary Artery, One Artery with Four or More Drug-eluting Intraluminal Devices, Open Approach
Ø2700DZ	Dilation of Coronary Artery, One Artery with Intraluminal Device, Open Approach
Ø2700EZ	Dilation of Coronary Artery, One Artery with Two Intraluminal Devices, Open Approach
Ø2700FZ	Dilation of Coronary Artery, One Artery with Three Intraluminal Devices, Open Approach
Ø2700GZ	Dilation of Coronary Artery, One Artery with Four or More Intraluminal Devices, Open Approach
Ø2700TZ	Dilation of Coronary Artery, One Artery with Radioactive Intraluminal Device, Open Approach
Ø2700ZZ	Dilation of Coronary Artery, One Artery, Open Approach
Ø27034Z	Dilation of Coronary Artery, One Artery with Drug-eluting Intraluminal Device, Percutaneous Approach
Ø27035Z	Dilation of Coronary Artery, One Artery with Two Drug-eluting Intraluminal Devices, Percutaneous Approach
Ø27036Z	Dilation of Coronary Artery, One Artery with Three Drug-eluting Intraluminal Devices, Percutaneous Approach
Ø27037Z	Dilation of Coronary Artery, One Artery with Four or More Drug-eluting Intraluminal Devices, Percutaneous Approach
Ø2703DZ	Dilation of Coronary Artery, One Artery with Intraluminal Device, Percutaneous Approach
Ø2703EZ	Dilation of Coronary Artery, One Artery with Two Intraluminal Devices, Percutaneous Approach
Ø2703FZ	Dilation of Coronary Artery, One Artery with Three Intraluminal Devices, Percutaneous Approach
Ø2703GZ	Dilation of Coronary Artery, One Artery with Four or More Intraluminal Devices, Percutaneous Approach
Ø2703TZ	Dilation of Coronary Artery, One Artery with Radioactive Intraluminal Device, Percutaneous Approach
Ø2703ZZ	Dilation of Coronary Artery, One Artery, Percutaneous Approach
Ø27044Z	Dilation of Coronary Artery, One Artery with Drug-eluting Intraluminal Device, Percutaneous Endoscopic Approach
Ø27045Z	Dilation of Coronary Artery, One Artery with Two Drug-eluting Intraluminal Devices, Percutaneous Endoscopic Approach
Ø27046Z	Dilation of Coronary Artery, One Artery with Three Drug-eluting Intraluminal Devices, Percutaneous Endoscopic Approach
Ø27047Z	Dilation of Coronary Artery, One Artery with Four or More Drug-eluting Intraluminal Devices, Percutaneous Endoscopic Approach
Ø2704DZ	Dilation of Coronary Artery, One Artery with Intraluminal Device, Percutaneous Endoscopic Approach
Ø2704EZ	Dilation of Coronary Artery, One Artery with Two Intraluminal Devices, Percutaneous Endoscopic Approach
Ø2704FZ	Dilation of Coronary Artery, One Artery with Three Intraluminal Devices, Percutaneous Endoscopic Approach
Ø2704GZ	Dilation of Coronary Artery, One Artery with Four or More Intraluminal Devices, Percutaneous Endoscopic Approach
Ø2704TZ	Dilation of Coronary Artery, One Artery with Radioactive Intraluminal Device, Percutaneous Endoscopic Approach
Ø2704ZZ	Dilation of Coronary Artery, One Artery, Percutaneous Endoscopic Approach

Table 3: Rows from table 00H

0   Medical and Surgical
0   Central Nervous System and Cranial Nerves
H   Insertion   Definition: Putting in a nonbiological appliance that monitors, assists, performs, or prevents a physiological function but does not physically take the place of a body part

Explanation: None

Body Part Character 4		Approach Character 5	Device Character 6	Qualifier Character 7
0 Brain Cerebrum Corpus callosum Encephalon		**0 Open**	**1 Radioactive Element** **2 Monitoring Device** **3 Infusion Device** **4 Radioactive Element, Cesium-131 Collagen Implant** **M Neurostimulator Lead** **Y Other Device**	**Z No Qualifier**
0 Brain Cerebrum Corpus callosum Encephalon		**3 Percutaneous** **4 Percutaneous Endoscopic**	**1 Radioactive Element** **2 Monitoring Device** **3 Infusion Device** **M Neurostimulator Lead** **Y Other Device**	**Z No Qualifier**
6 Cerebral Ventricle Aqueduct of Sylvius Cerebral aqueduct (Sylvius) Choroid plexus Ependyma Foramen of Monro (intraventricular) Fourth ventricle Interventricular foramen (Monro) Left lateral ventricle Right lateral ventricle Third ventricle	**E Cranial Nerve** **U Spinal Canal** Epidural space, spinal Extradural space, spinal Subarachnoid space, spinal Subdural space, spinal Vertebral canal **V Spinal Cord** Dorsal root ganglion	**0 Open** **3 Percutaneous** **4 Percutaneous Endoscopic**	**1 Radioactive Element** **2 Monitoring Device** **3 Infusion Device** **M Neurostimulator Lead** **Y Other Device**	**Z No Qualifier**

Table 3 is split into three rows; values of characters must all be selected from within the same row of the table. Rows 1 and 2 have the same body part (character 4) value of 0 Brain and the same qualifier value (character 7) of Z No Qualifier. However, the approach (character 5) values are not the same for these two rows, and there is one additional device (character 6) value in row 1 that is not included in row 2. As shown in row 1, body part value Brain (0) with device value Radioactive Element, Cesium-131 Collagen Implant (4) can only be used with approach value Open (0). In other words, code 00H034Z would be invalid as the approach value 3 is only applicable to row 2 and the device value 4 is only applicable to row 1. It would be inappropriate to build a code for body part 0 if all of the values are not contained in its own row.

Note: In this manual, there are instances in which some tables due to length must be continued on the next page. Each section must be used separately and value selection must be made within the same row of the table.

Character Meanings

In each section, each character has a specific meaning, and this character meaning remains constant within that section. Character meaning tables have been provided at the beginning of each body system in the Medical and Surgical section (0) and the Obstetric section (1) to help the user identify the character members available within that section. These tables have purple headers, unlike the official code tables that have green headers and **SHOULD NOT** be used to build a PCS code. Following is an excerpt of a character meaning table.

Table 4: Rows from Central Nervous System and Cranial Nerves - Character Meanings Table

Operation–Character 3	Body Part–Character 4	Approach–Character 5	Device–Character 6	Qualifier–Character 7
1 Bypass	0 Brain	0 Open	0 Drainage Device	0 Nasopharynx
2 Change	1 Cerebral Meninges	3 Percutaneous	1 Radioactive Element	1 Mastoid Sinus
5 Destruction	2 Dura Mater	4 Percutaneous Endoscopic	2 Monitoring Device	2 Atrium
7 Dilation	3 Epidural Space, Intracranial	X External	3 Infusion Device	3 Blood Vessel
8 Division	4 Subdural Space, Intracranial		4 Radioactive Element, Cesium-131 Collagen Implant	4 Pleural Cavity
9 Drainage	5 Subarachnoid Space, Intracranial		7 Autologous Tissue Substitute	5 Intestine
B Excision	6 Cerebral Ventricle		J Synthetic Substitute	6 Peritoneal Cavity
C Extirpation	7 Cerebral Hemisphere		K Nonautologous Tissue Substitute	7 Urinary Tract
D Extraction	8 Basal Ganglia		M Neurostimulator Lead	8 Bone Marrow
F Fragmentation	9 Thalamus		Y Other Device	9 Fallopian Tube
H Insertion	A Hypothalamus		Z No Device	A Subgaleal space
J Inspection	B Pons			B Cerebral Cisterns

Sections

The first character of the procedure code always specifies the section. There are 17 sections within the PCS manual, listed below.

Medical and Surgical Section
Ø   Medical and Surgical

Medical and Surgical-related Sections
1   Obstetrics
2   Placement
3   Administration
4   Measurement and Monitoring
5   Extracorporeal or Systemic Assistance and Performance
6   Extracorporeal or Systemic Therapies
7   Osteopathic
8   Other Procedures
9   Chiropractic

Ancillary Sections
B   Imaging
C   Nuclear Medicine
D   Radiation Therapy
F   Physical Rehabilitation and Diagnostic Audiology
G   Mental Health
H   Substance Abuse Treatment

New Technology Section
X   New Technology

Medical and Surgical Section (Ø)

The Medical and Surgical section contains codes for the vast majority of procedures typically reported in an inpatient setting.

Character Meaning

The seven characters for Medical and Surgical procedures have the following meaning:

Character	Meaning
1	Section
2	Body System
3	Root Operation
4	Body Part
5	Approach
6	Device
7	Qualifier

Section (Character 1)

Medical and Surgical procedure codes all have a first character value of Ø.

Body Systems (Character 2)

The second character represents the body system—the general physiological system or anatomical region where the procedure is being performed.

Body Systems
Ø   Central Nervous System and Cranial Nerves
1   Peripheral Nervous System
2   Heart and Great Vessels
3   Upper Arteries
4   Lower Arteries
5   Upper Veins
6   Lower Veins
7   Lymphatic and Hemic Systems
8   Eye
9   Ear, Nose, Sinus
B   Respiratory System
C   Mouth and Throat
D   Gastrointestinal System
F   Hepatobiliary System and Pancreas
G   Endocrine System
H   Skin and Breast
J   Subcutaneous Tissue and Fascia
K   Muscles
L   Tendons
M   Bursae and Ligaments
N   Head and Facial Bones
P   Upper Bones
Q   Lower Bones
R   Upper Joints
S   Lower Joints
T   Urinary System
U   Female Reproductive System
V   Male Reproductive System
W   Anatomical Regions, General
X   Anatomical Regions, Upper Extremities
Y   Anatomical Regions, Lower Extremities

Root Operations (Character 3)

The third character represents the root operation, or the primary objective, of the procedure. There are 31 different root operations in this section, each with its own precise definition.

- *Alteration:* Modifying the natural anatomic structure of a body part without affecting the function of the body part

- *Bypass:* Altering the route of passage of the contents of a tubular body part

- *Change:* Taking out or off a device from a body part and putting back an identical or similar device in or on the same body part without cutting or puncturing the skin or a mucous membrane

- *Control:* Stopping, or attempting to stop, postprocedural or other acute bleeding

- *Creation:* Putting in or on biological or synthetic material to form a new body part that to the extent possible replicates the anatomic structure or function of an absent body part

- *Destruction:* Physical eradication of all or a portion of a body part by the direct use of energy, force, or a destructive agent

- *Detachment:* Cutting off all or a portion of the upper or lower extremities

- *Dilation:* Expanding an orifice or the lumen of a tubular body part

- *Division:* Cutting into a body part without draining fluids and/or gases from the body part in order to separate or transect a body part

- *Drainage:* Taking or letting out fluids and/or gases from a body part

- *Excision:* Cutting out or off, without replacement, a portion of a body part

- *Extirpation:* Taking or cutting out solid matter from a body part

- *Extraction:* Pulling or stripping out or off all or a portion of a body part by the use of force

- *Fragmentation:* Breaking solid matter in a body part into pieces

- *Fusion:* Joining together portions of an articular body part rendering the articular body part immobile

- *Insertion:* Putting in a nonbiological appliance that monitors, assists, performs, or prevents a physiological function but does not physically take the place of a body part

- *Inspection:* Visually and/or manually exploring a body part

- *Map:* Locating the route of passage of electrical impulses and/or locating functional areas in a body part

- *Occlusion:* Completely closing an orifice or lumen of a tubular body part

- *Reattachment:* Putting back in or on all or a portion of a separated body part to its normal location or other suitable location

- *Release:* Freeing a body part from an abnormal physical constraint by cutting or by use of force

- *Removal:* Taking out or off a device from a body part

- *Repair:* Restoring, to the extent possible, a body part to its normal anatomic structure and function

- *Replacement:* Putting in or on biological or synthetic material that physically takes the place and/or function of all or a portion of a body part

- *Reposition:* Moving to its normal location or other suitable location all or a portion of a body part

- *Resection:* Cutting out or off, without replacement, all of a body part

- *Restriction:* Partially closing an orifice or lumen of a tubular body part

- *Revision:* Correcting, to the extent possible, a portion of a malfunctioning device or the position of a displaced device

- *Supplement:* Putting in or on biological or synthetic material that physically reinforces and/or augments the function of a portion of a body part

- *Transfer:* Moving, without taking out, all or a portion of a body part to another location to take over the function of all or a portion of a body part

- *Transplantation:* Putting in or on all or a portion of a living body part taken from another individual or animal to physically take the place and/or function of all or a portion of a similar body part

The standardized level of specificity designed into ICD-10-PCS restricts the use of broadly applicable "not otherwise specified (NOS)" or "unspecified code" options in the system. A minimal level of specificity is required to construct a valid code. "Not elsewhere classified (NEC)"

options are provided in ICD-10-PCS but only for specific, limited use. The root operation Repair in the Medical and Surgical section functions as a "not elsewhere classified" option. Repair is used only when the procedure performed is not one of the other specific root operations in the Medical and Surgical section.

Appendixes B and C provide additional subcategorization, explanations, and representative examples of the Medical and Surgical section root operations.

Body Part (Character 4)
The fourth character represents the body part, or specific anatomical site where the procedure was performed. The body system (second character) provides only a general indication of the procedure site. The body part and body system values, together, provide a precise description of the procedure site.

Approach (Character 5)
The fifth character represents the approach, or the technique used to reach the procedure site. There are seven different approach values in this section.

- *Open*: Cutting through the skin or mucous membrane and any other body layers necessary to expose the site of the procedure

- *Percutaneous*: Entry, by puncture or minor incision, of instrumentation through the skin or mucous membrane and any other body layers necessary to reach the site of the procedure

- *Percutaneous Endoscopic*: Entry, by puncture or minor incision, of instrumentation through the skin or mucous membrane and any other body layers necessary to reach and visualize the site of the procedure

- *Via Natural or Artificial Opening*: Entry of instrumentation through a natural or artificial external opening to reach the site of the procedure

- *Via Natural or Artificial Opening Endoscopic*: Entry of instrumentation through a natural or artificial external opening to reach and visualize the site of the procedure

- *Via Natural or Artificial Opening with Percutaneous Endoscopic Assistance:* Entry of instrumentation through a natural or artificial external opening and entry, by puncture or minor incision, of instrumentation through the skin or mucous membrane and any other body layers necessary to aid in the performance of the procedure

- *External*: Procedures performed directly on the skin or mucous membrane and procedures performed indirectly by the application of external force through the skin or mucous membrane

Appendix A provides definitions and comparisons of the components (access location, method, and type of instrumentation) for each approach and provides an example and illustration.

Device (Character 6)
The sixth character represents a device. Broad categories of devices found in this section include:

- Grafts (e.g., skin)

- Prostheses (e.g., hip joint)

- Implants (e.g., internal fixation device, mesh)

- Simple or Mechanical Appliances (e.g., drainage device, IUD)

- Electronic Appliances (e.g., pacemaker, monitoring device)

Depending on the procedure performed, there may or may not be a device left in place at the end of the procedure. For procedures that do not utilize a device, the value of *No Device* is available. For devices that cannot be categorized into one of the current values, many tables also have a device value of *Other Device*. This value is intended to be used temporarily until a more specific value can be added to the classification. No categories of medical or surgical devices are permanently classified to *Other Device*.

Instruments used to visualize the procedure site are specified in the fifth-character approach, not the sixth-character device value. Materials that are incidental to a procedure such as clips, ligatures, and sutures are not specified in the device character.

Appendix F compares the general device types and provides examples of each.

Appendix G provides an aggregation table that crosswalks specific device character values used for specific root operations to more general device character values used when the root operation represents an entire family of devices.

Qualifier (Character 7)

The seventh character is a qualifier that captures additional attributes of the procedure, where applicable.

Medical and Surgical Section Principles

In developing the Medical and Surgical procedure codes, several specific principles were followed.

Composite Terms Are Not Root Operations

Composite terms such as colonoscopy, sigmoidectomy, or appendectomy do not describe root operations, but they do specify multiple components of a specific root operation. In ICD-10-PCS, the components of a procedure are defined separately by the characters making up the complete code. The only component of a procedure specified in the root operation is the objective of the procedure. With each complete code the underlying objective of the procedure is specified by the root operation (third character), the precise part is specified by the body part (fourth character), and the method used to reach and visualize the procedure site is specified by the approach (fifth character). While colonoscopy, sigmoidectomy, and appendectomy are included in the Index, they do not constitute root operations in the Tables section. The objective of colonoscopy is the visualization of the colon and the root operation (character 3) is *Inspection*. Character 4 specifies the body part, which in this case is part of the colon. These composite terms, like colonoscopy or appendectomy, are included as cross-reference only. The index provides the correct root operation reference. Examples of other types of composite terms not representative of root operations are *partial* sigmoidectomy, *total* hysterectomy, and *partial* hip replacement. Always refer to the correct root operation in the Index and Tables section.

Root Operation Based on Objective of Procedure

The root operation is based on the objective of the procedure, such as *Resection* of transverse colon or *Dilation* of an artery. The assignment of the root operation is based on the procedure actually performed, which may or may not have been the intended procedure. If the intended procedure is modified or discontinued (e.g., excision instead of resection is performed), the root operation is determined by the procedure actually performed. If the desired result is not attained after completing the procedure (i.e., the artery does not remain expanded

after the dilation procedure), the root operation is still determined by the procedure actually performed.

Examples:

- Dilating the urethra is coded as *Dilation* since the objective of the procedure is to dilate the urethra. If dilation of the urethra includes putting in an intraluminal stent, the root operation remains *Dilation* and not *Insertion* of the intraluminal device because the underlying objective of the procedure is dilation of the urethra. The stent is identified by the intraluminal device value in the sixth character of the dilation procedure code.

- If the objective is solely to put a radioactive element in the urethra, then the procedure is coded to the root operation *Insertion*, with the radioactive element identified in the sixth character of the code.

- If the objective of the procedure is to correct a malfunctioning or displaced device, then the procedure is coded to the root operation *Revision*. In the root operation *Revision*, the original device being revised is identified in the device character. *Revision* is typically performed on mechanical appliances (e.g., pacemaker) or materials used in replacement procedures (e.g., synthetic substitute). Typical revision procedures include adjustment of pacemaker position and correction of malfunctioning knee prosthesis.

Combination Procedures Are Coded Separately

If multiple procedures as defined by distinct objectives are performed during an operative episode, then multiple codes are used. For example, obtaining the vein graft used for coronary bypass surgery is coded as a separate procedure from the bypass itself.

Redo of Procedures

The complete or partial redo of the original procedure is coded to the root operation that identifies the procedure performed rather than *Revision*.

Example:

A complete redo of a hip replacement procedure that requires putting in a new prosthesis is coded to the root operation *Replacement* rather than *Revision*.

The correction of complications arising from the original procedure, other than device complications, is coded to the procedure performed. Correction of a malfunctioning or displaced device would be coded to the root operation *Revision*.

Example:

A procedure to control hemorrhage arising from the original procedure is coded to *Control* rather than *Revision*.

Examples of Procedures Coded in the Medical Surgical Section

The following are examples of procedures from the Medical and Surgical section, coded in ICD-10-PCS.

- Suture of skin laceration, left lower arm: 0HQEXZZ

- Laparoscopic appendectomy: 0DTJ4ZZ

- Sigmoidoscopy with biopsy: 0DBN8ZX

- Tracheostomy with tracheostomy tube: 0B110F4

Obstetrics Section (1)

The Obstetrics section includes codes for procedures performed on the products of conception only. Procedures on pregnant females are coded in the Medical and Surgical section (e.g., episiotomy). The term "products of conception" refers to all physical components of a pregnancy, including the fetus, amnion, umbilical cord, and placenta. There is no differentiation of the products of conception based on gestational age. Thus, the diagnosis code, not the procedure code, specifies the products of conception as a zygote, embryo, or fetus, or of the trimester of the pregnancy.

Character Meanings

The seven characters in the Obstetrics section have the same meaning as in the Medical and Surgical section.

Character	Meaning
1	Section
2	Body System
3	Root Operation
4	Body Part
5	Approach
6	Device
7	Qualifier

Section (Character 1)

Obstetrics procedure codes have a first character value of *1*.

Body System (Character 2)

The second character represents the body system. There is only one value used in this section: *Pregnancy*.

Root Operation (Character 3)

The third character represents the root operation, or the primary objective, of the procedure. There are 12 values available in this section. Ten of these values specify root operations as defined in the Medical and Surgical section and include *Change, Drainage, Extraction, Insertion, Inspection, Removal, Repair, Reposition, Resection,* and *Transplantation*. The other two values are specific to this section only and are defined as follows:

- *Abortion*: Artificially terminating a pregnancy
- *Delivery*: Assisting the passage of the products of conception from the genital canal

A cesarean section is not a separate root operation because the underlying objective is *Extraction* (i.e., pulling out all or a portion of a body part).

Body Part (Character 4)

The fourth character represents the body part, which in this section is specific to the products of conception. The three values available are as follows:

- *Products of conception*
- *Products of conception, retained*
- *Products of conception, ectopic*

Approach (Character 5)

The fifth character represents the approach, as defined in the Medical and Surgical section.

Device (Character 6)

The sixth character represents a device used during the procedure, where applicable.

Qualifier (Character 7)

The seventh character is a qualifier that captures additional attributes of the procedure, where applicable.

Placement Section (2)

The Placement section includes codes for procedures that put a device in an orifice or on a body region, without making an incision or a puncture.

Character Meanings

The seven characters in the Placement section have the following meaning:

Character	Meaning
1	Section
2	Body System
3	Root Operation
4	Body Region
5	Approach
6	Device
7	Qualifier

Section (Character 1)

Placement procedure codes have a first character value of *2*.

Body System (Character 2)

The second character contains two values specifying either *Anatomical Regions* or *Anatomical Orifices*.

Root Operation (Character 3)

The third character represents the root operation, or the primary objective, of the procedure. There are seven values available in this section. Two of the values specify root operations as defined in the Medical and Surgical section and include *Change* and *Removal*. The other five values are specific to this section only and are defined as follows:

- *Compression*: Putting pressure on a body region
- *Dressing*: Putting material on a body region for protection
- *Immobilization*: Limiting or preventing motion of an external body region
- *Packing*: Putting material in a body region or orifice
- *Traction*: Exerting a pulling force on a body region in a distal direction

Body Region (Character 4)

The fourth character represents the specific body region or orifice. The body system (second character) provides only a general indication of the procedure site. The body region values and body system values, together, precisely describe the procedure site.

Approach (Character 5)

The fifth character represents the approach. Since all placement procedures are performed directly or indirectly on the skin or mucous membrane, the approach value is always *External*.

Device (Character 6)

The sixth character represents a device placed during the procedure, where applicable.

Except for devices used for fractures and dislocations, devices in this section are off the shelf and do not require any extensive design, fabrication, or fitting.

Qualifier (Character 7)

The seventh character is a qualifier. Because there are currently no specific qualifier values in this section, the value is always *No Qualifier.*

Administration Section (3)

The Administration section includes infusions, injections, and transfusions, as well as other related procedures, such as irrigation and tattooing. All codes in this section define procedures in which a diagnostic or therapeutic substance is given to the patient.

Character Meanings

The seven characters in the Administration section have the following meaning:

Character	Meaning
1	Section
2	Body System
3	Root Operation
4	Body System/Region
5	Approach
6	Substance
7	Qualifier

Section (Character 1)

Administration procedure codes have a first character value of *3*.

Body System (Character 2)

The second character can represent the general physiological system, anatomical region, or device to which a substance is being administered. The three values available in this section are *Indwelling Device, Physiological Systems and Anatomical Regions,* and *Circulatory System.*

Root Operation (Character 3)

The third character represents the root operation, or the primary objective, of the procedure. There are three values available in this section.

- *Introduction*: Putting in or on a therapeutic, diagnostic, nutritional, physiological, or prophylactic substance except blood or blood products
- *Irrigation*: Putting in or on a cleansing substance
- *Transfusion*: Putting in blood or blood products

Body/System Region (Character 4)

The fourth character represents the body system/region. The fourth character identifies the site where the substance is administered, not the site where the substance administered takes effect. Sites include *Skin and Mucous Membranes, Subcutaneous Tissue,* and *Muscle.* These differentiate intradermal, subcutaneous, and intramuscular injections, respectively. Other sites include *Eye, Respiratory Tract, Peritoneal Cavity,* and *Epidural Space.*

The body systems/regions for arteries and veins are *Peripheral Artery, Central Artery, Peripheral Vein,* and *Central Vein*. The *Peripheral Artery* or *Vein* is typically used when a substance is introduced locally into an artery or vein. For example, chemotherapy is the introduction of an antineoplastic substance into a peripheral artery or vein by a percutaneous approach. In general, the substance introduced into a peripheral artery or vein has a systemic effect.

The *Central Artery* or *Vein* is typically used when the site where the substance is introduced is distant from the point of entry into the artery or vein. For example, the introduction of a substance directly at the site of a clot within an artery or vein using a catheter is coded as an introduction of a thrombolytic substance into a central artery or vein by a percutaneous approach. In general, the substance introduced into a central artery or vein has a local effect.

Approach (Character 5)

The fifth character represents the approach, as defined in the Medical and Surgical section. The approach for intradermal, subcutaneous, and intramuscular introductions (i.e., injections) is *Percutaneous*. If a catheter is placed to introduce a substance into an internal site within the circulatory system, then the approach is also *Percutaneous*. For example, if a catheter is used to introduce contrast directly into the heart for angiography, then the procedure would be coded as a percutaneous introduction of contrast into the heart.

Substance (Character 6)

The sixth character represents the substance being introduced. Most of the values capture broad categories of substances to which several specific substances may be categorized.

Qualifier (Character 7)

The seventh character is a qualifier. The substance value (second character) provides the broad category to which a substance is classified. The qualifier and substance values, together, precisely describe the substance administered. Not every substance administered has its own unique qualifier.

Measurement and Monitoring Section (4)

The Measurement and Monitoring section represents procedures for determining the level of a physiological or physical function.

Character Meanings

The seven characters in the Measurement and Monitoring section have the following meaning:

Character	Meaning
1	Section
2	Body System
3	Root Operation
4	Body System
5	Approach
6	Function/Device
7	Qualifier

Section (Character 1)

Measurement and Monitoring procedure codes have a first character value of *4*.

Body System (Character 2)

The second character represents the body system or device being measured or monitored. There are two values available in this section, *Physiological Systems* and *Physiological Devices*.

Root Operation (Character 3)

The third character represents the root operation, or the primary objective, of the procedure. There are two values available in this section.

- *Measurement*: Determining the level of a physiological or physical function at a point in time

- *Monitoring*: Determining the level of a physiological or physical function repetitively over a period of time

Body System (Character 4)

The fourth character represents the specific body system measured or monitored.

Approach (Character 5)

The fifth character represents the approach, as defined in the Medical and Surgical section.

Function/Device (Character 6)

The sixth character represents the physiological or physical function, or the device function being measured or monitored.

Qualifier (Character 7)

The seventh character is a qualifier, which captures additional attributes of the procedure, where applicable.

Extracorporeal or Systemic Assistance and Performance Section (5)

The Extracorporeal or Systemic Assistance and Performance section describes procedures performed in a critical care setting, such as mechanical ventilation and cardioversion. It also includes other procedures, such as hemodialysis and hyperbaric oxygen treatment.

The procedures described in this section are meant to be temporary; that is, the equipment is used only for the duration of the procedure. The equipment resides primarily outside the body, though it may interface with the body via a tube or other means. Although parts of the equipment may be attached or inserted into the patient, such as lines or catheters, these are not coded as separate device insertion procedures.

Character Meanings

The seven characters in the Extracorporeal or Systemic Assistance and Performance section have the following meaning:

Character	Meaning
1	Section
2	Body System
3	Root Operation
4	Body System
5	Duration
6	Function
7	Qualifier

Section (Character 1)

Extracorporeal or Systemic Assistance and Performance procedure codes have a first character value of *5*.

Body System (Character 2)

The second character represents the body system. There is one value available in this section, *Physiological Systems*.

Root Operation (Character 3)

The third character represents the root operation, or the primary objective, of the procedure. There are three values available in this section.

- *Assistance*: Taking over a portion of a physiological function by extracorporeal means

- *Performance*: Completely taking over a physiological function by extracorporeal means

- *Restoration*: Returning, or attempting to return, a physiological function to its natural state by extracorporeal means

The root operation *Restoration* contains a single procedure code that identifies extracorporeal cardioversion.

Body System (Character 4)

The fourth character represents the body system for which support of a physiological function is required.

Duration (Character 5)

The fifth character specifies the duration of the procedure.

Function (Character 6)

The sixth character represents the physiological function assisted or performed (e.g., oxygenation, ventilation) during the procedure.

Qualifier (Character 7)

The seventh character is a qualifier, which captures additional attributes of the procedure, where applicable, such as the type of equipment used to support or assist a physiological function.

Extracorporeal or Systemic Therapies Section (6)

The Extracorporeal or Systemic Therapies section describes procedures in which equipment outside the body is used for a therapeutic purpose that does not involve the assistance or performance of a physiological function. For procedures such as hypothermia, for which the therapy is not applied to a specific body system but the entire body, a fourth character for *None* is used.

Character Meanings

The seven characters in the Extracorporeal or Systemic Therapies section have the following meaning:

Character	Meaning
1	Section
2	Body System
3	Root Operation
4	Body System
5	Duration
6	Qualifier
7	Qualifier

Section (Character 1)

Extracorporeal or Systemic Therapy procedure codes have a first character value of *6*.

Body System (Character 2)

The second character represents the body system. There is one value available in this section, *Physiological Systems*.

Root Operation (Character 3)

The third character represents the root operation, or the primary objective, of the procedure. There are 11 values available in this section.

- *Atmospheric Control*: Extracorporeal control of atmospheric pressure and composition

- *Decompression*: Extracorporeal elimination of undissolved gas from body fluids

  Decompression involves only one type of procedure: treatment for decompression sickness (the bends) in a hyperbaric chamber.

- *Electromagnetic Therapy*: Extracorporeal treatment by electromagnetic rays

- *Hyperthermia*: Extracorporeal raising of body temperature

  The term hyperthermia is used to describe both a temperature imbalance treatment and also as an adjunct radiation treatment for cancer. When treating the temperature imbalance, it is coded to this section; for the cancer treatment, it is coded in the Radiation Therapy section.

- *Hypothermia*: Extracorporeal lowering of body temperature

- *Perfusion*: Extracorporeal treatment by diffusion of therapeutic fluid

- *Pheresis*: Extracorporeal separation of blood products

  Pheresis may be used for two main purposes: to treat diseases when too much of a blood component is produced (e.g., leukemia) and to remove a blood product such as platelets from a donor, for transfusion into another patient.

- *Phototherapy*: Extracorporeal treatment by light rays

Phototherapy involves using a machine that exposes the blood to light rays outside the body, recirculates it, and then returns it to the body.

- *Shock Wave Therapy*: Extracorporeal treatment by shock waves

- *Ultrasound Therapy*: Extracorporeal treatment by ultrasound

- *Ultraviolet Light Therapy*: Extracorporeal treatment by ultraviolet light

Body System (Character 4)

The fourth character represents the body system on which the extracorporeal or systemic therapy is performed (e.g., skin, circulatory).

Duration (Character 5)

The fifth character specifies the duration of the procedure. There are two values available in this section, *Single* or *Multiple*.

Qualifier (Characters 6 and 7)

The sixth and seventh characters are qualifiers. The qualifier captures additional attributes of the procedure, where applicable.

Osteopathic Section (7)

Character Meanings

The seven characters in the Osteopathic section have the following meaning:

Character	Meaning
1	Section
2	Body System
3	Root Operation
4	Body Region
5	Approach
6	Method
7	Qualifier

Section (Character 1)

Osteopathic procedure codes have a first character value of *7*.

Body System (Character 2)

The second character represents the body system. There is one value available in this section, *Anatomical Regions*.

Root Operation (Character 3)

The third character represents the root operation, or the primary objective, of the procedure. There is one value available in this section.

- *Treatment*: Manual treatment to eliminate or alleviate somatic dysfunction and related disorders

Body Region (Character 4)

The fourth character represents the body region. The body system (second character) indicates only the anatomical region involved in the procedure. The body region values and body system value, together, precisely describe the procedure site.

Approach (Character 5)

The fifth character represents the approach. There is only one value available in this section, *External*.

Method (Character 6)

The sixth character represents the method used to carry out the osteopathic treatment.

Qualifier (Character 7)

The seventh character is a qualifier. Because there are currently no specific qualifier values in this section, the value is always *None*.

Other Procedures Section (8)

The Other Procedures section contains codes for procedures not included in the other medical and surgical-related sections, including computer- and robotic-assisted procedures.

Character Meanings

The seven characters in the Other Procedures section have the following meaning:

Character	Meaning
1	Section
2	Body System
3	Root Operation
4	Body Region
5	Approach
6	Method
7	Qualifier

Section (Character 1)

Other Procedures section codes have a first character value of *8*.

Body System (Character 2)

The second character represents the body system/region or a device. There are two values available in this section, *Physiological Systems and Anatomical Regions* and *Indwelling Device*.

Root Operation (Character 3)

The third character represents the root operation, or the primary objective, of the procedure. There is one value available in this section.

- *Other Procedures*: Methodologies that attempt to remediate or cure a disorder or disease.

Body Region (Character 4)

The fourth character contains specified body-region values, and also the body-region value *None*.

Approach (Character 5)

The fifth character represents the approach, as defined in the Medical and Surgical section.

Method (Character 6)

The sixth character specifies the method (e.g., *Acupuncture, Therapeutic Massage*).

Qualifier (Character 7)

The seventh character is a qualifier. The qualifier is used to capture additional attributes of the procedure, where applicable.

Chiropractic Section (9)

Character Meanings

The seven characters in the Chiropractic section have the following meaning:

Character	Meaning
1	Section
2	Body System
3	Root Operation
4	Body Region
5	Approach
6	Method
7	Qualifier

Section (Character 1)

Chiropractic section procedure codes have a first character value of *9*.

Body System (Character 2)

The second character represents the body region. There is one value available in this section, *Anatomical Regions*.

Root Operation (Character 3)

The third character represents the root operation, or the primary objective, of the procedure. There is one value available in this section.

- *Manipulation:* Manual procedure that involves a directed thrust to move a joint past the physiological range of motion, without exceeding the anatomical limit.

Body Region (Character 4)

The fourth character represents the body region on which the chiropractic manipulation is performed.

Approach (Character 5)

The fifth character represents the approach. There is only one value available in this section, *External*.

Method (Character 6)

The sixth character represents the method by which the manipulation is accomplished.

Qualifier (Character 7)

The seventh character is a qualifier. Because there are currently no specific qualifier values in this section, the value is always *None*.

Imaging Section (B)

The Imaging section contains codes for procedures such as plain radiography, fluoroscopy, CT, MRI, and ultrasound.

Procedures such as PET, uptakes, and scans are in the Nuclear Medicine section. Therapeutic radiation, for the treatment of cancer, is in the Radiation Therapy section.

Character Meanings

The seven characters in Imaging procedures have the following meaning:

Character	Meaning
1	Section
2	Body System
3	Root Type
4	Body Part
5	Contrast
6	Qualifier
7	Qualifier

Section (Character 1)

Imaging procedure codes have a first character value of *B*.

Body System (Character 2)

The second character represents the general body system where the imaging is being performed. The available values mimic those that are found in the Medical and Surgical section but may not be exact matches.

Root Type (Character 3)

The third character represents the root type. The section title, *Imaging,* essentially identifies the root operation, while the values for the third character describe the type of imaging being performed. There are six root types in this section.

- *Computerized Tomography (CT Scan)*: Computer reformatted digital display of multiplanar images developed from the capture of multiple exposures of external ionizing radiation

- *Fluoroscopy*: Single plane or bi-plane real time display of an image developed from the capture of external ionizing radiation on a fluorescent screen. The image may also be stored by either digital or analog means

- *Magnetic Resonance Imaging (MRI)*: Computer reformatted digital display of multiplanar images developed from the capture of radiofrequency signals emitted by nuclei in a body site excited within a magnetic field

- *Other Imaging:* Other specified modality for visualizing a body part

- *Plain Radiography*: Planar display of an image developed from the capture of external ionizing radiation on photographic or photoconductive plate

- *Ultrasonography*: Real time display of images of anatomy or flow information developed from the capture of reflected and attenuated high frequency sound waves

Body Part (Character 4)

The fourth character represents the body part, or specific anatomical site where the procedure was performed. The body system (second character) provides only a general indication of the procedure site. The body part and body system values, together, precisely describe the procedure site.

Contrast (Character 5)

The fifth character represents the type of contrast or enhancing material utilized to facilitate the procedure, when applicable.

Qualifier (Character 6)

The sixth character is a qualifier. The most common qualifier, *Unenhanced and Enhanced,* describes an image taken without contrast (unenhanced) followed by an image with contrast (enhanced). Other qualifier values describe other noncontrast material or technology used to facilitate the imaging.

Qualifier (Character 7)

The seventh character is a qualifier. The qualifier is used to capture additional attributes of the procedure, where applicable.

Nuclear Medicine Section (C)

The Nuclear Medicine section is organized like the Imaging section. Procedures captured in this section describe the introduction of radioactive material into the body to create an image, to diagnose or treat pathological conditions, or to assess metabolic functions.

The introduction of encapsulated radioactive material for the treatment of cancer is included in the Radiation Therapy section.

Character Meanings

The seven characters in the Nuclear Medicine section have the following meaning:

Character	Meaning
1	Section
2	Body System
3	Root Type
4	Body Part
5	Radionuclide
6	Qualifier
7	Qualifier

Section (Character 1)

Nuclear Medicine procedure codes have a first character value of *C*.

Body System (Character 2)

The second character represents the general body system or anatomical region to which the nuclear medicine procedure is performed.

Root Type (Character 3)

The third character represents the root type. The section title, *Nuclear Medicine*, essentially identifies the root operation, while the third character value describes the type of nuclear medicine being performed. There are seven root types available in this section.

- *Nonimaging Nuclear Medicine Assay:* Introduction of radioactive materials into the body for the study of body fluids and blood elements, by the detection of radioactive emissions

- *Nonimaging Nuclear Medicine Probe:* Introduction of radioactive materials into the body for the study of distribution and fate of certain substances by the detection of radioactive emissions; or alternatively, measurement of absorption of radioactive emissions from an external source

- *Nonimaging Nuclear Medicine Uptake:* Introduction of radioactive materials into the body for measurements of organ function, from the detection of radioactive emissions

- *Planar Nuclear Medicine Imaging*: Introduction of radioactive materials into the body for single-plane display of images developed from the capture of radioactive emissions
- *Positron Emission Tomography (PET) Imaging:* Introduction of radioactive materials into the body for three dimensional display of images developed from the simultaneous capture, 180 degrees apart, of radioactive emissions
- *Systemic Nuclear Medicine Therapy:* Introduction of unsealed radioactive materials into the body for treatment
- *Tomographic (Tomo) Nuclear Medicine Imaging*: Introduction of radioactive materials into the body for three dimensional display of images developed from the capture of radioactive emissions

Body Part (Character 4)
The fourth character represents the specific body part or region being studied, imaged, or treated. The body system (second character) provides only a general indication of the procedure site. The body part and body system values, together, provide a precise description of the procedure site.

Radionuclide (Character 5)
The fifth character represents the type of radioactive material utilized to facilitate the procedure, when applicable. The *Other Radionuclide* value is used for radioactive material that has been newly approved but does not yet have its own unique value in the coding system.

If more than one radioactive material is given to perform the procedure, more than one code is used.

Qualifier (Characters 6 and 7)
The sixth and seventh characters are qualifiers. Because there are currently no specific qualifier values in this section, the value is always *None*.

Radiation Therapy Section (D)
The Radiation Therapy section contains procedures performed for cancer treatment.

Character Meanings
The seven characters in the Radiation Therapy section have the following meaning:

Character	Meaning
1	Section
2	Body System
3	Modality
4	Treatment Site
5	Modality Qualifier
6	Isotope
7	Qualifier

Section (Character 1)
Radiation therapy procedure codes have a first character value of *D*.

Body System (Character 2)
The second character represents the general body system or anatomical region to which radiation therapy is being applied.

Modality (Character 3)
The third character represents the type of radiation, or modality, being used. There are four values available in this section.

- *Beam Radiation*
- *Brachytherapy*
- *Stereotactic Radiosurgery*
- *Other Radiation*

Treatment Site (Character 4)
The fourth character represents the specific body part or region being irradiated. The body system (second character) provides only a general indication of the procedure site. The treatment site and body system values, together, precisely describe the procedure site.

Modality Qualifier (Character 5)
The fifth character represents specific methods or materials unique to a particular type of radiation therapy. The modality (third character) and modality qualifier values, together, precisely describe the therapy performed.

Isotope (Character 6)
The sixth character represents the specific radioactive isotope introduced into the body, if applicable.

Qualifier (Character 7)
The seventh character is a qualifier. Besides the value of *None*, this section contains two other values, *Intraoperative* and *Unidirectional Source*.

Physical Rehabilitation and Diagnostic Audiology Section (F)
Character Meanings
The seven characters in the Physical Rehabilitation and Diagnostic Audiology section have the following meaning:

Character	Meaning
1	Section
2	Section Qualifier
3	Root Type
4	Body System/Region
5	Type Qualifier
6	Equipment
7	Qualifier

Section (Character 1)
Physical Rehabilitation and Diagnostic Audiology procedure codes have a first character value of *F*.

Section Qualifier (Character 2)
The second character qualifies which of the two services described in the section (character 1) is being represented. Therefore, only two values are available, *Rehabilitation* or *Diagnostic Audiology*.

Root Type (Character 3)
The third character represents the root type. The section qualifier (second character) identifies the root operation, while the third-character value describes the type of rehabilitation or diagnostic

audiology being performed. There are 14 root types available in this section, each classified into four general categories.

Assessment: Used to evaluate a patient's level of function to determine the type and timing of treatment required. Assessment procedures focus on the faculties of hearing and speech, on various aspects of body function, and on the patient's quality of life, such as muscle performance, neuromotor development, and reintegration skills.

There are six root type values available for assessment.

- *Speech Assessment:* Measurement of speech and related functions
- *Motor and/or Nerve Function Assessment:* Measurement of motor, nerve, and related functions
- *Activities of Daily Living Assessment:* Measurement of functional level for activities of daily living
- *Hearing Assessment:* Measurement of hearing and related functions
- *Hearing Aid Assessment:* Measurement of the appropriateness and/or effectiveness of a hearing device
- *Vestibular Assessment:* Measurement of the vestibular system and related functions

Treatment: Use of specific activities or methods to develop, improve, and/or restore the performance of necessary functions, compensate for dysfunction and/or minimize debilitation. Procedures include swallowing dysfunction exercises, bathing and showering techniques, wound management, gait training, and a host of activities typically associated with rehabilitation.

There are six root type values available for treatment.

- *Speech Treatment:* Application of techniques to improve, augment, or compensate for speech and related functional impairment
- *Motor Treatment:* Exercise or activities to increase or facilitate motor function
- *Activities of Daily Living Treatment:* Exercise or activities to facilitate functional competence for activities of daily living
- *Hearing Treatment:* Application of techniques to improve, augment, or compensate for hearing and related functional impairment
- *Cochlear Implant Treatment:* Application of techniques to improve the communication abilities of individuals with cochlear implant
- *Vestibular Treatment:* Application of techniques to improve, augment, or compensate for vestibular and related functional impairment

Caregiver Training: Educating a caregiver with the skills and knowledge needed to interact with and assist the patient.

There is only one root type value available for caregiver training.

- *Caregiver Training:* Training in activities to support patient's optimal level of function

Fitting(s): Design, fabrication, modification, selection, and/or application of splint, orthosis, prosthesis, hearing aids, and/or other rehabilitation device. The fifth character used in Device Fitting procedures describes the device being fitted rather than the method used to fit the device. Definitions of devices, when provided, are in the definitions portion of the ICD-10-PCS tables and index, under section F, character 5.

There is only one root type value available for fittings.

- *Device Fitting:* Fitting of a device designed to facilitate or support achievement of a higher level of function

Body System/Region (Character 4)
The fourth character represents the body system and body region, where applicable, that requires rehabilitation. For diagnostic audiology procedures, this value is always *None*.

Type Qualifier (Character 5)
The fifth character represents a type qualifier. The root type (third character) and type qualifier values, together, precisely describe the procedure performed.

Equipment (Character 6)
The sixth character represents any equipment used to facilitate the procedure. The values provided are broad categories that may capture several specific types of equipment.

Qualifier (Character 7)
The seventh character is a qualifier. As there are currently no specific qualifier values in this section, the value is always *None*.

Mental Health Section (G)
Character Meanings
The seven characters in the Mental Health section have the following meaning:

Character	Meaning
1	Section
2	Body System
3	Type
4	Qualifier
5	Qualifier
6	Qualifier
7	Qualifier

Section (Character 1)
Mental health procedure codes have a first character value of *G*.

Body System (Character 2)
The second character is always represented by the value of *None*. As mental health care manages the psychological aspects of a patient's health, there is no specific body system or region that can be represented in this section.

Type (Character 3)
The third character represents the type of procedure. There are 12 values available in this section.

- *Psychological Tests:* The administration and interpretation of standardized psychological tests and measurement instruments for the assessment of psychological function
- *Crisis Intervention:* Treatment of a traumatized, acutely disturbed, or distressed individual for the purpose of short-term stabilization
- *Medication Management:* Monitoring and adjusting the use of medications for the treatment of a mental health disorder

- *Individual Psychotherapy:* Treatment of an individual with a mental health disorder by behavioral, cognitive, psychoanalytic, psychodynamic, or psychophysiological means to improve functioning or well-being

- *Counseling:* The application of psychological methods to treat an individual with normal developmental issues and psychological problems in order to increase function, improve well-being, alleviate distress, maladjustment, or resolve crises

- *Family Psychotherapy:* Treatment that includes one or more family members of an individual with a mental health disorder by behavioral, cognitive, psychoanalytic, psychodynamic, or psychophysiological means to improve functioning or well-being

- *Electroconvulsive Therapy:* The application of controlled electrical voltages to treat a mental health disorder

- *Biofeedback:* Provision of information from the monitoring and regulating of physiological processes in conjunction with cognitive-behavioral techniques to improve patient functioning or well-being

- *Hypnosis:* Induction of a state of heightened suggestibility by auditory, visual, and tactile techniques to elicit an emotional or behavioral response

- *Narcosynthesis:* Administration of intravenous barbiturates in order to release suppressed or repressed thoughts

- *Group Psychotherapy:* Treatment of two or more individuals with a mental health disorder by behavioral, cognitive, psychoanalytic, psychodynamic, or psychophysiological means to improve functioning or well-being

- *Light Therapy:* Application of specialized light treatments to improve functioning or well-being

Qualifier (Character 4)
The fourth character is a qualifier. This value represents the specific technique used to evaluate or treat a patient's mental health. In conjunction with the type (third character), the qualifier value precisely describes the procedure.

Qualifier (Characters 5, 6, and 7)
The fifth, sixth, and seventh characters are qualifiers. As there are currently no specific qualifier values in this section, the value is always *None*.

Substance Abuse Treatment Section (H)
Character Meanings
The seven characters in the Substance Abuse Treatment section have the following meaning:

Character	Meaning
1	Section
2	Body System
3	Type
4	Qualifier
5	Qualifier
6	Qualifier
7	Qualifier

Section (Character 1)
Substance Abuse Treatment codes have a first character value of *H*.

Body System (Character 2)
The second character is always represented by the value of *None*. As the substance abuse treatment section describes management of the psychological aspects of a patient's health, there is no specific body system or region that can be represented in this section.

Type (Character 3)
The third character represents the specific type of treatment. There are seven values available in this section.

- *Detoxification Services:* Detoxification from alcohol and/or drugs

- *Individual Counseling:* The application of psychological methods to treat an individual with addictive behavior

- *Group Counseling:* The application of psychological methods to treat two or more individuals with addictive behavior

- *Individual Psychotherapy:* Treatment of an individual with addictive behavior by behavioral, cognitive, psychoanalytic, psychodynamic, or psychophysiological means

- *Family Counseling:* The application of psychological methods that includes one or more family members to treat an individual with addictive behavior

- *Medication Management:* Monitoring and adjusting the use of replacement medications for the treatment of addiction

- *Pharmacotherapy:* The use of replacement medications for the treatment of addiction

Qualifier (Character 4)
The fourth character is a qualifier. The qualifier value further characterizes the type (character 3) of treatment being rendered, where applicable.

Qualifier (Characters 5, 6, and 7)
The fifth, sixth, and seventh characters are qualifiers. As there are currently no specific qualifier values in this section, the value is always *None*.

New Technology Section (X)
General Information
Section X New Technology is a section added to ICD-10-PCS beginning October 1, 2015. The new section provides a place for codes that uniquely identify procedures requested via the New Technology Application Process or that capture other new technologies not currently classified in ICD-10-PCS.

Section X does not introduce any new coding concepts or unusual guidelines for correct coding. In fact, Section X codes maintain continuity with the other sections in ICD-10-PCS by using the same root operation and body part values as their closest counterparts in other sections of ICD-10-PCS. For example, the codes for the infusion of Sarilumab, use the same root operation (Introduction) and body part values (Central Vein and Peripheral Vein) in section X as the infusion codes in section 3 Administration, which are their closest counterparts in the other sections of ICD-10-PCS.

Character Meanings

The seven characters in the new technology section have the following meaning:

Character	Meaning
1	Section
2	Body System
3	Root Operation
4	Body Part
5	Approach
6	Device/Substance/Technology
7	Qualifier

Section (Character 1)

New technology procedure codes have a first character value of *X*.

Body System (Character 2)

The second character values for body system combine the uses of body system, body region, and physiological system as specified in other sections in ICD-10-PCS.

Root Operation (Character 3)

The third character utilizes the same root operation values as their counterparts in other sections of ICD-10-PCS.

Body Part (Character 4)

The fourth character represents the same body part values as their closest counterparts in other sections of ICD-10-PCS.

Approach (Character 5)

The fifth character represents the approach, as defined in the Medical and Surgical section.

Device/Substance/Technology (Character 6)

The sixth character represents the key feature of the new technology procedure. It may be specified as a new device, a new substance, or other new technology. Examples of sixth character values are *Robotic Waterjet Ablation, Interbody Fusion Device, Customizable,* and *Nafamostat Anticoagulant.*

Qualifier (Character 7)

The seventh character qualifier is used exclusively to specify the new technology group, a number or letter that changes each year that new technology codes are added to the system. For example, Section X codes added for the first year have the seventh character value 1, *New Technology Group 1*, and the next year that Section X codes are added have the seventh character value 2, *New Technology Group 2*, and so on. Changing the seventh character value to a unique letter or number every year that there are new codes in the new technology section allows the ICD-10-PCS to "recycle" the values in the third, fourth, and sixth characters as needed.

New Technology Coding Instruction

Section X codes are standalone codes. They are not supplemental codes. Section X codes fully represent the specific procedure described in the code title, and do not require any additional codes from other sections of ICD-10-PCS. When section X contains a code title which describes a specific new technology procedure, only that X code is reported for the procedure. There is no need to report a broader, non-specific code in another section of ICD-10-PCS.

For example, code XW033G5 Introduction of Sarilumab into Peripheral Vein, Percutaneous Approach, New Technology Group 5, would be reported to indicate that Sarilumab was administered via peripheral vein. A separate code from table 3E0 in the Administration section of ICD-10-PCS would not be reported in addition to this code. The X section code fully identifies the administration of the sarilumab, and no additional code is needed.

The New Technology section codes are easily found by looking in the ICD-10-PCS Index or the Tables. In the Index, the name of the new technology device, substance or technology for a section X code is included as a main term. In addition, all codes in section X are listed under the main term New Technology. The new technology code index entry for sarilumab is shown below.

Sarilumab XW0

New Technology
   Sarilumab XW0

ICD-10-PCS Index and Tabular Format

The *ICD-10-PCS: The Complete Official Code Set* is based on the official version of the International Classification of Diseases, 10th Revision, Procedure Classification System, issued by the U.S. Department of Health and Human Services, Centers for Medicare and Medicaid Services. This book is consistent with the content of the government's version of ICD-10-PCS and follows their official format.

Index

The Alphabetic Index can be used to locate the appropriate table containing all the information necessary to construct a procedure code, however, the PCS tables should always be consulted to find the most appropriate valid code. Users may choose a valid code directly from the tables—he or she need not consult the index before proceeding to the tables to complete the code.

Main Terms

The Alphabetic Index reflects the structure of the tables. Therefore, the index is organized as an alphabetic listing. The index:

- Is based on the value of the third character
- Contains common procedure terms
- Lists anatomic sites
- Uses device terms

The main terms in the Alphabetic Index are root operations, root procedure types, or common procedure names. In addition, anatomic sites from the Body Part Key and device terms from the Device Key have been added for ease of use.

Examples:

> *Resection* (root operation)
>
> *Fluoroscopy* (root type)
>
> *Prostatectomy* (common procedure name)
>
> *Brachiocephalic artery* (body part)
>
> *Bard® Dulex™ mesh* (device)

The index provides at least the first three or four values of the code, and some entries may provide complete valid codes. However, the user should always consult the appropriate table to verify that the most appropriate valid code has been selected.

Root Operation and Procedure Type Main Terms

For the *Medical and Surgical* and related sections, the root operation values are used as main terms in the index. The subterms under the root operation main terms are body parts. For the Ancillary section of the tables, the main terms in the index are the general type of procedure performed.

Examples:

> **Biofeedback** GZC9ZZZ
> **Destruction**
>   Acetabulum
>   Left ØQ55
>   Right ØQ54
>   Adenoids ØC5Q
>   Ampulla of Vater ØF5C
> **Planar Nuclear Medicine Imaging**
>   Abdomen CW1Ø

See Reference

The second type of term in the index uses common procedure names, such as "appendectomy" or "fundoplication." These common terms are listed as main terms with a "see" reference noting the PCS root operations that are possible valid code tables based on the objective of the procedure.

Examples:

> **Tendonectomy**
>   *see* Excision, Tendons ØLB
>   *see* Resection, Tendons ØLT

Use Reference

The index also lists anatomic sites from the Body Part Key and device terms from the Device Key. These terms are listed with a "use" reference. The purpose of these references is to act as an additional reference to the terms located in the Appendix Keys. The term provided is the Body Part value or Device value to be selected when constructing a procedure code using the code tables. This type of index reference is not intended to direct the user to another term in the index, but to provide guidance regarding character value selection. Therefore, "use" references generally do not refer to specific valid code tables.

Examples:

> **CoAxia NeuroFlo catheter**
>   *use* Intraluminal Device
> **Epitrochlear lymph node**
>   *use* Lymphatic, Left Upper Extremity
>   *use* Lymphatic, Right Upper Extremity
> **SynCardia Total Artificial Heart**
>   *use* Synthetic Substitute

Code Tables

ICD-10-PCS contains 17 sections of Code Tables organized by general type of procedure. The first three characters of a procedure code define each table. The tables consist of columns providing the possible last four characters of codes and rows providing valid values for each character. Within a PCS table, valid codes include all combinations of choices in characters 4 through 7 contained in the same row of the table. All seven characters must be specified to form a valid code.

There are three main sections of tables:

- Medical and Surgical section:
  - *Medical and Surgical* (Ø)
- Medical and Surgical-related sections:
  - *Obstetrics* (1)
  - *Placement* (2)
  - *Administration* (3)
  - *Measurement and Monitoring* (4)
  - *Extracorporeal or Systemic Assistance and Performance* (5)
  - *Extracorporeal or Systemic Therapies* (6)
  - *Osteopathic* (7)
  - *Other Procedures* (8)
  - *Chiropractic* (9)

- Ancillary sections:
  - — *Imaging* (B)
  - — *Nuclear Medicine* (C)
  - — *Radiation Therapy* (D)
  - — *Physical Rehabilitation and Diagnostic Audiology* (F)
  - — *Mental Health* (G)
  - — *Substance Abuse Treatment* (H)
- New Technology section:
  - — *New Technology* (X)

The first three character values define each table. The root operation or root type designated for each table is accompanied by its official definition.

Example:

Table 00F provides codes for procedures on the central nervous system that involve breaking up of solid matter into pieces:

Character 1, Section	0: Medical and Surgical
Character 2, Body System	0: Central Nervous System and Cranial Nerves
Character 3, Root Operation	F: Fragmentation: Breaking solid matter in a body part into pieces

Tables are arranged numerically, then alphabetically.

When reviewing tables, the user should keep in mind that:

- Some tables may cover multiple pages in the code book—to ensure maximum clarity about character choices, valid entries do not split rows between pages. For instance, the entire table of valid characters completing a code beginning with 4A1 is split between two pages, but the split is between, not within, rows. This means that all the valid sixth and seventh characters for, say, body system *Arterial* (3) and approach *External* (X) are contained on one page.
- Individual entries may be listed in several horizontal "selection" lines.
- When a table is continued onto another page, a note to this effect has been added in red.

Body Part Definitions:

An exclusive Optum feature in the tables is the incorporation of the body part definitions provided in appendix E into the Medical and Surgical section (0) tables under their appropriate body part characters in the first column (character 4). This provides the user a direct reference to all anatomical descriptions, terms, and sites that could be coded to that particular body part value.

Paired body parts typically have values for the right and left side and in some cases a value for bilateral. These paired body parts often have the same list of inclusive body part definitions. When there are paired body parts with the same body part definitions, the first listed body part (usually the right side) contains the list of body part definitions while the second listed body part (usually the left side) contains a *See* instruction. This *See* instruction references the body part value that contains the body part definitions. In the table below, body part value P – Upper Eyelid, Left is followed by a *See* instruction that states *See N Upper Eyelid, Right*. All body part descriptions under value N also apply to body part value P.

Example:

0　**Medical and Surgical**
8　**Eye**
M　**Reattachment**　　Definition: Putting back in or on all or a portion of a separated body part to its normal location or other suitable location
　　　　　　　　　　　　　Explanation: Vascular circulation and nervous pathways may or may not be reestablished

Body Part Character 4	Approach Character 5	Device Character 6	Qualifier Character 7
N **Upper Eyelid, Right** Lateral canthus Levator palpebrae superioris muscle Orbicularis oculi muscle Superior tarsal plate **P** **Upper Eyelid, Left** *See N Upper Eyelid, Right* **Q** **Lower Eyelid, Right** Inferior tarsal plate Medial canthus **R** **Lower Eyelid, Left** *See Q Lower Eyelid, Right*	**X** External	**Z** No Device	**Z** No Qualifier

ICD-10-PCS Additional Features

Use of Official Sources

Color-coding, symbol, and other annotations in this manual that identify coding and reimbursement issues are derived from various official federal government sources, including the *Federal Register*, volume 87, number 90, May 10, 2022 ("Hospital Inpatient Prospective Payment Systems for Acute Care Hospitals and the Long Term Care Hospital Prospective Payment System and Proposed Policy Changes and Fiscal Year 2023 Rates; Proposed Rule") and the proposed, version 40, MS-DRG Grouper software, Definitions Manual files and Medicare Code Editor (MCE) files published with the fiscal 2023 IPPS proposed rule. For the most current files related to IPPS, please refer to the following:

- FY2023 IPPS Final Rule
  https://www.cms.gov/Medicare/Medicare-Fee-for-Service-Payment/AcuteInpatientPPS/IPPS-Regulations-and-Notices

- FY2023 Final Version 40, MS-DRG Grouper software
  https://www.cms.gov/Medicare/Medicare-Fee-for-Service-Payment/AcuteInpatientPPS/MS-DRG-Classifications-and-Software

Table Notations

Many tables in ICD-10-PCS contain color or symbol annotations that may aid in code selection, provide clinical or coding information, or alert the coder to reimbursement issues affected by the PCS code assignment. These annotations may be displayed on or next to a character 4, character 6, or character 7 value. Please note that some values may have more than one annotation; this is true most often with the character 4 value.

Refer to the color/symbol legend at the bottom of each page in the tables section for an abridged description of each color and symbol.

Annotation Box

An annotation box has been appended to all tables that contain color-coding or symbol annotations. The color bar or symbol attached to a character value is provided in the box, as well as a list of the valid PCS code(s) to which that edit applies. The box may also list conditional criteria that must be met to satisfy the edit.

For example, see Table 00F. Four character 4 body part values have a gray color bar. In the annotation box below the table, the gray color bar is defined as "Non-OR," or a nonoperating room procedure edit. Following the Non-OR annotation are the PCS codes that are considered nonoperating room procedures from that row of Table 00F.

Bracketed Code Notation

The use of bracketed codes is an efficient convention to provide all valid character value alternatives for a specific set of circumstances. The character values in the brackets correspond to the valid values for the character in the position the bracket appears.

Examples:

In the annotation box for Table 00F the Noncovered Procedure edit (NC) applies to codes represented in the bracketed code 00F[3,4,5,6]XZZ.

> 00F[3,4,5,6]XZZ   Fragmentation in (Central Nervous System and Cranial Nerves), External Approach

The valid fourth character values (body part) that may be selected for this specific circumstance are as follows:

3	Epidural Space, Intracranial
4	Subdural Space, Intracranial
5	Subarachnoid Space, Intracranial
6	Cerebral Ventricle

The fragmentation of matter in the spinal canal, Body Part value U, is not included in the noncovered procedure code edit.

Color-Coding/Symbols

New and Revised Text

Changes within the ICD-10-PCS tables, since the last published edition of this manual, are highlighted in two ways:

- **Red font** identifies new or revised text effective April 1, 2022.

- **Green font** identifies new or revised text effective October 1, 2022.

Medicare Code Edits

Medicare administrative contractors (MACs) and many payers use Medicare code edits to check the coding accuracy on claims. The coding edits provided in this manual include only those directly related to ICD-10-PCS codes used for acute care hospital inpatient admissions. These edits are based on the proposed, version 40, Medicare Code Editor (MCE) files published with the fiscal 2023 IPPS proposed rule.

The PCS related Medicare code edits are listed below:

- Invalid procedure code

- *Sex conflict

- *Questionable obstetric admission

- *Noncovered procedure

- *Limited coverage procedure

Starred edits above that are related to PCS issues are identified in this manual by symbols as described below.

Sex Edit Symbols

The sex edit symbols below are used to detect inconsistencies between the patient's sex and the procedure. The symbols below most often appear to the right of the body part (character 4) value but may also be found to the right of the qualifier (character 7) value:

♂   Male procedure only

♀   Female procedure only

QA Questionable Obstetric Admission

An inpatient admission is considered questionable when a vaginal or cesarean delivery code is assigned without a corresponding secondary diagnosis code describing the outcome of delivery. Both a delivery (ICD-10-PCS) code and an outcome-of-delivery (ICD-10-CM) code must be present to avoid errors in MS-DRG assignment. This symbol is found only in the Obstetrics Section, appearing to the right of the body part (character 4) value.

NC **Noncovered Procedure**

Medicare does not cover all procedures. However, some noncovered procedures, due to the presence of certain diagnoses, are reimbursed.

LC **Limited Coverage**

For certain procedures whose medical complexity and serious nature incur extraordinary associated costs, Medicare limits coverage to a portion of the cost. The limited coverage edit indicates the type of limited coverage.

ICD-10 MS-DRG Definitions Manual Edits

An MS-DRG is assigned based on specific patient attributes, such as principal diagnosis, secondary diagnoses, procedures, and discharge status. The attributes (edits) provided in this manual include only those directly related to ICD-10-PCS codes used for acute care hospital inpatient admissions. These edits are based on the proposed, version 40, MS-DRG Grouper software and Definitions Manual published with the fiscal 2023 IPPS proposed rule.

Non-Operating Room Procedures Not Affecting MS-DRG Assignment

In the Medical and Surgical section (ØØ1-ØYW) and the Obstetric section (1Ø2-1ØY) tables **only,** ICD-10-PCS procedures codes that DO NOT affect MS-DRG assignment are identified by a **gray color bar** over the body part (character 4) value and are considered non-operating room (non-OR) procedures.

NOTE: The majority of the ICD-10-PCS codes in the Medical and Surgical-Related, Ancillary and New Technology section tables are non-operating room procedures that do not typically affect MS-DRG assignment. Only the Valid Operating Room and DRG Non-Operating Room procedures are highlighted in these sections, *see* Non-Operating Room Procedures Affecting MS-DRG Assignment and Valid OR Procedure description below.

Non-Operating Room Procedures Affecting MS-DRG Assignment

Some ICD-10-PCS procedure codes, although considered non-operating room procedures, may still affect MS-DRG assignment. In all sections of the ICD-10-PCS book, these procedures are identified by a **purple color bar** over the body part (character 4) value.

Valid OR Procedure

In the Medical and Surgical-Related (2WØ-9WB), Ancillary (BØØ-HZ9) and New Technology (X2A-XYØ) section tables **only**, any codes that are considered a valid operating room procedure are identified with a **blue color bar** over the body part (character 4) value and will affect MS-DRG assignment. All codes without a color bar (blue or purple) are considered non-operating room procedures.

Hospital-Acquired Condition Related Procedures

Procedures associated with hospital-acquired conditions (HAC) are identified with the **yellow color bar** over the body part (character 4) value. Appendix K provides each specific HAC category and its associated ICD-10-CM and ICD-10-PCS codes.

Combination Only

Some ICD-10-PCS procedure codes that describe non-operating room procedures can group to a specific MS-DRG but only when used in combination with certain other ICD-10-PCS procedure codes. Such codes are designated by a **red color bar** over the body part (character 4) value.

⊞ **Combination Member**

A combination member, which can be either a valid operating room procedure or a non-operating room procedure, is an ICD-10-PCS procedure code that can influence MS-DRG assignment either on its own or in combination with other specific ICD-10-PCS procedure codes. Combination member codes are designated by a plus sign (⊞) to the right of the body part (character 4) value.

Note: In the few instances when a code is both a combination member and a non-operating room procedure affecting the MS-DRG assignment, the body part (character 4) value will have a purple color bar and the combination member icon.

See Appendix L for Procedure Combinations

Under certain circumstances, more than one procedure code is needed in order to group to a specific MS-DRG. When codes within a table have been identified as a Combination Only (**red color bar**) or Combination Member (⊞) code, there is also a footnote instructing the coder to *see Appendix L*. Appendix L contains tables that identify the other procedure codes needed in the combination and the title and number of the MS-DRG to which the combination will group.

Other Table Notations

AHA Coding Clinic:

Official citations from AHA's *Coding Clinic for ICD-10-CM/PCS* have been provided at the beginning of each section, when applicable. Each specific citation is listed below a header identifying the table to which that particular *Coding Clinic* citation applies. The citations appear in purple type with the year, quarter, and page of the reference as well as the title of the question as it appears in that *Coding Clinic's* table of contents. *Coding Clinic* citations included in this edition have been updated through second quarter 2022.

NT **New Technology Add-on Payment**

This symbol identifies procedure codes that involve new technologies or medical services that have qualified for a new technology add-on payment (NTAP). CMS provides incremental payment, in addition to the DRG payment, for technologies that have received the NTAP designation. This symbol appears to the right of the sixth character value.

Note: Only specific brand or trade named devices, substances, or technologies receive NTAP approval. The sixth character value in the PCS table provides a generalized description that may be applicable to several brand or trade names. Unless otherwise specified in the annotation box, refer to appendix H or I to determine the specific brand or trade name of the device, substance, or technology that is applicable to the new technology add-on payment. New technology add-on payments are not exclusive to the New Technology (X) section.

Appendixes

The resources described below have been included as appendixes for *ICD-10-PCS The Complete Official Code Set*. These resources further instruct the coder on the appropriate application of the ICD-10-PCS code set.

Appendix A: Components of the Medical and Surgical Approach Definitions

This resource further defines the approach characters used in the Medical and Surgical (Ø) section. Complementing the detailed definition of the approach, additional information includes whether or not instrumentation is a part of the approach, the typical access location, the method used to initiate the approach, related procedural examples, and illustrations all of which will help the user determine the appropriate approach value.

Appendix B: Root Operation Definitions

This resource is a compilation of all root operations found in the Medical and Surgical-related sections (Ø-9) of this PCS manual. It provides a definition and in some cases a more detailed explanation of the root operation, to better reflect the purpose or objective. Examples of related procedure(s) may also be provided.

Appendix C: Comparison of Medical and Surgical Root Operations

The Medical and Surgical (Ø) section root operations are divided into groups that share similar attributes. These groups, and the root operations in each group, are listed in this resource along with information identifying the target of the root operation, the action used to perform the root operation, any clarification or further explanation on the objective of the root operation, and procedure examples.

Appendix D: Body Part Key

When an anatomical term or description is provided in the documentation but does not have a specific body part character within a table, the user can reference this resource to search for the anatomical description or site noted in the documentation to determine if there is a specific PCS body part character (character 4) to which the anatomical description or site could be coded.

Appendix E: Body Part Definitions

This resource is the reverse look-up of the Body Part Key. Each table in the Medical and Surgical section (Ø) of the PCS manual contains anatomical terms linked to a body part character or value, for example, in Table ØBB the Body Part (character 4) of 1 is Trachea. The body part Trachea may have anatomical structures or descriptions that may be used in procedure documentation instead of the term trachea. The Body Part Definitions list other anatomical structures or synonyms that are included in specific ICD-10-PCS body part values. According to the body part definitions, in the example above, cricoid cartilage is included in the Trachea (character 1) body part.

Appendix F: Device Classification

This resource provides an explanation of how a device is defined in the ICD-10-PCS classification along with two tables. The first table groups devices used in the ICD-10-PCS tables into general categories, including a definition of each device type and related examples. The second table provides definitions of transplant and grafting tissue types and associated terminology that may be found in the documentation.

Appendix G: Device Key and Aggregation Table

The Device Key helps users code the appropriate PCS sixth character for device. Devices are listed alphabetically by brand name or commonly used medical terminology and are translated to the appropriate PCS language or value. The key also reflects the body system where the device is located. For example, a SAPIEN valve used for transaortic valve replacement translates to Zooplastic Tissue in Heart and Great Vessels.

The following symbol **NT** has been placed next to those devices that have received an NTAP (new technology add-on payment) designation. When the code for this device is applied to an inpatient encounter, CMS provides incremental payment in addition to the DRG payment.

The Aggregation Table crosswalks specific device character value definitions for specific root operations in a specific body system to the more general device character value to be used when the root operation covers a wide range of body parts and the device character represents an entire family of devices.

Appendix H: Device Definitions

This resource is a reverse look-up to the Device Key. The user may reference this resource to see all the specific devices that may be grouped to a particular device character (character 6).

Example:

The operative report states, "An internal fixation device was used to repair a fractured femur. Kirschner wire, bone screws and neutralization plate all used and left in the bone at the end of the procedure. "

Although PCS requires all devices left in the body to be coded and the operative report lists three different devices, a check in the device definitions shows that all of these devices are included in the PCS value "Internal Fixation Device" and require only one code.

The following symbol **NT** has been placed next to those devices that have received an NTAP (new technology add-on payment) designation. When the code for this device is applied to an inpatient encounter, CMS provides incremental payment in addition to the DRG payment.

Appendix I: Substance Key/Substance Definitions

The Substance Key lists substances by trade name or synonym and relates them to a PCS character in the Administration (3) or New Technology (X) section in the Substance (sixth character) or Qualifier (seventh character) column.

The Substance Definitions table is the reverse look-up of the substance key, relating all substance categories, the sixth- or seventh character values, to all trade name or synonyms that may be classified to that particular character.

The following symbol **NT** has been placed next to those substances/technologies that have received an NTAP (new technology add-on payment) designation. When the code for this substance/technology is applied to an inpatient encounter, CMS provides incremental payment in addition to the DRG payment.

Appendix J: Sections B-H Character Definitions

In each ancillary section (B-H) the characters in a particular column may have different meanings depending on which section the user is working from. This resource provides the values for the characters in these sections as well as a definition of the character value.

Appendix K: Hospital Acquired Conditions

Hospital acquired conditions (HACs) are conditions that are considered reasonably preventable when occurring during the hospital admission and may prevent a case from grouping to a higher-paying MS-DRG. In certain instances the HACs are conditional, requiring a specific ICD-10-CM diagnosis code in combination with a specific ICD-10-PCS procedure code. This resource identifies these conditional HACs, listing the diagnosis and procedure codes that, in combination, may trigger a HAC edit. All codes, ICD-10-CM and ICD-10-PCS, are listed with their full descriptions.

Appendix L: Procedure Combination Tables

The procedure combination tables provided in this resource illustrate certain procedure combinations that must occur in order to assign a specific MS-DRG.

Appendix M: Coding Exercises and Answers

This resource provides the coding exercises with answers, and in some cases a brief explanation as to the reason that particular code was used.

ICD-10-PCS Official Guidelines for Coding and Reporting 2023

Narrative changes appear in **bold** text.

The Centers for Medicare and Medicaid Services (CMS) and the National Center for Health Statistics (NCHS), two departments within the U.S. Federal Government's Department of Health and Human Services (DHHS) provide the following guidelines for coding and reporting using the International Classification of Diseases, 10th Revision, Procedure Coding System (ICD-10-PCS). These guidelines should be used as a companion document to the official version of the ICD-10-PCS as published on the CMS website. The ICD-10-PCS is a procedure classification published by the United States for classifying procedures performed in hospital inpatient health care settings.

These guidelines have been approved by the four organizations that make up the Cooperating Parties for the ICD-10-PCS: the American Hospital Association (AHA), the American Health Information Management Association (AHIMA), CMS, and NCHS.

These guidelines are a set of rules that have been developed to accompany and complement the official conventions and instructions provided within the ICD-10-PCS itself. They are intended to provide direction that is applicable in most circumstances. However, there may be unique circumstances where exceptions are applied. The instructions and conventions of the classification take precedence over guidelines. These guidelines are based on the coding and sequencing instructions in the Tables, Index and Definitions of ICD-10-PCS, but provide additional instruction. Adherence to these guidelines when assigning ICD-10-PCS procedure codes is required under the Health Insurance Portability and Accountability Act (HIPAA). The procedure codes have been adopted under HIPAA for hospital inpatient healthcare settings. A joint effort between the healthcare provider and the coder is essential to achieve complete and accurate documentation, code assignment, and reporting of diagnoses and procedures. These guidelines have been developed to assist both the healthcare provider and the coder in identifying those procedures that are to be reported. The importance of consistent, complete documentation in the medical record cannot be overemphasized. Without such documentation accurate coding cannot be achieved.

Conventions

A1. ICD-10-PCS codes are composed of seven characters. Each character is an axis of classification that specifies information about the procedure performed. Within a defined code range, a character specifies the same type of information in that axis of classification.

> *Example:*
> The fifth axis of classification specifies the approach in sections Ø through 4 and 7 through 9 of the system.

A2. One of 34 possible values can be assigned to each axis of classification in the seven-character code: they are the numbers Ø through 9 and the alphabet (except I and O because they are easily confused with the numbers 1 and Ø). The number of unique values used in an axis of classification differs as needed.

> *Example:*
> Where the fifth axis of classification specifies the approach, seven different approach values are currently used to specify the approach.

A3. The valid values for an axis of classification can be added to as needed.

> *Example:*
> If a significantly distinct type of device is used in a new procedure, a new device value can be added to the system.

A4. As with words in their context, the meaning of any single value is a combination of its axis of classification and any preceding values on which it may be dependent.

> *Example:*
> The meaning of a body part value in the Medical and Surgical section is always dependent on the body system value. The body part value Ø in the Central Nervous body system specifies Brain and the body part value Ø in the Peripheral Nervous body system specifies Cervical Plexus.

A5. As the system is expanded to become increasingly detailed, over time more values will depend on preceding values for their meaning.

> *Example:*
> In the Lower Joints body system, the device value 3 in the root operation Insertion specifies Infusion Device and the device value 3 in the root operation Replacement specifies Ceramic Synthetic Substitute.

A6. The purpose of the alphabetic index is to locate the appropriate table that contains all information necessary to construct a procedure code. The PCS Tables should always be consulted to find the most appropriate valid code.

A7. It is not required to consult the index first before proceeding to the tables to complete the code. A valid code may be chosen directly from the tables.

A8. All seven characters must be specified to be a valid code. If the documentation is incomplete for coding purposes, the physician should be queried for the necessary information.

A9. Within a PCS table, valid codes include all combinations of choices in characters 4 through 7 contained in the same row of the table. In the example below, ØJHT3VZ is a valid code, and ØJHW3VZ is *not* a valid code.

Section:	Ø	**Medical and Surgical**
Body System:	J	**Subcutaneous Tissue and Fascia**
Operation:	H	**Insertion** Putting in a nonbiological appliance that monitors, assists, performs, or prevents a physiological function but does not physically take the place of a body part

	Body Part		Approach		Device		Qualifier
S	Subcutaneous Tissue and Fascia, Head and Neck	Ø	Open	1	Radioactive Element	Z	No Qualifier
V	Subcutaneous Tissue and Fascia, Upper Extremity	3	Percutaneous	3	Infusion Device		
W	Subcutaneous Tissue and Fascia, Lower Extremity			Y	Other Device		
T	Subcutaneous Tissue and Fascia, Trunk	Ø	Open	1	Radioactive Element	Z	No Qualifier
		3	Percutaneous	3	Infusion Device		
				V	Infusion Pump		
				Y	Other Device		

A10. "And," when used in a code description, means "and/or," except when used to describe a combination of multiple body parts for which separate values exist for each body part (e.g., Skin and Subcutaneous Tissue used as a qualifier, where there are separate body part values for "Skin" and "Subcutaneous Tissue").

Example:
Lower Arm and Wrist Muscle means lower arm and/or wrist muscle.

A11. Many of the terms used to construct PCS codes are defined within the system. It is the coder's responsibility to determine what the documentation in the medical record equates to in the PCS definitions. The physician is not expected to use the terms used in PCS code descriptions, nor is the coder required to query the physician when the correlation between the documentation and the defined PCS terms is clear.

Example:
When the physician documents "partial resection" the coder can independently correlate "partial resection" to the root operation Excision without querying the physician for clarification.

Medical and Surgical Section Guidelines (section Ø)

B2. Body System

General guidelines

B2.1a. The procedure codes in Anatomical Regions, General, Anatomical Regions, Upper Extremities and Anatomical Regions, Lower Extremities can be used when the procedure is performed on an anatomical region rather than a specific body part, or on the rare occasion when no information is available to support assignment of a code to a specific body part.

Examples:
Chest tube drainage of the pleural cavity is coded to the root operation Drainage found in the body system Anatomical Regions, General.

Suture repair of the abdominal wall is coded to the root operation Repair in the body system Anatomical Regions, General.

Amputation of the foot is coded to the root operation Detachment in the body system Anatomical Regions, Lower Extremities.

B2.1b. Where the general body part values "upper" and "lower" are provided as an option in the Upper Arteries, Lower Arteries, Upper Veins, Lower Veins, Muscles and Tendons body systems, "upper" or "lower" specifies body parts located above or below the diaphragm respectively.

Example:
Vein body parts above the diaphragm are found in the Upper Veins body system; vein body parts below the diaphragm are found in the Lower Veins body system.

B3. Root Operation

General guidelines

B3.1a. In order to determine the appropriate root operation, the full definition of the root operation as contained in the PCS Tables must be applied.

B3.1b. Components of a procedure specified in the root operation definition or explanation as integral to that root operation are not coded separately. Procedural steps necessary to reach the operative site

and close the operative site, including anastomosis of a tubular body part, are also not coded separately.

Examples:
Resection of a joint as part of a joint replacement procedure is included in the root operation definition of Replacement and is not coded separately.

Laparotomy performed to reach the site of an open liver biopsy is not coded separately.

In a resection of sigmoid colon with anastomosis of descending colon to rectum, the anastomosis is not coded separately.

Multiple procedures

B3.2. During the same operative episode, multiple procedures are coded if:

a. The same root operation is performed on different body parts as defined by distinct values of the body part character.

Examples:
Diagnostic excision of liver and pancreas are coded separately.

Excision of lesion in the ascending colon and excision of lesion in the transverse colon are coded separately.

b. The same root operation is repeated in multiple body parts, and those body parts are separate and distinct body parts classified to a single ICD-10-PCS body part value.

Examples:
Excision of the sartorius muscle and excision of the gracilis muscle are both included in the upper leg muscle body part value, and multiple procedures are coded.

Extraction of multiple toenails are coded separately.

c. Multiple root operations with distinct objectives are performed on the same body part.

Example:
Destruction of sigmoid lesion and bypass of sigmoid colon are coded separately.

d. The intended root operation is attempted using one approach but is converted to a different approach.

Example:
Laparoscopic cholecystectomy converted to an open cholecystectomy is coded as percutaneous endoscopic Inspection and open Resection.

Discontinued or incomplete procedures

B3.3. If the intended procedure is discontinued or otherwise not completed, code the procedure to the root operation performed. If a procedure is discontinued before any other root operation is performed, code the root operation Inspection of the body part or anatomical region inspected.

Example:
A planned aortic valve replacement procedure is discontinued after the initial thoracotomy and before any incision is made in the heart muscle, when the patient becomes hemodynamically unstable. This procedure is coded as an open Inspection of the mediastinum.

Biopsy procedures

B3.4a. Biopsy procedures are coded using the root operations Excision, Extraction, or Drainage and the qualifier Diagnostic.

Examples:
Fine needle aspiration biopsy of fluid in the lung is coded to the root operation Drainage with the qualifier Diagnostic.

Biopsy of bone marrow is coded to the root operation Extraction with the qualifier Diagnostic.

Lymph node sampling for biopsy is coded to the root operation Excision with the qualifier Diagnostic.

Biopsy followed by more definitive treatment

B3.4b. If a diagnostic Excision, Extraction, or Drainage procedure (biopsy) is followed by a more definitive procedure, such as Destruction, Excision or Resection at the same procedure site, both the biopsy and the more definitive treatment are coded.

Example:
Biopsy of breast followed by partial mastectomy at the same procedure site, both the biopsy and the partial mastectomy procedure are coded.

Overlapping body layers

B3.5. If root operations such as Excision, Extraction, Repair or Inspection are performed on overlapping layers of the musculoskeletal system, the body part specifying the deepest layer is coded.

Example:
Excisional debridement that includes skin and subcutaneous tissue and muscle is coded to the muscle body part.

Bypass procedures

B3.6a. Bypass procedures are coded by identifying the body part bypassed "from" and the body part bypassed "to." The fourth character body part specifies the body part bypassed from, and the qualifier specifies the body part bypassed to.

Example:
Bypass from stomach to jejunum, stomach is the body part and jejunum is the qualifier.

B3.6b. Coronary artery bypass procedures are coded differently than other bypass procedures as described in the previous guideline. Rather than identifying the body part bypassed from, the body part identifies the number of coronary arteries bypassed to, and the qualifier specifies the vessel bypassed from.

Example:
Aortocoronary artery bypass of the left anterior descending coronary artery and the obtuse marginal coronary artery is classified in the body part axis of classification as two coronary arteries, and the qualifier specifies the aorta as the body part bypassed from.

B3.6c. If multiple coronary arteries are bypassed, a separate procedure is coded for each coronary artery that uses a different device and/or qualifier.

Example:
Aortocoronary artery bypass and internal mammary coronary artery bypass are coded separately.

Control vs. more specific root operations

B3.7. The root operation Control is defined as, "Stopping, or attempting to stop, postprocedural or other acute bleeding." Control is the root operation coded when the procedure performed to achieve hemostasis, beyond what would be considered integral to a procedure, utilizes techniques (e.g. cautery, application of substances or pressure, suturing or ligation or clipping of bleeding points at the site) that are not described by a more specific root operation definition, such as Bypass, Detachment, Excision, Extraction, Reposition, Replacement, or Resection. If a more specific root operation definition applies to the procedure performed, then the more specific root operation is coded instead of Control.

Example:
Silver nitrate cautery to treat acute nasal bleeding is coded to the root operation Control.

Example:
Liquid embolization of the right internal iliac artery to treat acute hematoma by stopping blood flow is coded to the root operation Occlusion.

Example:
Suctioning of residual blood to achieve hemostasis during a transbronchial cryobiopsy is considered integral to the cryobiopsy procedure and is not coded separately.

Excision vs. Resection

B3.8. PCS contains specific body parts for anatomical subdivisions of a body part, such as lobes of the lungs or liver and regions of the intestine. Resection of the specific body part is coded whenever all of the body part is cut out or off, rather than coding Excision of a less specific body part.

Example:
Left upper lung lobectomy is coded to Resection of Upper Lung Lobe, Left rather than Excision of Lung, Left.

Excision for graft

B3.9. If an autograft is obtained from a different procedure site in order to complete the objective of the procedure, a separate procedure is coded, except when the seventh character qualifier value in the ICD-10-PCS table fully specifies the site from which the autograft was obtained.

Examples:
Coronary bypass with excision of saphenous vein graft, excision of saphenous vein is coded separately.

Replacement of breast with autologous deep inferior epigastric artery perforator (DIEP) flap, excision of the DIEP flap is not coded separately. The seventh character qualifier value Deep Inferior Epigastric Artery Perforator Flap in the Replacement table fully specifies the site of the autograft harvest.

Fusion procedures of the spine

B3.10a. The body part coded for a spinal vertebral joint(s) rendered immobile by a spinal fusion procedure is classified by the level of the spine (e.g. thoracic). There are distinct body part values for a single vertebral joint and for multiple vertebral joints at each spinal level.

Example:
Body part values specify Lumbar Vertebral Joint, Lumbar Vertebral Joints, 2 or More and Lumbosacral Vertebral Joint.

B3.10b. If multiple vertebral joints are fused, a separate procedure is coded for each vertebral joint that uses a different device and/or qualifier.

Example:
Fusion of lumbar vertebral joint, posterior approach, anterior column and fusion of lumbar vertebral joint, posterior approach, posterior column are coded separately.

B3.10c. Combinations of devices and materials are often used on a vertebral joint to render the joint immobile. When combinations of devices are used on the same vertebral joint, the device value coded for the procedure is as follows:

- If an interbody fusion device is used to render the joint immobile (containing bone graft or bone graft substitute), the procedure is coded with the device value Interbody Fusion Device

- If bone graft is the *only* device used to render the joint immobile, the procedure is coded with the device value Nonautologous Tissue Substitute or Autologous Tissue Substitute

- If a mixture of autologous and nonautologous bone graft (with or without biological or synthetic extenders or binders) is used to render the joint immobile, code the procedure with the device value Autologous Tissue Substitute

Examples:
Fusion of a vertebral joint using a cage style interbody fusion device containing morsellized bone graft is coded to the device Interbody Fusion Device.

Fusion of a vertebral joint using a bone dowel interbody fusion device made of cadaver bone and packed with a mixture of local morsellized bone and demineralized bone matrix is coded to the device Interbody Fusion Device.

Fusion of a vertebral joint using both autologous bone graft and bone bank bone graft is coded to the device Autologous Tissue Substitute.

Inspection procedures

B3.11a. Inspection of a body part(s) performed in order to achieve the objective of a procedure is not coded separately.

Example:
Fiberoptic bronchoscopy performed for irrigation of bronchus, only the irrigation procedure is coded.

B3.11b. If multiple tubular body parts are inspected, the most distal body part (the body part furthest from the starting point of the inspection) is coded. If multiple non-tubular body parts in a region are inspected, the body part that specifies the entire area inspected is coded.

Examples:
Cystoureteroscopy with inspection of bladder and ureters is coded to the ureter body part value.

Exploratory laparotomy with general inspection of abdominal contents is coded to the peritoneal cavity body part value.

B3.11c. When both an Inspection procedure and another procedure are performed on the same body part during the same episode, if the Inspection procedure is performed using a different approach than the other procedure, the Inspection procedure is coded separately.

Example:
Endoscopic Inspection of the duodenum is coded separately when open Excision of the duodenum is performed during the same procedural episode.

Occlusion vs. Restriction for vessel embolization procedures

B3.12. If the objective of an embolization procedure is to completely close a vessel, the root operation Occlusion is coded. If the objective of an embolization procedure is to narrow the lumen of a vessel, the root operation Restriction is coded.

Examples:
Tumor embolization is coded to the root operation Occlusion, because the objective of the procedure is to cut off the blood supply to the vessel.

Embolization of a cerebral aneurysm is coded to the root operation Restriction, because the objective of the procedure is not to close off the vessel entirely, but to narrow the lumen of the vessel at the site of the aneurysm where it is abnormally wide.

Release procedures

B3.13. In the root operation Release, the body part value coded is the body part being freed and not the tissue being manipulated or cut to free the body part.

Example:
Lysis of intestinal adhesions is coded to the specific intestine body part value.

Release vs. Division

B3.14. If the sole objective of the procedure is freeing a body part without cutting the body part, the root operation is Release. If the sole objective of the procedure is separating or transecting a body part, the root operation is Division.

Examples:
Freeing a nerve root from surrounding scar tissue to relieve pain is coded to the root operation Release.

Severing a nerve root to relieve pain is coded to the root operation Division.

Reposition for fracture treatment

B3.15. Reduction of a displaced fracture is coded to the root operation Reposition and the application of a cast or splint in conjunction with the Reposition procedure is not coded separately. Treatment of a nondisplaced fracture is coded to the procedure performed.

Examples:
Casting of a nondisplaced fracture is coded to the root operation Immobilization in the Placement section.

Putting a pin in a nondisplaced fracture is coded to the root operation Insertion.

Transplantation vs. Administration

B3.16. Putting in a mature and functioning living body part taken from another individual or animal is coded to the root operation Transplantation. Putting in autologous or nonautologous cells is coded to the Administration section.

Example:
Putting in autologous or nonautologous bone marrow, pancreatic islet cells or stem cells is coded to the Administration section.

Transfer procedures using multiple tissue layers

B3.17. The root operation Transfer contains qualifiers that can be used to specify when a transfer flap is composed of more than one tissue layer, such as a musculocutaneous flap. For procedures involving transfer of multiple tissue layers including skin, subcutaneous tissue, fascia or muscle, the procedure is coded to the body part value that describes the deepest tissue layer in the flap, and the qualifier can be used to describe the other tissue layer(s) in the transfer flap.

Example:
A musculocutaneous flap transfer is coded to the appropriate body part value in the body system Muscles, and the qualifier is used to describe the additional tissue layer(s) in the transfer flap.

Excision/Resection followed by replacement

B3.18. If an excision or resection of a body part is followed by a replacement procedure, code both procedures to identify each distinct objective, except when the excision or resection is considered integral and preparatory for the replacement procedure.

Examples:
Mastectomy followed by reconstruction, both resection and replacement of the breast are coded to fully capture the distinct objectives of the procedures performed.

Maxillectomy with obturator reconstruction, both excision and replacement of the maxilla are coded to fully capture the distinct objectives of the procedures performed.

Excisional debridement of tendon with skin graft, both the excision of the tendon and the replacement of the skin with a graft are coded to fully capture the distinct objectives of the procedures performed.

Esophagectomy followed by reconstruction with colonic interposition, both the resection and the transfer of the large intestine to function as the esophagus are coded to fully capture the distinct objectives of the procedures performed.

Examples:
Resection of a joint as part of a joint replacement procedure is considered integral and preparatory for the replacement of the joint and the resection is not coded separately.

Resection of a valve as part of a valve replacement procedure is considered integral and preparatory for the valve replacement and the resection is not coded separately.

Detachment procedures of extremities

B3.19. The root operation Detachment contains qualifiers that can be used to specify the level where the extremity was amputated. These qualifiers are dependent on the body part value in the "upper extremities" and "lower extremities" body systems. For procedures involving the detachment of all or part of the upper or lower extremities, the procedure is coded to the body part value that describes the site of the detachment.

Example:
An amputation at the proximal portion of the shaft of the tibia and fibula is coded to the Lower leg body part value in the body system Anatomical Regions, Lower Extremities, and the qualifier High is used to specify the level where the extremity was detached.

The following definitions were developed for the Detachment qualifiers

Body Part	Qualifier	Definition
Upper arm and upper leg	1	High: Amputation at the proximal portion of the shaft of the humerus or femur
	2	Mid: Amputation at the middle portion of the shaft of the humerus or femur
	3	Low: Amputation at the distal portion of the shaft of the humerus or femur
Lower arm and lower leg	1	High: Amputation at the proximal portion of the shaft of the radius/ulna or tibia/fibula
	2	Mid: Amputation at the middle portion of the shaft of the radius/ulna or tibia/fibula
	3	Low: Amputation at the distal portion of the shaft of the radius/ulna or tibia/fibula
Hand and Foot	0	Complete*
	4	Complete 1st Ray
	5	Complete 2nd Ray
	6	Complete 3rd Ray
	7	Complete 4th Ray
	8	Complete 5th Ray
	9	Partial 1st Ray
	B	Partial 2nd Ray
	C	Partial 3rd Ray
	D	Partial 4th Ray
	F	Partial 5th Ray

Body Part	Qualifier	Definition
Thumb, finger, or toe	0	Complete: Amputation at the metacarpophalangeal/metatarsal-phalangeal joint
	1	High: Amputation anywhere along the proximal phalanx
	2	Mid: Amputation through the proximal interphalangeal joint or anywhere along the middle phalanx
	3	Low: Amputation through the distal interphalangeal joint or anywhere along the distal phalanx

*When coding amputation of Hand and Foot, the following definitions are followed:

- **Complete: Amputation through the carpometacarpal joint of the hand, or through the tarsal-metatarsal joint of the foot.**

- **Partial: Amputation anywhere along the shaft or head of the metacarpal bone of the hand, or of the metatarsal bone of the foot.**

B4. Body Part

General guidelines

B4.1a. If a procedure is performed on a portion of a body part that does not have a separate body part value, code the body part value corresponding to the whole body part.

Example:
A procedure performed on the alveolar process of the mandible is coded to the mandible body part.

B4.1b. If the prefix "peri" is combined with a body part to identify the site of the procedure, and the site of the procedure is not further specified, then the procedure is coded to the body part named. This guideline applies only when a more specific body part value is not available.

Examples:
A procedure site identified as perirenal is coded to the kidney body part when the site of the procedure is not further specified.

A procedure site described in the documentation as peri-urethral, and the documentation also indicates that it is the vulvar tissue and not the urethral tissue that is the site of the procedure, then the procedure is coded to the vulva body part.

A procedure site documented as involving the periosteum is coded to the corresponding bone body part.

B4.1c. If a single vascular procedure is performed on a continuous section of an arterial or venous body part, code the body part value corresponding to the anatomically most proximal (closest to the heart) portion of the arterial or venous body part.

Example:
A procedure performed on a continuous section of artery from the femoral artery to the external iliac artery with the point of entry at the femoral artery is coded to the external iliac body part.

A procedure performed on a continuous section of artery from the femoral artery to the external iliac artery with the point of entry at the external iliac artery is also coded to the external iliac artery body part.

Branches of body parts

B4.2. Where a specific branch of a body part does not have its own body part value in PCS, the body part is typically coded to the closest proximal branch that has a specific body part value. In the cardiovascular body systems, if a general body part is available in the correct root operation table, and coding to a proximal branch would require assigning a code in a different body system, the procedure is coded using the general body part value.

> *Examples:*
>
> A procedure performed on the mandibular branch of the trigeminal nerve is coded to the trigeminal nerve body part value.
>
> Occlusion of the bronchial artery is coded to the body part value Upper Artery in the body system Upper Arteries, and not to the body part value Thoracic Aorta, Descending in the body system Heart and Great Vessels.

Bilateral body part values

B4.3. Bilateral body part values are available for a limited number of body parts. If the identical procedure is performed on contralateral body parts, and a bilateral body part value exists for that body part, a single procedure is coded using the bilateral body part value. If no bilateral body part value exists, each procedure is coded separately using the appropriate body part value.

> *Examples:*
>
> The identical procedure performed on both fallopian tubes is coded once using the body part value Fallopian Tube, Bilateral.
>
> The identical procedure performed on both knee joints is coded twice using the body part values Knee Joint, Right and Knee Joint, Left.

Coronary arteries

B4.4. The coronary arteries are classified as a single body part that is further specified by number of arteries treated. One procedure code specifying multiple arteries is used when the same procedure is performed, including the same device and qualifier values.

> *Examples:*
>
> Angioplasty of two distinct coronary arteries with placement of two stents is coded as Dilation of Coronary Artery, Two Arteries with Two Intraluminal Devices.
>
> Angioplasty of two distinct coronary arteries, one with stent placed and one without, is coded separately as Dilation of Coronary Artery, One Artery with Intraluminal Device, and Dilation of Coronary Artery, One Artery with no device.

Tendons, ligaments, bursae and fascia near a joint

B4.5. Procedures performed on tendons, ligaments, bursae and fascia supporting a joint are coded to the body part in the respective body system that is the focus of the procedure. Procedures performed on joint structures themselves are coded to the body part in the joint body systems.

> *Examples:*
>
> Repair of the anterior cruciate ligament of the knee is coded to the knee bursa and ligament body part in the bursae and ligaments body system.
>
> Knee arthroscopy with shaving of articular cartilage is coded to the knee joint body part in the Lower Joints body system.

Skin, subcutaneous tissue and fascia overlying a joint

B4.6. If a procedure is performed on the skin, subcutaneous tissue or fascia overlying a joint, the procedure is coded to the following body part:

- Shoulder is coded to Upper Arm
- Elbow is coded to Lower Arm
- Wrist is coded to Lower Arm
- Hip is coded to Upper Leg
- Knee is coded to Lower Leg
- Ankle is coded to Foot

Fingers and toes

B4.7. If a body system does not contain a separate body part value for fingers, procedures performed on the fingers are coded to the body part value for the hand. If a body system does not contain a separate body part value for toes, procedures performed on the toes are coded to the body part value for the foot.

> *Example:*
>
> Excision of finger muscle is coded to one of the hand muscle body part values in the Muscles body system.

Upper and lower intestinal tract

B4.8. In the Gastrointestinal body system, the general body part values Upper Intestinal Tract and Lower Intestinal Tract are provided as an option for the root operations such as Change, Insertion, Inspection, Removal and Revision. Upper Intestinal Tract includes the portion of the gastrointestinal tract from the esophagus down to and including the duodenum, and Lower Intestinal Tract includes the portion of the gastrointestinal tract from the jejunum down to and including the rectum and anus.

> *Example:*
>
> In the root operation Change table, change of a device in the jejunum is coded using the body part Lower Intestinal Tract.

B5. Approach

Open approach with percutaneous endoscopic assistance

B5.2a. Procedures performed using the open approach with percutaneous endoscopic assistance are coded to the approach Open.

> *Example:*
>
> Laparoscopic-assisted sigmoidectomy is coded to the approach Open.

Percutaneous endoscopic approach with extension of incision

B5.2b. Procedures performed using the percutaneous endoscopic approach, with incision or extension of an incision to assist in the removal of all or a portion of a body part or to anastomose a tubular body part to complete the procedure, are coded to the approach value Percutaneous Endoscopic.

> *Examples:*
>
> Laparoscopic sigmoid colectomy with extension of stapling port for removal of specimen and direct anastomosis is coded to the approach value percutaneous endoscopic.
>
> Laparoscopic nephrectomy with midline incision for removing the resected kidney is coded to the approach value percutaneous endoscopic.
>
> Robotic-assisted laparoscopic prostatectomy with extension of incision for removal of the resected prostate is coded to the approach value percutaneous endoscopic.

External approach

B5.3a. Procedures performed within an orifice on structures that are visible without the aid of any instrumentation are coded to the approach External.

> *Example:*
> Resection of tonsils is coded to the approach External.

B5.3b. Procedures performed indirectly by the application of external force through the intervening body layers are coded to the approach External.

> *Example:*
> Closed reduction of fracture is coded to the approach External.

Percutaneous procedure via device

B5.4. Procedures performed percutaneously via a device placed for the procedure are coded to the approach Percutaneous.

> *Example:*
> Fragmentation of kidney stone performed via percutaneous nephrostomy is coded to the approach Percutaneous.

B6. Device

General guidelines

B6.1a. A device is coded only if a device remains after the procedure is completed. If no device remains, the device value No Device is coded. In limited root operations, the classification provides the qualifier values Temporary and Intraoperative, for specific procedures involving clinically significant devices, where the purpose of the device is to be utilized for a brief duration during the procedure or current inpatient stay. If a device that is intended to remain after the procedure is completed requires removal before the end of the operative episode in which it was inserted (for example, the device size is inadequate or **an event documented as a** complication occurs), both the insertion and removal of the device should be coded.

B6.1b. Materials such as sutures, ligatures, radiological markers and temporary post-operative wound drains are considered integral to the performance of a procedure and are not coded as devices.

B6.1c. Procedures performed on a device only and not on a body part are specified in the root operations Change, Irrigation, Removal and Revision, and are coded to the procedure performed.

> *Example:*
> Irrigation of percutaneous nephrostomy tube is coded to the root operation Irrigation of indwelling device in the Administration section.

Drainage device

B6.2. A separate procedure to put in a drainage device is coded to the root operation Drainage with the device value Drainage Device.

Obstetric Section Guidelines (section 1)

C. Obstetrics Section

Products of conception

C1. Procedures performed on the products of conception are coded to the Obstetrics section. Procedures performed on the pregnant female other than the products of conception are coded to the appropriate root operation in the Medical and Surgical section.

> *Examples:*
> Amniocentesis is coded to the products of conception body part in the Obstetrics section.

Repair of obstetric urethral laceration is coded to the urethra body part in the Medical and Surgical section.

Procedures following delivery or abortion

C2. Procedures performed following a delivery or abortion for curettage of the endometrium or evacuation of retained products of conception are all coded in the Obstetrics section, to the root operation Extraction and the body part Products of Conception, Retained.

Diagnostic or therapeutic dilation and curettage performed during times other than the postpartum or post-abortion period are all coded in the Medical and Surgical section, to the root operation Extraction and the body part Endometrium.

Radiation Therapy Section Guidelines (section D)

D. Radiation Therapy Section

Brachytherapy

D1.a. Brachytherapy is coded to the modality Brachytherapy in the Radiation Therapy section. When a radioactive brachytherapy source is left in the body at the end of the procedure, it is coded separately to the root operation Insertion with the device value Radioactive Element.

> *Example:*
> Brachytherapy with implantation of a low dose rate brachytherapy source left in the body at the end of the procedure is coded to the applicable treatment site in section D, Radiation Therapy, with the modality Brachytherapy, the modality qualifier value Low Dose Rate, and the applicable isotope value and qualifier value. The implantation of the brachytherapy source is coded separately to the device value Radioactive Element in the appropriate Insertion table of the Medical and Surgical section. The Radiation Therapy section code identifies the specific modality and isotope of the brachytherapy, and the root operation Insertion code identifies the implantation of the brachytherapy source that remains in the body at the end of the procedure.

> *Exception:*
> Implantation of Cesium-131 brachytherapy seeds embedded in a collagen matrix to the treatment site after resection of brain tumor is coded to the root operation Insertion with the device value Radioactive Element, Cesium-131 Collagen Implant. The procedure is coded to the root operation Insertion only, because the device value identifies both the implantation of the radioactive element and a specific brachytherapy isotope that is not included in the Radiation Therapy section tables.

D1.b. A separate procedure to place a temporary applicator for delivering the brachytherapy is coded to the root operation Insertion and the device value Other Device.

> *Examples:*
> Intrauterine brachytherapy applicator placed as a separate procedure from the brachytherapy procedure is coded to Insertion of Other Device, and the brachytherapy is coded separately using the modality Brachytherapy in the Radiation Therapy section.

> Intrauterine brachytherapy applicator placed concomitantly with delivery of the brachytherapy dose is coded with a single code using the modality Brachytherapy in the Radiation Therapy section.

New Technology Section Guidelines (section X)

E. New Technology Section

General guidelines

E1.a. Section X codes fully represent the specific procedure described in the code title, and do not require additional codes from other sections of ICD-10-PCS. When section X contains a code title which fully describes a specific new technology procedure, and it is the only procedure performed, only the section X code is reported for the procedure. There is no need to report an additional code in another section of ICD-10-PCS.

Example:
XWØ43A6 Introduction of Cefiderocol Anti-infective into Central Vein, Percutaneous Approach, New Technology Group 6, can be coded to indicate that Cefiderocol Anti-infective was administered via a central vein. A separate code from table 3EØ in the Administration section of ICD-10-PCS is not coded in addition to this code.

E1.b. When multiple procedures are performed, New Technology section X codes are coded following the multiple procedures guideline.

Examples:
Dual filter cerebral embolic filtration used during transcatheter aortic valve replacement (TAVR), X2A5312 Cerebral Embolic Filtration, Dual Filter in Innominate Artery and Left Common Carotid Artery, Percutaneous Approach, New Technology Group 2, is coded for the cerebral embolic filtration, along with an ICD-10-PCS code for the TAVR procedure.

An extracorporeal flow reversal circuit for embolic neuroprotection placed during a transcarotid arterial revascularization procedure, a code from table X2A, Assistance of the Cardiovascular System is coded for the use of the extracorporeal flow reversal circuit, along with an ICD-10-PCS code for the transcarotid arterial revascularization procedure.

F. Selection of Principal Procedure

The following instructions should be applied in the selection of principal procedure and clarification on the importance of the relation to the principal diagnosis when more than one procedure is performed:

1. Procedure performed for definitive treatment of both principal diagnosis and secondary diagnosis

   a. Sequence procedure performed for definitive treatment most related to principal diagnosis as principal procedure.

2. Procedure performed for definitive treatment and diagnostic procedures performed for both principal diagnosis and secondary diagnosis.

   a. Sequence procedure performed for definitive treatment most related to principal diagnosis as principal procedure

3. A diagnostic procedure was performed for the principal diagnosis and a procedure is performed for definitive treatment of a secondary diagnosis.

   a. Sequence diagnostic procedure as principal procedure, since the procedure most related to the principal diagnosis takes precedence.

4. No procedures performed that are related to principal diagnosis; procedures performed for definitive treatment and diagnostic procedures were performed for secondary diagnosis

   a. Sequence procedure performed for definitive treatment of secondary diagnosis as principal procedure, since there are no procedures (definitive or nondefinitive treatment) related to principal diagnosis.

# #

3f (Aortic) Bioprosthesis valve *use* Zooplastic Tissue in Heart and Great Vessels

A

Abdominal aortic plexus *use* Abdominal Sympathetic Nerve
Abdominal cavity *use* Peritoneal Cavity
Abdominal esophagus *use* Esophagus, Lower
Abdominohysterectomy *see* Resection, Uterus ØUT9
Abdominoplasty
 see Alteration, Abdominal Wall ØWØF
 see Repair, Abdominal Wall ØWQF
 see Supplement, Abdominal Wall ØWUF
Abductor hallucis muscle
 use Foot Muscle, Left
 use Foot Muscle, Right
ABECMA® *use* Idecabtagene Vicleucel Immunotherapy
AbioCor® Total Replacement Heart *use* Synthetic Substitute
Ablation
 see Control bleeding in
 see Destruction
Abortion
 Abortifacient 10A07ZX
 Laminaria 10A07ZW
 Products of Conception 10A0
 Vacuum 10A07Z6
Abrasion *see* Extraction
Absolute Pro Vascular (OTW) Self-Expanding Stent System *use* Intraluminal Device
Accelerate PhenoTest™ BC XXE5XN6
Accessory cephalic vein
 use Cephalic Vein, Left
 use Cephalic Vein, Right
Accessory obturator nerve *use* Lumbar Plexus
Accessory phrenic nerve *use* Phrenic Nerve
Accessory spleen *use* Spleen
Acculink (RX) Carotid Stent System *use* Intraluminal Device
Acellular Hydrated Dermis *use* Nonautologous Tissue Substitute
Acetabular cup *use* Liner in Lower Joints
Acetabulectomy
 see Excision, Lower Bones ØQB
 see Resection, Lower Bones ØQT
Acetabulofemoral joint
 use Hip Joint, Left
 use Hip Joint, Right
Acetabuloplasty
 see Repair, Lower Bones ØQQ
 see Replacement, Lower Bones ØQR
 see Supplement, Lower Bones ØQU
Achilles tendon
 use Lower Leg Tendon, Left
 use Lower Leg Tendon, Right
Achillorrhaphy *see* Repair, Tendons ØLQ
Achillotenotomy, achillotomy
 see Division, Tendons ØL8
 see Drainage, Tendons ØL9
Acoustic Pulse Thrombolysis *see* Fragmentation, Artery
Acromioclavicular ligament
 use Shoulder Bursa and Ligament, Left
 use Shoulder Bursa and Ligament, Right
Acromion (process)
 use Scapula, Left
 use Scapula, Right
Acromionectomy
 see Excision, Upper Joints ØRB
 see Resection, Upper Joints ØRT
Acromioplasty
 see Repair, Upper Joints ØRQ
 see Replacement, Upper Joints ØRR
 see Supplement, Upper Joints ØRU
ACTEMRA® *use* Tocilizumab
Activa PC neurostimulator *use* Stimulator Generator, Multiple Array in ØJH
Activa RC neurostimulator *use* Stimulator Generator, Multiple Array Rechargeable in ØJH
Activa SC neurostimulator *use* Stimulator Generator, Single Array in ØJH
Activities of Daily Living Assessment F02

Activities of Daily Living Treatment F08
ACUITY™ Steerable Lead
 use Cardiac Lead, Defibrillator in 02H
 use Cardiac Lead, Pacemaker in 02H
Acupuncture
 Breast
  Anesthesia 8E0H300
  No Qualifier 8E0H30Z
 Integumentary System
  Anesthesia 8E0H300
  No Qualifier 8E0H30Z
Adductor brevis muscle
 use Upper Leg Muscle, Left
 use Upper Leg Muscle, Right
Adductor hallucis muscle
 use Foot Muscle, Left
 use Foot Muscle, Right
Adductor longus muscle
 use Upper Leg Muscle, Left
 use Upper Leg Muscle, Right
Adductor magnus muscle
 use Upper Leg Muscle, Left
 use Upper Leg Muscle, Right
Adenohypophysis *use* Pituitary Gland
Adenoidectomy
 see Excision, Adenoids ØCBQ
 see Resection, Adenoids ØCTQ
Adenoidotomy *see* Drainage, Adenoids ØC9Q
Adhesiolysis *see* Release
Administration
 Blood products *see* Transfusion
 Other substance *see* Introduction of substance in or on
Adrenalectomy
 see Excision, Endocrine System ØGB
 see Resection, Endocrine System ØGT
Adrenalorrhaphy *see* Repair, Endocrine System ØGQ
Adrenalotomy *see* Drainage, Endocrine System ØG9
Advancement
 see Reposition
 see Transfer
Advisa (MRI) *use* Pacemaker, Dual Chamber in ØJH
afami-cel *use* Afamitresgene Autoleucel Immunotherapy
Afamitresgene Autoleucel Immunotherapy XW0
AFX® Endovascular AAA System *use* Intraluminal Device
Aidoc Briefcase for PE (pulmonary embolism) XXE3X27
AIGISRx Antibacterial Envelope *use* Anti-Infective Envelope
Alar ligament of axis *use* Head and Neck Bursa and Ligament
Alfapump® system *use* Other Device
Alfieri Stitch Valvuloplasty *see* Restriction, Valve, Mitral 02VG
Alimentation *see* Introduction of substance in or on
ALPPS (Associating liver partition and portal vein ligation)
 see Division, Hepatobiliary System and Pancreas ØF8
 see Resection, Hepatobiliary System and Pancreas ØFT
Alteration
 Abdominal Wall ØWØF
 Ankle Region
  Left ØYØL
  Right ØYØK
 Arm
  Lower
   Left ØXØF
   Right ØXØD
  Upper
   Left ØXØ9
   Right ØXØ8
 Axilla
  Left ØXØ5
  Right ØXØ4
 Back
  Lower ØWØL
  Upper ØWØK
 Breast
  Bilateral ØHØV
  Left ØHØU
  Right ØHØT
 Buttock
  Left ØYØ1

Alteration — *continued*
 Buttock — *continued*
  Right ØYØØ
 Chest Wall ØWØ8
 Ear
  Bilateral Ø9Ø2
  Left Ø9Ø1
  Right Ø9ØØ
 Elbow Region
  Left ØXØC
  Right ØXØB
 Extremity
  Lower
   Left ØYØB
   Right ØYØ9
  Upper
   Left ØXØ7
   Right ØXØ6
 Eyelid
  Lower
   Left Ø8ØR
   Right Ø8ØQ
  Upper
   Left Ø8ØP
   Right Ø8ØN
 Face ØWØ2
 Head ØWØØ
 Jaw
  Lower ØWØ5
  Upper ØWØ4
 Knee Region
  Left ØYØG
  Right ØYØF
 Leg
  Lower
   Left ØYØJ
   Right ØYØH
  Upper
   Left ØYØD
   Right ØYØC
 Lip
  Lower ØCØ1X
  Upper ØCØØX
 Nasal Mucosa and Soft Tissue Ø9ØK
 Neck ØWØ6
 Perineum
  Female ØWØN
  Male ØWØM
 Shoulder Region
  Left ØXØ3
  Right ØXØ2
 Subcutaneous Tissue and Fascia
  Abdomen ØJØ8
  Back ØJØ7
  Buttock ØJØ9
  Chest ØJØ6
  Face ØJØ1
  Lower Arm
   Left ØJØH
   Right ØJØG
  Lower Leg
   Left ØJØP
   Right ØJØN
  Neck
   Left ØJØ5
   Right ØJØ4
  Upper Arm
   Left ØJØF
   Right ØJØD
  Upper Leg
   Left ØJØM
   Right ØJØL
 Wrist Region
  Left ØXØH
  Right ØXØG
Alveolar process of mandible
 use Mandible, Left
 use Mandible, Right
Alveolar process of maxilla *use* Maxilla
Alveolectomy
 see Excision, Head and Facial Bones ØNB
 see Resection, Head and Facial Bones ØNT
Alveoloplasty
 see Repair, Head and Facial Bones ØNQ
 see Replacement, Head and Facial Bones ØNR
 see Supplement, Head and Facial Bones ØNU
Alveolotomy
 see Division, Head and Facial Bones ØN8

Alveolotomy — *continued*
see Drainage, Head and Facial Bones ØN9
Ambulatory cardiac monitoring 4A12X45
Amivantamab Monoclonal Antibody XWØ
Amniocentesis *see* Drainage, Products of Conception 1Ø9Ø
Amnioinfusion *see* Introduction of substance in or on, Products of Conception 3EØE
Amnioscopy 1ØJØ8ZZ
Amniotomy *see* Drainage, Products of Conception 1Ø9Ø
AMPLATZER® Muscular VSD Occluder *use* Synthetic Substitute
Amputation *see* Detachment
AMS 8ØØ® Urinary Control System *use* Artificial Sphincter in Urinary System
Anal orifice *use* Anus
Analog radiography *see* Plain Radiography
Analog radiology *see* Plain Radiography
Anastomosis *see* Bypass
Anatomical snuffbox
use Lower Arm and Wrist Muscle, Left
use Lower Arm and Wrist Muscle, Right
Andexanet Alfa, Factor Xa Inhibitor Reversal Agent *use* Coagulation Factor Xa, Inactivated
Andexxa *use* Coagulation Factor Xa, Inactivated
AneuRx® AAA Advantage® *use* Intraluminal Device
Angiectomy
see Excision, Heart and Great Vessels Ø2B
see Excision, Lower Arteries Ø4B
see Excision, Lower Veins Ø6B
see Excision, Upper Arteries Ø3B
see Excision, Upper Veins Ø5B
Angiocardiography
Combined right and left heart *see* Fluoroscopy, Heart, Right and Left B216
Left Heart *see* Fluoroscopy, Heart, Left B215
Right Heart *see* Fluoroscopy, Heart, Right B214
SPY system intravascular fluorescence *see* Monitoring, Physiological Systems 4A1
Angiography
see Computerized Tomography (CT Scan), Artery
see Fluoroscopy, Artery
see Magnetic Resonance Imaging (MRI), Artery
see Plain Radiography, Artery
Angioplasty
see Dilation, Heart and Great Vessels Ø27
see Dilation, Lower Arteries Ø47
see Dilation, Upper Arteries Ø37
see Repair, Heart and Great Vessels Ø2Q
see Repair, Lower Arteries Ø4Q
see Repair, Upper Arteries Ø3Q
see Replacement, Heart and Great Vessels Ø2R
see Replacement, Lower Arteries Ø4R
see Replacement, Upper Arteries Ø3R
see Supplement, Heart and Great Vessels Ø2U
see Supplement, Lower Arteries Ø4U
see Supplement, Upper Arteries Ø3U
Angiorrhaphy
see Repair, Heart and Great Vessels Ø2Q
see Repair, Lower Arteries Ø4Q
see Repair, Upper Arteries Ø3Q
Angioscopy Ø2JY4ZZ, Ø3JY4ZZ, Ø4JY4ZZ
Angiotensin II *use* Synthetic Human Angiotensin II
Angiotripsy
see Occlusion, Lower Arteries Ø4L
see Occlusion, Upper Arteries Ø3L
Angular artery *use* Face Artery
Angular vein
use Face Vein, Left
use Face Vein, Right
Annular ligament
use Elbow Bursa and Ligament, Left
use Elbow Bursa and Ligament, Right
Annuloplasty
see Repair, Heart and Great Vessels Ø2Q
see Supplement, Heart and Great Vessels Ø2U
Annuloplasty ring *use* Synthetic Substitute
Anoplasty
see Repair, Anus ØDQQ
see Supplement, Anus ØDUQ
Anorectal junction *use* Rectum
Anoscopy ØDJD8ZZ
Ansa cervicalis *use* Cervical Plexus
Antabuse therapy HZ93ZZZ

Antebrachial fascia
use Subcutaneous Tissue and Fascia, Left Lower Arm
use Subcutaneous Tissue and Fascia, Right Lower Arm
Anterior cerebral artery *use* Intracranial Artery
Anterior cerebral vein *use* Intracranial Vein
Anterior choroidal artery *use* Intracranial Artery
Anterior circumflex humeral artery
use Axillary Artery, Left
use Axillary Artery, Right
Anterior communicating artery *use* Intracranial Artery
Anterior cruciate ligament (ACL)
use Knee Bursa and Ligament, Left
use Knee Bursa and Ligament, Right
Anterior crural nerve *use* Femoral Nerve
Anterior facial vein
use Face Vein, Left
use Face Vein, Right
Anterior intercostal artery
use Internal Mammary Artery, Left
use Internal Mammary Artery, Right
Anterior interosseous nerve *use* Median Nerve
Anterior lateral malleolar artery
use Anterior Tibial Artery, Left
use Anterior Tibial Artery, Right
Anterior lingual gland *use* Minor Salivary Gland
Anterior (pectoral) lymph node
use Lymphatic, Left Axillary
use Lymphatic, Right Axillary
Anterior medial malleolar artery
use Anterior Tibial Artery, Left
use Anterior Tibial Artery, Right
Anterior spinal artery
use Vertebral Artery, Left
use Vertebral Artery, Right
Anterior tibial recurrent artery
use Anterior Tibial Artery, Left
use Anterior Tibial Artery, Right
Anterior ulnar recurrent artery
use Ulnar Artery, Left
use Ulnar Artery, Right
Anterior vagal trunk *use* Vagus Nerve
Anterior vertebral muscle
use Neck Muscle, Left
use Neck Muscle, Right
Antibacterial Envelope (TYRX) (AIGISRx) *use* Anti-Infective Envelope
Antibiotic-eluting Bone Void Filler XWØVØP7
Antigen-free air conditioning *see* Atmospheric Control, Physiological Systems 6AØ
Antihelix
use External Ear, Bilateral
use External Ear, Left
use External Ear, Right
Antimicrobial envelope *use* Anti-Infective Envelope
Anti-SARS-CoV-2 hyperimmune globulin *use* Hyperimmune Globulin
Antitragus
use External Ear, Bilateral
use External Ear, Left
use External Ear, Right
Antrostomy *see* Drainage, Ear, Nose, Sinus Ø99
Antrotomy *see* Drainage, Ear, Nose, Sinus Ø99
Antrum of Highmore
use Maxillary Sinus, Left
use Maxillary Sinus, Right
Aortic annulus *use* Aortic Valve
Aortic arch *use* Thoracic Aorta, Ascending/Arch
Aortic intercostal artery *use* Upper Artery
Aortography
see Fluoroscopy, Lower Arteries B41
see Fluoroscopy, Upper Arteries B31
see Plain Radiography, Lower Arteries B4Ø
see Plain Radiography, Upper Arteries B3Ø
Aortoplasty
see Repair, Aorta, Abdominal Ø4QØ
see Repair, Aorta, Thoracic, Ascending/Arch Ø2QX
see Repair, Aorta, Thoracic, Descending Ø2QW
see Replacement, Aorta, Abdominal Ø4RØ
see Replacement, Aorta, Thoracic, Ascending/Arch Ø2RX
see Replacement, Aorta, Thoracic, Descending Ø2RW
see Supplement, Aorta, Abdominal Ø4UØ

Aortoplasty — *continued*
see Supplement, Aorta, Thoracic, Ascending/Arch Ø2UX
see Supplement, Aorta, Thoracic, Descending Ø2UW
Apalutamide Antineoplastic XWØDXJ5
Apical (subclavicular) lymph node
use Lymphatic, Left Axillary
use Lymphatic, Right Axillary
ApiFix® Minimally Invasive Deformity Correction (MID-C) System *use* Posterior (Dynamic) Distraction Device in New Technology
Apneustic center *use* Pons
Appendectomy
see Excision, Appendix ØDBJ
see Resection, Appendix ØDTJ
Appendicolysis *see* Release, Appendix ØDNJ
Appendicotomy *see* Drainage, Appendix ØD9J
Application *see* Introduction of substance in or on
aprevo™ *use* Interbody Fusion Device, Customizable in New Technology
Aquablation therapy, prostate XV5Ø8A4
Aquapheresis 6A55ØZ3
Aqueduct of Sylvius *use* Cerebral Ventricle
Aqueous humour
use Anterior Chamber, Left
use Anterior Chamber, Right
Arachnoid mater, intracranial *use* Cerebral Meninges
Arachnoid mater, spinal *use* Spinal Meninges
Arcuate artery
use Foot Artery, Left
use Foot Artery, Right
Areola
use Nipple, Left
use Nipple, Right
AROM (artificial rupture of membranes) 1Ø9Ø7ZC
Arterial canal (duct) *use* Pulmonary Artery, Left
Arterial pulse tracing *see* Measurement, Arterial 4AØ3
Arteriectomy
see Excision, Heart and Great Vessels Ø2B
see Excision, Lower Arteries Ø4B
see Excision, Upper Arteries Ø3B
Arteriography
see Fluoroscopy, Heart B21
see Fluoroscopy, Lower Arteries B41
see Fluoroscopy, Upper Arteries B31
see Plain Radiography, Heart B2Ø
see Plain Radiography, Lower Arteries B4Ø
see Plain Radiography, Upper Arteries B3Ø
Arterioplasty
see Repair, Heart and Great Vessels Ø2Q
see Repair, Lower Arteries Ø4Q
see Repair, Upper Arteries Ø3Q
see Replacement, Heart and Great Vessels Ø2R
see Replacement, Lower Arteries Ø4R
see Replacement, Upper Arteries Ø3R
see Supplement, Heart and Great Vessels Ø2U
see Supplement, Lower Arteries Ø4U
see Supplement, Upper Arteries Ø3U
Arteriorrhaphy
see Repair, Heart and Great Vessels Ø2Q
see Repair, Lower Arteries Ø4Q
see Repair, Upper Arteries Ø3Q
Arterioscopy
see Inspection, Artery, Lower Ø4JY
see Inspection, Artery, Upper Ø3JY
see Inspection, Great Vessel Ø2JY
Arthrectomy
see Excision, Lower Joints ØSB
see Excision, Upper Joints ØRB
see Resection, Lower Joints ØST
see Resection, Upper Joints ØRT
Arthrocentesis
see Drainage, Lower Joints ØS9
see Drainage, Upper Joints ØR9
Arthrodesis
see Fusion, Lower Joints ØSG
see Fusion, Upper Joints ØRG
Arthrography
see Plain Radiography, Non-Axial Lower Bones BQØ
see Plain Radiography, Non-Axial Upper Bones BPØ
see Plain Radiography, Skull and Facial Bones BNØ
Arthrolysis
see Release, Lower Joints ØSN
see Release, Upper Joints ØRN

Arthropexy
see Repair, Lower Joints ØSQ
see Repair, Upper Joints ØRQ
see Reposition, Lower Joints ØSS
see Reposition, Upper Joints ØRS
Arthroplasty
see Repair, Lower Joints ØSQ
see Repair, Upper Joints ØRQ
see Replacement, Lower Joints ØSR
see Replacement, Upper Joints ØRR
see Supplement, Lower Joints ØSU
see Supplement, Upper Joints ØRU
Arthroplasty, radial head
see Replacement, Radius, Left ØPRJ
see Replacement, Radius, Right ØPRH
Arthroscopy
see Inspection, Lower Joints ØSJ
see Inspection, Upper Joints ØRJ
Arthrotomy
see Drainage, Lower Joints ØS9
see Drainage, Upper Joints ØR9
Articulating Spacer (Antibiotic) use Articulating
Spacer in Lower Joints
Artificial anal sphincter (AAS) use Artificial Sphincter
in Gastrointestinal System
Artificial bowel sphincter (neosphincter) use Artifi-
cial Sphincter in Gastrointestinal System
Artificial Sphincter
Insertion of device in
Anus ØDHQ
Bladder ØTHB
Bladder Neck ØTHC
Urethra ØTHD
Removal of device from
Anus ØDPQ
Bladder ØTPB
Urethra ØTPD
Revision of device in
Anus ØDWQ
Bladder ØTWB
Urethra ØTWD
Artificial urinary sphincter (AUS) use Artificial
Sphincter in Urinary System
Aryepiglottic fold use Larynx
Arytenoid cartilage use Larynx
Arytenoid muscle
use Neck Muscle, Left
use Neck Muscle, Right
Arytenoidectomy see Excision, Larynx ØCBS
Arytenoidopexy see Repair, Larynx ØCQS
Ascenda Intrathecal Catheter use Infusion Device
Ascending aorta use Thoracic Aorta, Ascending/Arch
Ascending palatine artery use Face Artery
Ascending pharyngeal artery
use External Carotid Artery, Left
use External Carotid Artery, Right
aScope™ Duodeno see New Technology, Hepatobiliary
System and Pancreas XFJ
Aspiration, fine needle
Fluid or gas see Drainage
Tissue biopsy
see Excision
see Extraction
Assessment
Activities of daily living see Activities of Daily Living
Assessment, Rehabilitation FØ2
Hearing see Hearing Assessment, Diagnostic Audi-
ology F13
Hearing aid see Hearing Aid Assessment, Diagnos-
tic Audiology F14
Intravascular perfusion, using indocyanine green
(ICG) dye see Monitoring, Physiological Sys-
tems 4A1
Motor function see Motor Function Assessment,
Rehabilitation FØ1
Nerve function see Motor Function Assessment,
Rehabilitation FØ1
Speech see Speech Assessment, Rehabilitation FØØ
Vestibular see Vestibular Assessment, Diagnostic
Audiology F15
Vocational see Activities of Daily Living Treatment,
Rehabilitation FØ8
Assistance
Cardiac
Continuous
Output
Balloon Pump 5AØ221Ø

Assistance — continued
Cardiac — continued
Continuous — continued
Output — continued
Impeller Pump 5AØ221D
Other Pump 5AØ2216
Pulsatile Compression 5AØ2215
Oxygenation, Supersaturated 5AØ222C
Intermittent
Balloon Pump 5AØ211Ø
Impeller Pump 5AØ211D
Other Pump 5AØ2116
Pulsatile Compression 5AØ2115
Circulatory
Continuous, Oxygenation, Hyperbaric
5AØ5221
Intermittent, Oxygenation, Hyperbaric
5AØ5121
Respiratory
24-96 Consecutive Hours
Continuous Negative Airway Pressure
5AØ9459
Continuous Positive Airway Pressure
5AØ9457
High Nasal Flow/Velocity 5AØ945A
Intermittent Negative Airway Pressure
5AØ945B
Intermittent Positive Airway Pressure
5AØ9458
No Qualifier 5AØ945Z
Continuous, Filtration 5AØ92ØZ
Greater than 96 Consecutive Hours
Continuous Negative Airway Pressure
5AØ9559
Continuous Positive Airway Pressure
5AØ9557
High Nasal Flow/Velocity 5AØ955A
Intermittent Negative Airway Pressure
5AØ955B
Intermittent Positive Airway Pressure
5AØ9558
No Qualifier 5AØ955Z
Less than 24 Consecutive Hours
Continuous Negative Airway Pressure
5AØ9359
Continuous Positive Airway Pressure
5AØ9357
High Nasal Flow/Velocity 5AØ935A
Intermittent Negative Airway Pressure
5AØ935B
Intermittent Positive Airway Pressure
5AØ9358
No Qualifier 5AØ935Z
**Associating liver partition and portal vein ligation
(ALPPS)**
see Division, Hepatobiliary System and Pancreas
ØF8
see Resection, Hepatobiliary System and Pancreas
ØFT
Assurant (Cobalt) stent use Intraluminal Device
Atezolizumab Antineoplastic XWØ
Atherectomy
see Extirpation, Heart and Great Vessels Ø2C
see Extirpation, Lower Arteries Ø4C
see Extirpation, Upper Arteries Ø3C
Atlantoaxial joint use Cervical Vertebral Joint
Atmospheric Control 6AØZ
AtriClip LAA Exclusion System use Extraluminal De-
vice
Atrioseptoplasty
see Repair, Heart and Great Vessels Ø2Q
see Replacement, Heart and Great Vessels Ø2R
see Supplement, Heart and Great Vessels Ø2U
Atrioventricular node use Conduction Mechanism
Atrium dextrum cordis use Atrium, Right
Atrium pulmonale use Atrium, Left
Attain Ability® lead Ø2H
use Cardiac Lead, Defibrillator in Ø2H
use Cardiac Lead, Pacemaker in Ø2H
Attain Starfix® (OTW) lead
use Cardiac Lead, Defibrillator in Ø2H
use Cardiac Lead, Pacemaker in Ø2H
Audiology, diagnostic
see Hearing Aid Assessment, Diagnostic Audiology
F14
see Hearing Assessment, Diagnostic Audiology
F13

Audiology, diagnostic — continued
see Vestibular Assessment, Diagnostic Audiology
F15
Audiometry see Hearing Assessment, Diagnostic Audiology F13
Auditory tube
use Eustachian Tube, Left
use Eustachian Tube, Right
Auerbach's (myenteric) plexus use Abdominal Sympathetic Nerve
Auricle
use External Ear, Bilateral
use External Ear, Left
use External Ear, Right
Auricularis muscle use Head Muscle
Autograft use Autologous Tissue Substitute
AutoLITT® System see Destruction
Autologous artery graft
use Autologous Arterial Tissue in Heart and Great
Vessels
use Autologous Arterial Tissue in Lower Arteries
use Autologous Arterial Tissue in Lower Veins
use Autologous Arterial Tissue in Upper Arteries
use Autologous Arterial Tissue in Upper Veins
Autologous vein graft
use Autologous Venous Tissue in Heart and Great
Vessels
use Autologous Venous Tissue in Lower Arteries
use Autologous Venous Tissue in Lower Veins
use Autologous Venous Tissue in Upper Arteries
use Autologous Venous Tissue in Upper Veins
Automated Chest Compression (ACC) 5A1221J
AutoPulse® Resuscitation System 5A1221J
Autotransfusion see Transfusion
Autotransplant
Adrenal tissue see Reposition, Endocrine System
ØGS
Kidney see Reposition, Urinary System ØTS
Pancreatic tissue see Reposition, Pancreas ØFSG
Parathyroid tissue see Reposition, Endocrine Sys-
tem ØGS
Thyroid tissue see Reposition, Endocrine System
ØGS
Tooth see Reattachment, Mouth and Throat ØCM
Avulsion see Extraction
AVYCAZ® (ceftazidime-avibactam) use Other Anti-
infective
Axial Lumbar Interbody Fusion System use Inter-
body Fusion Device in Lower Joints
AxiaLIF® System use Interbody Fusion Device in Lower
Joints
Axicabtagene Ciloleucel use Axicabtagene Ciloleucel
Immunotherapy
Axicabtagene Ciloleucel Immunotherapy XWØ
Axillary fascia
use Subcutaneous Tissue and Fascia, Left Upper
Arm
use Subcutaneous Tissue and Fascia, Right Upper
Arm
Axillary nerve use Brachial Plexus
AZEDRA® use Iobenguane I-131 Antineoplastic

B

BAK/C® Interbody Cervical Fusion System use Inter-
body Fusion Device in Upper Joints
BAL (bronchial alveolar lavage), diagnostic see
Drainage, Respiratory System ØB9
Balanoplasty
see Repair, Penis ØVQS
see Supplement, Penis ØVUS
Balloon atrial septostomy (BAS) Ø2163Z7
Balloon Pump
Continuous, Output 5AØ221Ø
Intermittent, Output 5AØ211Ø
Bamlanivimab Monoclonal Antibody XWØ
Bandage, Elastic see Compression
Banding
see Occlusion
see Restriction
Banding, esophageal varices see Occlusion, Vein,
Esophageal Ø6L3
Banding, laparoscopic (adjustable) gastric
Initial procedure ØDV64CZ
Surgical correction see Revision of device in,
Stomach ØDW6

Bard® Composix® Kugel® patch use Synthetic Substitute
Bard® Composix® (E/X) (LP) mesh use Synthetic Substitute
Bard® Dulex™ mesh use Synthetic Substitute
Bard® Ventralex™ hernia patch use Synthetic Substitute
Baricitinib XW0
Barium swallow see Fluoroscopy, Gastrointestinal System BD1
Baroreflex Activation Therapy® (BAT®)
    use Stimulator Generator in Subcutaneous Tissue and Fascia
    use Stimulator Lead in Upper Arteries
Barricaid® Annular Closure Device (ACD) use Synthetic Substitute
Bartholin's (greater vestibular) gland use Vestibular Gland
Basal (internal) cerebral vein use Intracranial Vein
Basal metabolic rate (BMR) see Measurement, Physiological Systems 4A0Z
Basal nuclei use Basal Ganglia
Base of Tongue use Pharynx
Basilar artery use Intracranial Artery
Basis pontis use Pons
Beam Radiation
    Abdomen DW03
        Intraoperative DW033Z0
    Adrenal Gland DG02
        Intraoperative DG023Z0
    Bile Ducts DF02
        Intraoperative DF023Z0
    Bladder DT02
        Intraoperative DT023Z0
    Bone
        Intraoperative DP0C3Z0
        Other DP0C
    Bone Marrow D700
        Intraoperative D7003Z0
    Brain D000
        Intraoperative D0003Z0
    Brain Stem D001
        Intraoperative D0013Z0
    Breast
        Left DM00
            Intraoperative DM003Z0
        Right DM01
            Intraoperative DM013Z0
    Bronchus DB01
        Intraoperative DB013Z0
    Cervix DU01
        Intraoperative DU013Z0
    Chest DW02
        Intraoperative DW023Z0
    Chest Wall DB07
        Intraoperative DB073Z0
    Colon DD05
        Intraoperative DD053Z0
    Diaphragm DB08
        Intraoperative DB083Z0
    Duodenum DD02
        Intraoperative DD023Z0
    Ear D900
        Intraoperative D9003Z0
    Esophagus DD00
        Intraoperative DD003Z0
    Eye D800
        Intraoperative D8003Z0
    Femur DP09
        Intraoperative DP093Z0
    Fibula DP0B
        Intraoperative DP0B3Z0
    Gallbladder DF01
        Intraoperative DF013Z0
    Gland
        Adrenal DG02
            Intraoperative DG023Z0
        Parathyroid DG04
            Intraoperative DG043Z0
        Pituitary DG00
            Intraoperative DG003Z0
        Thyroid DG05
            Intraoperative DG053Z0
    Glands
        Intraoperative D9063Z0
        Salivary D906
    Head and Neck DW01
        Intraoperative DW013Z0

Beam Radiation — continued
    Hemibody DW04
        Intraoperative DW043Z0
    Humerus DP06
        Intraoperative DP063Z0
    Hypopharynx D903
        Intraoperative D9033Z0
    Ileum DD04
        Intraoperative DD043Z0
    Jejunum DD03
        Intraoperative DD033Z0
    Kidney DT00
        Intraoperative DT003Z0
    Larynx D90B
        Intraoperative D90B3Z0
    Liver DF00
        Intraoperative DF003Z0
    Lung DB02
        Intraoperative DB023Z0
    Lymphatics
        Abdomen D706
            Intraoperative D7063Z0
        Axillary D704
            Intraoperative D7043Z0
        Inguinal D708
            Intraoperative D7083Z0
        Neck D703
            Intraoperative D7033Z0
        Pelvis D707
            Intraoperative D7073Z0
        Thorax D705
            Intraoperative D7053Z0
    Mandible DP03
        Intraoperative DP033Z0
    Maxilla DP02
        Intraoperative DP023Z0
    Mediastinum DB06
        Intraoperative DB063Z0
    Mouth D904
        Intraoperative D9043Z0
    Nasopharynx D90D
        Intraoperative D90D3Z0
    Neck and Head DW01
        Intraoperative DW013Z0
    Nerve
        Intraoperative D0073Z0
        Peripheral D007
    Nose D901
        Intraoperative D9013Z0
    Oropharynx D90F
        Intraoperative D90F3Z0
    Ovary DU00
        Intraoperative DU003Z0
    Palate
        Hard D908
            Intraoperative D9083Z0
        Soft D909
            Intraoperative D9093Z0
    Pancreas DF03
        Intraoperative DF033Z0
    Parathyroid Gland DG04
        Intraoperative DG043Z0
    Pelvic Bones DP08
        Intraoperative DP083Z0
    Pelvic Region DW06
        Intraoperative DW063Z0
    Pineal Body DG01
        Intraoperative DG013Z0
    Pituitary Gland DG00
        Intraoperative DG003Z0
    Pleura DB05
        Intraoperative DB053Z0
    Prostate DV00
        Intraoperative DV003Z0
    Radius DP07
        Intraoperative DP073Z0
    Rectum DD07
        Intraoperative DD073Z0
    Rib DP05
        Intraoperative DP053Z0
    Sinuses D907
        Intraoperative D9073Z0
    Skin
        Abdomen DH08
            Intraoperative DH083Z0
        Arm DH04
            Intraoperative DH043Z0
        Back DH07
            Intraoperative DH073Z0

Beam Radiation — continued
    Skin — continued
        Buttock DH09
            Intraoperative DH093Z0
        Chest DH06
            Intraoperative DH063Z0
        Face DH02
            Intraoperative DH023Z0
        Leg DH0B
            Intraoperative DH0B3Z0
        Neck DH03
            Intraoperative DH033Z0
    Skull DP00
        Intraoperative DP003Z0
    Spinal Cord D006
        Intraoperative D0063Z0
    Spleen D702
        Intraoperative D7023Z0
    Sternum DP04
        Intraoperative DP043Z0
    Stomach DD01
        Intraoperative DD013Z0
    Testis DV01
        Intraoperative DV013Z0
    Thymus D701
        Intraoperative D7013Z0
    Thyroid Gland DG05
        Intraoperative DG053Z0
    Tibia DP0B
        Intraoperative DP0B3Z0
    Tongue D905
        Intraoperative D9053Z0
    Trachea DB00
        Intraoperative DB003Z0
    Ulna DP07
        Intraoperative DP073Z0
    Ureter DT01
        Intraoperative DT013Z0
    Urethra DT03
        Intraoperative DT033Z0
    Uterus DU02
        Intraoperative DU023Z0
    Whole Body DW05
        Intraoperative DW053Z0
Bedside swallow F00ZJWZ
Berlin Heart Ventricular Assist Device use Implantable Heart Assist System in Heart and Great Vessels
Betibeglogene Autotemcel XW1
beti-cel use Betibeglogene Autotemcel
Bezlotoxumab infusion see Introduction with qualifier Other Therapeutic Monoclonal Antibody
Biceps brachii muscle
    use Upper Arm Muscle, Left
    use Upper Arm Muscle, Right
Biceps femoris muscle
    use Upper Leg Muscle, Left
    use Upper Leg Muscle, Right
Bicipital aponeurosis
    use Subcutaneous Tissue and Fascia, Left Lower Arm
    use Subcutaneous Tissue and Fascia, Right Lower Arm
Bicuspid valve use Mitral Valve
Bili light therapy see Phototherapy, Skin 6A60
Bioactive embolization coil(s) use Intraluminal Device, Bioactive in Upper Arteries
Bioengineered Allogeneic Construct, Skin XHRPXF7
Biofeedback GZC9ZZZ
BioFire® FilmArray® Pneumonia Panel XXEBXQ6
Biopsy
    see Drainage with qualifier Diagnostic
    see Excision with qualifier Diagnostic
    see Extraction with qualifier Diagnostic
BiPAP see Assistance, Respiratory 5A09
Bisection see Division
Biventricular external heart assist system use Short-term External Heart Assist System in Heart and Great Vessels
Blepharectomy
    see Excision, Eye 08B
    see Resection, Eye 08T
Blepharoplasty
    see Repair, Eye 08Q
    see Replacement, Eye 08R
    see Reposition, Eye 08S
    see Supplement, Eye 08U
Blepharorrhaphy see Repair, Eye 08Q

Blepharotomy *see* Drainage, Eye Ø89
Blinatumomab *use* Other Antineoplastic
BLINCYTO® (blinatumomab) *use* Other Antineoplastic
Block, Nerve, anesthetic injection 3E0T3BZ
Blood glucose monitoring system *use* Monitoring Device
Blood pressure *see* Measurement, Arterial 4A03
BMR (basal metabolic rate) *see* Measurement, Physiological Systems 4A0Z
Body of femur
   use Femoral Shaft, Left
   use Femoral Shaft, Right
Body of fibula
   use Fibula, Left
   use Fibula, Right
Bone anchored hearing device
   use Hearing Device, Bone Conduction in Ø9H
   use Hearing Device in Head and Facial Bones
Bone bank bone graft *use* Nonautologous Tissue Substitute
Bone Growth Stimulator
   Insertion of device in
      Bone
         Facial ØNHW
         Lower ØQHY
         Nasal ØNHB
         Upper ØPHY
      Skull ØNHØ
   Removal of device from
      Bone
         Facial ØNPW
         Lower ØQPY
         Nasal ØNPB
         Upper ØPPY
      Skull ØNPØ
   Revision of device in
      Bone
         Facial ØNWW
         Lower ØQWY
         Nasal ØNWB
         Upper ØPWY
      Skull ØNWØ
Bone marrow transplant *see* Transfusion, Circulatory 3Ø2
Bone morphogenetic protein 2 (BMP 2) *use* Recombinant Bone Morphogenetic Protein
Bone screw (interlocking) (lag) (pedicle) (recessed)
   use Internal Fixation Device in Head and Facial Bones
   use Internal Fixation Device in Lower Bones
   use Internal Fixation Device in Upper Bones
Bony labyrinth
   use Inner Ear, Left
   use Inner Ear, Right
Bony orbit
   use Orbit, Left
   use Orbit, Right
Bony vestibule
   use Inner Ear, Left
   use Inner Ear, Right
Botallo's duct *use* Pulmonary Artery, Left
Bovine pericardial valve *use* Zooplastic Tissue in Heart and Great Vessels
Bovine pericardium graft *use* Zooplastic Tissue in Heart and Great Vessels
BP (blood pressure) *see* Measurement, Arterial 4A03
Brachial (lateral) lymph node
   use Lymphatic, Left Axillary
   use Lymphatic, Right Axillary
Brachialis muscle
   use Upper Arm Muscle, Left
   use Upper Arm Muscle, Right
Brachiocephalic artery *use* Innominate Artery
Brachiocephalic trunk *use* Innominate Artery
Brachiocephalic vein
   use Innominate Vein, Left
   use Innominate Vein, Right
Brachioradialis muscle
   use Lower Arm and Wrist Muscle, Left
   use Lower Arm and Wrist Muscle, Right
Brachytherapy
   Abdomen DW13
   Adrenal Gland DG12
   Back
      Lower DW1LBB
      Upper DW1KBB
   Bile Ducts DF12

Brachytherapy — *continued*
   Bladder DT12
   Bone Marrow D71Ø
   Brain DØ1Ø
   Brain Stem DØ11
   Breast
      Left DM1Ø
      Right DM11
   Bronchus DB11
   Cervix DU11
   Chest DW12
   Chest Wall DB17
   Colon DD15
   Cranial Cavity DW1ØBB
   Diaphragm DB18
   Duodenum DD12
   Ear D91Ø
   Esophagus DD1Ø
   Extremity
      Lower DW1YBB
      Upper DW1XBB
   Eye D81Ø
   Gallbladder DF11
   Gastrointestinal Tract DW1PBB
   Genitourinary Tract DW1RBB
   Gland
      Adrenal DG12
      Parathyroid DG14
      Pituitary DG1Ø
      Thyroid DG15
   Glands, Salivary D916
   Head and Neck DW11
   Hypopharynx D913
   Ileum DD14
   Jejunum DD13
   Kidney DT1Ø
   Larynx D91B
   Liver DF1Ø
   Lung DB12
   Lymphatics
      Abdomen D716
      Axillary D714
      Inguinal D718
      Neck D713
      Pelvis D717
      Thorax D715
   Mediastinum DB16
   Mouth D914
   Nasopharynx D91D
   Neck and Head DW11
   Nerve, Peripheral DØ17
   Nose D911
   Oropharynx D91F
   Ovary DU1Ø
   Palate
      Hard D918
      Soft D919
   Pancreas DF13
   Parathyroid Gland DG14
   Pelvic Region DW16
   Pineal Body DG11
   Pituitary Gland DG1Ø
   Pleura DB15
   Prostate DV1Ø
   Rectum DD17
   Respiratory Tract DW1QBB
   Sinuses D917
   Spinal Cord DØ16
   Spleen D712
   Stomach DD11
   Testis DV11
   Thymus D711
   Thyroid Gland DG15
   Tongue D915
   Trachea DB1Ø
   Ureter DT11
   Urethra DT13
   Uterus DU12
Brachytherapy, CivaSheet®
   see Brachytherapy with qualifier Unidirectional Source
   see Insertion with device Radioactive Element
Brachytherapy seeds *use* Radioactive Element
Brain Electrical Activity, Computer-aided Semiologic Analysis XXE0X48
Breast procedures, skin only *use* Skin, Chest
Brexanolone XWØ

Brexucabtagene Autoleucel *use* Brexucabtagene Autoleucel Immunotherapy
Brexucabtagene Autoleucel Immunotherapy XWØ
Breyanzi® *use* Lisocabtagene Maraleucel Immunotherapy
Broad Consortium Microbiota-based Live Biotherapeutic Suspension XWØH7X8
Broad ligament *use* Uterine Supporting Structure
Bromelain-enriched Proteolytic Enzyme XWØ
Bronchial artery *use* Upper Artery
Bronchography
   see Fluoroscopy, Respiratory System BB1
   see Plain Radiography, Respiratory System BBØ
Bronchoplasty
   see Repair, Respiratory System ØBQ
   see Supplement, Respiratory System ØBU
Bronchorrhaphy *see* Repair, Respiratory System ØBQ
Bronchoscopy ØBJØ8ZZ
Bronchotomy *see* Drainage, Respiratory System ØB9
Bronchus Intermedius *use* Main Bronchus, Right
BRYAN® Cervical Disc System *use* Synthetic Substitute
Buccal gland *use* Buccal Mucosa
Buccinator lymph node *use* Lymphatic, Head
Buccinator muscle *use* Facial Muscle
Buckling, scleral with implant *see* Supplement, Eye Ø8U
Bulbospongiosus muscle *use* Perineum Muscle
Bulbourethral (Cowper's) gland *use* Urethra
Bundle of His *use* Conduction Mechanism
Bundle of Kent *use* Conduction Mechanism
Bunionectomy *see* Excision, Lower Bones ØQB
Bursectomy
   see Excision, Bursae and Ligaments ØMB
   see Resection, Bursae and Ligaments ØMT
Bursocentesis *see* Drainage, Bursae and Ligaments ØM9
Bursography
   see Plain Radiography, Non-Axial Lower Bones BQØ
   see Plain Radiography, Non-Axial Upper Bones BPØ
Bursotomy
   see Division, Bursae and Ligaments ØM8
   see Drainage, Bursae and Ligaments ØM9
BVS 5ØØØ Ventricular Assist Device *use* Short-term External Heart Assist System in Heart and Great Vessels
Bypass
   Anterior Chamber
      Left Ø8133
      Right Ø8123
   Aorta
      Abdominal Ø41Ø
      Thoracic
         Ascending/Arch Ø21X
         Descending Ø21W
   Artery
      Anterior Tibial
         Left Ø41Q
         Right Ø41P
      Axillary
         Left Ø316Ø
         Right Ø315Ø
      Brachial
         Left Ø318
         Right Ø317
      Common Carotid
         Left Ø31JØ
         Right Ø31HØ
      Common Iliac
         Left Ø41D
         Right Ø41C
      Coronary
         Four or More Arteries Ø213
         One Artery Ø210
         Three Arteries Ø212
         Two Arteries Ø211
      External Carotid
         Left Ø31NØ
         Right Ø31MØ
      External Iliac
         Left Ø41J
         Right Ø41H
      Femoral
         Left Ø41L
         Right Ø41K
      Foot
         Left Ø41W
         Right Ø41V

Bypass — *continued*
  Artery — *continued*
    Hepatic 0413
    Innominate 03120
    Internal Carotid
      Left 031L0
      Right 031K0
    Internal Iliac
      Left 041F
      Right 041E
    Intracranial 031G0
    Peroneal
      Left 041U
      Right 041T
    Popliteal
      Left 041N
      Right 041M
    Posterior Tibial
      Left 041S
      Right 041R
    Pulmonary
      Left 021R
      Right 021Q
    Pulmonary Trunk 021P
    Radial
      Left 031C
      Right 031B
    Splenic 0414
    Subclavian
      Left 03140
      Right 03130
    Temporal
      Left 031T0
      Right 031S0
    Ulnar
      Left 031A
      Right 0319
  Atrium
    Left 0217
    Right 0216
  Bladder 0T1B
  Cavity, Cranial 0W110J
  Cecum 0D1H
  Cerebral Ventricle 0016
  Colon
    Ascending 0D1K
    Descending 0D1M
    Sigmoid 0D1N
    Transverse 0D1L
  Duct
    Common Bile 0F19
    Cystic 0F18
    Hepatic
      Common 0F17
      Left 0F16
      Right 0F15
    Lacrimal
      Left 081Y
      Right 081X
    Pancreatic 0F1D
      Accessory 0F1F
  Duodenum 0D19
  Ear
    Left 091E0
    Right 091D0
  Esophagus 0D15
    Lower 0D13
    Middle 0D12
    Upper 0D11
  Fallopian Tube
    Left 0U16
    Right 0U15
  Gallbladder 0F14
  Ileum 0D1B
  Intestine
    Large 0D1E
    Small 0D18
  Jejunum 0D1A
  Kidney Pelvis
    Left 0T14
    Right 0T13
  Pancreas 0F1G
  Pelvic Cavity 0W1J
  Peritoneal Cavity 0W1G
  Pleural Cavity
    Left 0W1B
    Right 0W19
  Spinal Canal 001U
  Stomach 0D16

Bypass — *continued*
  Trachea 0B11
  Ureter
    Left 0T17
    Right 0T16
  Ureters, Bilateral 0T18
  Vas Deferens
    Bilateral 0V1Q
    Left 0V1P
    Right 0V1N
  Vein
    Axillary
      Left 0518
      Right 0517
    Azygos 0510
    Basilic
      Left 051C
      Right 051B
    Brachial
      Left 051A
      Right 0519
    Cephalic
      Left 051F
      Right 051D
    Colic 0617
    Common Iliac
      Left 061D
      Right 061C
    Esophageal 0613
    External Iliac
      Left 061G
      Right 061F
    External Jugular
      Left 051Q
      Right 051P
    Face
      Left 051V
      Right 051T
    Femoral
      Left 061N
      Right 061M
    Foot
      Left 061V
      Right 061T
    Gastric 0612
    Hand
      Left 051H
      Right 051G
    Hemiazygos 0511
    Hepatic 0614
    Hypogastric
      Left 061J
      Right 061H
    Inferior Mesenteric 0616
    Innominate
      Left 0514
      Right 0513
    Internal Jugular
      Left 051N
      Right 051M
    Intracranial 051L
    Portal 0618
    Renal
      Left 061B
      Right 0619
    Saphenous
      Left 061Q
      Right 061P
    Splenic 0611
    Subclavian
      Left 0516
      Right 0515
    Superior Mesenteric 0615
    Vertebral
      Left 051S
      Right 051R
  Vena Cava
    Inferior 0610
    Superior 021V
  Ventricle
    Left 021L
    Right 021K
Bypass, cardiopulmonary 5A1221Z

C

Caesarean section *see* Extraction, Products of Conception 10D0

Calcaneocuboid joint
  use Tarsal Joint, Left
  use Tarsal Joint, Right
Calcaneocuboid ligament
  use Foot Bursa and Ligament, Left
  use Foot Bursa and Ligament, Right
Calcaneofibular ligament
  use Ankle Bursa and Ligament, Left
  use Ankle Bursa and Ligament, Right
Calcaneus
  use Tarsal, Left
  use Tarsal, Right
Cannulation
  see Bypass
  see Dilation
  see Drainage
  see Irrigation
Canthorrhaphy *see* Repair, Eye 08Q
Canthotomy *see* Release, Eye 08N
Capitate bone
  use Carpal, Left
  use Carpal, Right
Caplacizumab XW0
Capsulectomy, lens *see* Excision, Eye 08B
Capsulorrhaphy, joint
  see Repair, Lower Joints 0SQ
  see Repair, Upper Joints 0RQ
Caption Guidance system X2JAX47
Cardia *use* Esophagogastric Junction
Cardiac contractility modulation lead *use* Cardiac Lead in Heart and Great Vessels
Cardiac event recorder *use* Monitoring Device
Cardiac Lead
  Defibrillator
    Atrium
      Left 02H7
      Right 02H6
    Pericardium 02HN
    Vein, Coronary 02H4
    Ventricle
      Left 02HL
      Right 02HK
  Insertion of device in
    Atrium
      Left 02H7
      Right 02H6
    Pericardium 02HN
    Vein, Coronary 02H4
    Ventricle
      Left 02HL
      Right 02HK
  Pacemaker
    Atrium
      Left 02H7
      Right 02H6
    Pericardium 02HN
    Vein, Coronary 02H4
    Ventricle
      Left 02HL
      Right 02HK
  Removal of device from, Heart 02PA
  Revision of device in, Heart 02WA
Cardiac plexus *use* Thoracic Sympathetic Nerve
Cardiac Resynchronization Defibrillator Pulse Generator
  Abdomen 0JH8
  Chest 0JH6
Cardiac Resynchronization Pacemaker Pulse Generator
  Abdomen 0JH8
  Chest 0JH6
Cardiac resynchronization therapy (CRT) lead
  use Cardiac Lead, Defibrillator in 02H
  use Cardiac Lead, Pacemaker in 02H
Cardiac Rhythm Related Device
  Insertion of device in
    Abdomen 0JH8
    Chest 0JH6
  Removal of device from, Subcutaneous Tissue and Fascia, Trunk 0JPT
  Revision of device in, Subcutaneous Tissue and Fascia, Trunk 0JWT
Cardiocentesis *see* Drainage, Pericardial Cavity 0W9D
Cardioesophageal junction *use* Esophagogastric Junction
Cardiolysis *see* Release, Heart and Great Vessels 02N

CardioMEMS® pressure sensor *use* Monitoring Device, Pressure Sensor in 02H

Cardiomyotomy *see* Division, Esophagogastric Junction 0D84

Cardioplegia *see* Introduction of substance in or on, Heart 3E08

Cardiorrhaphy *see* Repair, Heart and Great Vessels 02Q

Cardioversion 5A2204Z

Caregiver Training F0FZ

Carmat total artificial heart (TAH) *use* Biologic with Synthetic Substitute, Autoregulated Electrohydraulic in 02R

Caroticotympanic artery
   use Internal Carotid Artery, Left
   use Internal Carotid Artery, Right

Carotid glomus
   use Carotid Bodies, Bilateral
   use Carotid Body, Left
   use Carotid Body, Right

Carotid sinus
   use Internal Carotid Artery, Left
   use Internal Carotid Artery, Right

Carotid (artery) sinus (baroreceptor) lead *use* Stimulator Lead in Upper Arteries

Carotid sinus nerve *use* Glossopharyngeal Nerve

Carotid WALLSTENT® Monorail® Endoprosthesis *use* Intraluminal Device

Carpectomy
   see Excision, Upper Bones 0PB
   see Resection, Upper Bones 0PT

Carpometacarpal ligament
   use Hand Bursa and Ligament, Left
   use Hand Bursa and Ligament, Right

CARVYKTI™ *use* Ciltacabtagene Autoleucel

Casirivimab (REGN10933) and Imdevimab (REGN10987) *use* REGN-COV2 Monoclonal Antibody

Casting *see* Immobilization

CAT scan *see* Computerized Tomography (CT Scan)

Catheterization
   see Dilation
   see Drainage
   see Insertion of device in
   see Irrigation
   Heart *see* Measurement, Cardiac 4A02
   Umbilical vein, for infusion 06H033T

Cauda equina *use* Lumbar Spinal Cord

Cauterization
   see Destruction
   see Repair

Cavernous plexus *use* Head and Neck Sympathetic Nerve

Cavoatrial junction *use* Superior Vena Cava

CBMA (Concentrated Bone Marrow Aspirate) *use* Other Substance

CBMA (Concentrated Bone Marrow Aspirate) injection *see* Introduction of substance in or on, Muscle 3E02

CD24Fc Immunomodulator XW0

Cecectomy
   see Excision, Cecum 0DBH
   see Resection, Cecum 0DTH

Cecocolostomy
   see Bypass, Gastrointestinal System 0D1
   see Drainage, Gastrointestinal System 0D9

Cecopexy
   see Repair, Cecum 0DQH
   see Reposition, Cecum 0DSH

Cecoplication *see* Restriction, Cecum 0DVH

Cecorrhaphy *see* Repair, Cecum 0DQH

Cecostomy
   see Bypass, Cecum 0D1H
   see Drainage, Cecum 0D9H

Cecotomy *see* Drainage, Cecum 0D9H

Cefiderocol Anti-infective XW0

Ceftazidime-avibactam *use* Other Anti-infective

Ceftolozane/Tazobactam Anti-infective XW0

Celiac ganglion *use* Abdominal Sympathetic Nerve

Celiac lymph node *use* Lymphatic, Aortic

Celiac (solar) plexus *use* Abdominal Sympathetic Nerve

Celiac trunk *use* Celiac Artery

Central axillary lymph node
   use Lymphatic, Left Axillary
   use Lymphatic, Right Axillary

Central venous pressure *see* Measurement, Venous 4A04

Centrimag® Blood Pump *use* Short-term External Heart Assist System in Heart and Great Vessels

Cephalogram BN00ZZZ

CERAMENT® G *use* Antibiotic-eluting Bone Void Filler

Ceramic on ceramic bearing surface *use* Synthetic Substitute, Ceramic in 0SR

Cerclage *see* Restriction

Cerebral aqueduct (Sylvius) *use* Cerebral Ventricle

Cerebral Embolic Filtration
   Dual Filter X2A5312
   Extracorporeal Flow Reversal Circuit X2A
   Single Deflection Filter X2A6325

Cerebrum *use* Brain

Cervical esophagus *use* Esophagus, Upper

Cervical facet joint
   use Cervical Vertebral Joint
   use Cervical Vertebral Joint, 2 or more

Cervical ganglion *use* Head and Neck Sympathetic Nerve

Cervical interspinous ligament *use* Head and Neck Bursa and Ligament

Cervical intertransverse ligament *use* Head and Neck Bursa and Ligament

Cervical Ligamentum Flavum *use* Head and Neck Bursa and Ligament

Cervical Lymph Node
   use Lymphatic, Left Neck
   use Lymphatic, Right Neck

Cervicectomy
   see Excision, Cervix 0UBC
   see Resection, Cervix 0UTC

Cervicothoracic facet joint *use* Cervicothoracic Vertebral Joint

Cesarean section *see* Extraction, Products of Conception 10D0

Cesium-131 Collagen Implant *use* Radioactive Element, Cesium-131 Collagen Implant in 00H

Change Device in
   Abdominal Wall 0W2FX
   Back
      Lower 0W2LX
      Upper 0W2KX
   Bladder 0T2BX
   Bone
      Facial 0N2WX
      Lower 0Q2YX
      Nasal 0N2BX
      Upper 0P2YX
   Bone Marrow 072TX
   Brain 0020X
   Breast
      Left 0H2UX
      Right 0H2TX
   Bursa and Ligament
      Lower 0M2YX
      Upper 0M2XX
   Cavity, Cranial 0W21X
   Chest Wall 0W28X
   Cisterna Chyli 072LX
   Diaphragm 0B2TX
   Duct
      Hepatobiliary 0F2BX
      Pancreatic 0F2DX
   Ear
      Left 092JX
      Right 092HX
   Epididymis and Spermatic Cord 0V2MX
   Extremity
      Lower
         Left 0Y2BX
         Right 0Y29X
      Upper
         Left 0X27X
         Right 0X26X
   Eye
      Left 0821X
      Right 0820X
   Face 0W22X
   Fallopian Tube 0U28X
   Gallbladder 0F24X
   Gland
      Adrenal 0G25X
      Endocrine 0G2SX
      Pituitary 0G20X
      Salivary 0C2AX
   Head 0W20X

Change Device in — *continued*
   Intestinal Tract
      Lower Intestinal Tract 0D2DXUZ
      Upper Intestinal Tract 0D20XUZ
   Jaw
      Lower 0W25X
      Upper 0W24X
   Joint
      Lower 0S2YX
      Upper 0R2YX
   Kidney 0T25X
   Larynx 0C2SX
   Liver 0F20X
   Lung
      Left 0B2LX
      Right 0B2KX
   Lymphatic 072NX
      Thoracic Duct 072KX
   Mediastinum 0W2CX
   Mesentery 0D2VX
   Mouth and Throat 0C2YX
   Muscle
      Lower 0K2YX
      Upper 0K2XX
   Nasal Mucosa and Soft Tissue 092KX
   Neck 0W26X
   Nerve
      Cranial 002EX
      Peripheral 012YX
   Omentum 0D2UX
   Ovary 0U23X
   Pancreas 0F2GX
   Parathyroid Gland 0G2RX
   Pelvic Cavity 0W2JX
   Penis 0V2SX
   Pericardial Cavity 0W2DX
   Perineum
      Female 0W2NX
      Male 0W2MX
   Peritoneal Cavity 0W2GX
   Peritoneum 0D2WX
   Pineal Body 0G21X
   Pleura 0B2QX
   Pleural Cavity
      Left 0W2BX
      Right 0W29X
   Products of Conception 10207
   Prostate and Seminal Vesicles 0V24X
   Retroperitoneum 0W2HX
   Scrotum and Tunica Vaginalis 0V28X
   Sinus 092YX
   Skin 0H2PX
   Skull 0N20X
   Spinal Canal 002UX
   Spleen 072PX
   Subcutaneous Tissue and Fascia
      Head and Neck 0J2SX
      Lower Extremity 0J2WX
      Trunk 0J2TX
      Upper Extremity 0J2VX
   Tendon
      Lower 0L2YX
      Upper 0L2XX
   Testis 0V2DX
   Thymus 072MX
   Thyroid Gland 0G2KX
   Trachea 0B21
   Tracheobronchial Tree 0B20X
   Ureter 0T29X
   Urethra 0T2DX
   Uterus and Cervix 0U2DXHZ
   Vagina and Cul-de-sac 0U2HXGZ
   Vas Deferens 0V2RX
   Vulva 0U2MX

Change Device in or on
   Abdominal Wall 2W03X
   Anorectal 2Y03X5Z
   Arm
      Lower
         Left 2W0DX
         Right 2W0CX
      Upper
         Left 2W0BX
         Right 2W0AX
   Back 2W05X
   Chest Wall 2W04X
   Ear 2Y02X5Z

Change Device in or on — *continued*
  Extremity
    Lower
      Left 2W0MX
      Right 2W0LX
    Upper
      Left 2W09X
      Right 2W08X
  Face 2W01X
  Finger
    Left 2W0KX
    Right 2W0JX
  Foot
    Left 2W0TX
    Right 2W0SX
  Genital Tract, Female 2Y04X5Z
  Hand
    Left 2W0FX
    Right 2W0EX
  Head 2W00X
  Inguinal Region
    Left 2W07X
    Right 2W06X
  Leg
    Lower
      Left 2W0RX
      Right 2W0QX
    Upper
      Left 2W0PX
      Right 2W0NX
  Mouth and Pharynx 2Y00X5Z
  Nasal 2Y01X5Z
  Neck 2W02X
  Thumb
    Left 2W0HX
    Right 2W0GX
  Toe
    Left 2W0VX
    Right 2W0UX
  Urethra 2Y05X5Z
Chemoembolization *see* Introduction of substance in or on
Chemosurgery, Skin 3E00XTZ
Chemothalamectomy *see* Destruction, Thalamus 0059
Chemotherapy, Infusion for Cancer *see* Introduction of substance in or on
Chest compression (CPR), external
  Manual 5A12012
  Mechanical 5A1221J
Chest x-ray *see* Plain Radiography, Chest BW03
Chiropractic Manipulation
  Abdomen 9WB9X
  Cervical 9WB1X
  Extremities
    Lower 9WB6X
    Upper 9WB7X
  Head 9WB0X
  Lumbar 9WB3X
  Pelvis 9WB5X
  Rib Cage 9WB8X
  Sacrum 9WB4X
  Thoracic 9WB2X
Choana *use* Nasopharynx
Cholangiogram
  see Fluoroscopy, Hepatobiliary System and Pancreas BF1
  see Plain Radiography, Hepatobiliary System and Pancreas BF0
Cholecystectomy
  see Excision, Gallbladder 0FB4
  see Resection, Gallbladder 0FT4
Cholecystojejunostomy
  see Bypass, Hepatobiliary System and Pancreas 0F1
  see Drainage, Hepatobiliary System and Pancreas 0F9
Cholecystopexy
  see Repair, Gallbladder 0FQ4
  see Reposition, Gallbladder 0FS4
Cholecystoscopy 0FJ44ZZ
Cholecystostomy
  see Bypass, Gallbladder 0F14
  see Drainage, Gallbladder 0F94
Cholecystotomy *see* Drainage, Gallbladder 0F94
Choledochectomy
  see Excision, Hepatobiliary System and Pancreas 0FB

Choledochectomy — *continued*
  see Resection, Hepatobiliary System and Pancreas 0FT
Choledocholithotomy *see* Extirpation, Duct, Common Bile 0FC9
Choledochoplasty
  see Repair, Hepatobiliary System and Pancreas 0FQ
  see Replacement, Hepatobiliary System and Pancreas 0FR
  see Supplement, Hepatobiliary System and Pancreas 0FU
Choledochoscopy 0FJB8ZZ
Choledochotomy *see* Drainage, Hepatobiliary System and Pancreas 0F9
Cholelithotomy *see* Extirpation, Hepatobiliary System and Pancreas 0FC
Chondrectomy
  see Excision, Lower Joints 0SB
  see Excision, Upper Joints 0RB
  Knee *see* Excision, Lower Joints 0SB
  Semilunar cartilage *see* Excision, Lower Joints 0SB
Chondroglossus muscle *use* Tongue, Palate, Pharynx Muscle
Chorda tympani *use* Facial Nerve
Chordotomy *see* Division, Central Nervous System and Cranial Nerves 008
Choroid plexus *use* Cerebral Ventricle
Choroidectomy
  see Excision, Eye 08B
  see Resection, Eye 08T
Ciliary body
  use Eye, Left
  use Eye, Right
Ciliary ganglion *use* Head and Neck Sympathetic Nerve
Ciltacabtagene Autoleucel XW0
cilta-cel *use* Ciltacabtagene Autoleucel
Circle of Willis *use* Intracranial Artery
Circumcision 0VTTXZZ
Circumflex iliac artery
  use Femoral Artery, Left
  use Femoral Artery, Right
CivaSheet® *use* Radioactive Element
CivaSheet® Brachytherapy
  see Brachytherapy with qualifier Unidirectional Source
  see Insertion with device Radioactive Element
Clamp and rod internal fixation system (CRIF)
  use Internal Fixation Device in Lower Bones
  use Internal Fixation Device in Upper Bones
Clamping *see* Occlusion
Claustrum *use* Basal Ganglia
Claviculectomy
  see Excision, Upper Bones 0PB
  see Resection, Upper Bones 0PT
Claviculotomy
  see Division, Upper Bones 0P8
  see Drainage, Upper Bones 0P9
Clipping, aneurysm
  see Occlusion using Extraluminal Device
  see Restriction using Extraluminal Device
Clitorectomy, clitoridectomy
  see Excision, Clitoris 0UBJ
  see Resection, Clitoris 0UTJ
Clolar *use* Clofarabine
Closure
  see Occlusion
  see Repair
Clysis *see* Introduction of substance in or on
Coagulation *see* Destruction
Coagulation Factor Xa, Inactivated XW0
Coagulation Factor Xa, (Recombinant) Inactivated *use* Coagulation Factor Xa, Inactivated
COALESCE® radiolucent interbody fusion device
  use Interbody Fusion Device in Lower Joints
  use Interbody Fusion Device in Upper Joints
CoAxia NeuroFlo catheter *use* Intraluminal Device
Cobalt/chromium head and polyethylene socket *use* Synthetic Substitute, Metal on Polyethylene in 0SR
Cobalt/chromium head and socket *use* Synthetic Substitute, Metal in 0SR
Coccygeal body *use* Coccygeal Glomus
Coccygeus muscle
  use Trunk Muscle, Left
  use Trunk Muscle, Right

Cochlea
  use Inner Ear, Left
  use Inner Ear, Right
Cochlear implant (CI), multiple channel (electrode)
  use Hearing Device, Multiple Channel Cochlear Prosthesis in 09H
Cochlear implant (CI), single channel (electrode)
  use Hearing Device, Single Channel Cochlear Prosthesis in 09H
Cochlear Implant Treatment F0BZ0
Cochlear nerve *use* Acoustic Nerve
COGNIS® CRT-D *use* Cardiac Resynchronization Defibrillator Pulse Generator in 0JH
COHERE® radiolucent interbody fusion device
  use Interbody Fusion Device in Lower Joints
  use Interbody Fusion Device in Upper Joints
Colectomy
  see Excision, Gastrointestinal System 0DB
  see Resection, Gastrointestinal System 0DT
Collapse *see* Occlusion
Collection from
  Breast, Breast Milk 8E0HX62
  Indwelling Device
    Circulatory System
      Blood 8C02X6K
      Other Fluid 8C02X6L
    Nervous System
      Cerebrospinal Fluid 8C01X6J
      Other Fluid 8C01X6L
  Integumentary System, Breast Milk 8E0HX62
  Reproductive System, Male, Sperm 8E0VX63
Colocentesis *see* Drainage, Gastrointestinal System 0D9
Colofixation
  see Repair, Gastrointestinal System 0DQ
  see Reposition, Gastrointestinal System 0DS
Cololysis *see* Release, Gastrointestinal System 0DN
Colonic Z-Stent® *use* Intraluminal Device
Colonoscopy 0DJD8ZZ
Colopexy
  see Repair, Gastrointestinal System 0DQ
  see Reposition, Gastrointestinal System 0DS
Coloplication *see* Restriction, Gastrointestinal System 0DV
Coloproctectomy
  see Excision, Gastrointestinal System 0DB
  see Resection, Gastrointestinal System 0DT
Coloproctostomy
  see Bypass, Gastrointestinal System 0D1
  see Drainage, Gastrointestinal System 0D9
Colopuncture *see* Drainage, Gastrointestinal System 0D9
Colorrhaphy *see* Repair, Gastrointestinal System 0DQ
Colostomy
  see Bypass, Gastrointestinal System 0D1
  see Drainage, Gastrointestinal System 0D9
Colpectomy
  see Excision, Vagina 0UBG
  see Resection, Vagina 0UTG
Colpocentesis *see* Drainage, Vagina 0U9G
Colpopexy
  see Repair, Vagina 0UQG
  see Reposition, Vagina 0USG
Colpoplasty
  see Repair, Vagina 0UQG
  see Supplement, Vagina 0UUG
Colporrhaphy *see* Repair, Vagina 0UQG
Colposcopy 0UJH8ZZ
Columella *use* Nasal Mucosa and Soft Tissue
Common digital vein
  use Foot Vein, Left
  use Foot Vein, Right
Common facial vein
  use Face Vein, Left
  use Face Vein, Right
Common fibular nerve *use* Peroneal Nerve
Common hepatic artery *use* Hepatic Artery
Common iliac (subaortic) lymph node *use* Lymphatic, Pelvis
Common interosseous artery
  use Ulnar Artery, Left
  use Ulnar Artery, Right
Common peroneal nerve *use* Peroneal Nerve
Complete (SE) stent *use* Intraluminal Device
Compression
  see Restriction
  Abdominal Wall 2W13X

Compression — *continued*
  Arm
    Lower
      Left 2W1DX
      Right 2W1CX
    Upper
      Left 2W1BX
      Right 2W1AX
  Back 2W15X
  Chest Wall 2W14X
  Extremity
    Lower
      Left 2W1MX
      Right 2W1LX
    Upper
      Left 2W19X
      Right 2W18X
  Face 2W11X
  Finger
    Left 2W1KX
    Right 2W1JX
  Foot
    Left 2W1TX
    Right 2W1SX
  Hand
    Left 2W1FX
    Right 2W1EX
  Head 2W10X
  Inguinal Region
    Left 2W17X
    Right 2W16X
  Leg
    Lower
      Left 2W1RX
      Right 2W1QX
    Upper
      Left 2W1PX
      Right 2W1NX
  Neck 2W12X
  Thumb
    Left 2W1HX
    Right 2W1GX
  Toe
    Left 2W1VX
    Right 2W1UX
Computer Assisted Procedure
  Extremity
    Lower
      No Qualifier 8E0YXBZ
      With Computerized Tomography
        8E0YXBG
      With Fluoroscopy 8E0YXBF
      With Magnetic Resonance Imaging
        8E0YXBH
    Upper
      No Qualifier 8E0XXBZ
      With Computerized Tomography
        8E0XXBG
      With Fluoroscopy 8E0XXBF
      With Magnetic Resonance Imaging
        8E0XXBH
  Head and Neck Region
    No Qualifier 8E09XBZ
    With Computerized Tomography 8E09XBG
    With Fluoroscopy 8E09XBF
    With Magnetic Resonance Imaging 8E09XBH
  Trunk Region
    No Qualifier 8E0WXBZ
    With Computerized Tomography 8E0WXBG
    With Fluoroscopy 8E0WXBF
    With Magnetic Resonance Imaging 8E0WXBH
Computer-aided Assessment, Intracranial Vascular Activity XXE0X07
Computer-aided Guidance, Transthoracic Echocardiography X2JAX47
Computer-aided Mechanical Aspiration X2C
Computer-aided Triage and Notification, Pulmonary Artery Flow XXE3X27
Computer-aided Valve Modeling and Notification, Coronary Artery Flow XXE3X68
Computer-assisted Intermittent Aspiration *see* New Technology, Cardiovascular System X2C
Computer-assisted Transcranial Magnetic Stimulation X0Z0X18
Computerized Tomography (CT Scan)
  Abdomen BW20
    Chest and Pelvis BW25
  Abdomen and Chest BW24

Computerized Tomography (CT Scan) — *continued*
  Abdomen and Pelvis BW21
  Airway, Trachea BB2F
  Ankle
    Left BQ2H
    Right BQ2G
  Aorta
    Abdominal B420
      Intravascular Optical Coherence
        B420Z2Z
    Thoracic B320
      Intravascular Optical Coherence
        B320Z2Z
  Arm
    Left BP2F
    Right BP2E
  Artery
    Celiac B421
      Intravascular Optical Coherence
        B421Z2Z
    Common Carotid
      Bilateral B325
      Intravascular Optical Coherence
        B325Z2Z
    Coronary
      Bypass Graft
        Intravascular Optical Coherence
          B223Z2Z
        Multiple B223
      Multiple B221
        Intravascular Optical Coherence
          B221Z2Z
    Internal Carotid
      Bilateral B328
      Intravascular Optical Coherence
        B328Z2Z
    Intracranial B32R
      Intravascular Optical Coherence
        B32RZ2Z
    Lower Extremity
      Bilateral B42H
        Intravascular Optical Coherence
          B42HZ2Z
      Left B42G
        Intravascular Optical Coherence
          B42GZ2Z
      Right B42F
        Intravascular Optical Coherence
          B42FZ2Z
    Pelvic B42C
      Intravascular Optical Coherence
        B42CZ2Z
    Pulmonary
      Left B32T
        Intravascular Optical Coherence
          B32TZ2Z
      Right B32S
        Intravascular Optical Coherence
          B32SZ2Z
    Renal
      Bilateral B428
        Intravascular Optical Coherence
          B428Z2Z
      Transplant B42M
        Intravascular Optical Coherence
          B42MZ2Z
    Superior Mesenteric B424
      Intravascular Optical Coherence
        B424Z2Z
    Vertebral
      Bilateral B32G
      Intravascular Optical Coherence
        B32GZ2Z
  Bladder BT20
  Bone
    Facial BN25
    Temporal BN2F
  Brain B020
  Calcaneus
    Left BQ2K
    Right BQ2J
  Cerebral Ventricle B028
  Chest, Abdomen and Pelvis BW25
  Chest and Abdomen BW24
  Cisterna B027
  Clavicle
    Left BP25
    Right BP24
  Coccyx BR2F

Computerized Tomography (CT Scan) — *continued*
  Colon BD24
  Ear B920
  Elbow
    Left BP2H
    Right BP2G
  Extremity
    Lower
      Left BQ2S
      Right BQ2R
    Upper
      Bilateral BP2V
      Left BP2U
      Right BP2T
  Eye
    Bilateral B827
    Left B826
    Right B825
  Femur
    Left BQ24
    Right BQ23
  Fibula
    Left BQ2C
    Right BQ2B
  Finger
    Left BP2S
    Right BP2R
  Foot
    Left BQ2M
    Right BQ2L
  Forearm
    Left BP2K
    Right BP2J
  Gland
    Adrenal, Bilateral BG22
    Parathyroid BG23
    Parotid, Bilateral B926
    Salivary, Bilateral B92D
    Submandibular, Bilateral B929
    Thyroid BG24
  Hand
    Left BP2P
    Right BP2N
  Hands and Wrists, Bilateral BP2Q
  Head BW28
  Head and Neck BW29
  Heart
    Intravascular Optical Coherence B226Z2Z
    Right and Left B226
  Hepatobiliary System, All BF2C
  Hip
    Left BQ21
    Right BQ20
  Humerus
    Left BP2B
    Right BP2A
  Intracranial Sinus B522
    Intravascular Optical Coherence B522Z2Z
  Joint
    Acromioclavicular, Bilateral BP23
    Finger
      Left BP2DZZZ
      Right BP2CZZZ
    Foot
      Left BQ2Y
      Right BQ2X
    Hand
      Left BP2DZZZ
      Right BP2CZZZ
    Sacroiliac BR2D
    Sternoclavicular
      Bilateral BP22
      Left BP21
      Right BP20
    Temporomandibular, Bilateral BN29
    Toe
      Left BQ2Y
      Right BQ2X
  Kidney
    Bilateral BT23
    Left BT22
    Right BT21
    Transplant BT29
  Knee
    Left BQ28
    Right BQ27
  Larynx B92J
  Leg
    Left BQ2F

Computerized Tomography (CT Scan) — continued

Leg — continued
Right BQ2D
Liver BF25
Liver and Spleen BF26
Lung, Bilateral BB24
Mandible BN26
Nasopharynx B92F
Neck BW2F
Neck and Head BW29
Orbit, Bilateral BN23
Oropharynx B92F
Pancreas BF27
Patella
Left BQ2W
Right BQ2V
Pelvic Region BW2G
Pelvis BR2C
Chest and Abdomen BW25
Pelvis and Abdomen BW21
Pituitary Gland B029
Prostate BV23
Ribs
Left BP2Y
Right BP2X
Sacrum BR2F
Scapula
Left BP27
Right BP26
Sella Turcica B029
Shoulder
Left BP29
Right BP28
Sinus
Intracranial B522
Intravascular Optical Coherence B522Z2Z
Paranasal B922
Skull BN20
Spinal Cord B02B
Spine
Cervical BR20
Lumbar BR29
Thoracic BR27
Spleen and Liver BF26
Thorax BP2W
Tibia
Left BQ2C
Right BQ2B
Toe
Left BQ2Q
Right BQ2P
Trachea BB2F
Tracheobronchial Tree
Bilateral BB29
Left BB28
Right BB27
Vein
Pelvic (Iliac)
Left B52G
Intravascular Optical Coherence B52GZ2Z
Right B52F
Intravascular Optical Coherence B52FZ2Z
Pelvic (Iliac) Bilateral B52H
Intravascular Optical Coherence B52HZ2Z
Portal B52T
Intravascular Optical Coherence B52TZ2Z
Pulmonary
Bilateral B52S
Intravascular Optical Coherence B52SZ2Z
Left B52R
Intravascular Optical Coherence B52RZ2Z
Right B52Q
Intravascular Optical Coherence B52QZ2Z
Renal
Bilateral B52L
Intravascular Optical Coherence B52LZ2Z
Left B52K
Intravascular Optical Coherence B52KZ2Z
Right B52J

Computerized Tomography (CT Scan) — continued

Vein — continued
Renal — continued
Right — continued
Intravascular Optical Coherence B52JZ2Z
Spanchnic B52T
Intravascular Optical Coherence B52TZ2Z
Vena Cava
Inferior B529
Intravascular Optical Coherence B529Z2Z
Superior B528
Intravascular Optical Coherence B528Z2Z
Ventricle, Cerebral B028
Wrist
Left BP2M
Right BP2L

Concerto II CRT-D *use* Cardiac Resynchronization Defibrillator Pulse Generator in 0JH

Condylectomy
see Excision, Head and Facial Bones 0NB
see Excision, Lower Bones 0QB
see Excision, Upper Bones 0PB

Condyloid process
use Mandible, Left
use Mandible, Right

Condylotomy
see Division, Head and Facial Bones 0N8
see Division, Lower Bones 0Q8
see Division, Upper Bones 0P8
see Drainage, Head and Facial Bones 0N9
see Drainage, Lower Bones 0Q9
see Drainage, Upper Bones 0P9

Condylysis
see Release, Head and Facial Bones 0NN
see Release, Lower Bones 0QN
see Release, Upper Bones 0PN

Conization, cervix *see* Excision, Cervix 0UBC

Conjunctivoplasty
see Repair, Eye 08Q
see Replacement, Eye 08R

CONSERVE® PLUS Total Resurfacing Hip System *use* Resurfacing Device in Lower Joints

Construction
Auricle, ear *see* Replacement, Ear, Nose, Sinus 09R
Ileal conduit *see* Bypass, Urinary System 0T1

Consulta CRT-D *use* Cardiac Resynchronization Defibrillator Pulse Generator in 0JH

Consulta CRT-P *use* Cardiac Resynchronization Pacemaker Pulse Generator in 0JH

Contact Radiation
Abdomen DWY37ZZ
Adrenal Gland DGY27ZZ
Bile Ducts DFY27ZZ
Bladder DTY27ZZ
Bone, Other DPYC7ZZ
Brain D0Y07ZZ
Brain Stem D0Y17ZZ
Breast
Left DMY07ZZ
Right DMY17ZZ
Bronchus DBY17ZZ
Cervix DUY17ZZ
Chest DWY27ZZ
Chest Wall DBY77ZZ
Colon DDY57ZZ
Diaphragm DBY87ZZ
Duodenum DDY27ZZ
Ear D9Y07ZZ
Esophagus DDY07ZZ
Eye D8Y07ZZ
Femur DPY97ZZ
Fibula DPYB7ZZ
Gallbladder DFY17ZZ
Gland
Adrenal DGY27ZZ
Parathyroid DGY47ZZ
Pituitary DGY07ZZ
Thyroid DGY57ZZ
Glands, Salivary D9Y67ZZ
Head and Neck DWY17ZZ
Hemibody DWY47ZZ
Humerus DPY67ZZ
Hypopharynx D9Y37ZZ
Ileum DDY47ZZ

Contact Radiation — continued

Jejunum DDY37ZZ
Kidney DTY07ZZ
Larynx D9YB7ZZ
Liver DFY07ZZ
Lung DBY27ZZ
Mandible DPY37ZZ
Maxilla DPY27ZZ
Mediastinum DBY67ZZ
Mouth D9Y47ZZ
Nasopharynx D9YD7ZZ
Neck and Head DWY17ZZ
Nerve, Peripheral D0Y77ZZ
Nose D9Y17ZZ
Oropharynx D9YF7ZZ
Ovary DUY07ZZ
Palate
Hard D9Y87ZZ
Soft D9Y97ZZ
Pancreas DFY37ZZ
Parathyroid Gland DGY47ZZ
Pelvic Bones DPY87ZZ
Pelvic Region DWY67ZZ
Pineal Body DGY17ZZ
Pituitary Gland DGY07ZZ
Pleura DBY57ZZ
Prostate DVY07ZZ
Radius DPY77ZZ
Rectum DDY77ZZ
Rib DPY57ZZ
Sinuses D9Y77ZZ
Skin
Abdomen DHY87ZZ
Arm DHY47ZZ
Back DHY77ZZ
Buttock DHY97ZZ
Chest DHY67ZZ
Face DHY27ZZ
Leg DHYB7ZZ
Neck DHY37ZZ
Skull DPY07ZZ
Spinal Cord D0Y67ZZ
Sternum DPY47ZZ
Stomach DDY17ZZ
Testis DVY17ZZ
Thyroid Gland DGY57ZZ
Tibia DPYB7ZZ
Tongue D9Y57ZZ
Trachea DBY07ZZ
Ulna DPY77ZZ
Ureter DTY17ZZ
Urethra DTY37ZZ
Uterus DUY27ZZ
Whole Body DWY57ZZ

ContaCT software (Measurement of intracranial arterial flow) 4A03X5D

CONTAK RENEWAL® 3 RF (HE) CRT-D *use* Cardiac Resynchronization Defibrillator Pulse Generator in 0JH

Contegra Pulmonary Valved Conduit *use* Zooplastic Tissue in Heart and Great Vessels

CONTEPO™ *use* Fosfomycin Anti-Infective

Continent ileostomy *see* Bypass, Ileum 0D1B

Continuous Glucose Monitoring (CGM) device *use* Monitoring Device

Continuous Negative Airway Pressure
24-96 Consecutive Hours, Ventilation 5A09459
Greater than 96 Consecutive Hours, Ventilation 5A09559
Less than 24 Consecutive Hours, Ventilation 5A09359

Continuous Positive Airway Pressure
24-96 Consecutive Hours, Ventilation 5A09457
Greater than 96 Consecutive Hours, Ventilation 5A09557
Less than 24 Consecutive Hours, Ventilation 5A09357

Continuous renal replacement therapy (CRRT) 5A1D90Z

Contraceptive Device
Change device in, Uterus and Cervix 0U2DXHZ
Insertion of device in
Cervix 0UHC
Subcutaneous Tissue and Fascia
Abdomen 0JH8
Chest 0JH6
Lower Arm
Left 0JHH

Contraceptive Device — *continued*
  Insertion of device in — *continued*
    Subcutaneous Tissue and Fascia — *contin-*
      ued
      Lower Arm — *continued*
        Right ØJHG
      Lower Leg
        Left ØJHP
        Right ØJHN
      Upper Arm
        Left ØJHF
        Right ØJHD
      Upper Leg
        Left ØJHM
        Right ØJHL
    Uterus ØUH9
  Removal of device from
    Subcutaneous Tissue and Fascia
      Lower Extremity ØJPW
      Trunk ØJPT
      Upper Extremity ØJPV
    Uterus and Cervix ØUPD
  Revision of device in
    Subcutaneous Tissue and Fascia
      Lower Extremity ØJWW
      Trunk ØJWT
      Upper Extremity ØJWV
    Uterus and Cervix ØUWD
Contractility Modulation Device
  Abdomen ØJH8
  Chest ØJH6
Control bleeding in
  Abdominal Wall ØW3F
  Ankle Region
    Left ØY3L
    Right ØY3K
  Arm
    Lower
      Left ØX3F
      Right ØX3D
    Upper
      Left ØX39
      Right ØX38
  Axilla
    Left ØX35
    Right ØX34
  Back
    Lower ØW3L
    Upper ØW3K
  Buttock
    Left ØY31
    Right ØY3Ø
  Cavity, Cranial ØW31
  Chest Wall ØW38
  Elbow Region
    Left ØX3C
    Right ØX3B
  Extremity
    Lower
      Left ØY3B
      Right ØY39
    Upper
      Left ØX37
      Right ØX36
  Face ØW32
  Femoral Region
    Left ØY38
    Right ØY37
  Foot
    Left ØY3N
    Right ØY3M
  Gastrointestinal Tract ØW3P
  Genitourinary Tract ØW3R
  Hand
    Left ØX3K
    Right ØX3J
  Head ØW3Ø
  Inguinal Region
    Left ØY36
    Right ØY35
  Jaw
    Lower ØW35
    Upper ØW34
  Knee Region
    Left ØY3G
    Right ØY3F
  Leg
    Lower
      Left ØY3J

Control bleeding in — *continued*
  Leg — *continued*
    Lower — *continued*
      Right ØY3H
    Upper
      Left ØY3D
      Right ØY3C
  Mediastinum ØW3C
  Nasal Mucosa and Soft Tissue Ø93K
  Neck ØW36
  Oral Cavity and Throat ØW33
  Pelvic Cavity ØW3J
  Pericardial Cavity ØW3D
  Perineum
    Female ØW3N
    Male ØW3M
  Peritoneal Cavity ØW3G
  Pleural Cavity
    Left ØW3B
    Right ØW39
  Respiratory Tract ØW3Q
  Retroperitoneum ØW3H
  Shoulder Region
    Left ØX33
    Right ØX32
  Wrist Region
    Left ØX3H
    Right ØX3G
Control bleeding using Tourniquet, External *see* Compression, Anatomical Regions 2W1
Control, Epistaxis *see* Control bleeding in, Nasal Mucosa and Soft Tissue Ø93K
Conus arteriosus *use* Ventricle, Right
Conus medullaris *use* Lumbar Spinal Cord
Convalescent Plasma (Nonautologous) *see* New Technology, Anatomical Regions XW1
Conversion
  Cardiac rhythm 5A22Ø4Z
  Gastrostomy to jejunostomy feeding device *see* Insertion of device in, Jejunum ØDHA
Cook Biodesign® Fistula Plug(s) *use* Nonautologous Tissue Substitute
Cook Biodesign® Hernia Graft(s) *use* Nonautologous Tissue Substitute
Cook Biodesign® Layered Graft(s) *use* Nonautologous Tissue Substitute
Cook Zenaprom™ Layered Graft(s) *use* Nonautologous Tissue Substitute
Cook Zenith AAA Endovascular Graft *use* Intraluminal Device
Cook Zenith® Fenestrated AAA Endovascular Graft
  use Intraluminal Device, Branched or Fenestrated, One or Two Arteries in Ø4V
  use Intraluminal Device, Branched or Fenestrated, Three or More Arteries in Ø4V
Coracoacromial ligament
  use Shoulder Bursa and Ligament, Left
  use Shoulder Bursa and Ligament, Right
Coracobrachialis muscle
  use Upper Arm Muscle, Left
  use Upper Arm Muscle, Right
Coracoclavicular ligament
  use Shoulder Bursa and Ligament, Left
  use Shoulder Bursa and Ligament, Right
Coracohumeral ligament
  use Shoulder Bursa and Ligament, Left
  use Shoulder Bursa and Ligament, Right
Coracoid process
  use Scapula, Left
  use Scapula, Right
Cordotomy *see* Division, Central Nervous System and Cranial Nerves ØØ8
Core needle biopsy *see* Excision with qualifier Diagnostic
CoreValve transcatheter aortic valve *use* Zooplastic Tissue in Heart and Great Vessels
Cormet Hip Resurfacing System *use* Resurfacing Device in Lower Joints
Corniculate cartilage *use* Larynx
CoRoent® XL *use* Interbody Fusion Device in Lower Joints
Coronary arteriography
  see Fluoroscopy, Heart B21
  see Plain Radiography, Heart B2Ø
Corox (OTW) Bipolar Lead
  use Cardiac Lead, Defibrillator in Ø2H
  use Cardiac Lead, Pacemaker in Ø2H

Corpus callosum *use* Brain
Corpus cavernosum *use* Penis
Corpus spongiosum *use* Penis
Corpus striatum *use* Basal Ganglia
Corrugator supercilii muscle *use* Facial Muscle
Cortical strip neurostimulator lead *use* Neurostimulator Lead in Central Nervous System and Cranial Nerves
Corvia IASD® *use* Synthetic Substitute
COSELA™ *use* Trilaciclib
Costatectomy
  see Excision, Upper Bones ØPB
  see Resection, Upper Bones ØPT
Costectomy
  see Excision, Upper Bones ØPB
  see Resection, Upper Bones ØPT
Costocervical trunk
  use Subclavian Artery, Left
  use Subclavian Artery, Right
Costochondrectomy
  see Excision, Upper Bones ØPB
  see Resection, Upper Bones ØPT
Costoclavicular ligament
  use Shoulder Bursa and Ligament, Left
  use Shoulder Bursa and Ligament, Right
Costosternoplasty
  see Repair, Upper Bones ØPQ
  see Replacement, Upper Bones ØPR
  see Supplement, Upper Bones ØPU
Costotomy
  see Division, Upper Bones ØP8
  see Drainage, Upper Bones ØP9
Costotransverse joint *use* Thoracic Vertebral Joint
Costotransverse ligament *use* Rib(s) Bursa and Ligament
Costovertebral joint *use* Thoracic Vertebral Joint
Costoxiphoid ligament *use* Sternum Bursa and Ligament
Counseling
  Family, for substance abuse, Other Family Counseling HZ63ZZZ
  Group
    12-Step HZ43ZZZ
    Behavioral HZ41ZZZ
    Cognitive HZ4ØZZZ
    Cognitive-Behavioral HZ42ZZZ
    Confrontational HZ48ZZZ
    Continuing Care HZ49ZZZ
    Infectious Disease
      Post-Test HZ4CZZZ
      Pre-Test HZ4CZZZ
    Interpersonal HZ44ZZZ
    Motivational Enhancement HZ47ZZZ
    Psychoeducation HZ46ZZZ
    Spiritual HZ4BZZZ
    Vocational HZ45ZZZ
  Individual
    12-Step HZ33ZZZ
    Behavioral HZ31ZZZ
    Cognitive HZ3ØZZZ
    Cognitive-Behavioral HZ32ZZZ
    Confrontational HZ38ZZZ
    Continuing Care HZ39ZZZ
    Infectious Disease
      Post-Test HZ3CZZZ
      Pre-Test HZ3CZZZ
    Interpersonal HZ34ZZZ
    Motivational Enhancement HZ37ZZZ
    Psychoeducation HZ36ZZZ
    Spiritual HZ3BZZZ
    Vocational HZ35ZZZ
  Mental Health Services
    Educational GZ6ØZZZ
    Other Counseling GZ63ZZZ
    Vocational GZ61ZZZ
Countershock, cardiac 5A22Ø4Z
COVID-19 Vaccine XWØ
COVID-19 Vaccine Booster XWØ
COVID-19 Vaccine Dose 1 XWØ
COVID-19 Vaccine Dose 2 XWØ
COVID-19 Vaccine Dose 3 XWØ
Cowper's (bulbourethral) gland *use* Urethra
CPAP (continuous positive airway pressure) *see* Assistance, Respiratory 5AØ9
Craniectomy
  see Excision, Head and Facial Bones ØNB
  see Resection, Head and Facial Bones ØNT

Cranioplasty
- *see* Repair, Head and Facial Bones ØNQ
- *see* Replacement, Head and Facial Bones ØNR
- *see* Supplement, Head and Facial Bones ØNU

Craniotomy
- *see* Division, Head and Facial Bones ØN8
- *see* Drainage, Central Nervous System and Cranial Nerves ØØ9
- *see* Drainage, Head and Facial Bones ØN9

Creation
- Perineum
  - Female ØW4NØ
  - Male ØW4MØ
- Valve
  - Aortic Ø24FØ
  - Mitral Ø24GØ
  - Tricuspid Ø24JØ

Cremaster muscle *use* Perineum Muscle

CRESEMBA® (isavuconazonium sulfate) *use* Other Anti-infective

Cribriform plate
- *use* Ethmoid Bone, Left
- *use* Ethmoid Bone, Right

Cricoid cartilage *use* Trachea

Cricoidectomy *see* Excision, Larynx ØCBS

Cricothyroid artery
- *use* Thyroid Artery, Left
- *use* Thyroid Artery, Right

Cricothyroid muscle
- *use* Neck Muscle, Left
- *use* Neck Muscle, Right

Crisis Intervention GZ2ZZZZ

CRRT (Continuous renal replacement therapy) 5A1D9ØZ

Crural fascia
- *use* Subcutaneous Tissue and Fascia, Left Upper Leg
- *use* Subcutaneous Tissue and Fascia, Right Upper Leg

Crushing, nerve
- Cranial *see* Destruction, Central Nervous System and Cranial Nerves ØØ5
- Peripheral *see* Destruction, Peripheral Nervous System Ø15

Cryoablation *see* Destruction

Cryotherapy *see* Destruction

Cryptorchidectomy
- *see* Excision, Male Reproductive System ØVB
- *see* Resection, Male Reproductive System ØVT

Cryptorchiectomy
- *see* Excision, Male Reproductive System ØVB
- *see* Resection, Male Reproductive System ØVT

Cryptotomy
- *see* Division, Gastrointestinal System ØD8
- *see* Drainage, Gastrointestinal System ØD9

CT scan *see* Computerized Tomography (CT Scan)

CT sialogram *see* Computerized Tomography (CT Scan), Ear, Nose, Mouth and Throat B92

Cubital lymph node
- *use* Lymphatic, Left Upper Extremity
- *use* Lymphatic, Right Upper Extremity

Cubital nerve *use* Ulnar Nerve

Cuboid bone
- *use* Tarsal, Left
- *use* Tarsal, Right

Cuboideonavicular joint
- *use* Tarsal Joint, Left
- *use* Tarsal Joint, Right

Culdocentesis *see* Drainage, Cul-de-sac ØU9F

Culdoplasty
- *see* Repair, Cul-de-sac ØUQF
- *see* Supplement, Cul-de-sac ØUUF

Culdoscopy ØUJH8ZZ

Culdotomy *see* Drainage, Cul-de-sac ØU9F

Culmen *use* Cerebellum

Cultured epidermal cell autograft *use* Autologous Tissue Substitute

Cuneiform cartilage *use* Larynx

Cuneonavicular joint
- *use* Joint, Tarsal, Left
- *use* Joint, Tarsal, Right

Cuneonavicular ligament
- *use* Foot Bursa and Ligament, Left
- *use* Foot Bursa and Ligament, Right

Curettage
- *see* Excision
- *see* Extraction

Cutaneous (transverse) cervical nerve *use* Cervical Plexus

CVP (central venous pressure) *see* Measurement, Venous 4AØ4

Cyclodiathermy *see* Destruction, Eye Ø85

Cyclophotocoagulation *see* Destruction, Eye Ø85

CYPHER® Stent *use* Intraluminal Device, Drug-eluting in Heart and Great Vessels

Cystectomy
- *see* Excision, Bladder ØTBB
- *see* Resection, Bladder ØTTB

Cystocele repair *see* Repair, Subcutaneous Tissue and Fascia, Pelvic Region ØJQC

Cystography
- *see* Fluoroscopy, Urinary System BT1
- *see* Plain Radiography, Urinary System BTØ

Cystolithotomy *see* Extirpation, Bladder ØTCB

Cystopexy
- *see* Repair, Bladder ØTQB
- *see* Reposition, Bladder ØTSB

Cystoplasty
- *see* Repair, Bladder ØTQB
- *see* Replacement, Bladder ØTRB
- *see* Supplement, Bladder ØTUB

Cystorrhaphy *see* Repair, Bladder ØTQB

Cystoscopy ØTJB8ZZ

Cystostomy *see* Bypass, Bladder ØT1B

Cystostomy Tube *use* Drainage Device

Cystotomy *see* Drainage, Bladder ØT9B

Cystourethrography
- *see* Fluoroscopy, Urinary System BT1
- *see* Plain Radiography, Urinary System BTØ

Cystourethroplasty
- *see* Repair, Urinary System ØTQ
- *see* Replacement, Urinary System ØTR
- *see* Supplement, Urinary System ØTU

Cytarabine and Daunorubicin Liposome Antineoplastic XWØ

D

Daratumumab and Hyaluronidase-fihj XWØ1318

Darzalex Faspro® *use* Daratumumab and Hyaluronidase-fihj

DBS lead *use* Neurostimulator Lead in Central Nervous System and Cranial Nerves

DeBakey Left Ventricular Assist Device *use* Implantable Heart Assist System in Heart and Great Vessels

Debridement
- Excisional *see* Excision
- Non-excisional *see* Extraction

Decompression, Circulatory 6A15

Decortication, lung
- *see* Extirpation, Respiratory System ØBC
- *see* Release, Respiratory System ØBN

Deep brain neurostimulator lead *use* Neurostimulator Lead in Central Nervous System and Cranial Nerves

Deep cervical fascia
- *use* Subcutaneous Tissue and Fascia, Left Neck
- *use* Subcutaneous Tissue and Fascia, Right Neck

Deep cervical vein
- *use* Vertebral Vein, Left
- *use* Vertebral Vein, Right

Deep circumflex iliac artery
- *use* External Iliac Artery, Left
- *use* External Iliac Artery, Right

Deep facial vein
- *use* Face Vein, Left
- *use* Face Vein, Right

Deep femoral artery
- *use* Femoral Artery, Left
- *use* Femoral Artery, Right

Deep femoral (profunda femoris) vein
- *use* Femoral Vein, Left
- *use* Femoral Vein, Right

Deep Inferior Epigastric Artery Perforator Flap
- Replacement
  - Bilateral ØHRVØ77
  - Left ØHRUØ77
  - Right ØHRTØ77
- Transfer
  - Left ØKXG
  - Right ØKXF

Deep palmar arch
- *use* Hand Artery, Left
- *use* Hand Artery, Right

Deep transverse perineal muscle *use* Perineum Muscle

DefenCath™ *use* Taurolidine Anti-infective and Heparin Anticoagulant

Deferential artery
- *use* Internal Iliac Artery, Left
- *use* Internal Iliac Artery, Right

Defibrillator Generator
- Abdomen ØJH8
- Chest ØJH6

Defibtech Automated Chest Compression (ACC) device 5A1221J

Defitelio *use* Other Substance

Defitelio® infusion *see* Introduction of substance in or on, Physiological Systems and Anatomical Regions 3EØ

Delivery
- Cesarean *see* Extraction, Products of Conception 1ØDØ
- Forceps *see* Extraction, Products of Conception 1ØDØ
- Manually assisted 1ØEØXZZ
- Products of Conception 1ØEØXZZ
- Vacuum assisted *see* Extraction, Products of Conception 1ØDØ

Delta frame external fixator
- *use* External Fixation Device, Hybrid in ØPH
- *use* External Fixation Device, Hybrid in ØPS
- *use* External Fixation Device, Hybrid in ØQH
- *use* External Fixation Device, Hybrid in ØQS

Delta III Reverse shoulder prosthesis *use* Synthetic Substitute, Reverse Ball and Socket in ØRR

Deltoid fascia
- *use* Subcutaneous Tissue and Fascia, Left Upper Arm
- *use* Subcutaneous Tissue and Fascia, Right Upper Arm

Deltoid ligament
- *use* Ankle Bursa and Ligament, Left
- *use* Ankle Bursa and Ligament, Right

Deltoid muscle
- *use* Shoulder Muscle, Left
- *use* Shoulder Muscle, Right

Deltopectoral (infraclavicular) lymph node
- *use* Lymphatic, Left Upper Extremity
- *use* Lymphatic, Right Upper Extremity

Denervation
- Cranial nerve *see* Destruction, Central Nervous System and Cranial Nerves ØØ5
- Peripheral nerve *see* Destruction, Peripheral Nervous System Ø15

Dens *use* Cervical Vertebra

Densitometry
- Plain Radiography
  - Femur
    - Left BQØ4ZZ1
    - Right BQØ3ZZ1
  - Hip
    - Left BQØ1ZZ1
    - Right BQØØZZ1
  - Spine
    - Cervical BRØØZZ1
    - Lumbar BRØ9ZZ1
    - Thoracic BRØ7ZZ1
    - Whole BRØGZZ1
- Ultrasonography
  - Elbow
    - Left BP4HZZ1
    - Right BP4GZZ1
  - Hand
    - Left BP4PZZ1
    - Right BP4NZZ1
  - Shoulder
    - Left BP49ZZ1
    - Right BP48ZZ1
  - Wrist
    - Left BP4MZZ1
    - Right BP4LZZ1

Denticulate (dentate) ligament *use* Spinal Meninges

Depressor anguli oris muscle *use* Facial Muscle

Depressor labii inferioris muscle *use* Facial Muscle

Depressor septi nasi muscle *use* Facial Muscle

Depressor supercilii muscle *use* Facial Muscle

Dermabrasion *see* Extraction, Skin and Breast ØHD

Dermis *use* Skin
Descending genicular artery
  use Femoral Artery, Left
  use Femoral Artery, Right
Destruction
  Acetabulum
    Left 0Q55
    Right 0Q54
  Adenoids 0C5Q
  Ampulla of Vater 0F5C
  Anal Sphincter 0D5R
  Anterior Chamber
    Left 08533ZZ
    Right 08523ZZ
  Anus 0D5Q
  Aorta
    Abdominal
    Thoracic
      Ascending/Arch 025X
      Descending 025W
  Aortic Body 0G5D
  Appendix 0D5J
  Artery
    Anterior Tibial
      Left 045Q
      Right 045P
    Axillary
      Left 0356
      Right 0355
    Brachial
      Left 0358
      Right 0357
    Celiac 0451
    Colic
      Left 0457
      Middle 0458
      Right 0456
    Common Carotid
      Left 035J
      Right 035H
    Common Iliac
      Left 045D
      Right 045C
    External Carotid
      Left 035N
      Right 035M
    External Iliac
      Left 045J
      Right 045H
    Face 035R
    Femoral
      Left 045L
      Right 045K
    Foot
      Left 045W
      Right 045V
    Gastric 0452
    Hand
      Left 035F
      Right 035D
    Hepatic 0453
    Inferior Mesenteric 045B
    Innominate 0352
    Internal Carotid
      Left 035L
      Right 035K
    Internal Iliac
      Left 045F
      Right 045E
    Internal Mammary
      Left 0351
      Right 0350
    Intracranial 035G
    Lower 045Y
    Peroneal
      Left 045U
      Right 045T
    Popliteal
      Left 045N
      Right 045M
    Posterior Tibial
      Left 045S
      Right 045R
    Pulmonary
      Left 025R
      Right 025Q
    Pulmonary Trunk 025P
    Radial
      Left 035C

Destruction — *continued*
  Artery — *continued*
    Radial — *continued*
      Right 035B
    Renal
      Left 045A
      Right 0459
    Splenic 0454
    Subclavian
      Left 0354
      Right 0353
    Superior Mesenteric 0455
    Temporal
      Left 035T
      Right 035S
    Thyroid
      Left 035V
      Right 035U
    Ulnar
      Left 035A
      Right 0359
    Upper 035Y
    Vertebral
      Left 035Q
      Right 035P
  Atrium
    Left 0257
    Right 0256
  Auditory Ossicle
    Left 095A
    Right 0959
  Basal Ganglia 0058
  Bladder 0T5B
  Bladder Neck 0T5C
  Bone
    Ethmoid
      Left 0N5G
      Right 0N5F
    Frontal 0N51
    Hyoid 0N5X
    Lacrimal
      Left 0N5J
      Right 0N5H
    Nasal 0N5B
    Occipital 0N57
    Palatine
      Left 0N5L
      Right 0N5K
    Parietal
      Left 0N54
      Right 0N53
    Pelvic
      Left 0Q53
      Right 0Q52
    Sphenoid 0N5C
    Temporal
      Left 0N56
      Right 0N55
    Zygomatic
      Left 0N5N
      Right 0N5M
  Brain 0050
  Breast
    Bilateral 0H5V
    Left 0H5U
    Right 0H5T
  Bronchus
    Lingula 0B59
    Lower Lobe
      Left 0B5B
      Right 0B56
    Main
      Left 0B57
      Right 0B53
    Middle Lobe, Right 0B55
    Upper Lobe
      Left 0B58
      Right 0B54
  Buccal Mucosa 0C54
  Bursa and Ligament
    Abdomen
      Left 0M5J
      Right 0M5H
    Ankle
      Left 0M5R
      Right 0M5Q
    Elbow
      Left 0M54
      Right 0M53

Destruction — *continued*
  Bursa and Ligament — *continued*
    Foot
      Left 0M5T
      Right 0M5S
    Hand
      Left 0M58
      Right 0M57
    Head and Neck 0M50
    Hip
      Left 0M5M
      Right 0M5L
    Knee
      Left 0M5P
      Right 0M5N
    Lower Extremity
      Left 0M5W
      Right 0M5V
    Perineum 0M5K
    Rib(s) 0M5G
    Shoulder
      Left 0M52
      Right 0M51
    Spine
      Lower 0M5D
      Upper 0M5C
    Sternum 0M5F
    Upper Extremity
      Left 0M5B
      Right 0M59
    Wrist
      Left 0M56
      Right 0M55
  Carina 0B52
  Carotid Bodies, Bilateral 0G58
  Carotid Body
    Left 0G56
    Right 0G57
  Carpal
    Left 0P5N
    Right 0P5M
  Cecum 0D5H
  Cerebellum 005C
  Cerebral Hemisphere 0057
  Cerebral Meninges 0051
  Cerebral Ventricle 0056
  Cervix 0U5C
  Chordae Tendineae 0259
  Choroid
    Left 085B
    Right 085A
  Cisterna Chyli 075L
  Clavicle
    Left 0P5B
    Right 0P59
  Clitoris 0U5J
  Coccygeal Glomus 0G5B
  Coccyx 0Q5S
  Colon
    Ascending 0D5K
    Descending 0D5M
    Sigmoid 0D5N
    Transverse 0D5L
  Conduction Mechanism 0258
  Conjunctiva
    Left 085TXZZ
    Right 085SXZZ
  Cord
    Bilateral 0V5H
    Left 0V5G
    Right 0V5F
  Cornea
    Left 0859XZZ
    Right 0858XZZ
  Cul-de-sac 0U5F
  Diaphragm 0B5T
  Disc
    Cervical Vertebral 0R53
    Cervicothoracic Vertebral 0R55
    Lumbar Vertebral 0S52
    Lumbosacral 0S54
    Thoracic Vertebral 0R59
    Thoracolumbar Vertebral 0R5B
  Duct
    Common Bile 0F59
    Cystic 0F58
    Hepatic
      Common 0F57
      Left 0F56

Destruction — *continued*
  Duct — *continued*
    Hepatic — *continued*
      Right ØF55
    Lacrimal
      Left Ø85Y
      Right Ø85X
    Pancreatic ØF5D
      Accessory ØF5F
    Parotid
      Left ØC5C
      Right ØC5B
  Duodenum ØD59
  Dura Mater ØØ52
  Ear
    External
      Left Ø951
      Right Ø950
    External Auditory Canal
      Left Ø954
      Right Ø953
    Inner
      Left Ø95E
      Right Ø95D
    Middle
      Left Ø956
      Right Ø955
  Endometrium ØU5B
  Epididymis
    Bilateral ØV5L
    Left ØV5K
    Right ØV5J
  Epiglottis ØC5R
  Esophagogastric Junction ØD54
  Esophagus ØD55
    Lower ØD53
    Middle ØD52
    Upper ØD51
  Eustachian Tube
    Left Ø95G
    Right Ø95F
  Eye
    Left Ø851XZZ
    Right Ø850XZZ
  Eyelid
    Lower
      Left Ø85R
      Right Ø85Q
    Upper
      Left Ø85P
      Right Ø85N
  Fallopian Tube
    Left ØU56
    Right ØU55
  Fallopian Tubes, Bilateral ØU57
  Femoral Shaft
    Left ØQ59
    Right ØQ58
  Femur
    Lower
      Left ØQ5C
      Right ØQ5B
    Upper
      Left ØQ57
      Right ØQ56
  Fibula
    Left ØQ5K
    Right ØQ5J
  Finger Nail ØH5QXZZ
  Gallbladder ØF54
  Gingiva
    Lower ØC56
    Upper ØC55
  Gland
    Adrenal
      Bilateral ØG54
      Left ØG52
      Right ØG53
    Lacrimal
      Left Ø85W
      Right Ø85V
    Minor Salivary ØC5J
    Parotid
      Left ØC59
      Right ØC58
    Pituitary ØG5Ø
    Sublingual
      Left ØC5F
      Right ØC5D

Destruction — *continued*
  Gland — *continued*
    Submaxillary
      Left ØC5H
      Right ØC5G
    Vestibular ØU5L
  Glenoid Cavity
    Left ØP58
    Right ØP57
  Glomus Jugulare ØG5C
  Humeral Head
    Left ØP5D
    Right ØP5C
  Humeral Shaft
    Left ØP5G
    Right ØP5F
  Hymen ØU5K
  Hypothalamus ØØ5A
  Ileocecal Valve ØD5C
  Ileum ØD5B
  Intestine
    Large ØD5E
      Left ØD5G
      Right ØD5F
    Small ØD58
  Iris
    Left Ø85D3ZZ
    Right Ø85C3ZZ
  Jejunum ØD5A
  Joint
    Acromioclavicular
      Left ØR5H
      Right ØR5G
    Ankle
      Left ØS5G
      Right ØS5F
    Carpal
      Left ØR5R
      Right ØR5Q
    Carpometacarpal
      Left ØR5T
      Right ØR5S
    Cervical Vertebral ØR51
    Cervicothoracic Vertebral ØR54
    Coccygeal ØS56
    Elbow
      Left ØR5M
      Right ØR5L
    Finger Phalangeal
      Left ØR5X
      Right ØR5W
    Hip
      Left ØS5B
      Right ØS59
    Knee
      Left ØS5D
      Right ØS5C
    Lumbar Vertebral ØS5Ø
    Lumbosacral ØS53
    Metacarpophalangeal
      Left ØR5V
      Right ØR5U
    Metatarsal-Phalangeal
      Left ØS5N
      Right ØS5M
    Occipital-cervical ØR5Ø
    Sacrococcygeal ØS55
    Sacroiliac
      Left ØS58
      Right ØS57
    Shoulder
      Left ØR5K
      Right ØR5J
    Sternoclavicular
      Left ØR5F
      Right ØR5E
    Tarsal
      Left ØS5J
      Right ØS5H
    Tarsometatarsal
      Left ØS5L
      Right ØS5K
    Temporomandibular
      Left ØR5D
      Right ØR5C
    Thoracic Vertebral ØR56
    Thoracolumbar Vertebral ØR5A
    Toe Phalangeal
      Left ØS5Q

Destruction — *continued*
  Joint — *continued*
    Toe Phalangeal — *continued*
      Right ØS5P
    Wrist
      Left ØR5P
      Right ØR5N
  Kidney
    Left ØT51
    Right ØT50
  Kidney Pelvis
    Left ØT54
    Right ØT53
  Larynx ØC5S
  Lens
    Left Ø85K3ZZ
    Right Ø85J3ZZ
  Lip
    Lower ØC51
    Upper ØC50
  Liver ØF5Ø
    Left Lobe ØF52
      Ultrasound-guided Cavitation XF52X08
    Right Lobe ØF51
      Ultrasound-guided Cavitation XF51X08
    Ultrasound-guided Cavitation XF50X08
  Lung
    Bilateral ØB5M
    Left ØB5L
    Lower Lobe
      Left ØB5J
      Right ØB5F
    Middle Lobe, Right ØB5D
    Right ØB5K
    Upper Lobe
      Left ØB5G
      Right ØB5C
  Lung Lingula ØB5H
  Lymphatic
    Aortic Ø75D
    Axillary
      Left Ø756
      Right Ø755
    Head Ø750
    Inguinal
      Left Ø75J
      Right Ø75H
    Internal Mammary
      Left Ø759
      Right Ø758
    Lower Extremity
      Left Ø75G
      Right Ø75F
    Mesenteric Ø75B
    Neck
      Left Ø752
      Right Ø751
    Pelvis Ø75C
    Thoracic Duct Ø75K
    Thorax Ø757
    Upper Extremity
      Left Ø754
      Right Ø753
  Mandible
    Left ØN5V
    Right ØN5T
  Maxilla ØN5R
  Medulla Oblongata ØØ5D
  Mesentery ØD5V
  Metacarpal
    Left ØP5Q
    Right ØP5P
  Metatarsal
    Left ØQ5P
    Right ØQ5N
  Muscle
    Abdomen
      Left ØK5L
      Right ØK5K
    Extraocular
      Left Ø85M
      Right Ø85L
    Facial ØK51
    Foot
      Left ØK5W
      Right ØK5V
    Hand
      Left ØK5D
      Right ØK5C

Destruction — continued
Muscle — continued
Head 0K50
Hip
   Left 0K5P
   Right 0K5N
Lower Arm and Wrist
   Left 0K5B
   Right 0K59
Lower Leg
   Left 0K5T
   Right 0K5S
Neck
   Left 0K53
   Right 0K52
Papillary 025D
Perineum 0K5M
Shoulder
   Left 0K56
   Right 0K55
Thorax
   Left 0K5J
   Right 0K5H
Tongue, Palate, Pharynx 0K54
Trunk
   Left 0K5G
   Right 0K5F
Upper Arm
   Left 0K58
   Right 0K57
Upper Leg
   Left 0K5R
   Right 0K5Q
Nasal Mucosa and Soft Tissue 095K
Nasopharynx 095N
Nerve
Abdominal Sympathetic 015M
Abducens 005L
Accessory 005R
Acoustic 005N
Brachial Plexus 0153
Cervical 0151
Cervical Plexus 0150
Facial 005M
Femoral 015D
Glossopharyngeal 005P
Head and Neck Sympathetic 015K
Hypoglossal 005S
Lumbar 015B
Lumbar Plexus 0159
Lumbar Sympathetic 015N
Lumbosacral Plexus 015A
Median 0155
Oculomotor 005H
Olfactory 005F
Optic 005G
Peroneal 015H
Phrenic 0152
Pudendal 015C
Radial 0156
Sacral 015R
Sacral Plexus 015Q
Sacral Sympathetic 015P
Sciatic 015F
Thoracic 0158
Thoracic Sympathetic 015L
Tibial 015G
Trigeminal 005K
Trochlear 005J
Ulnar 0154
Vagus 005Q
Nipple
Left 0H5X
Right 0H5W
Omentum 0D5U
Orbit
Left 0N5Q
Right 0N5P
Ovary
Bilateral 0U52
Left 0U51
Right 0U50
Palate
Hard 0C52
Soft 0C53
Pancreas 0F5G
Para-aortic Body 0G59
Paraganglion Extremity 0G5F
Parathyroid Gland 0G5R

Destruction — continued
Parathyroid Gland — continued
Inferior
   Left 0G5P
   Right 0G5N
Multiple 0G5Q
Superior
   Left 0G5M
   Right 0G5L
Patella
Left 0Q5F
Right 0Q5D
Penis 0V5S
Pericardium 025N
Peritoneum 0D5W
Phalanx
Finger
   Left 0P5V
   Right 0P5T
Thumb
   Left 0P5S
   Right 0P5R
Toe
   Left 0Q5R
   Right 0Q5Q
Pharynx 0C5M
Pineal Body 0G51
Pleura
Left 0B5P
Right 0B5N
Pons 005B
Prepuce 0V5T
Prostate 0V50
Robotic Waterjet Ablation XV508A4
Radius
Left 0P5J
Right 0P5H
Rectum 0D5P
Retina
Left 085F3ZZ
Right 085E3ZZ
Retinal Vessel
Left 085H3ZZ
Right 085G3ZZ
Ribs
1 to 2 0P51
3 or More 0P52
Sacrum 0Q51
Scapula
Left 0P56
Right 0P55
Sclera
Left 0857XZZ
Right 0856XZZ
Scrotum 0V55
Septum
Atrial 0255
Nasal 095M
Ventricular 025M
Sinus
Accessory 095P
Ethmoid
   Left 095V
   Right 095U
Frontal
   Left 095T
   Right 095S
Mastoid
   Left 095C
   Right 095B
Maxillary
   Left 095R
   Right 095Q
Sphenoid
   Left 095X
   Right 095W
Skin
Abdomen 0H57XZ
Back 0H56XZ
Buttock 0H58XZ
Chest 0H55XZ
Ear
   Left 0H53XZ
   Right 0H52XZ
Face 0H51XZ
Foot
   Left 0H5NXZ
   Right 0H5MXZ

Destruction — continued
Skin — continued
Hand
   Left 0H5GXZ
   Right 0H5FXZ
Inguinal 0H5AXZ
Lower Arm
   Left 0H5EXZ
   Right 0H5DXZ
Lower Leg
   Left 0H5LXZ
   Right 0H5KXZ
Neck 0H54XZ
Perineum 0H59XZ
Scalp 0H50XZ
Upper Arm
   Left 0H5CXZ
   Right 0H5BXZ
Upper Leg
   Left 0H5JXZ
   Right 0H5HXZ
Skull 0N50
Spinal Cord
Cervical 005W
Lumbar 005Y
Thoracic 005X
Spinal Meninges 005T
Spleen 075P
Sternum 0P50
Stomach 0D56
   Pylorus 0D57
Subcutaneous Tissue and Fascia
Abdomen 0J58
Back 0J57
Buttock 0J59
Chest 0J56
Face 0J51
Foot
   Left 0J5R
   Right 0J5Q
Hand
   Left 0J5K
   Right 0J5J
Lower Arm
   Left 0J5H
   Right 0J5G
Lower Leg
   Left 0J5P
   Right 0J5N
Neck
   Left 0J55
   Right 0J54
Pelvic Region 0J5C
Perineum 0J5B
Scalp 0J50
Upper Arm
   Left 0J5F
   Right 0J5D
Upper Leg
   Left 0J5M
   Right 0J5L
Tarsal
Left 0Q5M
Right 0Q5L
Tendon
Abdomen
   Left 0L5G
   Right 0L5F
Ankle
   Left 0L5T
   Right 0L5S
Foot
   Left 0L5W
   Right 0L5V
Hand
   Left 0L58
   Right 0L57
Head and Neck 0L50
Hip
   Left 0L5K
   Right 0L5J
Knee
   Left 0L5R
   Right 0L5Q
Lower Arm and Wrist
   Left 0L56
   Right 0L55
Lower Leg
   Left 0L5P

Destruction — *continued*
  Tendon — *continued*
    Lower Leg — *continued*
      Right 0L5N
    Perineum 0L5H
    Shoulder
      Left 0L52
      Right 0L51
    Thorax
      Left 0L5D
      Right 0L5C
    Trunk
      Left 0L5B
      Right 0L59
    Upper Arm
      Left 0L54
      Right 0L53
    Upper Leg
      Left 0L5M
      Right 0L5L
  Testis
    Bilateral 0V5C
    Left 0V5B
    Right 0V59
  Thalamus 0059
  Thymus 075M
  Thyroid Gland 0G5K
    Left Lobe 0G5G
    Right Lobe 0G5H
  Tibia
    Left 0Q5H
    Right 0Q5G
  Toe Nail 0H5RXZZ
  Tongue 0C57
  Tonsils 0C5P
  Tooth
    Lower 0C5X
    Upper 0C5W
  Trachea 0B51
  Tunica Vaginalis
    Left 0V57
    Right 0V56
  Turbinate, Nasal 095L
  Tympanic Membrane
    Left 0958
    Right 0957
  Ulna
    Left 0P5L
    Right 0P5K
  Ureter
    Left 0T57
    Right 0T56
  Urethra 0T5D
  Uterine Supporting Structure 0U54
  Uterus 0U59
  Uvula 0C5N
  Vagina 0U5G
  Valve
    Aortic 025F
    Mitral 025G
    Pulmonary 025H
    Tricuspid 025J
  Vas Deferens
    Bilateral 0V5Q
    Left 0V5P
    Right 0V5N
  Vein
    Axillary
      Left 0558
      Right 0557
    Azygos 0550
    Basilic
      Left 055C
      Right 055B
    Brachial
      Left 055A
      Right 0559
    Cephalic
      Left 055F
      Right 055D
    Colic 0657
    Common Iliac
      Left 065D
      Right 065C
    Coronary 0254
    Esophageal 0653
    External Iliac
      Left 065G
      Right 065F

Destruction — *continued*
  Vein — *continued*
    External Jugular
      Left 055Q
      Right 055P
    Face
      Left 055V
      Right 055T
    Femoral
      Left 065N
      Right 065M
    Foot
      Left 065V
      Right 065T
    Gastric 0652
    Hand
      Left 055H
      Right 055G
    Hemiazygos 0551
    Hepatic 0654
    Hypogastric
      Left 065J
      Right 065H
    Inferior Mesenteric 0656
    Innominate
      Left 0554
      Right 0553
    Internal Jugular
      Left 055N
      Right 055M
    Intracranial 055L
    Lower 065Y
    Portal 0658
    Pulmonary
      Left 025T
      Right 025S
    Renal
      Left 065B
      Right 0659
    Saphenous
      Left 065Q
      Right 065P
    Splenic 0651
    Subclavian
      Left 0556
      Right 0555
    Superior Mesenteric 0655
    Upper 055Y
    Vertebral
      Left 055S
      Right 055R
  Vena Cava
    Inferior 0650
    Superior 025V
  Ventricle
    Left 025L
    Right 025K
  Vertebra
    Cervical 0P53
    Lumbar 0Q50
    Thoracic 0P54
  Vesicle
    Bilateral 0V53
    Left 0V52
    Right 0V51
  Vitreous
    Left 08553ZZ
    Right 08543ZZ
  Vocal Cord
    Left 0C5V
    Right 0C5T
  Vulva 0U5M

Detachment
  Arm
    Lower
      Left 0X6F0Z
      Right 0X6D0Z
    Upper
      Left 0X690Z
      Right 0X680Z
  Elbow Region
    Left 0X6C0ZZ
    Right 0X6B0ZZ
  Femoral Region
    Left 0Y680ZZ
    Right 0Y670ZZ
  Finger
    Index
      Left 0X6P0Z

Detachment — *continued*
  Finger — *continued*
    Index — *continued*
      Right 0X6N0Z
    Little
      Left 0X6W0Z
      Right 0X6V0Z
    Middle
      Left 0X6R0Z
      Right 0X6Q0Z
    Ring
      Left 0X6T0Z
      Right 0X6S0Z
  Foot
    Left 0Y6N0Z
    Right 0Y6M0Z
  Forequarter
    Left 0X610ZZ
    Right 0X600ZZ
  Hand
    Left 0X6K0Z
    Right 0X6J0Z
  Hindquarter
    Bilateral 0Y640ZZ
    Left 0Y630ZZ
    Right 0Y620ZZ
  Knee Region
    Left 0Y6G0ZZ
    Right 0Y6F0ZZ
  Leg
    Lower
      Left 0Y6J0Z
      Right 0Y6H0Z
    Upper
      Left 0Y6D0Z
      Right 0Y6C0Z
  Shoulder Region
    Left 0X630ZZ
    Right 0X620ZZ
  Thumb
    Left 0X6M0Z
    Right 0X6L0Z
  Toe
    1st
      Left 0Y6Q0Z
      Right 0Y6P0Z
    2nd
      Left 0Y6S0Z
      Right 0Y6R0Z
    3rd
      Left 0Y6U0Z
      Right 0Y6T0Z
    4th
      Left 0Y6W0Z
      Right 0Y6V0Z
    5th
      Left 0Y6Y0Z
      Right 0Y6X0Z

Determination, Mental status GZ14ZZZ
Detorsion
  see Release
  see Reposition
Detoxification Services, for substance abuse HZ2ZZZZ
Device Fitting F0DZ
Diagnostic Audiology *see* Audiology, Diagnostic
Diagnostic imaging *see* Imaging, Diagnostic
Diagnostic radiology *see* Imaging, Diagnostic
Dialysis
  Hemodialysis *see* Performance, Urinary 5A1D
  Peritoneal 3E1M39Z
Diaphragma sellae *use* Dura Mater
Diaphragmatic pacemaker generator *use* Stimulator Generator in Subcutaneous Tissue and Fascia
Diaphragmatic Pacemaker Lead
  Insertion of device in, Diaphragm 0BHT
  Removal of device from, Diaphragm 0BPT
  Revision of device in, Diaphragm 0BWT
Digital radiography, plain *see* Plain Radiography
Dilation
  Ampulla of Vater 0F7C
  Anus 0D7Q
  Aorta
    Abdominal
    Thoracic
      Ascending/Arch 027X
      Descending 027W

Dilation — continued
  Artery
    Anterior Tibial
      Left 047Q
        Sustained Release Drug-eluting
          Intraluminal Device
          X27Q385
          Four or More X27Q3C5
          Three X27Q3B5
          Two X27Q395
      Right 047P
        Sustained Release Drug-eluting
          Intraluminal Device
          X27P385
          Four or More X27P3C5
          Three X27P3B5
          Two X27P395
    Axillary
      Left 0376
      Right 0375
    Brachial
      Left 0378
      Right 0377
    Celiac 0471
    Colic
      Left 0477
      Middle 0478
      Right 0476
    Common Carotid
      Left 037J
      Right 037H
    Common Iliac
      Left 047D
      Right 047C
    Coronary
      Four or More Arteries 0273
      One Artery 0270
      Three Arteries 0272
      Two Arteries 0271
    External Carotid
      Left 037N
      Right 037M
    External Iliac
      Left 047J
      Right 047H
    Face 037R
    Femoral
      Left 047L
        Sustained Release Drug-eluting
          Intraluminal Device
          X27J385
          Four or More X27J3C5
          Three X27J3B5
          Two X27J395
      Right 047K
        Sustained Release Drug-eluting
          Intraluminal Device
          X27H385
          Four or More X27H3C5
          Three X27H3B5
          Two X27H395
    Foot
      Left 047W
      Right 047V
    Gastric 0472
    Hand
      Left 037F
      Right 037D
    Hepatic 0473
    Inferior Mesenteric 047B
    Innominate 0372
    Internal Carotid
      Left 037L
      Right 037K
    Internal Iliac
      Left 047F
      Right 047E
    Internal Mammary
      Left 0371
      Right 0370
    Intracranial 037G
    Lower 047Y
    Peroneal
      Left 047U
        Sustained Release Drug-eluting
          Intraluminal Device
          X27U385
          Four or More X27U3C5
          Three X27U3B5

Dilation — continued
  Artery — continued
    Peroneal — continued
      Left — continued
        Sustained Release Drug-eluting In-
          traluminal Device — contin-
          ued
          Two X27U395
      Right 047T
        Sustained Release Drug-eluting
          Intraluminal Device
          X27T385
          Four or More X27T3C5
          Three X27T3B5
          Two X27T395
    Popliteal
      Left 047N
      Left Distal
        Sustained Release Drug-eluting
          Intraluminal Device
          X27N385
          Four or More X27N3C5
          Three X27N3B5
          Two X27N395
      Left Proximal
        Sustained Release Drug-eluting
          Intraluminal Device
          X27L385
          Four or More X27L3C5
          Three X27L3B5
          Two X27L395
      Right 047M
      Right Distal
        Sustained Release Drug-eluting
          Intraluminal Device
          X27M385
          Four or More X27M3C5
          Three X27M3B5
          Two X27M395
      Right Proximal
        Sustained Release Drug-eluting
          Intraluminal Device
          X27K385
          Four or More X27K3C5
          Three X27K3B5
          Two X27K395
    Posterior Tibial
      Left 047S
        Sustained Release Drug-eluting
          Intraluminal Device
          X27S385
          Four or More X27S3C5
          Three X27S3B5
          Two X27S395
      Right 047R
        Sustained Release Drug-eluting
          Intraluminal Device
          X27R385
          Four or More X27R3C5
          Three X27R3B5
          Two X27R395
    Pulmonary
      Left 027R
      Right 027Q
    Pulmonary Trunk 027P
    Radial
      Left 037C
      Right 037B
    Renal
      Left 047A
      Right 0479
    Splenic 0474
    Subclavian
      Left 0374
      Right 0373
    Superior Mesenteric 0475
    Temporal
      Left 037T
      Right 037S
    Thyroid
      Left 037V
      Right 037U
    Ulnar
      Left 037A
      Right 0379
    Upper 037Y
    Vertebral
      Left 037Q
      Right 037P

Dilation — continued
  Bladder 0T7B
  Bladder Neck 0T7C
  Bronchus
    Lingula 0B79
    Lower Lobe
      Left 0B7B
      Right 0B76
    Main
      Left 0B77
      Right 0B73
    Middle Lobe, Right 0B75
    Upper Lobe
      Left 0B78
      Right 0B74
  Carina 0B72
  Cecum 0D7H
  Cerebral Ventricle 0076
  Cervix 0U7C
  Colon
    Ascending 0D7K
    Descending 0D7M
    Sigmoid 0D7N
    Transverse 0D7L
  Duct
    Common Bile 0F79
    Cystic 0F78
    Hepatic
      Common 0F77
      Left 0F76
      Right 0F75
    Lacrimal
      Left 087Y
      Right 087X
    Pancreatic 0F7D
      Accessory 0F7F
    Parotid
      Left 0C7C
      Right 0C7B
  Duodenum 0D79
  Esophagogastric Junction 0D74
  Esophagus 0D75
    Lower 0D73
    Middle 0D72
    Upper 0D71
  Eustachian Tube
    Left 097G
    Right 097F
  Fallopian Tube
    Left 0U76
    Right 0U75
  Fallopian Tubes, Bilateral 0U77
  Hymen 0U7K
  Ileocecal Valve 0D7C
  Ileum 0D7B
  Intestine
    Large 0D7E
      Left 0D7G
      Right 0D7F
    Small 0D78
  Jejunum 0D7A
  Kidney Pelvis
    Left 0T74
    Right 0T73
  Larynx 0C7S
  Pharynx 0C7M
  Rectum 0D7P
  Stomach 0D76
    Pylorus 0D77
  Trachea 0B71
  Ureter
    Left 0T77
    Right 0T76
  Ureters, Bilateral 0T78
  Urethra 0T7D
  Uterus 0U79
  Vagina 0U7G
  Valve
    Aortic 027F
    Mitral 027G
    Pulmonary 027H
    Tricuspid 027J
  Vas Deferens
    Bilateral 0V7Q
    Left 0V7P
    Right 0V7N
  Vein
    Axillary
      Left 0578

Dilation — *continued*
  Vein — *continued*
    Axillary — *continued*
      Right 0577
    Azygos 0570
    Basilic
      Left 057C
      Right 057B
    Brachial
      Left 057A
      Right 0579
    Cephalic
      Left 057F
      Right 057D
    Colic 0677
    Common Iliac
      Left 067D
      Right 067C
    Esophageal 0673
    External Iliac
      Left 067G
      Right 067F
    External Jugular
      Left 057Q
      Right 057P
    Face
      Left 057V
      Right 057T
    Femoral
      Left 067N
      Right 067M
    Foot
      Left 067V
      Right 067T
    Gastric 0672
    Hand
      Left 057H
      Right 057G
    Hemiazygos 0571
    Hepatic 0674
    Hypogastric
      Left 067J
      Right 067H
    Inferior Mesenteric 0676
    Innominate
      Left 0574
      Right 0573
    Internal Jugular
      Left 057N
      Right 057M
    Intracranial 057L
    Lower 067Y
    Portal 0678
    Pulmonary
      Left 027T
      Right 027S
    Renal
      Left 067B
      Right 0679
    Saphenous
      Left 067Q
      Right 067P
    Splenic 0671
    Subclavian
      Left 0576
      Right 0575
    Superior Mesenteric 0675
    Upper 057Y
    Vertebral
      Left 057S
      Right 057R
  Vena Cava
    Inferior 0670
    Superior 027V
  Ventricle
    Left 027L
    Right 027K
Direct Lateral Interbody Fusion (DLIF) device *use*
  Interbody Fusion Device in Lower Joints
Disarticulation *see* Detachment
Discectomy, diskectomy
  see Excision, Lower Joints 0SB
  see Excision, Upper Joints 0RB
  see Resection, Lower Joints 0ST
  see Resection, Upper Joints 0RT
Discography
  see Fluoroscopy, Axial Skeleton, Except Skull and
    Facial Bones BR1

Discography — *continued*
  see Plain Radiography, Axial Skeleton, Except Skull
    and Facial Bones BR0
Dismembered pyeloplasty *see* Repair, Kidney Pelvis
Distal humerus
  use Humeral Shaft, Left
  use Humeral Shaft, Right
Distal humerus, involving joint
  use Elbow Joint, Left
  use Elbow Joint, Right
Distal radioulnar joint
  use Wrist Joint, Left
  use Wrist Joint, Right
Diversion *see* Bypass
Diverticulectomy *see* Excision, Gastrointestinal System
  0DB
Division
  Acetabulum
    Left 0Q85
    Right 0Q84
  Anal Sphincter 0D8R
  Basal Ganglia 0088
  Bladder Neck 0T8C
  Bone
    Ethmoid
      Left 0N8G
      Right 0N8F
    Frontal 0N81
    Hyoid 0N8X
    Lacrimal
      Left 0N8J
      Right 0N8H
    Nasal 0N8B
    Occipital 0N87
    Palatine
      Left 0N8L
      Right 0N8K
    Parietal
      Left 0N84
      Right 0N83
    Pelvic
      Left 0Q83
      Right 0Q82
    Sphenoid 0N8C
    Temporal
      Left 0N86
      Right 0N85
    Zygomatic
      Left 0N8N
      Right 0N8M
  Brain 0080
  Bursa and Ligament
    Abdomen
      Left 0M8J
      Right 0M8H
    Ankle
      Left 0M8R
      Right 0M8Q
    Elbow
      Left 0M84
      Right 0M83
    Foot
      Left 0M8T
      Right 0M8S
    Hand
      Left 0M88
      Right 0M87
    Head and Neck 0M80
    Hip
      Left 0M8M
      Right 0M8L
    Knee
      Left 0M8P
      Right 0M8N
    Lower Extremity
      Left 0M8W
      Right 0M8V
    Perineum 0M8K
    Rib(s) 0M8G
    Shoulder
      Left 0M82
      Right 0M81
    Spine
      Lower 0M8D
      Upper 0M8C
    Sternum 0M8F
    Upper Extremity
      Left 0M8B

Division — *continued*
  Bursa and Ligament — *continued*
    Upper Extremity — *continued*
      Right 0M89
    Wrist
      Left 0M86
      Right 0M85
  Carpal
    Left 0P8N
    Right 0P8M
  Cerebral Hemisphere 0087
  Chordae Tendineae 0289
  Clavicle
    Left 0P8B
    Right 0P89
  Coccyx 0Q8S
  Conduction Mechanism 0288
  Esophagogastric Junction 0D84
  Femoral Shaft
    Left 0Q89
    Right 0Q88
  Femur
    Lower
      Left 0Q8C
      Right 0Q8B
    Upper
      Left 0Q87
      Right 0Q86
  Fibula
    Left 0Q8K
    Right 0Q8J
  Gland, Pituitary 0G80
  Glenoid Cavity
    Left 0P88
    Right 0P87
  Humeral Head
    Left 0P8D
    Right 0P8C
  Humeral Shaft
    Left 0P8G
    Right 0P8F
  Hymen 0U8K
  Kidneys, Bilateral 0T82
  Liver 0F80
    Left Lobe 0F82
    Right Lobe 0F81
  Mandible
    Left 0N8V
    Right 0N8T
  Maxilla 0N8R
  Metacarpal
    Left 0P8Q
    Right 0P8P
  Metatarsal
    Left 0Q8P
    Right 0Q8N
  Muscle
    Abdomen
      Left 0K8L
      Right 0K8K
    Facial 0K81
    Foot
      Left 0K8W
      Right 0K8V
    Hand
      Left 0K8D
      Right 0K8C
    Head 0K80
    Hip
      Left 0K8P
      Right 0K8N
    Lower Arm and Wrist
      Left 0K8B
      Right 0K89
    Lower Leg
      Left 0K8T
      Right 0K8S
    Neck
      Left 0K83
      Right 0K82
    Papillary 028D
    Perineum 0K8M
    Shoulder
      Left 0K86
      Right 0K85
    Thorax
      Left 0K8J
      Right 0K8H
    Tongue, Palate, Pharynx 0K84

▽ **Subterms under main terms may continue to next column or page**

Division — *continued*

Muscle — *continued*

Trunk
  Left ØK8G
  Right ØK8F
Upper Arm
  Left ØK88
  Right ØK87
Upper Leg
  Left ØK8R
  Right ØK8Q

Nerve

Abdominal Sympathetic Ø18M
Abducens ØØ8L
Accessory ØØ8R
Acoustic ØØ8N
Brachial Plexus Ø183
Cervical Ø181
Cervical Plexus Ø18Ø
Facial ØØ8M
Femoral Ø18D
Glossopharyngeal ØØ8P
Head and Neck Sympathetic Ø18K
Hypoglossal ØØ8S
Lumbar Ø18B
Lumbar Plexus Ø189
Lumbar Sympathetic Ø18N
Lumbosacral Plexus Ø18A
Median Ø185
Oculomotor ØØ8H
Olfactory ØØ8F
Optic ØØ8G
Peroneal Ø18H
Phrenic Ø182
Pudendal Ø18C
Radial Ø186
Sacral Ø18R
Sacral Plexus Ø18Q
Sacral Sympathetic Ø18P
Sciatic Ø18F
Thoracic Ø188
Thoracic Sympathetic Ø18L
Tibial Ø18G
Trigeminal ØØ8K
Trochlear ØØ8J
Ulnar Ø184
Vagus ØØ8Q

Orbit

Left ØN8Q
Right ØN8P

Ovary

Bilateral ØU82
Left ØU81
Right ØU8Ø

Pancreas ØF8G

Patella

Left ØQ8F
Right ØQ8D

Perineum, Female ØW8NXZZ

Phalanx

Finger
  Left ØP8V
  Right ØP8T
Thumb
  Left ØP8S
  Right ØP8R
Toe
  Left ØQ8R
  Right ØQ8Q

Radius

Left ØP8J
Right ØP8H

Ribs

1 to 2 ØP81
3 or More ØP82

Sacrum ØQ81

Scapula

Left ØP86
Right ØP85

Skin

Abdomen ØH87XZZ
Back ØH86XZZ
Buttock ØH88XZZ
Chest ØH85XZZ
Ear
  Left ØH83XZZ
  Right ØH82XZZ
Face ØH81XZZ

Division — *continued*

Skin — *continued*

Foot
  Left ØH8NXZZ
  Right ØH8MXZZ
Hand
  Left ØH8GXZZ
  Right ØH8FXZZ
Inguinal ØH8AXZZ
Lower Arm
  Left ØH8EXZZ
  Right ØH8DXZZ
Lower Leg
  Left ØH8LXZZ
  Right ØH8KXZZ
Neck ØH84XZZ
Perineum ØH89XZZ
Scalp ØH8ØXZZ
Upper Arm
  Left ØH8CXZZ
  Right ØH8BXZZ
Upper Leg
  Left ØH8JXZZ
  Right ØH8HXZZ

Skull ØN8Ø

Spinal Cord

Cervical ØØ8W
Lumbar ØØ8Y
Thoracic ØØ8X

Sternum ØP8Ø

Stomach, Pylorus ØD87

Subcutaneous Tissue and Fascia

Abdomen ØJ88
Back ØJ87
Buttock ØJ89
Chest ØJ86
Face ØJ81
Foot
  Left ØJ8R
  Right ØJ8Q
Hand
  Left ØJ8K
  Right ØJ8J
Head and Neck ØJ8S
Lower Arm
  Left ØJ8H
  Right ØJ8G
Lower Extremity ØJ8W
Lower Leg
  Left ØJ8P
  Right ØJ8N
Neck
  Left ØJ85
  Right ØJ84
Pelvic Region ØJ8C
Perineum ØJ8B
Scalp ØJ8Ø
Trunk ØJ8T
Upper Arm
  Left ØJ8F
  Right ØJ8D
Upper Extremity ØJ8V
Upper Leg
  Left ØJ8M
  Right ØJ8L

Tarsal

Left ØQ8M
Right ØQ8L

Tendon

Abdomen
  Left ØL8G
  Right ØL8F
Ankle
  Left ØL8T
  Right ØL8S
Foot
  Left ØL8W
  Right ØL8V
Hand
  Left ØL88
  Right ØL87
Head and Neck ØL8Ø
Hip
  Left ØL8K
  Right ØL8J
Knee
  Left ØL8R
  Right ØL8Q

Division — *continued*

Tendon — *continued*

Lower Arm and Wrist
  Left ØL86
  Right ØL85
Lower Leg
  Left ØL8P
  Right ØL8N
Perineum ØL8H
Shoulder
  Left ØL82
  Right ØL81
Thorax
  Left ØL8D
  Right ØL8C
Trunk
  Left ØL8B
  Right ØL89
Upper Arm
  Left ØL84
  Right ØL83
Upper Leg
  Left ØL8M
  Right ØL8L

Thyroid Gland Isthmus ØG8J

Tibia

Left ØQ8H
Right ØQ8G

Turbinate, Nasal Ø98L

Ulna

Left ØP8L
Right ØP8K

Uterine Supporting Structure ØU84

Vertebra

Cervical ØP83
Lumbar ØQ8Ø
Thoracic ØP84

Doppler study *see* Ultrasonography
Dorsal digital nerve *use* Radial Nerve
Dorsal metacarpal vein
  use Hand Vein, Left
  use Hand Vein, Right
Dorsal metatarsal artery
  use Foot Artery, Left
  use Foot Artery, Right
Dorsal metatarsal vein
  use Foot Vein, Left
  use Foot Vein, Right
Dorsal root ganglion
  use Cervical Spinal Cord
  use Lumbar Spinal Cord
  use Spinal Cord
  use Thoracic Spinal Cord
Dorsal scapular artery
  use Subclavian Artery, Left
  use Subclavian Artery, Right
Dorsal scapular nerve *use* Brachial Plexus
Dorsal venous arch
  use Foot Vein, Left
  use Foot Vein, Right
Dorsalis pedis artery
  use Anterior Tibial Artery, Left
  use Anterior Tibial Artery, Right
DownStream® System 5AØ512C, 5AØ522C
Drainage
Abdominal Wall ØW9F
Acetabulum
  Left ØQ95
  Right ØQ94
Adenoids ØC9Q
Ampulla of Vater ØF9C
Anal Sphincter ØD9R
Ankle Region
  Left ØY9L
  Right ØY9K
Anterior Chamber
  Left Ø893
  Right Ø892
Anus ØD9Q
Aorta, Abdominal Ø49Ø
Aortic Body ØG9D
Appendix ØD9J
Arm
  Lower
    Left ØX9F
    Right ØX9D
  Upper
    Left ØX99

Index

Drainage — continued
   Arm — continued
      Upper — continued
         Right 0X98
   Artery
      Anterior Tibial
         Left 049Q
         Right 049P
      Axillary
         Left 0396
         Right 0395
      Brachial
         Left 0398
         Right 0397
      Celiac 0491
      Colic
         Left 0497
         Middle 0498
         Right 0496
      Common Carotid
         Left 039J
         Right 039H
      Common Iliac
         Left 049D
         Right 049C
      External Carotid
         Left 039N
         Right 039M
      External Iliac
         Left 049J
         Right 049H
      Face 039R
      Femoral
         Left 049L
         Right 049K
      Foot
         Left 049W
         Right 049V
      Gastric 0492
      Hand
         Left 039F
         Right 039D
      Hepatic 0493
      Inferior Mesenteric 049B
      Innominate 0392
      Internal Carotid
         Left 039L
         Right 039K
      Internal Iliac
         Left 049F
         Right 049E
      Internal Mammary
         Left 0391
         Right 0390
      Intracranial 039G
      Lower 049Y
      Peroneal
         Left 049U
         Right 049T
      Popliteal
         Left 049N
         Right 049M
      Posterior Tibial
         Left 049S
         Right 049R
      Radial
         Left 039C
         Right 039B
      Renal
         Left 049A
         Right 0499
      Splenic 0494
      Subclavian
         Left 0394
         Right 0393
      Superior Mesenteric 0495
      Temporal
         Left 039T
         Right 039S
      Thyroid
         Left 039V
         Right 039U
      Ulnar
         Left 039A
         Right 0399
      Upper 039Y
      Vertebral
         Left 039Q
         Right 039P

Drainage — continued
   Auditory Ossicle
      Left 099A
      Right 0999
   Axilla
      Left 0X95
      Right 0X94
   Back
      Lower 0W9L
      Upper 0W9K
   Basal Ganglia 0098
   Bladder 0T9B
   Bladder Neck 0T9C
   Bone
      Ethmoid
         Left 0N9G
         Right 0N9F
      Frontal 0N91
      Hyoid 0N9X
      Lacrimal
         Left 0N9J
         Right 0N9H
      Nasal 0N9B
      Occipital 0N97
      Palatine
         Left 0N9L
         Right 0N9K
      Parietal
         Left 0N94
         Right 0N93
      Pelvic
         Left 0Q93
         Right 0Q92
      Sphenoid 0N9C
      Temporal
         Left 0N96
         Right 0N95
      Zygomatic
         Left 0N9N
         Right 0N9M
   Bone Marrow 079T
   Brain 0090
   Breast
      Bilateral 0H9V
      Left 0H9U
      Right 0H9T
   Bronchus
      Lingula 0B99
      Lower Lobe
         Left 0B9B
         Right 0B96
      Main
         Left 0B97
         Right 0B93
      Middle Lobe, Right 0B95
      Upper Lobe
         Left 0B98
         Right 0B94
   Buccal Mucosa 0C94
   Bursa and Ligament
      Abdomen
         Left 0M9J
         Right 0M9H
      Ankle
         Left 0M9R
         Right 0M9Q
      Elbow
         Left 0M94
         Right 0M93
      Foot
         Left 0M9T
         Right 0M9S
      Hand
         Left 0M98
         Right 0M97
      Head and Neck 0M90
      Hip
         Left 0M9M
         Right 0M9L
      Knee
         Left 0M9P
         Right 0M9N
      Lower Extremity
         Left 0M9W
         Right 0M9V
      Perineum 0M9K
      Rib(s) 0M9G
      Shoulder
         Left 0M92

Drainage — continued
   Bursa and Ligament — continued
      Shoulder — continued
         Right 0M91
      Spine
         Lower 0M9D
         Upper 0M9C
      Sternum 0M9F
      Upper Extremity
         Left 0M9B
         Right 0M99
      Wrist
         Left 0M96
         Right 0M95
   Buttock
      Left 0Y91
      Right 0Y90
   Carina 0B92
   Carotid Bodies, Bilateral 0G98
   Carotid Body
      Left 0G96
      Right 0G97
   Carpal
      Left 0P9N
      Right 0P9M
   Cavity, Cranial 0W91
   Cecum 0D9H
   Cerebellum 009C
   Cerebral Hemisphere 0097
   Cerebral Meninges 0091
   Cerebral Ventricle 0096
   Cervix 0U9C
   Chest Wall 0W98
   Choroid
      Left 089B
      Right 089A
   Cisterna Chyli 079L
   Clavicle
      Left 0P9B
      Right 0P99
   Clitoris 0U9J
   Coccygeal Glomus 0G9B
   Coccyx 0Q9S
   Colon
      Ascending 0D9K
      Descending 0D9M
      Sigmoid 0D9N
      Transverse 0D9L
   Conjunctiva
      Left 089T
      Right 089S
   Cord
      Bilateral 0V9H
      Left 0V9G
      Right 0V9F
   Cornea
      Left 0899
      Right 0898
   Cul-de-sac 0U9F
   Diaphragm 0B9T
   Disc
      Cervical Vertebral 0R93
      Cervicothoracic Vertebral 0R95
      Lumbar Vertebral 0S92
      Lumbosacral 0S94
      Thoracic Vertebral 0R99
      Thoracolumbar Vertebral 0R9B
   Duct
      Common Bile 0F99
      Cystic 0F98
      Hepatic
         Common 0F97
         Left 0F96
         Right 0F95
      Lacrimal
         Left 089Y
         Right 089X
      Pancreatic 0F9D
         Accessory 0F9F
      Parotid
         Left 0C9C
         Right 0C9B
   Duodenum 0D99
   Dura Mater 0092
   Ear
      External
         Left 0991
         Right 0990

Drainage — Drainage

Drainage — *continued*
  Ear — *continued*
    External Auditory Canal
      Left 0994
      Right 0993
    Inner
      Left 099E
      Right 099D
    Middle
      Left 0996
      Right 0995
  Elbow Region
    Left 0X9C
    Right 0X9B
  Epididymis
    Bilateral 0V9L
    Left 0V9K
    Right 0V9J
  Epidural Space, Intracranial 0093
  Epiglottis 0C9R
  Esophagogastric Junction 0D94
  Esophagus 0D95
    Lower 0D93
    Middle 0D92
    Upper 0D91
  Eustachian Tube
    Left 099G
    Right 099F
  Extremity
    Lower
      Left 0Y9B
      Right 0Y99
    Upper
      Left 0X97
      Right 0X96
  Eye
    Left 0891
    Right 0890
  Eyelid
    Lower
      Left 089R
      Right 089Q
    Upper
      Left 089P
      Right 089N
  Face 0W92
  Fallopian Tube
    Left 0U96
    Right 0U95
  Fallopian Tubes, Bilateral 0U97
  Femoral Region
    Left 0Y98
    Right 0Y97
  Femoral Shaft
    Left 0Q99
    Right 0Q98
  Femur
    Lower
      Left 0Q9C
      Right 0Q9B
    Upper
      Left 0Q97
      Right 0Q96
  Fibula
    Left 0Q9K
    Right 0Q9J
  Finger Nail 0H9Q
  Foot
    Left 0Y9N
    Right 0Y9M
  Gallbladder 0F94
  Gingiva
    Lower 0C96
    Upper 0C95
  Gland
    Adrenal
      Bilateral 0G94
      Left 0G92
      Right 0G93
    Lacrimal
      Left 089W
      Right 089V
    Minor Salivary 0C9J
    Parotid
      Left 0C99
      Right 0C98
    Pituitary 0G90
    Sublingual
      Left 0C9F

Drainage — *continued*
  Gland — *continued*
    Sublingual — *continued*
      Right 0C9D
    Submaxillary
      Left 0C9H
      Right 0C9G
    Vestibular 0U9L
  Glenoid Cavity
    Left 0P98
    Right 0P97
  Glomus Jugulare 0G9C
  Hand
    Left 0X9K
    Right 0X9J
  Head 0W90
  Humeral Head
    Left 0P9D
    Right 0P9C
  Humeral Shaft
    Left 0P9G
    Right 0P9F
  Hymen 0U9K
  Hypothalamus 009A
  Ileocecal Valve 0D9C
  Ileum 0D9B
  Inguinal Region
    Left 0Y96
    Right 0Y95
  Intestine
    Large 0D9E
      Left 0D9G
      Right 0D9F
    Small 0D98
  Iris
    Left 089D
    Right 089C
  Jaw
    Lower 0W95
    Upper 0W94
  Jejunum 0D9A
  Joint
    Acromioclavicular
      Left 0R9H
      Right 0R9G
    Ankle
      Left 0S9G
      Right 0S9F
    Carpal
      Left 0R9R
      Right 0R9Q
    Carpometacarpal
      Left 0R9T
      Right 0R9S
    Cervical Vertebral 0R91
    Cervicothoracic Vertebral 0R94
    Coccygeal 0S96
    Elbow
      Left 0R9M
      Right 0R9L
    Finger Phalangeal
      Left 0R9X
      Right 0R9W
    Hip
      Left 0S9B
      Right 0S99
    Knee
      Left 0S9D
      Right 0S9C
    Lumbar Vertebral 0S90
    Lumbosacral 0S93
    Metacarpophalangeal
      Left 0R9V
      Right 0R9U
    Metatarsal-Phalangeal
      Left 0S9N
      Right 0S9M
    Occipital-cervical 0R90
    Sacrococcygeal 0S95
    Sacroiliac
      Left 0S98
      Right 0S97
    Shoulder
      Left 0R9K
      Right 0R9J
    Sternoclavicular
      Left 0R9F
      Right 0R9E

Drainage — *continued*
  Joint — *continued*
    Tarsal
      Left 0S9J
      Right 0S9H
    Tarsometatarsal
      Left 0S9L
      Right 0S9K
    Temporomandibular
      Left 0R9D
      Right 0R9C
    Thoracic Vertebral 0R96
    Thoracolumbar Vertebral 0R9A
    Toe Phalangeal
      Left 0S9Q
      Right 0S9P
    Wrist
      Left 0R9P
      Right 0R9N
  Kidney
    Left 0T91
    Right 0T90
  Kidney Pelvis
    Left 0T94
    Right 0T93
  Knee Region
    Left 0Y9G
    Right 0Y9F
  Larynx 0C9S
  Leg
    Lower
      Left 0Y9J
      Right 0Y9H
    Upper
      Left 0Y9D
      Right 0Y9C
  Lens
    Left 089K
    Right 089J
  Lip
    Lower 0C91
    Upper 0C90
  Liver 0F90
    Left Lobe 0F92
    Right Lobe 0F91
  Lung
    Bilateral 0B9M
    Left 0B9L
    Lower Lobe
      Left 0B9J
      Right 0B9F
    Middle Lobe, Right 0B9D
    Right 0B9K
    Upper Lobe
      Left 0B9G
      Right 0B9C
  Lung Lingula 0B9H
  Lymphatic
    Aortic 079D
    Axillary
      Left 0796
      Right 0795
    Head 0790
    Inguinal
      Left 079J
      Right 079H
    Internal Mammary
      Left 0799
      Right 0798
    Lower Extremity
      Left 079G
      Right 079F
    Mesenteric 079B
    Neck
      Left 0792
      Right 0791
    Pelvis 079C
    Thoracic Duct 079K
    Thorax 0797
    Upper Extremity
      Left 0794
      Right 0793
  Mandible
    Left 0N9V
    Right 0N9T
  Maxilla 0N9R
  Mediastinum 0W9C
  Medulla Oblongata 009D
  Mesentery 0D9V

Drainage — *continued*
Metacarpal
  Left 0P9Q
  Right 0P9P
Metatarsal
  Left 0Q9P
  Right 0Q9N
Muscle
  Abdomen
    Left 0K9L
    Right 0K9K
  Extraocular
    Left 089M
    Right 089L
  Facial 0K91
  Foot
    Left 0K9W
    Right 0K9V
  Hand
    Left 0K9D
    Right 0K9C
  Head 0K90
  Hip
    Left 0K9P
    Right 0K9N
  Lower Arm and Wrist
    Left 0K9B
    Right 0K99
  Lower Leg
    Left 0K9T
    Right 0K9S
  Neck
    Left 0K93
    Right 0K92
  Perineum 0K9M
  Shoulder
    Left 0K96
    Right 0K95
  Thorax
    Left 0K9J
    Right 0K9H
  Tongue, Palate, Pharynx 0K94
  Trunk
    Left 0K9G
    Right 0K9F
  Upper Arm
    Left 0K98
    Right 0K97
  Upper Leg
    Left 0K9R
    Right 0K9Q
Nasal Mucosa and Soft Tissue 099K
Nasopharynx 099N
Neck 0W96
Nerve
  Abdominal Sympathetic 019M
  Abducens 009L
  Accessory 009R
  Acoustic 009N
  Brachial Plexus 0193
  Cervical 0191
  Cervical Plexus 0190
  Facial 009M
  Femoral 019D
  Glossopharyngeal 009P
  Head and Neck Sympathetic 019K
  Hypoglossal 009S
  Lumbar 019B
  Lumbar Plexus 0199
  Lumbar Sympathetic 019N
  Lumbosacral Plexus 019A
  Median 0195
  Oculomotor 009H
  Olfactory 009F
  Optic 009G
  Peroneal 019H
  Phrenic 0192
  Pudendal 019C
  Radial 0196
  Sacral 019R
  Sacral Plexus 019Q
  Sacral Sympathetic 019P
  Sciatic 019F
  Thoracic 0198
  Thoracic Sympathetic 019L
  Tibial 019G
  Trigeminal 009K
  Trochlear 009J
  Ulnar 0194

Drainage — *continued*
Nerve — *continued*
  Vagus 009Q
Nipple
  Left 0H9X
  Right 0H9W
Omentum 0D9U
Oral Cavity and Throat 0W93
Orbit
  Left 0N9Q
  Right 0N9P
Ovary
  Bilateral 0U92
  Left 0U91
  Right 0U90
Palate
  Hard 0C92
  Soft 0C93
Pancreas 0F9G
Para-aortic Body 0G99
Paraganglion Extremity 0G9F
Parathyroid Gland 0G9R
  Inferior
    Left 0G9P
    Right 0G9N
  Multiple 0G9Q
  Superior
    Left 0G9M
    Right 0G9L
Patella
  Left 0Q9F
  Right 0Q9D
Pelvic Cavity 0W9J
Penis 0V9S
Pericardial Cavity 0W9D
Perineum
  Female 0W9N
  Male 0W9M
Peritoneal Cavity 0W9G
Peritoneum 0D9W
Phalanx
  Finger
    Left 0P9V
    Right 0P9T
  Thumb
    Left 0P9S
    Right 0P9R
  Toe
    Left 0Q9R
    Right 0Q9Q
Pharynx 0C9M
Pineal Body 0G91
Pleura
  Left 0B9P
  Right 0B9N
Pleural Cavity
  Left 0W9B
  Right 0W99
Pons 009B
Prepuce 0V9T
Products of Conception
  Amniotic Fluid
    Diagnostic 1090
    Therapeutic 1090
  Fetal Blood 1090
  Fetal Cerebrospinal Fluid 1090
  Fetal Fluid, Other 1090
  Fluid, Other 1090
Prostate 0V90
Radius
  Left 0P9J
  Right 0P9H
Rectum 0D9P
Retina
  Left 089F
  Right 089E
Retinal Vessel
  Left 089H
  Right 089G
Retroperitoneum 0W9H
Ribs
  1 to 2 0P91
  3 or More 0P92
Sacrum 0Q91
Scapula
  Left 0P96
  Right 0P95
Sclera
  Left 0897

Drainage — *continued*
Sclera — *continued*
  Right 0896
Scrotum 0V95
Septum, Nasal 099M
Shoulder Region
  Left 0X93
  Right 0X92
Sinus
  Accessory 099P
  Ethmoid
    Left 099V
    Right 099U
  Frontal
    Left 099T
    Right 099S
  Mastoid
    Left 099C
    Right 099B
  Maxillary
    Left 099R
    Right 099Q
  Sphenoid
    Left 099X
    Right 099W
Skin
  Abdomen 0H97
  Back 0H96
  Buttock 0H98
  Chest 0H95
  Ear
    Left 0H93
    Right 0H92
  Face 0H91
  Foot
    Left 0H9N
    Right 0H9M
  Hand
    Left 0H9G
    Right 0H9F
  Inguinal 0H9A
  Lower Arm
    Left 0H9E
    Right 0H9D
  Lower Leg
    Left 0H9L
    Right 0H9K
  Neck 0H94
  Perineum 0H99
  Scalp 0H90
  Upper Arm
    Left 0H9C
    Right 0H9B
  Upper Leg
    Left 0H9J
    Right 0H9H
Skull 0N90
Spinal Canal 009U
Spinal Cord
  Cervical 009W
  Lumbar 009Y
  Thoracic 009X
Spinal Meninges 009T
Spleen 079P
Sternum 0P90
Stomach 0D96
  Pylorus 0D97
Subarachnoid Space, Intracranial 0095
Subcutaneous Tissue and Fascia
  Abdomen 0J98
  Back 0J97
  Buttock 0J99
  Chest 0J96
  Face 0J91
  Foot
    Left 0J9R
    Right 0J9Q
  Hand
    Left 0J9K
    Right 0J9J
  Lower Arm
    Left 0J9H
    Right 0J9G
  Lower Leg
    Left 0J9P
    Right 0J9N
  Neck
    Left 0J95
    Right 0J94

Drainage — *continued*

Subcutaneous Tissue and Fascia — *continued*
Pelvic Region ØJ9C
Perineum ØJ9B
Scalp ØJ9Ø
Upper Arm
Left ØJ9F
Right ØJ9D
Upper Leg
Left ØJ9M
Right ØJ9L
Subdural Space, Intracranial ØØ94
Tarsal
Left ØQ9M
Right ØQ9L
Tendon
Abdomen
Left ØL9G
Right ØL9F
Ankle
Left ØL9T
Right ØL9S
Foot
Left ØL9W
Right ØL9V
Hand
Left ØL98
Right ØL97
Head and Neck ØL9Ø
Hip
Left ØL9K
Right ØL9J
Knee
Left ØL9R
Right ØL9Q
Lower Arm and Wrist
Left ØL96
Right ØL95
Lower Leg
Left ØL9P
Right ØL9N
Perineum ØL9H
Shoulder
Left ØL92
Right ØL91
Thorax
Left ØL9D
Right ØL9C
Trunk
Left ØL9B
Right ØL99
Upper Arm
Left ØL94
Right ØL93
Upper Leg
Left ØL9M
Right ØL9L
Testis
Bilateral ØV9C
Left ØV9B
Right ØV99
Thalamus ØØ99
Thymus Ø79M
Thyroid Gland ØG9K
Left Lobe ØG9G
Right Lobe ØG9H
Tibia
Left ØQ9H
Right ØQ9G
Toe Nail ØH9R
Tongue ØC97
Tonsils ØC9P
Tooth
Lower ØC9X
Upper ØC9W
Trachea ØB91
Tunica Vaginalis
Left ØV97
Right ØV96
Turbinate, Nasal Ø99L
Tympanic Membrane
Left Ø998
Right Ø997
Ulna
Left ØP9L
Right ØP9K
Ureter
Left ØT97
Right ØT96

Drainage — *continued*

Ureters, Bilateral ØT98
Urethra ØT9D
Uterine Supporting Structure ØU94
Uterus ØU99
Uvula ØC9N
Vagina ØU9G
Vas Deferens
Bilateral ØV9Q
Left ØV9P
Right ØV9N
Vein
Axillary
Left Ø598
Right Ø597
Azygos Ø59Ø
Basilic
Left Ø59C
Right Ø59B
Brachial
Left Ø59A
Right Ø599
Cephalic
Left Ø59F
Right Ø59D
Colic Ø697
Common Iliac
Left Ø69D
Right Ø69C
Esophageal Ø693
External Iliac
Left Ø69G
Right Ø69F
External Jugular
Left Ø59Q
Right Ø59P
Face
Left Ø59V
Right Ø59T
Femoral
Left Ø69N
Right Ø69M
Foot
Left Ø69V
Right Ø69T
Gastric Ø692
Hand
Left Ø59H
Right Ø59G
Hemiazygos Ø591
Hepatic Ø694
Hypogastric
Left Ø69J
Right Ø69H
Inferior Mesenteric Ø696
Innominate
Left Ø594
Right Ø593
Internal Jugular
Left Ø59N
Right Ø59M
Intracranial Ø59L
Lower Ø69Y
Portal Ø698
Renal
Left Ø69B
Right Ø699
Saphenous
Left Ø69Q
Right Ø69P
Splenic Ø691
Subclavian
Left Ø596
Right Ø595
Superior Mesenteric Ø695
Upper Ø59Y
Vertebral
Left Ø59S
Right Ø59R
Vena Cava, Inferior Ø69Ø
Vertebra
Cervical ØP93
Lumbar ØQ9Ø
Thoracic ØP94
Vesicle
Bilateral ØV93
Left ØV92
Right ØV91

Drainage — *continued*

Vitreous
Left Ø895
Right Ø894
Vocal Cord
Left ØC9V
Right ØC9T
Vulva ØU9M
Wrist Region
Left ØX9H
Right ØX9G
Dressing
Abdominal Wall 2W23X4Z
Arm
Lower
Left 2W2DX4Z
Right 2W2CX4Z
Upper
Left 2W2BX4Z
Right 2W2AX4Z
Back 2W25X4Z
Chest Wall 2W24X4Z
Extremity
Lower
Left 2W2MX4Z
Right 2W2LX4Z
Upper
Left 2W29X4Z
Right 2W28X4Z
Face 2W21X4Z
Finger
Left 2W2KX4Z
Right 2W2JX4Z
Foot
Left 2W2TX4Z
Right 2W2SX4Z
Hand
Left 2W2FX4Z
Right 2W2EX4Z
Head 2W20X4Z
Inguinal Region
Left 2W27X4Z
Right 2W26X4Z
Leg
Lower
Left 2W2RX4Z
Right 2W2QX4Z
Upper
Left 2W2PX4Z
Right 2W2NX4Z
Neck 2W22X4Z
Thumb
Left 2W2HX4Z
Right 2W2GX4Z
Toe
Left 2W2VX4Z
Right 2W2UX4Z
Driver stent (RX) (OTW) *use* Intraluminal Device
Drotrecogin alfa, infusion *see* Introduction of Recombinant Human-activated Protein C
Duct of Santorini *use* Pancreatic Duct, Accessory
Duct of Wirsung *use* Pancreatic Duct
Ductogram, mammary *see* Plain Radiography, Skin, Subcutaneous Tissue and Breast BHØ
Ductography, mammary *see* Plain Radiography, Skin, Subcutaneous Tissue and Breast BHØ
Ductus deferens
use Vas Deferens
use Vas Deferens, Bilateral
use Vas Deferens, Left
use Vas Deferens, Right
Duodenal ampulla *use* Ampulla of Vater
Duodenectomy
see Excision, Duodenum ØDB9
see Resection, Duodenum ØDT9
Duodenocholedochotomy *see* Drainage, Gallbladder ØF94
Duodenocystostomy
see Bypass, Gallbladder ØF14
see Drainage, Gallbladder ØF94
Duodenoenterostomy
see Bypass, Gastrointestinal System ØD1
see Drainage, Gastrointestinal System ØD9
Duodenojejunal flexure *use* Jejunum
Duodenolysis *see* Release, Duodenum ØDN9
Duodenorrhaphy *see* Repair, Duodenum ØDQ9

Duodenoscopy, single-use (aScope™ Duodeno) (EXALT™ Model D) see New Technology, Hepatobiliary System and Pancreas XFJ

Duodenostomy
  see Bypass, Duodenum ØD19
  see Drainage, Duodenum ØD99

Duodenotomy see Drainage, Duodenum ØD99

Dura mater, intracranial use Dura Mater

Dura mater, spinal use Spinal Meninges

DuraGraft® Endothelial Damage Inhibitor use Endothelial Damage Inhibitor

DuraHeart Left Ventricular Assist System use Implantable Heart Assist System in Heart and Great Vessels

Dural venous sinus use Intracranial Vein

Durata® Defibrillation Lead use Cardiac Lead, Defibrillator in Ø2H

Durvalumab Antineoplastic XWØ

DynaClip® (Forte)
  use Internal Fixation Device, Sustained Compression in ØRG
  use Internal Fixation Device, Sustained Compression in ØSG

DynaNail® (Hybrid) (Mini)
  use Internal Fixation Device, Sustained Compression in ØRG
  use Internal Fixation Device, Sustained Compression in ØSG

Dynesys® Dynamic Stabilization System
  use Spinal Stabilization Device, Pedicle-Based in ØRH
  use Spinal Stabilization Device, Pedicle-Based in ØSH

E

Earlobe
  use Ear, External, Bilateral
  use Ear, External, Left
  use Ear, External, Right

ECCO2R (Extracorporeal Carbon Dioxide Removal) 5A0920Z

Echocardiogram see Ultrasonography, Heart B24

Echography see Ultrasonography

EchoTip® Insight™ Portosystemic Pressure Gradient Measurement System 4A044B2

ECMO see Performance, Circulatory 5A15

ECMO, intraoperative see Performance, Circulatory 5A15A

Eculizumab XWØ

EDWARDS INTUITY Elite valve system (rapid deployment technique) see Replacement, Valve, Aortic Ø2RF

EEG (electroencephalogram) see Measurement, Central Nervous 4A00

EGD (esophagogastroduodenoscopy) ØDJ08ZZ

Eighth cranial nerve use Acoustic Nerve

Ejaculatory duct
  use Vas Deferens
  use Vas Deferens, Bilateral
  use Vas Deferens, Left
  use Vas Deferens, Right

EKG (electrocardiogram) see Measurement, Cardiac 4A02

EKOS® EkoSonic® Endovascular System see Fragmentation, Artery

Eladocagene exuparvovec XWØQ316

Electrical bone growth stimulator (EBGS)
  use Bone Growth Stimulator in Head and Facial Bones
  use Bone Growth Stimulator in Lower Bones
  use Bone Growth Stimulator in Upper Bones

Electrical muscle stimulation (EMS) lead use Stimulator Lead in Muscles

Electrocautery
  Destruction see Destruction
  Repair see Repair

Electroconvulsive Therapy
  Bilateral-Multiple Seizure GZB3ZZZ
  Bilateral-Single Seizure GZB2ZZZ
  Electroconvulsive Therapy, Other GZB4ZZZ
  Unilateral-Multiple Seizure GZB1ZZZ
  Unilateral-Single Seizure GZB0ZZZ

Electroencephalogram (EEG) see Measurement, Central Nervous 4A00

Electromagnetic Therapy
  Central Nervous 6A22
  Urinary 6A21

Electronic muscle stimulator lead use Stimulator Lead in Muscles

Electrophysiologic stimulation (EPS) see Measurement, Cardiac 4A02

Electroshock therapy see Electroconvulsive Therapy

Elevation, bone fragments, skull see Reposition, Head and Facial Bones ØNS

Eleventh cranial nerve use Accessory Nerve

Ellipsys® vascular access system see New Technology, Cardiovascular System X2K

E-Luminexx™ (Biliary) (Vascular) Stent use Intraluminal Device

Eluvia™ Drug-Eluting Vascular Stent System
  use Intraluminal Device, Sustained Release Drug-eluting in New Technology
  use Intraluminal Device, Sustained Release Drug-eluting, Two in New Technology
  use Intraluminal Device, Sustained Release Drug-eluting, Three in New Technology
  use Intraluminal Device, Sustained Release Drug-eluting, Four or More in New Technology

ELZONRIS™ use Tagraxofusp-erzs Antineoplastic

Embolectomy see Extirpation

Embolization
  see Occlusion
  see Restriction

Embolization coil(s) use Intraluminal Device

EMG (electromyogram) see Measurement, Musculoskeletal 4A0F

Encephalon use Brain

Endarterectomy
  see Extirpation, Lower Arteries Ø4C
  see Extirpation, Upper Arteries Ø3C

Endeavor® (III) (IV) (Sprint) Zotarolimus-eluting Coronary Stent System use Intraluminal Device, Drug-eluting in Heart and Great Vessels

EndoAVF procedure, using magnetic-guided radiofrequency see Bypass, Upper Arteries Ø31

EndoAVF procedure, using thermal resistance energy see New Technology, Cardiovascular System X2K

Endologix AFX® Endovascular AAA System use Intraluminal Device

EndoSure® sensor use Monitoring Device, Pressure Sensor in Ø2H

ENDOTAK RELIANCE® (G) Defibrillation Lead use Cardiac Lead, Defibrillator in Ø2H

Endothelial damage inhibitor, applied to vein graft XY0VX83

Endotracheal tube (cuffed) (double-lumen) use Intraluminal Device, Endotracheal Airway in Respiratory System

Endovascular fistula creation, using magnetic-guided radiofrequency see Bypass, Upper Arteries Ø31

Endovascular fistula creation, using thermal resistance energy see New Technology, Cardiovascular System X2K

Endurant® Endovascular Stent Graft use Intraluminal Device

Endurant® II AAA Stent Graft System use Intraluminal Device

Engineered Allogeneic Thymus Tissue XW020D8

Engineered Chimeric Antigen Receptor T-cell Immunotherapy
  Allogeneic XWØ
  Autologous XWØ

Enlargement
  see Dilation
  see Repair

EnRhythm use Pacemaker, Dual Chamber in ØJH

ENROUTE® Transcarotid Neuroprotection System see New Technology, Cardiovascular System X2A

ENSPRYNG™ use Satralizumab-mwge

Enterorrhaphy see Repair, Gastrointestinal System ØDQ

Enterra gastric neurostimulator use Stimulator Generator, Multiple Array in ØJH

Enucleation
  Eyeball see Resection, Eye Ø8T
  Eyeball with prosthetic implant see Replacement, Eye Ø8R

Ependyma use Cerebral Ventricle

Epicel® cultured epidermal autograft use Autologous Tissue Substitute

Epic™ Stented Tissue Valve (aortic) use Zooplastic Tissue in Heart and Great Vessels

Epidermis use Skin

Epididymectomy
  see Excision, Male Reproductive System ØVB
  see Resection, Male Reproductive System ØVT

Epididymoplasty
  see Repair, Male Reproductive System ØVQ
  see Supplement, Male Reproductive System ØVU

Epididymorrhaphy see Repair, Male Reproductive System ØVQ

Epididymotomy see Drainage, Male Reproductive System ØV9

Epidural space, spinal use Spinal Canal

Epiphysiodesis
  see Insertion of device in, Lower Bones ØQH
  see Insertion of device in, Upper Bones ØPH
  see Repair, Lower Bones ØQQ
  see Repair, Upper Bones ØPQ

Epiploic foramen use Peritoneum

Epiretinal Visual Prosthesis
  Left Ø8H105Z
  Right Ø8H005Z

Episiorrhaphy see Repair, Perineum, Female ØWQN

Episiotomy see Division, Perineum, Female ØW8N

Epithalamus use Thalamus

Epitrochlear lymph node
  use Lymphatic, Left Upper Extremity
  use Lymphatic, Right Upper Extremity

EPS (electrophysiologic stimulation) see Measurement, Cardiac 4A02

Eptifibatide, infusion see Introduction of Platelet Inhibitor

ERCP (endoscopic retrograde cholangiopancreatography) see Fluoroscopy, Hepatobiliary System and Pancreas BF1

Erdafitinib Antineoplastic XWØDXL5

Erector spinae muscle
  use Trunk Muscle, Left
  use Trunk Muscle, Right

ERLEADA™ use Apalutamide Antineoplastic

Esketamine Hydrochloride XW097M5

Esophageal artery use Upper Artery

Esophageal obturator airway (EOA) use Intraluminal Device, Airway in Gastrointestinal System

Esophageal plexus use Thoracic Sympathetic Nerve

Esophagectomy
  see Excision, Gastrointestinal System ØDB
  see Resection, Gastrointestinal System ØDT

Esophagocoloplasty
  see Repair, Gastrointestinal System ØDQ
  see Supplement, Gastrointestinal System ØDU

Esophagoenterostomy
  see Bypass, Gastrointestinal System ØD1
  see Drainage, Gastrointestinal System ØD9

Esophagoesophagostomy
  see Bypass, Gastrointestinal System ØD1
  see Drainage, Gastrointestinal System ØD9

Esophagogastrectomy
  see Excision, Gastrointestinal System ØDB
  see Resection, Gastrointestinal System ØDT

Esophagogastroduodenoscopy (EGD) ØDJ08ZZ

Esophagogastroplasty
  see Repair, Gastrointestinal System ØDQ
  see Supplement, Gastrointestinal System ØDU

Esophagogastroscopy ØDJ68ZZ

Esophagogastrostomy
  see Bypass, Gastrointestinal System ØD1
  see Drainage, Gastrointestinal System ØD9

Esophagojejunoplasty see Supplement, Gastrointestinal System ØDU

Esophagojejunostomy
  see Bypass, Gastrointestinal System ØD1
  see Drainage, Gastrointestinal System ØD9

Esophagomyotomy see Division, Esophagogastric Junction ØD84

Esophagoplasty
  see Repair, Gastrointestinal System ØDQ
  see Replacement, Esophagus ØDR5
  see Supplement, Gastrointestinal System ØDU

Esophagoplication see Restriction, Gastrointestinal System ØDV

Esophagorrhaphy see Repair, Gastrointestinal System ØDQ

Esophagoscopy 0DJ08ZZ
Esophagotomy *see* Drainage, Gastrointestinal System 0D9
Esteem® implantable hearing system *use* Hearing Device in Ear, Nose, Sinus
ESWL (extracorporeal shock wave lithotripsy) *see* Fragmentation
Etesevimab Monoclonal Antibody XW0
Ethmoidal air cell
  use Ethmoid Sinus, Left
  use Ethmoid Sinus, Right
Ethmoidectomy
  see Excision, Ear, Nose, Sinus 09B
  see Excision, Head and Facial Bones 0NB
  see Resection, Ear, Nose, Sinus 09T
  see Resection, Head and Facial Bones 0NT
Ethmoidotomy *see* Drainage, Ear, Nose, Sinus 099
Evacuation
  Hematoma *see* Extirpation
  Other Fluid *see* Drainage
Evera (XT) (S) (DR/VR) *use* Defibrillator Generator in 0JH
Everolimus-eluting coronary stent *use* Intraluminal Device, Drug-eluting in Heart and Great Vessels
Evisceration
  Eyeball *see* Resection, Eye 08T
  Eyeball with prosthetic implant *see* Replacement, Eye 08R
EVUSHELD™ *use* Tixagevimab and Cilgavimab Monoclonal Antibody
EXALT™ Model D Single-Use Duodenoscope *see* New Technology, Hepatobiliary System and Pancreas XFJ
Examination *see* Inspection
Exchange *see* Change device in
Excision
  Abdominal Wall 0WBF
  Acetabulum
    Left 0QB5
    Right 0QB4
  Adenoids 0CBQ
  Ampulla of Vater 0FBC
  Anal Sphincter 0DBR
  Ankle Region
    Left 0YBL
    Right 0YBK
  Anus 0DBQ
  Aorta
    Abdominal
    Thoracic
      Ascending/Arch 02BX
      Descending 02BW
  Aortic Body 0GBD
  Appendix 0DBJ
  Arm
    Lower
      Left 0XBF
      Right 0XBD
    Upper
      Left 0XB9
      Right 0XB8
  Artery
    Anterior Tibial
      Left 04BQ
      Right 04BP
    Axillary
      Left 03B6
      Right 03B5
    Brachial
      Left 03B8
      Right 03B7
    Celiac 04B1
    Colic
      Left 04B7
      Middle 04B8
      Right 04B6
    Common Carotid
      Left 03BJ
      Right 03BH
    Common Iliac
      Left 04BD
      Right 04BC
    External Carotid
      Left 03BN
      Right 03BM
    External Iliac
      Left 04BJ
      Right 04BH

Excision — *continued*
  Artery — *continued*
    Face 03BR
    Femoral
      Left 04BL
      Right 04BK
    Foot
      Left 04BW
      Right 04BV
    Gastric 04B2
    Hand
      Left 03BF
      Right 03BD
    Hepatic 04B3
    Inferior Mesenteric 04BB
    Innominate 03B2
    Internal Carotid
      Left 03BL
      Right 03BK
    Internal Iliac
      Left 04BF
      Right 04BE
    Internal Mammary
      Left 03B1
      Right 03B0
    Intracranial 03BG
    Lower 04BY
    Peroneal
      Left 04BU
      Right 04BT
    Popliteal
      Left 04BN
      Right 04BM
    Posterior Tibial
      Left 04BS
      Right 04BR
    Pulmonary
      Left 02BR
      Right 02BQ
    Pulmonary Trunk 02BP
    Radial
      Left 03BC
      Right 03BB
    Renal
      Left 04BA
      Right 04B9
    Splenic 04B4
    Subclavian
      Left 03B4
      Right 03B3
    Superior Mesenteric 04B5
    Temporal
      Left 03BT
      Right 03BS
    Thyroid
      Left 03BV
      Right 03BU
    Ulnar
      Left 03BA
      Right 03B9
    Upper 03BY
    Vertebral
      Left 03BQ
      Right 03BP
  Atrium
    Left 02B7
    Right 02B6
  Auditory Ossicle
    Left 09BA
    Right 09B9
  Axilla
    Left 0XB5
    Right 0XB4
  Back
    Lower 0WBL
    Upper 0WBK
  Basal Ganglia 00B8
  Bladder 0TBB
  Bladder Neck 0TBC
  Bone
    Ethmoid
      Left 0NBG
      Right 0NBF
    Frontal 0NB1
    Hyoid 0NBX
    Lacrimal
      Left 0NBJ
      Right 0NBH
    Nasal 0NBB

Excision — *continued*
  Bone — *continued*
    Occipital 0NB7
    Palatine
      Left 0NBL
      Right 0NBK
    Parietal
      Left 0NB4
      Right 0NB3
    Pelvic
      Left 0QB3
      Right 0QB2
    Sphenoid 0NBC
    Temporal
      Left 0NB6
      Right 0NB5
    Zygomatic
      Left 0NBN
      Right 0NBM
  Brain 00B0
  Breast
    Bilateral 0HBV
    Left 0HBU
    Right 0HBT
    Supernumerary 0HBY
  Bronchus
    Lingula 0BB9
    Lower Lobe
      Left 0BBB
      Right 0BB6
    Main
      Left 0BB7
      Right 0BB3
    Middle Lobe, Right 0BB5
    Upper Lobe
      Left 0BB8
      Right 0BB4
  Buccal Mucosa 0CB4
  Bursa and Ligament
    Abdomen
      Left 0MBJ
      Right 0MBH
    Ankle
      Left 0MBR
      Right 0MBQ
    Elbow
      Left 0MB4
      Right 0MB3
    Foot
      Left 0MBT
      Right 0MBS
    Hand
      Left 0MB8
      Right 0MB7
    Head and Neck 0MB0
    Hip
      Left 0MBM
      Right 0MBL
    Knee
      Left 0MBP
      Right 0MBN
    Lower Extremity
      Left 0MBW
      Right 0MBV
    Perineum 0MBK
    Rib(s) 0MBG
    Shoulder
      Left 0MB2
      Right 0MB1
    Spine
      Lower 0MBD
      Upper 0MBC
    Sternum 0MBF
    Upper Extremity
      Left 0MBB
      Right 0MB9
    Wrist
      Left 0MB6
      Right 0MB5
  Buttock
    Left 0YB1
    Right 0YB0
  Carina 0BB2
  Carotid Bodies, Bilateral 0GB8
  Carotid Body
    Left 0GB6
    Right 0GB7
  Carpal
    Left 0PBN

Excision — *continued*
Carpal — *continued*
  Right ØPBM
Cecum ØDBH
Cerebellum ØØBC
Cerebral Hemisphere ØØB7
Cerebral Meninges ØØB1
Cerebral Ventricle ØØB6
Cervix ØUBC
Chest Wall ØWB8
Chordae Tendineae Ø2B9
Choroid
  Left Ø8BB
  Right Ø8BA
Cisterna Chyli Ø7BL
Clavicle
  Left ØPBB
  Right ØPB9
Clitoris ØUBJ
Coccygeal Glomus ØGBB
Coccyx ØQBS
Colon
  Ascending ØDBK
  Descending ØDBM
  Sigmoid ØDBN
  Transverse ØDBL
Conduction Mechanism Ø2B8
Conjunctiva
  Left Ø8BTXZ
  Right Ø8BSXZ
Cord
  Bilateral ØVBH
  Left ØVBG
  Right ØVBF
Cornea
  Left Ø8B9XZ
  Right Ø8B8XZ
Cul-de-sac ØUBF
Diaphragm ØBBT
Disc
  Cervical Vertebral ØRB3
  Cervicothoracic Vertebral ØRB5
  Lumbar Vertebral ØSB2
  Lumbosacral ØSB4
  Thoracic Vertebral ØRB9
  Thoracolumbar Vertebral ØRBB
Duct
  Common Bile ØFB9
  Cystic ØFB8
  Hepatic
    Common ØFB7
    Left ØFB6
    Right ØFB5
  Lacrimal
    Left Ø8BY
    Right Ø8BX
  Pancreatic ØFBD
    Accessory ØFBF
  Parotid
    Left ØCBC
    Right ØCBB
Duodenum ØDB9
Dura Mater ØØB2
Ear
  External
    Left Ø9B1
    Right Ø9BØ
  External Auditory Canal
    Left Ø9B4
    Right Ø9B3
  Inner
    Left Ø9BE
    Right Ø9BD
  Middle
    Left Ø9B6
    Right Ø9B5
Elbow Region
  Left ØXBC
  Right ØXBB
Epididymis
  Bilateral ØVBL
  Left ØVBK
  Right ØVBJ
Epiglottis ØCBR
Esophagogastric Junction ØDB4
Esophagus ØDB5
  Lower ØDB3
  Middle ØDB2
  Upper ØDB1

Excision — *continued*
Eustachian Tube
  Left Ø9BG
  Right Ø9BF
Extremity
  Lower
    Left ØYBB
    Right ØYB9
  Upper
    Left ØXB7
    Right ØXB6
Eye
  Left Ø8B1
  Right Ø8BØ
Eyelid
  Lower
    Left Ø8BR
    Right Ø8BQ
  Upper
    Left Ø8BP
    Right Ø8BN
Face ØWB2
Fallopian Tube
  Left ØUB6
  Right ØUB5
Fallopian Tubes, Bilateral ØUB7
Femoral Region
  Left ØYB8
  Right ØYB7
Femoral Shaft
  Left ØQB9
  Right ØQB8
Femur
  Lower
    Left ØQBC
    Right ØQBB
  Upper
    Left ØQB7
    Right ØQB6
Fibula
  Left ØQBK
  Right ØQBJ
Finger Nail ØHBQXZ
Floor of mouth *see* Excision, Oral Cavity and Throat
  ØWB3
Foot
  Left ØYBN
  Right ØYBM
Gallbladder ØFB4
Gingiva
  Lower ØCB6
  Upper ØCB5
Gland
  Adrenal
    Bilateral ØGB4
    Left ØGB2
    Right ØGB3
  Lacrimal
    Left Ø8BW
    Right Ø8BV
  Minor Salivary ØCBJ
  Parotid
    Left ØCB9
    Right ØCB8
  Pituitary ØGBØ
  Sublingual
    Left ØCBF
    Right ØCBD
  Submaxillary
    Left ØCBH
    Right ØCBG
  Vestibular ØUBL
Glenoid Cavity
  Left ØPB8
  Right ØPB7
Glomus Jugulare ØGBC
Hand
  Left ØXBK
  Right ØXBJ
Head ØWBØ
Humeral Head
  Left ØPBD
  Right ØPBC
Humeral Shaft
  Left ØPBG
  Right ØPBF
Hymen ØUBK
Hypothalamus ØØBA
Ileocecal Valve ØDBC

Excision — *continued*
Ileum ØDBB
Inguinal Region
  Left ØYB6
  Right ØYB5
Intestine
  Large ØDBE
    Left ØDBG
    Right ØDBF
  Small ØDB8
Iris
  Left Ø8BD3Z
  Right Ø8BC3Z
Jaw
  Lower ØWB5
  Upper ØWB4
Jejunum ØDBA
Joint
  Acromioclavicular
    Left ØRBH
    Right ØRBG
  Ankle
    Left ØSBG
    Right ØSBF
  Carpal
    Left ØRBR
    Right ØRBQ
  Carpometacarpal
    Left ØRBT
    Right ØRBS
  Cervical Vertebral ØRB1
  Cervicothoracic Vertebral ØRB4
  Coccygeal ØSB6
  Elbow
    Left ØRBM
    Right ØRBL
  Finger Phalangeal
    Left ØRBX
    Right ØRBW
  Hip
    Left ØSBB
    Right ØSB9
  Knee
    Left ØSBD
    Right ØSBC
  Lumbar Vertebral ØSBØ
  Lumbosacral ØSB3
  Metacarpophalangeal
    Left ØRBV
    Right ØRBU
  Metatarsal-Phalangeal
    Left ØSBN
    Right ØSBM
  Occipital-cervical ØRBØ
  Sacrococcygeal ØSB5
  Sacroiliac
    Left ØSB8
    Right ØSB7
  Shoulder
    Left ØRBK
    Right ØRBJ
  Sternoclavicular
    Left ØRBF
    Right ØRBE
  Tarsal
    Left ØSBJ
    Right ØSBH
  Tarsometatarsal
    Left ØSBL
    Right ØSBK
  Temporomandibular
    Left ØRBD
    Right ØRBC
  Thoracic Vertebral ØRB6
  Thoracolumbar Vertebral ØRBA
  Toe Phalangeal
    Left ØSBQ
    Right ØSBP
  Wrist
    Left ØRBP
    Right ØRBN
Kidney
  Left ØTB1
  Right ØTBØ
Kidney Pelvis
  Left ØTB4
  Right ØTB3
Knee Region
  Left ØYBG

Excision — *continued*
  Knee Region — *continued*
    Right 0YBF
  Larynx 0CBS
  Leg
    Lower
      Left 0YBJ
      Right 0YBH
    Upper
      Left 0YBD
      Right 0YBC
  Lens
    Left 08BK3Z
    Right 08BJ3Z
  Lip
    Lower 0CB1
    Upper 0CB0
  Liver 0FB0
    Left Lobe 0FB2
    Right Lobe 0FB1
  Lung
    Bilateral 0BBM
    Left 0BBL
    Lower Lobe
      Left 0BBJ
      Right 0BBF
    Middle Lobe, Right 0BBD
    Right 0BBK
    Upper Lobe
      Left 0BBG
      Right 0BBC
  Lung Lingula 0BBH
  Lymphatic
    Aortic 07BD
    Axillary
      Left 07B6
      Right 07B5
    Head 07B0
    Inguinal
      Left 07BJ
      Right 07BH
    Internal Mammary
      Left 07B9
      Right 07B8
    Lower Extremity
      Left 07BG
      Right 07BF
    Mesenteric 07BB
    Neck
      Left 07B2
      Right 07B1
    Pelvis 07BC
    Thoracic Duct 07BK
    Thorax 07B7
    Upper Extremity
      Left 07B4
      Right 07B3
  Mandible
    Left 0NBV
    Right 0NBT
  Maxilla 0NBR
  Mediastinum 0WBC
  Medulla Oblongata 00BD
  Mesentery 0DBV
  Metacarpal
    Left 0PBQ
    Right 0PBP
  Metatarsal
    Left 0QBP
    Right 0QBN
  Muscle
    Abdomen
      Left 0KBL
      Right 0KBK
    Extraocular
      Left 08BM
      Right 08BL
    Facial 0KB1
    Foot
      Left 0KBW
      Right 0KBV
    Hand
      Left 0KBD
      Right 0KBC
    Head 0KB0
    Hip
      Left 0KBP
      Right 0KBN

Excision — *continued*
  Muscle — *continued*
    Lower Arm and Wrist
      Left 0KBB
      Right 0KB9
    Lower Leg
      Left 0KBT
      Right 0KBS
    Neck
      Left 0KB3
      Right 0KB2
    Papillary 02BD
    Perineum 0KBM
    Shoulder
      Left 0KB6
      Right 0KB5
    Thorax
      Left 0KBJ
      Right 0KBH
    Tongue, Palate, Pharynx 0KB4
    Trunk
      Left 0KBG
      Right 0KBF
    Upper Arm
      Left 0KB8
      Right 0KB7
    Upper Leg
      Left 0KBR
      Right 0KBQ
  Nasal Mucosa and Soft Tissue 09BK
  Nasopharynx 09BN
  Neck 0WB6
  Nerve
    Abdominal Sympathetic 01BM
    Abducens 00BL
    Accessory 00BR
    Acoustic 00BN
    Brachial Plexus 01B3
    Cervical 01B1
    Cervical Plexus 01B0
    Facial 00BM
    Femoral 01BD
    Glossopharyngeal 00BP
    Head and Neck Sympathetic 01BK
    Hypoglossal 00BS
    Lumbar 01BB
    Lumbar Plexus 01B9
    Lumbar Sympathetic 01BN
    Lumbosacral Plexus 01BA
    Median 01B5
    Oculomotor 00BH
    Olfactory 00BF
    Optic 00BG
    Peroneal 01BH
    Phrenic 01B2
    Pudendal 01BC
    Radial 01B6
    Sacral 01BR
    Sacral Plexus 01BQ
    Sacral Sympathetic 01BP
    Sciatic 01BF
    Thoracic 01B8
    Thoracic Sympathetic 01BL
    Tibial 01BG
    Trigeminal 00BK
    Trochlear 00BJ
    Ulnar 01B4
    Vagus 00BQ
  Nipple
    Left 0HBX
    Right 0HBW
  Omentum 0DBU
  Oral Cavity and Throat 0WB3
  Orbit
    Left 0NBQ
    Right 0NBP
  Ovary
    Bilateral 0UB2
    Left 0UB1
    Right 0UB0
  Palate
    Hard 0CB2
    Soft 0CB3
  Pancreas 0FBG
  Para-aortic Body 0GB9
  Paraganglion Extremity 0GBF
  Parathyroid Gland 0GBR
    Inferior
      Left 0GBP

Excision — *continued*
  Parathyroid Gland — *continued*
    Inferior — *continued*
      Right 0GBN
    Multiple 0GBQ
    Superior
      Left 0GBM
      Right 0GBL
  Patella
    Left 0QBF
    Right 0QBD
  Penis 0VBS
  Pericardium 02BN
  Perineum
    Female 0WBN
    Male 0WBM
  Peritoneum 0DBW
  Phalanx
    Finger
      Left 0PBV
      Right 0PBT
    Thumb
      Left 0PBS
      Right 0PBR
    Toe
      Left 0QBR
      Right 0QBQ
  Pharynx 0CBM
  Pineal Body 0GB1
  Pleura
    Left 0BBP
    Right 0BBN
  Pons 00BB
  Prepuce 0VBT
  Prostate 0VB0
  Radius
    Left 0PBJ
    Right 0PBH
  Rectum 0DBP
  Retina
    Left 08BF3Z
    Right 08BE3Z
  Retroperitoneum 0WBH
  Ribs
    1 to 2 0PB1
    3 or More 0PB2
  Sacrum 0QB1
  Scapula
    Left 0PB6
    Right 0PB5
  Sclera
    Left 08B7XZ
    Right 08B6XZ
  Scrotum 0VB5
  Septum
    Atrial 02B5
    Nasal 09BM
    Ventricular 02BM
  Shoulder Region
    Left 0XB3
    Right 0XB2
  Sinus
    Accessory 09BP
    Ethmoid
      Left 09BV
      Right 09BU
    Frontal
      Left 09BT
      Right 09BS
    Mastoid
      Left 09BC
      Right 09BB
    Maxillary
      Left 09BR
      Right 09BQ
    Sphenoid
      Left 09BX
      Right 09BW
  Skin
    Abdomen 0HB7XZ
    Back 0HB6XZ
    Buttock 0HB8XZ
    Chest 0HB5XZ
    Ear
      Left 0HB3XZ
      Right 0HB2XZ
    Face 0HB1XZ
    Foot
      Left 0HBNXZ

Excision — *continued*
  Skin — *continued*
    Foot — *continued*
      Right 0HBMXZ
    Hand
      Left 0HBGXZ
      Right 0HBFXZ
    Inguinal 0HBAXZ
    Lower Arm
      Left 0HBEXZ
      Right 0HBDXZ
    Lower Leg
      Left 0HBLXZ
      Right 0HBKXZ
    Neck 0HB4XZ
    Perineum 0HB9XZ
    Scalp 0HB0XZ
    Upper Arm
      Left 0HBCXZ
      Right 0HBBXZ
    Upper Leg
      Left 0HBJXZ
      Right 0HBHXZ
  Skull 0NB0
  Spinal Cord
    Cervical 00BW
    Lumbar 00BY
    Thoracic 00BX
  Spinal Meninges 00BT
  Spleen 07BP
  Sternum 0PB0
  Stomach 0DB6
    Pylorus 0DB7
  Subcutaneous Tissue and Fascia
    Abdomen 0JB8
    Back 0JB7
    Buttock 0JB9
    Chest 0JB6
    Face 0JB1
    Foot
      Left 0JBR
      Right 0JBQ
    Hand
      Left 0JBK
      Right 0JBJ
    Lower Arm
      Left 0JBH
      Right 0JBG
    Lower Leg
      Left 0JBP
      Right 0JBN
    Neck
      Left 0JB5
      Right 0JB4
    Pelvic Region 0JBC
    Perineum 0JBB
    Scalp 0JB0
    Upper Arm
      Left 0JBF
      Right 0JBD
    Upper Leg
      Left 0JBM
      Right 0JBL
  Tarsal
    Left 0QBM
    Right 0QBL
  Tendon
    Abdomen
      Left 0LBG
      Right 0LBF
    Ankle
      Left 0LBT
      Right 0LBS
    Foot
      Left 0LBW
      Right 0LBV
    Hand
      Left 0LB8
      Right 0LB7
    Head and Neck 0LB0
    Hip
      Left 0LBK
      Right 0LBJ
    Knee
      Left 0LBR
      Right 0LBQ
    Lower Arm and Wrist
      Left 0LB6
      Right 0LB5

Excision — *continued*
  Tendon — *continued*
    Lower Leg
      Left 0LBP
      Right 0LBN
    Perineum 0LBH
    Shoulder
      Left 0LB2
      Right 0LB1
    Thorax
      Left 0LBD
      Right 0LBC
    Trunk
      Left 0LBB
      Right 0LB9
    Upper Arm
      Left 0LB4
      Right 0LB3
    Upper Leg
      Left 0LBM
      Right 0LBL
  Testis
    Bilateral 0VBC
    Left 0VBB
    Right 0VB9
  Thalamus 00B9
  Thymus 07BM
  Thyroid Gland
    Left Lobe 0GBG
    Right Lobe 0GBH
  Thyroid Gland Isthmus 0GBJ
  Tibia
    Left 0QBH
    Right 0QBG
  Toe Nail 0HBRXZ
  Tongue 0CB7
  Tonsils 0CBP
  Tooth
    Lower 0CBX
    Upper 0CBW
  Trachea 0BB1
  Tunica Vaginalis
    Left 0VB7
    Right 0VB6
  Turbinate, Nasal 09BL
  Tympanic Membrane
    Left 09B8
    Right 09B7
  Ulna
    Left 0PBL
    Right 0PBK
  Ureter
    Left 0TB7
    Right 0TB6
  Urethra 0TBD
  Uterine Supporting Structure 0UB4
  Uterus 0UB9
  Uvula 0CBN
  Vagina 0UBG
  Valve
    Aortic 02BF
    Mitral 02BG
    Pulmonary 02BH
    Tricuspid 02BJ
  Vas Deferens
    Bilateral 0VBQ
    Left 0VBP
    Right 0VBN
  Vein
    Axillary
      Left 05B8
      Right 05B7
    Azygos 05B0
    Basilic
      Left 05BC
      Right 05BB
    Brachial
      Left 05BA
      Right 05B9
    Cephalic
      Left 05BF
      Right 05BD
    Colic 06B7
    Common Iliac
      Left 06BD
      Right 06BC
    Coronary 02B4
    Esophageal 06B3

Excision — *continued*
  Vein — *continued*
    External Iliac
      Left 06BG
      Right 06BF
    External Jugular
      Left 05BQ
      Right 05BP
    Face
      Left 05BV
      Right 05BT
    Femoral
      Left 06BN
      Right 06BM
    Foot
      Left 06BV
      Right 06BT
    Gastric 06B2
    Hand
      Left 05BH
      Right 05BG
    Hemiazygos 05B1
    Hepatic 06B4
    Hypogastric
      Left 06BJ
      Right 06BH
    Inferior Mesenteric 06B6
    Innominate
      Left 05B4
      Right 05B3
    Internal Jugular
      Left 05BN
      Right 05BM
    Intracranial 05BL
    Lower 06BY
    Portal 06B8
    Pulmonary
      Left 02BT
      Right 02BS
    Renal
      Left 06BB
      Right 06B9
    Saphenous
      Left 06BQ
      Right 06BP
    Splenic 06B1
    Subclavian
      Left 05B6
      Right 05B5
    Superior Mesenteric 06B5
    Upper 05BY
    Vertebral
      Left 05BS
      Right 05BR
  Vena Cava
    Inferior 06B0
    Superior 02BV
  Ventricle
    Left 02BL
    Right 02BK
  Vertebra
    Cervical 0PB3
    Lumbar 0QB0
    Thoracic 0PB4
  Vesicle
    Bilateral 0VB3
    Left 0VB2
    Right 0VB1
  Vitreous
    Left 08B53Z
    Right 08B43Z
  Vocal Cord
    Left 0CBV
    Right 0CBT
  Vulva 0UBM
  Wrist Region
    Left 0XBH
    Right 0XBG
EXCLUDER® AAA Endoprosthesis
  use Intraluminal Device
  use Intraluminal Device, Branched or Fenestrated, One or Two Arteries in 04V
  use Intraluminal Device, Branched or Fenestrated, Three or More Arteries in 04V
EXCLUDER® IBE Endoprosthesis *use* Intraluminal Device, Branched or Fenestrated, One or Two Arteries in 04V
Exclusion, Left atrial appendage (LAA) *see* Occlusion, Atrium, Left 02L7

Exercise, rehabilitation see Motor Treatment, Rehabilitation F07
Exploration see Inspection
Express® Biliary SD Monorail® Premounted Stent System use Intraluminal Device
Express® (LD) Premounted Stent System use Intraluminal Device
Express® SD Renal Monorail® Premounted Stent System use Intraluminal Device
Ex-PRESS™ mini glaucoma shunt use Synthetic Substitute
Extensor carpi radialis muscle
　use Lower Arm and Wrist Muscle, Left
　use Lower Arm and Wrist Muscle, Right
Extensor carpi ulnaris muscle
　use Lower Arm and Wrist Muscle, Left
　use Lower Arm and Wrist Muscle, Right
Extensor digitorum brevis muscle
　use Foot Muscle, Left
　use Foot Muscle, Right
Extensor digitorum longus muscle
　use Lower Leg Muscle, Left
　use Lower Leg Muscle, Right
Extensor hallucis brevis muscle
　use Foot Muscle, Left
　use Foot Muscle, Right
Extensor hallucis longus muscle
　use Lower Leg Muscle, Left
　use Lower Leg Muscle, Right
External anal sphincter use Anal Sphincter
External auditory meatus
　use External Auditory Canal, Left
　use External Auditory Canal, Right
External fixator
　use External Fixation Device in Head and Facial Bones
　use External Fixation Device in Lower Bones
　use External Fixation Device in Lower Joints
　use External Fixation Device in Upper Bones
　use External Fixation Device in Upper Joints
External maxillary artery use Face Artery
External naris use Nasal Mucosa and Soft Tissue
External oblique aponeurosis use Subcutaneous Tissue and Fascia, Trunk
External oblique muscle
　use Abdomen Muscle, Left
　use Abdomen Muscle, Right
External popliteal nerve use Peroneal Nerve
External pudendal artery
　use Femoral Artery, Left
　use Femoral Artery, Right
External pudendal vein
　use Saphenous Vein, Left
　use Saphenous Vein, Right
External urethral sphincter use Urethra
Extirpation
　Acetabulum
　　Left 0QC5
　　Right 0QC4
　Adenoids 0CCQ
　Ampulla of Vater 0FCC
　Anal Sphincter 0DCR
　Anterior Chamber
　　Left 08C3
　　Right 08C2
　Anus 0DCQ
　Aorta
　　Abdominal 04C0
　　Thoracic
　　　Ascending/Arch 02CX
　　　Descending 02CW
　Aortic Body 0GCD
　Appendix 0DCJ
　Artery
　　Anterior Tibial
　　　Left 04CQ
　　　Right 04CP
　　Axillary
　　　Left 03C6
　　　Right 03C5
　　Brachial
　　　Left 03C8
　　　Right 03C7
　　Celiac 04C1
　　Colic
　　　Left 04C7
　　　Middle 04C8

Extirpation — continued
　Artery — continued
　　Colic — continued
　　　Right 04C6
　　Common Carotid
　　　Left 03CJ
　　　Right 03CH
　　Common Iliac
　　　Left 04CD
　　　Right 04CC
　　Coronary
　　　Four or More Arteries 02C3
　　　One Artery 02C0
　　　Three Arteries 02C2
　　　Two Arteries 02C1
　　External Carotid
　　　Left 03CN
　　　Right 03CM
　　External Iliac
　　　Left 04CJ
　　　Right 04CH
　　Face 03CR
　　Femoral
　　　Left 04CL
　　　Right 04CK
　　Foot
　　　Left 04CW
　　　Right 04CV
　　Gastric 04C2
　　Hand
　　　Left 03CF
　　　Right 03CD
　　Hepatic 04C3
　　Inferior Mesenteric 04CB
　　Innominate 03C2
　　Internal Carotid
　　　Left 03CL
　　　Right 03CK
　　Internal Iliac
　　　Left 04CF
　　　Right 04CE
　　Internal Mammary
　　　Left 03C1
　　　Right 03C0
　　Intracranial 03CG
　　Lower 04CY
　　Peroneal
　　　Left 04CU
　　　Right 04CT
　　Popliteal
　　　Left 04CN
　　　Right 04CM
　　Posterior Tibial
　　　Left 04CS
　　　Right 04CR
　　Pulmonary
　　　Left 02CR
　　　Right 02CQ
　　Pulmonary Trunk 02CP
　　Radial
　　　Left 03CC
　　　Right 03CB
　　Renal
　　　Left 04CA
　　　Right 04C9
　　Splenic 04C4
　　Subclavian
　　　Left 03C4
　　　Right 03C3
　　Superior Mesenteric 04C5
　　Temporal
　　　Left 03CT
　　　Right 03CS
　　Thyroid
　　　Left 03CV
　　　Right 03CU
　　Ulnar
　　　Left 03CA
　　　Right 03C9
　　Upper 03CY
　　Vertebral
　　　Left 03CQ
　　　Right 03CP
　Atrium
　　Left 02C7
　　Right 02C6
　Auditory Ossicle
　　Left 09CA
　　Right 09C9

Extirpation — continued
　Basal Ganglia 00C8
　Bladder 0TCB
　Bladder Neck 0TCC
　Bone
　　Ethmoid
　　　Left 0NCG
　　　Right 0NCF
　　Frontal 0NC1
　　Hyoid 0NCX
　　Lacrimal
　　　Left 0NCJ
　　　Right 0NCH
　　Nasal 0NCB
　　Occipital 0NC7
　　Palatine
　　　Left 0NCL
　　　Right 0NCK
　　Parietal
　　　Left 0NC4
　　　Right 0NC3
　　Pelvic
　　　Left 0QC3
　　　Right 0QC2
　　Sphenoid 0NCC
　　Temporal
　　　Left 0NC6
　　　Right 0NC5
　　Zygomatic
　　　Left 0NCN
　　　Right 0NCM
　Brain 00C0
　Breast
　　Bilateral 0HCV
　　Left 0HCU
　　Right 0HCT
　Bronchus
　　Lingula 0BC9
　　Lower Lobe
　　　Left 0BCB
　　　Right 0BC6
　　Main
　　　Left 0BC7
　　　Right 0BC3
　　Middle Lobe, Right 0BC5
　　Upper Lobe
　　　Left 0BC8
　　　Right 0BC4
　Buccal Mucosa 0CC4
　Bursa and Ligament
　　Abdomen
　　　Left 0MCJ
　　　Right 0MCH
　　Ankle
　　　Left 0MCR
　　　Right 0MCQ
　　Elbow
　　　Left 0MC4
　　　Right 0MC3
　　Foot
　　　Left 0MCT
　　　Right 0MCS
　　Hand
　　　Left 0MC8
　　　Right 0MC7
　　Head and Neck 0MC0
　　Hip
　　　Left 0MCM
　　　Right 0MCL
　　Knee
　　　Left 0MCP
　　　Right 0MCN
　　Lower Extremity
　　　Left 0MCW
　　　Right 0MCV
　　Perineum 0MCK
　　Rib(s) 0MCG
　　Shoulder
　　　Left 0MC2
　　　Right 0MC1
　　Spine
　　　Lower 0MCD
　　　Upper 0MCC
　　Sternum 0MCF
　　Upper Extremity
　　　Left 0MCB
　　　Right 0MC9
　　Wrist
　　　Left 0MC6

Extirpation — *continued*
  Bursa and Ligament — *continued*
    Wrist — *continued*
      Right ØMC5
  Carina ØBC2
  Carotid Bodies, Bilateral ØGC8
  Carotid Body
    Left ØGC6
    Right ØGC7
  Carpal
    Left ØPCN
    Right ØPCM
  Cavity, Cranial ØWC1
  Cecum ØDCH
  Cerebellum ØØCC
  Cerebral Hemisphere ØØC7
  Cerebral Meninges ØØC1
  Cerebral Ventricle ØØC6
  Cervix ØUCC
  Chordae Tendineae Ø2C9
  Choroid
    Left Ø8CB
    Right Ø8CA
  Cisterna Chyli Ø7CL
  Clavicle
    Left ØPCB
    Right ØPC9
  Clitoris ØUCJ
  Coccygeal Glomus ØGCB
  Coccyx ØQCS
  Colon
    Ascending ØDCK
    Descending ØDCM
    Sigmoid ØDCN
    Transverse ØDCL
  Computer-aided Mechanical Aspiration X2C
  Conduction Mechanism Ø2C8
  Conjunctiva
    Left Ø8CTXZZ
    Right Ø8CSXZZ
  Cord
    Bilateral ØVCH
    Left ØVCG
    Right ØVCF
  Cornea
    Left Ø8C9XZZ
    Right Ø8C8XZZ
  Cul-de-sac ØUCF
  Diaphragm ØBCT
  Disc
    Cervical Vertebral ØRC3
    Cervicothoracic Vertebral ØRC5
    Lumbar Vertebral ØSC2
    Lumbosacral ØSC4
    Thoracic Vertebral ØRC9
    Thoracolumbar Vertebral ØRCB
  Duct
    Common Bile ØFC9
    Cystic ØFC8
    Hepatic
      Common ØFC7
      Left ØFC6
      Right ØFC5
    Lacrimal
      Left Ø8CY
      Right Ø8CX
    Pancreatic ØFCD
      Accessory ØFCF
    Parotid
      Left ØCCC
      Right ØCCB
  Duodenum ØDC9
  Dura Mater ØØC2
  Ear
    External
      Left Ø9C1
      Right Ø9CØ
    External Auditory Canal
      Left Ø9C4
      Right Ø9C3
    Inner
      Left Ø9CE
      Right Ø9CD
    Middle
      Left Ø9C6
      Right Ø9C5
  Endometrium ØUCB
  Epididymis
    Bilateral ØVCL

Extirpation — *continued*
  Epididymis — *continued*
    Left ØVCK
    Right ØVCJ
  Epidural Space, Intracranial ØØC3
  Epiglottis ØCCR
  Esophagogastric Junction ØDC4
  Esophagus ØDC5
    Lower ØDC3
    Middle ØDC2
    Upper ØDC1
  Eustachian Tube
    Left Ø9CG
    Right Ø9CF
  Eye
    Left Ø8C1XZZ
    Right Ø8CØXZZ
  Eyelid
    Lower
      Left Ø8CR
      Right Ø8CQ
    Upper
      Left Ø8CP
      Right Ø8CN
  Fallopian Tube
    Left ØUC6
    Right ØUC5
  Fallopian Tubes, Bilateral ØUC7
  Femoral Shaft
    Left ØQC9
    Right ØQC8
  Femur
    Lower
      Left ØQCC
      Right ØQCB
    Upper
      Left ØQC7
      Right ØQC6
  Fibula
    Left ØQCK
    Right ØQCJ
  Finger Nail ØHCQXZZ
  Gallbladder ØFC4
  Gastrointestinal Tract ØWCP
  Genitourinary Tract ØWCR
  Gingiva
    Lower ØCC6
    Upper ØCC5
  Gland
    Adrenal
      Bilateral ØGC4
      Left ØGC2
      Right ØGC3
    Lacrimal
      Left Ø8CW
      Right Ø8CV
    Minor Salivary ØCCJ
    Parotid
      Left ØCC9
      Right ØCC8
    Pituitary ØGCØ
    Sublingual
      Left ØCCF
      Right ØCCD
    Submaxillary
      Left ØCCH
      Right ØCCG
    Vestibular ØUCL
  Glenoid Cavity
    Left ØPC8
    Right ØPC7
  Glomus Jugulare ØGCC
  Humeral Head
    Left ØPCD
    Right ØPCC
  Humeral Shaft
    Left ØPCG
    Right ØPCF
  Hymen ØUCK
  Hypothalamus ØØCA
  Ileocecal Valve ØDCC
  Ileum ØDCB
  Intestine
    Large ØDCE
      Left ØDCG
      Right ØDCF
    Small ØDC8
  Iris
    Left Ø8CD

Extirpation — *continued*
  Iris — *continued*
    Right Ø8CC
  Jaw
    Lower ØWC5
    Upper ØWC4
  Jejunum ØDCA
  Joint
    Acromioclavicular
      Left ØRCH
      Right ØRCG
    Ankle
      Left ØSCG
      Right ØSCF
    Carpal
      Left ØRCR
      Right ØRCQ
    Carpometacarpal
      Left ØRCT
      Right ØRCS
    Cervical Vertebral ØRC1
    Cervicothoracic Vertebral ØRC4
    Coccygeal ØSC6
    Elbow
      Left ØRCM
      Right ØRCL
    Finger Phalangeal
      Left ØRCX
      Right ØRCW
    Hip
      Left ØSCB
      Right ØSC9
    Knee
      Left ØSCD
      Right ØSCC
    Lumbar Vertebral ØSCØ
    Lumbosacral ØSC3
    Metacarpophalangeal
      Left ØRCV
      Right ØRCU
    Metatarsal-Phalangeal
      Left ØSCN
      Right ØSCM
    Occipital-cervical ØRCØ
    Sacrococcygeal ØSC5
    Sacroiliac
      Left ØSC8
      Right ØSC7
    Shoulder
      Left ØRCK
      Right ØRCJ
    Sternoclavicular
      Left ØRCF
      Right ØRCE
    Tarsal
      Left ØSCJ
      Right ØSCH
    Tarsometatarsal
      Left ØSCL
      Right ØSCK
    Temporomandibular
      Left ØRCD
      Right ØRCC
    Thoracic Vertebral ØRC6
    Thoracolumbar Vertebral ØRCA
    Toe Phalangeal
      Left ØSCQ
      Right ØSCP
    Wrist
      Left ØRCP
      Right ØRCN
  Kidney
    Left ØTC1
    Right ØTCØ
  Kidney Pelvis
    Left ØTC4
    Right ØTC3
  Larynx ØCCS
  Lens
    Left Ø8CK
    Right Ø8CJ
  Lip
    Lower ØCC1
    Upper ØCCØ
  Liver ØFCØ
    Left Lobe ØFC2
    Right Lobe ØFC1
  Lung
    Bilateral ØBCM

▼ **Subterms under main terms may continue to next column or page**

Extirpation — continued
  Lung — continued
    Left 0BCL
    Lower Lobe
      Left 0BCJ
      Right 0BCF
    Middle Lobe, Right 0BCD
    Right 0BCK
    Upper Lobe
      Left 0BCG
      Right 0BCC
  Lung Lingula 0BCH
  Lymphatic
    Aortic 07CD
    Axillary
      Left 07C6
      Right 07C5
    Head 07C0
    Inguinal
      Left 07CJ
      Right 07CH
    Internal Mammary
      Left 07C9
      Right 07C8
    Lower Extremity
      Left 07CG
      Right 07CF
    Mesenteric 07CB
    Neck
      Left 07C2
      Right 07C1
    Pelvis 07CC
    Thoracic Duct 07CK
    Thorax 07C7
    Upper Extremity
      Left 07C4
      Right 07C3
  Mandible
    Left 0NCV
    Right 0NCT
  Maxilla 0NCR
  Mediastinum 0WCC
  Medulla Oblongata 00CD
  Mesentery 0DCV
  Metacarpal
    Left 0PCQ
    Right 0PCP
  Metatarsal
    Left 0QCP
    Right 0QCN
  Muscle
    Abdomen
      Left 0KCL
      Right 0KCK
    Extraocular
      Left 08CM
      Right 08CL
    Facial 0KC1
    Foot
      Left 0KCW
      Right 0KCV
    Hand
      Left 0KCD
      Right 0KCC
    Head 0KC0
    Hip
      Left 0KCP
      Right 0KCN
    Lower Arm and Wrist
      Left 0KCB
      Right 0KC9
    Lower Leg
      Left 0KCT
      Right 0KCS
    Neck
      Left 0KC3
      Right 0KC2
    Papillary 02CD
    Perineum 0KCM
    Shoulder
      Left 0KC6
      Right 0KC5
    Thorax
      Left 0KCJ
      Right 0KCH
    Tongue, Palate, Pharynx 0KC4
    Trunk
      Left 0KCG
      Right 0KCF

Extirpation — continued
  Muscle — continued
    Upper Arm
      Left 0KC8
      Right 0KC7
    Upper Leg
      Left 0KCR
      Right 0KCQ
  Nasal Mucosa and Soft Tissue 09CK
  Nasopharynx 09CN
  Nerve
    Abdominal Sympathetic 01CM
    Abducens 00CL
    Accessory 00CR
    Acoustic 00CN
    Brachial Plexus 01C3
    Cervical 01C1
    Cervical Plexus 01C0
    Facial 00CM
    Femoral 01CD
    Glossopharyngeal 00CP
    Head and Neck Sympathetic 01CK
    Hypoglossal 00CS
    Lumbar 01CB
    Lumbar Plexus 01C9
    Lumbar Sympathetic 01CN
    Lumbosacral Plexus 01CA
    Median 01C5
    Oculomotor 00CH
    Olfactory 00CF
    Optic 00CG
    Peroneal 01CH
    Phrenic 01C2
    Pudendal 01CC
    Radial 01C6
    Sacral 01CR
    Sacral Plexus 01CQ
    Sacral Sympathetic 01CP
    Sciatic 01CF
    Thoracic 01C8
    Thoracic Sympathetic 01CL
    Tibial 01CG
    Trigeminal 00CK
    Trochlear 00CJ
    Ulnar 01C4
    Vagus 00CQ
  Nipple
    Left 0HCX
    Right 0HCW
  Omentum 0DCU
  Oral Cavity and Throat 0WC3
  Orbit
    Left 0NCQ
    Right 0NCP
  Orbital Atherectomy see Extirpation, Heart and
      Great Vessels 02C
  Ovary
    Bilateral 0UC2
    Left 0UC1
    Right 0UC0
  Palate
    Hard 0CC2
    Soft 0CC3
  Pancreas 0FCG
  Para-aortic Body 0GC9
  Paraganglion Extremity 0GCF
  Parathyroid Gland 0GCR
    Inferior
      Left 0GCP
      Right 0GCN
    Multiple 0GCQ
    Superior
      Left 0GCM
      Right 0GCL
  Patella
    Left 0QCF
    Right 0QCD
  Pelvic Cavity 0WCJ
  Penis 0VCS
  Pericardial Cavity 0WCD
  Pericardium 02CN
  Peritoneal Cavity 0WCG
  Peritoneum 0DCW
  Phalanx
    Finger
      Left 0PCV
      Right 0PCT
    Thumb
      Left 0PCS

Extirpation — continued
  Phalanx — continued
    Thumb — continued
      Right 0PCR
    Toe
      Left 0QCR
      Right 0QCQ
  Pharynx 0CCM
  Pineal Body 0GC1
  Pleura
    Left 0BCP
    Right 0BCN
  Pleural Cavity
    Left 0WCB
    Right 0WC9
  Pons 00CB
  Prepuce 0VCT
  Prostate 0VC0
  Radius
    Left 0PCJ
    Right 0PCH
  Rectum 0DCP
  Respiratory Tract 0WCQ
  Retina
    Left 08CF
    Right 08CE
  Retinal Vessel
    Left 08CH
    Right 08CG
  Retroperitoneum 0WCH
  Ribs
    1 to 2 0PC1
    3 or More 0PC2
  Sacrum 0QC1
  Scapula
    Left 0PC6
    Right 0PC5
  Sclera
    Left 08C7XZZ
    Right 08C6XZZ
  Scrotum 0VC5
  Septum
    Atrial 02C5
    Nasal 09CM
    Ventricular 02CM
  Sinus
    Accessory 09CP
    Ethmoid
      Left 09CV
      Right 09CU
    Frontal
      Left 09CT
      Right 09CS
    Mastoid
      Left 09CC
      Right 09CB
    Maxillary
      Left 09CR
      Right 09CQ
    Sphenoid
      Left 09CX
      Right 09CW
  Skin
    Abdomen 0HC7XZZ
    Back 0HC6XZZ
    Buttock 0HC8XZZ
    Chest 0HC5XZZ
    Ear
      Left 0HC3XZZ
      Right 0HC2XZZ
    Face 0HC1XZZ
    Foot
      Left 0HCNXZZ
      Right 0HCMXZZ
    Hand
      Left 0HCGXZZ
      Right 0HCFXZZ
    Inguinal 0HCAXZZ
    Lower Arm
      Left 0HCEXZZ
      Right 0HCDXZZ
    Lower Leg
      Left 0HCLXZZ
      Right 0HCKXZZ
    Neck 0HC4XZZ
    Perineum 0HC9XZZ
    Scalp 0HC0XZZ
    Upper Arm
      Left 0HCCXZZ

Extirpation — *continued*
  Skin — *continued*
    Upper Arm — *continued*
      Right 0HCBXZZ
    Upper Leg
      Left 0HCJXZZ
      Right 0HCHXZZ
  Spinal Canal 00CU
  Spinal Cord
    Cervical 00CW
    Lumbar 00CY
    Thoracic 00CX
  Spinal Meninges 00CT
  Spleen 07CP
  Sternum 0PC0
  Stomach 0DC6
    Pylorus 0DC7
  Subarachnoid Space, Intracranial 00C5
  Subcutaneous Tissue and Fascia
    Abdomen 0JC8
    Back 0JC7
    Buttock 0JC9
    Chest 0JC6
    Face 0JC1
    Foot
      Left 0JCR
      Right 0JCQ
    Hand
      Left 0JCK
      Right 0JCJ
    Lower Arm
      Left 0JCH
      Right 0JCG
    Lower Leg
      Left 0JCP
      Right 0JCN
    Neck
      Left 0JC5
      Right 0JC4
    Pelvic Region 0JCC
    Perineum 0JCB
    Scalp 0JC0
    Upper Arm
      Left 0JCF
      Right 0JCD
    Upper Leg
      Left 0JCM
      Right 0JCL
  Subdural Space, Intracranial 00C4
  Tarsal
    Left 0QCM
    Right 0QCL
  Tendon
    Abdomen
      Left 0LCG
      Right 0LCF
    Ankle
      Left 0LCT
      Right 0LCS
    Foot
      Left 0LCW
      Right 0LCV
    Hand
      Left 0LC8
      Right 0LC7
    Head and Neck 0LC0
    Hip
      Left 0LCK
      Right 0LCJ
    Knee
      Left 0LCR
      Right 0LCQ
    Lower Arm and Wrist
      Left 0LC6
      Right 0LC5
    Lower Leg
      Left 0LCP
      Right 0LCN
    Perineum 0LCH
    Shoulder
      Left 0LC2
      Right 0LC1
    Thorax
      Left 0LCD
      Right 0LCC
    Trunk
      Left 0LCB
      Right 0LC9

Extirpation — *continued*
  Tendon — *continued*
    Upper Arm
      Left 0LC4
      Right 0LC3
    Upper Leg
      Left 0LCM
      Right 0LCL
  Testis
    Bilateral 0VCC
    Left 0VCB
    Right 0VC9
  Thalamus 00C9
  Thymus 07CM
  Thyroid Gland 0GCK
    Left Lobe 0GCG
    Right Lobe 0GCH
  Tibia
    Left 0QCH
    Right 0QCG
  Toe Nail 0HCRXZZ
  Tongue 0CC7
  Tonsils 0CCP
  Tooth
    Lower 0CCX
    Upper 0CCW
  Trachea 0BC1
  Tunica Vaginalis
    Left 0VC7
    Right 0VC6
  Turbinate, Nasal 09CL
  Tympanic Membrane
    Left 09C8
    Right 09C7
  Ulna
    Left 0PCL
    Right 0PCK
  Ureter
    Left 0TC7
    Right 0TC6
  Urethra 0TCD
  Uterine Supporting Structure 0UC4
  Uterus 0UC9
  Uvula 0CCN
  Vagina 0UCG
  Valve
    Aortic 02CF
    Mitral 02CG
    Pulmonary 02CH
    Tricuspid 02CJ
  Vas Deferens
    Bilateral 0VCQ
    Left 0VCP
    Right 0VCN
  Vein
    Axillary
      Left 05C8
      Right 05C7
    Azygos 05C0
    Basilic
      Left 05CC
      Right 05CB
    Brachial
      Left 05CA
      Right 05C9
    Cephalic
      Left 05CF
      Right 05CD
    Colic 06C7
    Common Iliac
      Left 06CD
      Right 06CC
    Coronary 02C4
    Esophageal 06C3
    External Iliac
      Left 06CG
      Right 06CF
    External Jugular
      Left 05CQ
      Right 05CP
    Face
      Left 05CV
      Right 05CT
    Femoral
      Left 06CN
      Right 06CM
    Foot
      Left 06CV
      Right 06CT

Extirpation — *continued*
  Vein — *continued*
    Gastric 06C2
    Hand
      Left 05CH
      Right 05CG
    Hemiazygos 05C1
    Hepatic 06C4
    Hypogastric
      Left 06CJ
      Right 06CH
    Inferior Mesenteric 06C6
    Innominate
      Left 05C4
      Right 05C3
    Internal Jugular
      Left 05CN
      Right 05CM
    Intracranial 05CL
    Lower 06CY
    Portal 06C8
    Pulmonary
      Left 02CT
      Right 02CS
    Renal
      Left 06CB
      Right 06C9
    Saphenous
      Left 06CQ
      Right 06CP
    Splenic 06C1
    Subclavian
      Left 05C6
      Right 05C5
    Superior Mesenteric 06C5
    Upper 05CY
    Vertebral
      Left 05CS
      Right 05CR
  Vena Cava
    Inferior 06C0
    Superior 02CV
  Ventricle
    Left 02CL
    Right 02CK
  Vertebra
    Cervical 0PC3
    Lumbar 0QC0
    Thoracic 0PC4
  Vesicle
    Bilateral 0VC3
    Left 0VC2
    Right 0VC1
  Vitreous
    Left 08C5
    Right 08C4
  Vocal Cord
    Left 0CCV
    Right 0CCT
  Vulva 0UCM

Extracorporeal Carbon Dioxide Removal (ECCO2R) 5A0920Z

Extracorporeal shock wave lithotripsy *see* Fragmentation

Extracranial-intracranial bypass (EC-IC) *see* Bypass, Upper Arteries 031

Extraction
  Acetabulum
    Left 0QD50ZZ
    Right 0QD40ZZ
  Ampulla of Vater 0FDC
  Anus 0DDQ
  Appendix 0DDJ
  Auditory Ossicle
    Left 09DA0ZZ
    Right 09D90ZZ
  Bone
    Ethmoid
      Left 0NDG0ZZ
      Right 0NDF0ZZ
    Frontal 0ND10ZZ
    Hyoid 0NDX0ZZ
    Lacrimal
      Left 0NDJ0ZZ
      Right 0NDH0ZZ
    Nasal 0NDB0ZZ
    Occipital 0ND70ZZ
    Palatine
      Left 0NDL0ZZ

▼ **Subterms under main terms may continue to next column or page**

Extraction — continued
Bone — continued
Palatine — continued
Right 0NDK0ZZ
Parietal
Left 0ND40ZZ
Right 0ND30ZZ
Pelvic
Left 0QD30ZZ
Right 0QD20ZZ
Sphenoid 0NDC0ZZ
Temporal
Left 0ND60ZZ
Right 0ND50ZZ
Zygomatic
Left 0NDN0ZZ
Right 0NDM0ZZ
Bone Marrow 07DT
Iliac 07DR
Sternum 07DQ
Vertebral 07DS
Brain 00D0
Breast
Bilateral 0HDV0ZZ
Left 0HDU0ZZ
Right 0HDT0ZZ
Supernumerary 0HDY0ZZ
Bronchus
Lingula 0BD9
Lower Lobe
Left 0BDB
Right 0BD6
Main
Left 0BD7
Right 0BD3
Middle Lobe, Right 0BD5
Upper Lobe
Left 0BD8
Right 0BD4
Bursa and Ligament
Abdomen
Left 0MDJ
Right 0MDH
Ankle
Left 0MDR
Right 0MDQ
Elbow
Left 0MD4
Right 0MD3
Foot
Left 0MDT
Right 0MDS
Hand
Left 0MD8
Right 0MD7
Head and Neck 0MD0
Hip
Left 0MDM
Right 0MDL
Knee
Left 0MDP
Right 0MDN
Lower Extremity
Left 0MDW
Right 0MDV
Perineum 0MDK
Rib(s) 0MDG
Shoulder
Left 0MD2
Right 0MD1
Spine
Lower 0MDD
Upper 0MDC
Sternum 0MDF
Upper Extremity
Left 0MDB
Right 0MD9
Wrist
Left 0MD6
Right 0MD5
Carina 0BD2
Carpal
Left 0PDN0ZZ
Right 0PDM0ZZ
Cecum 0DDH
Cerebellum 00DC
Cerebral Hemisphere 00D7
Cerebral Meninges 00D1
Cisterna Chyli 07DL

Extraction — continued
Clavicle
Left 0PDB0ZZ
Right 0PD90ZZ
Coccyx 0QDS0ZZ
Colon
Ascending 0DDK
Descending 0DDM
Sigmoid 0DDN
Transverse 0DDL
Cornea
Left 08D9XZ
Right 08D8XZ
Duct
Common Bile 0FD9
Cystic 0FD8
Hepatic
Common 0FD7
Left 0FD6
Right 0FD5
Pancreatic 0FDD
Accessory 0FDF
Duodenum 0DD9
Dura Mater 00D2
Endometrium 0UDB
Esophagogastric Junction 0DD4
Esophagus 0DD5
Lower 0DD3
Middle 0DD2
Upper 0DD1
Femoral Shaft
Left 0QD90ZZ
Right 0QD80ZZ
Femur
Lower
Left 0QDC0ZZ
Right 0QDB0ZZ
Upper
Left 0QD70ZZ
Right 0QD60ZZ
Fibula
Left 0QDK0ZZ
Right 0QDJ0ZZ
Finger Nail 0HDQXZZ
Gallbladder 0FD4
Glenoid Cavity
Left 0PD80ZZ
Right 0PD70ZZ
Hair 0HDSXZZ
Humeral Head
Left 0PDD0ZZ
Right 0PDC0ZZ
Humeral Shaft
Left 0PDG0ZZ
Right 0PDF0ZZ
Ileocecal Valve 0DDC
Ileum 0DDB
Intestine
Large 0DDE
Left 0DDG
Right 0DDF
Small 0DD8
Jejunum 0DDA
Kidney
Left 0TD1
Right 0TD0
Lens
Left 08DK3ZZ
Right 08DJ3ZZ
Liver 0FD0
Left Lobe 0FD2
Right Lobe 0FD1
Lung
Bilateral 0BDM
Left 0BDL
Lower Lobe
Left 0BDJ
Right 0BDF
Middle Lobe, Right 0BDD
Right 0BDK
Upper Lobe
Left 0BDG
Right 0BDC
Lung Lingula 0BDH
Lymphatic
Aortic 07DD
Axillary
Left 07D6
Right 07D5

Extraction — continued
Lymphatic — continued
Head 07D0
Inguinal
Left 07DJ
Right 07DH
Internal Mammary
Left 07D9
Right 07D8
Lower Extremity
Left 07DG
Right 07DF
Mesenteric 07DB
Neck
Left 07D2
Right 07D1
Pelvis 07DC
Thoracic Duct 07DK
Thorax 07D7
Upper Extremity
Left 07D4
Right 07D3
Mandible
Left 0NDV0ZZ
Right 0NDT0ZZ
Maxilla 0NDR0ZZ
Metacarpal
Left 0PDQ0ZZ
Right 0PDP0ZZ
Metatarsal
Left 0QDP0ZZ
Right 0QDN0ZZ
Muscle
Abdomen
Left 0KDL0ZZ
Right 0KDK0ZZ
Facial 0KD10ZZ
Foot
Left 0KDW0ZZ
Right 0KDV0ZZ
Hand
Left 0KDD0ZZ
Right 0KDC0ZZ
Head 0KD00ZZ
Hip
Left 0KDP0ZZ
Right 0KDN0ZZ
Lower Arm and Wrist
Left 0KDB0ZZ
Right 0KD90ZZ
Lower Leg
Left 0KDT0ZZ
Right 0KDS0ZZ
Neck
Left 0KD30ZZ
Right 0KD20ZZ
Perineum 0KDM0ZZ
Shoulder
Left 0KD60ZZ
Right 0KD50ZZ
Thorax
Left 0KDJ0ZZ
Right 0KDH0ZZ
Tongue, Palate, Pharynx 0KD40ZZ
Trunk
Left 0KDG0ZZ
Right 0KDF0ZZ
Upper Arm
Left 0KD80ZZ
Right 0KD70ZZ
Upper Leg
Left 0KDR0ZZ
Right 0KDQ0ZZ
Nerve
Abdominal Sympathetic 01DM
Abducens 00DL
Accessory 00DR
Acoustic 00DN
Brachial Plexus 01D3
Cervical 01D1
Cervical Plexus 01D0
Facial 00DM
Femoral 01DD
Glossopharyngeal 00DP
Head and Neck Sympathetic 01DK
Hypoglossal 00DS
Lumbar 01DB
Lumbar Plexus 01D9
Lumbar Sympathetic 01DN

Extraction — *continued*
  Nerve — *continued*
    Lumbosacral Plexus 01DA
    Median 01D5
    Oculomotor 00DH
    Olfactory 00DF
    Optic 00DG
    Peroneal 01DH
    Phrenic 01D2
    Pudendal 01DC
    Radial 01D6
    Sacral 01DR
    Sacral Plexus 01DQ
    Sacral Sympathetic 01DP
    Sciatic 01DF
    Thoracic 01D8
    Thoracic Sympathetic 01DL
    Tibial 01DG
    Trigeminal 00DK
    Trochlear 00DJ
    Ulnar 01D4
    Vagus 00DQ
  Orbit
    Left 0NDQ0ZZ
    Right 0NDP0ZZ
  Ova 0UDN
  Pancreas 0FDG
  Patella
    Left 0QDF0ZZ
    Right 0QDD0ZZ
  Phalanx
    Finger
      Left 0PDV0ZZ
      Right 0PDT0ZZ
    Thumb
      Left 0PDS0ZZ
      Right 0PDR0ZZ
    Toe
      Left 0QDR0ZZ
      Right 0QDQ0ZZ
  Pleura
    Left 0BDP
    Right 0BDN
  Products of Conception
    Ectopic 10D2
    Extraperitoneal 10D00Z2
    High 10D00Z0
    High Forceps 10D07Z5
    Internal Version 10D07Z7
    Low 10D00Z1
    Low Forceps 10D07Z3
    Mid Forceps 10D07Z4
    Other 10D07Z8
    Retained 10D1
    Vacuum 10D07Z6
  Radius
    Left 0PDJ0ZZ
    Right 0PDH0ZZ
  Rectum 0DDP
  Ribs
    1 to 2 0PD10ZZ
    3 or More 0PD20ZZ
  Sacrum 0QD10ZZ
  Scapula
    Left 0PD60ZZ
    Right 0PD50ZZ
  Septum, Nasal 09DM
  Sinus
    Accessory 09DP
    Ethmoid
      Left 09DV
      Right 09DU
    Frontal
      Left 09DT
      Right 09DS
    Mastoid
      Left 09DC
      Right 09DB
    Maxillary
      Left 09DR
      Right 09DQ
    Sphenoid
      Left 09DX
      Right 09DW
  Skin
    Abdomen 0HD7XZZ
    Back 0HD6XZZ
    Buttock 0HD8XZZ
    Chest 0HD5XZZ

Extraction — *continued*
  Skin — *continued*
    Ear
      Left 0HD3XZZ
      Right 0HD2XZZ
    Face 0HD1XZZ
    Foot
      Left 0HDNXZZ
      Right 0HDMXZZ
    Hand
      Left 0HDGXZZ
      Right 0HDFXZZ
    Inguinal 0HDAXZZ
    Lower Arm
      Left 0HDEXZZ
      Right 0HDDXZZ
    Lower Leg
      Left 0HDLXZZ
      Right 0HDKXZZ
    Neck 0HD4XZZ
    Perineum 0HD9XZZ
    Scalp 0HD0XZZ
    Upper Arm
      Left 0HDCXZZ
      Right 0HDBXZZ
    Upper Leg
      Left 0HDJXZZ
      Right 0HDHXZZ
  Skull 0ND00ZZ
  Spinal Meninges 00DT
  Spleen 07DP
  Sternum 0PD00ZZ
  Stomach 0DD6
    Pylorus 0DD7
  Subcutaneous Tissue and Fascia
    Abdomen 0JD8
    Back 0JD7
    Buttock 0JD9
    Chest 0JD6
    Face 0JD1
    Foot
      Left 0JDR
      Right 0JDQ
    Hand
      Left 0JDK
      Right 0JDJ
    Lower Arm
      Left 0JDH
      Right 0JDG
    Lower Leg
      Left 0JDP
      Right 0JDN
    Neck
      Left 0JD5
      Right 0JD4
    Pelvic Region 0JDC
    Perineum 0JDB
    Scalp 0JD0
    Upper Arm
      Left 0JDF
      Right 0JDD
    Upper Leg
      Left 0JDM
      Right 0JDL
  Tarsal
    Left 0QDM0ZZ
    Right 0QDL0ZZ
  Tendon
    Abdomen
      Left 0LDG0ZZ
      Right 0LDF0ZZ
    Ankle
      Left 0LDT0ZZ
      Right 0LDS0ZZ
    Foot
      Left 0LDW0ZZ
      Right 0LDV0ZZ
    Hand
      Left 0LD80ZZ
      Right 0LD70ZZ
    Head and Neck 0LD00ZZ
    Hip
      Left 0LDK0ZZ
      Right 0LDJ0ZZ
    Knee
      Left 0LDR0ZZ
      Right 0LDQ0ZZ
    Lower Arm and Wrist
      Left 0LD60ZZ

Extraction — *continued*
  Tendon — *continued*
    Lower Arm and Wrist — *continued*
      Right 0LD50ZZ
    Lower Leg
      Left 0LDP0ZZ
      Right 0LDN0ZZ
    Perineum 0LDH0ZZ
    Shoulder
      Left 0LD20ZZ
      Right 0LD10ZZ
    Thorax
      Left 0LDD0ZZ
      Right 0LDC0ZZ
    Trunk
      Left 0LDB0ZZ
      Right 0LD90ZZ
    Upper Arm
      Left 0LD40ZZ
      Right 0LD30ZZ
    Upper Leg
      Left 0LDM0ZZ
      Right 0DLL0ZZ
  Thymus 07DM
  Tibia
    Left 0QDH0ZZ
    Right 0QDG0ZZ
  Toe Nail 0HDRXZZ
  Tooth
    Lower 0CDXXZ
    Upper 0CDWXZ
  Trachea 0BD1
  Turbinate, Nasal 09DL
  Tympanic Membrane
    Left 09D8
    Right 09D7
  Ulna
    Left 0PDL0ZZ
    Right 0PDK0ZZ
  Vein
    Basilic
      Left 05DC
      Right 05DB
    Brachial
      Left 05DA
      Right 05D9
    Cephalic
      Left 05DF
      Right 05DD
    Femoral
      Left 06DN
      Right 06DM
    Foot
      Left 06DV
      Right 06DT
    Hand
      Left 05DH
      Right 05DG
    Lower 06DY
    Saphenous
      Left 06DQ
      Right 06DP
    Upper 05DY
  Vertebra
    Cervical 0PD30ZZ
    Lumbar 0QD00ZZ
    Thoracic 0PD40ZZ
  Vocal Cord
    Left 0CDV
    Right 0CDT

Extradural space, intracranial *use* Epidural Space, Intracranial
Extradural space, spinal *use* Spinal Canal
EXtreme Lateral Interbody Fusion (XLIF) device
  use Interbody Fusion Device in Lower Joints

F

Face lift *see* Alteration, Face 0W02
Facet replacement spinal stabilization device
  use Spinal Stabilization Device, Facet Replacement in 0RH
  use Spinal Stabilization Device, Facet Replacement in 0SH
Facial artery *use* Face Artery
Factor Xa Inhibitor Reversal Agent, Andexanet Alfa *use* Coagulation Factor Xa, Inactivated
False vocal cord *use* Larynx

Falx cerebri *use* Dura Mater
Fascia lata
    use Subcutaneous Tissue and Fascia, Left Upper Leg
    use Subcutaneous Tissue and Fascia, Right Upper Leg
Fasciaplasty, fascioplasty
    see Repair, Subcutaneous Tissue and Fascia ØJQ
    see Replacement, Subcutaneous Tissue and Fascia ØJR
Fasciectomy *see* Excision, Subcutaneous Tissue and Fascia ØJB
Fasciorrhaphy *see* Repair, Subcutaneous Tissue and Fascia ØJQ
Fasciotomy
    see Division, Subcutaneous Tissue and Fascia ØJ8
    see Drainage, Subcutaneous Tissue and Fascia ØJ9
    see Release
Feeding Device
    Change device in
        Lower Intestinal Tract ØD2DXUZ
        Upper Intestinal Tract ØD20XUZ
    Insertion of device in
        Duodenum ØDH9
        Esophagus ØDH5
        Ileum ØDHB
        Intestine, Small ØDH8
        Jejunum ØDHA
        Stomach ØDH6
    Removal of device from
        Esophagus ØDP5
        Intestinal Tract
            Lower Intestinal Tract ØDPD
            Upper Intestinal Tract ØDPØ
        Stomach ØDP6
    Revision of device in
        Intestinal Tract
            Lower Intestinal Tract ØDWD
            Upper Intestinal Tract ØDWØ
        Stomach ØDW6
        Upper Intestinal Tract ØDWØ
Femoral head
    use Upper Femur, Left
    use Upper Femur, Right
Femoral lymph node
    use Lymphatic, Left Lower Extremity
    use Lymphatic, Right Lower Extremity
Femoropatellar joint
    use Knee Joint, Left
    use Knee Joint, Left, Tibial Surface
    use Knee Joint, Right
    use Knee Joint, Right, Femoral Surface
Femorotibial joint
    use Knee Joint, Left
    use Knee Joint, Left, Tibial Surface
    use Knee Joint, Right
    use Knee Joint, Right, Tibial Surface
FETROJA® *use* Cefiderocol Anti-infective
FGS (fluorescence-guided surgery) *see* Fluorescence Guided Procedure
Fibular artery
    use Peroneal Artery, Left
    use Peroneal Artery, Right
Fibular sesamoid
    use Metatarsal, Left
    use Metatarsal, Right
Fibularis brevis muscle
    use Lower Leg Muscle, Left
    use Lower Leg Muscle, Right
Fibularis longus muscle
    use Lower Leg Muscle, Left
    use Lower Leg Muscle, Right
Fifth cranial nerve *use* Trigeminal Nerve
Filum terminale *use* Spinal Meninges
Fimbriectomy
    see Excision, Female Reproductive System ØUB
    see Resection, Female Reproductive System ØUT
Fine needle aspiration
    Fluid or gas *see* Drainage
    Tissue biopsy
        see Excision
        see Extraction
First cranial nerve *use* Olfactory Nerve
First intercostal nerve *use* Brachial Plexus
Fistulization
    see Bypass
    see Drainage

Fistulization — *continued*
    see Repair
Fitting
    Arch bars, for fracture reduction *see* Reposition, Mouth and Throat ØCS
    Arch bars, for immobilization *see* Immobilization, Face 2W31
    Artificial limb *see* Device Fitting, Rehabilitation FØD
    Hearing aid *see* Device Fitting, Rehabilitation FØD
    Ocular prosthesis FØDZ8UZ
    Prosthesis, limb *see* Device Fitting, Rehabilitation FØD
    Prosthesis, ocular FØDZ8UZ
Fixation, bone
    External, with fracture reduction *see* Reposition
    External, without fracture reduction *see* Insertion
    Internal, with fracture reduction *see* Reposition
    Internal, without fracture reduction *see* Insertion
FLAIR® Endovascular Stent Graft *use* Intraluminal Device
Flexible Composite Mesh *use* Synthetic Substitute
Flexor carpi radialis muscle
    use Lower Arm and Wrist Muscle, Left
    use Lower Arm and Wrist Muscle, Right
Flexor carpi ulnaris muscle
    use Lower Arm and Wrist Muscle, Left
    use Lower Arm and Wrist Muscle, Right
Flexor digitorum brevis muscle
    use Foot Muscle, Left
    use Foot Muscle, Right
Flexor digitorum longus muscle
    use Lower Leg Muscle, Left
    use Lower Leg Muscle, Right
Flexor hallucis brevis muscle
    use Foot Muscle, Left
    use Foot Muscle, Right
Flexor hallucis longus muscle
    use Lower Leg Muscle, Left
    use Lower Leg Muscle, Right
Flexor pollicis longus muscle
    use Lower Arm and Wrist Muscle, Left
    use Lower Arm and Wrist Muscle, Right
Flow Diverter embolization device *use* Intraluminal Device, Flow Diverter in Ø3V
FlowSense Noninvasive Thermal Sensor 4BØØXWØ
Fluorescence Guided Procedure
    Extremity
        Lower 8EØY
        Upper 8EØX
    Head and Neck Region 8EØ9
        Aminolevulinic Acid 8EØ90EM
        No Qualifier 8EØ90EZ
    Trunk Region 8EØW
Fluorescent Pyrazine, Kidney XT25XE5
Fluoroscopy
    Abdomen and Pelvis BW11
    Airway, Upper BB1DZZZ
    Ankle
        Left BQ1H
        Right BQ1G
    Aorta
        Abdominal B41Ø
            Laser, Intraoperative B41Ø
        Thoracic B31Ø
            Laser, Intraoperative B31Ø
        Thoraco-Abdominal B31P
            Laser, Intraoperative B31P
    Aorta and Bilateral Lower Extremity Arteries B41D
        Laser, Intraoperative B41D
    Arm
        Left BP1FZZZ
        Right BP1EZZZ
    Artery
        Brachiocephalic-Subclavian
            Laser, Intraoperative B311
            Right B311
        Bronchial B31L
            Laser, Intraoperative B31L
        Bypass Graft, Other B21F
        Cervico-Cerebral Arch B31Q
            Laser, Intraoperative B31Q
        Common Carotid
            Bilateral B315
               Laser, Intraoperative B315
            Left B314
               Laser, Intraoperative B314

Fluoroscopy — *continued*
    Artery — *continued*
        Common Carotid — *continued*
            Right B313
               Laser, Intraoperative B313
        Coronary
            Bypass Graft
               Multiple B213
                  Laser, Intraoperative B213
               Single B212
                  Laser, Intraoperative B212
            Multiple B211
               Laser, Intraoperative B211
            Single B21Ø
               Laser, Intraoperative B21Ø
        External Carotid
            Bilateral B31C
               Laser, Intraoperative B31C
            Left B31B
               Laser, Intraoperative B31B
            Right B319
               Laser, Intraoperative B319
        Hepatic B412
            Laser, Intraoperative B412
        Inferior Mesenteric B415
            Laser, Intraoperative B415
        Intercostal B31L
            Laser, Intraoperative B31L
        Internal Carotid
            Bilateral B318
               Laser, Intraoperative B318
            Left B317
               Laser, Intraoperative B317
            Right B316
               Laser, Intraoperative B316
        Internal Mammary Bypass Graft
            Left B218
            Right B217
        Intra-Abdominal
            Laser, Intraoperative B41B
            Other B41B
        Intracranial B31R
            Laser, Intraoperative B31R
        Lower
            Laser, Intraoperative B41J
            Other B41J
        Lower Extremity
            Bilateral and Aorta B41D
               Laser, Intraoperative B41D
            Left B41G
               Laser, Intraoperative B41G
            Right B41F
               Laser, Intraoperative B41F
        Lumbar B419
            Laser, Intraoperative B419
        Pelvic B41C
            Laser, Intraoperative B41C
        Pulmonary
            Left B31T
               Laser, Intraoperative B31T
            Right B31S
               Laser, Intraoperative B31S
        Pulmonary Trunk B31U
            Laser, Intraoperative B31U
        Renal
            Bilateral B418
               Laser, Intraoperative B418
            Left B417
               Laser, Intraoperative B417
            Right B416
               Laser, Intraoperative B416
        Spinal B31M
            Laser, Intraoperative B31M
        Splenic B413
            Laser, Intraoperative B413
        Subclavian
            Laser, Intraoperative B312
            Left B312
        Superior Mesenteric B414
            Laser, Intraoperative B414
        Upper
            Laser, Intraoperative B31N
            Other B31N
        Upper Extremity
            Bilateral B31K
               Laser, Intraoperative B31K
            Left B31J
               Laser, Intraoperative B31J
            Right B31H

Fluoroscopy — *continued*
Artery — *continued*
Upper Extremity — *continued*
Right — *continued*
Laser, Intraoperative B31H
Vertebral
Bilateral B31G
Laser, Intraoperative B31G
Left B31F
Laser, Intraoperative B31F
Right B31D
Laser, Intraoperative B31D
Bile Duct BF1Ø
Pancreatic Duct and Gallbladder BF14
Bile Duct and Gallbladder BF13
Biliary Duct BF11
Bladder BT1Ø
Kidney and Ureter BT14
Left BT1F
Right BT1D
Bladder and Urethra BT1B
Bowel, Small BD1
Calcaneus
Left BQ1KZZZ
Right BQ1JZZZ
Clavicle
Left BP15ZZZ
Right BP14ZZZ
Coccyx BR1F
Colon BD14
Corpora Cavernosa BV1Ø
Dialysis Fistula B51W
Dialysis Shunt B51W
Diaphragm BB16ZZZ
Disc
Cervical BR11
Lumbar BR13
Thoracic BR12
Duodenum BD19
Elbow
Left BP1H
Right BP1G
Epiglottis B91G
Esophagus BD11
Extremity
Lower BW1C
Upper BW1J
Facet Joint
Cervical BR14
Lumbar BR16
Thoracic BR15
Fallopian Tube
Bilateral BU12
Left BU11
Right BU1Ø
Fallopian Tube and Uterus BU18
Femur
Left BQ14ZZZ
Right BQ13ZZZ
Finger
Left BP1SZZZ
Right BP1RZZZ
Foot
Left BQ1MZZZ
Right BQ1LZZZ
Forearm
Left BP1KZZZ
Right BP1JZZZ
Gallbladder BF12
Bile Duct and Pancreatic Duct BF14
Gallbladder and Bile Duct BF13
Gastrointestinal, Upper BD1
Hand
Left BP1PZZZ
Right BP1NZZZ
Head and Neck BW19
Heart
Left B215
Right B214
Right and Left B216
Hip
Left BQ11
Right BQ1Ø
Humerus
Left BP1BZZZ
Right BP1AZZZ
Ileal Diversion Loop BT1C
Ileal Loop, Ureters and Kidney BT1G
Intracranial Sinus B512

Fluoroscopy — *continued*
Joint
Acromioclavicular, Bilateral BP13ZZZ
Finger
Left BP1D
Right BP1C
Foot
Left BQ1Y
Right BQ1X
Hand
Left BP1D
Right BP1C
Lumbosacral BR1B
Sacroiliac BR1D
Sternoclavicular
Bilateral BP12ZZZ
Left BP11ZZZ
Right BP1ØZZZ
Temporomandibular
Bilateral BN19
Left BN18
Right BN17
Thoracolumbar BR18
Toe
Left BQ1Y
Right BQ1X
Kidney
Bilateral BT13
Ileal Loop and Ureter BT1G
Left BT12
Right BT11
Ureter and Bladder BT14
Left BT1F
Right BT1D
Knee
Left BQ18
Right BQ17
Larynx B91J
Leg
Left BQ1FZZZ
Right BQ1DZZZ
Liver BF15
Lung
Bilateral BB14ZZZ
Left BB13ZZZ
Right BB12ZZZ
Mediastinum BB1CZZZ
Mouth BD1B
Neck and Head BW19
Oropharynx BD1B
Pancreatic Duct BF1
Gallbladder and Bile Buct BF14
Patella
Left BQ1WZZZ
Right BQ1VZZZ
Pelvis BR1C
Pelvis and Abdomen BW11
Pharynix B91G
Ribs
Left BP1YZZZ
Right BP1XZZZ
Sacrum BR1F
Scapula
Left BP17ZZZ
Right BP16ZZZ
Shoulder
Left BP19
Right BP18
Sinus, Intracranial B512
Spinal Cord BØ1B
Spine
Cervical BR1Ø
Lumbar BR19
Thoracic BR17
Whole BR1G
Sternum BR1H
Stomach BD12
Toe
Left BQ1QZZZ
Right BQ1PZZZ
Tracheobronchial Tree
Bilateral BB19YZZ
Left BB18YZZ
Right BB17YZZ
Ureter
Ileal Loop and Kidney BT1G
Kidney and Bladder BT14
Left BT1F
Right BT1D

Fluoroscopy — *continued*
Ureter — *continued*
Left BT17
Right BT16
Urethra BT15
Urethra and Bladder BT1B
Uterus BU16
Uterus and Fallopian Tube BU18
Vagina BU19
Vasa Vasorum BV18
Vein
Cerebellar B511
Cerebral B511
Epidural B51Ø
Jugular
Bilateral B515
Left B514
Right B513
Lower Extremity
Bilateral B51D
Left B51C
Right B51B
Other B51V
Pelvic (Iliac)
Left B51G
Right B51F
Pelvic (Iliac) Bilateral B51H
Portal B51T
Pulmonary
Bilateral B51S
Left B51R
Right B51Q
Renal
Bilateral B51L
Left B51K
Right B51J
Spanchnic B51T
Subclavian
Left B517
Right B516
Upper Extremity
Bilateral B51P
Left B51N
Right B51M
Vena Cava
Inferior B519
Superior B518
Wrist
Left BP1M
Right BP1L
Fluoroscopy, laser intraoperative
see Fluoroscopy, Heart B21
see Fluoroscopy, Lower Arteries B41
see Fluoroscopy, Upper Arteries B31
Flushing *see* Irrigation
Foley catheter *use* Drainage Device
Fontan completion procedure Stage II *see* Bypass, Vena Cava, Inferior Ø61Ø
Foramen magnum *use* Occipital Bone
Foramen of Monro (intraventricular) *use* Cerebral Ventricle
Foreskin *use* Prepuce
Formula™ Balloon-Expandable Renal Stent System *use* Intraluminal Device
Fosfomycin Anti-infective XWØ
Fosfomycin injection *use* Fosfomycin Anti-infective
Fossa of Rosenmuller *use* Nasopharynx
Fostamatinib XWØ
Fourth cranial nerve *use* Trochlear Nerve
Fourth ventricle *use* Cerebral Ventricle
Fovea
use Retina, Left
use Retina, Right
Fragmentation
Ampulla of Vater ØFFC
Anus ØDFQ
Appendix ØDFJ
Artery
Anterior Tibial
Left Ø4FQ3Z
Right Ø4FP3Z
Axillary
Left Ø3F63Z
Right Ø3F53Z
Brachial
Left Ø3F83Z
Right Ø3F73Z

Fragmentation — *continued*
  Artery — *continued*
    Common Iliac
      Left 04FD3Z
      Right 04FC3Z
    Coronary
      Four or More Arteries 02F33ZZ
      One Artery 02F03ZZ
      Three Arteries 02F23ZZ
      Two Arteries 02F13ZZ
    External Iliac
      Left 04FJ3Z
      Right 04FH3Z
    Femoral
      Left 04FL3Z
      Right 04FK3Z
    Innominate 03F23Z
    Internal Iliac
      Left 04FF3Z
      Right 04FE3Z
    Intracranial 03FG3Z
    Lower 04FY3Z
    Peroneal
      Left 04FU3Z
      Right 04FT3Z
    Popliteal
      Left 04FN3Z
      Right 04FM3Z
    Posterior Tibial
      Left 04FS3Z
      Right 04FR3Z
    Pulmonary
      Left 02FR3Z
      Right 02FQ3Z
    Pulmonary Trunk 02FP3Z
    Radial
      Left 03FC3Z
      Right 03FB3Z
    Subclavian
      Left 03F43Z
      Right 03F33Z
    Ulnar
      Left 03FA3Z
      Right 03F93Z
    Upper 03FY3Z
  Bladder 0TFB
  Bladder Neck 0TFC
  Bronchus
    Lingula 0BF9
    Lower Lobe
      Left 0BFB
      Right 0BF6
    Main
      Left 0BF7
      Right 0BF3
    Middle Lobe, Right 0BF5
    Upper Lobe
      Left 0BF8
      Right 0BF4
  Carina 0BF2
  Cavity, Cranial 0WF1
  Cecum 0DFH
  Cerebral Ventricle 00F6
  Colon
    Ascending 0DFK
    Descending 0DFM
    Sigmoid 0DFN
    Transverse 0DFL
  Duct
    Common Bile 0FF9
    Cystic 0FF8
    Hepatic
      Common 0FF7
      Left 0FF6
      Right 0FF5
    Pancreatic 0FFD
      Accessory 0FFF
    Parotid
      Left 0CFC
      Right 0CFB
  Duodenum 0DF9
  Epidural Space, Intracranial 00F3
  Esophagus 0DF5
  Fallopian Tube
    Left 0UF6
    Right 0UF5
  Fallopian Tubes, Bilateral 0UF7
  Gallbladder 0FF4
  Gastrointestinal Tract 0WFP

Fragmentation — *continued*
  Genitourinary Tract 0WFR
  Ileum 0DFB
  Intestine
    Large 0DFE
      Left 0DFG
      Right 0DFF
    Small 0DF8
  Jejunum 0DFA
  Kidney Pelvis
    Left 0TF4
    Right 0TF3
  Mediastinum 0WFC
  Oral Cavity and Throat 0WF3
  Pelvic Cavity 0WFJ
  Pericardial Cavity 0WFD
  Pericardium 02FN
  Peritoneal Cavity 0WFG
  Pleural Cavity
    Left 0WFB
    Right 0WF9
  Rectum 0DFP
  Respiratory Tract 0WFQ
  Spinal Canal 00FU
  Stomach 0DF6
  Subarachnoid Space, Intracranial 00F5
  Subdural Space, Intracranial 00F4
  Trachea 0BF1
  Ureter
    Left 0TF7
    Right 0TF6
  Urethra 0TFD
  Uterus 0UF9
  Vein
    Axillary
      Left 05F83Z
      Right 05F73Z
    Basilic
      Left 05FC3Z
      Right 05FB3Z
    Brachial
      Left 05FA3Z
      Right 05F93Z
    Cephalic
      Left 05FF3Z
      Right 05FD3Z
    Common Iliac
      Left 06FD3Z
      Right 06FC3Z
    External Iliac
      Left 06FG3Z
      Right 06FF3Z
    Femoral
      Left 06FN3Z
      Right 06FM3Z
    Hypogastric
      Left 06FJ3Z
      Right 06FH3Z
    Innominate
      Left 05F43Z
      Right 05F33Z
    Lower 06FY3Z
    Pulmonary
      Left 02FT3Z
      Right 02FS3Z
    Saphenous
      Left 06FQ3Z
      Right 06FP3Z
    Subclavian
      Left 05F63Z
      Right 05F53Z
    Upper 05FY3Z
  Vitreous
    Left 08F5
    Right 08F4
Fragmentation, Ultrasonic *see* Fragmentation, Artery
Freestyle (Stentless) Aortic Root Bioprosthesis *use* Zooplastic Tissue in Heart and Great Vessels
Frenectomy
  see Excision, Mouth and Throat 0CB
  see Resection, Mouth and Throat 0CT
Frenoplasty, frenuloplasty
  see Repair, Mouth and Throat 0CQ
  see Replacement, Mouth and Throat 0CR
  see Supplement, Mouth and Throat 0CU
Frenotomy
  see Drainage, Mouth and Throat 0C9
  see Release, Mouth and Throat 0CN

Frenulotomy
  see Drainage, Mouth and Throat 0C9
  see Release, Mouth and Throat 0CN
Frenulum labii inferioris *use* Lower Lip
Frenulum labii superioris *use* Upper Lip
Frenulum linguae *use* Tongue
Frenulumectomy
  see Excision, Mouth and Throat 0CB
  see Resection, Mouth and Throat 0CT
Frontal lobe *use* Cerebral Hemisphere
Frontal vein
  use Face Vein, Left
  use Face Vein, Right
Frozen elephant trunk (FET) technique, aortic arch replacement
  see New Technology, Cardiovascular System X2R
  see Replacement, Heart and Great Vessels 02R
Frozen elephant trunk (FET) technique, thoracic aorta restriction
  see New Technology, Cardiovascular System X2V
  see Restriction, Heart and Great Vessels 02V
FUJIFILM EP-7000X System for Oxygen Saturation Endoscopic Imaging (OXEI) *see* New Technology, Gastrointestinal System XD2
Fulguration *see* Destruction
Fundoplication, gastroesophageal *see* Restriction, Esophagogastric Junction 0DV4
Fundus uteri *use* Uterus
Fusion
  Acromioclavicular
    Left 0RGH
    Right 0RGG
  Ankle
    Left 0SGG
    Right 0SGF
  Carpal
    Left 0RGR
    Right 0RGQ
  Carpometacarpal
    Left 0RGT
    Right 0RGS
  Cervical Vertebral 0RG1
    2 or more 0RG2
  Cervicothoracic Vertebral 0RG4
  Coccygeal 0SG6
  Elbow
    Left 0RGM
    Right 0RGL
  Finger Phalangeal
    Left 0RGX
    Right 0RGW
  Hip
    Left 0SGB
    Right 0SG9
  Knee
    Left 0SGD
    Right 0SGC
  Lumbar Vertebral 0SG0
    2 or more 0SG1
      Interbody Fusion Device, Customizable XRGC
      Interbody Fusion Device, Customizable XRGB
  Lumbosacral 0SG3
    Interbody Fusion Device, Customizable XRGD
  Metacarpophalangeal
    Left 0RGV
    Right 0RGU
  Metatarsal-Phalangeal
    Left 0SGN
    Right 0SGM
  Occipital-cervical 0RG0
  Sacrococcygeal 0SG5
  Sacroiliac
    Internal Fixation Device with Tulip Connector XRG
    Left 0SG8
    Right 0SG7
  Shoulder
    Left 0RGK
    Right 0RGJ
  Sternoclavicular
    Left 0RGF
    Right 0RGE
  Tarsal
    Left 0SGJ
    Right 0SGH
  Tarsometatarsal
    Left 0SGL

Fusion — *continued*
Tarsometatarsal — *continued*
Right 0SGK
Temporomandibular
Left 0RGD
Right 0RGC
Thoracic Vertebral 0RG6
2 to 7 0RG7
8 or more 0RG8
Thoracolumbar Vertebral 0RGA
Interbody Fusion Device, Customizable XRGA
Toe Phalangeal
Left 0SGQ
Right 0SGP
Wrist
Left 0RGP
Right 0RGN
Fusion screw (compression) (lag) (locking)
use Internal Fixation Device in Lower Joints
use Internal Fixation Device in Upper Joints

G

Gait training *see* Motor Treatment, Rehabilitation F07
Galea aponeurotica *use* Subcutaneous Tissue and Fascia, Scalp
Gammaglobulin *use* Globulin
GammaTile™ *use* Radioactive Element, Cesium-131 Collagen Implant in 00H
GAMUNEX-C, for COVID-19 treatment *use* High-Dose Intravenous Immune Globulin
Ganglion impar (ganglion of Walther) *use* Sacral Sympathetic Nerve
Ganglionectomy
Destruction of lesion *see* Destruction
Excision of lesion *see* Excision
Gasserian ganglion *use* Trigeminal Nerve
Gastrectomy
Partial *see* Excision, Stomach 0DB6
Total *see* Resection, Stomach 0DT6
Vertical (sleeve) *see* Excision, Stomach 0DB6
Gastric electrical stimulation (GES) lead *use* Stimulator Lead in Gastrointestinal System
Gastric lymph node *use* Lymphatic, Aortic
Gastric pacemaker lead *use* Stimulator Lead in Gastrointestinal System
Gastric plexus *use* Abdominal Sympathetic Nerve
Gastrocnemius muscle
use Lower Leg Muscle, Left
use Lower Leg Muscle, Right
Gastrocolic ligament *use* Omentum
Gastrocolic omentum *use* Omentum
Gastrocolostomy
see Bypass, Gastrointestinal System 0D1
see Drainage, Gastrointestinal System 0D9
Gastroduodenal artery *use* Hepatic Artery
Gastroduodenectomy
see Excision, Gastrointestinal System 0DB
see Resection, Gastrointestinal System 0DT
Gastroduodenoscopy 0DJ08ZZ
Gastroenteroplasty
see Repair, Gastrointestinal System 0DQ
see Supplement, Gastrointestinal System 0DU
Gastroenterostomy
see Bypass, Gastrointestinal System 0D1
see Drainage, Gastrointestinal System 0D9
Gastroesophageal (GE) junction *use* Esophagogastric Junction
Gastrogastrostomy
see Bypass, Stomach 0D16
see Drainage, Stomach 0D96
Gastrohepatic omentum *use* Omentum
Gastrojejunostomy
see Bypass, Stomach 0D16
see Drainage, Stomach 0D96
Gastrolysis *see* Release, Stomach 0DN6
Gastropexy
see Repair, Stomach 0DQ6
see Reposition, Stomach 0DS6
Gastrophrenic ligament *use* Omentum
Gastroplasty
see Repair, Stomach 0DQ6
see Supplement, Stomach 0DU6
Gastroplication *see* Restriction, Stomach 0DV6
Gastropylorectomy *see* Excision, Gastrointestinal System 0DB

Gastrorrhaphy *see* Repair, Stomach 0DQ6
Gastroscopy 0DJ68ZZ
Gastrosplenic ligament *use* Omentum
Gastrostomy
see Bypass, Stomach 0D16
see Drainage, Stomach 0D96
Gastrotomy *see* Drainage, Stomach 0D96
Gemellus muscle
use Hip Muscle, Left
use Hip Muscle, Right
Geniculate ganglion *use* Facial Nerve
Geniculate nucleus *use* Thalamus
Genioglossus muscle *use* Tongue, Palate, Pharynx Muscle
Genioplasty *see* Alteration, Jaw, Lower 0W05
Genitofemoral nerve *use* Lumbar Plexus
GIAPREZA™ *use* Synthetic Human Angiotensin II
Gilteritinib Antineoplastic XW0DXV5
Gingivectomy *see* Excision, Mouth and Throat 0CB
Gingivoplasty
see Repair, Mouth and Throat 0CQ
see Replacement, Mouth and Throat 0CR
see Supplement, Mouth and Throat 0CU
Glans penis *use* Prepuce
Glenohumeral joint
use Shoulder Joint, Left
use Shoulder Joint, Right
Glenohumeral ligament
use Shoulder Bursa and Ligament, Left
use Shoulder Bursa and Ligament, Right
Glenoid fossa (of scapula)
use Glenoid Cavity, Left
use Glenoid Cavity, Right
Glenoid ligament (labrum)
use Shoulder Joint, Left
use Shoulder Joint, Right
Globus pallidus *use* Basal Ganglia
Glomectomy
see Excision, Endocrine System 0GB
see Resection, Endocrine System 0GT
Glossectomy
see Excision, Tongue 0CB7
see Resection, Tongue 0CT7
Glossoepiglottic fold *use* Epiglottis
Glossopexy
see Repair, Tongue 0CQ7
see Reposition, Tongue 0CS7
Glossoplasty
see Repair, Tongue 0CQ7
see Replacement, Tongue 0CR7
see Supplement, Tongue 0CU7
Glossorrhaphy *see* Repair, Tongue 0CQ7
Glossotomy *see* Drainage, Tongue 0C97
Glottis *use* Larynx
Gluteal Artery Perforator Flap
Replacement
Bilateral 0HRV079
Left 0HRU079
Right 0HRT079
Transfer
Left 0KXG
Right 0KXF
Gluteal lymph node *use* Lymphatic, Pelvis
Gluteal vein
use Hypogastric Vein, Left
use Hypogastric Vein, Right
Gluteus maximus muscle
use Hip Muscle, Left
use Hip Muscle, Right
Gluteus medius muscle
use Hip Muscle, Left
use Hip Muscle, Right
Gluteus minimus muscle
use Hip Muscle, Left
use Hip Muscle, Right
GORE EXCLUDER® AAA Endoprosthesis
use Intraluminal Device
use Intraluminal Device, Branched or Fenestrated, One or Two Arteries in 04V
use Intraluminal Device, Branched or Fenestrated, Three or More Arteries in 04V
GORE EXCLUDER® IBE Endoprosthesis *use* Intraluminal Device, Branched or Fenestrated, One or Two Arteries in 04V
GORE TAG® Thoracic Endoprosthesis *use* Intraluminal Device

GORE® DUALMESH® *use* Synthetic Substitute
Gracilis muscle
use Upper Leg Muscle, Left
use Upper Leg Muscle, Right
Graft
see Replacement
see Supplement
Great auricular nerve *use* Cervical Plexus
Great cerebral vein *use* Intracranial Vein
Great(er) saphenous vein
use Saphenous Vein, Left
use Saphenous Vein, Right
Greater alar cartilage *use* Nasal Mucosa and Soft Tissue
Greater occipital nerve *use* Cervical Nerve
Greater Omentum *use* Omentum
Greater splanchnic nerve *use* Thoracic Sympathetic Nerve
Greater superficial petrosal nerve *use* Facial Nerve
Greater trochanter
use Upper Femur, Left
use Upper Femur, Right
Greater tuberosity
use Humeral Head, Left
use Humeral Head, Right
Greater vestibular (Bartholin's) gland *use* Vestibular Gland
Greater wing *use* Sphenoid Bone
GS-5734 *use* Remdesivir Anti-infective
Guedel airway *use* Intraluminal Device, Airway in Mouth and Throat
Guidance, catheter placement
EKG *see* Measurement, Physiological Systems 4A0
Fluoroscopy *see* Fluoroscopy, Veins B51
Ultrasound *see* Ultrasonography, Veins B54

H

Hallux
use 1st Toe, Left
use 1st Toe, Right
Hamate bone
use Carpal, Left
use Carpal, Right
Hancock Bioprosthesis (aortic) (mitral) valve *use* Zooplastic Tissue in Heart and Great Vessels
Hancock Bioprosthetic Valved Conduit *use* Zooplastic Tissue in Heart and Great Vessels
Harmony™ transcatheter pulmonary valve (TPV) placement 02RH38M
Harvesting, Stem Cells *see* Pheresis, Circulatory 6A55
hdIVIG (high-dose intravenous immunoglobulin), for COVID-19 treatment *use* High-Dose Intravenous Immune Globulin
Head of fibula
use Fibula, Left
use Fibula, Right
Hearing Aid Assessment F14Z
Hearing Assessment F13Z
Hearing Device
Bone Conduction
Left 09HE
Right 09HD
Insertion of device in
Left 0NH6
Right 0NH5
Multiple Channel Cochlear Prosthesis
Left 09HE
Right 09HD
Removal of device from, Skull 0NP0
Revision of device in, Skull 0NW0
Single Channel Cochlear Prosthesis
Left 09HE
Right 09HD
Hearing Treatment F09Z
Heart Assist System
Implantable
Insertion of device in, Heart 02HA
Removal of device from, Heart 02PA
Revision of device in, Heart 02WA
Short-term External
Insertion of device in, Heart 02HA
Removal of device from, Heart 02PA
Revision of device in, Heart 02WA
HeartMate 3™ LVAS *use* Implantable Heart Assist System in Heart and Great Vessels

HeartMate II® Left Ventricular Assist Device (LVAD)
  use Implantable Heart Assist System in Heart and Great Vessels
HeartMate XVE® Left Ventricular Assist Device (LVAD) *use* Implantable Heart Assist System in Heart and Great Vessels
HeartMate® implantable heart assist system *see* Insertion of device in, Heart Ø2HA
Helix
  use Ear, External, Bilateral
  use Ear, External, Left
  use Ear, External, Right
Hematopoietic cell transplant (HCT) *see* Transfusion, Circulatory 3Ø2
Hemicolectomy *see* Resection, Gastrointestinal System ØDT
Hemicystectomy *see* Excision, Urinary System ØTB
Hemigastrectomy *see* Excision, Gastrointestinal System ØDB
Hemiglossectomy *see* Excision, Mouth and Throat ØCB
Hemilaminectomy
  see Excision, Lower Bones ØQB
  see Excision, Upper Bones ØPB
Hemilaminotomy
  see Drainage, Lower Bones ØQ9
  see Drainage, Upper Bones ØP9
  see Excision, Lower Bones ØQB
  see Excision, Upper Bones ØPB
  see Release, Central Nervous System and Cranial Nerves ØØN
  see Release, Lower Bones ØQN
  see Release, Peripheral Nervous System Ø1N
  see Release, Upper Bones ØPN
Hemilaryngectomy *see* Excision, Larynx ØCBS
Hemimandibulectomy *see* Excision, Head and Facial Bones ØNB
Hemimaxillectomy *see* Excision, Head and Facial Bones ØNB
Hemipylorectomy *see* Excision, Gastrointestinal System ØDB
Hemispherectomy
  see Excision, Central Nervous System and Cranial Nerves ØØB
  see Resection, Central Nervous System and Cranial Nerves ØØT
Hemithyroidectomy
  see Excision, Endocrine System ØGB
  see Resection, Endocrine System ØGT
Hemodialysis *see* Performance, Urinary 5A1D
Hemolung® Respiratory Assist System (RAS) 5AØ92ØZ
Hemospray® Endoscopic Hemostat *use* Mineral-based Topical Hemostatic Agent
Hepatectomy
  see Excision, Hepatobiliary System and Pancreas ØFB
  see Resection, Hepatobiliary System and Pancreas ØFT
Hepatic artery proper *use* Hepatic Artery
Hepatic flexure *use* Transverse Colon
Hepatic lymph node *use* Lymphatic, Aortic
Hepatic plexus *use* Abdominal Sympathetic Nerve
Hepatic portal vein *use* Portal Vein
Hepaticoduodenostomy
  see Bypass, Hepatobiliary System and Pancreas ØF1
  see Drainage, Hepatobiliary System and Pancreas ØF9
Hepaticotomy *see* Drainage, Hepatobiliary System and Pancreas ØF9
Hepatocholedochostomy *see* Drainage, Duct, Common Bile ØF99
Hepatogastric ligament *use* Omentum
Hepatopancreatic ampulla *use* Ampulla of Vater
Hepatopexy
  see Repair, Hepatobiliary System and Pancreas ØFQ
  see Reposition, Hepatobiliary System and Pancreas ØFS
Hepatorrhaphy *see* Repair, Hepatobiliary System and Pancreas ØFQ
Hepatotomy *see* Drainage, Hepatobiliary System and Pancreas ØF9
Herculink (RX) Elite Renal Stent System *use* Intraluminal Device
Herniorrhaphy
  see Repair, Anatomical Regions, General ØWQ

Herniorrhaphy — *continued*
  see Repair, Anatomical Regions, Lower Extremities ØYQ
  With synthetic substitute
    see Supplement, Anatomical Regions, General ØWU
    see Supplement, Anatomical Regions, Lower Extremities ØYU
HIG (hyperimmune globulin), for COVID-19 treatment *use* Hyperimmune Globulin
High-Dose Intravenous Immune Globulin, for COVID-19 treatment XW1
High-dose intravenous immunoglobulin (hdIVIG), for COVID-19 treatment *use* High-Dose Intravenous Immune Globulin
Hip (joint) liner *use* Liner in Lower Joints
HIPEC (hyperthermic intraperitoneal chemotherapy) 3EØM3ØY
HistoSonics® System *see* New Technology, Hepatobiliary System and Pancreas XF5
Histotripsy, liver *see* New Technology, Hepatobiliary System and Pancreas XF5
hIVIG (hyperimmune intravenous immunoglobulin), for COVID-19 treatment *use* Hyperimmune Globulin
Holter Monitoring 4A12X45
Holter valve ventricular shunt *use* Synthetic Substitute
Human angiotensin II, synthetic *use* Synthetic Human Angiotensin II
Humeroradial joint
  use Elbow Joint, Left
  use Elbow Joint, Right
Humeroulnar joint
  use Elbow Joint, Left
  use Elbow Joint, Right
Humerus, distal
  use Humeral Shaft, Left
  use Humeral Shaft, Right
Hydrocelectomy *see* Excision, Male Reproductive System ØVB
Hydrotherapy
  Assisted exercise in pool *see* Motor Treatment, Rehabilitation FØ7
  Whirlpool *see* Activities of Daily Living Treatment, Rehabilitation FØ8
Hymenectomy
  see Excision, Hymen ØUBK
  see Resection, Hymen ØUTK
Hymenoplasty
  see Repair, Hymen ØUQK
  see Supplement, Hymen ØUUK
Hymenorrhaphy *see* Repair, Hymen ØUQK
Hymenotomy
  see Division, Hymen ØU8K
  see Drainage, Hymen ØU9K
Hyoglossus muscle *use* Tongue, Palate, Pharynx Muscle
Hyoid artery
  use Thyroid Artery, Left
  use Thyroid Artery, Right
Hyperalimentation *see* Introduction of substance in or on
Hyperbaric oxygenation
  Decompression sickness treatment *see* Decompression, Circulatory 6A15
  Other treatment *see* Assistance, Circulatory 5AØ5
Hyperimmune globulin *use* Globulin
Hyperimmune Globulin, for COVID-19 treatment XW1
Hyperimmune intravenous immunoglobulin (hIVIG), for COVID-19 treatment *use* Hyperimmune Globulin
Hyperthermia
  Radiation Therapy
    Abdomen DWY38ZZ
    Adrenal Gland DGY28ZZ
    Bile Ducts DFY28ZZ
    Bladder DTY28ZZ
    Bone Marrow D7YØ8ZZ
    Bone, Other DPYC8ZZ
    Brain DØYØ8ZZ
    Brain Stem DØY18ZZ
    Breast
      Left DMYØ8ZZ
      Right DMY18ZZ
    Bronchus DBY18ZZ

Hyperthermia — *continued*
  Radiation Therapy — *continued*
    Cervix DUY18ZZ
    Chest DWY28ZZ
    Chest Wall DBY78ZZ
    Colon DDY58ZZ
    Diaphragm DBY88ZZ
    Duodenum DDY28ZZ
    Ear D9YØ8ZZ
    Esophagus DDYØ8ZZ
    Eye D8YØ8ZZ
    Femur DPY98ZZ
    Fibula DPYB8ZZ
    Gallbladder DFY18ZZ
    Gland
      Adrenal DGY28ZZ
      Parathyroid DGY48ZZ
      Pituitary DGYØ8ZZ
      Thyroid DGY58ZZ
    Glands, Salivary D9Y68ZZ
    Head and Neck DWY18ZZ
    Hemibody DWY48ZZ
    Humerus DPY68ZZ
    Hypopharynx D9Y38ZZ
    Ileum DDY48ZZ
    Jejunum DDY38ZZ
    Kidney DTYØ8ZZ
    Larynx D9YB8ZZ
    Liver DFY98ZZ
    Lung DBY28ZZ
    Lymphatics
      Abdomen D7Y68ZZ
      Axillary D7Y48ZZ
      Inguinal D7Y88ZZ
      Neck D7Y38ZZ
      Pelvis D7Y78ZZ
      Thorax D7Y58ZZ
    Mandible DPY38ZZ
    Maxilla DPY28ZZ
    Mediastinum DBY68ZZ
    Mouth D9Y48ZZ
    Nasopharynx D9YD8ZZ
    Neck and Head DWY18ZZ
    Nerve, Peripheral DØY78ZZ
    Nose D9Y18ZZ
    Oropharynx D9YF8ZZ
    Ovary DUYØ8ZZ
    Palate
      Hard D9Y88ZZ
      Soft D9Y98ZZ
    Pancreas DFY38ZZ
    Parathyroid Gland DGY48ZZ
    Pelvic Bones DPY88ZZ
    Pelvic Region DWY68ZZ
    Pineal Body DGY18ZZ
    Pituitary Gland DGYØ8ZZ
    Pleura DBY58ZZ
    Prostate DVYØ8ZZ
    Radius DPY78ZZ
    Rectum DDY78ZZ
    Rib DPY58ZZ
    Sinuses D9Y78ZZ
    Skin
      Abdomen DHY88ZZ
      Arm DHY48ZZ
      Back DHY78ZZ
      Buttock DHY98ZZ
      Chest DHY68ZZ
      Face DHY28ZZ
      Leg DHYB8ZZ
      Neck DHY38ZZ
    Skull DPYØ8ZZ
    Spinal Cord DØY68ZZ
    Spleen D7Y28ZZ
    Sternum DPY48ZZ
    Stomach DDY18ZZ
    Testis DVY18ZZ
    Thymus D7Y18ZZ
    Thyroid Gland DGY58ZZ
    Tibia DPYB8ZZ
    Tongue D9Y58ZZ
    Trachea DBYØ8ZZ
    Ulna DPY78ZZ
    Ureter DTY18ZZ
    Urethra DTY38ZZ
    Uterus DUY28ZZ
    Whole Body DWY58ZZ
  Whole Body 6A3Z

Hyperthermic Intraperitoneal Chemotherapy (HIPEC) 3E0M30Y
Hypnosis GZFZZZZ
Hypogastric artery
　use Internal Iliac Artery, Left
　use Internal Iliac Artery, Right
Hypopharynx *use* Pharynx
Hypophysectomy
　see Excision, Gland, Pituitary 0GB0
　see Resection, Gland, Pituitary 0GT0
Hypophysis *use* Pituitary Gland
Hypothalamotomy *see* Destruction, Thalamus 0059
Hypothenar muscle
　use Hand Muscle, Left
　use Hand Muscle, Right
Hypothermia, Whole Body 6A4Z
Hysterectomy
　Supracervical *see* Resection, Uterus 0UT9
　Total *see* Resection, Uterus 0UT9
Hysterolysis *see* Release, Uterus 0UN9
Hysteropexy
　see Repair, Uterus 0UQ9
　see Reposition, Uterus 0US9
Hysteroplasty *see* Repair, Uterus 0UQ9
Hysterorrhaphy *see* Repair, Uterus 0UQ9
Hysteroscopy 0UJD8ZZ
Hysterotomy *see* Drainage, Uterus 0U99
Hysterotrachelectomy
　see Resection, Cervix 0UTC
　see Resection, Uterus 0UT9
Hysterotracheloplasty *see* Repair, Uterus 0UQ9
Hysterotrachelorrhaphy *see* Repair, Uterus 0UQ9

I

IABP (Intra-aortic balloon pump) *see* Assistance, Cardiac 5A02
IAEMT (Intraoperative anesthetic effect monitoring and titration) *see* Monitoring, Central Nervous 4A10
IASD® (InterAtrial Shunt Device), Corvia *use* Synthetic Substitute
Idarucizumab, Pradaxa® (dabigatran) reversal agent *use* Other Therapeutic Substance
Idecabtagene Vicleucel *use* Idecabtagene Vicleucel Immunotherapy
Idecabtagene Vicleucel Immunotherapy XW0
Ide-cel *use* Idecabtagene Vicleucel Immunotherapy
iFuse Bedrock™ Granite Implant System *use* Internal Fixation Device with Tulip Connector in New Technology
IGIV-C, for COVID-19 treatment *use* Hyperimmune Globulin
IHD (Intermittent hemodialysis) 5A1D70Z
Ileal artery *use* Superior Mesenteric Artery
Ileectomy
　see Excision, Ileum 0DBB
　see Resection, Ileum 0DTB
Ileocolic artery *use* Superior Mesenteric Artery
Ileocolic vein *use* Colic Vein
Ileopexy
　see Repair, Ileum 0DQB
　see Reposition, Ileum 0DSB
Ileorrhaphy *see* Repair, Ileum 0DQB
Ileoscopy 0DJD8ZZ
Ileostomy
　see Bypass, Ileum 0D1B
　see Drainage, Ileum 0D9B
Ileotomy *see* Drainage, Ileum 0D9B
Ileoureterostomy *see* Bypass, Urinary System 0T1
Iliac crest
　use Pelvic Bone, Left
　use Pelvic Bone, Right
Iliac fascia
　use Subcutaneous Tissue and Fascia, Left Upper Leg
　use Subcutaneous Tissue and Fascia, Right Upper Leg
Iliac lymph node *use* Lymphatic, Pelvis
Iliacus muscle
　use Hip Muscle, Left
　use Hip Muscle, Right
Iliofemoral ligament
　use Hip Bursa and Ligament, Left
　use Hip Bursa and Ligament, Right
Iliohypogastric nerve *use* Lumbar Plexus

Ilioinguinal nerve *use* Lumbar Plexus
Iliolumbar artery
　use Internal Iliac Artery, Left
　use Internal Iliac Artery, Right
Iliolumbar ligament *use* Lower Spine Bursa and Ligament
Iliotibial tract (band)
　use Subcutaneous Tissue and Fascia, Left Upper Leg
　use Subcutaneous Tissue and Fascia, Right Upper Leg
Ilium
　use Pelvic Bone, Left
　use Pelvic Bone, Right
Ilizarov external fixator
　use External Fixation Device, Ring in 0PH
　use External Fixation Device, Ring in 0PS
　use External Fixation Device, Ring in 0QH
　use External Fixation Device, Ring in 0QS
Ilizarov-Vecklich device
　use External Fixation Device, Limb Lengthening in 0PH
　use External Fixation Device, Limb Lengthening in 0QH
Imaging, diagnostic
　see Computerized Tomography (CT Scan)
　see Fluoroscopy
　see Magnetic Resonance Imaging (MRI)
　see Plain Radiography
　see Ultrasonography
Imdevimab (REGN10987) and Casirivimab (REGN10933) *use* REGN-COV2 Monoclonal Antibody
IMFINZI® *use* Durvalumab Antineoplastic
Imipenem-cilastatin-relebactam Anti-infective XW0
IMI/REL *use* Imipenem-cilastatin-relebactam Anti-infective
Immobilization
　Abdominal Wall 2W33X
　Arm
　　Lower
　　　Left 2W3DX
　　　Right 2W3CX
　　Upper
　　　Left 2W3BX
　　　Right 2W3AX
　Back 2W35X
　Chest Wall 2W34X
　Extremity
　　Lower
　　　Left 2W3MX
　　　Right 2W3LX
　　Upper
　　　Left 2W39X
　　　Right 2W38X
　Face 2W31X
　Finger
　　Left 2W3KX
　　Right 2W3JX
　Foot
　　Left 2W3TX
　　Right 2W3SX
　Hand
　　Left 2W3FX
　　Right 2W3EX
　Head 2W30X
　Inguinal Region
　　Left 2W37X
　　Right 2W36X
　Leg
　　Lower
　　　Left 2W3RX
　　　Right 2W3QX
　　Upper
　　　Left 2W3PX
　　　Right 2W3NX
　Neck 2W32X
　Thumb
　　Left 2W3HX
　　Right 2W3GX
　Toe
　　Left 2W3VX
　　Right 2W3UX
Immunization *see* Introduction of Serum, Toxoid, and Vaccine
Immunoglobulin *use* Globulin

Immunotherapy *see* Introduction of Immunotherapeutic Substance
Immunotherapy, antineoplastic
　Interferon *see* Introduction of Low-dose Interleukin-2
　Interleukin-2, high-dose *see* Introduction of High-dose Interleukin-2
　Interleukin-2, low-dose *see* Introduction of Low-dose Interleukin-2
　Monoclonal antibody *see* Introduction of Monoclonal Antibody
　Proleukin, high-dose *see* Introduction of High-dose Interleukin-2
　Proleukin, low-dose *see* Introduction of Low-dose Interleukin-2
Impella® heart pump *use* Short-term External Heart Assist System in Heart and Great Vessels
Impeller Pump
　Continuous, Output 5A0221D
　Intermittent, Output 5A0211D
Implantable cardioverter-defibrillator (ICD) *use* Defibrillator Generator in 0JH
Implantable drug infusion pump (anti-spasmodic) (chemotherapy) (pain) *use* Infusion Device, Pump in Subcutaneous Tissue and Fascia
Implantable glucose monitoring device *use* Monitoring Device
Implantable hemodynamic monitor (IHM) *use* Monitoring Device, Hemodynamic in 0JH
Implantable hemodynamic monitoring system (IHMS) *use* Monitoring Device, Hemodynamic in 0JH
Implantable Miniature Telescope™ (IMT) *use* Synthetic Substitute, Intraocular Telescope in 08R
Implantation
　see Insertion
　see Replacement
Implanted (venous)(access) port *use* Vascular Access Device, Totally Implantable in Subcutaneous Tissue and Fascia
IMV (intermittent mandatory ventilation) *see* Assistance, Respiratory 5A09
In Vitro Fertilization 8E0ZXY1
Incision, abscess *see* Drainage
Incudectomy
　see Excision, Ear, Nose, Sinus 09B
　see Resection, Ear, Nose, Sinus 09T
Incudopexy
　see Repair, Ear, Nose, Sinus 09Q
　see Reposition, Ear, Nose, Sinus 09S
Incus
　use Auditory Ossicle, Left
　use Auditory Ossicle, Right
Induction of labor
　Artificial rupture of membranes *see* Drainage, Pregnancy 109
　Oxytocin *see* Introduction of Hormone
InDura, intrathecal catheter (1P) (spinal) *use* Infusion Device
Inebilizumab-cdon XW0
Inferior cardiac nerve *use* Thoracic Sympathetic Nerve
Inferior cerebellar vein *use* Intracranial Vein
Inferior cerebral vein *use* Intracranial Vein
Inferior epigastric artery
　use External Iliac Artery, Left
　use External Iliac Artery, Right
Inferior epigastric lymph node *use* Lymphatic, Pelvis
Inferior genicular artery
　use Popliteal Artery, Left
　use Popliteal Artery, Right
Inferior gluteal artery
　use Internal Iliac Artery, Left
　use Internal Iliac Artery, Right
Inferior gluteal nerve *use* Sacral Plexus
Inferior hypogastric plexus *use* Abdominal Sympathetic Nerve
Inferior labial artery *use* Face Artery
Inferior longitudinal muscle *use* Tongue, Palate, Pharynx Muscle
Inferior mesenteric ganglion *use* Abdominal Sympathetic Nerve
Inferior mesenteric lymph node *use* Lymphatic, Mesenteric
Inferior mesenteric plexus *use* Abdominal Sympathetic Nerve
Inferior oblique muscle
　use Extraocular Muscle, Left

Inferior oblique muscle — *continued*
  use Extraocular Muscle, Right
Inferior pancreaticoduodenal artery *use* Superior
  Mesenteric Artery
Inferior phrenic artery *use* Abdominal Aorta
Inferior rectus muscle
  use Extraocular Muscle, Left
  use Extraocular Muscle, Right
Inferior suprarenal artery
  use Renal Artery, Left
  use Renal Artery, Right
Inferior tarsal plate
  use Lower Eyelid, Left
  use Lower Eyelid, Right
Inferior thyroid vein
  use Innominate Vein, Left
  use Innominate Vein, Right
Inferior tibiofibular joint
  use Ankle Joint, Left
  use Ankle Joint, Right
Inferior turbinate *use* Nasal Turbinate
Inferior ulnar collateral artery
  use Brachial Artery, Left
  use Brachial Artery, Right
Inferior vesical artery
  use Internal Iliac Artery, Left
  use Internal Iliac Artery, Right
Infraauricular lymph node *use* Lymphatic, Head
Infraclavicular (deltopectoral) lymph node
  use Lymphatic, Left Upper Extremity
  use Lymphatic, Right Upper Extremity
Infrahyoid muscle
  use Neck Muscle, Left
  use Neck Muscle, Right
Infraparotid lymph node *use* Lymphatic, Head
Infraspinatus fascia
  use Subcutaneous Tissue and Fascia, Left Upper
    Arm
  use Subcutaneous Tissue and Fascia, Right Upper
    Arm
Infraspinatus muscle
  use Shoulder Muscle, Left
  use Shoulder Muscle, Right
Infundibulopelvic ligament *use* Uterine Supporting
  Structure
Infusion *see* Introduction of substance in or on
Infusion Device, Pump
  Insertion of device in
    Abdomen ØJH8
    Back ØJH7
    Chest ØJH6
    Lower Arm
      Left ØJHH
      Right ØJHG
    Lower Leg
      Left ØJHP
      Right ØJHN
    Trunk ØJHT
    Upper Arm
      Left ØJHF
      Right ØJHD
    Upper Leg
      Left ØJHM
      Right ØJHL
  Removal of device from
    Lower Extremity ØJPW
    Trunk ØJPT
    Upper Extremity ØJPV
  Revision of device in
    Lower Extremity ØJWW
    Trunk ØJWT
    Upper Extremity ØJWV
Infusion, glucarpidase
  Central Vein 3EØ43GQ
  Peripheral Vein 3EØ33GQ
Inguinal canal
  use Inguinal Region, Bilateral
  use Inguinal Region, Left
  use Inguinal Region, Right
Inguinal triangle
  use Inguinal Region, Bilateral
  use Inguinal Region, Left
  use Inguinal Region, Right
Injection *see* Introduction of substance in or on
Injection reservoir, port *use* Vascular Access Device,
  Totally Implantable in Subcutaneous Tissue and
  Fascia

Injection reservoir, pump *use* Infusion Device, Pump
  in Subcutaneous Tissue and Fascia
Insemination, artificial 3EØP7LZ
Insertion
  Antimicrobial envelope *see* Introduction of Anti-
    infective
  Aqueous drainage shunt
    see Bypass, Eye Ø81
    see Drainage, Eye Ø89
  Bone, Pelvic, Internal Fixation Device with Tulip
    Connector XNH
  Joint
    Lumbar Vertebral, Posterior Spinal Motion
      Preservation Device XRHBØ18
    Lumbosacral, Posterior Spinal Motion
      Preservation Device XRHDØ18
  Neurostimulator Lead, Sphenopalatine Ganglion
    XØHK3Q8
  Neurostimulator Lead with Paired Stimulation
    System XØHQ3R8
  Products of Conception 1ØHØ
  Spinal Stabilization Device
    see Insertion of device in, Lower Joints ØSH
    see Insertion of device in, Upper Joints ØRH
Insertion of device in
  Abdominal Wall ØWHF
  Acetabulum
    Left ØQH5
    Right ØQH4
  Anal Sphincter ØDHR
  Ankle Region
    Left ØYHL
    Right ØYHK
  Anus ØDHQ
  Aorta
    Abdominal Ø4HØ
    Thoracic
      Ascending/Arch Ø2HX
      Descending Ø2HW
  Arm
    Lower
      Left ØXHF
      Right ØXHD
    Upper
      Left ØXH9
      Right ØXH8
  Artery
    Anterior Tibial
      Left Ø4HQ
      Right Ø4HP
    Axillary
      Left Ø3H6
      Right Ø3H5
    Brachial
      Left Ø3H8
      Right Ø3H7
    Celiac Ø4H1
    Colic
      Left Ø4H7
      Middle Ø4H8
      Right Ø4H6
    Common Carotid
      Left Ø3HJ
      Right Ø3HH
    Common Iliac
      Left Ø4HD
      Right Ø4HC
    Coronary
      Four or More Arteries Ø2H3
      One Artery Ø2HØ
      Three Arteries Ø2H2
      Two Arteries Ø2H1
    External Carotid
      Left Ø3HN
      Right Ø3HM
    External Iliac
      Left Ø4HJ
      Right Ø4HH
    Face Ø3HR
    Femoral
      Left Ø4HL
      Right Ø4HK
    Foot
      Left Ø4HW
      Right Ø4HV
    Gastric Ø4H2
    Hand
      Left Ø3HF

Insertion of device in — *continued*
  Artery — *continued*
    Hand — *continued*
      Right Ø3HD
    Hepatic Ø4H3
    Inferior Mesenteric Ø4HB
    Innominate Ø3H2
    Internal Carotid
      Left Ø3HL
      Right Ø3HK
    Internal Iliac
      Left Ø4HF
      Right Ø4HE
    Internal Mammary
      Left Ø3H1
      Right Ø3HØ
    Intracranial Ø3HG
    Lower Ø4HY
    Peroneal
      Left Ø4HU
      Right Ø4HT
    Popliteal
      Left Ø4HN
      Right Ø4HM
    Posterior Tibial
      Left Ø4HS
      Right Ø4HR
    Pulmonary
      Left Ø2HR
      Right Ø2HQ
    Pulmonary Trunk Ø2HP
    Radial
      Left Ø3HC
      Right Ø3HB
    Renal
      Left Ø4HA
      Right Ø4H9
    Splenic Ø4H4
    Subclavian
      Left Ø3H4
      Right Ø3H3
    Superior Mesenteric Ø4H5
    Temporal
      Left Ø3HT
      Right Ø3HS
    Thyroid
      Left Ø3HV
      Right Ø3HU
    Ulnar
      Left Ø3HA
      Right Ø3H9
    Upper Ø3HY
    Vertebral
      Left Ø3HQ
      Right Ø3HP
  Atrium
    Left Ø2H7
    Right Ø2H6
  Axilla
    Left ØXH5
    Right ØXH4
  Back
    Lower ØWHL
    Upper ØWHK
  Bladder ØTHB
  Bladder Neck ØTHC
  Bone
    Ethmoid
      Left ØNHG
      Right ØNHF
    Facial ØNHW
    Frontal ØNH1
    Hyoid ØNHX
    Lacrimal
      Left ØNHJ
      Right ØNHH
    Lower ØQHY
    Nasal ØNHB
    Occipital ØNH7
    Palatine
      Left ØNHL
      Right ØNHK
    Parietal
      Left ØNH4
      Right ØNH3
    Pelvic
      Left ØQH3
      Right ØQH2
    Sphenoid ØNHC

Insertion of device in — *continued*
  Bone — *continued*
    Temporal
      Left ØNH6
      Right ØNH5
    Upper ØPHY
    Zygomatic
      Left ØNHN
      Right ØNHM
  Bone Marrow Ø7HT
  Brain ØØHØ
  Breast
    Bilateral ØHHV
    Left ØHHU
    Right ØHHT
  Bronchus
    Lingula ØBH9
    Lower Lobe
      Left ØBHB
      Right ØBH6
    Main
      Left ØBH7
      Right ØBH3
    Middle Lobe, Right ØBH5
    Upper Lobe
      Left ØBH8
      Right ØBH4
  Bursa and Ligament
    Lower ØMHY
    Upper ØMHX
  Buttock
    Left ØYH1
    Right ØYHØ
  Carpal
    Left ØPHN
    Right ØPHM
  Cavity, Cranial ØWH1
  Cerebral Ventricle ØØH6
  Cervix ØUHC
  Chest Wall ØWH8
  Cisterna Chyli Ø7HL
  Clavicle
    Left ØPHB
    Right ØPH9
  Coccyx ØQHS
  Cul-de-sac ØUHF
  Diaphragm ØBHT
  Disc
    Cervical Vertebral ØRH3
    Cervicothoracic Vertebral ØRH5
    Lumbar Vertebral ØSH2
    Lumbosacral ØSH4
    Thoracic Vertebral ØRH9
    Thoracolumbar Vertebral ØRHB
  Duct
    Hepatobiliary ØFHB
    Pancreatic ØFHD
  Duodenum ØDH9
  Ear
    Inner
      Left Ø9HE
      Right Ø9HD
    Left Ø9HJ
    Right Ø9HH
  Elbow Region
    Left ØXHC
    Right ØXHB
  Epididymis and Spermatic Cord ØVHM
  Esophagus ØDH5
  Extremity
    Lower
      Left ØYHB
      Right ØYH9
    Upper
      Left ØXH7
      Right ØXH6
  Eye
    Left Ø8H1
    Right Ø8HØ
  Face ØWH2
  Fallopian Tube ØUH8
  Femoral Region
    Left ØYH8
    Right ØYH7
  Femoral Shaft
    Left ØQH9
    Right ØQH8

Insertion of device in — *continued*
  Femur
    Lower
      Left ØQHC
      Right ØQHB
    Upper
      Left ØQH7
      Right ØQH6
  Fibula
    Left ØQHK
    Right ØQHJ
  Foot
    Left ØYHN
    Right ØYHM
  Gallbladder ØFH4
  Gastrointestinal Tract ØWHP
  Genitourinary Tract ØWHR
  Gland
    Endocrine ØGHS
    Salivary ØCHA
  Glenoid Cavity
    Left ØPH8
    Right ØPH7
  Hand
    Left ØXHK
    Right ØXHJ
  Head ØWHØ
  Heart Ø2HA
  Humeral Head
    Left ØPHD
    Right ØPHC
  Humeral Shaft
    Left ØPHG
    Right ØPHF
  Ileum ØDHB
  Inguinal Region
    Left ØYH6
    Right ØYH5
  Intestinal Tract
    Lower Intestinal Tract ØDHD
    Upper Intestinal Tract ØDHØ
  Intestine
    Large ØDHE
    Small ØDH8
  Jaw
    Lower ØWH5
    Upper ØWH4
  Jejunum ØDHA
  Joint
    Acromioclavicular
      Left ØRHH
      Right ØRHG
    Ankle
      Left ØSHG
      Right ØSHF
    Carpal
      Left ØRHR
      Right ØRHQ
    Carpometacarpal
      Left ØRHT
      Right ØRHS
    Cervical Vertebral ØRH1
    Cervicothoracic Vertebral ØRH4
    Coccygeal ØSH6
    Elbow
      Left ØRHM
      Right ØRHL
    Finger Phalangeal
      Left ØRHX
      Right ØRHW
    Hip
      Left ØSHB
      Right ØSH9
    Knee
      Left ØSHD
      Right ØSHC
    Lumbar Vertebral ØSHØ
    Lumbosacral ØSH3
    Metacarpophalangeal
      Left ØRHV
      Right ØRHU
    Metatarsal-Phalangeal
      Left ØSHN
      Right ØSHM
    Occipital-cervical ØRHØ
    Sacrococcygeal ØSH5
    Sacroiliac
      Left ØSH8
      Right ØSH7

Insertion of device in — *continued*
  Joint — *continued*
    Shoulder
      Left ØRHK
      Right ØRHJ
    Sternoclavicular
      Left ØRHF
      Right ØRHE
    Tarsal
      Left ØSHJ
      Right ØSHH
    Tarsometatarsal
      Left ØSHL
      Right ØSHK
    Temporomandibular
      Left ØRHD
      Right ØRHC
    Thoracic Vertebral ØRH6
    Thoracolumbar Vertebral ØRHA
    Toe Phalangeal
      Left ØSHQ
      Right ØSHP
    Wrist
      Left ØRHP
      Right ØRHN
  Kidney ØTH5
  Knee Region
    Left ØYHG
    Right ØYHF
  Larynx ØCHS
  Leg
    Lower
      Left ØYHJ
      Right ØYHH
    Upper
      Left ØYHD
      Right ØYHC
  Liver ØFHØ
    Left Lobe ØFH2
    Right Lobe ØFH1
  Lung
    Left ØBHL
    Right ØBHK
  Lymphatic Ø7HN
    Thoracic Duct Ø7HK
  Mandible
    Left ØNHV
    Right ØNHT
  Maxilla ØNHR
  Mediastinum ØWHC
  Metacarpal
    Left ØPHQ
    Right ØPHP
  Metatarsal
    Left ØQHP
    Right ØQHN
  Mouth and Throat ØCHY
  Muscle
    Lower ØKHY
    Upper ØKHX
  Nasal Mucosa and Soft Tissue Ø9HK
  Nasopharynx Ø9HN
  Neck ØWH6
  Nerve
    Cranial ØØHE
    Peripheral Ø1HY
  Nipple
    Left ØHHX
    Right ØHHW
  Oral Cavity and Throat ØWH3
  Orbit
    Left ØNHQ
    Right ØNHP
  Ovary ØUH3
  Pancreas ØFHG
  Patella
    Left ØQHF
    Right ØQHD
  Pelvic Cavity ØWHJ
  Penis ØVHS
  Pericardial Cavity ØWHD
  Pericardium Ø2HN
  Perineum
    Female ØWHN
    Male ØWHM
  Peritoneal Cavity ØWHG
  Phalanx
    Finger
      Left ØPHV

Insertion of device in — *continued*
  Phalanx — *continued*
    Finger — *continued*
      Right ØPHT
    Thumb
      Left ØPHS
      Right ØPHR
    Toe
      Left ØQHR
      Right ØQHQ
  Pleura ØBHQ
  Pleural Cavity
    Left ØWHB
    Right ØWH9
  Prostate ØVHØ
  Prostate and Seminal Vesicles ØVH4
  Radius
    Left ØPHJ
    Right ØPHH
  Rectum ØDHP
  Respiratory Tract ØWHQ
  Retroperitoneum ØWHH
  Ribs
    1 to 2 ØPH1
    3 or More ØPH2
  Sacrum ØQH1
  Scapula
    Left ØPH6
    Right ØPH5
  Scrotum and Tunica Vaginalis ØVH8
  Shoulder Region
    Left ØXH3
    Right ØXH2
  Sinus Ø9HY
  Skin ØHHPXYZ
  Skull ØNHØ
  Spinal Canal ØØHU
  Spinal Cord ØØHV
  Spleen Ø7HP
  Sternum ØPHØ
  Stomach ØDH6
  Subcutaneous Tissue and Fascia
    Abdomen ØJH8
    Back ØJH7
    Buttock ØJH9
    Chest ØJH6
    Face ØJH1
    Foot
      Left ØJHR
      Right ØJHQ
    Hand
      Left ØJHK
      Right ØJHJ
    Head and Neck ØJHS
    Lower Arm
      Left ØJHH
      Right ØJHG
    Lower Extremity ØJHW
    Lower Leg
      Left ØJHP
      Right ØJHN
    Neck
      Left ØJH5
      Right ØJH4
    Pelvic Region ØJHC
    Perineum ØJHB
    Scalp ØJHØ
    Trunk ØJHT
    Upper Arm
      Left ØJHF
      Right ØJHD
    Upper Extremity ØJHV
    Upper Leg
      Left ØJHM
      Right ØJHL
  Tarsal
    Left ØQHM
    Right ØQHL
  Tendon
    Lower ØLHY
    Upper ØLHX
  Testis ØVHD
  Thymus Ø7HM
  Tibia
    Left ØQHH
    Right ØQHG
  Tongue ØCH7
  Trachea ØBH1
  Tracheobronchial Tree ØBHØ

Insertion of device in — *continued*
  Ulna
    Left ØPHL
    Right ØPHK
  Ureter ØTH9
  Urethra ØTHD
  Uterus ØUH9
  Uterus and Cervix ØUHD
  Vagina ØUHG
  Vagina and Cul-de-sac ØUHH
  Vas Deferens ØVHR
  Vein
    Axillary
      Left Ø5H8
      Right Ø5H7
    Azygos Ø5HØ
    Basilic
      Left Ø5HC
      Right Ø5HB
    Brachial
      Left Ø5HA
      Right Ø5H9
    Cephalic
      Left Ø5HF
      Right Ø5HD
    Colic Ø6H7
    Common Iliac
      Left Ø6HD
      Right Ø6HC
    Coronary Ø2H4
    Esophageal Ø6H3
    External Iliac
      Left Ø6HG
      Right Ø6HF
    External Jugular
      Left Ø5HQ
      Right Ø5HP
    Face
      Left Ø5HV
      Right Ø5HT
    Femoral
      Left Ø6HN
      Right Ø6HM
    Foot
      Left Ø6HV
      Right Ø6HT
    Gastric Ø6H2
    Hand
      Left Ø5HH
      Right Ø5HG
    Hemiazygos Ø5H1
    Hepatic Ø6H4
    Hypogastric
      Left Ø6HJ
      Right Ø6HH
    Inferior Mesenteric Ø6H6
    Innominate
      Left Ø5H4
      Right Ø5H3
    Internal Jugular
      Left Ø5HN
      Right Ø5HM
    Intracranial Ø5HL
    Lower Ø6HY
    Portal Ø6H8
    Pulmonary
      Left Ø2HT
      Right Ø2HS
    Renal
      Left Ø6HB
      Right Ø6H9
    Saphenous
      Left Ø6HQ
      Right Ø6HP
    Splenic Ø6H1
    Subclavian
      Left Ø5H6
      Right Ø5H5
    Superior Mesenteric Ø6H5
    Upper Ø5HY
    Vertebral
      Left Ø5HS
      Right Ø5HR
  Vena Cava
    Inferior Ø6HØ
    Superior Ø2HV
  Ventricle
    Left Ø2HL
    Right Ø2HK

Insertion of device in — *continued*
  Vertebra
    Cervical ØPH3
    Lumbar ØQHØ
    Thoracic ØPH4
  Wrist Region
    Left ØXHH
    Right ØXHG
Inspection
  Abdominal Wall ØWJF
  Ankle Region
    Left ØYJL
    Right ØYJK
  Arm
    Lower
      Left ØXJF
      Right ØXJD
    Upper
      Left ØXJ9
      Right ØXJ8
  Artery
    Lower Ø4JY
    Upper Ø3JY
  Axilla
    Left ØXJ5
    Right ØXJ4
  Back
    Lower ØWJL
    Upper ØWJK
  Bladder ØTJB
  Bone
    Facial ØNJW
    Lower ØQJY
    Nasal ØNJB
    Upper ØPJY
  Bone Marrow Ø7JT
  Brain ØØJØ
  Breast
    Left ØHJU
    Right ØHJT
  Bursa and Ligament
    Lower ØMJY
    Upper ØMJX
  Buttock
    Left ØYJ1
    Right ØYJØ
  Cavity, Cranial ØWJ1
  Chest Wall ØWJ8
  Cisterna Chyli Ø7JL
  Diaphragm ØBJT
  Disc
    Cervical Vertebral ØRJ3
    Cervicothoracic Vertebral ØRJ5
    Lumbar Vertebral ØSJ2
    Lumbosacral ØSJ4
    Thoracic Vertebral ØRJ9
    Thoracolumbar Vertebral ØRJB
  Duct
    Hepatobiliary ØFJB
    Pancreatic ØFJD
  Ear
    Inner
      Left Ø9JE
      Right Ø9JD
    Left Ø9JJ
    Right Ø9JH
  Elbow Region
    Left ØXJC
    Right ØXJB
  Epididymis and Spermatic Cord ØVJM
  Extremity
    Lower
      Left ØYJB
      Right ØYJ9
    Upper
      Left ØXJ7
      Right ØXJ6
  Eye
    Left Ø8J1XZZ
    Right Ø8JØXZZ
  Face ØWJ2
  Fallopian Tube ØUJ8
  Femoral Region
    Bilateral ØYJE
    Left ØYJ8
    Right ØYJ7
  Finger Nail ØHJQXZZ
  Foot
    Left ØYJN

Inspection — *continued*
  Foot — *continued*
    Right 0YJM
  Gallbladder 0FJ4
  Gastrointestinal Tract 0WJP
  Genitourinary Tract 0WJR
  Gland
    Adrenal 0GJ5
    Endocrine 0GJS
    Pituitary 0GJ0
    Salivary 0CJA
  Great Vessel 02JY
  Hand
    Left 0XJK
    Right 0XJJ
  Head 0WJ0
  Heart 02JA
  Inguinal Region
    Bilateral 0YJA
    Left 0YJ6
    Right 0YJ5
  Intestinal Tract
    Lower Intestinal Tract 0DJD
    Upper Intestinal Tract 0DJ0
  Jaw
    Lower 0WJ5
    Upper 0WJ4
  Joint
    Acromioclavicular
      Left 0RJH
      Right 0RJG
    Ankle
      Left 0SJG
      Right 0SJF
    Carpal
      Left 0RJR
      Right 0RJQ
    Carpometacarpal
      Left 0RJT
      Right 0RJS
    Cervical Vertebral 0RJ1
    Cervicothoracic Vertebral 0RJ4
    Coccygeal 0SJ6
    Elbow
      Left 0RJM
      Right 0RJL
    Finger Phalangeal
      Left 0RJX
      Right 0RJW
    Hip
      Left 0SJB
      Right 0SJ9
    Knee
      Left 0SJD
      Right 0SJC
    Lumbar Vertebral 0SJ0
    Lumbosacral 0SJ3
    Metacarpophalangeal
      Left 0RJV
      Right 0RJU
    Metatarsal-Phalangeal
      Left 0SJN
      Right 0SJM
    Occipital-cervical 0RJ0
    Sacrococcygeal 0SJ5
    Sacroiliac
      Left 0SJ8
      Right 0SJ7
    Shoulder
      Left 0RJK
      Right 0RJJ
    Sternoclavicular
      Left 0RJF
      Right 0RJE
    Tarsal
      Left 0SJJ
      Right 0SJH
    Tarsometatarsal
      Left 0SJL
      Right 0SJK
    Temporomandibular
      Left 0RJD
      Right 0RJC
    Thoracic Vertebral 0RJ6
    Thoracolumbar Vertebral 0RJA
    Toe Phalangeal
      Left 0SJQ
      Right 0SJP

Inspection — *continued*
  Joint — *continued*
    Wrist
      Left 0RJP
      Right 0RJN
  Kidney 0TJ5
  Knee Region
    Left 0YJG
    Right 0YJF
  Larynx 0CJS
  Leg
    Lower
      Left 0YJJ
      Right 0YJH
    Upper
      Left 0YJD
      Right 0YJC
  Lens
    Left 08JKXZZ
    Right 08JJXZZ
  Liver 0FJ0
  Lung
    Left 0BJL
    Right 0BJK
  Lymphatic 07JN
    Thoracic Duct 07JK
  Mediastinum 0WJC
  Mesentery 0DJV
  Mouth and Throat 0CJY
  Muscle
    Extraocular
      Left 08JM
      Right 08JL
    Lower 0KJY
    Upper 0KJX
  Nasal Mucosa and Soft Tissue 09JK
  Neck 0WJ6
  Nerve
    Cranial 00JE
    Peripheral 01JY
  Omentum 0DJU
  Oral Cavity and Throat 0WJ3
  Ovary 0UJ3
  Pancreas 0FJG
  Parathyroid Gland 0GJR
  Pelvic Cavity 0WJJ
  Penis 0VJS
  Pericardial Cavity 0WJD
  Perineum
    Female 0WJN
    Male 0WJM
  Peritoneal Cavity 0WJG
  Peritoneum 0DJW
  Pineal Body 0GJ1
  Pleura 0BJQ
  Pleural Cavity
    Left 0WJB
    Right 0WJ9
  Products of Conception 10J0
    Ectopic 10J2
    Retained 10J1
  Prostate and Seminal Vesicles 0VJ4
  Respiratory Tract 0WJQ
  Retroperitoneum 0WJH
  Scrotum and Tunica Vaginalis 0VJ8
  Shoulder Region
    Left 0XJ3
    Right 0XJ2
  Sinus 09JY
  Skin 0HJPXZZ
  Skull 0NJ0
  Spinal Canal 00JU
  Spinal Cord 00JV
  Spleen 07JP
  Stomach 0DJ6
  Subcutaneous Tissue and Fascia
    Head and Neck 0JJS
    Lower Extremity 0JJW
    Trunk 0JJT
    Upper Extremity 0JJV
  Tendon
    Lower 0LJY
    Upper 0LJX
  Testis 0VJD
  Thymus 07JM
  Thyroid Gland 0GJK
  Toe Nail 0HJRXZZ
  Trachea 0BJ1
  Tracheobronchial Tree 0BJ0

Inspection — *continued*
  Tympanic Membrane
    Left 09J8
    Right 09J7
  Ureter 0TJ9
  Urethra 0TJD
  Uterus and Cervix 0UJD
  Vagina and Cul-de-sac 0UJH
  Vas Deferens 0VJR
  Vein
    Lower 06JY
    Upper 05JY
  Vulva 0UJM
  Wrist Region
    Left 0XJH
    Right 0XJG
Instillation *see* Introduction of substance in or on
Insufflation *see* Introduction of substance in or on
Interatrial septum *use* Atrial Septum
InterAtrial Shunt Device IASD®, Corvia *use* Synthetic Substitute
Interbody fusion (spine) cage
  use Interbody Fusion Device in Lower Joints
  use Interbody Fusion Device in Upper Joints
Interbody Fusion Device, Customizable
  Lumbar Vertebral XRGB
    2 or more XRGC
  Lumbosacral XRGD
  Thoracolumbar Vertebral XRGA
Intercarpal joint
  use Carpal Joint, Left
  use Carpal Joint, Right
Intercarpal ligament
  use Hand Bursa and Ligament, Left
  use Hand Bursa and Ligament, Right
INTERCEPT Blood System for Plasma Pathogen Reduced Cryoprecipitated Fibrinogen Complex *use* Pathogen Reduced Cryoprecipitated Fibrinogen Complex
INTERCEPT Fibrinogen Complex *use* Pathogen Reduced Cryoprecipitated Fibrinogen Complex
Interclavicular ligament
  use Shoulder Bursa and Ligament, Left
  use Shoulder Bursa and Ligament, Right
Intercostal lymph node *use* Lymphatic, Thorax
Intercostal muscle
  use Thorax Muscle, Left
  use Thorax Muscle, Right
Intercostal nerve *use* Thoracic Nerve
Intercostobrachial nerve *use* Thoracic Nerve
Intercuneiform joint
  use Tarsal Joint, Left
  use Tarsal Joint, Right
Intercuneiform ligament
  use Foot Bursa and Ligament, Left
  use Foot Bursa and Ligament, Right
Intermediate bronchus *use* Main Bronchus, Right
Intermediate cuneiform bone
  use Tarsal, Left
  use Tarsal, Right
Intermittent Coronary Sinus Occlusion X2A7358
Intermittent hemodialysis (IHD) 5A1D70Z
Intermittent mandatory ventilation *see* Assistance, Respiratory 5A09
Intermittent Negative Airway Pressure
  24-96 Consecutive Hours, Ventilation 5A0945B
  Greater than 96 Consecutive Hours, Ventilation 5A0955B
  Less than 24 Consecutive Hours, Ventilation 5A0935B
Intermittent Positive Airway Pressure
  24-96 Consecutive Hours, Ventilation 5A09458
  Greater than 96 Consecutive Hours, Ventilation 5A09558
  Less than 24 Consecutive Hours, Ventilation 5A09358
Intermittent positive pressure breathing *see* Assistance, Respiratory 5A09
Internal anal sphincter *use* Anal Sphincter
Internal carotid artery, intracranial portion *use* Intracranial Artery
Internal carotid plexus *use* Head and Neck Sympathetic Nerve
Internal (basal) cerebral vein *use* Intracranial Vein
Internal Fixation Device with Tulip Connector
  Fusion, Joint, Sacroiliac XRG
  Insertion, Bone, Pelvic XNH

▽ Subterms under main terms may continue to next column or page

Internal iliac vein
use Hypogastric Vein, Left
use Hypogastric Vein, Right
Internal maxillary artery
use External Carotid Artery, Left
use External Carotid Artery, Right
Internal naris *use* Nasal Mucosa and Soft Tissue
Internal oblique muscle
use Abdomen Muscle, Left
use Abdomen Muscle, Right
Internal pudendal artery
use Internal Iliac Artery, Left
use Internal Iliac Artery, Right
Internal pudendal vein
use Hypogastric Vein, Left
use Hypogastric Vein, Right
Internal thoracic artery
use Internal Mammary Artery, Left
use Internal Mammary Artery, Right
use Subclavian Artery, Left
use Subclavian Artery, Right
Internal urethral sphincter *use* Urethra
Interphalangeal (IP) joint
use Finger Phalangeal Joint, Left
use Finger Phalangeal Joint, Right
use Toe Phalangeal Joint, Left
use Toe Phalangeal Joint, Right
Interphalangeal ligament
use Foot Bursa and Ligament, Left
use Foot Bursa and Ligament, Right
use Hand Bursa and Ligament, Left
use Hand Bursa and Ligament, Right
Interrogation, cardiac rhythm related device
Interrogation only *see* Measurement, Cardiac 4B02
With cardiac function testing *see* Measurement, Cardiac 4A02
Interruption *see* Occlusion
Interspinalis muscle
use Trunk Muscle, Left
use Trunk Muscle, Right
Interspinous ligament, cervical *use* Head and Neck Bursa and Ligament
Interspinous ligament, lumbar *use* Lower Spine Bursa and Ligament
Interspinous ligament, thoracic *use* Upper Spine Bursa and Ligament
Interspinous process spinal stabilization device
use Spinal Stabilization Device, Interspinous Process in 0RH
use Spinal Stabilization Device, Interspinous Process in 0SH
InterStim® Therapy lead *use* Neurostimulator Lead in Peripheral Nervous System
InterStim™ II Therapy neurostimulator *use* Stimulator Generator, Single Array in 0JH
InterStim™ Micro Therapy neurostimulator *use* Stimulator Generator, Single Array Rechargeable in 0JH
Intertransversarius muscle
use Trunk Muscle, Left
use Trunk Muscle, Right
Intertransverse ligament, cervical *use* Head and Neck Bursa and Ligament
Intertransverse ligament, lumbar *use* Lower Spine Bursa and Ligament
Intertransverse ligament, thoracic *use* Upper Spine Bursa and Ligament
Interventricular foramen (Monro) *use* Cerebral Ventricle
Interventricular septum *use* Ventricular Septum
Intestinal lymphatic trunk *use* Cisterna Chyli
Intracranial Arterial Flow, Whole Blood mRNA XXE5XT7
Intraluminal Device
Airway
Esophagus 0DH5
Mouth and Throat 0CHY
Nasopharynx 09HN
Bioactive
Occlusion
Common Carotid
Left 03LJ
Right 03LH
External Carotid
Left 03LN
Right 03LM

Intraluminal Device — *continued*
Bioactive — *continued*
Occlusion — *continued*
Internal Carotid
Left 03LL
Right 03LK
Intracranial 03LG
Vertebral
Left 03LQ
Right 03LP
Restriction
Common Carotid
Left 03VJ
Right 03VH
External Carotid
Left 03VN
Right 03VM
Internal Carotid
Left 03VL
Right 03VK
Intracranial 03VG
Vertebral
Left 03VQ
Right 03VP
Endobronchial Valve
Lingula 0BH9
Lower Lobe
Left 0BHB
Right 0BH6
Main
Left 0BH7
Right 0BH3
Middle Lobe, Right 0BH5
Upper Lobe
Left 0BH8
Right 0BH4
Endotracheal Airway
Change device in, Trachea 0B21XEZ
Insertion of device in, Trachea 0BH1
Pessary
Change device in, Vagina and Cul-de-sac 0U2HXGZ
Insertion of device in
Cul-de-sac 0UHF
Vagina 0UHG
Intramedullary (IM) rod (nail)
use Internal Fixation Device, Intramedullary in Lower Bones
use Internal Fixation Device, Intramedullary in Upper Bones
Intramedullary skeletal kinetic distractor (ISKD)
use Internal Fixation Device, Intramedullary in Lower Bones
use Internal Fixation Device, Intramedullary in Upper Bones
Intraocular Telescope
Left 08RK30Z
Right 08RJ30Z
Intraoperative Radiation Therapy (IORT)
Anus DDY8CZZ
Bile Ducts DFY2CZZ
Bladder DTY2CZZ
Brain D0Y0CZZ
Brain Stem D0Y1CZZ
Cervix DUY1CZZ
Colon DDY5CZZ
Duodenum DDY2CZZ
Gallbladder DFY1CZZ
Ileum DDY4CZZ
Jejunum DDY3CZZ
Kidney DTY0CZZ
Larynx D9YBCZZ
Liver DFY0CZZ
Mouth D9Y4CZZ
Nasopharynx D9YDCZZ
Nerve, Peripheral D0Y7CZZ
Ovary DUY0CZZ
Pancreas DFY3CZZ
Pharynx D9YCCZZ
Prostate DVY0CZZ
Rectum DDY7CZZ
Spinal Cord D0Y6CZZ
Stomach DDY1CZZ
Ureter DTY1CZZ
Urethra DTY3CZZ
Uterus DUY2CZZ
Intra.OX 8E02XDZ

Intrauterine Device (IUD) *use* Contraceptive Device in Female Reproductive System
Intravascular fluorescence angiography (IFA) *see* Monitoring, Physiological Systems 4A1
Intravascular Lithotripsy (IVL) *see* Fragmentation
Intravascular ultrasound assisted thrombolysis *see* Fragmentation, Artery
Introduction of substance in or on
Artery
Central 3E06
Analgesics 3E06
Anesthetic, Intracirculatory 3E06
Antiarrhythmic 3E06
Anti-infective 3E06
Anti-inflammatory 3E06
Antineoplastic 3E06
Destructive Agent 3E06
Diagnostic Substance, Other 3E06
Electrolytic Substance 3E06
Hormone 3E06
Hypnotics 3E06
Immunotherapeutic 3E06
Nutritional Substance 3E06
Platelet Inhibitor 3E06
Radioactive Substance 3E06
Sedatives 3E06
Serum 3E06
Thrombolytic 3E06
Toxoid 3E06
Vaccine 3E06
Vasopressor 3E06
Water Balance Substance 3E06
Coronary 3E07
Diagnostic Substance, Other 3E07
Platelet Inhibitor 3E07
Thrombolytic 3E07
Peripheral 3E05
Analgesics 3E05
Anesthetic, Intracirculatory 3E05
Antiarrhythmic 3E05
Anti-infective 3E05
Anti-inflammatory 3E05
Antineoplastic 3E05
Destructive Agent 3E05
Diagnostic Substance, Other 3E05
Electrolytic Substance 3E05
Hormone 3E05
Hypnotics 3E05
Immunotherapeutic 3E05
Nutritional Substance 3E05
Platelet Inhibitor 3E05
Radioactive Substance 3E05
Sedatives 3E05
Serum 3E05
Thrombolytic 3E05
Toxoid 3E05
Vaccine 3E05
Vasopressor 3E05
Water Balance Substance 3E05
Biliary Tract 3E0J
Analgesics 3E0J
Anesthetic Agent 3E0J
Anti-infective 3E0J
Anti-inflammatory 3E0J
Antineoplastic 3E0J
Destructive Agent 3E0J
Diagnostic Substance, Other 3E0J
Electrolytic Substance 3E0J
Gas 3E0J
Hypnotics 3E0J
Islet Cells, Pancreatic 3E0J
Nutritional Substance 3E0J
Radioactive Substance 3E0J
Sedatives 3E0J
Water Balance Substance 3E0J
Bone 3E0V
Analgesics 3E0V3NZ
Anesthetic Agent 3E0V3BZ
Anti-infective 3E0V32
Anti-inflammatory 3E0V33Z
Antineoplastic 3E0V30
Destructive Agent 3E0V3TZ
Diagnostic Substance, Other 3E0V3KZ
Electrolytic Substance 3E0V37Z
Hypnotics 3E0V3NZ
Nutritional Substance 3E0V36Z
Radioactive Substance 3E0V3HZ
Sedatives 3E0V3NZ
Water Balance Substance 3E0V37Z

Introduction of substance in or on — *continued*
  Bone Marrow 3E0A3GC
    Antineoplastic 3E0A30
  Brain 3E0Q
    Analgesics 3E0Q
    Anesthetic Agent 3E0Q
    Anti-infective 3E0Q
    Anti-inflammatory 3E0Q
    Antineoplastic 3E0Q
    Destructive Agent 3E0Q
    Diagnostic Substance, Other 3E0Q
    Electrolytic Substance 3E0Q
    Gas 3E0Q
    Hypnotics 3E0Q
    Nutritional Substance 3E0Q
    Radioactive Substance 3E0Q
    Sedatives 3E0Q
    Stem Cells
      Embryonic 3E0Q
      Somatic 3E0Q
    Water Balance Substance 3E0Q
  Cranial Cavity 3E0Q
    Analgesics 3E0Q
    Anesthetic Agent 3E0Q
    Anti-infective 3E0Q
    Anti-inflammatory 3E0Q
    Antineoplastic 3E0Q
    Destructive Agent 3E0Q
    Diagnostic Substance, Other 3E0Q
    Electrolytic Substance 3E0Q
    Gas 3E0Q
    Hypnotics 3E0Q
    Nutritional Substance 3E0Q
    Radioactive Substance 3E0Q
    Sedatives 3E0Q
    Stem Cells
      Embryonic 3E0Q
      Somatic 3E0Q
    Water Balance Substance 3E0Q
  Ear 3E0B
    Analgesics 3E0B
    Anesthetic Agent 3E0B
    Anti-infective 3E0B
    Anti-inflammatory 3E0B
    Antineoplastic 3E0B
    Destructive Agent 3E0B
    Diagnostic Substance, Other 3E0B
    Hypnotics 3E0B
    Radioactive Substance 3E0B
    Sedatives 3E0B
  Epidural Space 3E0S3GC
    Analgesics 3E0S3NZ
    Anesthetic Agent 3E0S3BZ
    Anti-infective 3E0S32
    Anti-inflammatory 3E0S33Z
    Antineoplastic 3E0S30
    Destructive Agent 3E0S3TZ
    Diagnostic Substance, Other 3E0S3KZ
    Electrolytic Substance 3E0S37Z
    Gas 3E0S
    Hypnotics 3E0S3NZ
    Nutritional Substance 3E0S36Z
    Radioactive Substance 3E0S3HZ
    Sedatives 3E0S3NZ
    Water Balance Substance 3E0S37Z
  Eye 3E0C
    Analgesics 3E0C
    Anesthetic Agent 3E0C
    Anti-infective 3E0C
    Anti-inflammatory 3E0C
    Antineoplastic 3E0C
    Destructive Agent 3E0C
    Diagnostic Substance, Other 3E0C
    Gas 3E0C
    Hypnotics 3E0C
    Pigment 3E0C
    Radioactive Substance 3E0C
    Sedatives 3E0C
  Gastrointestinal Tract
    Lower 3E0H
      Analgesics 3E0H
      Anesthetic Agent 3E0H
      Anti-infective 3E0H
      Anti-inflammatory 3E0H
      Antineoplastic 3E0H
      Destructive Agent 3E0H
      Diagnostic Substance, Other 3E0H
      Electrolytic Substance 3E0H
      Gas 3E0H

Introduction of substance in or on — *continued*
  Gastrointestinal Tract — *continued*
    Lower — *continued*
      Hypnotics 3E0H
      Nutritional Substance 3E0H
      Radioactive Substance 3E0H
      Sedatives 3E0H
      Water Balance Substance 3E0H
    Upper 3E0G
      Analgesics 3E0G
      Anesthetic Agent 3E0G
      Anti-infective 3E0G
      Anti-inflammatory 3E0G
      Antineoplastic 3E0G
      Destructive Agent 3E0G
      Diagnostic Substance, Other 3E0G
      Electrolytic Substance 3E0G
      Gas 3E0G
      Hypnotics 3E0G
      Nutritional Substance 3E0G
      Radioactive Substance 3E0G
      Sedatives 3E0G
      Water Balance Substance 3E0G
  Genitourinary Tract 3E0K
    Analgesics 3E0K
    Anesthetic Agent 3E0K
    Anti-infective 3E0K
    Anti-inflammatory 3E0K
    Antineoplastic 3E0K
    Destructive Agent 3E0K
    Diagnostic Substance, Other 3E0K
    Electrolytic Substance 3E0K
    Gas 3E0K
    Hypnotics 3E0K
    Nutritional Substance 3E0K
    Radioactive Substance 3E0K
    Sedatives 3E0K
    Water Balance Substance 3E0K
  Heart 3E08
    Diagnostic Substance, Other 3E08
    Platelet Inhibitor 3E08
    Thrombolytic 3E08
  Joint 3E0U
    Analgesics 3E0U3NZ
    Anesthetic Agent 3E0U3BZ
    Anti-infective 3E0U
    Anti-inflammatory 3E0U33Z
    Antineoplastic 3E0U30
    Destructive Agent 3E0U3TZ
    Diagnostic Substance, Other 3E0U3KZ
    Electrolytic Substance 3E0U37Z
    Gas 3E0U3SF
    Hypnotics 3E0U3NZ
    Nutritional Substance 3E0U36Z
    Radioactive Substance 3E0U3HZ
    Sedatives 3E0U3NZ
    Water Balance Substance 3E0U37Z
  Lymphatic 3E0W3GC
    Analgesics 3E0W3NZ
    Anesthetic Agent 3E0W3BZ
    Anti-infective 3E0W32
    Anti-inflammatory 3E0W33Z
    Antineoplastic 3E0W30
    Destructive Agent 3E0W3TZ
    Diagnostic Substance, Other 3E0W3KZ
    Electrolytic Substance 3E0W37Z
    Hypnotics 3E0W3NZ
    Nutritional Substance 3E0W36Z
    Radioactive Substance 3E0W3HZ
    Sedatives 3E0W3NZ
    Water Balance Substance 3E0W37Z
  Mouth 3E0D
    Analgesics 3E0D
    Anesthetic Agent 3E0D
    Antiarrhythmic 3E0D
    Anti-infective 3E0D
    Anti-inflammatory 3E0D
    Antineoplastic 3E0D
    Destructive Agent 3E0D
    Diagnostic Substance, Other 3E0D
    Electrolytic Substance 3E0D
    Hypnotics 3E0D
    Nutritional Substance 3E0D
    Radioactive Substance 3E0D
    Sedatives 3E0D
    Serum 3E0D
    Toxoid 3E0D
    Vaccine 3E0D
    Water Balance Substance 3E0D

Introduction of substance in or on — *continued*
  Mucous Membrane 3E00XGC
    Analgesics 3E00XNZ
    Anesthetic Agent 3E00XBZ
    Anti-infective 3E00X2
    Anti-inflammatory 3E00X3Z
    Antineoplastic 3E00X0
    Destructive Agent 3E00XTZ
    Diagnostic Substance, Other 3E00XKZ
    Hypnotics 3E00XNZ
    Pigment 3E00XMZ
    Sedatives 3E00XNZ
    Serum 3E00X4Z
    Toxoid 3E00X4Z
    Vaccine 3E00X4Z
  Muscle 3E023GC
    Analgesics 3E023NZ
    Anesthetic Agent 3E023BZ
    Anti-infective 3E0232
    Anti-inflammatory 3E0233Z
    Antineoplastic 3E0230
    Destructive Agent 3E023TZ
    Diagnostic Substance, Other 3E023KZ
    Electrolytic Substance 3E0237Z
    Hypnotics 3E023NZ
    Nutritional Substance 3E0236Z
    Radioactive Substance 3E023HZ
    Sedatives 3E023NZ
    Serum 3E0234Z
    Toxoid 3E0234Z
    Vaccine 3E0234Z
    Water Balance Substance 3E0237Z
  Nerve
    Cranial 3E0X3GC
      Anesthetic Agent 3E0X3BZ
      Anti-inflammatory 3E0X33Z
      Destructive Agent 3E0X3TZ
    Peripheral 3E0T3GC
      Anesthetic Agent 3E0T3BZ
      Anti-inflammatory 3E0T33Z
      Destructive Agent 3E0T3TZ
    Plexus 3E0T3GC
      Anesthetic Agent 3E0T3BZ
      Anti-inflammatory 3E0T33Z
      Destructive Agent 3E0T3TZ
  Nose 3E09
    Analgesics 3E09
    Anesthetic Agent 3E09
    Anti-infective 3E09
    Anti-inflammatory 3E09
    Antineoplastic 3E09
    Destructive Agent 3E09
    Diagnostic Substance, Other 3E09
    Hypnotics 3E09
    Radioactive Substance 3E09
    Sedatives 3E09
    Serum 3E09
    Toxoid 3E09
    Vaccine 3E09
  Pancreatic Tract 3E0J
    Analgesics 3E0J
    Anesthetic Agent 3E0J
    Anti-infective 3E0J
    Anti-inflammatory 3E0J
    Antineoplastic 3E0J
    Destructive Agent 3E0J
    Diagnostic Substance, Other 3E0J
    Electrolytic Substance 3E0J
    Gas 3E0J
    Hypnotics 3E0J
    Islet Cells, Pancreatic 3E0J
    Nutritional Substance 3E0J
    Radioactive Substance 3E0J
    Sedatives 3E0J
    Water Balance Substance 3E0J
  Pericardial Cavity 3E0Y
    Analgesics 3E0Y3NZ
    Anesthetic Agent 3E0Y3BZ
    Anti-infective 3E0Y32
    Anti-inflammatory 3E0Y33Z
    Antineoplastic 3E0Y
    Destructive Agent 3E0Y3TZ
    Diagnostic Substance, Other 3E0Y3KZ
    Electrolytic Substance 3E0Y37Z
    Gas 3E0Y
    Hypnotics 3E0Y3NZ
    Nutritional Substance 3E0Y36Z
    Radioactive Substance 3E0Y3HZ
    Sedatives 3E0Y3NZ

Introduction of substance in or on — *continued*

Pericardial Cavity — *continued*
  Water Balance Substance 3E0Y37Z
Peritoneal Cavity 3E0M
  Adhesion Barrier 3E0M
  Analgesics 3E0M3NZ
  Anesthetic Agent 3E0M3BZ
  Anti-infective 3E0M32
  Anti-inflammatory 3E0M33Z
  Antineoplastic 3E0M
  Destructive Agent 3E0M3TZ
  Diagnostic Substance, Other 3E0M3KZ
  Electrolytic Substance 3E0M37Z
  Gas 3E0M
  Hypnotics 3E0M3NZ
  Nutritional Substance 3E0M36Z
  Radioactive Substance 3E0M3HZ
  Sedatives 3E0M3NZ
  Water Balance Substance 3E0M37Z
Pharynx 3E0D
  Analgesics 3E0D
  Anesthetic Agent 3E0D
  Antiarrhythmic 3E0D
  Anti-infective 3E0D
  Anti-inflammatory 3E0D
  Antineoplastic 3E0D
  Destructive Agent 3E0D
  Diagnostic Substance, Other 3E0D
  Electrolytic Substance 3E0D
  Hypnotics 3E0D
  Nutritional Substance 3E0D
  Radioactive Substance 3E0D
  Sedatives 3E0D
  Serum 3E0D
  Toxoid 3E0D
  Vaccine 3E0D
  Water Balance Substance 3E0D
Pleural Cavity 3E0L
  Adhesion Barrier 3E0L
  Analgesics 3E0L3NZ
  Anesthetic Agent 3E0L3BZ
  Anti-infective 3E0L32
  Anti-inflammatory 3E0L33Z
  Antineoplastic 3E0L
  Destructive Agent 3E0L3TZ
  Diagnostic Substance, Other 3E0L3KZ
  Electrolytic Substance 3E0L37Z
  Gas 3E0L
  Hypnotics 3E0L3NZ
  Nutritional Substance 3E0L36Z
  Radioactive Substance 3E0L3HZ
  Sedatives 3E0L3NZ
  Water Balance Substance 3E0L37Z
Products of Conception 3E0E
  Analgesics 3E0E
  Anesthetic Agent 3E0E
  Anti-infective 3E0E
  Anti-inflammatory 3E0E
  Antineoplastic 3E0E
  Destructive Agent 3E0E
  Diagnostic Substance, Other 3E0E
  Electrolytic Substance 3E0E
  Gas 3E0E
  Hypnotics 3E0E
  Nutritional Substance 3E0E
  Radioactive Substance 3E0E
  Sedatives 3E0E
  Water Balance Substance 3E0E
Reproductive
  Female 3E0P
    Adhesion Barrier 3E0P
    Analgesics 3E0P
    Anesthetic Agent 3E0P
    Anti-infective 3E0P
    Anti-inflammatory 3E0P
    Antineoplastic 3E0P
    Destructive Agent 3E0P
    Diagnostic Substance, Other 3E0P
    Electrolytic Substance 3E0P
    Gas 3E0P
    Hormone 3E0P
    Hypnotics 3E0P
    Nutritional Substance 3E0P
    Ovum, Fertilized 3E0P
    Radioactive Substance 3E0P
    Sedatives 3E0P
    Sperm 3E0P
    Water Balance Substance 3E0P
  Male 3E0N

Introduction of substance in or on — *continued*

Reproductive — *continued*
  Male — *continued*
    Analgesics 3E0N
    Anesthetic Agent 3E0N
    Anti-infective 3E0N
    Anti-inflammatory 3E0N
    Antineoplastic 3E0N
    Destructive Agent 3E0N
    Diagnostic Substance, Other 3E0N
    Electrolytic Substance 3E0N
    Gas 3E0N
    Hypnotics 3E0N
    Nutritional Substance 3E0N
    Radioactive Substance 3E0N
    Sedatives 3E0N
    Water Balance Substance 3E0N
Respiratory Tract 3E0F
  Analgesics 3E0F
  Anesthetic Agent 3E0F
  Anti-infective 3E0F
  Anti-inflammatory 3E0F
  Antineoplastic 3E0F
  Destructive Agent 3E0F
  Diagnostic Substance, Other 3E0F
  Electrolytic Substance 3E0F
  Gas 3E0F
  Hypnotics 3E0F
  Nutritional Substance 3E0F
  Radioactive Substance 3E0F
  Sedatives 3E0F
  Water Balance Substance 3E0F
Skin 3E00XGC
  Analgesics 3E00XNZ
  Anesthetic Agent 3E00XBZ
  Anti-infective 3E00X2
  Anti-inflammatory 3E00X3Z
  Antineoplastic 3E00X0
  Destructive Agent 3E00XTZ
  Diagnostic Substance, Other 3E00XKZ
  Hypnotics 3E00XNZ
  Pigment 3E00XMZ
  Sedatives 3E00XNZ
  Serum 3E00X4Z
  Toxoid 3E00X4Z
  Vaccine 3E00X4Z
Spinal Canal 3E0R3GC
  Analgesics 3E0R3NZ
  Anesthetic Agent 3E0R3BZ
  Anti-infective 3E0R32
  Anti-inflammatory 3E0R33Z
  Antineoplastic 3E0R30
  Destructive Agent 3E0R3TZ
  Diagnostic Substance, Other 3E0R3KZ
  Electrolytic Substance 3E0R37Z
  Gas 3E0R
  Hypnotics 3E0R3NZ
  Nutritional Substance 3E0R36Z
  Radioactive Substance 3E0R3HZ
  Sedatives 3E0R3NZ
  Stem Cells
    Embryonic 3E0R
    Somatic 3E0R
  Water Balance Substance 3E0R37Z
Subcutaneous Tissue 3E013GC
  Analgesics 3E013NZ
  Anesthetic Agent 3E013BZ
  Anti-infective 3E01
  Anti-inflammatory 3E0133Z
  Antineoplastic 3E0130
  Destructive Agent 3E013TZ
  Diagnostic Substance, Other 3E013KZ
  Electrolytic Substance 3E0137Z
  Hormone 3E013V
  Hypnotics 3E013NZ
  Nutritional Substance 3E0136Z
  Radioactive Substance 3E013HZ
  Sedatives 3E013NZ
  Serum 3E0134Z
  Toxoid 3E0134Z
  Vaccine 3E0134Z
  Water Balance Substance 3E0137Z
Vein
  Central 3E04
    Analgesics 3E04
    Anesthetic, Intracirculatory 3E04
    Antiarrhythmic 3E04
    Anti-infective 3E04
    Anti-inflammatory 3E04

Introduction of substance in or on — *continued*

Vein — *continued*
  Central — *continued*
    Antineoplastic 3E04
    Destructive Agent 3E04
    Diagnostic Substance, Other 3E04
    Electrolytic Substance 3E04
    Hormone 3E04
    Hypnotics 3E04
    Immunotherapeutic 3E04
    Nutritional Substance 3E04
    Platelet Inhibitor 3E04
    Radioactive Substance 3E04
    Sedatives 3E04
    Serum 3E04
    Thrombolytic 3E04
    Toxoid 3E04
    Vaccine 3E04
    Vasopressor 3E04
    Water Balance Substance 3E04
  Peripheral 3E03
    Analgesics 3E03
    Anesthetic, Intracirculatory 3E03
    Antiarrhythmic 3E03
    Anti-infective 3E03
    Anti-inflammatory 3E03
    Antineoplastic 3E03
    Destructive Agent 3E03
    Diagnostic Substance, Other 3E03
    Electrolytic Substance 3E03
    Hormone 3E03
    Hypnotics 3E03
    Immunotherapeutic 3E03
    Islet Cells, Pancreatic 3E03
    Nutritional Substance 3E03
    Platelet Inhibitor 3E03
    Radioactive Substance 3E03
    Sedatives 3E03
    Serum 3E03
    Thrombolytic 3E03
    Toxoid 3E03
    Vaccine 3E03
    Vasopressor 3E03
    Water Balance Substance 3E03

Intubation
Airway
  see Insertion of device in, Esophagus 0DH5
  see Insertion of device in, Mouth and Throat 0CHY
  see Insertion of device in, Trachea 0BH1
Drainage device *see* Drainage
Feeding Device *see* Insertion of device in, Gastrointestinal System 0DH
INTUITY Elite valve system, EDWARDS (rapid deployment technique) *see* Replacement, Valve, Aortic 02RF
Iobenguane I-131 Antineoplastic XW0
Iobenguane I-131, High Specific Activity (HSA) *use* Iobenguane I-131 Antineoplastic
IPPB (intermittent positive pressure breathing) *see* Assistance, Respiratory 5A09
IRE (Irreversible Electroporation) *see* Destruction, Hepatobiliary System and Pancreas 0F5
Iridectomy
  see Excision, Eye 08B
  see Resection, Eye 08T
Iridoplasty
  see Repair, Eye 08Q
  see Replacement, Eye 08R
  see Supplement, Eye 08U
Iridotomy *see* Drainage, Eye 089
Irreversible Electroporation (IRE) *see* Destruction, Hepatobiliary System and Pancreas 0F5
Irrigation
Biliary Tract, Irrigating Substance 3E1J
Brain, Irrigating Substance 3E1Q38Z
Cranial Cavity, Irrigating Substance 3E1Q38Z
Ear, Irrigating Substance 3E1B
Epidural Space, Irrigating Substance 3E1S38Z
Eye, Irrigating Substance 3E1C
Gastrointestinal Tract
  Lower, Irrigating Substance 3E1H
  Upper, Irrigating Substance 3E1G
Genitourinary Tract, Irrigating Substance 3E1K
Irrigating Substance 3C1ZX8Z
Joint, Irrigating Substance 3E1U
Mucous Membrane, Irrigating Substance 3E10
Nose, Irrigating Substance 3E19

Irrigation — *continued*
  Pancreatic Tract, Irrigating Substance 3E1J
  Pericardial Cavity, Irrigating Substance 3E1Y38Z
  Peritoneal Cavity
    Dialysate 3E1M39Z
    Irrigating Substance 3E1M
  Pleural Cavity, Irrigating Substance 3E1L38Z
  Reproductive
    Female, Irrigating Substance 3E1P
    Male, Irrigating Substance 3E1N
  Respiratory Tract, Irrigating Substance 3E1F
  Skin, Irrigating Substance 3E10
  Spinal Canal, Irrigating Substance 3E1R38Z
Isavuconazole (isavuconazonium sulfate) *use* Other Anti-infective
Ischemic Stroke System (ISS500) *use* Neurostimulator Lead in New Technology
Ischiatic nerve *use* Sciatic Nerve
Ischiocavernosus muscle *use* Perineum Muscle
Ischiofemoral ligament
  use Hip Bursa and Ligament, Left
  use Hip Bursa and Ligament, Right
Ischium
  use Pelvic Bone, Left
  use Pelvic Bone, Right
ISC-REST kit
  ISCDx XXE5XT7
  QIAGEN Access Anti-SARS-CoV-2 Total Test XXE5XV7
  QIAstat-Dx Respiratory SARS-CoV-2 Panel XXE97U7
Isolation 8E0ZXY6
Isotope Administration, Other Radiation, Whole Body DWY5G
ISS500 (Ischemic Stroke System) *use* Neurostimulator Lead in New Technology
Itrel (3) (4) neurostimulator *use* Stimulator Generator, Single Array in 0JH

J

Jakafi® *use* Ruxolitinib
Jejunal artery *use* Superior Mesenteric Artery
Jejunectomy
  see Excision, Jejunum 0DBA
  see Resection, Jejunum 0DTA
Jejunocolostomy
  see Bypass, Gastrointestinal System 0D1
  see Drainage, Gastrointestinal System 0D9
Jejunopexy
  see Repair, Jejunum 0DQA
  see Reposition, Jejunum 0DSA
Jejunostomy
  see Bypass, Jejunum 0D1A
  see Drainage, Jejunum 0D9A
Jejunotomy *see* Drainage, Jejunum 0D9A
Joint fixation plate
  use Internal Fixation Device in Lower Joints
  use Internal Fixation Device in Upper Joints
Joint liner (insert) *use* Liner in Lower Joints
Joint spacer (antibiotic)
  use Spacer in Lower Joints
  use Spacer in Upper Joints
Jugular body *use* Glomus Jugulare
Jugular lymph node
  use Lymphatic, Left Neck
  use Lymphatic, Right Neck

K

Kappa *use* Pacemaker, Dual Chamber in 0JH
Kcentra *use* 4-Factor Prothrombin Complex Concentrate
Keratectomy, kerectomy
  see Excision, Eye 08B
  see Resection, Eye 08T
Keratocentesis *see* Drainage, Eye 089
Keratoplasty
  see Repair, Eye 08Q
  see Replacement, Eye 08R
  see Supplement, Eye 08U
Keratotomy
  see Drainage, Eye 089
  see Repair, Eye 08Q
KEVZARA® *use* Sarilumab

Keystone Heart TriGuard 3™ CEPD (cerebral embolic protection device) X2A6325
Kirschner wire (K-wire)
  use Internal Fixation Device in Head and Facial Bones
  use Internal Fixation Device in Lower Bones
  use Internal Fixation Device in Lower Joints
  use Internal Fixation Device in Upper Bones
  use Internal Fixation Device in Upper Joints
Knee (implant) insert *use* Liner in Lower Joints
KUB x-ray *see* Plain Radiography, Kidney, Ureter and Bladder BT04
Kuntscher nail
  use Internal Fixation Device, Intramedullary in Lower Bones
  use Internal Fixation Device, Intramedullary in Upper Bones
KYMRIAH® *use* Tisagenlecleucel Immunotherapy

L

Labia majora *use* Vulva
Labia minora *use* Vulva
Labial gland
  use Lower Lip
  use Upper Lip
Labiectomy
  see Excision, Female Reproductive System 0UB
  see Resection, Female Reproductive System 0UT
Lacrimal canaliculus
  use Lacrimal Duct, Left
  use Lacrimal Duct, Right
Lacrimal punctum
  use Lacrimal Duct, Left
  use Lacrimal Duct, Right
Lacrimal sac
  use Lacrimal Duct, Left
  use Lacrimal Duct, Right
LAGB (laparoscopic adjustable gastric banding)
  Initial procedure 0DV64CZ
  Surgical correction *see* Revision of device in, Stomach 0DW6
Laminectomy
  see Excision, Lower Bones 0QB
  see Excision, Upper Bones 0PB
  see Release, Central Nervous System and Cranial Nerves 00N
  see Release, Peripheral Nervous System 01N
Laminotomy
  see Drainage, Lower Bones 0Q9
  see Drainage, Upper Bones 0P9
  see Excision, Lower Bones 0QB
  see Excision, Upper Bones 0PB
  see Release, Central Nervous System and Cranial Nerves 00N
  see Release, Lower Bones 0QN
  see Release, Peripheral Nervous System 01N
  see Release, Upper Bones 0PN
Laparoscopic-assisted transanal pull-through
  see Excision, Gastrointestinal System 0DB
  see Resection, Gastrointestinal System 0DT
Laparoscopy *see* Inspection
Laparotomy
  Drainage *see* Drainage, Peritoneal Cavity 0W9G
  Exploratory *see* Inspection, Peritoneal Cavity 0WJG
LAP-BAND® adjustable gastric banding system *use* Extraluminal Device
Laryngectomy
  see Excision, Larynx 0CBS
  see Resection, Larynx 0CTS
Laryngocentesis *see* Drainage, Larynx 0C9S
Laryngogram *see* Fluoroscopy, Larynx B91J
Laryngopexy *see* Repair, Larynx 0CQS
Laryngopharynx *use* Pharynx
Laryngoplasty
  see Repair, Larynx 0CQS
  see Replacement, Larynx 0CRS
  see Supplement, Larynx 0CUS
Laryngorrhaphy *see* Repair, Larynx 0CQS
Laryngoscopy 0CJS8ZZ
Laryngotomy *see* Drainage, Larynx 0C9S
Laser Interstitial Thermal Therapy
  Ampulla of Vater 0F5C
  Anus 0D5Q
  Aortic Body 0G5D
  Appendix 0D5J

Laser Interstitial Thermal Therapy — *continued*
  Brain 0050
  Breast
    Bilateral 0H5V
    Left 0H5U
    Right 0H5T
  Carotid Bodies, Bilateral 0G58
  Carotid Body
    Left 0G56
    Right 0G57
  Cecum 0D5H
  Coccygeal Glomus 0G5B
  Colon
    Ascending 0D5K
    Descending 0D5M
    Sigmoid 0D5N
    Transverse 0D5L
  Duct
    Common Bile 0F59
    Cystic 0F58
    Hepatic
      Common 0F57
      Left 0F56
      Right 0F55
    Pancreatic 0F5D
      Accessory 0F5F
  Duodenum 0D59
  Esophagogastric Junction 0D54
  Esophagus 0D55
    Lower 0D53
    Middle 0D52
    Upper 0D51
  Gallbladder 0F54
  Gland
    Adrenal
      Bilateral 0G54
      Left 0G52
      Right 0G53
    Pituitary 0G50
  Glomus Jugulare 0G5C
  Ileocecal Valve 0D5C
  Ileum 0D5B
  Intestine
    Large 0D5E
      Left 0D5G
      Right 0D5F
    Small 0D58
  Jejunum 0D5A
  Liver 0F50
    Left Lobe 0F52
    Right Lobe 0F51
  Lung
    Bilateral 0B5M
    Left 0B5L
    Lower Lobe
      Left 0B5J
      Right 0B5F
    Middle Lobe, Right 0B5D
    Right 0B5K
    Upper Lobe
      Left 0B5G
      Right 0B5C
  Lung Lingula 0B5H
  Pancreas 0F5G
  Para-aortic Body 0G59
  Paraganglion Extremity 0G5F
  Parathyroid Gland 0G5R
    Inferior
      Left 0G5P
      Right 0G5N
    Multiple 0G5Q
    Superior
      Left 0G5M
      Right 0G5L
  Pineal Body 0G51
  Prostate 0V50
  Rectum 0D5P
  Spinal Cord
    Cervical 005W
    Lumbar 005Y
    Thoracic 005X
  Stomach 0D56
    Pylorus 0D57
  Thyroid Gland 0G5K
    Left Lobe 0G5G
    Right Lobe 0G5H
Lateral canthus
  use Upper Eyelid, Left
  use Upper Eyelid, Right

Lateral collateral ligament (LCL)
　use Knee Bursa and Ligament, Left
　use Knee Bursa and Ligament, Right
Lateral condyle of femur
　use Lower Femur, Left
　use Lower Femur, Right
Lateral condyle of tibia
　use Tibia, Left
　use Tibia, Right
Lateral cuneiform bone
　use Tarsal, Left
　use Tarsal, Right
Lateral epicondyle of femur
　use Lower Femur, Left
　use Lower Femur, Right
Lateral epicondyle of humerus
　use Humeral Shaft, Left
　use Humeral Shaft, Right
Lateral femoral cutaneous nerve *use* Lumbar Plexus
Lateral (brachial) lymph node
　use Lymphatic, Left Axillary
　use Lymphatic, Right Axillary
Lateral malleolus
　use Fibula, Left
　use Fibula, Right
Lateral meniscus
　use Knee Joint, Left
　use Knee Joint, Right
Lateral nasal cartilage *use* Nasal Mucosa and Soft
　　Tissue
Lateral plantar artery
　use Foot Artery, Left
　use Foot Artery, Right
Lateral plantar nerve *use* Tibial Nerve
Lateral rectus muscle
　use Extraocular Muscle, Left
　use Extraocular Muscle, Right
Lateral sacral artery
　use Internal Iliac Artery, Left
　use Internal Iliac Artery, Right
Lateral sacral vein
　use Hypogastric Vein, Left
　use Hypogastric Vein, Right
Lateral sural cutaneous nerve *use* Peroneal Nerve
Lateral tarsal artery
　use Foot Artery, Left
　use Foot Artery, Right
Lateral temporomandibular ligament *use* Head and
　　Neck Bursa and Ligament
Lateral thoracic artery
　use Axillary Artery, Left
　use Axillary Artery, Right
Latissimus dorsi muscle
　use Trunk Muscle, Left
　use Trunk Muscle, Right
Latissimus Dorsi Myocutaneous Flap
　Replacement
　　Bilateral 0HRV075
　　Left 0HRU075
　　Right 0HRT075
　Transfer
　　Left 0KXG
　　Right 0KXF
Lavage
　see Irrigation
　Bronchial alveolar, diagnostic *see* Drainage, Respiratory System 0B9
Least splanchnic nerve *use* Thoracic Sympathetic
　　Nerve
Lefamulin Anti-infective XW0
Left ascending lumbar vein *use* Hemiazygos Vein
Left atrioventricular valve *use* Mitral Valve
Left auricular appendix *use* Atrium, Left
Left colic vein *use* Colic Vein
Left coronary sulcus *use* Heart, Left
Left gastric artery *use* Gastric Artery
Left gastroepiploic artery *use* Splenic Artery
Left gastroepiploic vein *use* Splenic Vein
Left inferior phrenic vein *use* Renal Vein, Left
Left inferior pulmonary vein *use* Pulmonary Vein,
　　Left
Left jugular trunk *use* Thoracic Duct
Left lateral ventricle *use* Cerebral Ventricle
Left ovarian vein *use* Renal Vein, Left
Left second lumbar vein *use* Renal Vein, Left
Left subclavian trunk *use* Thoracic Duct

Left subcostal vein *use* Hemiazygos Vein
Left superior pulmonary vein *use* Pulmonary Vein,
　　Left
Left suprarenal vein *use* Renal Vein, Left
Left testicular vein *use* Renal Vein, Left
Lengthening
　Bone, with device *see* Insertion of Limb Lengthening Device
　Muscle, by incision *see* Division, Muscles 0K8
　Tendon, by incision *see* Division, Tendons 0L8
Leptomeninges, intracranial *use* Cerebral Meninges
Leptomeninges, spinal *use* Spinal Meninges
Leronlimab Monoclonal Antibody XW013K6
Lesser alar cartilage *use* Nasal Mucosa and Soft Tissue
Lesser occipital nerve *use* Cervical Plexus
Lesser Omentum *use* Omentum
Lesser saphenous vein
　use Saphenous Vein, Left
　use Saphenous Vein, Right
Lesser splanchnic nerve *use* Thoracic Sympathetic
　　Nerve
Lesser trochanter
　use Upper Femur, Left
　use Upper Femur, Right
Lesser tuberosity
　use Humeral Head, Left
　use Humeral Head, Right
Lesser wing *use* Sphenoid Bone
Leukopheresis, therapeutic *see* Pheresis, Circulatory
　　6A55
Levator anguli oris muscle *use* Facial Muscle
Levator ani muscle *use* Perineum Muscle
Levator labii superioris alaeque nasi muscle *use*
　　Facial Muscle
Levator labii superioris muscle *use* Facial Muscle
Levator palpebrae superioris muscle
　use Upper Eyelid, Left
　use Upper Eyelid, Right
Levator scapulae muscle
　use Neck Muscle, Left
　use Neck Muscle, Right
Levator veli palatini muscle *use* Tongue, Palate,
　　Pharynx Muscle
Levatores costarum muscle
　use Thorax Muscle, Left
　use Thorax Muscle, Right
Lifeline ARM Automated Chest Compression (ACC)
　device 5A1221J
LifeStent® (Flexstar) (XL) Vascular Stent System
　use Intraluminal Device
Lifileucel *use* Lifileucel Immunotherapy
Lifileucel Immunotherapy XW0
Ligament of head of fibula
　use Knee Bursa and Ligament, Left
　use Knee Bursa and Ligament, Right
Ligament of the lateral malleolus
　use Ankle Bursa and Ligament, Left
　use Ankle Bursa and Ligament, Right
Ligamentum flavum, cervical *use* Head and Neck
　　Bursa and Ligament
Ligamentum flavum, lumbar *use* Lower Spine Bursa
　　and Ligament
Ligamentum flavum, thoracic *use* Upper Spine Bursa
　　and Ligament
LigaPASS 2.0™ PJK Prevention System *use* Posterior
　　Vertebral Tether in New Technology
Ligation *see* Occlusion
Ligation, hemorrhoid *see* Occlusion, Lower Veins,
　　Hemorrhoidal Plexus
Light Therapy GZJZZZZ
Liner
　Removal of device from
　　Hip
　　　Left 0SPB09Z
　　　Right 0SP909Z
　　Knee
　　　Left 0SPD09Z
　　　Right 0SPC09Z
　Revision of device in
　　Hip
　　　Left 0SWB09Z
　　　Right 0SW909Z
　　Knee
　　　Left 0SWD09Z
　　　Right 0SWC09Z

Liner — *continued*
　Supplement
　　Hip
　　　Left 0SUB09Z
　　　　Acetabular Surface 0SUE09Z
　　　　Femoral Surface 0SUS09Z
　　　Right 0SU909Z
　　　　Acetabular Surface 0SUA09Z
　　　　Femoral Surface 0SUR09Z
　　Knee
　　　Left 0SUD09
　　　　Femoral Surface 0SUU09Z
　　　　Tibial Surface 0SUW09Z
　　　Right 0SUC09
　　　　Femoral Surface 0SUT09Z
　　　　Tibial Surface 0SUV09Z
Lingual artery
　use External Carotid Artery, Left
　use External Carotid Artery, Right
Lingual tonsil *use* Pharynx
Lingulectomy, lung
　see Excision, Lung Lingula 0BBH
　see Resection, Lung Lingula 0BTH
Lisocabtagene Maraleucel *use* Lisocabtagene Maraleucel Immunotherapy
Lisocabtagene Maraleucel Immunotherapy XW0
Lithoplasty *see* Fragmentation
Lithotripsy
　see Fragmentation
　With removal of fragments *see* Extirpation
LITT (laser interstitial thermal therapy)
　see Destruction
　see Laser Interstitial Thermal Therapy
LIVIAN™ CRT-D *use* Cardiac Resynchronization Defibrillator Pulse Generator in 0JH
LIVTENCITY™ *use* Maribavir Anti-infective
Lobectomy
　see Excision, Central Nervous System and Cranial
　　Nerves 00B
　see Excision, Endocrine System 0GB
　see Excision, Hepatobiliary System and Pancreas
　　0FB
　see Excision, Respiratory System 0BB
　see Resection, Endocrine System 0GT
　see Resection, Hepatobiliary System and Pancreas
　　0FT
　see Resection, Respiratory System 0BT
Lobotomy *see* Division, Brain 0080
Localization
　see Imaging
　see Map
Locus ceruleus *use* Pons
Long thoracic nerve *use* Brachial Plexus
Loop ileostomy *see* Bypass, Ileum 0D1B
Loop recorder, implantable *use* Monitoring Device
Lower GI series *see* Fluoroscopy, Colon BD14
Lower Respiratory Fluid Nucleic Acid-base Microbial Detection XXEBXQ6
LTX Regional Anticoagulant *use* Nafamostat Anticoagulant
LUCAS® Chest Compression System 5A1221J
Lumbar artery *use* Abdominal Aorta
Lumbar facet joint *use* Lumbar Vertebral Joint
Lumbar ganglion *use* Lumbar Sympathetic Nerve
Lumbar lymph node *use* Lymphatic, Aortic
Lumbar lymphatic trunk *use* Cisterna Chyli
Lumbar splanchnic nerve *use* Lumbar Sympathetic
　　Nerve
Lumbosacral facet joint *use* Lumbosacral Joint
Lumbosacral trunk *use* Lumbar Nerve
Lumpectomy *see* Excision
Lunate bone
　use Carpal, Left
　use Carpal, Right
Lunotriquetral ligament
　use Hand Bursa and Ligament, Left
　use Hand Bursa and Ligament, Right
Lurbinectedin XW0
Lymphadenectomy
　see Excision, Lymphatic and Hemic Systems 07B
　see Resection, Lymphatic and Hemic Systems 07T
Lymphadenotomy *see* Drainage, Lymphatic and Hemic
　　Systems 079
Lymphangiectomy
　see Excision, Lymphatic and Hemic Systems 07B
　see Resection, Lymphatic and Hemic Systems 07T

Lymphangiogram *see* Plain Radiography, Lymphatic System B70
Lymphangioplasty
  see Repair, Lymphatic and Hemic Systems Ø7Q
  see Supplement, Lymphatic and Hemic Systems Ø7U
Lymphangiorrhaphy *see* Repair, Lymphatic and Hemic Systems Ø7Q
Lymphangiotomy *see* Drainage, Lymphatic and Hemic Systems Ø79
Lysis *see* Release

M

Macula XXE5XR7
  use Retina, Left
  use Retina, Right
MAGEC® Spinal Bracing and Distraction System
  use Magnetically Controlled Growth Rod(s) in New Technology
Magnet extraction, ocular foreign body *see* Extirpation, Eye Ø8C
Magnetic Resonance Imaging (MRI)
  Abdomen BW3Ø
  Ankle
    Left BQ3H
    Right BQ3G
  Aorta
    Abdominal B43Ø
    Thoracic B33Ø
  Arm
    Left BP3F
    Right BP3E
  Artery
    Celiac B431
    Cervico-Cerebral Arch B33Q
    Common Carotid, Bilateral B335
    Coronary
      Bypass Graft, Multiple B233
      Multiple B231
    Internal Carotid, Bilateral B338
    Intracranial B33R
    Lower Extremity
      Bilateral B43H
      Left B43G
      Right B43F
    Pelvic B43C
    Renal, Bilateral B438
    Spinal B33M
    Superior Mesenteric B434
    Upper Extremity
      Bilateral B33K
      Left B33J
      Right B33H
    Vertebral, Bilateral B33G
  Bladder BT3Ø
  Brachial Plexus BW3P
  Brain BØ3Ø
  Breast
    Bilateral BH32
    Left BH31
    Right BH3Ø
  Calcaneus
    Left BQ3K
    Right BQ3J
  Chest BW33Y
  Coccyx BR3F
  Connective Tissue
    Lower Extremity BL31
    Upper Extremity BL3Ø
  Corpora Cavernosa BV3Ø
  Disc
    Cervical BR31
    Lumbar BR33
    Thoracic BR32
  Ear B93Ø
  Elbow
    Left BP3H
    Right BP3G
  Eye
    Bilateral B837
    Left B836
    Right B835
  Femur
    Left BQ34
    Right BQ33
  Fetal Abdomen BY33

Magnetic Resonance Imaging (MRI) — *continued*
  Fetal Extremity BY35
  Fetal Head BY3Ø
  Fetal Heart BY31
  Fetal Spine BY34
  Fetal Thorax BY32
  Fetus, Whole BY36
  Foot
    Left BQ3M
    Right BQ3L
  Forearm
    Left BP3K
    Right BP3J
  Gland
    Adrenal, Bilateral BG32
    Parathyroid BG33
    Parotid, Bilateral B936
    Salivary, Bilateral B93D
    Submandibular, Bilateral B939
    Thyroid BG34
  Head BW38
  Heart, Right and Left B236
  Hip
    Left BQ31
    Right BQ3Ø
  Intracranial Sinus B532
  Joint
    Finger
      Left BP3D
      Right BP3C
    Hand
      Left BP3D
      Right BP3C
    Temporomandibular, Bilateral BN39
  Kidney
    Bilateral BT33
    Left BT32
    Right BT31
    Transplant BT39
  Knee
    Left BQ38
    Right BQ37
  Larynx B93J
  Leg
    Left BQ3F
    Right BQ3D
  Liver BF35
  Liver and Spleen BF36
  Lung Apices BB3G
  Lung, Bilateral, Hyperpolarized Xenon 129 (Xe-129) BB34Z3Z
  Nasopharynx B93F
  Neck BW3F
  Nerve
    Acoustic BØ3C
    Brachial Plexus BW3P
  Oropharynx B93F
  Ovary
    Bilateral BU35
    Left BU34
    Right BU33
  Ovary and Uterus BU3C
  Pancreas BF37
  Patella
    Left BQ3W
    Right BQ3V
  Pelvic Region BW3G
  Pelvis BR3C
  Pituitary Gland BØ39
  Plexus, Brachial BW3P
  Prostate BV33
  Retroperitoneum BW3H
  Sacrum BR3F
  Scrotum BV34
  Sella Turcica BØ39
  Shoulder
    Left BP39
    Right BP38
  Sinus
    Intracranial B532
    Paranasal B932
  Spinal Cord BØ3B
  Spine
    Cervical BR3Ø
    Lumbar BR39
    Thoracic BR37
  Spleen and Liver BF36
  Subcutaneous Tissue
    Abdomen BH3H

Magnetic Resonance Imaging (MRI) — *continued*
  Subcutaneous Tissue — *continued*
    Extremity
      Lower BH3J
      Upper BH3F
    Head BH3D
    Neck BH3D
    Pelvis BH3H
    Thorax BH3G
  Tendon
    Lower Extremity BL33
    Upper Extremity BL32
  Testicle
    Bilateral BV37
    Left BV36
    Right BV35
  Toe
    Left BQ3Q
    Right BQ3P
  Uterus BU36
    Pregnant BU3B
  Uterus and Ovary BU3C
  Vagina BU39
  Vein
    Cerebellar B531
    Cerebral B531
    Jugular, Bilateral B535
    Lower Extremity
      Bilateral B53D
      Left B53C
      Right B53B
    Other B53V
    Pelvic (Iliac) Bilateral B53H
    Portal B53T
    Pulmonary, Bilateral B53S
    Renal, Bilateral B53L
    Spanchnic B53T
    Upper Extremity
      Bilateral B53P
      Left B53N
      Right B53M
  Vena Cava
    Inferior B539
    Superior B538
  Wrist
    Left BP3M
    Right BP3L
Magnetically Controlled Growth Rod(s)
  Cervical XNS3
  Lumbar XNS4
  Thoracic XNS3
Magnetic-guided radiofrequency endovascular fistula
  Radial Artery, Left Ø31C3ZF
  Radial Artery, Right Ø31B3ZF
  Ulnar Artery, Left Ø31A3ZF
  Ulnar Artery, Right Ø3193ZF
Magnus Neuromodulation System (MNS) XØZØX18
Malleotomy *see* Drainage, Ear, Nose, Sinus Ø99
Malleus
  use Auditory Ossicle, Left
  use Auditory Ossicle, Right
Mammaplasty, mammoplasty
  see Alteration, Skin and Breast ØHØ
  see Repair, Skin and Breast ØHQ
  see Replacement, Skin and Breast ØHR
  see Supplement, Skin and Breast ØHU
Mammary duct
  use Breast, Bilateral
  use Breast, Left
  use Breast, Right
Mammary gland
  use Breast, Bilateral
  use Breast, Left
  use Breast, Right
Mammectomy
  see Excision, Skin and Breast ØHB
  see Resection, Skin and Breast ØHT
Mammillary body *use* Hypothalamus
Mammography *see* Plain Radiography, Skin, Subcutaneous Tissue and Breast BHØ
Mammotomy *see* Drainage, Skin and Breast ØH9
Mandibular nerve *use* Trigeminal Nerve
Mandibular notch
  use Mandible, Left
  use Mandible, Right
Mandibulectomy
  see Excision, Head and Facial Bones ØNB

▼ **Subterms under main terms may continue to next column or page**

Mandibulectomy — *continued*
  see Resection, Head and Facial Bones ØNT
Manipulation
  Adhesions *see* Release
  Chiropractic *see* Chiropractic Manipulation
Manual removal, retained placenta *see* Extraction,
    Products of Conception, Retained 1ØD1
Manubrium *use* Sternum
Map
  Basal Ganglia ØØK8
  Brain ØØKØ
  Cerebellum ØØKC
  Cerebral Hemisphere ØØK7
  Conduction Mechanism Ø2K8
  Hypothalamus ØØKA
  Medulla Oblongata ØØKD
  Pons ØØKB
  Thalamus ØØK9
Mapping
  Doppler ultrasound *see* Ultrasonography
  Electrocardiogram only *see* Measurement, Cardiac
    4AØ2
Maribavir Anti-infective XWØ
Mark IV Breathing Pacemaker System *use* Stimulator
    Generator in Subcutaneous Tissue and Fascia
MarrowStim™ PAD Kit for CBMA (Concentrated Bone
    Marrow Aspirate) *use* Other Substance
**MarrowStim™ PAD Kit, for injection of concentrat-
    ed bone marrow aspirate** *see* Introduction of
    substance in or on, Muscle 3EØ2
Marsupialization
  see Drainage
  see Excision
Massage, cardiac
  External 5A12Ø12
  Open Ø2QAØZZ
Masseter muscle *use* Head Muscle
Masseteric fascia *use* Subcutaneous Tissue and Fascia,
    Face
Mastectomy
  see Excision, Skin and Breast ØHB
  see Resection, Skin and Breast ØHT
Mastoid air cells
  use Mastoid Sinus, Left
  use Mastoid Sinus, Right
Mastoid (postauricular) lymph node
  use Lymphatic, Left Neck
  use Lymphatic, Right Neck
Mastoid process
  use Temporal Bone, Left
  use Temporal Bone, Right
Mastoidectomy
  see Excision, Ear, Nose, Sinus Ø9B
  see Resection, Ear, Nose, Sinus Ø9T
Mastoidotomy *see* Drainage, Ear, Nose, Sinus Ø99
Mastopexy
  see Repair, Skin and Breast ØHQ
  see Reposition, Skin and Breast ØHS
Mastorrhaphy *see* Repair, Skin and Breast ØHQ
Mastotomy *see* Drainage, Skin and Breast ØH9
Maxillary artery
  use External Carotid Artery, Left
  use External Carotid Artery, Right
Maxillary nerve *use* Trigeminal Nerve
Maximo II DR (VR) *use* Defibrillator Generator in ØJH
Maximo II DR CRT-D *use* Cardiac Resynchronization
    Defibrillator Pulse Generator in ØJH
Measurement
  Arterial
    Flow
      Coronary 4AØ3
      Intracranial 4AØ3X5D
      Peripheral 4AØ3
      Pulmonary 4AØ3
    Pressure
      Coronary 4AØ3
      Peripheral 4AØ3
      Pulmonary 4AØ3
      Thoracic, Other 4AØ3
    Pulse
      Coronary 4AØ3
      Peripheral 4AØ3
      Pulmonary 4AØ3
    Saturation, Peripheral 4AØ3
    Sound, Peripheral 4AØ3
  Biliary
    Flow 4AØC

Measurement — *continued*
  Biliary — *continued*
    Pressure 4AØC
  Cardiac
    Action Currents 4AØ2
    Defibrillator 4BØ2XTZ
    Electrical Activity 4AØ2
      Guidance 4AØ2X4A
      No Qualifier 4AØ2X4Z
    Output 4AØ2
    Pacemaker 4BØ2XSZ
    Rate 4AØ2
    Rhythm 4AØ2
    Sampling and Pressure
      Bilateral 4AØ2
      Left Heart 4AØ2
      Right Heart 4AØ2
    Sound 4AØ2
    Total Activity, Stress 4AØ2XM4
  Central Nervous
    Cerebrospinal Fluid Shunt, Wireless Sensor
      4BØØXWØ
    Conductivity 4AØØ
    Electrical Activity 4AØØ
    Pressure 4AØØØBZ
      Intracranial 4AØØ
    Saturation, Intracranial 4AØØ
    Stimulator 4BØØXVZ
    Temperature, Intracranial 4AØØ
  Circulatory, Volume 4AØ5XLZ
  Gastrointestinal
    Motility 4AØB
    Pressure 4AØB
    Secretion 4AØB
  Lower Respiratory Fluid Nucleic Acid-base Micro-
    bial Detection XXEBXQ6
  Lymphatic
    Flow 4AØ6
    Pressure 4AØ6
  Metabolism 4AØZ
  Musculoskeletal
    Contractility 4AØF
    Pressure 4AØF3BE
    Stimulator 4BØFXVZ
  Olfactory, Acuity 4AØ8XØZ
  Peripheral Nervous
    Conductivity
      Motor 4AØ1
      Sensory 4AØ1
    Electrical Activity 4AØ1
    Stimulator 4BØ1XVZ
  Positive Blood Culture Fluorescence Hybridization
    for Organism Identification, Concentration
    and Susceptibility XXE5XN6
  Products of Conception
    Cardiac
      Electrical Activity 4AØH
      Rate 4AØH
      Rhythm 4AØH
      Sound 4AØH
    Nervous
      Conductivity 4AØJ
      Electrical Activity 4AØJ
      Pressure 4AØJ
  Respiratory
    Capacity 4AØ9
    Flow 4AØ9
    Pacemaker 4BØ9XSZ
    Rate 4AØ9
    Resistance 4AØ9
    Total Activity 4AØ9
    Volume 4AØ9
  Sleep 4AØZXQZ
  Temperature 4AØZ
  Urinary
    Contractility 4AØD
    Flow 4AØD
    Pressure 4AØD
    Resistance 4AØD
    Volume 4AØD
  Venous
    Flow
      Central 4AØ4
      Peripheral 4AØ4
      Portal 4AØ4
      Pulmonary 4AØ4
    Pressure
      Central 4AØ4
      Peripheral 4AØ4

Measurement — *continued*
  Venous — *continued*
    Pressure — *continued*
      Portal 4AØ4
      Pulmonary 4AØ4
    Pulse
      Central 4AØ4
      Peripheral 4AØ4
      Portal 4AØ4
      Pulmonary 4AØ4
    Saturation, Peripheral 4AØ4
  Visual
    Acuity 4AØ7XØZ
    Mobility 4AØ7X7Z
    Pressure 4AØ7XBZ
  Whole Blood Nucleic Acid-base Microbial Detection
    XXE5XM5
Meatoplasty, urethra *see* Repair, Urethra ØTQD
Meatotomy *see* Drainage, Urinary System ØT9
Mechanical chest compression (mCPR) 5A1221J
**Mechanical Initial Specimen Diversion Technique
    Using Active Negative Pressure (blood collec-
    tion)** XXE5XR7
Mechanical ventilation *see* Performance, Respiratory
    5A19
Medial canthus
  use Lower Eyelid, Left
  use Lower Eyelid, Right
Medial collateral ligament (MCL)
  use Knee Bursa and Ligament, Left
  use Knee Bursa and Ligament, Right
Medial condyle of femur
  use Lower Femur, Left
  use Lower Femur, Right
Medial condyle of tibia
  use Tibia, Left
  use Tibia, Right
Medial cuneiform bone
  use Tarsal, Left
  use Tarsal, Right
Medial epicondyle of femur
  use Lower Femur, Left
  use Lower Femur, Right
Medial epicondyle of humerus
  use Humeral Shaft, Left
  use Humeral Shaft, Right
Medial malleolus
  use Tibia, Left
  use Tibia, Right
Medial meniscus
  use Knee Joint, Left
  use Knee Joint, Right
Medial plantar artery
  use Foot Artery, Left
  use Foot Artery, Right
Medial plantar nerve *use* Tibial Nerve
Medial popliteal nerve *use* Tibial Nerve
Medial rectus muscle
  use Extraocular Muscle, Left
  use Extraocular Muscle, Right
Medial sural cutaneous nerve *use* Tibial Nerve
Median antebrachial vein
  use Basilic Vein, Left
  use Basilic Vein, Right
Median cubital vein
  use Basilic Vein, Left
  use Basilic Vein, Right
Median sacral artery *use* Abdominal Aorta
Mediastinal cavity *use* Mediastinum
Mediastinal lymph node *use* Lymphatic, Thorax
Mediastinal space *use* Mediastinum
Mediastinoscopy ØWJC4ZZ
Medication Management GZ3ZZZZ
  for substance abuse
    Antabuse HZ83ZZZ
    Bupropion HZ87ZZZ
    Clonidine HZ86ZZZ
    Levo-alpha-acetyl-methadol (LAAM)
      HZ82ZZZ
    Methadone Maintenance HZ81ZZZ
    Naloxone HZ85ZZZ
    Naltrexone HZ84ZZZ
    Nicotine Replacement HZ80ZZZ
    Other Replacement Medication HZ89ZZZ
    Psychiatric Medication HZ88ZZZ
Meditation 8EØZXY5

Medtronic Endurant® II AAA stent graft system use Intraluminal Device

Meissner's (submucous) plexus use Abdominal Sympathetic Nerve

Melody® transcatheter pulmonary valve use Zooplastic Tissue in Heart and Great Vessels

Membranous urethra use Urethra

Meningeorrhaphy
  see Repair, Cerebral Meninges 00Q1
  see Repair, Spinal Meninges 00QT

Meniscectomy, knee
  see Excision, Joint, Knee, Left 0SBD
  see Excision, Joint, Knee, Right 0SBC

Mental foramen
  use Mandible, Left
  use Mandible, Right

Mentalis muscle use Facial Muscle

Mentoplasty see Alteration, Jaw, Lower 0W05

Meropenem-vaborbactam Anti-infective XW0

Mesenterectomy see Excision, Mesentery 0DBV

Mesenteriorrhaphy, mesenterorrhaphy see Repair, Mesentery 0DQV

Mesenteriplication see Repair, Mesentery 0DQV

Mesoappendix use Mesentery

Mesocolon use Mesentery

Metacarpal ligament
  use Hand Bursa and Ligament, Left
  use Hand Bursa and Ligament, Right

Metacarpophalangeal ligament
  use Hand Bursa and Ligament, Left
  use Hand Bursa and Ligament, Right

Metal on metal bearing surface use Synthetic Substitute, Metal in 0SR

Metatarsal ligament
  use Foot Bursa and Ligament, Left
  use Foot Bursa and Ligament, Right

Metatarsectomy
  see Excision, Lower Bones 0QB
  see Resection, Lower Bones 0QT

Metatarsophalangeal (MTP) joint
  use Metatarsal-Phalangeal Joint, Left
  use Metatarsal-Phalangeal Joint, Right

Metatarsophalangeal ligament
  use Foot Bursa and Ligament, Left
  use Foot Bursa and Ligament, Right

Metathalamus use Thalamus

Micro-Driver stent (RX) (OTW) use Intraluminal Device

MicroMed HeartAssist use Implantable Heart Assist System in Heart and Great Vessels

Micrus CERECYTE Microcoil use Intraluminal Device, Bioactive in Upper Arteries

Midcarpal joint
  use Carpal Joint, Left
  use Carpal Joint, Right

Middle cardiac nerve use Thoracic Sympathetic Nerve

Middle cerebral artery use Intracranial Artery

Middle cerebral vein use Intracranial Vein

Middle colic vein use Colic Vein

Middle genicular artery
  use Popliteal Artery, Left
  use Popliteal Artery, Right

Middle hemorrhoidal vein
  use Hypogastric Vein, Left
  use Hypogastric Vein, Right

Middle rectal artery
  use Internal Iliac Artery, Left
  use Internal Iliac Artery, Right

Middle suprarenal artery use Abdominal Aorta

Middle temporal artery
  use Temporal Artery, Left
  use Temporal Artery, Right

Middle turbinate use Nasal Turbinate

Mineral-based Topical Hemostatic Agent XW0

MIRODERM™ Biologic Wound Matrix use Nonautologous Tissue Substitute

MIRODERM™ skin graft see Replacement, Skin and Breast 0HR

MitraClip valve repair system use Synthetic Substitute

Mitral annulus use Mitral Valve

Mitroflow® Aortic Pericardial Heart Valve use Zooplastic Tissue in Heart and Great Vessels

MNS (Magnus Neuromodulation System) X0Z0X18

Mobilization, adhesions see Release

Molar gland use Buccal Mucosa

MolecuLight i:X® wound imaging see Other Imaging, Anatomical Regions BW5

Monitoring
  Arterial
    Flow
      Coronary 4A13
      Peripheral 4A13
      Pulmonary 4A13
    Pressure
      Coronary 4A13
      Peripheral 4A13
      Pulmonary 4A13
    Pulse
      Coronary 4A13
      Peripheral 4A13
      Pulmonary 4A13
    Saturation, Peripheral 4A13
    Sound, Peripheral 4A13
  Cardiac
    Electrical Activity 4A12
      Ambulatory 4A12X45
      No Qualifier 4A12X4Z
    Output 4A12
    Rate 4A12
    Rhythm 4A12
    Sound 4A12
    Total Activity, Stress 4A12XM4
    Vascular Perfusion, Indocyanine Green Dye 4A12XSH
  Central Nervous
    Conductivity 4A10
    Electrical Activity
      Intraoperative 4A10
      No Qualifier 4A10
    Pressure 4A100BZ
      Intracranial 4A10
    Saturation, Intracranial 4A10
    Temperature, Intracranial 4A10
  Gastrointestinal
    Motility 4A1B
    Pressure 4A1B
    Secretion 4A1B
    Vascular Perfusion, Indocyanine Green Dye 4A1BXSH
  Kidney, Fluorescent Pyrazine XT25XE5
  Lymphatic
    Flow
      Indocyanine Green Dye 4A16
      No Qualifier 4A16
    Pressure 4A16
  Oxygen Saturation Endoscopic Imaging (OXEI) XD2
  Peripheral Nervous
    Conductivity
      Motor 4A11
      Sensory 4A11
    Electrical Activity
      Intraoperative 4A11
      No Qualifier 4A11
  Products of Conception
    Cardiac
      Electrical Activity 4A1H
      Rate 4A1H
      Rhythm 4A1H
      Sound 4A1H
    Nervous
      Conductivity 4A1J
      Electrical Activity 4A1J
      Pressure 4A1J
  Respiratory
    Capacity 4A19
    Flow 4A19
    Rate 4A19
    Resistance 4A19
    Volume 4A19
  Skin and Breast, Vascular Perfusion, Indocyanine Green Dye 4A1GXSH
  Sleep 4A1ZXQZ
  Temperature 4A1Z
  Urinary
    Contractility 4A1D
    Flow 4A1D
    Pressure 4A1D
    Resistance 4A1D
    Volume 4A1D
  Venous
    Flow
      Central 4A14
      Peripheral 4A14
      Portal 4A14

Monitoring — continued
  Venous — continued
    Flow — continued
      Pulmonary 4A14
    Pressure
      Central 4A14
      Peripheral 4A14
      Portal 4A14
      Pulmonary 4A14
    Pulse
      Central 4A14
      Peripheral 4A14
      Portal 4A14
      Pulmonary 4A14
    Saturation
      Central 4A14
      Portal 4A14
      Pulmonary 4A14

Monitoring Device, Hemodynamic
  Abdomen 0JH8
  Chest 0JH6

Mosaic Bioprosthesis (aortic) (mitral) valve use Zooplastic Tissue in Heart and Great Vessels

Mosunetuzumab Antineoplastic XW0

Motor Function Assessment F01

Motor Treatment F07

MR Angiography
  see Magnetic Resonance Imaging (MRI), Heart B23
  see Magnetic Resonance Imaging (MRI), Lower Arteries B43
  see Magnetic Resonance Imaging (MRI), Upper Arteries B33

MULTI-LINK (VISION) (MINI-VISION) (ULTRA) Coronary Stent System use Intraluminal Device

Multiple sleep latency test 4A0ZXQZ

Musculocutaneous nerve use Brachial Plexus

Musculopexy
  see Repair, Muscles 0KQ
  see Reposition, Muscles 0KS

Musculophrenic artery
  use Internal Mammary Artery, Left
  use Internal Mammary Artery, Right

Musculoplasty
  see Repair, Muscles 0KQ
  see Supplement, Muscles 0KU

Musculorrhaphy see Repair, Muscles 0KQ

Musculospiral nerve use Radial Nerve

Myectomy
  see Excision, Muscles 0KB
  see Resection, Muscles 0KT

Myelencephalon use Medulla Oblongata

Myelogram
  CT see Computerized Tomography (CT Scan), Central Nervous System B02
  MRI see Magnetic Resonance Imaging (MRI), Central Nervous System B03

Myenteric (Auerbach's) plexus use Abdominal Sympathetic Nerve

Myocardial Bridge Release see Release, Artery, Coronary

Myomectomy see Excision, Female Reproductive System 0UB

Myometrium use Uterus

Myopexy
  see Repair, Muscles 0KQ
  see Reposition, Muscles 0KS

Myoplasty
  see Repair, Muscles 0KQ
  see Supplement, Muscles 0KU

Myorrhaphy see Repair, Muscles 0KQ

Myoscopy see Inspection, Muscles 0KJ

Myotomy
  see Division, Muscles 0K8
  see Drainage, Muscles 0K9

Myringectomy
  see Excision, Ear, Nose, Sinus 09B
  see Resection, Ear, Nose, Sinus 09T

Myringoplasty
  see Repair, Ear, Nose, Sinus 09Q
  see Replacement, Ear, Nose, Sinus 09R
  see Supplement, Ear, Nose, Sinus 09U

Myringostomy see Drainage, Ear, Nose, Sinus 099

Myringotomy see Drainage, Ear, Nose, Sinus 099

Subterms under main terms may continue to next column or page

N

NA-1 (Nerinitide) *use* Nerinitide
Nafamostat Anticoagulant XY0YX37
Nail bed
  use Finger Nail
  use Toe Nail
Nail plate
  use Finger Nail
  use Toe Nail
nanoLOCK™ interbody fusion device
  use Interbody Fusion Device in Lower Joints
  use Interbody Fusion Device in Upper Joints
Narcosynthesis GZGZZZZ
Narsoplimab Monoclonal Antibody XW0
Nasal cavity *use* Nasal Mucosa and Soft Tissue
Nasal concha *use* Nasal Turbinate
Nasalis muscle *use* Facial Muscle
Nasolacrimal duct
  use Lacrimal Duct, Left
  use Lacrimal Duct, Right
Nasopharyngeal airway (NPA) *use* Intraluminal Device, Airway in Ear, Nose, Sinus
Navicular bone
  use Tarsal, Left
  use Tarsal, Right
Near Infrared Spectroscopy, Circulatory System 8E02
Neck of femur
  use Upper Femur, Left
  use Upper Femur, Right
Neck of humerus (anatomical) (surgical)
  use Humeral Head, Left
  use Humeral Head, Right
Nelli® Seizure Monitoring System XXE0X48
Neovasc Reducer™ *use* Reduction Device in New Technology
Nephrectomy
  see Excision, Urinary System 0TB
  see Resection, Urinary System 0TT
Nephrolithotomy *see* Extirpation, Urinary System 0TC
Nephrolysis *see* Release, Urinary System 0TN
Nephropexy
  see Repair, Urinary System 0TQ
  see Reposition, Urinary System 0TS
Nephroplasty
  see Repair, Urinary System 0TQ
  see Supplement, Urinary System 0TU
Nephropyeloureterostomy
  see Bypass, Urinary System 0T1
  see Drainage, Urinary System 0T9
Nephrorrhaphy *see* Repair, Urinary System 0TQ
Nephroscopy, transurethral 0TJ58ZZ
Nephrostomy
  see Bypass, Urinary System 0T1
  see Drainage, Urinary System 0T9
Nephrotomography
  see Fluoroscopy, Urinary System BT1
  see Plain Radiography, Urinary System BT0
Nephrotomy
  see Division, Urinary System 0T8
  see Drainage, Urinary System 0T9
Nerinitide XW0
Nerve conduction study
  see Measurement, Central Nervous 4A00
  see Measurement, Peripheral Nervous 4A01
Nerve Function Assessment F01
Nerve to the stapedius *use* Facial Nerve
Nesiritide *use* Human B-Type Natriuretic Peptide
Neurectomy
  see Excision, Central Nervous System and Cranial Nerves 00B
  see Excision, Peripheral Nervous System 01B
Neurexeresis
  see Extraction, Central Nervous System and Cranial Nerves 00D
  see Extraction, Peripheral Nervous System 01D
NeuroBlate™ System *see* Destruction
Neurohypophysis *use* Pituitary Gland
Neurolysis
  see Release, Central Nervous System and Cranial Nerves 00N
  see Release, Peripheral Nervous System 01N
Neuromuscular electrical stimulation (NEMS) lead
  use Stimulator Lead in Muscles

Neurophysiologic monitoring *see* Monitoring, Central Nervous 4A10
Neuroplasty
  see Repair, Central Nervous System and Cranial Nerves 00Q
  see Repair, Peripheral Nervous System 01Q
  see Supplement, Central Nervous System and Cranial Nerves 00U
  see Supplement, Peripheral Nervous System 01U
Neurorrhaphy
  see Repair, Central Nervous System and Cranial Nerves 00Q
  see Repair, Peripheral Nervous System 01Q
Neurostimulator Generator
  Insertion of device in, Skull 0NH00NZ
  Removal of device from, Skull 0NP00NZ
  Revision of device in, Skull 0NW00NZ
Neurostimulator generator, multiple channel *use* Stimulator Generator, Multiple Array in 0JH
Neurostimulator generator, multiple channel rechargeable *use* Stimulator Generator, Multiple Array Rechargeable in 0JH
Neurostimulator generator, single channel *use* Stimulator Generator, Single Array in 0JH
Neurostimulator generator, single channel rechargeable *use* Stimulator Generator, Single Array Rechargeable in 0JH
Neurostimulator Lead
  Insertion of device in
    Brain 00H0
    Cerebral Ventricle 00H6
    Nerve
      Cranial 00HE
      Peripheral 01HY
    Spinal Canal 00HU
    Spinal Cord 00HV
    Vein
      Azygos 05H0
      Innominate
        Left 05H4
        Right 05H3
  Removal of device from
    Brain 00P0
    Cerebral Ventricle 00P6
    Nerve
      Cranial 00PE
      Peripheral 01PY
    Spinal Canal 00PU
    Spinal Cord 00PV
    Vein
      Azygos 05P0
      Innominate
        Left 05P4
        Right 05P3
  Revision of device in
    Brain 00W0
    Cerebral Ventricle 00W6
    Nerve
      Cranial 00WE
      Peripheral 01WY
    Spinal Canal 00WU
    Spinal Cord 00WV
    Vein
      Azygos 05W0
      Innominate
        Left 05W4
        Right 05W3
    Sphenopalatine Ganglion, Insertion X0HK3Q8
Neurostimulator Lead in Oropharynx XWHD7Q7
Neurostimulator Lead with Paired Stimulation System, Insertion X0HQ3R8
Neurotomy
  see Division, Central Nervous System and Cranial Nerves 008
  see Division, Peripheral Nervous System 018
Neurotripsy
  see Destruction, Central Nervous System and Cranial Nerves 005
  see Destruction, Peripheral Nervous System 015
Neutralization plate
  use Internal Fixation Device in Head and Facial Bones
  use Internal Fixation Device in Lower Bones
  use Internal Fixation Device in Upper Bones
New Technology
  Afamitresgene Autoleucel Immunotherapy XW0
  Amivantamab Monoclonal Antibody XW0
  Antibiotic-eluting Bone Void Filler XW0V0P7

New Technology — *continued*
  Aorta
    Thoracic Arch using Branched Synthetic Substitute with Intraluminal Device X2RX0N7
    Thoracic Descending using Branched Synthetic Substitute with Intraluminal Device X2VW0N7
  Apalutamide Antineoplastic XW0DXJ5
  Atezolizumab Antineoplastic XW0
  Axicabtagene Ciloleucel Immunotherapy XW0
  Bamlanivimab Monoclonal Antibody XW0
  Baricitinib XW0
  Betibeglogene Autotemcel XW1
  Bioengineered Allogeneic Construct, Skin XHRPXF7
  Brain Electrical Activity, Computer-aided Semiologic Analysis XXE0X48
  Brexanolone XW0
  Brexucabtagene Autoleucel Immunotherapy XW0
  Broad Consortium Microbiota-based Live Biotherapeutic Suspension XW0H7X8
  Bromelain-enriched Proteolytic Enzyme XW0
  Caplacizumab XW0
  CD24Fc Immunomodulator XW0
  Cefiderocol Anti-infective XW0
  Ceftolozane/Tazobactam Anti-infective XW0
  Cerebral Embolic Filtration
    Dual Filter X2A5312
    Extracorporeal Flow Reversal Circuit X2A
    Single Deflection Filter X2A6325
  Ciltacabtagene Autoleucel XW0
  Coagulation Factor Xa, Inactivated XW0
  Computer-aided Assessment, Intracranial Vascular Activity XXE0X07
  Computer-aided Guidance, Transthoracic Echocardiography X2JAX47
  Computer-aided Mechanical Aspiration X2C
  Computer-aided Triage and Notification, Pulmonary Artery Flow XXE3X27
  Computer-aided Valve Modeling and Notification, Coronary Artery Flow XXE3X68
  Computer-assisted Transcranial Magnetic Stimulation X0Z0X18
  Coronary Sinus, Reduction Device X2V73Q7
  COVID-19 Vaccine XW0
  COVID-19 Vaccine Booster XW0
  COVID-19 Vaccine Dose 1 XW0
  COVID-19 Vaccine Dose 2 XW0
  COVID-19 Vaccine Dose 3 XW0
  Cytarabine and Daunorubicin Liposome Antineoplastic XW0
  Daratumumab and Hyaluronidase-fihj XW01318
  Destruction
    Liver
      Left Lobe, Ultrasound-guided Cavitation XF52X08
      Right Lobe, Ultrasound-guided Cavitation XF51X08
      Ultrasound-guided Cavitation XF50X08
    Prostate, Robotic Waterjet Ablation XV508A4
  Dilation
    Anterior Tibial
      Left
        Sustained Release Drug-eluting Intraluminal Device X27Q385
        Four or More X27Q3C5
        Three X27Q3B5
        Two X27Q395
      Right
        Sustained Release Drug-eluting Intraluminal Device X27P385
        Four or More X27P3C5
        Three X27P3B5
        Two X27P395
    Femoral
      Left
        Sustained Release Drug-eluting Intraluminal Device X27J385
        Four or More X27J3C5
        Three X27J3B5
        Two X27J395
      Right
        Sustained Release Drug-eluting Intraluminal Device X27H385
        Four or More X27H3C5

New Technology — *continued*
 Dilation — *continued*
  Femoral — *continued*
   Right — *continued*
    Three X27H3B5
    Two X27H395
  Peroneal
   Left
    Sustained Release Drug-eluting
     Intraluminal Device
     X27U385
    Four or More X27U3C5
    Three X27U3B5
    Two X27U395
   Right
    Sustained Release Drug-eluting
     Intraluminal Device
     X27T385
    Four or More X27T3C5
    Three X27T3B5
    Two X27T395
  Popliteal
   Left Distal
    Sustained Release Drug-eluting
     Intraluminal Device
     X27N385
    Four or More X27N3C5
    Three X27N3B5
    Two X27N395
   Left Proximal
    Sustained Release Drug-eluting
     Intraluminal Device
     X27L385
    Four or More X27L3C5
    Three X27L3B5
    Two X27L395
   Right Distal
    Sustained Release Drug-eluting
     Intraluminal Device
     X27M385
    Four or More X27M3C5
    Three X27M3B5
    Two X27M395
   Right Proximal
    Sustained Release Drug-eluting
     Intraluminal Device
     X27K385
    Four or More X27K3C5
    Three X27K3B5
    Two X27K395
  Posterior Tibial
   Left
    Sustained Release Drug-eluting
     Intraluminal Device
     X27S385
    Four or More X27S3C5
    Three X27S3B5
    Two X27S395
   Right
    Sustained Release Drug-eluting
     Intraluminal Device
     X27R385
    Four or More X27R3C5
    Three X27R3B5
    Two X27R395
 Durvalumab Antineoplastic XW0
 Eculizumab XW0
 Eladocagene exuparvovec XW0Q316
 Endothelial Damage Inhibitor XY0VX83
 Engineered Allogeneic Thymus Tissue XW020D8
 Engineered Chimeric Antigen Receptor T-cell Im-
  munotherapy
  Allogeneic XW0
  Autologous XW0
 Erdafitinib Antineoplastic XW0DXL5
 Esketamine Hydrochloride XW097M5
 Etesevimab Monoclonal Antibody XW0
 Fosfomycin Anti-infective XW0
 Fostamatinib XW0
 Fusion
  Lumbar Vertebral
   2 or more, Interbody Fusion Device,
    Customizable XRGC
   Interbody Fusion Device, Customizable
    XRGB
  Lumbosacral, Interbody Fusion Device, Cus-
   tomizable XRGD
  Sacroiliac, Internal Fixation Device with Tulip
   Connector XRG

New Technology — *continued*
 Fusion — *continued*
  Thoracolumbar Vertebral, Interbody Fusion
   Device, Customizable XRGA
 Gilteritinib Antineoplastic XW0DXV5
 High-Dose Intravenous Immune Globulin, for
  COVID-19 treatment XW1
 Hyperimmune Globulin, for COVID-19 treatment
  XW1
 Idecabtagene Vicleucel Immunotherapy XW0
 Imipenem-cilastatin-relebactam Anti-infective
  XW0
 Inebilizumab-cdon XW0
 Insertion
  Bone, Pelvic, Internal Fixation Device with
   Tulip Connector XNH
  Joint
   Lumbar Vertebral, Posterior Spinal Mo-
    tion Preservation Device
    XRHB018
   Lumbosacral, Posterior Spinal Motion
    Preservation Device XRHD018
  Neurostimulator Lead, Sphenopalatine Gan-
   glion X0HK3Q8
  Neurostimulator Lead with Paired Stimula-
   tion System X0HQ3R8
 Intermittent Coronary Sinus Occlusion X2A7358
 Intracranial Arterial Flow, Whole Blood mRNA
  XXE5XT7
 Iobenguane I-131 Antineoplastic XW0
 Kidney, Fluorescent Pyrazine XT25XE5
 Lefamulin Anti-infective XW0
 Leronlimab Monoclonal Antibody XW013K6
 Lifileucel Immunotherapy XW0
 Lisocabtagene Maraleucel Immunotherapy XW0
 Lower Respiratory Fluid Nucleic Acid-base Micro-
  bial Detection XXEBXQ6
 Lurbinectedin XW0
 Maribavir Anti-infective XW0
 Mechanical Initial Specimen Diversion Technique
  Using Active Negative Pressure (blood col-
  lection) XXE5XR7
 Meropenem-vaborbactam Anti-infective XW0
 Mineral-based Topical Hemostatic Agent XW0
 Mosunetuzumab Antineoplastic XW0
 Nafamostat Anticoagulant XY0YX37
 Narsoplimab Monoclonal Antibody XW0
 Nerinitide XW0
 Neurostimulator Lead in Oropharynx XWHD7Q7
 Omadacycline Anti-infective XW0
 Omidubicel XW1
 Other New Technology Monoclonal Antibody XW0
 Other New Technology Therapeutic Substance
  XW0
 OTL-103 XW1
 OTL-200 XW1
 Oxygen Saturation Endoscopic Imaging (OXEI) XD2
 Plasma, Convalescent (Nonautologous) XW1
 Plazomicin Anti-infective XW0
 Positive Blood Culture Fluorescence Hybridization
  for Organism Identification, Concentration
  and Susceptibility XXE5XN6
 Quantitative Flow Ratio Analysis, Coronary Artery
  Flow XXE3X58
 Radial artery arteriovenous fistula, using Thermal
  Resistance Energy X2K
 REGN-COV2 Monoclonal Antibody XW0
 Remdesivir Anti-infective XW0
 Replacement
  Lateral Meniscus Synthetic Substitute XRR
  Medial Meniscus Synthetic Substitute XRR
 Reposition
  Cervical, Magnetically Controlled Growth
   Rod(s) XNS3
  Lumbar
   Magnetically Controlled Growth Rod(s)
    XNS0
   Posterior (Dynamic) Distraction Device
    XNS0
  Thoracic
   Magnetically Controlled Growth Rod(s)
    XNS4
   Posterior (Dynamic) Distraction Device
    XNS4
 Ruxolitinib XW0DXT5
 Sarilumab XW0
 SARS-CoV-2 Antibody Detection, Serum/Plasma
  Nanoparticle Fluorescence XXE5XV7

New Technology — *continued*
 SARS-CoV-2 Polymerase Chain Reaction, Nasopha-
  ryngeal Fluid XXE97U7
 Satralizumab-mwge XW01397
 Single-use Duodenoscope XFJ
 Single-use Oversleeve with Intraoperative Colonic
  Irrigation XDPH8K7
 Spesolimab Monoclonal Antibody XW0
 Supplement
  Bursa and Ligament, Spine, Posterior Verte-
   bral Tether XKU
  Vertebra
   Lumbar, Mechanically Expandable
    (Paired) Synthetic Substitute
    XNU0356
   Thoracic, Mechanically Expandable
    (Paired) Synthetic Substitute
    XNU4356
 Synthetic Human Angiotensin II XW0
 Tabelecleucel Immunotherapy XW0
 Tagraxofusp-erzs Antineoplastic XW0
 Taurolidine Anti-infective and Heparin Anticoagu-
  lant XY0YX28
 Teclistamab Antineoplastic XW01348
 Terlipressin XW0
 Tisagenlecleucel Immunotherapy XW0
 Tixagevimab and Cilgavimab Monoclonal Antibody
  XW023X7
 Tocilizumab XW0
 Treosulfan XW0
 Trilaciclib XW0
 Uridine Triacetate XW0DX82
 Venetoclax Antineoplastic XW0DXR5
 Whole Blood Nucleic Acid-base Microbial Detection
  XXE5XM5
 Whole Blood Reverse Transcription and Quantita-
  tive Real-time Polymerase Chain Reaction
  XXE5X38
NexoBrid™ *use* Bromelain-enriched Proteolytic Enzyme
Ninth cranial nerve *use* Glossopharyngeal Nerve
NIRS (Near Infrared Spectroscopy) *see* Physiological
 Systems and Anatomical Regions 8E0
Nitinol framed polymer mesh *use* Synthetic Substi-
 tute
Niyad™ *use* Nafamostat Anticoagulant
Nonimaging Nuclear Medicine Assay
 Bladder, Kidneys and Ureters CT63
 Blood C763
 Kidneys, Ureters and Bladder CT63
 Lymphatics and Hematologic System C76YYZZ
 Ureters, Kidneys and Bladder CT63
 Urinary System CT6YYZZ
Nonimaging Nuclear Medicine Probe
 Abdomen CW50
 Abdomen and Chest CW54
 Abdomen and Pelvis CW51
 Brain C050
 Central Nervous System C05YYZZ
 Chest CW53
 Chest and Abdomen CW54
 Chest and Neck CW56
 Extremity
  Lower CP5PZZZ
  Upper CP5NZZZ
 Head and Neck CW5B
 Heart C25YYZZ
  Right and Left C256
 Lymphatics
  Head C75J
  Head and Neck C755
  Lower Extremity C75P
  Neck C75K
  Pelvic C75D
  Trunk C75M
  Upper Chest C75L
  Upper Extremity C75N
 Lymphatics and Hematologic System C75YYZZ
 Musculoskeletal System, Other CP5YYZZ
 Neck and Chest CW56
 Neck and Head CW5B
 Pelvic Region CW5J
 Pelvis and Abdomen CW51
 Spine CP55ZZZ
Nonimaging Nuclear Medicine Uptake
 Endocrine System CG4YYZZ
 Gland, Thyroid CG42
Non-tunneled central venous catheter *use* Infusion
 Device

▽ Subterms under main terms may continue to next column or page

Nostril *use* Nasal Mucosa and Soft Tissue
Novacor Left Ventricular Assist Device *use* Implantable Heart Assist System in Heart and Great Vessels
Novation® Ceramic AHS® (Articulation Hip System) *use* Synthetic Substitute, Ceramic in ØSR
Nuclear medicine
  see Nonimaging Nuclear Medicine Assay
  see Nonimaging Nuclear Medicine Probe
  see Nonimaging Nuclear Medicine Uptake
  see Planar Nuclear Medicine Imaging
  see Positron Emission Tomographic (PET) Imaging
  see Systemic Nuclear Medicine Therapy
  see Tomographic (Tomo) Nuclear Medicine Imaging
Nuclear scintigraphy *see* Nuclear Medicine
NUsurface® Meniscus Implant
  use Synthetic Substitute, Lateral Meniscus in New Technology
  use Synthetic Substitute, Medial Meniscus in New Technology
Nutrition, concentrated substances
  Enteral infusion 3EØG36Z
  Parenteral (peripheral) infusion *see* Introduction of Nutritional Substance
NUZYRA™ *use* Omadacycline Anti-infective

O

Obliteration *see* Destruction
Obturator artery
  use Internal Iliac Artery, Left
  use Internal Iliac Artery, Right
Obturator lymph node *use* Lymphatic, Pelvis
Obturator muscle
  use Hip Muscle, Left
  use Hip Muscle, Right
Obturator nerve *use* Lumbar Plexus
Obturator vein
  use Hypogastric Vein, Left
  use Hypogastric Vein, Right
Obtuse margin *use* Heart, Left
Occipital artery
  use External Carotid Artery, Left
  use External Carotid Artery, Right
Occipital lobe *use* Cerebral Hemisphere
Occipital lymph node
  use Lymphatic, Left Neck
  use Lymphatic, Right Neck
Occipitofrontalis muscle *use* Facial Muscle
Occlusion
  Ampulla of Vater ØFLC
  Anus ØDLQ
  Aorta
    Abdominal 04LØ
    Thoracic, Descending 02LW3DJ
  Artery
    Anterior Tibial
      Left 04LQ
      Right 04LP
    Axillary
      Left 03L6
      Right 03L5
    Brachial
      Left 03L8
      Right 03L7
    Celiac 04L1
    Colic
      Left 04L7
      Middle 04L8
      Right 04L6
    Common Carotid
      Left 03LJ
      Right 03LH
    Common Iliac
      Left 04LD
      Right 04LC
    External Carotid
      Left 03LN
      Right 03LM
    External Iliac
      Left 04LJ
      Right 04LH
    Face 03LR
    Femoral
      Left 04LL
      Right 04LK

Occlusion — *continued*
  Artery — *continued*
    Foot
      Left 04LW
      Right 04LV
    Gastric 04L2
    Hand
      Left 03LF
      Right 03LD
    Hepatic 04L3
    Inferior Mesenteric 04LB
    Innominate 03L2
    Internal Carotid
      Left 03LL
      Right 03LK
    Internal Iliac
      Left 04LF
      Right 04LE
    Internal Mammary
      Left 03L1
      Right 03LØ
    Intracranial 03LG
    Lower 04LY
    Peroneal
      Left 04LU
      Right 04LT
    Popliteal
      Left 04LN
      Right 04LM
    Posterior Tibial
      Left 04LS
      Right 04LR
    Pulmonary
      Left 02LR
      Right 02LQ
    Pulmonary Trunk 02LP
    Radial
      Left 03LC
      Right 03LB
    Renal
      Left 04LA
      Right 04L9
    Splenic 04L4
    Subclavian
      Left 03L4
      Right 03L3
    Superior Mesenteric 04L5
    Temporal
      Left 03LT
      Right 03LS
    Thyroid
      Left 03LV
      Right 03LU
    Ulnar
      Left 03LA
      Right 03L9
    Upper 03LY
    Vertebral
      Left 03LQ
      Right 03LP
  Atrium, Left 02L7
  Bladder ØTLB
  Bladder Neck ØTLC
  Bronchus
    Lingula ØBL9
    Lower Lobe
      Left ØBLB
      Right ØBL6
    Main
      Left ØBL7
      Right ØBL3
    Middle Lobe, Right ØBL5
    Upper Lobe
      Left ØBL8
      Right ØBL4
  Carina ØBL2
  Cecum ØDLH
  Cisterna Chyli 07LL
  Colon
    Ascending ØDLK
    Descending ØDLM
    Sigmoid ØDLN
    Transverse ØDLL
  Cord
    Bilateral ØVLH
    Left ØVLG
    Right ØVLF
  Cul-de-sac ØULF

Occlusion — *continued*
  Duct
    Common Bile ØFL9
    Cystic ØFL8
    Hepatic
      Common ØFL7
      Left ØFL6
      Right ØFL5
    Lacrimal
      Left 08LY
      Right 08LX
    Pancreatic ØFLD
      Accessory ØFLF
    Parotid
      Left ØCLC
      Right ØCLB
  Duodenum ØDL9
  Esophagogastric Junction ØDL4
  Esophagus ØDL5
    Lower ØDL3
    Middle ØDL2
    Upper ØDL1
  Fallopian Tube
    Left ØUL6
    Right ØUL5
  Fallopian Tubes, Bilateral ØUL7
  Ileocecal Valve ØDLC
  Ileum ØDLB
  Intestine
    Large ØDLE
      Left ØDLG
      Right ØDLF
    Small ØDL8
  Jejunum ØDLA
  Kidney Pelvis
    Left ØTL4
    Right ØTL3
  Left atrial appendage (LAA) *see* Occlusion, Atrium, Left 02L7
  Lymphatic
    Aortic 07LD
    Axillary
      Left 07L6
      Right 07L5
    Head 07LØ
    Inguinal
      Left 07LJ
      Right 07LH
    Internal Mammary
      Left 07L9
      Right 07L8
    Lower Extremity
      Left 07LG
      Right 07LF
    Mesenteric 07LB
    Neck
      Left 07L2
      Right 07L1
    Pelvis 07LC
    Thoracic Duct 07LK
    Thorax 07L7
    Upper Extremity
      Left 07L4
      Right 07L3
  Rectum ØDLP
  Stomach ØDL6
    Pylorus ØDL7
  Trachea ØBL1
  Ureter
    Left ØTL7
    Right ØTL6
  Urethra ØTLD
  Vagina ØULG
  Valve, Pulmonary 02LH
  Vas Deferens
    Bilateral ØVLQ
    Left ØVLP
    Right ØVLN
  Vein
    Axillary
      Left 05L8
      Right 05L7
    Azygos 05LØ
    Basilic
      Left 05LC
      Right 05LB
    Brachial
      Left 05LA
      Right 05L9

Occlusion — *continued*
  Vein — *continued*
    Cephalic
      Left 05LF
      Right 05LD
    Colic 06L7
    Common Iliac
      Left 06LD
      Right 06LC
    Esophageal 06L3
    External Iliac
      Left 06LG
      Right 06LF
    External Jugular
      Left 05LQ
      Right 05LP
    Face
      Left 05LV
      Right 05LT
    Femoral
      Left 06LN
      Right 06LM
    Foot
      Left 06LV
      Right 06LT
    Gastric 06L2
    Hand
      Left 05LH
      Right 05LG
    Hemiazygos 05L1
    Hepatic 06L4
    Hypogastric
      Left 06LJ
      Right 06LH
    Inferior Mesenteric 06L6
    Innominate
      Left 05L4
      Right 05L3
    Internal Jugular
      Left 05LN
      Right 05LM
    Intracranial 05LL
    Lower 06LY
    Portal 06L8
    Pulmonary
      Left 02LT
      Right 02LS
    Renal
      Left 06LB
      Right 06L9
    Saphenous
      Left 06LQ
      Right 06LP
    Splenic 06L1
    Subclavian
      Left 05L6
      Right 05L5
    Superior Mesenteric 06L5
    Upper 05LY
    Vertebral
      Left 05LS
      Right 05LR
  Vena Cava
    Inferior 06L0
    Superior 02LV
Occlusion, REBOA (resuscitative endovascular balloon occlusion of the aorta)
  02LW3DJ
  04L03DJ
Occupational therapy *see* Activities of Daily Living Treatment, Rehabilitation F08
Octagam 10%, for COVID-19 treatment *use* High-Dose Intravenous Immune Globulin
Odentectomy
  see Excision, Mouth and Throat 0CB
  see Resection, Mouth and Throat 0CT
Odontoid process *use* Cervical Vertebra
Olecranon bursa
  use Elbow Bursa and Ligament, Left
  use Elbow Bursa and Ligament, Right
Olecranon process
  use Ulna, Left
  use Ulna, Right
Olfactory bulb *use* Olfactory Nerve
Olumiant® *use* Baricitinib
Omadacycline Anti-infective XW0
Omentectomy, omentumectomy
  see Excision, Gastrointestinal System 0DB

Omentectomy, omentumectomy — *continued*
  see Resection, Gastrointestinal System 0DT
Omentofixation *see* Repair, Gastrointestinal System 0DQ
Omentoplasty
  see Repair, Gastrointestinal System 0DQ
  see Replacement, Gastrointestinal System 0DR
  see Supplement, Gastrointestinal System 0DU
Omentorrhaphy *see* Repair, Gastrointestinal System 0DQ
Omentotomy *see* Drainage, Gastrointestinal System 0D9
Omidubicel XW1
Omnilink Elite Vascular Balloon Expandable Stent System *use* Intraluminal Device
Onychectomy
  see Excision, Skin and Breast 0HB
  see Resection, Skin and Breast 0HT
Onychoplasty
  see Repair, Skin and Breast 0HQ
  see Replacement, Skin and Breast 0HR
Onychotomy *see* Drainage, Skin and Breast 0H9
Oophorectomy
  see Excision, Female Reproductive System 0UB
  see Resection, Female Reproductive System 0UT
Oophoropexy
  see Repair, Female Reproductive System 0UQ
  see Reposition, Female Reproductive System 0US
Oophoroplasty
  see Repair, Female Reproductive System 0UQ
  see Supplement, Female Reproductive System 0UU
Oophororrhaphy *see* Repair, Female Reproductive System 0UQ
Oophorostomy *see* Drainage, Female Reproductive System 0U9
Oophorotomy
  see Division, Female Reproductive System 0U8
  see Drainage, Female Reproductive System 0U9
Oophorrhaphy *see* Repair, Female Reproductive System 0UQ
Open Pivot Aortic Valve Graft (AVG) *use* Synthetic Substitute
Open Pivot (mechanical) Valve *use* Synthetic Substitute
Ophthalmic artery *use* Intracranial Artery
Ophthalmic nerve *use* Trigeminal Nerve
Ophthalmic vein *use* Intracranial Vein
Opponensplasty
  Tendon replacement *see* Replacement, Tendons 0LR
  Tendon transfer *see* Transfer, Tendons 0LX
Optic chiasma *use* Optic Nerve
Optic disc
  use Retina, Left
  use Retina, Right
Optic foramen *use* Sphenoid Bone
Optical coherence tomography, intravascular *see* Computerized Tomography (CT Scan)
Optimizer™ III implantable pulse generator *use* Contractility Modulation Device in 0JH
Orbicularis oculi muscle
  use Upper Eyelid, Left
  use Upper Eyelid, Right
Orbicularis oris muscle *use* Facial Muscle
Orbital Atherectomy *see* Extirpation, Heart and Great Vessels 02C
Orbital fascia *use* Subcutaneous Tissue and Fascia, Face
Orbital portion of ethmoid bone
  use Orbit, Left
  use Orbit, Right
Orbital portion of frontal bone
  use Orbit, Left
  use Orbit, Right
Orbital portion of lacrimal bone
  use Orbit, Left
  use Orbit, Right
Orbital portion of maxilla
  use Orbit, Left
  use Orbit, Right
Orbital portion of palatine bone
  use Orbit, Left
  use Orbit, Right
Orbital portion of sphenoid bone
  use Orbit, Left
  use Orbit, Right

Orbital portion of zygomatic bone
  use Orbit, Left
  use Orbit, Right
Orchectomy, orchidectomy, orchiectomy
  see Excision, Male Reproductive System 0VB
  see Resection, Male Reproductive System 0VT
Orchidoplasty, orchioplasty
  see Repair, Male Reproductive System 0VQ
  see Replacement, Male Reproductive System 0VR
  see Supplement, Male Reproductive System 0VU
Orchidorrhaphy, orchiorrhaphy *see* Repair, Male Reproductive System 0VQ
Orchidotomy, orchiotomy, orchotomy *see* Drainage, Male Reproductive System 0V9
Orchiopexy
  see Repair, Male Reproductive System 0VQ
  see Reposition, Male Reproductive System 0VS
Oropharyngeal airway (OPA) *use* Intraluminal Device, Airway in Mouth and Throat
Oropharynx *use* Pharynx
Ossiculectomy
  see Excision, Ear, Nose, Sinus 09B
  see Resection, Ear, Nose, Sinus 09T
Ossiculotomy *see* Drainage, Ear, Nose, Sinus 099
Ostectomy
  see Excision, Head and Facial Bones 0NB
  see Excision, Lower Bones 0QB
  see Excision, Upper Bones 0PB
  see Resection, Head and Facial Bones 0NT
  see Resection, Lower Bones 0QT
  see Resection, Upper Bones 0PT
Osteoclasis
  see Division, Head and Facial Bones 0N8
  see Division, Lower Bones 0Q8
  see Division, Upper Bones 0P8
Osteolysis
  see Release, Head and Facial Bones 0NN
  see Release, Lower Bones 0QN
  see Release, Upper Bones 0PN
Osteopathic Treatment
  Abdomen 7W09X
  Cervical 7W01X
  Extremity
    Lower 7W06X
    Upper 7W07X
  Head 7W00X
  Lumbar 7W03X
  Pelvis 7W05X
  Rib Cage 7W08X
  Sacrum 7W04X
  Thoracic 7W02X
Osteopexy
  see Repair, Head and Facial Bones 0NQ
  see Repair, Lower Bones 0QQ
  see Repair, Upper Bones 0PQ
  see Reposition, Head and Facial Bones 0NS
  see Reposition, Lower Bones 0QS
  see Reposition, Upper Bones 0PS
Osteoplasty
  see Repair, Head and Facial Bones 0NQ
  see Repair, Lower Bones 0QQ
  see Repair, Upper Bones 0PQ
  see Replacement, Head and Facial Bones 0NR
  see Replacement, Lower Bones 0QR
  see Replacement, Upper Bones 0PR
  see Supplement, Head and Facial Bones 0NU
  see Supplement, Lower Bones 0QU
  see Supplement, Upper Bones 0PU
Osteorrhaphy
  see Repair, Head and Facial Bones 0NQ
  see Repair, Lower Bones 0QQ
  see Repair, Upper Bones 0PQ
Osteotomy, ostotomy
  see Division, Head and Facial Bones 0N8
  see Division, Lower Bones 0Q8
  see Division, Upper Bones 0P8
  see Drainage, Head and Facial Bones 0N9
  see Drainage, Lower Bones 0Q9
  see Drainage, Upper Bones 0P9
Other Imaging
  Bile Duct and Gallbladder, Indocyanine Green Dye, Intraoperative BF5320Ø
  Bile Duct, Indocyanine Green Dye, Intraoperative BF50200
  Extremity
    Lower BW5CZ1Z
    Upper BW5JZ1Z

Subterms under main terms may continue to next column or page

Other Imaging — *continued*
  Gallbladder and Bile Duct, Indocyanine Green Dye, Intraoperative BF53200
  Gallbladder, Indocyanine Green Dye, Intraoperative BF52200
  Head and Neck BW59Z1Z
  Hepatobiliary System, All, Indocyanine Green Dye, Intraoperative BF5C200
  Liver and Spleen, Indocyanine Green Dye, Intraoperative BF56200
  Liver, Indocyanine Green Dye, Intraoperative BF55200
  Neck and Head BW59Z1Z
  Pancreas, Indocyanine Green Dye, Intraoperative BF57200
  Spleen and Liver, Indocyanine Green Dye, Intraoperative BF56200
  Trunk BW52Z1Z

Other New Technology Monoclonal Antibody XW0
Other New Technology Therapeutic Substance XW0
Otic ganglion *use* Head and Neck Sympathetic Nerve
OTL-101 *use* Hematopoietic Stem/Progenitor Cells, Genetically Modified
OTL-103 XW1
OTL-200 XW1
Otoplasty
  see Repair, Ear, Nose, Sinus 09Q
  see Replacement, Ear, Nose, Sinus 09R
  see Supplement, Ear, Nose, Sinus 09U
Otoscopy *see* Inspection, Ear, Nose, Sinus 09J
Oval window
  use Middle Ear, Left
  use Middle Ear, Right
Ovarian artery *use* Abdominal Aorta
Ovarian ligament *use* Uterine Supporting Structure
Ovariectomy
  see Excision, Female Reproductive System 0UB
  see Resection, Female Reproductive System 0UT
Ovariocentesis *see* Drainage, Female Reproductive System 0U9
Ovariopexy
  see Repair, Female Reproductive System 0UQ
  see Reposition, Female Reproductive System 0US
Ovariotomy
  see Division, Female Reproductive System 0U8
  see Drainage, Female Reproductive System 0U9
Ovatio™ CRT-D *use* Cardiac Resynchronization Defibrillator Pulse Generator in 0JH
Oversewing
  Gastrointestinal ulcer *see* Repair, Gastrointestinal System 0DQ
  Pleural bleb *see* Repair, Respiratory System 0BQ
Oviduct
  use Fallopian Tube, Left
  use Fallopian Tube, Right
Oximetry, Fetal pulse 10H073Z
OXINIUM *use* Synthetic Substitute, Oxidized Zirconium on Polyethylene in 0SR
Oxygen Saturation Endoscopic Imaging (OXEI) XD2
Oxygenation
  Extracorporeal membrane (ECMO) *see* Performance, Circulatory 5A15
  Hyperbaric *see* Assistance, Circulatory 5A05
  Supersaturated *see* Assistance, Circulatory 5A05

P

Pacemaker
  Dual Chamber
    Abdomen 0JH8
    Chest 0JH6
  Intracardiac
    Insertion of device in
      Atrium
        Left 02H7
        Right 02H6
      Vein, Coronary 02H4
      Ventricle
        Left 02HL
        Right 02HK
    Removal of device from, Heart 02PA
    Revision of device in, Heart 02WA
  Single Chamber
    Abdomen 0JH8
    Chest 0JH6

Pacemaker — *continued*
  Single Chamber Rate Responsive
    Abdomen 0JH8
    Chest 0JH6
Packing
  Abdominal Wall 2W43X5Z
  Anorectal 2Y43X5Z
  Arm
    Lower
      Left 2W4DX5Z
      Right 2W4CX5Z
    Upper
      Left 2W4BX5Z
      Right 2W4AX5Z
  Back 2W45X5Z
  Chest Wall 2W44X5Z
  Ear 2Y42X5Z
  Extremity
    Lower
      Left 2W4MX5Z
      Right 2W4LX5Z
    Upper
      Left 2W49X5Z
      Right 2W48X5Z
  Face 2W41X5Z
  Finger
    Left 2W4KX5Z
    Right 2W4JX5Z
  Foot
    Left 2W4TX5Z
    Right 2W4SX5Z
  Genital Tract, Female 2Y44X5Z
  Hand
    Left 2W4FX5Z
    Right 2W4EX5Z
  Head 2W40X5Z
  Inguinal Region
    Left 2W47X5Z
    Right 2W46X5Z
  Leg
    Lower
      Left 2W4RX5Z
      Right 2W4QX5Z
    Upper
      Left 2W4PX5Z
      Right 2W4NX5Z
  Mouth and Pharynx 2Y40X5Z
  Nasal 2Y41X5Z
  Neck 2W42X5Z
  Thumb
    Left 2W4HX5Z
    Right 2W4GX5Z
  Toe
    Left 2W4VX5Z
    Right 2W4UX5Z
  Urethra 2Y45X5Z
Paclitaxel-eluting coronary stent *use* Intraluminal Device, Drug-eluting in Heart and Great Vessels
Paclitaxel-eluting peripheral stent
  use Intraluminal Device, Drug-eluting in Lower Arteries
  use Intraluminal Device, Drug-eluting in Upper Arteries
Palatine gland *use* Buccal Mucosa
Palatine tonsil *use* Tonsils
Palatine uvula *use* Uvula
Palatoglossal muscle *use* Tongue, Palate, Pharynx Muscle
Palatopharyngeal muscle *use* Tongue, Palate, Pharynx Muscle
Palatoplasty
  see Repair, Mouth and Throat 0CQ
  see Replacement, Mouth and Throat 0CR
  see Supplement, Mouth and Throat 0CU
Palatorrhaphy *see* Repair, Mouth and Throat 0CQ
Palmar cutaneous nerve
  use Median Nerve
  use Radial Nerve
Palmar (volar) digital vein
  use Hand Vein, Left
  use Hand Vein, Right
Palmar fascia (aponeurosis)
  use Subcutaneous Tissue and Fascia, Left Hand
  use Subcutaneous Tissue and Fascia, Right Hand
Palmar interosseous muscle
  use Hand Muscle, Left
  use Hand Muscle, Right

Palmar (volar) metacarpal vein
  use Hand Vein, Left
  use Hand Vein, Right
Palmar ulnocarpal ligament
  use Wrist Bursa and Ligament, Left
  use Wrist Bursa and Ligament, Right
Palmaris longus muscle
  use Lower Arm and Wrist Muscle, Left
  use Lower Arm and Wrist Muscle, Right
Pancreatectomy
  see Excision, Pancreas 0FBG
  see Resection, Pancreas 0FTG
Pancreatic artery *use* Splenic Artery
Pancreatic plexus *use* Abdominal Sympathetic Nerve
Pancreatic vein *use* Splenic Vein
Pancreaticoduodenostomy *see* Bypass, Hepatobiliary System and Pancreas 0F1
Pancreaticosplenic lymph node *use* Lymphatic, Aortic
Pancreatogram, endoscopic retrograde *see* Fluoroscopy, Pancreatic Duct BF18
Pancreatolithotomy *see* Extirpation, Pancreas 0FCG
Pancreatotomy
  see Division, Pancreas 0F8G
  see Drainage, Pancreas 0F9G
Panniculectomy
  see Excision, Skin, Abdomen 0HB7
  see Excision, Subcutaneous Tissue and Fascia, Abdomen 0JB8
Paraaortic lymph node *use* Lymphatic, Aortic
Paracentesis
  Eye *see* Drainage, Eye 089
  Peritoneal Cavity *see* Drainage, Peritoneal Cavity 0W9G
  Tympanum *see* Drainage, Ear, Nose, Sinus 099
Parapharyngeal space *use* Neck
Pararectal lymph node *use* Lymphatic, Mesenteric
Parasternal lymph node *use* Lymphatic, Thorax
Parathyroidectomy
  see Excision, Endocrine System 0GB
  see Resection, Endocrine System 0GT
Paratracheal lymph node *use* Lymphatic, Thorax
Paraurethral (Skene's) gland *use* Vestibular Gland
Parenteral nutrition, total *see* Introduction of Nutritional Substance
Parietal lobe *use* Cerebral Hemisphere
Parotid lymph node *use* Lymphatic, Head
Parotid plexus *use* Facial Nerve
Parotidectomy
  see Excision, Mouth and Throat 0CB
  see Resection, Mouth and Throat 0CT
Pars flaccida
  use Tympanic Membrane, Left
  use Tympanic Membrane, Right
Partial joint replacement
  Hip *see* Replacement, Lower Joints 0SR
  Knee *see* Replacement, Lower Joints 0SR
  Shoulder *see* Replacement, Upper Joints 0RR
Partially absorbable mesh *use* Synthetic Substitute
Patch, blood, spinal 3E0R3GC
Patellapexy
  see Repair, Lower Bones 0QQ
  see Reposition, Lower Bones 0QS
Patellaplasty
  see Repair, Lower Bones 0QQ
  see Replacement, Lower Bones 0QR
  see Supplement, Lower Bones 0QU
Patellar ligament
  use Knee Bursa and Ligament, Left
  use Knee Bursa and Ligament, Right
Patellar tendon
  use Knee Tendon, Left
  use Knee Tendon, Right
Patellectomy
  see Excision, Lower Bones 0QB
  see Resection, Lower Bones 0QT
Patellofemoral joint
  use Knee Joint, Left
  use Knee Joint, Left, Femoral Surface
  use Knee Joint, Right
  use Knee Joint, Right, Femoral Surface
pAVF (percutaneous arteriovenous fistula), using magnetic-guided radiofrequency *see* Bypass, Upper Arteries 031

pAVF (percutaneous arteriovenous fistula), using thermal resistance energy see New Technology, Cardiovascular System X2K

Pectineus muscle
use Upper Leg Muscle, Left
use Upper Leg Muscle, Right

Pectoral fascia use Subcutaneous Tissue and Fascia, Chest

Pectoral (anterior) lymph node
use Lymphatic Left, Axillary
use Lymphatic Right, Axillary

Pectoralis major muscle
use Thorax Muscle, Left
use Thorax Muscle, Right

Pectoralis minor muscle
use Thorax Muscle, Left
use Thorax Muscle, Right

Pedicle-based dynamic stabilization device
use Spinal Stabilization Device, Pedicle-Based in ØSH
use Spinal Stabilization Device, Pedicle-Based in ØRH

PEEP (positive end expiratory pressure) see Assistance, Respiratory 5AØ9

PEG (percutaneous endoscopic gastrostomy) ØDH63UZ

PEJ (percutaneous endoscopic jejunostomy) ØDHA3UZ

Pelvic splanchnic nerve
use Abdominal Sympathetic Nerve
use Sacral Sympathetic Nerve

Penectomy
see Excision, Male Reproductive System ØVB
see Resection, Male Reproductive System ØVT

Penile urethra use Urethra

Penumbra Indigo® Aspiration System see New Technology, Cardiovascular System X2C

PERCEPT™ PC neurostimulator use Stimulator Generator, Multiple Array in ØJH

Perceval sutureless valve (rapid deployment technique) see Replacement, Valve, Aortic Ø2RF

Percutaneous endoscopic gastrojejunostomy (PEG/J) tube use Feeding Device in Gastrointestinal System

Percutaneous endoscopic gastrostomy (PEG) tube use Feeding Device in Gastrointestinal System

Percutaneous nephrostomy catheter use Drainage Device

Percutaneous transluminal coronary angioplasty (PTCA) see Dilation, Heart and Great Vessels Ø27

Performance
Biliary
Multiple, Filtration 5A1C6ØZ
Single, Filtration 5A1CØØZ
Cardiac
Continuous
Output 5A1221Z
Pacing 5A1223Z
Intermittent, Pacing 5A1213Z
Single, Output, Manual 5A12Ø12
Circulatory
Continuous
Central Membrane 5A1522F
Peripheral Veno-arterial Membrane 5A1522G
Peripheral Veno-venous Membrane 5A1522H
Intraoperative
Central Membrane 5A15A2F
Peripheral Veno-arterial Membrane 5A15A2G
Peripheral Veno-venous Membrane 5A15A2H
Respiratory
24-96 Consecutive Hours, Ventilation 5A1945Z
Greater than 96 Consecutive Hours, Ventilation 5A1955Z
Less than 24 Consecutive Hours, Ventilation 5A1935Z
Single, Ventilation, Nonmechanical 5A19Ø54
Urinary
Continuous, Greater than 18 hours per day, Filtration 5A1D9ØZ
Intermittent, Less than 6 Hours Per Day, Filtration 5A1D7ØZ

Performance — continued
Urinary — continued
Prolonged Intermittent, 6-18 hours per day, Filtration 5A1D8ØZ

Perfusion see Introduction of substance in or on

Perfusion, donor organ
Heart 6AB5ØBZ
Kidney(s) 6ABTØBZ
Liver 6ABFØBZ
Lung(s) 6ABBØBZ

Perianal skin use Skin, Perineum

Pericardiectomy
see Excision, Pericardium Ø2BN
see Resection, Pericardium Ø2TN

Pericardiocentesis see Drainage, Pericardial Cavity ØW9D

Pericardiolysis see Release, Pericardium Ø2NN

Pericardiophrenic artery
use Internal Mammary Artery, Left
use Internal Mammary Artery, Right

Pericardioplasty
see Repair, Pericardium Ø2QN
see Replacement, Pericardium Ø2RN
see Supplement, Pericardium Ø2UN

Pericardiorrhaphy see Repair, Pericardium Ø2QN

Pericardiostomy see Drainage, Pericardial Cavity ØW9D

Pericardiotomy see Drainage, Pericardial Cavity ØW9D

Perimetrium use Uterus

Peripheral Intravascular Lithotripsy (Peripheral IVL) see Fragmentation

Peripheral parenteral nutrition see Introduction of Nutritional Substance

Peripherally inserted central catheter (PICC) use Infusion Device

Peritoneal dialysis 3E1M39Z

Peritoneocentesis
see Drainage, Peritoneal Cavity ØW9G
see Drainage, Peritoneum ØD9W

Peritoneoplasty
see Repair, Peritoneum ØDQW
see Replacement, Peritoneum ØDRW
see Supplement, Peritoneum ØDUW

Peritoneoscopy ØDJW4ZZ

Peritoneotomy see Drainage, Peritoneum ØD9W

Peritoneumectomy see Excision, Peritoneum ØDBW

Peroneus brevis muscle
use Lower Leg Muscle, Left
use Lower Leg Muscle, Right

Peroneus longus muscle
use Lower Leg Muscle, Left
use Lower Leg Muscle, Right

Pessary ring use Intraluminal Device, Pessary in Female Reproductive System

PET scan see Positron Emission Tomographic (PET) Imaging

Petrous part of temoporal bone
use Temporal Bone, Left
use Temporal Bone, Right

Phacoemulsification, lens
With IOL implant see Replacement, Eye Ø8R
Without IOL implant see Extraction, Eye Ø8D

Phagenyx® System XWHD7Q7

Phalangectomy
see Excision, Lower Bones ØQB
see Excision, Upper Bones ØPB
see Resection, Lower Bones ØQT
see Resection, Upper Bones ØPT

Phallectomy
see Excision, Penis ØVBS
see Resection, Penis ØVTS

Phalloplasty
see Repair, Penis ØVQS
see Supplement, Penis ØVUS

Phallotomy see Drainage, Penis ØV9S

Pharmacotherapy, for substance abuse
Antabuse HZ93ZZZ
Bupropion HZ97ZZZ
Clonidine HZ96ZZZ
Levo-alpha-acetyl-methadol (LAAM) HZ92ZZZ
Methadone Maintenance HZ91ZZZ
Naloxone HZ95ZZZ
Naltrexone HZ94ZZZ
Nicotine Replacement HZ90ZZZ
Psychiatric Medication HZ98ZZZ
Replacement Medication, Other HZ99ZZZ

Pharyngeal constrictor muscle use Tongue, Palate, Pharynx Muscle

Pharyngeal plexus use Vagus Nerve

Pharyngeal recess use Nasopharynx

Pharyngeal tonsil use Adenoids

Pharyngogram see Fluoroscopy, Pharynix B91G

Pharyngoplasty
see Repair, Mouth and Throat ØCQ
see Replacement, Mouth and Throat ØCR
see Supplement, Mouth and Throat ØCU

Pharyngorrhaphy see Repair, Mouth and Throat ØCQ

Pharyngotomy see Drainage, Mouth and Throat ØC9

Pharyngotympanic tube
use Eustachian Tube, Left
use Eustachian Tube, Right

Pheresis
Erythrocytes 6A55
Leukocytes 6A55
Plasma 6A55
Platelets 6A55
Stem Cells
Cord Blood 6A55
Hematopoietic 6A55

Phlebectomy
see Excision, Lower Veins Ø6B
see Excision, Upper Veins Ø5B
see Extraction, Lower Veins Ø6D
see Extraction, Upper Veins Ø5D

Phlebography
see Plain Radiography, Veins B5Ø
Impedance 4AØ4X51

Phleborrhaphy
see Repair, Lower Veins Ø6Q
see Repair, Upper Veins Ø5Q

Phlebotomy
see Drainage, Lower Veins Ø69
see Drainage, Upper Veins Ø59

Photocoagulation
For Destruction see Destruction
For Repair see Repair

Photopheresis, therapeutic see Phototherapy, Circulatory 6A65

Phototherapy
Circulatory 6A65
Skin 6A6Ø
Ultraviolet light see Ultraviolet Light Therapy, Physiological Systems 6A8

Phrenectomy, phrenoneurectomy see Excision, Nerve, Phrenic Ø1B2

Phrenemphraxis see Destruction, Nerve, Phrenic Ø152

Phrenic nerve stimulator generator use Stimulator Generator in Subcutaneous Tissue and Fascia

Phrenic nerve stimulator lead use Diaphragmatic Pacemaker Lead in Respiratory System

Phreniclasis see Destruction, Nerve, Phrenic Ø152

Phrenicoexeresis see Extraction, Nerve, Phrenic Ø1D2

Phrenicotomy see Division, Nerve, Phrenic Ø182

Phrenicotripsy see Destruction, Nerve, Phrenic Ø152

Phrenoplasty
see Repair, Respiratory System ØBQ
see Supplement, Respiratory System ØBU

Phrenotomy see Drainage, Respiratory System ØB9

Physiatry see Motor Treatment, Rehabilitation FØ7

Physical medicine see Motor Treatment, Rehabilitation FØ7

Physical therapy see Motor Treatment, Rehabilitation FØ7

PHYSIOMESH™ Flexible Composite Mesh use Synthetic Substitute

Pia mater, intracranial use Cerebral Meninges

Pia mater, spinal use Spinal Meninges

PiCSO® Impulse System X2A7358

Pinealectomy
see Excision, Pineal Body ØGB1
see Resection, Pineal Body ØGT1

Pinealoscopy ØGJ14ZZ

Pinealotomy see Drainage, Pineal Body ØG91

Pinna
use External Ear, Bilateral
use External Ear, Left
use External Ear, Right

Pipeline™ (Flex) embolization device use Intraluminal Device, Flow Diverter in Ø3V

Piriform recess (sinus) use Pharynx

Piriformis muscle
use Hip Muscle, Left
use Hip Muscle, Right

PIRRT (Prolonged intermittent renal replacement therapy) 5A1D8ØZ

Pisiform bone
    use Carpal, Left
    use Carpal, Right

Pisohamate ligament
    use Hand Bursa and Ligament, Left
    use Hand Bursa and Ligament, Right

Pisometacarpal ligament
    use Hand Bursa and Ligament, Left
    use Hand Bursa and Ligament, Right

Pituitectomy
    see Excision, Gland, Pituitary ØGBØ
    see Resection, Gland, Pituitary ØGTØ

Plain film radiology *see* Plain Radiography

Plain Radiography
    Abdomen BW00ZZZ
    Abdomen and Pelvis BW01ZZZ
    Abdominal Lymphatic
        Bilateral B701
        Unilateral B700
    Airway, Upper BB0DZZZ
    Ankle
        Left BQ0H
        Right BQ0G
    Aorta
        Abdominal B400
        Thoracic B300
        Thoraco-Abdominal B30P
    Aorta and Bilateral Lower Extremity Arteries B40D
    Arch
        Bilateral BN0DZZZ
        Left BN0CZZZ
        Right BN0BZZZ
    Arm
        Left BP0FZZZ
        Right BP0EZZZ
    Artery
        Brachiocephalic-Subclavian, Right B301
        Bronchial B30L
        Bypass Graft, Other B20F
        Cervico-Cerebral Arch B30Q
        Common Carotid
            Bilateral B305
            Left B304
            Right B303
        Coronary
            Bypass Graft
                Multiple B203
                Single B202
            Multiple B201
            Single B200
        External Carotid
            Bilateral B30C
            Left B30B
            Right B309
        Hepatic B402
        Inferior Mesenteric B405
        Intercostal B30L
        Internal Carotid
            Bilateral B308
            Left B307
            Right B306
        Internal Mammary Bypass Graft
            Left B208
            Right B207
        Intra-Abdominal, Other B40B
        Intracranial B30R
        Lower Extremity
            Bilateral and Aorta B40D
            Left B40G
            Right B40F
        Lower, Other B40J
        Lumbar B409
        Pelvic B40C
        Pulmonary
            Left B30T
            Right B30S
        Renal
            Bilateral B408
            Left B407
            Right B406
            Transplant B40M
        Spinal B30M
        Splenic B403
        Subclavian, Left B302
        Superior Mesenteric B404
        Upper Extremity
            Bilateral B30K
            Left B30J

Plain Radiography — *continued*
    Artery — *continued*
        Upper Extremity — *continued*
            Right B30H
        Upper, Other B30N
        Vertebral
            Bilateral B30G
            Left B30F
            Right B30D
    Bile Duct BF00
    Bile Duct and Gallbladder BF03
    Bladder BT00
        Kidney and Ureter BT04
    Bladder and Urethra BT0B
    Bone
        Facial BN05ZZZ
        Nasal BN04ZZZ
    Bones, Long, All BW0BZZZ
    Breast
        Bilateral BH02ZZZ
        Left BH01ZZZ
        Right BH00ZZZ
    Calcaneus
        Left BQ0KZZZ
        Right BQ0JZZZ
    Chest BW03ZZZ
    Clavicle
        Left BP05ZZZ
        Right BP04ZZZ
    Coccyx BR0FZZZ
    Corpora Cavernosa BV00
    Dialysis Fistula B50W
    Dialysis Shunt B50W
    Disc
        Cervical BR01
        Lumbar BR03
        Thoracic BR02
    Duct
        Lacrimal
            Bilateral B802
            Left B801
            Right B800
        Mammary
            Multiple
                Left BH06
                Right BH05
            Single
                Left BH04
                Right BH03
    Elbow
        Left BP0H
        Right BP0G
    Epididymis
        Left BV02
        Right BV01
    Extremity
        Lower BW0CZZZ
        Upper BW0JZZZ
    Eye
        Bilateral B807ZZZ
        Left B806ZZZ
        Right B805ZZZ
    Facet Joint
        Cervical BR04
        Lumbar BR06
        Thoracic BR05
    Fallopian Tube
        Bilateral BU02
        Left BU01
        Right BU00
    Fallopian Tube and Uterus BU08
    Femur
        Left, Densitometry BQ04ZZ1
        Right, Densitometry BQ03ZZ1
    Finger
        Left BP0SZZZ
        Right BP0RZZZ
    Foot
        Left BQ0MZZZ
        Right BQ0LZZZ
    Forearm
        Left BP0KZZZ
        Right BP0JZZZ
    Gallbladder and Bile Duct BF03
    Gland
        Parotid
            Bilateral B906
            Left B905
            Right B904

Plain Radiography — *continued*
    Gland — *continued*
        Salivary
            Bilateral B90D
            Left B90C
            Right B90B
        Submandibular
            Bilateral B909
            Left B908
            Right B907
    Hand
        Left BP0PZZZ
        Right BP0NZZZ
    Heart
        Left B205
        Right B204
        Right and Left B206
    Hepatobiliary System, All BF0C
    Hip
        Left BQ01
            Densitometry BQ01ZZ1
        Right BQ00
            Densitometry BQ00ZZ1
    Humerus
        Left BP0BZZZ
        Right BP0AZZZ
    Ileal Diversion Loop BT0C
    Intracranial Sinus B502
    Joint
        Acromioclavicular, Bilateral BP03ZZZ
        Finger
            Left BP0D
            Right BP0C
        Foot
            Left BQ0Y
            Right BQ0X
        Hand
            Left BP0D
            Right BP0C
        Lumbosacral BR0BZZZ
        Sacroiliac BR0D
        Sternoclavicular
            Bilateral BP02ZZZ
            Left BP01ZZZ
            Right BP00ZZZ
        Temporomandibular
            Bilateral BN09
            Left BN08
            Right BN07
        Thoracolumbar BR08ZZZ
        Toe
            Left BQ0Y
            Right BQ0X
    Kidney
        Bilateral BT03
        Left BT02
        Right BT01
        Ureter and Bladder BT04
    Knee
        Left BQ08
        Right BQ07
    Leg
        Left BQ0FZZZ
        Right BQ0DZZZ
    Lymphatic
        Head B704
        Lower Extremity
            Bilateral B70B
            Left B709
            Right B708
        Neck B704
        Pelvic B70C
        Upper Extremity
            Bilateral B707
            Left B706
            Right B705
    Mandible BN06ZZZ
    Mastoid B90HZZZ
    Nasopharynx B90FZZZ
    Optic Foramina
        Left B804ZZZ
        Right B803ZZZ
    Orbit
        Bilateral BN03ZZZ
        Left BN02ZZZ
        Right BN01ZZZ
    Oropharynx B90FZZZ
    Patella
        Left BQ0WZZZ

Plain Radiography — *continued*
Patella — *continued*
Right BQ0VZZZ
Pelvis BR0CZZZ
Pelvis and Abdomen BW01ZZZ
Prostate BV03
Retroperitoneal Lymphatic
Bilateral B701
Unilateral B700
Ribs
Left BP0YZZZ
Right BP0XZZZ
Sacrum BR0FZZZ
Scapula
Left BP07ZZZ
Right BP06ZZZ
Shoulder
Left BP09
Right BP08
Sinus
Intracranial B502
Paranasal B902ZZZ
Skull BN00ZZZ
Spinal Cord B00B
Spine
Cervical, Densitometry BR00ZZ1
Lumbar, Densitometry BR09ZZ1
Thoracic, Densitometry BR07ZZ1
Whole, Densitometry BR0GZZ1
Sternum BR0HZZZ
Teeth
All BN0JZZZ
Multiple BN0HZZZ
Testicle
Left BV06
Right BV05
Toe
Left BQ0QZZZ
Right BQ0PZZZ
Tooth, Single BN0GZZZ
Tracheobronchial Tree
Bilateral BB09YZZ
Left BB08YZZ
Right BB07YZZ
Ureter
Bilateral BT08
Kidney and Bladder BT04
Left BT07
Right BT06
Urethra BT05
Urethra and Bladder BT0B
Uterus BU06
Uterus and Fallopian Tube BU08
Vagina BU09
Vasa Vasorum BV08
Vein
Cerebellar B501
Cerebral B501
Epidural B500
Jugular
Bilateral B505
Left B504
Right B503
Lower Extremity
Bilateral B50D
Left B50C
Right B50B
Other B50V
Pelvic (Iliac)
Left B50G
Right B50F
Pelvic (Iliac) Bilateral B50H
Portal B50T
Pulmonary
Bilateral B50S
Left B50R
Right B50Q
Renal
Bilateral B50L
Left B50K
Right B50J
Spanchnic B50T
Subclavian
Left B507
Right B506
Upper Extremity
Bilateral B50P
Left B50N
Right B50M

Plain Radiography — *continued*
Vena Cava
Inferior B509
Superior B508
Whole Body BW0KZZZ
Infant BW0MZZZ
Whole Skeleton BW0LZZZ
Wrist
Left BP0M
Right BP0L
Planar Nuclear Medicine Imaging
Abdomen CW10
Abdomen and Chest CW14
Abdomen and Pelvis CW11
Anatomical Region, Other CW1ZZZZ
Anatomical Regions, Multiple CW1YYZZ
Bladder and Ureters CT1H
Bladder, Kidneys and Ureters CT13
Blood C713
Bone Marrow C710
Brain C010
Breast CH1YYZZ
Bilateral CH12
Left CH11
Right CH10
Bronchi and Lungs CB12
Central Nervous System C01YYZZ
Cerebrospinal Fluid C015
Chest CW13
Chest and Abdomen CW14
Chest and Neck CW16
Digestive System CD1YYZZ
Ducts, Lacrimal, Bilateral C819
Ear, Nose, Mouth and Throat C91YYZZ
Endocrine System CG1YYZZ
Extremity
Lower CW1D
Bilateral CP1F
Left CP1D
Right CP1C
Upper CW1M
Bilateral CP1B
Left CP19
Right CP18
Eye C81YYZZ
Gallbladder CF14
Gastrointestinal Tract CD17
Upper CD15
Gland
Adrenal, Bilateral CG14
Parathyroid CG11
Thyroid CG12
Glands, Salivary, Bilateral C91B
Head and Neck CW1B
Heart C21YYZZ
Right and Left C216
Hepatobiliary System, All CF1C
Hepatobiliary System and Pancreas CF1YYZZ
Kidneys, Ureters and Bladder CT13
Liver CF15
Liver and Spleen CF16
Lungs and Bronchi CB12
Lymphatics
Head C71J
Head and Neck C715
Lower Extremity C71P
Neck C71K
Pelvic C71D
Trunk C71M
Upper Chest C71L
Upper Extremity C71N
Lymphatics and Hematologic System C71YYZZ
Musculoskeletal System
All CP1Z
Other CP1YYZZ
Myocardium C21G
Neck and Chest CW16
Neck and Head CW1B
Pancreas and Hepatobiliary System CF1YYZZ
Pelvic Region CW1J
Pelvis CP16
Pelvis and Abdomen CW11
Pelvis and Spine CP17
Reproductive System, Male CV1YYZZ
Respiratory System CB1YYZZ
Skin CH1YYZZ
Skull CP11
Spine CP15
Spine and Pelvis CP17

Planar Nuclear Medicine Imaging — *continued*
Spleen C712
Spleen and Liver CF16
Subcutaneous Tissue CH1YYZZ
Testicles, Bilateral CV19
Thorax CP14
Ureters and Bladder CT1H
Ureters, Kidneys and Bladder CT13
Urinary System CT1YYZZ
Veins C51YYZZ
Central C51R
Lower Extremity
Bilateral C51D
Left C51C
Right C51B
Upper Extremity
Bilateral C51Q
Left C51P
Right C51N
Whole Body CW1N
Plantar digital vein
use Foot Vein, Left
use Foot Vein, Right
Plantar fascia (aponeurosis)
use Subcutaneous Tissue and Fascia, Left Foot
use Subcutaneous Tissue and Fascia, Right Foot
Plantar metatarsal vein
use Foot Vein, Left
use Foot Vein, Right
Plantar venous arch
use Foot Vein, Left
use Foot Vein, Right
Plaque Radiation
Abdomen DWY3FZZ
Adrenal Gland DGY2FZZ
Anus DDY8FZZ
Bile Ducts DFY2FZZ
Bladder DTY2FZZ
Bone Marrow D7Y0FZZ
Bone, Other DPYCFZZ
Brain D0Y0FZZ
Brain Stem D0Y1FZZ
Breast
Left DMY0FZZ
Right DMY1FZZ
Bronchus DBY1FZZ
Cervix DUY1FZZ
Chest DWY2FZZ
Chest Wall DBY7FZZ
Colon DDY5FZZ
Diaphragm DBY8FZZ
Duodenum DDY2FZZ
Ear D9Y0FZZ
Esophagus DDY0FZZ
Eye D8Y0FZZ
Femur DPY9FZZ
Fibula DPYBFZZ
Gallbladder DFY1FZZ
Gland
Adrenal DGY2FZZ
Parathyroid DGY4FZZ
Pituitary DGY0FZZ
Thyroid DGY5FZZ
Glands, Salivary D9Y6FZZ
Head and Neck DWY1FZZ
Hemibody DWY4FZZ
Humerus DPY6FZZ
Ileum DDY4FZZ
Jejunum DDY3FZZ
Kidney DTY0FZZ
Larynx D9YBFZZ
Liver DFY0FZZ
Lung DBY2FZZ
Lymphatics
Abdomen D7Y6FZZ
Axillary D7Y4FZZ
Inguinal D7Y8FZZ
Neck D7Y3FZZ
Pelvis D7Y7FZZ
Thorax D7Y5FZZ
Mandible DPY3FZZ
Maxilla DPY2FZZ
Mediastinum DBY6FZZ
Mouth D9Y4FZZ
Nasopharynx D9YDFZZ
Neck and Head DWY1FZZ
Nerve, Peripheral D0Y7FZZ
Nose D9Y1FZZ

Plaque Radiation — *continued*
Ovary DUY0FZZ
Palate
  Hard D9Y8FZZ
  Soft D9Y9FZZ
Pancreas DFY3FZZ
Parathyroid Gland DGY4FZZ
Pelvic Bones DPY8FZZ
Pelvic Region DWY6FZZ
Pharynx D9YCFZZ
Pineal Body DGY1FZZ
Pituitary Gland DGY0FZZ
Pleura DBY5FZZ
Prostate DVY0FZZ
Radius DPY7FZZ
Rectum DDY7FZZ
Rib DPY5FZZ
Sinuses D9Y7FZZ
Skin
  Abdomen DHY8FZZ
  Arm DHY4FZZ
  Back DHY7FZZ
  Buttock DHY9FZZ
  Chest DHY6FZZ
  Face DHY2FZZ
  Foot DHYCFZZ
  Hand DHY5FZZ
  Leg DHYBFZZ
  Neck DHY3FZZ
Skull DPY0FZZ
Spinal Cord D0Y6FZZ
Spleen D7Y2FZZ
Sternum DPY4FZZ
Stomach DDY1FZZ
Testis DVY1FZZ
Thymus D7Y1FZZ
Thyroid Gland DGY5FZZ
Tibia DPYBFZZ
Tongue D9Y5FZZ
Trachea DBY0FZZ
Ulna DPY7FZZ
Ureter DTY1FZZ
Urethra DTY3FZZ
Uterus DUY2FZZ
Whole Body DWY5FZZ
Plasma, Convalescent (Nonautologous) XW1
Plasmapheresis, therapeutic *see* Pheresis, Physiological Systems 6A5
Plateletpheresis, therapeutic *see* Pheresis, Physiological Systems 6A5
Platysma muscle
use Neck Muscle, Left
use Neck Muscle, Right
Plazomicin Anti-infective XW0
Pleurectomy
see Excision, Respiratory System 0BB
see Resection, Respiratory System 0BT
Pleurocentesis *see* Drainage, Anatomical Regions, General 0W9
Pleurodesis, pleurosclerosis
Chemical injection *see* Introduction of Substance in or on, Pleural Cavity 3E0L
Surgical *see* Destruction, Respiratory System 0B5
Pleurolysis *see* Release, Respiratory System 0BN
Pleuroscopy 0BJQ4ZZ
Pleurotomy *see* Drainage, Respiratory System 0B9
Plica semilunaris
use Conjunctiva, Left
use Conjunctiva, Right
Plication *see* Restriction
Pneumectomy
see Excision, Respiratory System 0BB
see Resection, Respiratory System 0BT
Pneumocentesis *see* Drainage, Respiratory System 0B9
Pneumogastric nerve *use* Vagus Nerve
Pneumolysis *see* Release, Respiratory System 0BN
Pneumonectomy *see* Resection, Respiratory System 0BT
Pneumonolysis *see* Release, Respiratory System 0BN
Pneumonopexy
see Repair, Respiratory System 0BQ
see Reposition, Respiratory System 0BS
Pneumonorrhaphy *see* Repair, Respiratory System 0BQ
Pneumonotomy *see* Drainage, Respiratory System 0B9
Pneumotaxic center *use* Pons
Pneumotomy *see* Drainage, Respiratory System 0B9

Pollicization *see* Transfer, Anatomical Regions, Upper Extremities 0XX
Polyclonal hyperimmune globulin *use* Globulin
Polyethylene socket *use* Synthetic Substitute, Polyethylene in 0SR
Polymethylmethacrylate (PMMA) *use* Synthetic Substitute
Polypectomy, gastrointestinal *see* Excision, Gastrointestinal System 0DB
Polypropylene mesh *use* Synthetic Substitute
Polysomnogram 4A1ZXQZ
Pontine tegmentum *use* Pons
Popliteal ligament
use Knee Bursa and Ligament, Left
use Knee Bursa and Ligament, Right
Popliteal lymph node
use Lymphatic, Left Lower Extremity
use Lymphatic, Right Lower Extremity
Popliteal vein
use Femoral Vein, Left
use Femoral Vein, Right
Popliteus muscle
use Lower Leg Muscle, Left
use Lower Leg Muscle, Right
Porcine (bioprosthetic) valve *use* Zooplastic Tissue in Heart and Great Vessels
Positive Blood Culture Fluorescence Hybridization for Organism Identification, Concentration and Susceptibility XXE5XN6
Positive end expiratory pressure *see* Performance, Respiratory 5A19
Positron Emission Tomographic (PET) Imaging
Brain C030
Bronchi and Lungs CB32
Central Nervous System C03YYZZ
Heart C23YYZZ
Lungs and Bronchi CB32
Myocardium C23G
Respiratory System CB3YYZZ
Whole Body CW3NYZZ
Positron emission tomography *see* Positron Emission Tomographic (PET) Imaging
Postauricular (mastoid) lymph node
use Lymphatic, Left Neck
use Lymphatic, Right Neck
Postcava *use* Inferior Vena Cava
Posterior auricular artery
use External Carotid Artery, Left
use External Carotid Artery, Right
Posterior auricular nerve *use* Facial Nerve
Posterior auricular vein
use External Jugular Vein, Left
use External Jugular Vein, Right
Posterior cerebral artery *use* Intracranial Artery
Posterior chamber
use Eye, Left
use Eye, Right
Posterior circumflex humeral artery
use Axillary Artery, Left
use Axillary Artery, Right
Posterior communicating artery *use* Intracranial Artery
Posterior cruciate ligament (PCL)
use Knee Bursa and Ligament, Left
use Knee Bursa and Ligament, Right
Posterior (Dynamic) Distraction Device
Lumbar XNS0
Thoracic XNS4
Posterior facial (retromandibular) vein
use Face Vein, Left
use Face Vein, Right
Posterior femoral cutaneous nerve *use* Sacral Plexus
Posterior inferior cerebellar artery (PICA) *use* Intracranial Artery
Posterior interosseous nerve *use* Radial Nerve
Posterior labial nerve *use* Pudendal Nerve
Posterior (subscapular) lymph node
use Lymphatic, Left Axillary
use Lymphatic, Right Axillary
Posterior scrotal nerve *use* Pudendal Nerve
Posterior spinal artery
use Vertebral Artery, Left
use Vertebral Artery, Right
Posterior tibial recurrent artery
use Anterior Tibial Artery, Left
use Anterior Tibial Artery, Right

Posterior ulnar recurrent artery
use Ulnar Artery, Left
use Ulnar Artery, Right
Posterior vagal trunk *use* Vagus Nerve
PPN (peripheral parenteral nutrition) *see* Introduction of Nutritional Substance
Praxbind® (idarucizumab), Pradaxa® (dabigatran) reversal agent *use* Other Therapeutic Substance
Preauricular lymph node *use* Lymphatic, Head
Precava *use* Superior Vena Cava
PRECICE intramedullary limb lengthening system
use Internal Fixation Device, Intramedullary Limb Lengthening in 0PH
use Internal Fixation Device, Intramedullary Limb Lengthening in 0QH
Precision TAVI™ Coronary Obstruction Module XXE3X68
Prepatellar bursa
use Knee Bursa and Ligament, Left
use Knee Bursa and Ligament, Right
Preputiotomy *see* Drainage, Male Reproductive System 0V9
Pressure support ventilation *see* Performance, Respiratory 5A19
PRESTIGE® Cervical Disc *use* Synthetic Substitute
Pretracheal fascia
use Subcutaneous Tissue and Fascia, Left Neck
use Subcutaneous Tissue and Fascia, Right Neck
Prevertebral fascia
use Subcutaneous Tissue and Fascia, Left Neck
use Subcutaneous Tissue and Fascia, Right Neck
PrimeAdvanced neurostimulator (SureScan) (MRI Safe) *use* Stimulator Generator, Multiple Array in 0JH
Princeps pollicis artery
use Hand Artery, Left
use Hand Artery, Right
Probing, duct
Diagnostic *see* Inspection
Dilation *see* Dilation
PROCEED™ Ventral Patch *use* Synthetic Substitute
Procerus muscle *use* Facial Muscle
Proctectomy
see Excision, Rectum 0DBP
see Resection, Rectum 0DTP
Proctoclysis *see* Introduction of substance in or on, Gastrointestinal Tract, Lower 3E0H
Proctocolectomy
see Excision, Gastrointestinal System 0DB
see Resection, Gastrointestinal System 0DT
Proctocolpoplasty
see Repair, Gastrointestinal System 0DQ
see Supplement, Gastrointestinal System 0DU
Proctoperineoplasty
see Repair, Gastrointestinal System 0DQ
see Supplement, Gastrointestinal System 0DU
Proctoperineorrhaphy *see* Repair, Gastrointestinal System 0DQ
Proctopexy
see Repair, Rectum 0DQP
see Reposition, Rectum 0DSP
Proctoplasty
see Repair, Rectum 0DQP
see Supplement, Rectum 0DUP
Proctorrhaphy *see* Repair, Rectum 0DQP
Proctoscopy 0DJD8ZZ
Proctosigmoidectomy
see Excision, Gastrointestinal System 0DB
see Resection, Gastrointestinal System 0DT
Proctosigmoidoscopy 0DJD8ZZ
Proctostomy *see* Drainage, Rectum 0D9P
Proctotomy *see* Drainage, Rectum 0D9P
Prodisc-C *use* Synthetic Substitute
Prodisc-L *use* Synthetic Substitute
Production, atrial septal defect *see* Excision, Septum, Atrial 02B5
Profunda brachii
use Brachial Artery, Left
use Brachial Artery, Right
Profunda femoris (deep femoral) vein
use Femoral Vein, Left
use Femoral Vein, Right
PROLENE Polypropylene Hernia System (PHS) *use* Synthetic Substitute
Prolonged intermittent renal replacement therapy (PIRRT) 5A1D80Z

Pronator quadratus muscle
  use Lower Arm and Wrist Muscle, Left
  use Lower Arm and Wrist Muscle, Right
Pronator teres muscle
  use Lower Arm and Wrist Muscle, Left
  use Lower Arm and Wrist Muscle, Right
Prostatectomy
  see Excision, Prostate 0VB0
  see Resection, Prostate 0VT0
Prostatic artery
  use Internal Iliac Artery, Left
  use Internal Iliac Artery, Right
Prostatic urethra *use* Urethra
Prostatomy, prostatotomy *see* Drainage, Prostate 0V90
Protecta XT CRT-D *use* Cardiac Resynchronization Defibrillator Pulse Generator in 0JH
Protecta XT DR (XT VR) *use* Defibrillator Generator in 0JH
Protege® RX Carotid Stent System *use* Intraluminal Device
Proximal radioulnar joint
  use Elbow Joint, Left
  use Elbow Joint, Right
Psoas muscle
  use Hip Muscle, Left
  use Hip Muscle, Right
PSV (pressure support ventilation) *see* Performance, Respiratory 5A19
Psychoanalysis GZ54ZZZ
Psychological Tests
  Cognitive Status GZ14ZZZ
  Developmental GZ10ZZZ
  Intellectual and Psychoeducational GZ12ZZZ
  Neurobehavioral Status GZ14ZZZ
  Neuropsychological GZ13ZZZ
  Personality and Behavioral GZ11ZZZ
Psychotherapy
  Family, Mental Health Services GZ72ZZZ
  Group GZHZZZZ
    Mental Health Services GZHZZZZ
  Individual
    see Psychotherapy, Individual, Mental Health Services
    for substance abuse
      12-Step HZ53ZZZ
      Behavioral HZ51ZZZ
      Cognitive HZ50ZZZ
      Cognitive-Behavioral HZ52ZZZ
      Confrontational HZ58ZZZ
      Interactive HZ55ZZZ
      Interpersonal HZ54ZZZ
      Motivational Enhancement HZ57ZZZ
      Psychoanalysis HZ5BZZZ
      Psychodynamic HZ5CZZZ
      Psychoeducation HZ56ZZZ
      Psychophysiological HZ5DZZZ
      Supportive HZ59ZZZ
  Mental Health Services
    Behavioral GZ51ZZZ
    Cognitive GZ52ZZZ
    Cognitive-Behavioral GZ58ZZZ
    Interactive GZ50ZZZ
    Interpersonal GZ53ZZZ
    Psychoanalysis GZ54ZZZ
    Psychodynamic GZ55ZZZ
    Psychophysiological GZ59ZZZ
    Supportive GZ56ZZZ
PTCA (percutaneous transluminal coronary angioplasty) *see* Dilation, Heart and Great Vessels 027
Pterygoid muscle *use* Head Muscle
Pterygoid process *use* Sphenoid Bone
Pterygopalatine (sphenopalatine) ganglion *use* Head and Neck Sympathetic Nerve
Pubis
  use Pelvic Bone, Left
  use Pelvic Bone, Right
Pubofemoral ligament
  use Hip Bursa and Ligament, Left
  use Hip Bursa and Ligament, Right
Pudendal nerve *use* Sacral Plexus
Pull-through, laparoscopic-assisted transanal
  see Excision, Gastrointestinal System 0DB
  see Resection, Gastrointestinal System 0DT
Pull-through, rectal *see* Resection, Rectum 0DTP
Pulmoaortic canal *use* Pulmonary Artery, Left
Pulmonary annulus *use* Pulmonary Valve

Pulmonary artery wedge monitoring *see* Monitoring, Arterial 4A13
Pulmonary plexus
  use Thoracic Sympathetic Nerve
  use Vagus Nerve
Pulmonic valve *use* Pulmonary Valve
Pulpectomy *see* Excision, Mouth and Throat 0CB
Pulverization *see* Fragmentation
Pulvinar *use* Thalamus
Pump reservoir *use* Infusion Device, Pump in Subcutaneous Tissue and Fascia
Punch biopsy *see* Excision with qualifier Diagnostic
Puncture *see* Drainage
Puncture, lumbar *see* Drainage, Spinal Canal 009U
Pure-Vu® System XDPH8K7
Pyelography
  see Fluoroscopy, Urinary System BT1
  see Plain Radiography, Urinary System BT0
Pyeloileostomy, urinary diversion *see* Bypass, Urinary System 0T1
Pyeloplasty
  see Repair, Urinary System 0TQ
  see Replacement, Urinary System 0TR
  see Supplement, Urinary System 0TU
Pyeloplasty, dismembered *see* Repair, Kidney Pelvis
Pyelorrhaphy *see* Repair, Urinary System 0TQ
Pyeloscopy 0TJ58ZZ
Pyelostomy
  see Bypass, Urinary System 0T1
  see Drainage, Urinary System 0T9
Pyelotomy *see* Drainage, Urinary System 0T9
Pylorectomy
  see Excision, Stomach, Pylorus 0DB7
  see Resection, Stomach, Pylorus 0DT7
Pyloric antrum *use* Stomach, Pylorus
Pyloric canal *use* Stomach, Pylorus
Pyloric sphincter *use* Stomach, Pylorus
Pylorodiosis *see* Dilation, Stomach, Pylorus 0D77
Pylorogastrectomy
  see Excision, Gastrointestinal System 0DB
  see Resection, Gastrointestinal System 0DT
Pyloroplasty
  see Repair, Stomach, Pylorus 0DQ7
  see Supplement, Stomach, Pylorus 0DU7
Pyloroscopy 0DJ68ZZ
Pylorotomy *see* Drainage, Stomach, Pylorus 0D97
Pyramidalis muscle
  use Abdomen Muscle, Left
  use Abdomen Muscle, Right

Q

QAngio XA® 3D XXE3X58
QFR® (Quantitative Flow Ratio) analysis of coronary angiography XXE3X58
Quadrangular cartilage *use* Nasal Septum
Quadrant resection of breast *see* Excision, Skin and Breast 0HB
Quadrate lobe *use* Liver
Quadratus femoris muscle
  use Hip Muscle, Left
  use Hip Muscle, Right
Quadratus lumborum muscle
  use Trunk Muscle, Left
  use Trunk Muscle, Right
Quadratus plantae muscle
  use Foot Muscle, Left
  use Foot Muscle, Right
Quadriceps (femoris)
  use Upper Leg Muscle, Left
  use Upper Leg Muscle, Right
Quantitative Flow Ratio Analysis, Coronary Artery Flow XXE3X58
Quarantine 8E0ZXY6

R

Radial artery arteriovenous fistula, using Thermal Resistance Energy X2K
Radial collateral carpal ligament
  use Wrist Bursa and Ligament, Left
  use Wrist Bursa and Ligament, Right
Radial collateral ligament
  use Elbow Bursa and Ligament, Left
  use Elbow Bursa and Ligament, Right

Radial notch
  use Ulna, Left
  use Ulna, Right
Radial recurrent artery
  use Radial Artery, Left
  use Radial Artery, Right
Radial vein
  use Brachial Vein, Left
  use Brachial Vein, Right
Radialis indicis
  use Hand Artery, Left
  use Hand Artery, Right
Radiation Therapy
  see Beam Radiation
  see Brachytherapy
  see Other Radiation
  see Stereotactic Radiosurgery
Radiation treatment *see* Radiation Therapy
Radiocarpal joint
  use Wrist Joint, Left
  use Wrist Joint, Right
Radiocarpal ligament
  use Wrist Bursa and Ligament, Left
  use Wrist Bursa and Ligament, Right
Radiography *see* Plain Radiography
Radiology, analog *see* Plain Radiography
Radiology, diagnostic *see* Imaging, Diagnostic
Radioulnar ligament
  use Wrist Bursa and Ligament, Left
  use Wrist Bursa and Ligament, Right
Range of motion testing *see* Motor Function Assessment, Rehabilitation F01
Rapid ASPECTS XXE0X07
REALIZE® Adjustable Gastric Band *use* Extraluminal Device
Reattachment
  Abdominal Wall 0WMF0ZZ
  Ampulla of Vater 0FMC
  Ankle Region
    Left 0YML0ZZ
    Right 0YMK0ZZ
  Arm
    Lower
      Left 0XMF0ZZ
      Right 0XMD0ZZ
    Upper
      Left 0XM90ZZ
      Right 0XM80ZZ
  Axilla
    Left 0XM50ZZ
    Right 0XM40ZZ
  Back
    Lower 0WML0ZZ
    Upper 0WMK0ZZ
  Bladder 0TMB
  Bladder Neck 0TMC
  Breast
    Bilateral 0HMVXZZ
    Left 0HMUXZZ
    Right 0HMTXZZ
  Bronchus
    Lingula 0BM90ZZ
    Lower Lobe
      Left 0BMB0ZZ
      Right 0BM60ZZ
    Main
      Left 0BM70ZZ
      Right 0BM30ZZ
    Middle Lobe, Right 0BM50ZZ
    Upper Lobe
      Left 0BM80ZZ
      Right 0BM40ZZ
  Bursa and Ligament
    Abdomen
      Left 0MMJ
      Right 0MMH
    Ankle
      Left 0MMR
      Right 0MMQ
    Elbow
      Left 0MM4
      Right 0MM3
    Foot
      Left 0MMT
      Right 0MMS
    Hand
      Left 0MM8
      Right 0MM7

Reattachment — *continued*
  Bursa and Ligament — *continued*
    Head and Neck 0MM0
    Hip
      Left 0MMM
      Right 0MML
    Knee
      Left 0MMP
      Right 0MMN
    Lower Extremity
      Left 0MMW
      Right 0MMV
    Perineum 0MMK
    Rib(s) 0MMG
    Shoulder
      Left 0MM2
      Right 0MM1
    Spine
      Lower 0MMD
      Upper 0MMC
    Sternum 0MMF
    Upper Extremity
      Left 0MMB
      Right 0MM9
    Wrist
      Left 0MM6
      Right 0MM5
  Buttock
    Left 0YM10ZZ
    Right 0YM00ZZ
  Carina 0BM20ZZ
  Cecum 0DMH
  Cervix 0UMC
  Chest Wall 0WM80ZZ
  Clitoris 0UMJXZZ
  Colon
    Ascending 0DMK
    Descending 0DMM
    Sigmoid 0DMN
    Transverse 0DML
  Cord
    Bilateral 0VMH
    Left 0VMG
    Right 0VMF
  Cul-de-sac 0UMF
  Diaphragm 0BMT0ZZ
  Duct
    Common Bile 0FM9
    Cystic 0FM8
    Hepatic
      Common 0FM7
      Left 0FM6
      Right 0FM5
    Pancreatic 0FMD
      Accessory 0FMF
  Duodenum 0DM9
  Ear
    Left 09M1XZZ
    Right 09M0XZZ
  Elbow Region
    Left 0XMC0ZZ
    Right 0XMB0ZZ
  Esophagus 0DM5
  Extremity
    Lower
      Left 0YMB0ZZ
      Right 0YM90ZZ
    Upper
      Left 0XM70ZZ
      Right 0XM60ZZ
  Eyelid
    Lower
      Left 08MRXZZ
      Right 08MQXZZ
    Upper
      Left 08MPXZZ
      Right 08MNXZZ
  Face 0WM20ZZ
  Fallopian Tube
    Left 0UM6
    Right 0UM5
  Fallopian Tubes, Bilateral 0UM7
  Femoral Region
    Left 0YM80ZZ
    Right 0YM70ZZ
  Finger
    Index
      Left 0XMP0ZZ
      Right 0XMN0ZZ

Reattachment — *continued*
  Finger — *continued*
    Little
      Left 0XMW0ZZ
      Right 0XMV0ZZ
    Middle
      Left 0XMR0ZZ
      Right 0XMQ0ZZ
    Ring
      Left 0XMT0ZZ
      Right 0XMS0ZZ
  Foot
    Left 0YMN0ZZ
    Right 0YMM0ZZ
  Forequarter
    Left 0XM10ZZ
    Right 0XM00ZZ
  Gallbladder 0FM4
  Gland
    Left 0GM2
    Right 0GM3
  Hand
    Left 0XMK0ZZ
    Right 0XMJ0ZZ
  Hindquarter
    Bilateral 0YM40ZZ
    Left 0YM30ZZ
    Right 0YM20ZZ
  Hymen 0UMK
  Ileum 0DMB
  Inguinal Region
    Left 0YM60ZZ
    Right 0YM50ZZ
  Intestine
    Large 0DME
      Left 0DMG
      Right 0DMF
    Small 0DM8
  Jaw
    Lower 0WM50ZZ
    Upper 0WM40ZZ
  Jejunum 0DMA
  Kidney
    Left 0TM1
    Right 0TM0
  Kidney Pelvis
    Left 0TM4
    Right 0TM3
  Kidneys, Bilateral 0TM2
  Knee Region
    Left 0YMG0ZZ
    Right 0YMF0ZZ
  Leg
    Lower
      Left 0YMJ0ZZ
      Right 0YMH0ZZ
    Upper
      Left 0YMD0ZZ
      Right 0YMC0ZZ
  Lip
    Lower 0CM10ZZ
    Upper 0CM00ZZ
  Liver 0FM0
    Left Lobe 0FM2
    Right Lobe 0FM1
  Lung
    Left 0BML0ZZ
    Lower Lobe
      Left 0BMJ0ZZ
      Right 0BMF0ZZ
    Middle Lobe, Right 0BMD0ZZ
    Right 0BMK0ZZ
    Upper Lobe
      Left 0BMG0ZZ
      Right 0BMC0ZZ
  Lung Lingula 0BMH0ZZ
  Muscle
    Abdomen
      Left 0KML
      Right 0KMK
    Facial 0KM1
    Foot
      Left 0KMW
      Right 0KMV
    Hand
      Left 0KMD
      Right 0KMC
    Head 0KM0

Reattachment — *continued*
  Muscle — *continued*
    Hip
      Left 0KMP
      Right 0KMN
    Lower Arm and Wrist
      Left 0KMB
      Right 0KM9
    Lower Leg
      Left 0KMT
      Right 0KMS
    Neck
      Left 0KM3
      Right 0KM2
    Perineum 0KMM
    Shoulder
      Left 0KM6
      Right 0KM5
    Thorax
      Left 0KMJ
      Right 0KMH
    Tongue, Palate, Pharynx 0KM4
    Trunk
      Left 0KMG
      Right 0KMF
    Upper Arm
      Left 0KM8
      Right 0KM7
    Upper Leg
      Left 0KMR
      Right 0KMQ
  Nasal Mucosa and Soft Tissue 09MKXZZ
  Neck 0WM60ZZ
  Nipple
    Left 0HMXXZZ
    Right 0HMWXZZ
  Ovary
    Bilateral 0UM2
    Left 0UM1
    Right 0UM0
  Palate, Soft 0CM30ZZ
  Pancreas 0FMG
  Parathyroid Gland 0GMR
    Inferior
      Left 0GMP
      Right 0GMN
    Multiple 0GMQ
    Superior
      Left 0GMM
      Right 0GML
  Penis 0VMSXZZ
  Perineum
    Female 0WMN0ZZ
    Male 0WMM0ZZ
  Rectum 0DMP
  Scrotum 0VM5XZZ
  Shoulder Region
    Left 0XM30ZZ
    Right 0XM20ZZ
  Skin
    Abdomen 0HM7XZZ
    Back 0HM6XZZ
    Buttock 0HM8XZZ
    Chest 0HM5XZZ
    Ear
      Left 0HM3XZZ
      Right 0HM2XZZ
    Face 0HM1XZZ
    Foot
      Left 0HMNXZZ
      Right 0HMMXZZ
    Hand
      Left 0HMGXZZ
      Right 0HMFXZZ
    Inguinal 0HMAXZZ
    Lower Arm
      Left 0HMEXZZ
      Right 0HMDXZZ
    Lower Leg
      Left 0HMLXZZ
      Right 0HMKXZZ
    Neck 0HM4XZZ
    Perineum 0HM9XZZ
    Scalp 0HM0XZZ
    Upper Arm
      Left 0HMCXZZ
      Right 0HMBXZZ
    Upper Leg
      Left 0HMJXZZ

Reattachment — *continued*
  Skin — *continued*
    Upper Leg — *continued*
      Right ØHMHXZZ
  Stomach ØDM6
  Tendon
    Abdomen
      Left ØLMG
      Right ØLMF
    Ankle
      Left ØLMT
      Right ØLMS
    Foot
      Left ØLMW
      Right ØLMV
    Hand
      Left ØLM8
      Right ØLM7
    Head and Neck ØLMØ
    Hip
      Left ØLMK
      Right ØLMJ
    Knee
      Left ØLMR
      Right ØLMQ
    Lower Arm and Wrist
      Left ØLM6
      Right ØLM5
    Lower Leg
      Left ØLMP
      Right ØLMN
    Perineum ØLMH
    Shoulder
      Left ØLM2
      Right ØLM1
    Thorax
      Left ØLMD
      Right ØLMC
    Trunk
      Left ØLMB
      Right ØLM9
    Upper Arm
      Left ØLM4
      Right ØLM3
    Upper Leg
      Left ØLMM
      Right ØLML
  Testis
    Bilateral ØVMC
    Left ØVMB
    Right ØVM9
  Thumb
    Left ØXMMØZZ
    Right ØXMLØZZ
  Thyroid Gland
    Left Lobe ØGMG
    Right Lobe ØGMH
  Toe
    1st
      Left ØYMQØZZ
      Right ØYMPØZZ
    2nd
      Left ØYMSØZZ
      Right ØYMRØZZ
    3rd
      Left ØYMUØZZ
      Right ØYMTØZZ
    4th
      Left ØYMWØZZ
      Right ØYMVØZZ
    5th
      Left ØYMYØZZ
      Right ØYMXØZZ
  Tongue ØCM7ØZZ
  Tooth
    Lower ØCMX
    Upper ØCMW
  Trachea ØBM1ØZZ
  Tunica Vaginalis
    Left ØVM7
    Right ØVM6
  Ureter
    Left ØTM7
    Right ØTM6
  Ureters, Bilateral ØTM8
  Urethra ØTMD
  Uterine Supporting Structure ØUM4
  Uterus ØUM9
  Uvula ØCMNØZZ

Reattachment — *continued*
  Vagina ØUMG
  Vulva ØUMMXZZ
  Wrist Region
    Left ØXMHØZZ
    Right ØXMGØZZ
REBOA (resuscitative endovascular balloon occlusion of the aorta)
  02LW3DJ
  04L03DJ
Rebound HRD® (Hernia Repair Device) *use* Synthetic Substitute
REBYOTA® *use* Broad Consortium Microbiota-based Live Biotherapeutic Suspension
RECELL® cell suspension autograft *see* Replacement, Skin and Breast ØHR
Recession
  see Repair
  see Reposition
Reclosure, disrupted abdominal wall ØWQFXZZ
Reconstruction
  see Repair
  see Replacement
  see Supplement
Rectectomy
  see Excision, Rectum ØDBP
  see Resection, Rectum ØDTP
Rectocele repair *see* Repair, Subcutaneous Tissue and Fascia, Pelvic Region ØJQC
Rectopexy
  see Repair, Gastrointestinal System ØDQ
  see Reposition, Gastrointestinal System ØDS
Rectoplasty
  see Repair, Gastrointestinal System ØDQ
  see Supplement, Gastrointestinal System ØDU
Rectorrhaphy *see* Repair, Gastrointestinal System ØDQ
Rectoscopy ØDJD8ZZ
Rectosigmoid junction *use* Sigmoid Colon
Rectosigmoidectomy
  see Excision, Gastrointestinal System ØDB
  see Resection, Gastrointestinal System ØDT
Rectostomy *see* Drainage, Rectum ØD9P
Rectotomy *see* Drainage, Rectum ØD9P
Rectus abdominis muscle
  use Abdomen Muscle, Left
  use Abdomen Muscle, Right
Rectus femoris muscle
  use Upper Leg Muscle, Left
  use Upper Leg Muscle, Right
Recurrent laryngeal nerve *use* Vagus Nerve
Reducer™ System *use* Reduction Device in New Technology
Reduction
  Dislocation *see* Reposition
  Fracture *see* Reposition
  Intussusception, intestinal *see* Reposition, Gastrointestinal System ØDS
  Mammoplasty *see* Excision, Skin and Breast ØHB
  Prolapse *see* Reposition
  Torsion *see* Reposition
  Volvulus, gastrointestinal *see* Reposition, Gastrointestinal System ØDS
Reduction Device, Coronary Sinus X2V73Q7
Refusion *see* Fusion
REGN-COV2 Monoclonal Antibody XWØ
Rehabilitation
  see Activities of Daily Living Assessment, Rehabilitation FØ2
  see Activities of Daily Living Treatment, Rehabilitation FØ8
  see Caregiver Training, Rehabilitation FØF
  see Cochlear Implant Treatment, Rehabilitation FØB
  see Device Fitting, Rehabilitation FØD
  see Hearing Treatment, Rehabilitation FØ9
  see Motor Function Assessment, Rehabilitation FØ1
  see Motor Treatment, Rehabilitation FØ7
  see Speech Assessment, Rehabilitation FØØ
  see Speech Treatment, Rehabilitation FØ6
  see Vestibular Treatment, Rehabilitation FØC
Reimplantation
  see Reattachment
  see Reposition
  see Transfer
Reinforcement
  see Repair

Reinforcement — *continued*
  see Supplement
Relaxation, scar tissue *see* Release
Release
  Acetabulum
    Left ØQN5
    Right ØQN4
  Adenoids ØCNQ
  Ampulla of Vater ØFNC
  Anal Sphincter ØDNR
  Anterior Chamber
    Left Ø8N33ZZ
    Right Ø8N23ZZ
  Anus ØDNQ
  Aorta
    Abdominal 04N0
    Thoracic
      Ascending/Arch 02NX
      Descending 02NW
  Aortic Body ØGND
  Appendix ØDNJ
  Artery
    Anterior Tibial
      Left 04NQ
      Right 04NP
    Axillary
      Left 03N6
      Right 03N5
    Brachial
      Left 03N8
      Right 03N7
    Celiac 04N1
    Colic
      Left 04N7
      Middle 04N8
      Right 04N6
    Common Carotid
      Left 03NJ
      Right 03NH
    Common Iliac
      Left 04ND
      Right 04NC
    Coronary
      Four or More Arteries 02N3
      One Artery 02N0
      Three Arteries 02N2
      Two Arteries 02N1
    External Carotid
      Left 03NN
      Right 03NM
    External Iliac
      Left 04NJ
      Right 04NH
    Face 03NR
    Femoral
      Left 04NL
      Right 04NK
    Foot
      Left 04NW
      Right 04NV
    Gastric 04N2
    Hand
      Left 03NF
      Right 03ND
    Hepatic 04N3
    Inferior Mesenteric 04NB
    Innominate 03N2
    Internal Carotid
      Left 03NL
      Right 03NK
    Internal Iliac
      Left 04NF
      Right 04NE
    Internal Mammary
      Left 03N1
      Right 03N0
    Intracranial 03NG
    Lower 04NY
    Peroneal
      Left 04NU
      Right 04NT
    Popliteal
      Left 04NN
      Right 04NM
    Posterior Tibial
      Left 04NS
      Right 04NR
    Pulmonary
      Left 02NR

▼ **Subterms under main terms may continue to next column or page**

Release — *continued*
  Artery — *continued*
    Pulmonary — *continued*
      Right 02NQ
    Pulmonary Trunk 02NP
    Radial
      Left 03NC
      Right 03NB
    Renal
      Left 04NA
      Right 04N9
    Splenic 04N4
    Subclavian
      Left 03N4
      Right 03N3
    Superior Mesenteric 04N5
    Temporal
      Left 03NT
      Right 03NS
    Thyroid
      Left 03NV
      Right 03NU
    Ulnar
      Left 03NA
      Right 03N9
    Upper 03NY
    Vertebral
      Left 03NQ
      Right 03NP
  Atrium
    Left 02N7
    Right 02N6
  Auditory Ossicle
    Left 09NA
    Right 09N9
  Basal Ganglia 00N8
  Bladder 0TNB
  Bladder Neck 0TNC
  Bone
    Ethmoid
      Left 0NNG
      Right 0NNF
    Frontal 0NN1
    Hyoid 0NNX
    Lacrimal
      Left 0NNJ
      Right 0NNH
    Nasal 0NNB
    Occipital 0NN7
    Palatine
      Left 0NNL
      Right 0NNK
    Parietal
      Left 0NN4
      Right 0NN3
    Pelvic
      Left 0QN3
      Right 0QN2
    Sphenoid 0NNC
    Temporal
      Left 0NN6
      Right 0NN5
    Zygomatic
      Left 0NNN
      Right 0NNM
  Brain 00N0
  Breast
    Bilateral 0HNV
    Left 0HNU
    Right 0HNT
  Bronchus
    Lingula 0BN9
    Lower Lobe
      Left 0BNB
      Right 0BN6
    Main
      Left 0BN7
      Right 0BN3
    Middle Lobe, Right 0BN5
    Upper Lobe
      Left 0BN8
      Right 0BN4
  Buccal Mucosa 0CN4
  Bursa and Ligament
    Abdomen
      Left 0MNJ
      Right 0MNH
    Ankle
      Left 0MNR

Release — *continued*
  Bursa and Ligament — *continued*
    Ankle — *continued*
      Right 0MNQ
    Elbow
      Left 0MN4
      Right 0MN3
    Foot
      Left 0MNT
      Right 0MNS
    Hand
      Left 0MN8
      Right 0MN7
    Head and Neck 0MN0
    Hip
      Left 0MNM
      Right 0MNL
    Knee
      Left 0MNP
      Right 0MNN
    Lower Extremity
      Left 0MNW
      Right 0MNV
    Perineum 0MNK
    Rib(s) 0MNG
    Shoulder
      Left 0MN2
      Right 0MN1
    Spine
      Lower 0MND
      Upper 0MNG
    Sternum 0MNF
    Upper Extremity
      Left 0MNB
      Right 0MN9
    Wrist
      Left 0MN6
      Right 0MN5
  Carina 0BN2
  Carotid Bodies, Bilateral 0GN8
  Carotid Body
    Left 0GN6
    Right 0GN7
  Carpal
    Left 0PNN
    Right 0PNM
  Cecum 0DNH
  Cerebellum 00NC
  Cerebral Hemisphere 00N7
  Cerebral Meninges 00N1
  Cerebral Ventricle 00N6
  Cervix 0UNC
  Chordae Tendineae 02N9
  Choroid
    Left 08NB
    Right 08NA
  Cisterna Chyli 07NL
  Clavicle
    Left 0PNB
    Right 0PN9
  Clitoris 0UNJ
  Coccygeal Glomus 0GNB
  Coccyx 0QNS
  Colon
    Ascending 0DNK
    Descending 0DNM
    Sigmoid 0DNN
    Transverse 0DNL
  Conduction Mechanism 02N8
  Conjunctiva
    Left 08NTXZZ
    Right 08NSXZZ
  Cord
    Bilateral 0VNH
    Left 0VNG
    Right 0VNF
  Cornea
    Left 08N9XZZ
    Right 08N8XZZ
  Cul-de-sac 0UNF
  Diaphragm 0BNT
  Disc
    Cervical Vertebral 0RN3
    Cervicothoracic Vertebral 0RN5
    Lumbar Vertebral 0SN2
    Lumbosacral 0SN4
    Thoracic Vertebral 0RN9
    Thoracolumbar Vertebral 0RNB

Release — *continued*
  Duct
    Common Bile 0FN9
    Cystic 0FN8
    Hepatic
      Common 0FN7
      Left 0FN6
      Right 0FN5
    Lacrimal
      Left 08NY
      Right 08NX
    Pancreatic 0FND
      Accessory 0FNF
    Parotid
      Left 0CNC
      Right 0CNB
  Duodenum 0DN9
  Dura Mater 00N2
  Ear
    External
      Left 09N1
      Right 09N0
    External Auditory Canal
      Left 09N4
      Right 09N3
    Inner
      Left 09NE
      Right 09ND
    Middle
      Left 09N6
      Right 09N5
  Epididymis
    Bilateral 0VNL
    Left 0VNK
    Right 0VNJ
  Epiglottis 0CNR
  Esophagogastric Junction 0DN4
  Esophagus 0DN5
    Lower 0DN3
    Middle 0DN2
    Upper 0DN1
  Eustachian Tube
    Left 09NG
    Right 09NF
  Eye
    Left 08N1XZZ
    Right 08N0XZZ
  Eyelid
    Lower
      Left 08NR
      Right 08NQ
    Upper
      Left 08NP
      Right 08NN
  Fallopian Tube
    Left 0UN6
    Right 0UN5
  Fallopian Tubes, Bilateral 0UN7
  Femoral Shaft
    Left 0QN9
    Right 0QN8
  Femur
    Lower
      Left 0QNC
      Right 0QNB
    Upper
      Left 0QN7
      Right 0QN6
  Fibula
    Left 0QNK
    Right 0QNJ
  Finger Nail 0HNQXZZ
  Gallbladder 0FN4
  Gingiva
    Lower 0CN6
    Upper 0CN5
  Gland
    Adrenal
      Bilateral 0GN4
      Left 0GN2
      Right 0GN3
    Lacrimal
      Left 08NW
      Right 08NV
    Minor Salivary 0CNJ
    Parotid
      Left 0CN9
      Right 0CN8
    Pituitary 0GN0

Release — *continued*
　Gland — *continued*
　　Sublingual
　　　Left ØCNF
　　　Right ØCND
　　Submaxillary
　　　Left ØCNH
　　　Right ØCNG
　　Vestibular ØUNL
　Glenoid Cavity
　　Left ØPN8
　　Right ØPN7
　Glomus Jugulare ØGNC
　Humeral Head
　　Left ØPND
　　Right ØPNC
　Humeral Shaft
　　Left ØPNG
　　Right ØPNF
　Hymen ØUNK
　Hypothalamus ØØNA
　Ileocecal Valve ØDNC
　Ileum ØDNB
　Intestine
　　Large ØDNE
　　　Left ØDNG
　　　Right ØDNF
　　Small ØDN8
　Iris
　　Left Ø8ND3ZZ
　　Right Ø8NC3ZZ
　Jejunum ØDNA
　Joint
　　Acromioclavicular
　　　Left ØRNH
　　　Right ØRNG
　　Ankle
　　　Left ØSNG
　　　Right ØSNF
　　Carpal
　　　Left ØRNR
　　　Right ØRNQ
　　Carpometacarpal
　　　Left ØRNT
　　　Right ØRNS
　　Cervical Vertebral ØRN1
　　Cervicothoracic Vertebral ØRN4
　　Coccygeal ØSN6
　　Elbow
　　　Left ØRNM
　　　Right ØRNL
　　Finger Phalangeal
　　　Left ØRNX
　　　Right ØRNW
　　Hip
　　　Left ØSNB
　　　Right ØSN9
　　Knee
　　　Left ØSND
　　　Right ØSNC
　　Lumbar Vertebral ØSNØ
　　Lumbosacral ØSN3
　　Metacarpophalangeal
　　　Left ØRNV
　　　Right ØRNU
　　Metatarsal-Phalangeal
　　　Left ØSNN
　　　Right ØSNM
　　Occipital-cervical ØRNØ
　　Sacrococcygeal ØSN5
　　Sacroiliac
　　　Left ØSN8
　　　Right ØSN7
　　Shoulder
　　　Left ØRNK
　　　Right ØRNJ
　　Sternoclavicular
　　　Left ØRNF
　　　Right ØRNE
　　Tarsal
　　　Left ØSNJ
　　　Right ØSNH
　　Tarsometatarsal
　　　Left ØSNL
　　　Right ØSNK
　　Temporomandibular
　　　Left ØRND
　　　Right ØRNC
　　Thoracic Vertebral ØRN6

Release — *continued*
　Joint — *continued*
　　Thoracolumbar Vertebral ØRNA
　　Toe Phalangeal
　　　Left ØSNQ
　　　Right ØSNP
　　Wrist
　　　Left ØRNP
　　　Right ØRNN
　Kidney
　　Left ØTN1
　　Right ØTNØ
　Kidney Pelvis
　　Left ØTN4
　　Right ØTN3
　Larynx ØCNS
　Lens
　　Left Ø8NK3ZZ
　　Right Ø8NJ3ZZ
　Lip
　　Lower ØCN1
　　Upper ØCNØ
　Liver ØFNØ
　　Left Lobe ØFN2
　　Right Lobe ØFN1
　Lung
　　Bilateral ØBNM
　　Left ØBNL
　　Lower Lobe
　　　Left ØBNJ
　　　Right ØBNF
　　Middle Lobe, Right ØBND
　　Right ØBNK
　　Upper Lobe
　　　Left ØBNG
　　　Right ØBNC
　Lung Lingula ØBNH
　Lymphatic
　　Aortic Ø7ND
　　Axillary
　　　Left Ø7N6
　　　Right Ø7N5
　　Head Ø7NØ
　　Inguinal
　　　Left Ø7NJ
　　　Right Ø7NH
　　Internal Mammary
　　　Left Ø7N9
　　　Right Ø7N8
　　Lower Extremity
　　　Left Ø7NG
　　　Right Ø7NF
　　Mesenteric Ø7NB
　　Neck
　　　Left Ø7N2
　　　Right Ø7N1
　　Pelvis Ø7NC
　　Thoracic Duct Ø7NK
　　Thorax Ø7N7
　　Upper Extremity
　　　Left Ø7N4
　　　Right Ø7N3
　Mandible
　　Left ØNNV
　　Right ØNNT
　Maxilla ØNNR
　Medulla Oblongata ØØND
　Mesentery ØDNV
　Metacarpal
　　Left ØPNQ
　　Right ØPNP
　Metatarsal
　　Left ØQNP
　　Right ØQNN
　Muscle
　　Abdomen
　　　Left ØKNL
　　　Right ØKNK
　　Extraocular
　　　Left Ø8NM
　　　Right Ø8NL
　　Facial ØKN1
　　Foot
　　　Left ØKNW
　　　Right ØKNV
　　Hand
　　　Left ØKND
　　　Right ØKNC
　　Head ØKNØ

Release — *continued*
　Muscle — *continued*
　　Hip
　　　Left ØKNP
　　　Right ØKNN
　　Lower Arm and Wrist
　　　Left ØKNB
　　　Right ØKN9
　　Lower Leg
　　　Left ØKNT
　　　Right ØKNS
　　Neck
　　　Left ØKN3
　　　Right ØKN2
　　Papillary Ø2ND
　　Perineum ØKNM
　　Shoulder
　　　Left ØKN6
　　　Right ØKN5
　　Thorax
　　　Left ØKNJ
　　　Right ØKNH
　　Tongue, Palate, Pharynx ØKN4
　　Trunk
　　　Left ØKNG
　　　Right ØKNF
　　Upper Arm
　　　Left ØKN8
　　　Right ØKN7
　　Upper Leg
　　　Left ØKNR
　　　Right ØKNQ
　Myocardial Bridge *see* Release, Artery, Coronary
　Nasal Mucosa and Soft Tissue Ø9NK
　Nasopharynx Ø9NN
　Nerve
　　Abdominal Sympathetic Ø1NM
　　Abducens ØØNL
　　Accessory ØØNR
　　Acoustic ØØNN
　　Brachial Plexus Ø1N3
　　Cervical Ø1N1
　　Cervical Plexus Ø1NØ
　　Facial ØØNM
　　Femoral Ø1ND
　　Glossopharyngeal ØØNP
　　Head and Neck Sympathetic Ø1NK
　　Hypoglossal ØØNS
　　Lumbar Ø1NB
　　Lumbar Plexus Ø1N9
　　Lumbar Sympathetic Ø1NN
　　Lumbosacral Plexus Ø1NA
　　Median Ø1N5
　　Oculomotor ØØNH
　　Olfactory ØØNF
　　Optic ØØNG
　　Peroneal Ø1NH
　　Phrenic Ø1N2
　　Pudendal Ø1NC
　　Radial Ø1N6
　　Sacral Ø1NR
　　Sacral Plexus Ø1NQ
　　Sacral Sympathetic Ø1NP
　　Sciatic Ø1NF
　　Thoracic Ø1N8
　　Thoracic Sympathetic Ø1NL
　　Tibial Ø1NG
　　Trigeminal ØØNK
　　Trochlear ØØNJ
　　Ulnar Ø1N4
　　Vagus ØØNQ
　Nipple
　　Left ØHNX
　　Right ØHNW
　Omentum ØDNU
　Orbit
　　Left ØNNQ
　　Right ØNNP
　Ovary
　　Bilateral ØUN2
　　Left ØUN1
　　Right ØUNØ
　Palate
　　Hard ØCN2
　　Soft ØCN3
　Pancreas ØFNG
　Para-aortic Body ØGN9
　Paraganglion Extremity ØGNF
　Parathyroid Gland ØGNR

Release — Release

Release — *continued*
  Parathyroid Gland — *continued*
    Inferior
      Left ØGNP
      Right ØGNN
    Multiple ØGNQ
    Superior
      Left ØGNM
      Right ØGNL
  Patella
    Left ØQNF
    Right ØQND
  Penis ØVNS
  Pericardium Ø2NN
  Peritoneum ØDNW
  Phalanx
    Finger
      Left ØPNV
      Right ØPNT
    Thumb
      Left ØPNS
      Right ØPNR
    Toe
      Left ØQNR
      Right ØQNQ
  Pharynx ØCNM
  Pineal Body ØGN1
  Pleura
    Left ØBNP
    Right ØBNN
  Pons ØØNB
  Prepuce ØVNT
  Prostate ØVNØ
  Radius
    Left ØPNJ
    Right ØPNH
  Rectum ØDNP
  Retina
    Left Ø8NF3ZZ
    Right Ø8NE3ZZ
  Retinal Vessel
    Left Ø8NH3ZZ
    Right Ø8NG3ZZ
  Ribs
    1 to 2 ØPN1
    3 or More ØPN2
  Sacrum ØQN1
  Scapula
    Left ØPN6
    Right ØPN5
  Sclera
    Left Ø8N7XZZ
    Right Ø8N6XZZ
  Scrotum ØVN5
  Septum
    Atrial Ø2N5
    Nasal Ø9NM
    Ventricular Ø2NM
  Sinus
    Accessory Ø9NP
    Ethmoid
      Left Ø9NV
      Right Ø9NU
    Frontal
      Left Ø9NT
      Right Ø9NS
    Mastoid
      Left Ø9NC
      Right Ø9NB
    Maxillary
      Left Ø9NR
      Right Ø9NQ
    Sphenoid
      Left Ø9NX
      Right Ø9NW
  Skin
    Abdomen ØHN7XZZ
    Back ØHN6XZZ
    Buttock ØHN8XZZ
    Chest ØHN5XZZ
    Ear
      Left ØHN3XZZ
      Right ØHN2XZZ
    Face ØHN1XZZ
    Foot
      Left ØHNNXZZ
      Right ØHNMXZZ
    Hand
      Left ØHNGXZZ

Release — *continued*
  Skin — *continued*
    Hand — *continued*
      Right ØHNFXZZ
    Inguinal ØHNAXZZ
    Lower Arm
      Left ØHNEXZZ
      Right ØHNDXZZ
    Lower Leg
      Left ØHNLXZZ
      Right ØHNKXZZ
    Neck ØHN4XZZ
    Perineum ØHN9XZZ
    Scalp ØHNØXZZ
    Upper Arm
      Left ØHNCXZZ
      Right ØHNBXZZ
    Upper Leg
      Left ØHNJXZZ
      Right ØHNHXZZ
  Spinal Cord
    Cervical ØØNW
    Lumbar ØØNY
    Thoracic ØØNX
  Spinal Meninges ØØNT
  Spleen Ø7NP
  Sternum ØPNØ
  Stomach ØDN6
    Pylorus ØDN7
  Subcutaneous Tissue and Fascia
    Abdomen ØJN8
    Back ØJN7
    Buttock ØJN9
    Chest ØJN6
    Face ØJN1
    Foot
      Left ØJNR
      Right ØJNQ
    Hand
      Left ØJNK
      Right ØJNJ
    Lower Arm
      Left ØJNH
      Right ØJNG
    Lower Leg
      Left ØJNP
      Right ØJNN
    Neck
      Left ØJN5
      Right ØJN4
    Pelvic Region ØJNC
    Perineum ØJNB
    Scalp ØJNØ
    Upper Arm
      Left ØJNF
      Right ØJND
    Upper Leg
      Left ØJNM
      Right ØJNL
  Tarsal
    Left ØQNM
    Right ØQNL
  Tendon
    Abdomen
      Left ØLNG
      Right ØLNF
    Ankle
      Left ØLNT
      Right ØLNS
    Foot
      Left ØLNW
      Right ØLNV
    Hand
      Left ØLN8
      Right ØLN7
    Head and Neck ØLNØ
    Hip
      Left ØLNK
      Right ØLNJ
    Knee
      Left ØLNR
      Right ØLNQ
    Lower Arm and Wrist
      Left ØLN6
      Right ØLN5
    Lower Leg
      Left ØLNP
      Right ØLNN
    Perineum ØLNH

Release — *continued*
  Tendon — *continued*
    Shoulder
      Left ØLN2
      Right ØLN1
    Thorax
      Left ØLND
      Right ØLNC
    Trunk
      Left ØLNB
      Right ØLN9
    Upper Arm
      Left ØLN4
      Right ØLN3
    Upper Leg
      Left ØLNM
      Right ØLNL
  Testis
    Bilateral ØVNC
    Left ØVNB
    Right ØVN9
  Thalamus ØØN9
  Thymus Ø7NM
  Thyroid Gland ØGNK
    Left Lobe ØGNG
    Right Lobe ØGNH
  Tibia
    Left ØQNH
    Right ØQNG
  Toe Nail ØHNRXZZ
  Tongue ØCN7
  Tonsils ØCNP
  Tooth
    Lower ØCNX
    Upper ØCNW
  Trachea ØBN1
  Tunica Vaginalis
    Left ØVN7
    Right ØVN6
  Turbinate, Nasal Ø9NL
  Tympanic Membrane
    Left Ø9N8
    Right Ø9N7
  Ulna
    Left ØPNL
    Right ØPNK
  Ureter
    Left ØTN7
    Right ØTN6
  Urethra ØTND
  Uterine Supporting Structure ØUN4
  Uterus ØUN9
  Uvula ØCNN
  Vagina ØUNG
  Valve
    Aortic Ø2NF
    Mitral Ø2NG
    Pulmonary Ø2NH
    Tricuspid Ø2NJ
  Vas Deferens
    Bilateral ØVNQ
    Left ØVNP
    Right ØVNN
  Vein
    Axillary
      Left Ø5N8
      Right Ø5N7
    Azygos Ø5NØ
    Basilic
      Left Ø5NC
      Right Ø5NB
    Brachial
      Left Ø5NA
      Right Ø5N9
    Cephalic
      Left Ø5NF
      Right Ø5ND
    Colic Ø6N7
    Common Iliac
      Left Ø6ND
      Right Ø6NC
    Coronary Ø2N4
    Esophageal Ø6N3
    External Iliac
      Left Ø6NG
      Right Ø6NF
    External Jugular
      Left Ø5NQ
      Right Ø5NP

Release — continued
  Vein — continued
    Face
      Left Ø5NV
      Right Ø5NT
    Femoral
      Left Ø6NN
      Right Ø6NM
    Foot
      Left Ø6NV
      Right Ø6NT
    Gastric Ø6N2
    Hand
      Left Ø5NH
      Right Ø5NG
    Hemiazygos Ø5N1
    Hepatic Ø6N4
    Hypogastric
      Left Ø6NJ
      Right Ø6NH
    Inferior Mesenteric Ø6N6
    Innominate
      Left Ø5N4
      Right Ø5N3
    Internal Jugular
      Left Ø5NN
      Right Ø5NM
    Intracranial Ø5NL
    Lower Ø6NY
    Portal Ø6N8
    Pulmonary
      Left Ø2NT
      Right Ø2NS
    Renal
      Left Ø6NB
      Right Ø6N9
    Saphenous
      Left Ø6NQ
      Right Ø6NP
    Splenic Ø6N1
    Subclavian
      Left Ø5N6
      Right Ø5N5
    Superior Mesenteric Ø6N5
    Upper Ø5NY
    Vertebral
      Left Ø5NS
      Right Ø5NR
  Vena Cava
    Inferior Ø6NØ
    Superior Ø2NV
  Ventricle
    Left Ø2NL
    Right Ø2NK
  Vertebra
    Cervical ØPN3
    Lumbar ØQNØ
    Thoracic ØPN4
  Vesicle
    Bilateral ØVN3
    Left ØVN2
    Right ØVN1
  Vitreous
    Left Ø8N53ZZ
    Right Ø8N43ZZ
  Vocal Cord
    Left ØCNV
    Right ØCNT
  Vulva ØUNM
Relocation see Reposition
Remdesivir Anti-infective XWØ
Removal
  Abdominal Wall 2W53X
  Anorectal 2Y53X5Z
  Arm
    Lower
      Left 2W5DX
      Right 2W5CX
    Upper
      Left 2W5BX
      Right 2W5AX
  Back 2W55X
  Chest Wall 2W54X
  Ear 2Y52X5Z
  Extremity
    Lower
      Left 2W5MX
      Right 2W5LX

Removal — continued
  Extremity — continued
    Upper
      Left 2W59X
      Right 2W58X
  Face 2W51X
  Finger
    Left 2W5KX
    Right 2W5JX
  Foot
    Left 2W5TX
    Right 2W5SX
  Genital Tract, Female 2Y54X5Z
  Hand
    Left 2W5FX
    Right 2W5EX
  Head 2W50X
  Inguinal Region
    Left 2W57X
    Right 2W56X
  Leg
    Lower
      Left 2W5RX
      Right 2W5QX
    Upper
      Left 2W5PX
      Right 2W5NX
  Mouth and Pharynx 2Y50X5Z
  Nasal 2Y51X5Z
  Neck 2W52X
  Thumb
    Left 2W5HX
    Right 2W5GX
  Toe
    Left 2W5VX
    Right 2W5UX
  Urethra 2Y55X5Z
Removal of device from
  Abdominal Wall ØWPF
  Acetabulum
    Left ØQP5
    Right ØQP4
  Anal Sphincter ØDPR
  Anus ØDPQ
  Artery
    Lower Ø4PY
    Upper Ø3PY
  Back
    Lower ØWPL
    Upper ØWPK
  Bladder ØTPB
  Bone
    Facial ØNPW
    Lower ØQPY
    Nasal ØNPB
    Pelvic
      Left ØQP3
      Right ØQP2
    Upper ØPPY
  Bone Marrow Ø7PT
  Brain ØØPØ
  Breast
    Left ØHPU
    Right ØHPT
  Bursa and Ligament
    Lower ØMPY
    Upper ØMPX
  Carpal
    Left ØPPN
    Right ØPPM
  Cavity, Cranial ØWP1
  Cerebral Ventricle ØØP6
  Chest Wall ØWP8
  Cisterna Chyli Ø7PL
  Clavicle
    Left ØPPB
    Right ØPP9
  Coccyx ØQPS
  Diaphragm ØBPT
  Disc
    Cervical Vertebral ØRP3
    Cervicothoracic Vertebral ØRP5
    Lumbar Vertebral ØSP2
    Lumbosacral ØSP4
    Thoracic Vertebral ØRP9
    Thoracolumbar Vertebral ØRPB
  Duct
    Hepatobiliary ØFPB
    Pancreatic ØFPD

Removal of device from — continued
  Ear
    Inner
      Left Ø9PJ
      Right Ø9PD
    Left Ø9PJ
    Right Ø9PH
  Epididymis and Spermatic Cord ØVPM
  Esophagus ØDP5
  Extremity
    Lower
      Left ØYPB
      Right ØYP9
    Upper
      Left ØXP7
      Right ØXP6
  Eye
    Left Ø8P1
    Right Ø8PØ
  Face ØWP2
  Fallopian Tube ØUP8
  Femoral Shaft
    Left ØQP9
    Right ØQP8
  Femur
    Lower
      Left ØQPC
      Right ØQPB
    Upper
      Left ØQP7
      Right ØQP6
  Fibula
    Left ØQPK
    Right ØQPJ
  Finger Nail ØHPQX
  Gallbladder ØFP4
  Gastrointestinal Tract ØWPP
  Genitourinary Tract ØWPR
  Gland
    Adrenal ØGP5
    Endocrine ØGPS
    Pituitary ØGPØ
    Salivary ØCPA
  Glenoid Cavity
    Left ØPP8
    Right ØPP7
  Great Vessel Ø2PY
  Hair ØHPSX
  Head ØWPØ
  Heart Ø2PA
  Humeral Head
    Left ØPPD
    Right ØPPC
  Humeral Shaft
    Left ØPPG
    Right ØPPF
  Intestinal Tract
    Lower Intestinal Tract ØDPD
    Upper Intestinal Tract ØDPØ
  Jaw
    Lower ØWP5
    Upper ØWP4
  Joint
    Acromioclavicular
      Left ØRPH
      Right ØRPG
    Ankle
      Left ØSPG
      Right ØSPF
    Carpal
      Left ØRPR
      Right ØRPQ
    Carpometacarpal
      Left ØRPT
      Right ØRPS
    Cervical Vertebral ØRP1
    Cervicothoracic Vertebral ØRP4
    Coccygeal ØSP6
    Elbow
      Left ØRPM
      Right ØRPL
    Finger Phalangeal
      Left ØRPX
      Right ØRPW
    Hip
      Left ØSPB
        Acetabular Surface ØSPE
        Femoral Surface ØSPS
      Right ØSP9

▽ **Subterms under main terms may continue to next column or page**

Removal of device from — *continued*
　Joint — *continued*
　　Hip — *continued*
　　　Right — *continued*
　　　　Acetabular Surface ØSPA
　　　　Femoral Surface ØSPR
　　　Knee
　　　　Left ØSPD
　　　　　Femoral Surface ØSPU
　　　　　Tibial Surface ØSPW
　　　　Right ØSPC
　　　　　Femoral Surface ØSPT
　　　　　Tibial Surface ØSPV
　　　Lumbar Vertebral ØSPØ
　　　Lumbosacral ØSP3
　　　Metacarpophalangeal
　　　　Left ØRPV
　　　　Right ØRPU
　　　Metatarsal-Phalangeal
　　　　Left ØSPN
　　　　Right ØSPM
　　　Occipital-cervical ØRPØ
　　　Sacrococcygeal ØSP5
　　　Sacroiliac
　　　　Left ØSP8
　　　　Right ØSP7
　　　Shoulder
　　　　Left ØRPK
　　　　Right ØRPJ
　　　Sternoclavicular
　　　　Left ØRPF
　　　　Right ØRPE
　　　Tarsal
　　　　Left ØSPJ
　　　　Right ØSPH
　　　Tarsometatarsal
　　　　Left ØSPL
　　　　Right ØSPK
　　　Temporomandibular
　　　　Left ØRPD
　　　　Right ØRPC
　　　Thoracic Vertebral ØRP6
　　　Thoracolumbar Vertebral ØRPA
　　　Toe Phalangeal
　　　　Left ØSPQ
　　　　Right ØSPP
　　　Wrist
　　　　Left ØRPP
　　　　Right ØRPN
　Kidney ØTP5
　Larynx ØCPS
　Lens
　　Left Ø8PK3
　　Right Ø8PJ3
　Liver ØFPØ
　Lung
　　Left ØBPL
　　Right ØBPK
　Lymphatic Ø7PN
　　Thoracic Duct Ø7PK
　Mediastinum ØWPC
　Mesentery ØDPV
　Metacarpal
　　Left ØPPQ
　　Right ØPPP
　Metatarsal
　　Left ØQPP
　　Right ØQPN
　Mouth and Throat ØCPY
　Muscle
　　Extraocular
　　　Left Ø8PM
　　　Right Ø8PL
　　Lower ØKPY
　　Upper ØKPX
　Nasal Mucosa and Soft Tissue Ø9PK
　Neck ØWP6
　Nerve
　　Cranial ØØPE
　　Peripheral Ø1PY
　Omentum ØDPU
　Ovary ØUP3
　Pancreas ØFPG
　Parathyroid Gland ØGPR
　Patella
　　Left ØQPF
　　Right ØQPD
　Pelvic Cavity ØWPJ
　Penis ØVPS

Removal of device from — *continued*
　Pericardial Cavity ØWPD
　Perineum
　　Female ØWPN
　　Male ØWPM
　Peritoneal Cavity ØWPG
　Peritoneum ØDPW
　Phalanx
　　Finger
　　　Left ØPPV
　　　Right ØPPT
　　Thumb
　　　Left ØPPS
　　　Right ØPPR
　　Toe
　　　Left ØQPR
　　　Right ØQPQ
　Pineal Body ØGP1
　Pleura ØBPQ
　Pleural Cavity
　　Left ØWPB
　　Right ØWP9
　Products of Conception 1ØPØ
　Prostate and Seminal Vesicles ØVP4
　Radius
　　Left ØPPJ
　　Right ØPPH
　Rectum ØDPP
　Respiratory Tract ØWPQ
　Retroperitoneum ØWPH
　Ribs
　　1 to 2 ØPP1
　　3 or More ØPP2
　Sacrum ØQP1
　Scapula
　　Left ØPP6
　　Right ØPP5
　Scrotum and Tunica Vaginalis ØVP8
　Sinus Ø9PY
　Skin ØHPPX
　Skull ØNPØ
　Spinal Canal ØØPU
　Spinal Cord ØØPV
　Spleen Ø7PP
　Sternum ØPPØ
　Stomach ØDP6
　Subcutaneous Tissue and Fascia
　　Head and Neck ØJPS
　　Lower Extremity ØJPW
　　Trunk ØJPT
　　Upper Extremity ØJPV
　Tarsal
　　Left ØQPM
　　Right ØQPL
　Tendon
　　Lower ØLPY
　　Upper ØLPX
　Testis ØVPD
　Thymus Ø7PM
　Thyroid Gland ØGPK
　Tibia
　　Left ØQPH
　　Right ØQPG
　Toe Nail ØHPRX
　Trachea ØBP1
　Tracheobronchial Tree ØBPØ
　Tympanic Membrane
　　Left Ø9P8
　　Right Ø9P7
　Ulna
　　Left ØPPL
　　Right ØPPK
　Ureter ØTP9
　Urethra ØTPD
　Uterus and Cervix ØUPD
　Vagina and Cul-de-sac ØUPH
　Vas Deferens ØVPR
　Vein
　　Azygos Ø5PØ
　　Innominate
　　　Left Ø5P4
　　　Right Ø5P3
　　Lower Ø6PY
　　Upper Ø5PY
　Vertebra
　　Cervical ØPP3
　　Lumbar ØQPØ
　　Thoracic ØPP4
　Vulva ØUPM

Renal calyx
　use Kidney
　use Kidney, Left
　use Kidney, Right
　use Kidneys, Bilateral
Renal capsule
　use Kidney
　use Kidney, Left
　use Kidney, Right
　use Kidneys, Bilateral
Renal cortex
　use Kidney
　use Kidney, Left
　use Kidney, Right
　use Kidneys, Bilateral
Renal dialysis *see* Performance, Urinary 5A1D
Renal nerve *use* Abdominal Sympathetic Nerve
Renal plexus *use* Abdominal Sympathetic Nerve
Renal segment
　use Kidney
　use Kidney, Left
　use Kidney, Right
　use Kidneys, Bilateral
Renal segmental artery
　use Renal Artery, Left
　use Renal Artery, Right
Reopening, operative site
　Control of bleeding *see* Control bleeding in
　Inspection only *see* Inspection
Repair
　Abdominal Wall ØWQF
　Acetabulum
　　Left ØQQ5
　　Right ØQQ4
　Adenoids ØCQQ
　Ampulla of Vater ØFQC
　Anal Sphincter ØDQR
　Ankle Region
　　Left ØYQL
　　Right ØYQK
　Anterior Chamber
　　Left Ø8Q33ZZ
　　Right Ø8Q23ZZ
　Anus ØDQQ
　Aorta
　　Abdominal Ø4QØ
　　Thoracic
　　　Ascending/Arch Ø2QX
　　　Descending Ø2QW
　Aortic Body ØGQD
　Appendix ØDQJ
　Arm
　　Lower
　　　Left ØXQF
　　　Right ØXQD
　　Upper
　　　Left ØXQ9
　　　Right ØXQ8
　Artery
　　Anterior Tibial
　　　Left Ø4QQ
　　　Right Ø4QP
　　Axillary
　　　Left Ø3Q6
　　　Right Ø3Q5
　　Brachial
　　　Left Ø3Q8
　　　Right Ø3Q7
　　Celiac Ø4Q1
　　Colic
　　　Left Ø4Q7
　　　Middle Ø4Q8
　　　Right Ø4Q6
　　Common Carotid
　　　Left Ø3QJ
　　　Right Ø3QH
　　Common Iliac
　　　Left Ø4QD
　　　Right Ø4QC
　　Coronary
　　　Four or More Arteries Ø2Q3
　　　One Artery Ø2QØ
　　　Three Arteries Ø2Q2
　　　Two Arteries Ø2Q1
　　External Carotid
　　　Left Ø3QN
　　　Right Ø3QM

Repair — *continued*
  Artery — *continued*
    External Iliac
      Left 04QJ
      Right 04QH
    Face 03QR
    Femoral
      Left 04QL
      Right 04QK
    Foot
      Left 04QW
      Right 04QV
    Gastric 04Q2
    Hand
      Left 03QF
      Right 03QD
    Hepatic 04Q3
    Inferior Mesenteric 04QB
    Innominate 03Q2
    Internal Carotid
      Left 03QL
      Right 03QK
    Internal Iliac
      Left 04QF
      Right 04QE
    Internal Mammary
      Left 03Q1
      Right 03Q0
    Intracranial 03QG
    Lower 04QY
    Peroneal
      Left 04QU
      Right 04QT
    Popliteal
      Left 04QN
      Right 04QM
    Posterior Tibial
      Left 04QS
      Right 04QR
    Pulmonary
      Left 02QR
      Right 02QQ
    Pulmonary Trunk 02QP
    Radial
      Left 03QC
      Right 03QB
    Renal
      Left 04QA
      Right 04Q9
    Splenic 04Q4
    Subclavian
      Left 03Q4
      Right 03Q3
    Superior Mesenteric 04Q5
    Temporal
      Left 03QT
      Right 03QS
    Thyroid
      Left 03QV
      Right 03QU
    Ulnar
      Left 03QA
      Right 03Q9
    Upper 03QY
    Vertebral
      Left 03QQ
      Right 03QP
  Atrium
    Left 02Q7
    Right 02Q6
  Auditory Ossicle
    Left 09QA
    Right 09Q9
  Axilla
    Left 0XQ5
    Right 0XQ4
  Back
    Lower 0WQL
    Upper 0WQK
  Basal Ganglia 00Q8
  Bladder 0TQB
  Bladder Neck 0TQC
  Bone
    Ethmoid
      Left 0NQG
      Right 0NQF
    Frontal 0NQ1
    Hyoid 0NQX

Repair — *continued*
  Bone — *continued*
    Lacrimal
      Left 0NQJ
      Right 0NQH
    Nasal 0NQB
    Occipital 0NQ7
    Palatine
      Left 0NQL
      Right 0NQK
    Parietal
      Left 0NQ4
      Right 0NQ3
    Pelvic
      Left 0QQ3
      Right 0QQ2
    Sphenoid 0NQC
    Temporal
      Left 0NQ6
      Right 0NQ5
    Zygomatic
      Left 0NQN
      Right 0NQM
  Brain 00Q0
  Breast
    Bilateral 0HQV
    Left 0HQU
    Right 0HQT
    Supernumerary 0HQY
  Bronchus
    Lingula 0BQ9
    Lower Lobe
      Left 0BQB
      Right 0BQ6
    Main
      Left 0BQ7
      Right 0BQ3
    Middle Lobe, Right 0BQ5
    Upper Lobe
      Left 0BQ8
      Right 0BQ4
  Buccal Mucosa 0CQ4
  Bursa and Ligament
    Abdomen
      Left 0MQJ
      Right 0MQH
    Ankle
      Left 0MQR
      Right 0MQQ
    Elbow
      Left 0MQ4
      Right 0MQ3
    Foot
      Left 0MQT
      Right 0MQS
    Hand
      Left 0MQ8
      Right 0MQ7
    Head and Neck 0MQ0
    Hip
      Left 0MQM
      Right 0MQL
    Knee
      Left 0MQP
      Right 0MQN
    Lower Extremity
      Left 0MQW
      Right 0MQV
    Perineum 0MQK
    Rib(s) 0MQG
    Shoulder
      Left 0MQ2
      Right 0MQ1
    Spine
      Lower 0MQD
      Upper 0MQC
    Sternum 0MQF
    Upper Extremity
      Left 0MQB
      Right 0MQ9
    Wrist
      Left 0MQ6
      Right 0MQ5
  Buttock
    Left 0YQ1
    Right 0YQ0
  Carina 0BQ2
  Carotid Bodies, Bilateral 0GQ8

Repair — *continued*
  Carotid Body
    Left 0GQ6
    Right 0GQ7
  Carpal
    Left 0PQN
    Right 0PQM
  Cecum 0DQH
  Cerebellum 00QC
  Cerebral Hemisphere 00Q7
  Cerebral Meninges 00Q1
  Cerebral Ventricle 00Q6
  Cervix 0UQC
  Chest Wall 0WQ8
  Chordae Tendineae 02Q9
  Choroid
    Left 08QB
    Right 08QA
  Cisterna Chyli 07QL
  Clavicle
    Left 0PQB
    Right 0PQ9
  Clitoris 0UQJ
  Coccygeal Glomus 0GQB
  Coccyx 0QQS
  Colon
    Ascending 0DQK
    Descending 0DQM
    Sigmoid 0DQN
    Transverse 0DQL
  Conduction Mechanism 02Q8
  Conjunctiva
    Left 08QTXZZ
    Right 08QSXZZ
  Cord
    Bilateral 0VQH
    Left 0VQG
    Right 0VQF
  Cornea
    Left 08Q9XZZ
    Right 08Q8XZZ
  Cul-de-sac 0UQF
  Diaphragm 0BQT
  Disc
    Cervical Vertebral 0RQ3
    Cervicothoracic Vertebral 0RQ5
    Lumbar Vertebral 0SQ2
    Lumbosacral 0SQ4
    Thoracic Vertebral 0RQ9
    Thoracolumbar Vertebral 0RQB
  Duct
    Common Bile 0FQ9
    Cystic 0FQ8
    Hepatic
      Common 0FQ7
      Left 0FQ6
      Right 0FQ5
    Lacrimal
      Left 08QY
      Right 08QX
    Pancreatic 0FQD
      Accessory 0FQF
    Parotid
      Left 0CQC
      Right 0CQB
  Duodenum 0DQ9
  Dura Mater 00Q2
  Ear
    External
      Bilateral 09Q2
      Left 09Q1
      Right 09Q0
    External Auditory Canal
      Left 09Q4
      Right 09Q3
    Inner
      Left 09QE
      Right 09QD
    Middle
      Left 09Q6
      Right 09Q5
  Elbow Region
    Left 0XQC
    Right 0XQB
  Epididymis
    Bilateral 0VQL
    Left 0VQK
    Right 0VQJ
  Epiglottis 0CQR

Subterms under main terms may continue to next column or page

Repair — *continued*
　Esophagogastric Junction ØDQ4
　Esophagus ØDQ5
　　Lower ØDQ3
　　Middle ØDQ2
　　Upper ØDQ1
　Eustachian Tube
　　Left Ø9QG
　　Right Ø9QF
　Extremity
　　Lower
　　　Left ØYQB
　　　Right ØYQ9
　　Upper
　　　Left ØXQ7
　　　Right ØXQ6
　Eye
　　Left Ø8Q1XZZ
　　Right Ø8Q0XZZ
　Eyelid
　　Lower
　　　Left Ø8QR
　　　Right Ø8QQ
　　Upper
　　　Left Ø8QP
　　　Right Ø8QN
　Face ØWQ2
　Fallopian Tube
　　Left ØUQ6
　　Right ØUQ5
　Fallopian Tubes, Bilateral ØUQ7
　Femoral Region
　　Bilateral ØYQE
　　Left ØYQ8
　　Right ØYQ7
　Femoral Shaft
　　Left ØQQ9
　　Right ØQQ8
　Femur
　　Lower
　　　Left ØQQC
　　　Right ØQQB
　　Upper
　　　Left ØQQ7
　　　Right ØQQ6
　Fibula
　　Left ØQQK
　　Right ØQQJ
　Finger
　　Index
　　　Left ØXQP
　　　Right ØXQN
　　Little
　　　Left ØXQW
　　　Right ØXQV
　　Middle
　　　Left ØXQR
　　　Right ØXQQ
　　Ring
　　　Left ØXQT
　　　Right ØXQS
　Finger Nail ØHQQXZZ
　Floor of mouth *see* Repair, Oral Cavity and Throat
　　ØWQ3
　Foot
　　Left ØYQN
　　Right ØYQM
　Gallbladder ØFQ4
　Gingiva
　　Lower ØCQ6
　　Upper ØCQ5
　Gland
　　Adrenal
　　　Bilateral ØGQ4
　　　Left ØGQ2
　　　Right ØGQ3
　　Lacrimal
　　　Left Ø8QW
　　　Right Ø8QV
　　Minor Salivary ØCQJ
　　Parotid
　　　Left ØCQ9
　　　Right ØCQ8
　　Pituitary ØGQ0
　　Sublingual
　　　Left ØCQF
　　　Right ØCQD
　　Submaxillary
　　　Left ØCQH

Repair — *continued*
　Gland — *continued*
　　Submaxillary — *continued*
　　　Right ØCQG
　　Vestibular ØUQL
　Glenoid Cavity
　　Left ØPQ8
　　Right ØPQ7
　Glomus Jugulare ØGQC
　Hand
　　Left ØXQK
　　Right ØXQJ
　Head ØWQ0
　Heart Ø2QA
　　Left Ø2QC
　　Right Ø2QB
　Humeral Head
　　Left ØPQD
　　Right ØPQC
　Humeral Shaft
　　Left ØPQG
　　Right ØPQF
　Hymen ØUQK
　Hypothalamus ØØQA
　Ileocecal Valve ØDQC
　Ileum ØDQB
　Inguinal Region
　　Bilateral ØYQA
　　Left ØYQ6
　　Right ØYQ5
　Intestine
　　Large ØDQE
　　　Left ØDQG
　　　Right ØDQF
　　Small ØDQ8
　Iris
　　Left Ø8QD3ZZ
　　Right Ø8QC3ZZ
　Jaw
　　Lower ØWQ5
　　Upper ØWQ4
　Jejunum ØDQA
　Joint
　　Acromioclavicular
　　　Left ØRQH
　　　Right ØRQG
　　Ankle
　　　Left ØSQG
　　　Right ØSQF
　　Carpal
　　　Left ØRQR
　　　Right ØRQQ
　　Carpometacarpal
　　　Left ØRQT
　　　Right ØRQS
　　Cervical Vertebral ØRQ1
　　Cervicothoracic Vertebral ØRQ4
　　Coccygeal ØSQ6
　　Elbow
　　　Left ØRQM
　　　Right ØRQL
　　Finger Phalangeal
　　　Left ØRQX
　　　Right ØRQW
　　Hip
　　　Left ØSQB
　　　Right ØSQ9
　　Knee
　　　Left ØSQD
　　　Right ØSQC
　　Lumbar Vertebral ØSQ0
　　Lumbosacral ØSQ3
　　Metacarpophalangeal
　　　Left ØRQV
　　　Right ØRQU
　　Metatarsal-Phalangeal
　　　Left ØSQN
　　　Right ØSQM
　　Occipital-cervical ØRQ0
　　Sacrococcygeal ØSQ5
　　Sacroiliac
　　　Left ØSQ8
　　　Right ØSQ7
　　Shoulder
　　　Left ØRQK
　　　Right ØRQJ
　　Sternoclavicular
　　　Left ØRQF
　　　Right ØRQE

Repair — *continued*
　Joint — *continued*
　　Tarsal
　　　Left ØSQJ
　　　Right ØSQH
　　Tarsometatarsal
　　　Left ØSQL
　　　Right ØSQK
　　Temporomandibular
　　　Left ØRQD
　　　Right ØRQC
　　Thoracic Vertebral ØRQ6
　　Thoracolumbar Vertebral ØRQA
　　Toe Phalangeal
　　　Left ØSQQ
　　　Right ØSQP
　　Wrist
　　　Left ØRQP
　　　Right ØRQN
　Kidney
　　Left ØTQ1
　　Right ØTQ0
　Kidney Pelvis
　　Left ØTQ4
　　Right ØTQ3
　Knee Region
　　Left ØYQG
　　Right ØYQF
　Larynx ØCQS
　Leg
　　Lower
　　　Left ØYQJ
　　　Right ØYQH
　　Upper
　　　Left ØYQD
　　　Right ØYQC
　Lens
　　Left Ø8QK3ZZ
　　Right Ø8QJ3ZZ
　Lip
　　Lower ØCQ1
　　Upper ØCQ0
　Liver ØFQ0
　　Left Lobe ØFQ2
　　Right Lobe ØFQ1
　Lung
　　Bilateral ØBQM
　　Left ØBQL
　　Lower Lobe
　　　Left ØBQJ
　　　Right ØBQF
　　Middle Lobe, Right ØBQD
　　Right ØBQK
　　Upper Lobe
　　　Left ØBQG
　　　Right ØBQC
　Lung Lingula ØBQH
　Lymphatic
　　Aortic Ø7QD
　　Axillary
　　　Left Ø7Q6
　　　Right Ø7Q5
　　Head Ø7Q0
　　Inguinal
　　　Left Ø7QJ
　　　Right Ø7QH
　　Internal Mammary
　　　Left Ø7Q9
　　　Right Ø7Q8
　　Lower Extremity
　　　Left Ø7QG
　　　Right Ø7QF
　　Mesenteric Ø7QB
　　Neck
　　　Left Ø7Q2
　　　Right Ø7Q1
　　Pelvis Ø7QC
　　Thoracic Duct Ø7QK
　　Thorax Ø7Q7
　　Upper Extremity
　　　Left Ø7Q4
　　　Right Ø7Q3
　Mandible
　　Left ØNQV
　　Right ØNQT
　Maxilla ØNQR
　Mediastinum ØWQC
　Medulla Oblongata ØØQD
　Mesentery ØDQV

Repair — continued
- Metacarpal
  - Left ØPQQ
  - Right ØPQP
- Metatarsal
  - Left ØQQP
  - Right ØQQN
- Muscle
  - Abdomen
    - Left ØKQL
    - Right ØKQK
  - Extraocular
    - Left Ø8QM
    - Right Ø8QL
  - Facial ØKQ1
  - Foot
    - Left ØKQW
    - Right ØKQV
  - Hand
    - Left ØKQD
    - Right ØKQC
  - Head ØKQØ
  - Hip
    - Left ØKQP
    - Right ØKQN
  - Lower Arm and Wrist
    - Left ØKQB
    - Right ØKQ9
  - Lower Leg
    - Left ØKQT
    - Right ØKQS
  - Neck
    - Left ØKQ3
    - Right ØKQ2
  - Papillary Ø2QD
  - Perineum ØKQM
  - Shoulder
    - Left ØKQ6
    - Right ØKQ5
  - Thorax
    - Left ØKQJ
    - Right ØKQH
  - Tongue, Palate, Pharynx ØKQ4
  - Trunk
    - Left ØKQG
    - Right ØKQF
  - Upper Arm
    - Left ØKQ8
    - Right ØKQ7
  - Upper Leg
    - Left ØKQR
    - Right ØKQQ
- Nasal Mucosa and Soft Tissue Ø9QK
- Nasopharynx Ø9QN
- Neck ØWQ6
- Nerve
  - Abdominal Sympathetic Ø1QM
  - Abducens ØØQL
  - Accessory ØØQR
  - Acoustic ØØQN
  - Brachial Plexus Ø1Q3
  - Cervical Ø1Q1
  - Cervical Plexus Ø1QØ
  - Facial ØØQM
  - Femoral Ø1QD
  - Glossopharyngeal ØØQP
  - Head and Neck Sympathetic Ø1QK
  - Hypoglossal ØØQS
  - Lumbar Ø1QB
  - Lumbar Plexus Ø1Q9
  - Lumbar Sympathetic Ø1QN
  - Lumbosacral Plexus Ø1QA
  - Median Ø1Q5
  - Oculomotor ØØQH
  - Olfactory ØØQF
  - Optic ØØQG
  - Peroneal Ø1QH
  - Phrenic Ø1Q2
  - Pudendal Ø1QC
  - Radial Ø1Q6
  - Sacral Ø1QR
  - Sacral Plexus Ø1QQ
  - Sacral Sympathetic Ø1QP
  - Sciatic Ø1QF
  - Thoracic Ø1Q8
  - Thoracic Sympathetic Ø1QL
  - Tibial Ø1QG
  - Trigeminal ØØQK
  - Trochlear ØØQJ

Repair — continued
- Nerve — continued
  - Ulnar Ø1Q4
  - Vagus ØØQQ
- Nipple
  - Left ØHQX
  - Right ØHQW
- Omentum ØDQU
- Oral Cavity and Throat ØWQ3
- Orbit
  - Left ØNQQ
  - Right ØNQP
- Ovary
  - Bilateral ØUQ2
  - Left ØUQ1
  - Right ØUQØ
- Palate
  - Hard ØCQ2
  - Soft ØCQ3
- Pancreas ØFQG
- Para-aortic Body ØGQ9
- Paraganglion Extremity ØGQF
- Parathyroid Gland ØGQR
  - Inferior
    - Left ØGQP
    - Right ØGQN
  - Multiple ØGQQ
  - Superior
    - Left ØGQM
    - Right ØGQL
- Patella
  - Left ØQQF
  - Right ØQQD
- Penis ØVQS
- Pericardium Ø2QN
- Perineum
  - Female ØWQN
  - Male ØWQM
- Peritoneum ØDQW
- Phalanx
  - Finger
    - Left ØPQV
    - Right ØPQT
  - Thumb
    - Left ØPQS
    - Right ØPQR
  - Toe
    - Left ØQQR
    - Right ØQQQ
- Pharynx ØCQM
- Pineal Body ØGQ1
- Pleura
  - Left ØBQP
  - Right ØBQN
- Pons ØØQB
- Prepuce ØVQT
- Products of Conception 1ØQØ
- Prostate ØVQØ
- Radius
  - Left ØPQJ
  - Right ØPQH
- Rectum ØDQP
- Retina
  - Left Ø8QF3ZZ
  - Right Ø8QE3ZZ
- Retinal Vessel
  - Left Ø8QH3ZZ
  - Right Ø8QG3ZZ
- Ribs
  - 1 to 2 ØPQ1
  - 3 or More ØPQ2
- Sacrum ØQQ1
- Scapula
  - Left ØPQ6
  - Right ØPQ5
- Sclera
  - Left Ø8Q7XZZ
  - Right Ø8Q6XZZ
- Scrotum ØVQ5
- Septum
  - Atrial Ø2Q5
  - Nasal Ø9QM
  - Ventricular Ø2QM
- Shoulder Region
  - Left ØXQ3
  - Right ØXQ2
- Sinus
  - Accessory Ø9QP

Repair — continued
- Sinus — continued
  - Ethmoid
    - Left Ø9QV
    - Right Ø9QU
  - Frontal
    - Left Ø9QT
    - Right Ø9QS
  - Mastoid
    - Left Ø9QC
    - Right Ø9QB
  - Maxillary
    - Left Ø9QR
    - Right Ø9QQ
  - Sphenoid
    - Left Ø9QX
    - Right Ø9QW
- Skin
  - Abdomen ØHQ7XZZ
  - Back ØHQ6XZZ
  - Buttock ØHQ8XZZ
  - Chest ØHQ5XZZ
  - Ear
    - Left ØHQ3XZZ
    - Right ØHQ2XZZ
  - Face ØHQ1XZZ
  - Foot
    - Left ØHQNXZZ
    - Right ØHQMXZZ
  - Hand
    - Left ØHQGXZZ
    - Right ØHQFXZZ
  - Inguinal ØHQAXZZ
  - Lower Arm
    - Left ØHQEXZZ
    - Right ØHQDXZZ
  - Lower Leg
    - Left ØHQLXZZ
    - Right ØHQKXZZ
  - Neck ØHQ4XZZ
  - Perineum ØHQ9XZZ
  - Scalp ØHQØXZZ
  - Upper Arm
    - Left ØHQCXZZ
    - Right ØHQBXZZ
  - Upper Leg
    - Left ØHQJXZZ
    - Right ØHQHXZZ
- Skull ØNQØ
- Spinal Cord
  - Cervical ØØQW
  - Lumbar ØØQY
  - Thoracic ØØQX
- Spinal Meninges ØØQT
- Spleen Ø7QP
- Sternum ØPQØ
- Stomach ØDQ6
  - Pylorus ØDQ7
- Subcutaneous Tissue and Fascia
  - Abdomen ØJQ8
  - Back ØJQ7
  - Buttock ØJQ9
  - Chest ØJQ6
  - Face ØJQ1
  - Foot
    - Left ØJQR
    - Right ØJQQ
  - Hand
    - Left ØJQK
    - Right ØJQJ
  - Lower Arm
    - Left ØJQH
    - Right ØJQG
  - Lower Leg
    - Left ØJQP
    - Right ØJQN
  - Neck
    - Left ØJQ5
    - Right ØJQ4
  - Pelvic Region ØJQC
  - Perineum ØJQB
  - Scalp ØJQØ
  - Upper Arm
    - Left ØJQF
    - Right ØJQD
  - Upper Leg
    - Left ØJQM
    - Right ØJQL

Repair — continued

Tarsal
Left 0QQM
Right 0QQL
Tendon
Abdomen
Left 0LQG
Right 0LQF
Ankle
Left 0LQT
Right 0LQS
Foot
Left 0LQW
Right 0LQV
Hand
Left 0LQ8
Right 0LQ7
Head and Neck 0LQ0
Hip
Left 0LQK
Right 0LQJ
Knee
Left 0LQR
Right 0LQQ
Lower Arm and Wrist
Left 0LQ6
Right 0LQ5
Lower Leg
Left 0LQP
Right 0LQN
Perineum 0LQH
Shoulder
Left 0LQ2
Right 0LQ1
Thorax
Left 0LQD
Right 0LQC
Trunk
Left 0LQB
Right 0LQ9
Upper Arm
Left 0LQ4
Right 0LQ3
Upper Leg
Left 0LQM
Right 0LQL
Testis
Bilateral 0VQC
Left 0VQB
Right 0VQ9
Thalamus 00Q9
Thumb
Left 0XQM
Right 0XQL
Thymus 07QM
Thyroid Gland 0GQK
Left Lobe 0GQG
Right Lobe 0GQH
Thyroid Gland Isthmus 0GQJ
Tibia
Left 0QQH
Right 0QQG
Toe
1st
Left 0YQQ
Right 0YQP
2nd
Left 0YQS
Right 0YQR
3rd
Left 0YQU
Right 0YQT
4th
Left 0YQW
Right 0YQV
5th
Left 0YQY
Right 0YQX
Toe Nail 0HQRXZZ
Tongue 0CQ7
Tonsils 0CQP
Tooth
Lower 0CQX
Upper 0CQW
Trachea 0BQ1
Tunica Vaginalis
Left 0VQ7
Right 0VQ6
Turbinate, Nasal 09QL

Repair — continued

Tympanic Membrane
Left 09Q8
Right 09Q7
Ulna
Left 0PQL
Right 0PQK
Ureter
Left 0TQ7
Right 0TQ6
Urethra 0TQD
Uterine Supporting Structure 0UQ4
Uterus 0UQ9
Uvula 0CQN
Vagina 0UQG
Valve
Aortic 02QF
Mitral 02QG
Pulmonary 02QH
Tricuspid 02QJ
Vas Deferens
Bilateral 0VQQ
Left 0VQP
Right 0VQN
Vein
Axillary
Left 05Q8
Right 05Q7
Azygos 05Q0
Basilic
Left 05QC
Right 05QB
Brachial
Left 05QA
Right 05Q9
Cephalic
Left 05QF
Right 05QD
Colic 06Q7
Common Iliac
Left 06QD
Right 06QC
Coronary 02Q4
Esophageal 06Q3
External Iliac
Left 06QG
Right 06QF
External Jugular
Left 05QQ
Right 05QP
Face
Left 05QV
Right 05QT
Femoral
Left 06QN
Right 06QM
Foot
Left 06QV
Right 06QT
Gastric 06Q2
Hand
Left 05QH
Right 05QG
Hemiazygos 05Q1
Hepatic 06Q4
Hypogastric
Left 06QJ
Right 06QH
Inferior Mesenteric 06Q6
Innominate
Left 05Q4
Right 05Q3
Internal Jugular
Left 05QN
Right 05QM
Intracranial 05QL
Lower 06QY
Portal 06Q8
Pulmonary
Left 02QT
Right 02QS
Renal
Left 06QB
Right 06Q9
Saphenous
Left 06QQ
Right 06QP
Splenic 06Q1

Repair — continued

Vein — continued
Subclavian
Left 05Q6
Right 05Q5
Superior Mesenteric 06Q5
Upper 05QY
Vertebral
Left 05QS
Right 05QR
Vena Cava
Inferior 06Q0
Superior 02QV
Ventricle
Left 02QL
Right 02QK
Vertebra
Cervical 0PQ3
Lumbar 0QQ0
Thoracic 0PQ4
Vesicle
Bilateral 0VQ3
Left 0VQ2
Right 0VQ1
Vitreous
Left 08Q53ZZ
Right 08Q43ZZ
Vocal Cord
Left 0CQV
Right 0CQT
Vulva 0UQM
Wrist Region
Left 0XQH
Right 0XQG

Repair, obstetric laceration, periurethral 0UQMXZZ

Replacement

Acetabulum
Left 0QR5
Right 0QR4
Ampulla of Vater 0FRC
Anal Sphincter 0DRR
Aorta
Abdominal 04R0
Thoracic
Ascending/Arch 02RX
Descending 02RW
Artery
Anterior Tibial
Left 04RQ
Right 04RP
Axillary
Left 03R6
Right 03R5
Brachial
Left 03R8
Right 03R7
Celiac 04R1
Colic
Left 04R7
Middle 04R8
Right 04R6
Common Carotid
Left 03RJ
Right 03RH
Common Iliac
Left 04RD
Right 04RC
External Carotid
Left 03RN
Right 03RM
External Iliac
Left 04RJ
Right 04RH
Face 03RR
Femoral
Left 04RL
Right 04RK
Foot
Left 04RW
Right 04RV
Gastric 04R2
Hand
Left 03RF
Right 03RD
Hepatic 04R3
Inferior Mesenteric 04RB
Innominate 03R2
Internal Carotid
Left 03RL

Replacement — *continued*
  Artery — *continued*
    Internal Carotid — *continued*
      Right Ø3RK
    Internal Iliac
      Left Ø4RF
      Right Ø4RE
    Internal Mammary
      Left Ø3R1
      Right Ø3RØ
    Intracranial Ø3RG
    Lower Ø4RY
    Peroneal
      Left Ø4RU
      Right Ø4RT
    Popliteal
      Left Ø4RN
      Right Ø4RM
    Posterior Tibial
      Left Ø4RS
      Right Ø4RR
    Pulmonary
      Left Ø2RR
      Right Ø2RQ
    Pulmonary Trunk Ø2RP
    Radial
      Left Ø3RC
      Right Ø3RB
    Renal
      Left Ø4RA
      Right Ø4R9
    Splenic Ø4R4
    Subclavian
      Left Ø3R4
      Right Ø3R3
    Superior Mesenteric Ø4R5
    Temporal
      Left Ø3RT
      Right Ø3RS
    Thyroid
      Left Ø3RV
      Right Ø3RU
    Ulnar
      Left Ø3RA
      Right Ø3R9
    Upper Ø3RY
    Vertebral
      Left Ø3RQ
      Right Ø3RP
  Atrium
    Left Ø2R7
    Right Ø2R6
  Auditory Ossicle
    Left Ø9RAØ
    Right Ø9R9Ø
  Bladder ØTRB
  Bladder Neck ØTRC
  Bone
    Ethmoid
      Left ØNRG
      Right ØNRF
    Frontal ØNR1
    Hyoid ØNRX
    Lacrimal
      Left ØNRJ
      Right ØNRH
    Nasal ØNRB
    Occipital ØNR7
    Palatine
      Left ØNRL
      Right ØNRK
    Parietal
      Left ØNR4
      Right ØNR3
    Pelvic
      Left ØQR3
      Right ØQR2
    Sphenoid ØNRC
    Temporal
      Left ØNR6
      Right ØNR5
    Zygomatic
      Left ØNRN
      Right ØNRM
  Breast
    Bilateral ØHRV
    Left ØHRU
    Right ØHRT

Replacement — *continued*
  Bronchus
    Lingula ØBR9
    Lower Lobe
      Left ØBRB
      Right ØBR6
    Main
      Left ØBR7
      Right ØBR3
    Middle Lobe, Right ØBR5
    Upper Lobe
      Left ØBR8
      Right ØBR4
  Buccal Mucosa ØCR4
  Bursa and Ligament
    Abdomen
      Left ØMRJ
      Right ØMRH
    Ankle
      Left ØMRR
      Right ØMRQ
    Elbow
      Left ØMR4
      Right ØMR3
    Foot
      Left ØMRT
      Right ØMRS
    Hand
      Left ØMR8
      Right ØMR7
    Head and Neck ØMRØ
    Hip
      Left ØMRM
      Right ØMRL
    Knee
      Left ØMRP
      Right ØMRN
    Lower Extremity
      Left ØMRW
      Right ØMRV
    Perineum ØMRK
    Rib(s) ØMRG
    Shoulder
      Left ØMR2
      Right ØMR1
    Spine
      Lower ØMRD
      Upper ØMRC
    Sternum ØMRF
    Upper Extremity
      Left ØMRB
      Right ØMR9
    Wrist
      Left ØMR6
      Right ØMR5
  Carina ØBR2
  Carpal
    Left ØPRN
    Right ØPRM
  Cerebral Meninges ØØR1
  Cerebral Ventricle ØØR6
  Chordae Tendineae Ø2R9
  Choroid
    Left Ø8RB
    Right Ø8RA
  Clavicle
    Left ØPRB
    Right ØPR9
  Coccyx ØQRS
  Conjunctiva
    Left Ø8RTX
    Right Ø8RSX
  Cornea
    Left Ø8R9
    Right Ø8R8
  Diaphragm ØBRT
  Disc
    Cervical Vertebral ØRR3Ø
    Cervicothoracic Vertebral ØRR5Ø
    Lumbar Vertebral ØSR2Ø
    Lumbosacral ØSR4Ø
    Thoracic Vertebral ØRR9Ø
    Thoracolumbar Vertebral ØRRBØ
  Duct
    Common Bile ØFR9
    Cystic ØFR8
    Hepatic
      Common ØFR7
      Left ØFR6

Replacement — *continued*
  Duct — *continued*
    Hepatic — *continued*
      Right ØFR5
    Lacrimal
      Left Ø8RY
      Right Ø8RX
    Pancreatic ØFRD
      Accessory ØFRF
    Parotid
      Left ØCRC
      Right ØCRB
  Dura Mater ØØR2
  Ear
    External
      Bilateral Ø9R2
      Left Ø9R1
      Right Ø9RØ
    Inner
      Left Ø9REØ
      Right Ø9RDØ
    Middle
      Left Ø9R6Ø
      Right Ø9R5Ø
  Epiglottis ØCRR
  Esophagus ØDR5
  Eye
    Left Ø8R1
    Right Ø8RØ
  Eyelid
    Lower
      Left Ø8RR
      Right Ø8RQ
    Upper
      Left Ø8RP
      Right Ø8RN
  Femoral Shaft
    Left ØQR9
    Right ØQR8
  Femur
    Lower
      Left ØQRC
      Right ØQRB
    Upper
      Left ØQR7
      Right ØQR6
  Fibula
    Left ØQRK
    Right ØQRJ
  Finger Nail ØHRQX
  Gingiva
    Lower ØCR6
    Upper ØCR5
  Glenoid Cavity
    Left ØPR8
    Right ØPR7
  Hair ØHRSX
  Heart Ø2RAØ
  Humeral Head
    Left ØPRD
    Right ØPRC
  Humeral Shaft
    Left ØPRG
    Right ØPRF
  Iris
    Left Ø8RD3
    Right Ø8RC3
  Joint
    Acromioclavicular
      Left ØRRHØ
      Right ØRRGØ
    Ankle
      Left ØSRG
      Right ØSRF
    Carpal
      Left ØRRRØ
      Right ØRRQØ
    Carpometacarpal
      Left ØRRTØ
      Right ØRRSØ
    Cervical Vertebral ØRR1Ø
    Cervicothoracic Vertebral ØRR4Ø
    Coccygeal ØSR6Ø
    Elbow
      Left ØRRMØ
      Right ØRRLØ
    Finger Phalangeal
      Left ØRRXØ
      Right ØRRWØ

▽ **Subterms under main terms may continue to next column or page**

Replacement — continued
Joint — continued
Hip
Left ØSRB
Acetabular Surface ØSRE
Femoral Surface ØSRS
Right ØSR9
Acetabular Surface ØSRA
Femoral Surface ØSRR
Knee
Left ØSRD
Femoral Surface ØSRU
Tibial Surface ØSRW
Right ØSRC
Femoral Surface ØSRT
Tibial Surface ØSRV
Lumbar Vertebral ØSR00
Lumbosacral ØSR30
Metacarpophalangeal
Left ØRRVØ
Right ØRRUØ
Metatarsal-Phalangeal
Left ØSRNØ
Right ØSRMØ
Occipital-cervical ØRR00
Sacrococcygeal ØSR50
Sacroiliac
Left ØSR8Ø
Right ØSR7Ø
Shoulder
Left ØRRK
Right ØRRJ
Sternoclavicular
Left ØRRFØ
Right ØRREØ
Tarsal
Left ØSRJØ
Right ØSRHØ
Tarsometatarsal
Left ØSRLØ
Right ØSRKØ
Temporomandibular
Left ØRRDØ
Right ØRRCØ
Thoracic Vertebral ØRR60
Thoracolumbar Vertebral ØRRAØ
Toe Phalangeal
Left ØSRQØ
Right ØSRPØ
Wrist
Left ØRRPØ
Right ØRRNØ
Kidney Pelvis
Left ØTR4
Right ØTR3
Larynx ØCRS
Lens
Left Ø8RK3ØZ
Right Ø8RJ3ØZ
Lip
Lower ØCR1
Upper ØCRØ
Mandible
Left ØNRV
Right ØNRT
Maxilla ØNRR
Mesentery ØDRV
Metacarpal
Left ØPRQ
Right ØPRP
Metatarsal
Left ØQRP
Right ØQRN
Muscle
Abdomen
Left ØKRL
Right ØKRK
Facial ØKR1
Foot
Left ØKRW
Right ØKRV
Hand
Left ØKRD
Right ØKRC
Head ØKR0
Hip
Left ØKRP
Right ØKRN

Replacement — continued
Muscle — continued
Lower Arm and Wrist
Left ØKRB
Right ØKR9
Lower Leg
Left ØKRT
Right ØKRS
Neck
Left ØKR3
Right ØKR2
Papillary Ø2RD
Perineum ØKRM
Shoulder
Left ØKR6
Right ØKR5
Thorax
Left ØKRJ
Right ØKRH
Tongue, Palate, Pharynx ØKR4
Trunk
Left ØKRG
Right ØKRF
Upper Arm
Left ØKR8
Right ØKR7
Upper Leg
Left ØKRR
Right ØKRQ
Nasal Mucosa and Soft Tissue Ø9RK
Nasopharynx Ø9RN
Nerve
Abducens ØØRL
Accessory ØØRR
Acoustic ØØRN
Cervical Ø1R1
Facial ØØRM
Femoral Ø1RD
Glossopharyngeal ØØRP
Hypoglossal ØØRS
Lumbar Ø1RB
Median Ø1R5
Oculomotor ØØRH
Olfactory ØØRF
Optic ØØRG
Peroneal Ø1RH
Phrenic Ø1R2
Pudendal Ø1RC
Radial Ø1R6
Sacral Ø1RR
Sciatic Ø1RF
Thoracic Ø1R8
Tibial Ø1RG
Trigeminal ØØRK
Trochlear ØØRJ
Ulnar Ø1R4
Vagus ØØRQ
Nipple
Left ØHRX
Right ØHRW
Omentum ØDRU
Orbit
Left ØNRQ
Right ØNRP
Palate
Hard ØCR2
Soft ØCR3
Patella
Left ØQRF
Right ØQRD
Pericardium Ø2RN
Peritoneum ØDRW
Phalanx
Finger
Left ØPRV
Right ØPRT
Thumb
Left ØPRS
Right ØPRR
Toe
Left ØQRR
Right ØQRQ
Pharynx ØCRM
Radius
Left ØPRJ
Right ØPRH
Retinal Vessel
Left Ø8RH3
Right Ø8RG3

Replacement — continued
Ribs
1 to 2 ØPR1
3 or More ØPR2
Sacrum ØQR1
Scapula
Left ØPR6
Right ØPR5
Sclera
Left Ø8R7X
Right Ø8R6X
Septum
Atrial Ø2R5
Nasal Ø9RM
Ventricular Ø2RM
Skin
Abdomen ØHR7
Back ØHR6
Buttock ØHR8
Chest ØHR5
Ear
Left ØHR3
Right ØHR2
Face ØHR1
Foot
Left ØHRN
Right ØHRM
Hand
Left ØHRG
Right ØHRF
Inguinal ØHRA
Lower Arm
Left ØHRE
Right ØHRD
Lower Leg
Left ØHRL
Right ØHRK
Neck ØHR4
Perineum ØHR9
Scalp ØHRØ
Upper Arm
Left ØHRC
Right ØHRB
Upper Leg
Left ØHRJ
Right ØHRH
Skull ØNRØ
Spinal Meninges ØØRT
Sternum ØPRØ
Subcutaneous Tissue and Fascia
Abdomen ØJR8
Back ØJR7
Buttock ØJR9
Chest ØJR6
Face ØJR1
Foot
Left ØJRR
Right ØJRQ
Hand
Left ØJRK
Right ØJRJ
Lower Arm
Left ØJRH
Right ØJRG
Lower Leg
Left ØJRP
Right ØJRN
Neck
Left ØJR5
Right ØJR4
Pelvic Region ØJRC
Perineum ØJRB
Scalp ØJRØ
Upper Arm
Left ØJRF
Right ØJRD
Upper Leg
Left ØJRM
Right ØJRL
Tarsal
Left ØQRM
Right ØQRL
Tendon
Abdomen
Left ØLRG
Right ØLRF
Ankle
Left ØLRT
Right ØLRS

Replacement — *continued*
Tendon — *continued*
Foot
Left ØLRW
Right ØLRV
Hand
Left ØLR8
Right ØLR7
Head and Neck ØLRØ
Hip
Left ØLRK
Right ØLRJ
Knee
Left ØLRR
Right ØLRQ
Lower Arm and Wrist
Left ØLR6
Right ØLR5
Lower Leg
Left ØLRP
Right ØLRN
Perineum ØLRH
Shoulder
Left ØLR2
Right ØLR1
Thorax
Left ØLRD
Right ØLRC
Trunk
Left ØLRB
Right ØLR9
Upper Arm
Left ØLR4
Right ØLR3
Upper Leg
Left ØLRM
Right ØLRL
Testis
Bilateral ØVRCØJZ
Left ØVRBØJZ
Right ØVR9ØJZ
Thumb
Left ØXRM
Right ØXRL
Tibia
Left ØQRH
Right ØQRG
Toe Nail ØHRRX
Tongue ØCR7
Tooth
Lower ØCRX
Upper ØCRW
Trachea ØBR1
Turbinate, Nasal Ø9RL
Tympanic Membrane
Left Ø9R8
Right Ø9R7
Ulna
Left ØPRL
Right ØPRK
Ureter
Left ØTR7
Right ØTR6
Urethra ØTRD
Uvula ØCRN
Valve
Aortic Ø2RF
Mitral Ø2RG
Pulmonary Ø2RH
Tricuspid Ø2RJ
Vein
Axillary
Left Ø5R8
Right Ø5R7
Azygos Ø5RØ
Basilic
Left Ø5RC
Right Ø5RB
Brachial
Left Ø5RA
Right Ø5R9
Cephalic
Left Ø5RF
Right Ø5RD
Colic Ø6R7
Common Iliac
Left Ø6RD
Right Ø6RC
Esophageal Ø6R3

Replacement — *continued*
Vein — *continued*
External Iliac
Left Ø6RG
Right Ø6RF
External Jugular
Left Ø5RQ
Right Ø5RP
Face
Left Ø5RV
Right Ø5RT
Femoral
Left Ø6RN
Right Ø6RM
Foot
Left Ø6RV
Right Ø6RT
Gastric Ø6R2
Hand
Left Ø5RH
Right Ø5RG
Hemiazygos Ø5R1
Hepatic Ø6R4
Hypogastric
Left Ø6RJ
Right Ø6RH
Inferior Mesenteric Ø6R6
Innominate
Left Ø5R4
Right Ø5R3
Internal Jugular
Left Ø5RN
Right Ø5RM
Intracranial Ø5RL
Lower Ø6RY
Portal Ø6R8
Pulmonary
Left Ø2RT
Right Ø2RS
Renal
Left Ø6RB
Right Ø6R9
Saphenous
Left Ø6RQ
Right Ø6RP
Splenic Ø6R1
Subclavian
Left Ø5R6
Right Ø5R5
Superior Mesenteric Ø6R5
Upper Ø5RY
Vertebral
Left Ø5RS
Right Ø5RR
Vena Cava
Inferior Ø6RØ
Superior Ø2RV
Ventricle
Left Ø2RL
Right Ø2RK
Vertebra
Cervical ØPR3
Lumbar ØQRØ
Thoracic ØPR4
Vitreous
Left Ø8R53
Right Ø8R43
Vocal Cord
Left ØCRV
Right ØCRT
Replacement, hip
Partial or total *see* Replacement, Lower Joints ØSR
Resurfacing only *see* Supplement, Lower Joints ØSU
Replacement, knee
Meniscus implant only *see* New Technology, Joints XRR
Partial or total *see* Replacement, Lower Joints ØSR
Replantation *see* Reposition
Replantation, scalp *see* Reattachment, Skin, Scalp ØHMØ
Reposition
Acetabulum
Left ØQS5
Right ØQS4
Ampulla of Vater ØFSC
Anus ØDSQ

Reposition — *continued*
Aorta
Abdominal Ø4SØ
Thoracic
Ascending/Arch Ø2SXØZZ
Descending Ø2SWØZZ
Artery
Anterior Tibial
Left Ø4SQ
Right Ø4SP
Axillary
Left Ø3S6
Right Ø3S5
Brachial
Left Ø3S8
Right Ø3S7
Celiac Ø4S1
Colic
Left Ø4S7
Middle Ø4S8
Right Ø4S6
Common Carotid
Left Ø3SJ
Right Ø3SH
Common Iliac
Left Ø4SD
Right Ø4SC
Coronary
One Artery Ø2SØØZZ
Two Arteries Ø2S1ØZZ
External Carotid
Left Ø3SN
Right Ø3SM
External Iliac
Left Ø4SJ
Right Ø4SH
Face Ø3SR
Femoral
Left Ø4SL
Right Ø4SK
Foot
Left Ø4SW
Right Ø4SV
Gastric Ø4S2
Hand
Left Ø3SF
Right Ø3SD
Hepatic Ø4S3
Inferior Mesenteric Ø4SB
Innominate Ø3S2
Internal Carotid
Left Ø3SL
Right Ø3SK
Internal Iliac
Left Ø4SF
Right Ø4SE
Internal Mammary
Left Ø3S1
Right Ø3SØ
Intracranial Ø3SG
Lower Ø4SY
Peroneal
Left Ø4SU
Right Ø4ST
Popliteal
Left Ø4SN
Right Ø4SM
Posterior Tibial
Left Ø4SS
Right Ø4SR
Pulmonary
Left Ø2SRØZZ
Right Ø2SQØZZ
Pulmonary Trunk Ø2SPØZZ
Radial
Left Ø3SC
Right Ø3SB
Renal
Left Ø4SA
Right Ø4S9
Splenic Ø4S4
Subclavian
Left Ø3S4
Right Ø3S3
Superior Mesenteric Ø4S5
Temporal
Left Ø3ST
Right Ø3SS

Reposition — continued
  Artery — continued
    Thyroid
      Left Ø3SV
      Right Ø3SU
    Ulnar
      Left Ø3SA
      Right Ø3S9
    Upper Ø3SY
    Vertebral
      Left Ø3SQ
      Right Ø3SP
  Auditory Ossicle
    Left Ø9SA
    Right Ø9S9
  Bladder ØTSB
  Bladder Neck ØTSC
  Bone
    Ethmoid
      Left ØNSG
      Right ØNSF
    Frontal ØNS1
    Hyoid ØNSX
    Lacrimal
      Left ØNSJ
      Right ØNSH
    Nasal ØNSB
    Occipital ØNS7
    Palatine
      Left ØNSL
      Right ØNSK
    Parietal
      Left ØNS4
      Right ØNS3
    Pelvic
      Left ØQS3
      Right ØQS2
    Sphenoid ØNSC
    Temporal
      Left ØNS6
      Right ØNS5
    Zygomatic
      Left ØNSN
      Right ØNSM
  Breast
    Bilateral ØHSVØZZ
    Left ØHSUØZZ
    Right ØHSTØZZ
  Bronchus
    Lingula ØBS9ØZZ
    Lower Lobe
      Left ØBSBØZZ
      Right ØBS6ØZZ
    Main
      Left ØBS7ØZZ
      Right ØBS3ØZZ
    Middle Lobe, Right ØBS5ØZZ
    Upper Lobe
      Left ØBS8ØZZ
      Right ØBS4ØZZ
  Bursa and Ligament
    Abdomen
      Left ØMSJ
      Right ØMSH
    Ankle
      Left ØMSR
      Right ØMSQ
    Elbow
      Left ØMS4
      Right ØMS3
    Foot
      Left ØMST
      Right ØMSS
    Hand
      Left ØMS8
      Right ØMS7
    Head and Neck ØMSØ
    Hip
      Left ØMSM
      Right ØMSL
    Knee
      Left ØMSP
      Right ØMSN
    Lower Extremity
      Left ØMSW
      Right ØMSV
    Perineum ØMSK
    Rib(s) ØMSG

Reposition — continued
  Bursa and Ligament — continued
    Shoulder
      Left ØMS2
      Right ØMS1
    Spine
      Lower ØMSD
      Upper ØMSC
    Sternum ØMSF
    Upper Extremity
      Left ØMSB
      Right ØMS9
    Wrist
      Left ØMS6
      Right ØMS5
  Carina ØBS2ØZZ
  Carpal
    Left ØPSN
    Right ØPSM
  Cecum ØDSH
  Cervix ØUSC
  Clavicle
    Left ØPSB
    Right ØPS9
  Coccyx ØQSS
  Colon
    Ascending ØDSK
    Descending ØDSM
    Sigmoid ØDSN
    Transverse ØDSL
  Cord
    Bilateral ØVSH
    Left ØVSG
    Right ØVSF
  Cul-de-sac ØUSF
  Diaphragm ØBSTØZZ
  Duct
    Common Bile ØFS9
    Cystic ØFS8
    Hepatic
      Common ØFS7
      Left ØFS6
      Right ØFS5
    Lacrimal
      Left Ø8SY
      Right Ø8SX
    Pancreatic ØFSD
      Accessory ØFSF
    Parotid
      Left ØCSC
      Right ØCSB
  Duodenum ØDS9
  Ear
    Bilateral Ø9S2
    Left Ø9S1
    Right Ø9SØ
  Epiglottis ØCSR
  Esophagus ØDS5
  Eustachian Tube
    Left Ø9SG
    Right Ø9SF
  Eyelid
    Lower
      Left Ø8SR
      Right Ø8SQ
    Upper
      Left Ø8SP
      Right Ø8SN
  Fallopian Tube
    Left ØUS6
    Right ØUS5
  Fallopian Tubes, Bilateral ØUS7
  Femoral Shaft
    Left ØQS9
    Right ØQS8
  Femur
    Lower
      Left ØQSC
      Right ØQSB
    Upper
      Left ØQS7
      Right ØQS6
  Fibula
    Left ØQSK
    Right ØQSJ
  Gallbladder ØFS4
  Gland
    Adrenal
      Left ØGS2

Reposition — continued
  Gland — continued
    Adrenal — continued
      Right ØGS3
    Lacrimal
      Left Ø8SW
      Right Ø8SV
  Glenoid Cavity
    Left ØPS8
    Right ØPS7
  Hair ØHSSXZZ
  Humeral Head
    Left ØPSD
    Right ØPSC
  Humeral Shaft
    Left ØPSG
    Right ØPSF
  Ileum ØDSB
  Intestine
    Large ØDSE
    Small ØDS8
  Iris
    Left Ø8SD3ZZ
    Right Ø8SC3ZZ
  Jejunum ØDSA
  Joint
    Acromioclavicular
      Left ØRSH
      Right ØRSG
    Ankle
      Left ØSSG
      Right ØSSF
    Carpal
      Left ØRSR
      Right ØRSQ
    Carpometacarpal
      Left ØRST
      Right ØRSS
    Cervical Vertebral ØRS1
    Cervicothoracic Vertebral ØRS4
    Coccygeal ØSS6
    Elbow
      Left ØRSM
      Right ØRSL
    Finger Phalangeal
      Left ØRSX
      Right ØRSW
    Hip
      Left ØSSB
      Right ØSS9
    Knee
      Left ØSSD
      Right ØSSC
    Lumbar Vertebral ØSSØ
    Lumbosacral ØSS3
    Metacarpophalangeal
      Left ØRSV
      Right ØRSU
    Metatarsal-Phalangeal
      Left ØSSN
      Right ØSSM
    Occipital-cervical ØRSØ
    Sacrococcygeal ØSS5
    Sacroiliac
      Left ØSS8
      Right ØSS7
    Shoulder
      Left ØRSK
      Right ØRSJ
    Sternoclavicular
      Left ØRSF
      Right ØRSE
    Tarsal
      Left ØSSJ
      Right ØSSH
    Tarsometatarsal
      Left ØSSL
      Right ØSSK
    Temporomandibular
      Left ØRSD
      Right ØRSC
    Thoracic Vertebral ØRS6
    Thoracolumbar Vertebral ØRSA
    Toe Phalangeal
      Left ØSSQ
      Right ØSSP
    Wrist
      Left ØRSP
      Right ØRSN

Reposition — *continued*

Kidney
  Left 0TS1
  Right 0TS0
Kidney Pelvis
  Left 0TS4
  Right 0TS3
Kidneys, Bilateral 0TS2
Lens
  Left 08SK3ZZ
  Right 08SJ3ZZ
Lip
  Lower 0CS1
  Upper 0CS0
Liver 0FS0
Lung
  Left 0BSL0ZZ
  Lower Lobe
    Left 0BSJ0ZZ
    Right 0BSF0ZZ
  Middle Lobe, Right 0BSD0ZZ
  Right 0BSK0ZZ
  Upper Lobe
    Left 0BSG0ZZ
    Right 0BSC0ZZ
Lung Lingula 0BSH0ZZ
Mandible
  Left 0NSV
  Right 0NST
Maxilla 0NSR
Metacarpal
  Left 0PSQ
  Right 0PSP
Metatarsal
  Left 0QSP
  Right 0QSN
Muscle
  Abdomen
    Left 0KSL
    Right 0KSK
  Extraocular
    Left 08SM
    Right 08SL
  Facial 0KS1
  Foot
    Left 0KSW
    Right 0KSV
  Hand
    Left 0KSD
    Right 0KSC
  Head 0KS0
  Hip
    Left 0KSP
    Right 0KSN
  Lower Arm and Wrist
    Left 0KSB
    Right 0KS9
  Lower Leg
    Left 0KST
    Right 0KSS
  Neck
    Left 0KS3
    Right 0KS2
  Perineum 0KSM
  Shoulder
    Left 0KS6
    Right 0KS5
  Thorax
    Left 0KSJ
    Right 0KSH
  Tongue, Palate, Pharynx 0KS4
  Trunk
    Left 0KSG
    Right 0KSF
  Upper Arm
    Left 0KS8
    Right 0KS7
  Upper Leg
    Left 0KSR
    Right 0KSQ
Nasal Mucosa and Soft Tissue 09SK
Nerve
  Abducens 00SL
  Accessory 00SR
  Acoustic 00SN
  Brachial Plexus 01S3
  Cervical 01S1
  Cervical Plexus 01S0
  Facial 00SM

Reposition — *continued*

Nerve — *continued*
  Femoral 01SD
  Glossopharyngeal 00SP
  Hypoglossal 00SS
  Lumbar 01SB
  Lumbar Plexus 01S9
  Lumbosacral Plexus 01SA
  Median 01S5
  Oculomotor 00SH
  Olfactory 00SF
  Optic 00SG
  Peroneal 01SH
  Phrenic 01S2
  Pudendal 01SC
  Radial 01S6
  Sacral 01SR
  Sacral Plexus 01SQ
  Sciatic 01SF
  Thoracic 01S8
  Tibial 01SG
  Trigeminal 00SK
  Trochlear 00SJ
  Ulnar 01S4
  Vagus 00SQ
Nipple
  Left 0HSXXZZ
  Right 0HSWXZZ
Orbit
  Left 0NSQ
  Right 0NSP
Ovary
  Bilateral 0US2
  Left 0US1
  Right 0US0
Palate
  Hard 0CS2
  Soft 0CS3
Pancreas 0FSG
Parathyroid Gland 0GSR
  Inferior
    Left 0GSP
    Right 0GSN
  Multiple 0GSQ
  Superior
    Left 0GSM
    Right 0GSL
Patella
  Left 0QSF
  Right 0QSD
Phalanx
  Finger
    Left 0PSV
    Right 0PST
  Thumb
    Left 0PSS
    Right 0PSR
  Toe
    Left 0QSR
    Right 0QSQ
Products of Conception 10S0
  Ectopic 10S2
Radius
  Left 0PSJ
  Right 0PSH
Rectum 0DSP
Retinal Vessel
  Left 08SH3ZZ
  Right 08SG3ZZ
Ribs
  1 to 2 0PS1
  3 or More 0PS2
Sacrum 0QS1
Scapula
  Left 0PS6
  Right 0PS5
Septum, Nasal 09SM
Sesamoid Bone(s) 1st Toe
  see Reposition, Metatarsal, Left 0QSP
  see Reposition, Metatarsal, Right 0QSN
Skull 0NS0
Spinal Cord
  Cervical 00SW
  Lumbar 00SY
  Thoracic 00SX
Spleen 07SP0ZZ
Sternum 0PS0
Stomach 0DS6

Reposition — *continued*

Tarsal
  Left 0QSM
  Right 0QSL
Tendon
  Abdomen
    Left 0LSG
    Right 0LSF
  Ankle
    Left 0LST
    Right 0LSS
  Foot
    Left 0LSW
    Right 0LSV
  Hand
    Left 0LS8
    Right 0LS7
  Head and Neck 0LS0
  Hip
    Left 0LSK
    Right 0LSJ
  Knee
    Left 0LSR
    Right 0LSQ
  Lower Arm and Wrist
    Left 0LS6
    Right 0LS5
  Lower Leg
    Left 0LSP
    Right 0LSN
  Perineum 0LSH
  Shoulder
    Left 0LS2
    Right 0LS1
  Thorax
    Left 0LSD
    Right 0LSC
  Trunk
    Left 0LSB
    Right 0LS9
  Upper Arm
    Left 0LS4
    Right 0LS3
  Upper Leg
    Left 0LSM
    Right 0LSL
Testis
  Bilateral 0VSC
  Left 0VSB
  Right 0VS9
Thymus 07SM0ZZ
Thyroid Gland
  Left Lobe 0GSG
  Right Lobe 0GSH
Tibia
  Left 0QSH
  Right 0QSG
Tongue 0CS7
Tooth
  Lower 0CSX
  Upper 0CSW
Trachea 0BS10ZZ
Turbinate, Nasal 09SL
Tympanic Membrane
  Left 09S8
  Right 09S7
Ulna
  Left 0PSL
  Right 0PSK
Ureter
  Left 0TS7
  Right 0TS6
Ureters, Bilateral 0TS8
Urethra 0TSD
Uterine Supporting Structure 0US4
Uterus 0US9
Uvula 0CSN
Vagina 0USG
Vein
  Axillary
    Left 05S8
    Right 05S7
  Azygos 05S0
  Basilic
    Left 05SC
    Right 05SB
  Brachial
    Left 05SA
    Right 05S9

Reposition — continued

Vein — continued
  Cephalic
    Left Ø5SF
    Right Ø5SD
  Colic Ø6S7
  Common Iliac
    Left Ø6SD
    Right Ø6SC
  Esophageal Ø6S3
  External Iliac
    Left Ø6SG
    Right Ø6SF
  External Jugular
    Left Ø5SQ
    Right Ø5SP
  Face
    Left Ø5SV
    Right Ø5ST
  Femoral
    Left Ø6SN
    Right Ø6SM
  Foot
    Left Ø6SV
    Right Ø6ST
  Gastric Ø6S2
  Hand
    Left Ø5SH
    Right Ø5SG
  Hemiazygos Ø5S1
  Hepatic Ø6S4
  Hypogastric
    Left Ø6SJ
    Right Ø6SH
  Inferior Mesenteric Ø6S6
  Innominate
    Left Ø5S4
    Right Ø5S3
  Internal Jugular
    Left Ø5SN
    Right Ø5SM
  Intracranial Ø5SL
  Lower Ø6SY
  Portal Ø6S8
  Pulmonary
    Left Ø2STØZZ
    Right Ø2SSØZZ
  Renal
    Left Ø6SB
    Right Ø6S9
  Saphenous
    Left Ø6SQ
    Right Ø6SP
  Splenic Ø6S1
  Subclavian
    Left Ø5S6
    Right Ø5S5
  Superior Mesenteric Ø6S5
  Upper Ø5SY
  Vertebral
    Left Ø5SS
    Right Ø5SR
Vena Cava
  Inferior Ø6SØ
  Superior Ø2SVØZZ
Vertebra
  Cervical ØPS3
    Magnetically Controlled Growth Rod(s) XNS3
  Lumbar ØQSØ
    Magnetically Controlled Growth Rod(s) XNSØ
    Posterior (Dynamic) Distraction Device XNSØ
  Thoracic ØPS4
    Magnetically Controlled Growth Rod(s) XNS4
    Posterior (Dynamic) Distraction Device XNS4
Vocal Cord
  Left ØCSV
  Right ØCST

Resection

Acetabulum
  Left ØQT5ØZZ
  Right ØQT4ØZZ
Adenoids ØCTQ
Ampulla of Vater ØFTC
Anal Sphincter ØDTR

Resection — continued

Anus ØDTQ
Aortic Body ØGTD
Appendix ØDTJ
Auditory Ossicle
  Left Ø9TA
  Right Ø9T9
Bladder ØTTB
Bladder Neck ØTTC
Bone
  Ethmoid
    Left ØNTGØZZ
    Right ØNTFØZZ
  Frontal ØNT1ØZZ
  Hyoid ØNTXØZZ
  Lacrimal
    Left ØNTJØZZ
    Right ØNTHØZZ
  Nasal ØNTBØZZ
  Occipital ØNT7ØZZ
  Palatine
    Left ØNTLØZZ
    Right ØNTKØZZ
  Parietal
    Left ØNT4ØZZ
    Right ØNT3ØZZ
  Pelvic
    Left ØQT3ØZZ
    Right ØQT2ØZZ
  Sphenoid ØNTCØZZ
  Temporal
    Left ØNT6ØZZ
    Right ØNT5ØZZ
  Zygomatic
    Left ØNTNØZZ
    Right ØNTMØZZ
Breast
  Bilateral ØHTVØZZ
  Left ØHTUØZZ
  Right ØHTTØZZ
  Supernumerary ØHTYØZZ
Bronchus
  Lingula ØBT9
  Lower Lobe
    Left ØBTB
    Right ØBT6
  Main
    Left ØBT7
    Right ØBT3
  Middle Lobe, Right ØBT5
  Upper Lobe
    Left ØBT8
    Right ØBT4
Bursa and Ligament
  Abdomen
    Left ØMTJ
    Right ØMTH
  Ankle
    Left ØMTR
    Right ØMTQ
  Elbow
    Left ØMT4
    Right ØMT3
  Foot
    Left ØMTT
    Right ØMTS
  Hand
    Left ØMT8
    Right ØMT7
  Head and Neck ØMTØ
  Hip
    Left ØMTM
    Right ØMTL
  Knee
    Left ØMTP
    Right ØMTN
  Lower Extremity
    Left ØMTW
    Right ØMTV
  Perineum ØMTK
  Rib(s) ØMTG
  Shoulder
    Left ØMT2
    Right ØMT1
  Spine
    Lower ØMTD
    Upper ØMTC
  Sternum ØMTF

Resection — continued

Bursa and Ligament — continued
  Upper Extremity
    Left ØMTB
    Right ØMT9
  Wrist
    Left ØMT6
    Right ØMT5
Carina ØBT2
Carotid Bodies, Bilateral ØGT8
Carotid Body
  Left ØGT6
  Right ØGT7
Carpal
  Left ØPTNØZZ
  Right ØPTMØZZ
Cecum ØDTH
Cerebral Hemisphere ØØT7
Cervix ØUTC
Chordae Tendineae Ø2T9
Cisterna Chyli Ø7TL
Clavicle
  Left ØPTBØZZ
  Right ØPT9ØZZ
Clitoris ØUTJ
Coccygeal Glomus ØGTB
Coccyx ØQTSØZZ
Colon
  Ascending ØDTK
  Descending ØDTM
  Sigmoid ØDTN
  Transverse ØDTL
Conduction Mechanism Ø2T8
Cord
  Bilateral ØVTH
  Left ØVTG
  Right ØVTF
Cornea
  Left Ø8T9XZZ
  Right Ø8T8XZZ
Cul-de-sac ØUTF
Diaphragm ØBTT
Disc
  Cervical Vertebral ØRT3ØZZ
  Cervicothoracic Vertebral ØRT5ØZZ
  Lumbar Vertebral ØST2ØZZ
  Lumbosacral ØST4ØZZ
  Thoracic Vertebral ØRT9ØZZ
  Thoracolumbar Vertebral ØRTBØZZ
Duct
  Common Bile ØFT9
  Cystic ØFT8
  Hepatic
    Common ØFT7
    Left ØFT6
    Right ØFT5
  Lacrimal
    Left Ø8TY
    Right Ø8TX
  Pancreatic ØFTD
    Accessory ØFTF
  Parotid
    Left ØCTCØZZ
    Right ØCTBØZZ
Duodenum ØDT9
Ear
  External
    Left Ø9T1
    Right Ø9TØ
  Inner
    Left Ø9TE
    Right Ø9TD
  Middle
    Left Ø9T6
    Right Ø9T5
Epididymis
  Bilateral ØVTL
  Left ØVTK
  Right ØVTJ
Epiglottis ØCTR
Esophagogastric Junction ØDT4
Esophagus ØDT5
  Lower ØDT3
  Middle ØDT2
  Upper ØDT1
Eustachian Tube
  Left Ø9TG
  Right Ø9TF

Resection — *continued*
Eye
  Left Ø8T1XZZ
  Right Ø8TØXZZ
Eyelid
  Lower
    Left Ø8TR
    Right Ø8TQ
  Upper
    Left Ø8TP
    Right Ø8TN
Fallopian Tube
  Left ØUT6
  Right ØUT5
Fallopian Tubes, Bilateral ØUT7
Femoral Shaft
  Left ØQT9ØZZ
  Right ØQT8ØZZ
Femur
  Lower
    Left ØQTCØZZ
    Right ØQTBØZZ
  Upper
    Left ØQT7ØZZ
    Right ØQT6ØZZ
Fibula
  Left ØQTKØZZ
  Right ØQTJØZZ
Finger Nail ØHTQXZZ
Gallbladder ØFT4
Gland
  Adrenal
    Bilateral ØGT4
    Left ØGT2
    Right ØGT3
  Lacrimal
    Left Ø8TW
    Right Ø8TV
  Minor Salivary ØCTJØZZ
  Parotid
    Left ØCT9ØZZ
    Right ØCT8ØZZ
  Pituitary ØGTØ
  Sublingual
    Left ØCTFØZZ
    Right ØCTDØZZ
  Submaxillary
    Left ØCTHØZZ
    Right ØCTGØZZ
  Vestibular ØUTL
Glenoid Cavity
  Left ØPT8ØZZ
  Right ØPT7ØZZ
Glomus Jugulare ØGTC
Humeral Head
  Left ØPTDØZZ
  Right ØPTCØZZ
Humeral Shaft
  Left ØPTGØZZ
  Right ØPTFØZZ
Hymen ØUTK
Ileocecal Valve ØDTC
Ileum ØDTB
Intestine
  Large ØDTE
    Left ØDTG
    Right ØDTF
  Small ØDT8
Iris
  Left Ø8TD3ZZ
  Right Ø8TC3ZZ
Jejunum ØDTA
Joint
  Acromioclavicular
    Left ØRTHØZZ
    Right ØRTGØZZ
  Ankle
    Left ØSTGØZZ
    Right ØSTFØZZ
  Carpal
    Left ØRTRØZZ
    Right ØRTQØZZ
  Carpometacarpal
    Left ØRTTØZZ
    Right ØRTSØZZ
  Cervicothoracic Vertebral ØRT4ØZZ
  Coccygeal ØST6ØZZ
  Elbow
    Left ØRTMØZZ

Resection — *continued*
Joint — *continued*
  Elbow — *continued*
    Right ØRTLØZZ
  Finger Phalangeal
    Left ØRTXØZZ
    Right ØRTWØZZ
  Hip
    Left ØSTBØZZ
    Right ØST9ØZZ
  Knee
    Left ØSTDØZZ
    Right ØSTCØZZ
  Metacarpophalangeal
    Left ØRTVØZZ
    Right ØRTUØZZ
  Metatarsal-Phalangeal
    Left ØSTNØZZ
    Right ØSTMØZZ
  Sacrococcygeal ØST5ØZZ
  Sacroiliac
    Left ØST8ØZZ
    Right ØST7ØZZ
  Shoulder
    Left ØRTKØZZ
    Right ØRTJØZZ
  Sternoclavicular
    Left ØRTFØZZ
    Right ØRTEØZZ
  Tarsal
    Left ØSTJØZZ
    Right ØSTHØZZ
  Tarsometatarsal
    Left ØSTLØZZ
    Right ØSTKØZZ
  Temporomandibular
    Left ØRTDØZZ
    Right ØRTCØZZ
  Toe Phalangeal
    Left ØSTQØZZ
    Right ØSTPØZZ
  Wrist
    Left ØRTPØZZ
    Right ØRTNØZZ
Kidney
  Left ØTT1
  Right ØTTØ
Kidney Pelvis
  Left ØTT4
  Right ØTT3
Kidneys, Bilateral ØTT2
Larynx ØCTS
Lens
  Left Ø8TK3ZZ
  Right Ø8TJ3ZZ
Lip
  Lower ØCT1
  Upper ØCTØ
Liver ØFTØ
  Left Lobe ØFT2
  Right Lobe ØFT1
Lung
  Bilateral ØBTM
  Left ØBTL
  Lower Lobe
    Left ØBTJ
    Right ØBTF
  Middle Lobe, Right ØBTD
  Right ØBTK
  Upper Lobe
    Left ØBTG
    Right ØBTC
Lung Lingula ØBTH
Lymphatic
  Aortic Ø7TD
  Axillary
    Left Ø7T6
    Right Ø7T5
  Head Ø7TØ
  Inguinal
    Left Ø7TJ
    Right Ø7TH
  Internal Mammary
    Left Ø7T9
    Right Ø7T8
  Lower Extremity
    Left Ø7TG
    Right Ø7TF
  Mesenteric Ø7TB

Resection — *continued*
Lymphatic — *continued*
  Neck
    Left Ø7T2
    Right Ø7T1
  Pelvis Ø7TC
  Thoracic Duct Ø7TK
  Thorax Ø7T7
  Upper Extremity
    Left Ø7T4
    Right Ø7T3
Mandible
  Left ØNTVØZZ
  Right ØNTTØZZ
Maxilla ØNTRØZZ
Metacarpal
  Left ØPTQØZZ
  Right ØPTPØZZ
Metatarsal
  Left ØQTPØZZ
  Right ØQTNØZZ
Muscle
  Abdomen
    Left ØKTL
    Right ØKTK
  Extraocular
    Left Ø8TM
    Right Ø8TL
  Facial ØKT1
  Foot
    Left ØKTW
    Right ØKTV
  Hand
    Left ØKTD
    Right ØKTC
  Head ØKTØ
  Hip
    Left ØKTP
    Right ØKTN
  Lower Arm and Wrist
    Left ØKTB
    Right ØKT9
  Lower Leg
    Left ØKTT
    Right ØKTS
  Neck
    Left ØKT3
    Right ØKT2
  Papillary Ø2TD
  Perineum ØKTM
  Shoulder
    Left ØKT6
    Right ØKT5
  Thorax
    Left ØKTJ
    Right ØKTH
  Tongue, Palate, Pharynx ØKT4
  Trunk
    Left ØKTG
    Right ØKTF
  Upper Arm
    Left ØKT8
    Right ØKT7
  Upper Leg
    Left ØKTR
    Right ØKTQ
Nasal Mucosa and Soft Tissue Ø9TK
Nasopharynx Ø9TN
Nipple
  Left ØHTXXZZ
  Right ØHTWXZZ
Omentum ØDTU
Orbit
  Left ØNTQØZZ
  Right ØNTPØZZ
Ovary
  Bilateral ØUT2
  Left ØUT1
  Right ØUTØ
Palate
  Hard ØCT2
  Soft ØCT3
Pancreas ØFTG
Para-aortic Body ØGT9
Paraganglion Extremity ØGTF
Parathyroid Gland ØGTR
  Inferior
    Left ØGTP
    Right ØGTN

Resection — *continued*
  Parathyroid Gland — *continued*
    Multiple ØGTQ
    Superior
      Left ØGTM
      Right ØGTL
  Patella
    Left ØQTFØZZ
    Right ØQTDØZZ
  Penis ØVTS
  Pericardium Ø2TN
  Phalanx
    Finger
      Left ØPTVØZZ
      Right ØPTTØZZ
    Thumb
      Left ØPTSØZZ
      Right ØPTRØZZ
    Toe
      Left ØQTRØZZ
      Right ØQTQØZZ
  Pharynx ØCTM
  Pineal Body ØGT1
  Prepuce ØVTT
  Products of Conception, Ectopic 1ØT2
  Prostate ØVTØ
  Radius
    Left ØPTJØZZ
    Right ØPTHØZZ
  Rectum ØDTP
  Ribs
    1 to 2 ØPT1ØZZ
    3 or More ØPT2ØZZ
  Scapula
    Left ØPT6ØZZ
    Right ØPT5ØZZ
  Scrotum ØVT5
  Septum
    Atrial Ø2T5
    Nasal Ø9TM
    Ventricular Ø2TM
  Sinus
    Accessory Ø9TP
    Ethmoid
      Left Ø9TV
      Right Ø9TU
    Frontal
      Left Ø9TT
      Right Ø9TS
    Mastoid
      Left Ø9TC
      Right Ø9TB
    Maxillary
      Left Ø9TR
      Right Ø9TQ
    Sphenoid
      Left Ø9TX
      Right Ø9TW
  Spleen Ø7TP
  Sternum ØPTØØZZ
  Stomach ØDT6
    Pylorus ØDT7
  Tarsal
    Left ØQTMØZZ
    Right ØQTLØZZ
  Tendon
    Abdomen
      Left ØLTG
      Right ØLTF
    Ankle
      Left ØLTT
      Right ØLTS
    Foot
      Left ØLTW
      Right ØLTV
    Hand
      Left ØLT8
      Right ØLT7
    Head and Neck ØLTØ
    Hip
      Left ØLTK
      Right ØLTJ
    Knee
      Left ØLTR
      Right ØLTQ
    Lower Arm and Wrist
      Left ØLT6
      Right ØLT5

Resection — *continued*
  Tendon — *continued*
    Lower Leg
      Left ØLTP
      Right ØLTN
    Perineum ØLTH
    Shoulder
      Left ØLT2
      Right ØLT1
    Thorax
      Left ØLTD
      Right ØLTC
    Trunk
      Left ØLTB
      Right ØLT9
    Upper Arm
      Left ØLT4
      Right ØLT3
    Upper Leg
      Left ØLTM
      Right ØLTL
  Testis
    Bilateral ØVTC
    Left ØVTB
    Right ØVT9
  Thymus Ø7TM
  Thyroid Gland ØGTK
    Left Lobe ØGTG
    Right Lobe ØGTH
  Thyroid Gland Isthmus ØGTJ
  Tibia
    Left ØQTHØZZ
    Right ØQTGØZZ
  Toe Nail ØHTRXZZ
  Tongue ØCT7
  Tonsils ØCTP
  Tooth
    Lower ØCTXØZ
    Upper ØCTWØZ
  Trachea ØBT1
  Tunica Vaginalis
    Left ØVT7
    Right ØVT6
  Turbinate, Nasal Ø9TL
  Tympanic Membrane
    Left Ø9T8
    Right Ø9T7
  Ulna
    Left ØPTLØZZ
    Right ØPTKØZZ
  Ureter
    Left ØTT7
    Right ØTT6
  Urethra ØTTD
  Uterine Supporting Structure ØUT4
  Uterus ØUT9
  Uvula ØCTN
  Vagina ØUTG
  Valve, Pulmonary Ø2TH
  Vas Deferens
    Bilateral ØVTQ
    Left ØVTP
    Right ØVTN
  Vesicle
    Bilateral ØVT3
    Left ØVT2
    Right ØVT1
  Vitreous
    Left Ø8T53ZZ
    Right Ø8T43ZZ
  Vocal Cord
    Left ØCTV
    Right ØCTT
  Vulva ØUTM
Resection, Left ventricular outflow tract obstruction (LVOT) *see* Dilation, Ventricle, Left Ø27L
Resection, Subaortic membrane (Left ventricular outflow tract obstruction) *see* Dilation, Ventricle, Left Ø27L
Restoration, Cardiac, Single, Rhythm 5A22Ø4Z
RestoreAdvanced neurostimulator (SureScan) (MRI Safe) *use* Stimulator Generator, Multiple Array Rechargeable in ØJH
RestoreSensor neurostimulator (SureScan) (MRI Safe) *use* Stimulator Generator, Multiple Array Rechargeable in ØJH

RestoreUltra neurostimulator (SureScan) (MRI Safe) *use* Stimulator Generator, Multiple Array Rechargeable in ØJH
Restriction
  Ampulla of Vater ØFVC
  Anus ØDVQ
  Aorta
    Abdominal Ø4VØ
      Intraluminal Device, Branched or Fenestrated Ø4VØ
    Thoracic
      Ascending/Arch, Intraluminal Device, Branched or Fenestrated Ø2VX
      Descending, Intraluminal Device, Branched or Fenestrated Ø2VW
  Artery
    Anterior Tibial
      Left Ø4VQ
      Right Ø4VP
    Axillary
      Left Ø3V6
      Right Ø3V5
    Brachial
      Left Ø3V8
      Right Ø3V7
    Celiac Ø4V1
    Colic
      Left Ø4V7
      Middle Ø4V8
      Right Ø4V6
    Common Carotid
      Left Ø3VJ
      Right Ø3VH
    Common Iliac
      Left Ø4VD
      Right Ø4VC
    External Carotid
      Left Ø3VN
      Right Ø3VM
    External Iliac
      Left Ø4VJ
      Right Ø4VH
    Face Ø3VR
    Femoral
      Left Ø4VL
      Right Ø4VK
    Foot
      Left Ø4VW
      Right Ø4VV
    Gastric Ø4V2
    Hand
      Left Ø3VF
      Right Ø3VD
    Hepatic Ø4V3
    Inferior Mesenteric Ø4VB
    Innominate Ø3V2
    Internal Carotid
      Left Ø3VL
      Right Ø3VK
    Internal Iliac
      Left Ø4VF
      Right Ø4VE
    Internal Mammary
      Left Ø3V1
      Right Ø3VØ
    Intracranial Ø3VG
    Lower Ø4VY
    Peroneal
      Left Ø4VU
      Right Ø4VT
    Popliteal
      Left Ø4VN
      Right Ø4VM
    Posterior Tibial
      Left Ø4VS
      Right Ø4VR
    Pulmonary
      Left Ø2VR
      Right Ø2VQ
    Pulmonary Trunk Ø2VP
    Radial
      Left Ø3VC
      Right Ø3VB
    Renal
      Left Ø4VA
      Right Ø4V9
    Splenic Ø4V4
    Subclavian
      Left Ø3V4

Restriction — *continued*
  Artery — *continued*
    Subclavian — *continued*
      Right 03V3
    Superior Mesenteric 04V5
    Temporal
      Left 03VT
      Right 03VS
    Thyroid
      Left 03VV
      Right 03VU
    Ulnar
      Left 03VA
      Right 03V9
    Upper 03VY
    Vertebral
      Left 03VQ
      Right 03VP
  Bladder 0TVB
  Bladder Neck 0TVC
  Bronchus
    Lingula 0BV9
    Lower Lobe
      Left 0BVB
      Right 0BV6
    Main
      Left 0BV7
      Right 0BV3
    Middle Lobe, Right 0BV5
    Upper Lobe
      Left 0BV8
      Right 0BV4
  Carina 0BV2
  Cecum 0DVH
  Cervix 0UVC
  Cisterna Chyli 07VL
  Colon
    Ascending 0DVK
    Descending 0DVM
    Sigmoid 0DVN
    Transverse 0DVL
  Duct
    Common Bile 0FV9
    Cystic 0FV8
    Hepatic
      Common 0FV7
      Left 0FV6
      Right 0FV5
    Lacrimal
      Left 08VY
      Right 08VX
    Pancreatic 0FVD
      Accessory 0FVF
    Parotid
      Left 0CVC
      Right 0CVB
  Duodenum 0DV9
  Esophagogastric Junction 0DV4
  Esophagus 0DV5
    Lower 0DV3
    Middle 0DV2
    Upper 0DV1
  Heart 02VA
  Ileocecal Valve 0DVC
  Ileum 0DVB
  Intestine
    Large 0DVE
      Left 0DVG
      Right 0DVF
    Small 0DV8
  Jejunum 0DVA
  Kidney Pelvis
    Left 0TV4
    Right 0TV3
  Lymphatic
    Aortic 07VD
    Axillary
      Left 07V6
      Right 07V5
    Head 07V0
    Inguinal
      Left 07VJ
      Right 07VH
    Internal Mammary
      Left 07V9
      Right 07V8
    Lower Extremity
      Left 07VG
      Right 07VF

Restriction — *continued*
  Lymphatic — *continued*
    Mesenteric 07VB
    Neck
      Left 07V2
      Right 07V1
    Pelvis 07VC
    Thoracic Duct 07VK
    Thorax 07V7
    Upper Extremity
      Left 07V4
      Right 07V3
  Rectum 0DVP
  Stomach 0DV6
    Pylorus 0DV7
  Trachea 0BV1
  Ureter
    Left 0TV7
    Right 0TV6
  Urethra 0TVD
  Valve, Mitral 02VG
  Vein
    Axillary
      Left 05V8
      Right 05V7
    Azygos 05V0
    Basilic
      Left 05VC
      Right 05VB
    Brachial
      Left 05VA
      Right 05V9
    Cephalic
      Left 05VF
      Right 05VD
    Colic 06V7
    Common Iliac
      Left 06VD
      Right 06VC
    Esophageal 06V3
    External Iliac
      Left 06VG
      Right 06VF
    External Jugular
      Left 05VQ
      Right 05VP
    Face
      Left 05VV
      Right 05VT
    Femoral
      Left 06VN
      Right 06VM
    Foot
      Left 06VV
      Right 06VT
    Gastric 06V2
    Hand
      Left 05VH
      Right 05VG
    Hemiazygos 05V1
    Hepatic 06V4
    Hypogastric
      Left 06VJ
      Right 06VH
    Inferior Mesenteric 06V6
    Innominate
      Left 05V4
      Right 05V3
    Internal Jugular
      Left 05VN
      Right 05VM
    Intracranial 05VL
    Lower 06VY
    Portal 06V8
    Pulmonary
      Left 02VT
      Right 02VS
    Renal
      Left 06VB
      Right 06V9
    Saphenous
      Left 06VQ
      Right 06VP
    Splenic 06V1
    Subclavian
      Left 05V6
      Right 05V5
    Superior Mesenteric 06V5
    Upper 05VY

Restriction — *continued*
  Vein — *continued*
    Vertebral
      Left 05VS
      Right 05VR
    Vena Cava
      Inferior 06V0
      Superior 02VV
    Ventricle, Left 02VL
Resurfacing Device
  Removal of device from
    Left 0SPB0BZ
    Right 0SP90BZ
  Revision of device in
    Left 0SWB0BZ
    Right 0SW90BZ
  Supplement
    Left 0SUB0BZ
      Acetabular Surface 0SUE0BZ
      Femoral Surface 0SUS0BZ
    Right 0SU90BZ
      Acetabular Surface 0SUA0BZ
      Femoral Surface 0SUR0BZ
Resuscitation
  Cardiopulmonary *see* Assistance, Cardiac 5A02
  Cardioversion 5A2204Z
  Defibrillation 5A2204Z
  Endotracheal intubation *see* Insertion of device in, Trachea 0BH1
  External chest compression, manual 5A12012
  External chest compression, mechanical 5A1221J
  Pulmonary 5A19054
Resuscitative endovascular balloon occlusion of the aorta (REBOA)
  02LW3DJ
  04L03DJ
Resuture, Heart valve prosthesis *see* Revision of device in, Heart and Great Vessels 02W
Retained placenta, manual removal *see* Extraction, Products of Conception, Retained 10D1
RETHYMIC® *use* Engineered Allogeneic Thymus Tissue
Retraining
  Cardiac *see* Motor Treatment, Rehabilitation F07
  Vocational *see* Activities of Daily Living Treatment, Rehabilitation F08
Retrogasserian rhizotomy *see* Division, Nerve, Trigeminal 008K
Retroperitoneal cavity *use* Retroperitoneum
Retroperitoneal lymph node *use* Lymphatic, Aortic
Retroperitoneal space *use* Retroperitoneum
Retropharyngeal lymph node
  use Lymphatic, Left Neck
  use Lymphatic, Right Neck
Retropharyngeal space *use* Neck
Retropubic space *use* Pelvic Cavity
Reveal (LINQ) (DX) (XT) *use* Monitoring Device
Reverse total shoulder replacement *see* Replacement, Upper Joints 0RR
Reverse® Shoulder Prosthesis *use* Synthetic Substitute, Reverse Ball and Socket in 0RR
Revision
  Correcting a portion of existing device *see* Revision of device in
  Removal of device without replacement *see* Removal of device from
  Replacement of existing device
    see Removal of device from
    see Root operation to place new device, e.g., Insertion, Replacement, Supplement
Revision of device in
  Abdominal Wall 0WWF
  Acetabulum
    Left 0QW5
    Right 0QW4
  Anal Sphincter 0DWR
  Anus 0DWQ
  Artery
    Lower 04WY
    Upper 03WY
  Auditory Ossicle
    Left 09WA
    Right 09W9
  Back
    Lower 0WWL
    Upper 0WWK
  Bladder 0TWB
  Bone
    Facial 0NWW

Revision of device in — *continued*
- Bone — *continued*
  - Lower 0QWY
  - Nasal 0NWB
  - Pelvic
    - Left 0QW3
    - Right 0QW2
  - Upper 0PWY
- Bone Marrow 07WT
- Brain 00W0
- Breast
  - Left 0HWU
  - Right 0HWT
- Bursa and Ligament
  - Lower 0MWY
  - Upper 0MWX
- Carpal
  - Left 0PWN
  - Right 0PWM
- Cavity, Cranial 0WW1
- Cerebral Ventricle 00W6
- Chest Wall 0WW8
- Cisterna Chyli 07WL
- Clavicle
  - Left 0PWB
  - Right 0PW9
- Coccyx 0QWS
- Diaphragm 0BWT
- Disc
  - Cervical Vertebral 0RW3
  - Cervicothoracic Vertebral 0RW5
  - Lumbar Vertebral 0SW2
  - Lumbosacral 0SW4
  - Thoracic Vertebral 0RW9
  - Thoracolumbar Vertebral 0RWB
- Duct
  - Hepatobiliary 0FWB
  - Pancreatic 0FWD
- Ear
  - Inner
    - Left 09WE
    - Right 09WD
  - Left 09WJ
  - Right 09WH
- Epididymis and Spermatic Cord 0VWM
- Esophagus 0DW5
- Extremity
  - Lower
    - Left 0YWB
    - Right 0YW9
  - Upper
    - Left 0XW7
    - Right 0XW6
- Eye
  - Left 08W1
  - Right 08W0
- Face 0WW2
- Fallopian Tube 0UW8
- Femoral Shaft
  - Left 0QW9
  - Right 0QW8
- Femur
  - Lower
    - Left 0QWC
    - Right 0QWB
  - Upper
    - Left 0QW7
    - Right 0QW6
- Fibula
  - Left 0QWK
  - Right 0QWJ
- Finger Nail 0HWQX
- Gallbladder 0FW4
- Gastrointestinal Tract 0WWP
- Genitourinary Tract 0WWR
- Gland
  - Adrenal 0GW5
  - Endocrine 0GWS
  - Pituitary 0GW0
  - Salivary 0CWA
- Glenoid Cavity
  - Left 0PW8
  - Right 0PW7
- Great Vessel 02WY
- Hair 0HWSX
- Head 0WW0
- Heart 02WA
- Humeral Head
  - Left 0PWD

Revision of device in — *continued*
- Humeral Head — *continued*
  - Right 0PWC
- Humeral Shaft
  - Left 0PWG
  - Right 0PWF
- Intestinal Tract
  - Lower Intestinal Tract 0DWD
  - Upper Intestinal Tract 0DW0
- Intestine
  - Large 0DWE
  - Small 0DW8
- Jaw
  - Lower 0WW5
  - Upper 0WW4
- Joint
  - Acromioclavicular
    - Left 0RWH
    - Right 0RWG
  - Ankle
    - Left 0SWG
    - Right 0SWF
  - Carpal
    - Left 0RWR
    - Right 0RWQ
  - Carpometacarpal
    - Left 0RWT
    - Right 0RWS
  - Cervical Vertebral 0RW1
  - Cervicothoracic Vertebral 0RW4
  - Coccygeal 0SW6
  - Elbow
    - Left 0RWM
    - Right 0RWL
  - Finger Phalangeal
    - Left 0RWX
    - Right 0RWW
  - Hip
    - Left 0SWB
      - Acetabular Surface 0SWE
      - Femoral Surface 0SWS
    - Right 0SW9
      - Acetabular Surface 0SWA
      - Femoral Surface 0SWR
  - Knee
    - Left 0SWD
      - Femoral Surface 0SWU
      - Tibial Surface 0SWW
    - Right 0SWC
      - Femoral Surface 0SWT
      - Tibial Surface 0SWV
  - Lumbar Vertebral 0SW0
  - Lumbosacral 0SW3
  - Metacarpophalangeal
    - Left 0RWV
    - Right 0RWU
  - Metatarsal-Phalangeal
    - Left 0SWN
    - Right 0SWM
  - Occipital-cervical 0RW0
  - Sacrococcygeal 0SW5
  - Sacroiliac
    - Left 0SW8
    - Right 0SW7
  - Shoulder
    - Left 0RWK
    - Right 0RWJ
  - Sternoclavicular
    - Left 0RWF
    - Right 0RWE
  - Tarsal
    - Left 0SWJ
    - Right 0SWH
  - Tarsometatarsal
    - Left 0SWL
    - Right 0SWK
  - Temporomandibular
    - Left 0RWD
    - Right 0RWC
  - Thoracic Vertebral 0RW6
  - Thoracolumbar Vertebral 0RWA
  - Toe Phalangeal
    - Left 0SWQ
    - Right 0SWP
  - Wrist
    - Left 0RWP
    - Right 0RWN
- Kidney 0TW5
- Larynx 0CWS

Revision of device in — *continued*
- Lens
  - Left 08WK
  - Right 08WJ
- Liver 0FW0
- Lung
  - Left 0BWL
  - Right 0BWK
- Lymphatic 07WN
  - Thoracic Duct 07WK
- Mediastinum 0WWC
- Mesentery 0DWV
- Metacarpal
  - Left 0PWQ
  - Right 0PWP
- Metatarsal
  - Left 0QWP
  - Right 0QWN
- Mouth and Throat 0CWY
- Muscle
  - Extraocular
    - Left 08WM
    - Right 08WL
  - Lower 0KWY
  - Upper 0KWX
- Nasal Mucosa and Soft Tissue 09WK
- Neck 0WW6
- Nerve
  - Cranial 00WE
  - Peripheral 01WY
- Omentum 0DWU
- Ovary 0UW3
- Pancreas 0FWG
- Parathyroid Gland 0GWR
- Patella
  - Left 0QWF
  - Right 0QWD
- Pelvic Cavity 0WWJ
- Penis 0VWS
- Pericardial Cavity 0WWD
- Perineum
  - Female 0WWN
  - Male 0WWM
- Peritoneal Cavity 0WWG
- Peritoneum 0DWW
- Phalanx
  - Finger
    - Left 0PWV
    - Right 0PWT
  - Thumb
    - Left 0PWS
    - Right 0PWR
  - Toe
    - Left 0QWR
    - Right 0QWQ
- Pineal Body 0GW1
- Pleura 0BWQ
- Pleural Cavity
  - Left 0WWB
  - Right 0WW9
- Prostate and Seminal Vesicles 0VW4
- Radius
  - Left 0PWJ
  - Right 0PWH
- Respiratory Tract 0WWQ
- Retroperitoneum 0WWH
- Ribs
  - 1 to 2 0PW1
  - 3 or More 0PW2
- Sacrum 0QW1
- Scapula
  - Left 0PW6
  - Right 0PW5
- Scrotum and Tunica Vaginalis 0VW8
- Septum
  - Atrial 02W5
  - Ventricular 02WM
- Sinus 09WY
- Skin 0HWPX
- Skull 0NW0
- Spinal Canal 00WU
- Spinal Cord 00WV
- Spleen 07WP
- Sternum 0PW0
- Stomach 0DW6
- Subcutaneous Tissue and Fascia
  - Head and Neck 0JWS
  - Lower Extremity 0JWW
  - Trunk 0JWT

Revision of device in — *continued*
  Subcutaneous Tissue and Fascia — *continued*
    Upper Extremity ØJWV
  Tarsal
    Left ØQWM
    Right ØQWL
  Tendon
    Lower ØLWY
    Upper ØLWX
  Testis ØVWD
  Thymus Ø7WM
  Thyroid Gland ØGWK
  Tibia
    Left ØQWH
    Right ØQWG
  Toe Nail ØHWRX
  Trachea ØBW1
  Tracheobronchial Tree ØBWØ
  Tympanic Membrane
    Left Ø9W8
    Right Ø9W7
  Ulna
    Left ØPWL
    Right ØPWK
  Ureter ØTW9
  Urethra ØTWD
  Uterus and Cervix ØUWD
  Vagina and Cul-de-sac ØUWH
  Valve
    Aortic Ø2WF
    Mitral Ø2WG
    Pulmonary Ø2WH
    Tricuspid Ø2WJ
  Vas Deferens ØVWR
  Vein
    Azygos Ø5WØ
    Innominate
      Left Ø5W4
      Right Ø5W3
    Lower Ø6WY
    Upper Ø5WY
  Vertebra
    Cervical ØPW3
    Lumbar ØQWØ
    Thoracic ØPW4
  Vulva ØUWM
Revo MRI™ SureScan® pacemaker *use* Pacemaker, Dual Chamber in ØJH
rhBMP-2 *use* Recombinant Bone Morphogenetic Protein
Rheos® System device *use* Stimulator Generator in Subcutaneous Tissue and Fascia
Rheos® System lead *use* Stimulator Lead in Upper Arteries
Rhinopharynx *use* Nasopharynx
Rhinoplasty
  see Alteration, Nasal Mucosa and Soft Tissue Ø9ØK
  see Repair, Nasal Mucosa and Soft Tissue Ø9QK
  see Replacement, Nasal Mucosa and Soft Tissue Ø9RK
  see Supplement, Nasal Mucosa and Soft Tissue Ø9UK
Rhinorrhaphy *see* Repair, Nasal Mucosa and Soft Tissue Ø9QK
Rhinoscopy Ø9JKXZZ
Rhizotomy
  see Division, Central Nervous System and Cranial Nerves ØØ8
  see Division, Peripheral Nervous System Ø18
Rhomboid major muscle
  use Trunk Muscle, Left
  use Trunk Muscle, Right
Rhomboid minor muscle
  use Trunk Muscle, Left
  use Trunk Muscle, Right
Rhythm electrocardiogram *see* Measurement, Cardiac 4AØ2
Rhytidectomy *see* Alteration, Face ØWØ2
Right ascending lumbar vein *use* Azygos Vein
Right atrioventricular valve *use* Tricuspid Valve
Right auricular appendix *use* Atrium, Right
Right colic vein *use* Colic Vein
Right coronary sulcus *use* Heart, Right
Right gastric artery *use* Gastric Artery
Right gastroepiploic vein *use* Superior Mesenteric Vein
Right inferior phrenic vein *use* Inferior Vena Cava

Right inferior pulmonary vein *use* Pulmonary Vein, Right
Right jugular trunk *use* Lymphatic, Right Neck
Right lateral ventricle *use* Cerebral Ventricle
Right lymphatic duct *use* Lymphatic, Right Neck
Right ovarian vein *use* Inferior Vena Cava
Right second lumbar vein *use* Inferior Vena Cava
Right subclavian trunk *use* Lymphatic, Right Neck
Right subcostal vein *use* Azygos Vein
Right superior pulmonary vein *use* Pulmonary Vein, Right
Right suprarenal vein *use* Inferior Vena Cava
Right testicular vein *use* Inferior Vena Cava
Rima glottidis *use* Larynx
Risorius muscle *use* Facial Muscle
RNS System lead *use* Neurostimulator Lead in Central Nervous System and Cranial Nerves
RNS system neurostimulator generator *use* Neurostimulator Generator in Head and Facial Bones
Robotic Assisted Procedure
  Extremity
    Lower 8EØY
    Upper 8EØX
  Head and Neck Region 8EØ9
  Trunk Region 8EØW
Robotic Waterjet Ablation, Destruction, Prostate XV5Ø8A4
Rotation of fetal head
  Forceps 1ØSØ7ZZ
  Manual 1ØSØXZZ
Round ligament of uterus *use* Uterine Supporting Structure
Round window
  use Inner Ear, Left
  use Inner Ear, Right
Roux-en-Y operation
  see Bypass, Gastrointestinal System ØD1
  see Bypass, Hepatobiliary System and Pancreas ØF1
Rupture
  Adhesions *see* Release
  Fluid collection *see* Drainage
Ruxolitinib XWØDXT5
RYBREVANT™ *use* Amivantamab Monoclonal Antibody

S

Sacral ganglion *use* Sacral Sympathetic Nerve
Sacral lymph node *use* Lymphatic, Pelvis
Sacral nerve modulation (SNM) lead *use* Stimulator Lead in Urinary System
Sacral neuromodulation lead *use* Stimulator Lead in Urinary System
Sacral splanchnic nerve *use* Sacral Sympathetic Nerve
Sacrectomy *see* Excision, Lower Bones ØQB
Sacrococcygeal ligament *use* Lower Spine Bursa and Ligament
Sacrococcygeal symphysis *use* Sacrococcygeal Joint
Sacroiliac ligament *use* Lower Spine Bursa and Ligament
Sacrospinous ligament *use* Lower Spine Bursa and Ligament
Sacrotuberous ligament *use* Lower Spine Bursa and Ligament
Salpingectomy
  see Excision, Female Reproductive System ØUB
  see Resection, Female Reproductive System ØUT
Salpingolysis *see* Release, Female Reproductive System ØUN
Salpingopexy
  see Repair, Female Reproductive System ØUQ
  see Reposition, Female Reproductive System ØUS
Salpingopharyngeus muscle *use* Tongue, Palate, Pharynx Muscle
Salpingoplasty
  see Repair, Female Reproductive System ØUQ
  see Supplement, Female Reproductive System ØUU
Salpingorrhaphy *see* Repair, Female Reproductive System ØUQ
Salpingoscopy ØUJ88ZZ
Salpingostomy *see* Drainage, Female Reproductive System ØU9
Salpingotomy *see* Drainage, Female Reproductive System ØU9
Salpinx
  use Fallopian Tube, Left

Salpinx — *continued*
  use Fallopian Tube, Right
Saphenous nerve *use* Femoral Nerve
SAPIEN transcatheter aortic valve *use* Zooplastic Tissue in Heart and Great Vessels
Sarilumab XWØ
SARS-CoV-2 Antibody Detection, Serum/Plasma Nanoparticle Fluorescence XXE5XV7
SARS-CoV-2 Polymerase Chain Reaction, Nasopharyngeal Fluid XXE97U7
Sartorius muscle
  use Upper Leg Muscle, Left
  use Upper Leg Muscle, Right
Satralizumab-mwge XWØ1397
SAVAL below-the-knee (BTK) drug-eluting stent system
  use Intraluminal Device, Sustained Release Drug-eluting in New Technology
  use Intraluminal Device, Sustained Release Drug-eluting, Two in New Technology
  use Intraluminal Device, Sustained Release Drug-eluting, Three in New Technology
  use Intraluminal Device, Sustained Release Drug-eluting, Four or More in New Technology
Scalene muscle
  use Neck Muscle, Left
  use Neck Muscle, Right
Scan
  Computerized Tomography (CT) *see* Computerized Tomography (CT Scan)
  Radioisotope *see* Planar Nuclear Medicine Imaging
Scaphoid bone
  use Carpal, Left
  use Carpal, Right
Scapholunate ligament
  use Wrist Bursa and Ligament, Left
  use Wrist Bursa and Ligament, Right
Scaphotrapezium ligament
  use Hand Bursa and Ligament, Left
  use Hand Bursa and Ligament, Right
Scapulectomy
  see Excision, Upper Bones ØPB
  see Resection, Upper Bones ØPT
Scapulopexy
  see Repair, Upper Bones ØPQ
  see Reposition, Upper Bones ØPS
Scarpa's (vestibular) ganglion *use* Acoustic Nerve
Sclerectomy *see* Excision, Eye Ø8B
Sclerotherapy, mechanical *see* Destruction
Sclerotherapy, via injection of sclerosing agent *see* Introduction, Destructive Agent
Sclerotomy *see* Drainage, Eye Ø89
Scrotectomy
  see Excision, Male Reproductive System ØVB
  see Resection, Male Reproductive System ØVT
Scrotoplasty
  see Repair, Male Reproductive System ØVQ
  see Supplement, Male Reproductive System ØVU
Scrotorrhaphy *see* Repair, Male Reproductive System ØVQ
Scrototomy *see* Drainage, Male Reproductive System ØV9
Sebaceous gland *use* Skin
Second cranial nerve *use* Optic Nerve
Section, cesarean *see* Extraction, Pregnancy 1ØD
Secura (DR) (VR) *use* Defibrillator Generator in ØJH
Sella turcica *use* Sphenoid Bone
Semicircular canal
  use Inner Ear, Left
  use Inner Ear, Right
Semimembranosus muscle
  use Upper Leg Muscle, Left
  use Upper Leg Muscle, Right
Semitendinosus muscle
  use Upper Leg Muscle, Left
  use Upper Leg Muscle, Right
Sentinel™ Cerebral Protection System (CPS) X2A5312
Seprafilm *use* Adhesion Barrier
Septal cartilage *use* Nasal Septum
Septectomy
  see Excision, Ear, Nose, Sinus Ø9B
  see Excision, Heart and Great Vessels Ø2B
  see Resection, Ear, Nose, Sinus Ø9T
  see Resection, Heart and Great Vessels Ø2T
SeptiCyte® RAPID XXE5X38

Septoplasty
  see Repair, Ear, Nose, Sinus 09Q
  see Repair, Heart and Great Vessels 02Q
  see Replacement, Ear, Nose, Sinus 09R
  see Replacement, Heart and Great Vessels 02R
  see Reposition, Ear, Nose, Sinus 09S
  see Supplement, Ear, Nose, Sinus 09U
  see Supplement, Heart and Great Vessels 02U
Septostomy, balloon atrial 02163Z7
Septotomy *see* Drainage, Ear, Nose, Sinus 099
Sequestrectomy, bone *see* Extirpation
Serratus anterior muscle
  use Thorax Muscle, Left
  use Thorax Muscle, Right
Serratus posterior muscle
  use Trunk Muscle, Left
  use Trunk Muscle, Right
Seventh cranial nerve *use* Facial Nerve
Shapshot_NIR 8E02XDZ
Sheffield hybrid external fixator
  use External Fixation Device, Hybrid in 0PH
  use External Fixation Device, Hybrid in 0PS
  use External Fixation Device, Hybrid in 0QH
  use External Fixation Device, Hybrid in 0QS
Sheffield ring external fixator
  use External Fixation Device, Ring in 0PH
  use External Fixation Device, Ring in 0PS
  use External Fixation Device, Ring in 0QH
  use External Fixation Device, Ring in 0QS
Shirodkar cervical cerclage 0UVC7ZZ
Shock Wave Therapy, Musculoskeletal 6A93
Shockwave Intravascular Lithotripsy (Shockwave IVL) *see* Fragmentation
Short gastric artery *use* Splenic Artery
Shortening
  see Excision
  see Repair
  see Reposition
Shunt creation *see* Bypass
Sialoadenectomy
  Complete *see* Resection, Mouth and Throat 0CT
  Partial *see* Excision, Mouth and Throat 0CB
Sialodochoplasty
  see Repair, Mouth and Throat 0CQ
  see Replacement, Mouth and Throat 0CR
  see Supplement, Mouth and Throat 0CU
Sialoectomy
  see Excision, Mouth and Throat 0CB
  see Resection, Mouth and Throat 0CT
Sialography *see* Plain Radiography, Ear, Nose, Mouth and Throat B90
Sialolithotomy *see* Extirpation, Mouth and Throat 0CC
S-ICD™ lead *use* Subcutaneous Defibrillator Lead in Subcutaneous Tissue and Fascia
Sigmoid artery *use* Inferior Mesenteric Artery
Sigmoid flexure *use* Sigmoid Colon
Sigmoid vein *use* Inferior Mesenteric Vein
Sigmoidectomy
  see Excision, Gastrointestinal System 0DB
  see Resection, Gastrointestinal System 0DT
Sigmoidorrhaphy *see* Repair, Gastrointestinal System 0DQ
Sigmoidoscopy 0DJD8ZZ
Sigmoidotomy *see* Drainage, Gastrointestinal System 0D9
Single lead pacemaker (atrium) (ventricle) *use* Pacemaker, Single Chamber in 0JH
Single lead rate responsive pacemaker (atrium) (ventricle) *use* Pacemaker, Single Chamber Rate Responsive in 0JH
Single-use Duodenoscope XFJ
Single-use Oversleeve with Intraoperative Colonic Irrigation XDPH8K7
Sinoatrial node *use* Conduction Mechanism
Sinogram
  Abdominal Wall *see* Fluoroscopy, Abdomen and Pelvis BW11
  Chest Wall *see* Plain Radiography, Chest BW03
  Retroperitoneum *see* Fluoroscopy, Abdomen and Pelvis BW11
Sinus venosus *use* Atrium, Right
Sinusectomy
  see Excision, Ear, Nose, Sinus 09B
  see Resection, Ear, Nose, Sinus 09T
Sinusoscopy 09JY4ZZ
Sinusotomy *see* Drainage, Ear, Nose, Sinus 099

Sirolimus-eluting coronary stent *use* Intraluminal Device, Drug-eluting in Heart and Great Vessels
Sixth cranial nerve *use* Abducens Nerve
Size reduction, breast *see* Excision, Skin and Breast 0HB
SJM Biocor® Stented Valve System *use* Zooplastic Tissue in Heart and Great Vessels
Skene's (paraurethral) gland *use* Vestibular Gland
Sling
  Fascial, orbicularis muscle (mouth) *see* Supplement, Muscle, Facial 0KU1
  Levator muscle, for urethral suspension *see* Reposition, Bladder Neck 0TSC
  Pubococcygeal, for urethral suspension *see* Reposition, Bladder Neck 0TSC
  Rectum *see* Reposition, Rectum 0DSP
Small bowel series *see* Fluoroscopy, Bowel, Small BD13
Small saphenous vein
  use Saphenous Vein, Left
  use Saphenous Vein, Right
Snapshot_NIR 8E02XDZ
Snaring, polyp, colon *see* Excision, Gastrointestinal System 0DB
Solar (celiac) plexus *use* Abdominal Sympathetic Nerve
Soleus muscle
  use Lower Leg Muscle, Left
  use Lower Leg Muscle, Right
Soliris® *use* Eculizumab
Spacer
  Insertion of device in
    Disc
      Lumbar Vertebral 0SH2
      Lumbosacral 0SH4
    Joint
      Acromioclavicular
        Left 0RHH
        Right 0RHG
      Ankle
        Left 0SHG
        Right 0SHF
      Carpal
        Left 0RHR
        Right 0RHQ
      Carpometacarpal
        Left 0RHT
        Right 0RHS
      Cervical Vertebral 0RH1
      Cervicothoracic Vertebral 0RH4
      Coccygeal 0SH6
      Elbow
        Left 0RHM
        Right 0RHL
      Finger Phalangeal
        Left 0RHX
        Right 0RHW
      Hip
        Left 0SHB
        Right 0SH9
      Knee
        Left 0SHD
        Right 0SHC
      Lumbar Vertebral 0SH0
      Lumbosacral 0SH3
      Metacarpophalangeal
        Left 0RHV
        Right 0RHU
      Metatarsal-Phalangeal
        Left 0SHN
        Right 0SHM
      Occipital-cervical 0RH0
      Sacrococcygeal 0SH5
      Sacroiliac
        Left 0SH8
        Right 0SH7
      Shoulder
        Left 0RHK
        Right 0RHJ
      Sternoclavicular
        Left 0RHF
        Right 0RHE
      Tarsal
        Left 0SHJ
        Right 0SHH
      Tarsometatarsal
        Left 0SHL
        Right 0SHK

Spacer — *continued*
  Insertion of device in — *continued*
    Joint — *continued*
      Temporomandibular
        Left 0RHD
        Right 0RHC
      Thoracic Vertebral 0RH6
      Thoracolumbar Vertebral 0RHA
      Toe Phalangeal
        Left 0SHQ
        Right 0SHP
      Wrist
        Left 0RHP
        Right 0RHN
  Removal of device from
    Acromioclavicular
      Left 0RPH
      Right 0RPG
    Ankle
      Left 0SPG
      Right 0SPF
    Carpal
      Left 0RPR
      Right 0RPQ
    Carpometacarpal
      Left 0RPT
      Right 0RPS
    Cervical Vertebral 0RP1
    Cervicothoracic Vertebral 0RP4
    Coccygeal 0SP6
    Elbow
      Left 0RPM
      Right 0RPL
    Finger Phalangeal
      Left 0RPX
      Right 0RPW
    Hip
      Left 0SPB
      Right 0SP9
    Knee
      Left 0SPD
      Right 0SPC
    Lumbar Vertebral 0SP0
    Lumbosacral 0SP3
    Metacarpophalangeal
      Left 0RPV
      Right 0RPU
    Metatarsal-Phalangeal
      Left 0SPN
      Right 0SPM
    Occipital-cervical 0RP0
    Sacrococcygeal 0SP5
    Sacroiliac
      Left 0SP8
      Right 0SP7
    Shoulder
      Left 0RPK
      Right 0RPJ
    Sternoclavicular
      Left 0RPF
      Right 0RPE
    Tarsal
      Left 0SPJ
      Right 0SPH
    Tarsometatarsal
      Left 0SPL
      Right 0SPK
    Temporomandibular
      Left 0RPD
      Right 0RPC
    Thoracic Vertebral 0RP6
    Thoracolumbar Vertebral 0RPA
    Toe Phalangeal
      Left 0SPQ
      Right 0SPP
    Wrist
      Left 0RPP
      Right 0RPN
  Revision of device in
    Acromioclavicular
      Left 0RWH
      Right 0RWG
    Ankle
      Left 0SWG
      Right 0SWF
    Carpal
      Left 0RWR
      Right 0RWQ

Spacer — *continued*
Revision of device in — *continued*
Carpometacarpal
Left ØRWT
Right ØRWS
Cervical Vertebral ØRW1
Cervicothoracic Vertebral ØRW4
Coccygeal ØSW6
Elbow
Left ØRWM
Right ØRWL
Finger Phalangeal
Left ØRWX
Right ØRWW
Hip
Left ØSWB
Right ØSW9
Knee
Left ØSWD
Right ØSWC
Lumbar Vertebral ØSWØ
Lumbosacral ØSW3
Metacarpophalangeal
Left ØRWV
Right ØRWU
Metatarsal-Phalangeal
Left ØSWN
Right ØSWM
Occipital-cervical ØRWØ
Sacrococcygeal ØSW5
Sacroiliac
Left ØSW8
Right ØSW7
Shoulder
Left ØRWK
Right ØRWJ
Sternoclavicular
Left ØRWF
Right ØRWE
Tarsal
Left ØSWJ
Right ØSWH
Tarsometatarsal
Left ØSWL
Right ØSWK
Temporomandibular
Left ØRWD
Right ØRWC
Thoracic Vertebral ØRW6
Thoracolumbar Vertebral ØRWA
Toe Phalangeal
Left ØSWQ
Right ØSWP
Wrist
Left ØRWP
Right ØRWN
Spacer, Articulating (Antibiotic) *use* Articulating Spacer in Lower Joints
Spacer, Static (Antibiotic) *use* Spacer in Lower Joints
Spectroscopy
Intravascular Near Infrared 8E023DZ
Near Infrared *see* Physiological Systems and Anatomical Regions 8EØ
Speech Assessment FØØ
Speech therapy *see* Speech Treatment, Rehabilitation FØ6
Speech Treatment FØ6
Spesolimab Monoclonal Antibody XWØ
Sphenoidectomy
see Excision, Ear, Nose, Sinus Ø9B
see Excision, Head and Facial Bones ØNB
see Resection, Ear, Nose, Sinus Ø9T
see Resection, Head and Facial Bones ØNT
Sphenoidotomy *see* Drainage, Ear, Nose, Sinus Ø99
Sphenomandibular ligament *use* Head and Neck Bursa and Ligament
Sphenopalatine (pterygopalatine) ganglion *use* Head and Neck Sympathetic Nerve
Sphincterorrhaphy, anal *see* Repair, Anal Sphincter ØDQR
Sphincterotomy, anal
see Division, Anal Sphincter ØD8R
see Drainage, Anal Sphincter ØD9R
Spinal cord neurostimulator lead *use* Neurostimulator Lead in Central Nervous System and Cranial Nerves

Spinal growth rods, magnetically controlled *use* Magnetically Controlled Growth Rod(s) in New Technology
Spinal nerve, cervical *use* Cervical Nerve
Spinal nerve, lumbar *use* Lumbar Nerve
Spinal nerve, sacral *use* Sacral Nerve
Spinal nerve, thoracic *use* Thoracic Nerve
Spinal Stabilization Device
Facet Replacement
Cervical Vertebral ØRH1
Cervicothoracic Vertebral ØRH4
Lumbar Vertebral ØSHØ
Lumbosacral ØSH3
Occipital-cervical ØRHØ
Thoracic Vertebral ØRH6
Thoracolumbar Vertebral ØRHA
Interspinous Process
Cervical Vertebral ØRH1
Cervicothoracic Vertebral ØRH4
Lumbar Vertebral ØSHØ
Lumbosacral ØSH3
Occipital-cervical ØRHØ
Thoracic Vertebral ØRH6
Thoracolumbar Vertebral ØRHA
Pedicle-Based
Cervical Vertebral ØRH1
Cervicothoracic Vertebral ØRH4
Lumbar Vertebral ØSHØ
Lumbosacral ØSH3
Occipital-cervical ØRHØ
Thoracic Vertebral ØRH6
Thoracolumbar Vertebral ØRHA
SpineJack® system *use* Synthetic Substitute, Mechanically Expandable (Paired) in New Technology
Spinous process
use Cervical Vertebra
use Lumbar Vertebra
use Thoracic Vertebra
Spiral ganglion *use* Acoustic Nerve
Spiration IBV™ Valve System *use* Intraluminal Device, Endobronchial Valve in Respiratory System
Splenectomy
see Excision, Lymphatic and Hemic Systems Ø7B
see Resection, Lymphatic and Hemic Systems Ø7T
Splenic flexure *use* Transverse Colon
Splenic plexus *use* Abdominal Sympathetic Nerve
Splenius capitis muscle *use* Head Muscle
Splenius cervicis muscle
use Neck Muscle, Left
use Neck Muscle, Right
Splenolysis *see* Release, Lymphatic and Hemic Systems Ø7N
Splenopexy
see Repair, Lymphatic and Hemic Systems Ø7Q
see Reposition, Lymphatic and Hemic Systems Ø7S
Splenoplasty *see* Repair, Lymphatic and Hemic Systems Ø7Q
Splenorrhaphy *see* Repair, Lymphatic and Hemic Systems Ø7Q
Splenotomy *see* Drainage, Lymphatic and Hemic Systems Ø79
Splinting, musculoskeletal *see* Immobilization, Anatomical Regions 2W3
SPRAVATO™ *use* Esketamine Hydrochloride
SPY PINPOINT fluorescence imaging system
see Monitoring, Physiological Systems 4A1
see Other Imaging, Hepatobiliary System and Pancreas BF5
SPY system intraoperative fluorescence cholangiography *see* Other Imaging, Hepatobiliary System and Pancreas BF5
SPY system intravascular fluorescence angiography *see* Monitoring, Physiological Systems 4A1
SSO2 (Supersaturated Oxygen) therapy, cardiac intra-arterial 5AØ222C
Staged hepatectomy
see Division, Hepatobiliary System and Pancreas ØF8
see Resection, Hepatobiliary System and Pancreas ØFT
Stapedectomy
see Excision, Ear, Nose, Sinus Ø9B
see Resection, Ear, Nose, Sinus Ø9T
Stapediolysis *see* Release, Ear, Nose, Sinus Ø9N
Stapedioplasty
see Repair, Ear, Nose, Sinus Ø9Q
see Replacement, Ear, Nose, Sinus Ø9R

Stapedioplasty — *continued*
see Supplement, Ear, Nose, Sinus Ø9U
Stapedotomy *see* Drainage, Ear, Nose, Sinus Ø99
Stapes
use Auditory Ossicle, Left
use Auditory Ossicle, Right
Static Spacer (Antibiotic) *use* Spacer in Lower Joints
STELARA® *use* Other New Technology Therapeutic Substance
Stellate ganglion *use* Head and Neck Sympathetic Nerve
Stem cell transplant *see* Transfusion, Circulatory 3Ø2
Stensen's duct
use Parotid Duct, Left
use Parotid Duct, Right
Stent, intraluminal (cardiovascular) (gastrointestinal) (hepatobiliary) (urinary) *use* Intraluminal Device
Stent retriever thrombectomy *see* Extirpation, Upper Arteries Ø3C
Stented tissue valve *use* Zooplastic Tissue in Heart and Great Vessels
Stereotactic Radiosurgery
Abdomen DW23
Adrenal Gland DG22
Bile Ducts DF22
Bladder DT22
Bone Marrow D72Ø
Brain DØ2Ø
Brain Stem DØ21
Breast
Left DM2Ø
Right DM21
Bronchus DB21
Cervix DU21
Chest DW22
Chest Wall DB27
Colon DD25
Diaphragm DB28
Duodenum DD22
Ear D92Ø
Esophagus DD2Ø
Eye D82Ø
Gallbladder DF21
Gamma Beam
Abdomen DW23JZZ
Adrenal Gland DG22JZZ
Bile Ducts DF22JZZ
Bladder DT22JZZ
Bone Marrow D72ØJZZ
Brain DØ2ØJZZ
Brain Stem DØ21JZZ
Breast
Left DM2ØJZZ
Right DM21JZZ
Bronchus DB21JZZ
Cervix DU21JZZ
Chest DW22JZZ
Chest Wall DB27JZZ
Colon DD25JZZ
Diaphragm DB28JZZ
Duodenum DD22JZZ
Ear D92ØJZZ
Esophagus DD2ØJZZ
Eye D82ØJZZ
Gallbladder DF21JZZ
Gland
Adrenal DG22JZZ
Parathyroid DG24JZZ
Pituitary DG2ØJZZ
Thyroid DG25JZZ
Glands, Salivary D926JZZ
Head and Neck DW21JZZ
Ileum DD24JZZ
Jejunum DD23JZZ
Kidney DT2ØJZZ
Larynx D92BJZZ
Liver DF2ØJZZ
Lung DB22JZZ
Lymphatics
Abdomen D726JZZ
Axillary D724JZZ
Inguinal D728JZZ
Neck D723JZZ
Pelvis D727JZZ
Thorax D725JZZ
Mediastinum DB26JZZ
Mouth D924JZZ

Stereotactic Radiosurgery — *continued*
  Gamma Beam — *continued*
    Nasopharynx D92DJZZ
    Neck and Head DW21JZZ
    Nerve, Peripheral D027JZZ
    Nose D921JZZ
    Ovary DU20JZZ
    Palate
      Hard D928JZZ
      Soft D929JZZ
    Pancreas DF23JZZ
    Parathyroid Gland DG24JZZ
    Pelvic Region DW26JZZ
    Pharynx D92CJZZ
    Pineal Body DG21JZZ
    Pituitary Gland DG20JZZ
    Pleura DB25JZZ
    Prostate DV20JZZ
    Rectum DD27JZZ
    Sinuses D927JZZ
    Spinal Cord D026JZZ
    Spleen D722JZZ
    Stomach DD21JZZ
    Testis DV21JZZ
    Thymus D721JZZ
    Thyroid Gland DG25JZZ
    Tongue D925JZZ
    Trachea DB20JZZ
    Ureter DT21JZZ
    Urethra DT23JZZ
    Uterus DU22JZZ
  Gland
    Adrenal DG22
    Parathyroid DG24
    Pituitary DG20
    Thyroid DG25
  Glands, Salivary D926
  Head and Neck DW21
  Ileum DD24
  Jejunum DD23
  Kidney DT20
  Larynx D92B
  Liver DF20
  Lung DB22
  Lymphatics
    Abdomen D726
    Axillary D724
    Inguinal D728
    Neck D723
    Pelvis D727
    Thorax D725
  Mediastinum DB26
  Mouth D924
  Nasopharynx D92D
  Neck and Head DW21
  Nerve, Peripheral D027
  Nose D921
  Other Photon
    Abdomen DW23DZZ
    Adrenal Gland DG22DZZ
    Bile Ducts DF22DZZ
    Bladder DT22DZZ
    Bone Marrow D720DZZ
    Brain D020DZZ
    Brain Stem D021DZZ
    Breast
      Left DM20DZZ
      Right DM21DZZ
    Bronchus DB21DZZ
    Cervix DU21DZZ
    Chest DW22DZZ
    Chest Wall DB27DZZ
    Colon DD25DZZ
    Diaphragm DB28DZZ
    Duodenum DD22DZZ
    Ear D920DZZ
    Esophagus DD20DZZ
    Eye D820DZZ
    Gallbladder DF21DZZ
    Gland
      Adrenal DG22DZZ
      Parathyroid DG24DZZ
      Pituitary DG20DZZ
      Thyroid DG25DZZ
    Glands, Salivary D926DZZ
    Head and Neck DW21DZZ
    Ileum DD24DZZ
    Jejunum DD23DZZ
    Kidney DT20DZZ

Stereotactic Radiosurgery — *continued*
  Other Photon — *continued*
    Larynx D92BDZZ
    Liver DF20DZZ
    Lung DB22DZZ
    Lymphatics
      Abdomen D726DZZ
      Axillary D724DZZ
      Inguinal D728DZZ
      Neck D723DZZ
      Pelvis D727DZZ
      Thorax D725DZZ
    Mediastinum DB26DZZ
    Mouth D924DZZ
    Nasopharynx D92DDZZ
    Neck and Head DW21DZZ
    Nerve, Peripheral D027DZZ
    Nose D921DZZ
    Ovary DU20DZZ
    Palate
      Hard D928DZZ
      Soft D929DZZ
    Pancreas DF23DZZ
    Parathyroid Gland DG24DZZ
    Pelvic Region DW26DZZ
    Pharynx D92CDZZ
    Pineal Body DG21DZZ
    Pituitary Gland DG20DZZ
    Pleura DB25DZZ
    Prostate DV20DZZ
    Rectum DD27DZZ
    Sinuses D927DZZ
    Spinal Cord D026DZZ
    Spleen D722DZZ
    Stomach DD21DZZ
    Testis DV21DZZ
    Thymus D721DZZ
    Thyroid Gland DG25DZZ
    Tongue D925DZZ
    Trachea DB20DZZ
    Ureter DT21DZZ
    Urethra DT23DZZ
    Uterus DU22DZZ
  Ovary DU20
  Palate
    Hard D928
    Soft D929
  Pancreas DF23
  Parathyroid Gland DG24
  Particulate
    Abdomen DW23HZZ
    Adrenal Gland DG22HZZ
    Bile Ducts DF22HZZ
    Bladder DT22HZZ
    Bone Marrow D720HZZ
    Brain D020HZZ
    Brain Stem D021HZZ
    Breast
      Left DM20HZZ
      Right DM21HZZ
    Bronchus DB21HZZ
    Cervix DU21HZZ
    Chest DW22HZZ
    Chest Wall DB27HZZ
    Colon DD25HZZ
    Diaphragm DB28HZZ
    Duodenum DD22HZZ
    Ear D920HZZ
    Esophagus DD20HZZ
    Eye D820HZZ
    Gallbladder DF21HZZ
    Gland
      Adrenal DG22HZZ
      Parathyroid DG24HZZ
      Pituitary DG20HZZ
      Thyroid DG25HZZ
    Glands, Salivary D926HZZ
    Head and Neck DW21HZZ
    Ileum DD24HZZ
    Jejunum DD23HZZ
    Kidney DT20HZZ
    Larynx D92BHZZ
    Liver DF20HZZ
    Lung DB22HZZ
    Lymphatics
      Abdomen D726HZZ
      Axillary D724HZZ
      Inguinal D728HZZ
      Neck D723HZZ

Stereotactic Radiosurgery — *continued*
  Particulate — *continued*
    Lymphatics — *continued*
      Pelvis D727HZZ
      Thorax D725HZZ
    Mediastinum DB26HZZ
    Mouth D924HZZ
    Nasopharynx D92DHZZ
    Neck and Head DW21HZZ
    Nerve, Peripheral D027HZZ
    Nose D921HZZ
    Ovary DU20HZZ
    Palate
      Hard D928HZZ
      Soft D929HZZ
    Pancreas DF23HZZ
    Parathyroid Gland DG24HZZ
    Pelvic Region DW26HZZ
    Pharynx D92CHZZ
    Pineal Body DG21HZZ
    Pituitary Gland DG20HZZ
    Pleura DB25HZZ
    Prostate DV20HZZ
    Rectum DD27HZZ
    Sinuses D927HZZ
    Spinal Cord D026HZZ
    Spleen D722HZZ
    Stomach DD21HZZ
    Testis DV21HZZ
    Thymus D721HZZ
    Thyroid Gland DG25HZZ
    Tongue D925HZZ
    Trachea DB20HZZ
    Ureter DT21HZZ
    Urethra DT23HZZ
    Uterus DU22HZZ
  Pelvic Region DW26
  Pharynx D92C
  Pineal Body DG21
  Pituitary Gland DG20
  Pleura DB25
  Prostate DV20
  Rectum DD27
  Sinuses D927
  Spinal Cord D026
  Spleen D722
  Stomach DD21
  Testis DV21
  Thymus D721
  Thyroid Gland DG25
  Tongue D925
  Trachea DB20
  Ureter DT21
  Urethra DT23
  Uterus DU22

Steripath® Micro™ Blood Collection System
  XXE5XR7

Sternoclavicular ligament
  use Shoulder Bursa and Ligament, Left
  use Shoulder Bursa and Ligament, Right

Sternocleidomastoid artery
  use Thyroid Artery, Left
  use Thyroid Artery, Right

Sternocleidomastoid muscle
  use Neck Muscle, Left
  use Neck Muscle, Right

Sternocostal ligament *use* Sternum Bursa and Ligament

Sternotomy
  see Division, Sternum 0P80
  see Drainage, Sternum 0P90

Stimulation, cardiac
  Cardioversion 5A2204Z
  Electrophysiologic testing *see* Measurement, Cardiac 4A02

Stimulator Generator
  Insertion of device in
    Abdomen 0JH8
    Back 0JH7
    Chest 0JH6
    Multiple Array
      Abdomen 0JH8
      Back 0JH7
      Chest 0JH6
    Multiple Array Rechargeable
      Abdomen 0JH8
      Back 0JH7
      Chest 0JH6

Stimulator Generator — *continued*
  Removal of device from, Subcutaneous Tissue and
    Fascia, Trunk ØJPT
  Revision of device in, Subcutaneous Tissue and
    Fascia, Trunk ØJWT
  Single Array
    Abdomen ØJH8
    Back ØJH7
    Chest ØJH6
  Single Array Rechargeable
    Abdomen ØJH8
    Back ØJH7
    Chest ØJH6
Stimulator Lead
  Insertion of device in
    Anal Sphincter ØDHR
    Artery
      Left Ø3HL
      Right Ø3HK
    Bladder ØTHB
    Muscle
      Lower ØKHY
      Upper ØKHX
    Stomach ØDH6
    Ureter ØTH9
  Removal of device from
    Anal Sphincter ØDPR
    Artery, Upper Ø3PY
    Bladder ØTPB
    Muscle
      Lower ØKPY
      Upper ØKPX
    Stomach ØDP6
    Ureter ØTP9
  Revision of device in
    Anal Sphincter ØDWR
    Artery, Upper Ø3WY
    Bladder ØTWB
    Muscle
      Lower ØKWY
      Upper ØKWX
    Stomach ØDW6
    Ureter ØTW9
Stoma
  Excision
    Abdominal Wall ØWBFXZ2
    Neck ØWB6XZ2
  Repair
    Abdominal Wall ØWQFXZ2
    Neck ØWQ6XZ2
Stomatoplasty
  see Repair, Mouth and Throat ØCQ
  see Replacement, Mouth and Throat ØCR
  see Supplement, Mouth and Throat ØCU
Stomatorrhaphy *see* Repair, Mouth and Throat ØCQ
StrataGraft® *use* Bioengineered Allogeneic Construct
Stratos LV *use* Cardiac Resynchronization Pacemaker
  Pulse Generator in ØJH
Stress test 4A02XM4, 4A12XM4
Stripping *see* Extraction
Study
  Electrophysiologic stimulation, cardiac *see* Measurement, Cardiac 4A02
  Ocular motility 4AØ7X7Z
  Pulmonary airway flow measurement *see* Measurement, Respiratory 4AØ9
  Visual acuity 4AØ7XØZ
Styloglossus muscle *use* Tongue, Palate, Pharynx
  Muscle
Stylomandibular ligament *use* Head and Neck Bursa
  and Ligament
Stylopharyngeus muscle *use* Tongue, Palate, Pharynx
  Muscle
Subacromial bursa
  use Shoulder Bursa and Ligament, Left
  use Shoulder Bursa and Ligament, Right
Subaortic (common iliac) lymph node *use* Lymphatic, Pelvis
Subarachnoid space, spinal *use* Spinal Canal
Subclavicular (apical) lymph node
  use Lymphatic, Left Axillary
  use Lymphatic, Right Axillary
Subclavius muscle
  use Thorax Muscle, Left
  use Thorax Muscle, Right
Subclavius nerve *use* Brachial Plexus
Subcostal artery *use* Upper Artery

Subcostal muscle
  use Thorax Muscle, Left
  use Thorax Muscle, Right
Subcostal nerve *use* Thoracic Nerve
Subcutaneous Defibrillator Lead
  Insertion of device in, Subcutaneous Tissue and
    Fascia, Chest ØJH6
  Removal of device from, Subcutaneous Tissue and
    Fascia, Trunk ØJPT
  Revision of device in, Subcutaneous Tissue and
    Fascia, Trunk ØJWT
Subcutaneous injection reservoir, port *use* Vascular
  Access Device, Totally Implantable in Subcutaneous Tissue and Fascia
Subcutaneous injection reservoir, pump *use* Infusion Device, Pump in Subcutaneous Tissue and
  Fascia
Subdermal progesterone implant *use* Contraceptive
  Device in Subcutaneous Tissue and Fascia
Subdural space, spinal *use* Spinal Canal
Submandibular ganglion
  use Facial Nerve
  use Head and Neck Sympathetic Nerve
Submandibular gland
  use Submaxillary Gland, Left
  use Submaxillary Gland, Right
Submandibular lymph node *use* Lymphatic, Head
Submandibular space *use* Subcutaneous Tissue and
  Fascia, Face
Submaxillary ganglion *use* Head and Neck Sympathetic Nerve
Submaxillary lymph node *use* Lymphatic, Head
Submental artery *use* Face Artery
Submental lymph node *use* Lymphatic, Head
Submucous (Meissner's) plexus *use* Abdominal
  Sympathetic Nerve
Suboccipital nerve *use* Cervical Nerve
Suboccipital venous plexus
  use Vertebral Vein, Left
  use Vertebral Vein, Right
Subparotid lymph node *use* Lymphatic, Head
Subscapular aponeurosis
  use Subcutaneous Tissue and Fascia, Left Upper
    Arm
  use Subcutaneous Tissue and Fascia, Right Upper
    Arm
Subscapular artery
  use Axillary Artery, Left
  use Axillary Artery, Right
Subscapular (posterior) lymph node
  use Lymphatic, Axillary, Left
  use Lymphatic, Axillary, Right
Subscapularis muscle
  use Shoulder Muscle, Left
  use Shoulder Muscle, Right
Substance Abuse Treatment
  Counseling
    Family, for substance abuse, Other Family
      Counseling HZ63ZZZ
    Group
      12-Step HZ43ZZZ
      Behavioral HZ41ZZZ
      Cognitive HZ40ZZZ
      Cognitive-Behavioral HZ42ZZZ
      Confrontational HZ48ZZZ
      Continuing Care HZ49ZZZ
      Infectious Disease
        Post-Test HZ4CZZZ
        Pre-Test HZ4CZZZ
      Interpersonal HZ44ZZZ
      Motivational Enhancement HZ47ZZZ
      Psychoeducation HZ46ZZZ
      Spiritual HZ4BZZZ
      Vocational HZ45ZZZ
    Individual
      12-Step HZ33ZZZ
      Behavioral HZ31ZZZ
      Cognitive HZ30ZZZ
      Cognitive-Behavioral HZ32ZZZ
      Confrontational HZ38ZZZ
      Continuing Care HZ39ZZZ
      Infectious Disease
        Post-Test HZ3CZZZ
        Pre-Test HZ3CZZZ
      Interpersonal HZ34ZZZ
      Motivational Enhancement HZ37ZZZ
      Psychoeducation HZ36ZZZ

Substance Abuse Treatment — *continued*
  Counseling — *continued*
    Individual — *continued*
      Spiritual HZ3BZZZ
      Vocational HZ35ZZZ
  Detoxification Services, for substance abuse
    HZ2ZZZZ
  Medication Management
    Antabuse HZ83ZZZ
    Bupropion HZ87ZZZ
    Clonidine HZ86ZZZ
    Levo-alpha-acetyl-methadol (LAAM)
      HZ82ZZZ
    Methadone Maintenance HZ81ZZZ
    Naloxone HZ85ZZZ
    Naltrexone HZ84ZZZ
    Nicotine Replacement HZ80ZZZ
    Other Replacement Medication HZ89ZZZ
    Psychiatric Medication HZ88ZZZ
  Pharmacotherapy
    Antabuse HZ93ZZZ
    Bupropion HZ97ZZZ
    Clonidine HZ96ZZZ
    Levo-alpha-acetyl-methadol (LAAM)
      HZ92ZZZ
    Methadone Maintenance HZ91ZZZ
    Naloxone HZ95ZZZ
    Naltrexone HZ94ZZZ
    Nicotine Replacement HZ90ZZZ
    Psychiatric Medication HZ98ZZZ
    Replacement Medication, Other HZ99ZZZ
  Psychotherapy
    12-Step HZ53ZZZ
    Behavioral HZ51ZZZ
    Cognitive HZ50ZZZ
    Cognitive-Behavioral HZ52ZZZ
    Confrontational HZ58ZZZ
    Interactive HZ55ZZZ
    Interpersonal HZ54ZZZ
    Motivational Enhancement HZ57ZZZ
    Psychoanalysis HZ5BZZZ
    Psychodynamic HZ5CZZZ
    Psychoeducation HZ56ZZZ
    Psychophysiological HZ5DZZZ
    Supportive HZ59ZZZ
Substantia nigra *use* Basal Ganglia
Subtalar (talocalcaneal) joint
  use Tarsal Joint, Left
  use Tarsal Joint, Right
Subtalar ligament
  use Foot Bursa and Ligament, Left
  use Foot Bursa and Ligament, Right
Subthalamic nucleus *use* Basal Ganglia
Suction curettage (D&C), nonobstetric *see* Extraction, Endometrium ØUDB
Suction curettage, obstetric post-delivery *see* Extraction, Products of Conception, Retained 1ØD1
Superficial circumflex iliac vein
  use Saphenous Vein, Left
  use Saphenous Vein, Right
Superficial epigastric artery
  use Femoral Artery, Left
  use Femoral Artery, Right
Superficial epigastric vein
  use Saphenous Vein, Left
  use Saphenous Vein, Right
Superficial Inferior Epigastric Artery Flap
  Replacement
    Bilateral ØHRVØ78
    Left ØHRUØ78
    Right ØHRTØ78
  Transfer
    Left ØKXG
    Right ØKXF
Superficial palmar arch
  use Hand Artery, Left
  use Hand Artery, Right
Superficial palmar venous arch
  use Hand Vein, Left
  use Hand Vein, Right
Superficial temporal artery
  use Temporal Artery, Left
  use Temporal Artery, Right
Superficial transverse perineal muscle *use* Perineum
  Muscle
Superior cardiac nerve *use* Thoracic Sympathetic
  Nerve
Superior cerebellar vein *use* Intracranial Vein

Superior cerebral vein *use* Intracranial Vein
Superior clunic (cluneal) nerve *use* Lumbar Nerve
Superior epigastric artery
    use Internal Mammary Artery, Left
    use Internal Mammary Artery, Right
Superior genicular artery
    use Popliteal Artery, Left
    use Popliteal Artery, Right
Superior gluteal artery
    use Internal Iliac Artery, Left
    use Internal Iliac Artery, Right
Superior gluteal nerve *use* Lumbar Plexus
Superior hypogastric plexus *use* Abdominal Sympathetic Nerve
Superior labial artery *use* Face Artery
Superior laryngeal artery
    use Thyroid Artery, Left
    use Thyroid Artery, Right
Superior laryngeal nerve *use* Vagus Nerve
Superior longitudinal muscle *use* Tongue, Palate, Pharynx Muscle
Superior mesenteric ganglion *use* Abdominal Sympathetic Nerve
Superior mesenteric lymph node *use* Lymphatic, Mesenteric
Superior mesenteric plexus *use* Abdominal Sympathetic Nerve
Superior oblique muscle
    use Extraocular Muscle, Left
    use Extraocular Muscle, Right
Superior olivary nucleus *use* Pons
Superior rectal artery *use* Inferior Mesenteric Artery
Superior rectal vein *use* Inferior Mesenteric Vein
Superior rectus muscle
    use Extraocular Muscle, Left
    use Extraocular Muscle, Right
Superior tarsal plate
    use Upper Eyelid, Left
    use Upper Eyelid, Right
Superior thoracic artery
    use Axillary Artery, Left
    use Axillary Artery, Right
Superior thyroid artery
    use External Carotid Artery, Left
    use External Carotid Artery, Right
    use Thyroid Artery, Left
    use Thyroid Artery, Right
Superior turbinate *use* Nasal Turbinate
Superior ulnar collateral artery
    use Brachial Artery, Left
    use Brachial Artery, Right
Superior vesical artery
    use Internal Iliac Artery, Left
    use Internal Iliac Artery, Right
Supersaturated Oxygen therapy 5A0512C, 5A0522C
Supersaturated Oxygen (SSO2) therapy, cardiac intra-arterial 5A0222C
Supplement
    Abdominal Wall 0WUF
    Acetabulum
        Left 0QU5
        Right 0QU4
    Ampulla of Vater 0FUC
    Anal Sphincter 0DUR
    Ankle Region
        Left 0YUL
        Right 0YUK
    Anus 0DUQ
    Aorta
        Abdominal 04U0
        Thoracic
            Ascending/Arch 02UX
            Descending 02UW
    Arm
        Lower
            Left 0XUF
            Right 0XUD
        Upper
            Left 0XU9
            Right 0XU8
    Artery
        Anterior Tibial
            Left 04UQ
            Right 04UP
        Axillary
            Left 03U6
            Right 03U5

Supplement — *continued*
    Artery — *continued*
        Brachial
            Left 03U8
            Right 03U7
        Celiac 04U1
        Colic
            Left 04U7
            Middle 04U8
            Right 04U6
        Common Carotid
            Left 03UJ
            Right 03UH
        Common Iliac
            Left 04UD
            Right 04UC
        Coronary
            Four or More Arteries 02U3
            One Artery 02U0
            Three Arteries 02U2
            Two Arteries 02U1
        External Carotid
            Left 03UN
            Right 03UM
        External Iliac
            Left 04UJ
            Right 04UH
        Face 03UR
        Femoral
            Left 04UL
            Right 04UK
        Foot
            Left 04UW
            Right 04UV
        Gastric 04U2
        Hand
            Left 03UF
            Right 03UD
        Hepatic 04U3
        Inferior Mesenteric 04UB
        Innominate 03U2
        Internal Carotid
            Left 03UL
            Right 03UK
        Internal Iliac
            Left 04UF
            Right 04UE
        Internal Mammary
            Left 03U1
            Right 03U0
        Intracranial 03UG
        Lower 04UY
        Peroneal
            Left 04UU
            Right 04UT
        Popliteal
            Left 04UN
            Right 04UM
        Posterior Tibial
            Left 04US
            Right 04UR
        Pulmonary
            Left 02UR
            Right 02UQ
        Pulmonary Trunk 02UP
        Radial
            Left 03UC
            Right 03UB
        Renal
            Left 04UA
            Right 04U9
        Splenic 04U4
        Subclavian
            Left 03U4
            Right 03U3
        Superior Mesenteric 04U5
        Temporal
            Left 03UT
            Right 03US
        Thyroid
            Left 03UV
            Right 03UU
        Ulnar
            Left 03UA
            Right 03U9
        Upper 03UY
        Vertebral
            Left 03UQ
            Right 03UP

Supplement — *continued*
    Atrium
        Left 02U7
        Right 02U6
    Auditory Ossicle
        Left 09UA
        Right 09U9
    Axilla
        Left 0XU5
        Right 0XU4
    Back
        Lower 0WUL
        Upper 0WUK
    Bladder 0TUB
    Bladder Neck 0TUC
    Bone
        Ethmoid
            Left 0NUG
            Right 0NUF
        Frontal 0NU1
        Hyoid 0NUX
        Lacrimal
            Left 0NUJ
            Right 0NUH
        Nasal 0NUB
        Occipital 0NU7
        Palatine
            Left 0NUL
            Right 0NUK
        Parietal
            Left 0NU4
            Right 0NU3
        Pelvic
            Left 0QU3
            Right 0QU2
        Sphenoid 0NUC
        Temporal
            Left 0NU6
            Right 0NU5
        Zygomatic
            Left 0NUN
            Right 0NUM
    Breast
        Bilateral 0HUV
        Left 0HUU
        Right 0HUT
    Bronchus
        Lingula 0BU9
        Lower Lobe
            Left 0BUB
            Right 0BU6
        Main
            Left 0BU7
            Right 0BU3
        Middle Lobe, Right 0BU5
        Upper Lobe
            Left 0BU8
            Right 0BU4
    Buccal Mucosa 0CU4
    Bursa and Ligament
        Abdomen
            Left 0MUJ
            Right 0MUH
        Ankle
            Left 0MUR
            Right 0MUQ
        Elbow
            Left 0MU4
            Right 0MU3
        Foot
            Left 0MUT
            Right 0MUS
        Hand
            Left 0MU8
            Right 0MU7
        Head and Neck 0MU0
        Hip
            Left 0MUM
            Right 0MUL
        Knee
            Left 0MUP
            Right 0MUN
        Lower Extremity
            Left 0MUW
            Right 0MUV
        Perineum 0MUK
        Rib(s) 0MUG
        Shoulder
            Left 0MU2

Supplement — *continued*
    Bursa and Ligament — *continued*
        Shoulder — *continued*
            Right ØMU1
        Spine
            Lower ØMUD
            Posterior Vertebral Tether XKU
            Upper ØMUC
        Sternum ØMUF
        Upper Extremity
            Left ØMUB
            Right ØMU9
        Wrist
            Left ØMU6
            Right ØMU5
    Buttock
        Left ØYU1
        Right ØYUØ
    Carina ØBU2
    Carpal
        Left ØPUN
        Right ØPUM
    Cecum ØDUH
    Cerebral Meninges ØØU1
    Cerebral Ventricle ØØU6
    Chest Wall ØWU8
    Chordae Tendineae Ø2U9
    Cisterna Chyli Ø7UL
    Clavicle
        Left ØPUB
        Right ØPU9
    Clitoris ØUUJ
    Coccyx ØQUS
    Colon
        Ascending ØDUK
        Descending ØDUM
        Sigmoid ØDUN
        Transverse ØDUL
    Cord
        Bilateral ØVUH
        Left ØVUG
        Right ØVUF
    Cornea
        Left Ø8U9
        Right Ø8U8
    Cul-de-sac ØUUF
    Diaphragm ØBUT
    Disc
        Cervical Vertebral ØRU3
        Cervicothoracic Vertebral ØRU5
        Lumbar Vertebral ØSU2
        Lumbosacral ØSU4
        Thoracic Vertebral ØRU9
        Thoracolumbar Vertebral ØRUB
    Duct
        Common Bile ØFU9
        Cystic ØFU8
        Hepatic
            Common ØFU7
            Left ØFU6
            Right ØFU5
        Lacrimal
            Left Ø8UY
            Right Ø8UX
        Pancreatic ØFUD
            Accessory ØFUF
    Duodenum ØDU9
    Dura Mater ØØU2
    Ear
        External
            Bilateral Ø9U2
            Left Ø9U1
            Right Ø9UØ
        Inner
            Left Ø9UE
            Right Ø9UD
        Middle
            Left Ø9U6
            Right Ø9U5
    Elbow Region
        Left ØXUC
        Right ØXUB
    Epididymis
        Bilateral ØVUL
        Left ØVUK
        Right ØVUJ
    Epiglottis ØCUR
    Esophagogastric Junction ØDU4
    Esophagus ØDU5

Supplement — *continued*
    Esophagus — *continued*
        Lower ØDU3
        Middle ØDU2
        Upper ØDU1
    Extremity
        Lower
            Left ØYUB
            Right ØYU9
        Upper
            Left ØXU7
            Right ØXU6
    Eye
        Left Ø8U1
        Right Ø8UØ
    Eyelid
        Lower
            Left Ø8UR
            Right Ø8UQ
        Upper
            Left Ø8UP
            Right Ø8UN
    Face ØWU2
    Fallopian Tube
        Left ØUU6
        Right ØUU5
    Fallopian Tubes, Bilateral ØUU7
    Femoral Region
        Bilateral ØYUE
        Left ØYU8
        Right ØYU7
    Femoral Shaft
        Left ØQU9
        Right ØQU8
    Femur
        Lower
            Left ØQUC
            Right ØQUB
        Upper
            Left ØQU7
            Right ØQU6
    Fibula
        Left ØQUK
        Right ØQUJ
    Finger
        Index
            Left ØXUP
            Right ØXUN
        Little
            Left ØXUW
            Right ØXUV
        Middle
            Left ØXUR
            Right ØXUQ
        Ring
            Left ØXUT
            Right ØXUS
    Foot
        Left ØYUN
        Right ØYUM
    Gingiva
        Lower ØCU6
        Upper ØCU5
    Glenoid Cavity
        Left ØPU8
        Right ØPU7
    Hand
        Left ØXUK
        Right ØXUJ
    Head ØWUØ
    Heart Ø2UA
    Humeral Head
        Left ØPUD
        Right ØPUC
    Humeral Shaft
        Left ØPUG
        Right ØPUF
    Hymen ØUUK
    Ileocecal Valve ØDUC
    Ileum ØDUB
    Inguinal Region
        Bilateral ØYUA
        Left ØYU6
        Right ØYU5
    Intestine
        Large ØDUE
            Left ØDUG
            Right ØDUF
        Small ØDU8

Supplement — *continued*
    Iris
        Left Ø8UD
        Right Ø8UC
    Jaw
        Lower ØWU5
        Upper ØWU4
    Jejunum ØDUA
    Joint
        Acromioclavicular
            Left ØRUH
            Right ØRUG
        Ankle
            Left ØSUG
            Right ØSUF
        Carpal
            Left ØRUR
            Right ØRUQ
        Carpometacarpal
            Left ØRUT
            Right ØRUS
        Cervical Vertebral ØRU1
        Cervicothoracic Vertebral ØRU4
        Coccygeal ØSU6
        Elbow
            Left ØRUM
            Right ØRUL
        Finger Phalangeal
            Left ØRUX
            Right ØRUW
        Hip
            Left ØSUB
                Acetabular Surface ØSUE
                Femoral Surface ØSUS
            Right ØSU9
                Acetabular Surface ØSUA
                Femoral Surface ØSUR
        Knee
            Left ØSUD
                Femoral Surface ØSUUØ9Z
                Tibial Surface ØSUWØ9Z
            Right ØSUC
                Femoral Surface ØSUTØ9Z
                Tibial Surface ØSUVØ9Z
        Lumbar Vertebral ØSUØ
        Lumbosacral ØSU3
        Metacarpophalangeal
            Left ØRUV
            Right ØRUU
        Metatarsal-Phalangeal
            Left ØSUN
            Right ØSUM
        Occipital-cervical ØRUØ
        Sacrococcygeal ØSU5
        Sacroiliac
            Left ØSU8
            Right ØSU7
        Shoulder
            Left ØRUK
            Right ØRUJ
        Sternoclavicular
            Left ØRUF
            Right ØRUE
        Tarsal
            Left ØSUJ
            Right ØSUH
        Tarsometatarsal
            Left ØSUL
            Right ØSUK
        Temporomandibular
            Left ØRUD
            Right ØRUC
        Thoracic Vertebral ØRU6
        Thoracolumbar Vertebral ØRUA
        Toe Phalangeal
            Left ØSUQ
            Right ØSUP
        Wrist
            Left ØRUP
            Right ØRUN
    Kidney Pelvis
        Left ØTU4
        Right ØTU3
    Knee Region
        Left ØYUG
        Right ØYUF
    Larynx ØCUS

Supplement — *continued*
Leg
  Lower
    Left ØYUJ
    Right ØYUH
  Upper
    Left ØYUD
    Right ØYUC
Lip
  Lower ØCU1
  Upper ØCUØ
Lymphatic
  Aortic Ø7UD
  Axillary
    Left Ø7U6
    Right Ø7U5
  Head Ø7UØ
  Inguinal
    Left Ø7UJ
    Right Ø7UH
  Internal Mammary
    Left Ø7U9
    Right Ø7U8
  Lower Extremity
    Left Ø7UG
    Right Ø7UF
  Mesenteric Ø7UB
  Neck
    Left Ø7U2
    Right Ø7U1
  Pelvis Ø7UC
  Thoracic Duct Ø7UK
  Thorax Ø7U7
  Upper Extremity
    Left Ø7U4
    Right Ø7U3
Mandible
  Left ØNUV
  Right ØNUT
Maxilla ØNUR
Mediastinum ØWUC
Mesentery ØDUV
Metacarpal
  Left ØPUQ
  Right ØPUP
Metatarsal
  Left ØQUP
  Right ØQUN
Muscle
  Abdomen
    Left ØKUL
    Right ØKUK
  Extraocular
    Left Ø8UM
    Right Ø8UL
  Facial ØKU1
  Foot
    Left ØKUW
    Right ØKUV
  Hand
    Left ØKUD
    Right ØKUC
  Head ØKUØ
  Hip
    Left ØKUP
    Right ØKUN
  Lower Arm and Wrist
    Left ØKUB
    Right ØKU9
  Lower Leg
    Left ØKUT
    Right ØKUS
  Neck
    Left ØKU3
    Right ØKU2
  Papillary Ø2UD
  Perineum ØKUM
  Shoulder
    Left ØKU6
    Right ØKU5
  Thorax
    Left ØKUJ
    Right ØKUH
  Tongue, Palate, Pharynx ØKU4
  Trunk
    Left ØKUG
    Right ØKUF
  Upper Arm
    Left ØKU8

Supplement — *continued*
Muscle — *continued*
  Upper Arm — *continued*
    Right ØKU7
  Upper Leg
    Left ØKUR
    Right ØKUQ
Nasal Mucosa and Soft Tissue Ø9UK
Nasopharynx Ø9UN
Neck ØWU6
Nerve
  Abducens ØØUL
  Accessory ØØUR
  Acoustic ØØUN
  Cervical Ø1U1
  Facial ØØUM
  Femoral Ø1UD
  Glossopharyngeal ØØUP
  Hypoglossal ØØUS
  Lumbar Ø1UB
  Median Ø1U5
  Oculomotor ØØUH
  Olfactory ØØUF
  Optic ØØUG
  Peroneal Ø1UH
  Phrenic Ø1U2
  Pudendal Ø1UC
  Radial Ø1U6
  Sacral Ø1UR
  Sciatic Ø1UF
  Thoracic Ø1U8
  Tibial Ø1UG
  Trigeminal ØØUK
  Trochlear ØØUJ
  Ulnar Ø1U4
  Vagus ØØUQ
Nipple
  Left ØHUX
  Right ØHUW
Omentum ØDUU
Orbit
  Left ØNUQ
  Right ØNUP
Palate
  Hard ØCU2
  Soft ØCU3
Patella
  Left ØQUF
  Right ØQUD
Penis ØVUS
Pericardium Ø2UN
Perineum
  Female ØWUN
  Male ØWUM
Peritoneum ØDUW
Phalanx
  Finger
    Left ØPUV
    Right ØPUT
  Thumb
    Left ØPUS
    Right ØPUR
  Toe
    Left ØQUR
    Right ØQUQ
Pharynx ØCUM
Prepuce ØVUT
Radius
  Left ØPUJ
  Right ØPUH
Rectum ØDUP
Retina
  Left Ø8UF
  Right Ø8UE
Retinal Vessel
  Left Ø8UH
  Right Ø8UG
Ribs
  1 to 2 ØPU1
  3 or More ØPU2
Sacrum ØQU1
Scapula
  Left ØPU6
  Right ØPU5
Scrotum ØVU5
Septum
  Atrial Ø2U5
  Nasal Ø9UM
  Ventricular Ø2UM

Supplement — *continued*
Shoulder Region
  Left ØXU3
  Right ØXU2
Sinus
  Accessory Ø9UP
  Ethmoid
    Left Ø9UV
    Right Ø9UU
  Frontal
    Left Ø9UT
    Right Ø9US
  Mastoid
    Left Ø9UC
    Right Ø9UB
  Maxillary
    Left Ø9UR
    Right Ø9UQ
  Sphenoid
    Left Ø9UX
    Right Ø9UW
Skull ØNUØ
Spinal Meninges ØØUT
Sternum ØPUØ
Stomach ØDU6
  Pylorus ØDU7
Subcutaneous Tissue and Fascia
  Abdomen ØJU8
  Back ØJU7
  Buttock ØJU9
  Chest ØJU6
  Face ØJU1
  Foot
    Left ØJUR
    Right ØJUQ
  Hand
    Left ØJUK
    Right ØJUJ
  Lower Arm
    Left ØJUH
    Right ØJUG
  Lower Leg
    Left ØJUP
    Right ØJUN
  Neck
    Left ØJU5
    Right ØJU4
  Pelvic Region ØJUC
  Perineum ØJUB
  Scalp ØJUØ
  Upper Arm
    Left ØJUF
    Right ØJUD
  Upper Leg
    Left ØJUM
    Right ØJUL
Tarsal
  Left ØQUM
  Right ØQUL
Tendon
  Abdomen
    Left ØLUG
    Right ØLUF
  Ankle
    Left ØLUT
    Right ØLUS
  Foot
    Left ØLUW
    Right ØLUV
  Hand
    Left ØLU8
    Right ØLU7
  Head and Neck ØLUØ
  Hip
    Left ØLUK
    Right ØLUJ
  Knee
    Left ØLUR
    Right ØLUQ
  Lower Arm and Wrist
    Left ØLU6
    Right ØLU5
  Lower Leg
    Left ØLUP
    Right ØLUN
  Perineum ØLUH
  Shoulder
    Left ØLU2
    Right ØLU1

Supplement — *continued*
  Tendon — *continued*
    Thorax
      Left 0LUD
      Right 0LUC
    Trunk
      Left 0LUB
      Right 0LU9
    Upper Arm
      Left 0LU4
      Right 0LU3
    Upper Leg
      Left 0LUM
      Right 0LUL
  Testis
    Bilateral 0VUC0
    Left 0VUB0
    Right 0VU90
  Thumb
    Left 0XUM
    Right 0XUL
  Tibia
    Left 0QUH
    Right 0QUG
  Toe
    1st
      Left 0YUQ
      Right 0YUP
    2nd
      Left 0YUS
      Right 0YUR
    3rd
      Left 0YUU
      Right 0YUT
    4th
      Left 0YUW
      Right 0YUV
    5th
      Left 0YUY
      Right 0YUX
  Tongue 0CU7
  Trachea 0BU1
  Tunica Vaginalis
    Left 0VU7
    Right 0VU6
  Turbinate, Nasal 09UL
  Tympanic Membrane
    Left 09U8
    Right 09U7
  Ulna
    Left 0PUL
    Right 0PUK
  Ureter
    Left 0TU7
    Right 0TU6
  Urethra 0TUD
  Uterine Supporting Structure 0UU4
  Uvula 0CUN
  Vagina 0UUG
  Valve
    Aortic 02UF
    Mitral 02UG
    Pulmonary 02UH
    Tricuspid 02UJ
  Vas Deferens
    Bilateral 0VUQ
    Left 0VUP
    Right 0VUN
  Vein
    Axillary
      Left 05U8
      Right 05U7
    Azygos 05U0
    Basilic
      Left 05UC
      Right 05UB
    Brachial
      Left 05UA
      Right 05U9
    Cephalic
      Left 05UF
      Right 05UD
    Colic 06U7
    Common Iliac
      Left 06UD
      Right 06UC
    Esophageal 06U3
    External Iliac
      Left 06UG

Supplement — *continued*
  Vein — *continued*
    External Iliac — *continued*
      Right 06UF
    External Jugular
      Left 05UQ
      Right 05UP
    Face
      Left 05UV
      Right 05UT
    Femoral
      Left 06UN
      Right 06UM
    Foot
      Left 06UV
      Right 06UT
    Gastric 06U2
    Hand
      Left 05UH
      Right 05UG
    Hemiazygos 05U1
    Hepatic 06U4
    Hypogastric
      Left 06UJ
      Right 06UH
    Inferior Mesenteric 06U6
    Innominate
      Left 05U4
      Right 05U3
    Internal Jugular
      Left 05UN
      Right 05UM
    Intracranial 05UL
    Lower 06UY
    Portal 06U8
    Pulmonary
      Left 02UT
      Right 02US
    Renal
      Left 06UB
      Right 06U9
    Saphenous
      Left 06UQ
      Right 06UP
    Splenic 06U1
    Subclavian
      Left 05U6
      Right 05U5
    Superior Mesenteric 06U5
    Upper 05UY
    Vertebral
      Left 05US
      Right 05UR
  Vena Cava
    Inferior 06U0
    Superior 02UV
  Ventricle
    Left 02UL
    Right 02UK
  Vertebra
    Cervical 0PU3
    Lumbar 0QU0
      Mechanically Expandable (Paired) Synthetic Substitute XNU0356
    Thoracic 0PU4
      Mechanically Expandable (Paired) Synthetic Substitute XNU4356
  Vesicle
    Bilateral 0VU3
    Left 0VU2
    Right 0VU1
  Vocal Cord
    Left 0CUV
    Right 0CUT
  Vulva 0UUM
  Wrist Region
    Left 0XUH
    Right 0XUG
Supraclavicular (Virchow's) lymph node
  use Lymphatic, Left Neck
  use Lymphatic, Right Neck
Supraclavicular nerve *use* Cervical Plexus
Suprahyoid lymph node *use* Lymphatic, Head
Suprahyoid muscle
  use Neck Muscle, Left
  use Neck Muscle, Right
Suprainguinal lymph node *use* Lymphatic, Pelvis

Supraorbital vein
  use Face Vein, Left
  use Face Vein, Right
Suprarenal gland
  use Adrenal Gland
  use Adrenal Gland, Bilateral
  use Adrenal Gland, Left
  use Adrenal Gland, Right
Suprarenal plexus *use* Abdominal Sympathetic Nerve
Suprascapular nerve *use* Brachial Plexus
Supraspinatus fascia
  use Subcutaneous Tissue and Fascia, Left Upper Arm
  use Subcutaneous Tissue and Fascia, Right Upper Arm
Supraspinatus muscle
  use Shoulder Muscle, Left
  use Shoulder Muscle, Right
Supraspinous ligament
  use Lower Spine Bursa and Ligament
  use Upper Spine Bursa and Ligament
Suprasternal notch *use* Sternum
Supratrochlear lymph node
  use Lymphatic, Left Upper Extremity
  use Lymphatic, Right Upper Extremity
Sural artery
  use Popliteal Artery, Left
  use Popliteal Artery, Right
Surpass Streamline™ Flow Diverter *use* Intraluminal Device, Flow Diverter in 03V
Suspension
  Bladder Neck *see* Reposition, Bladder Neck 0TSC
  Kidney *see* Reposition, Urinary System 0TS
  Urethra *see* Reposition, Urinary System 0TS
  Urethrovesical *see* Reposition, Bladder Neck 0TSC
  Uterus *see* Reposition, Uterus 0US9
  Vagina *see* Reposition, Vagina 0USG
Sustained Release Drug-eluting Intraluminal Device
  Dilation
    Anterior Tibial
      Left X27Q385
      Right X27P385
    Femoral
      Left X27J385
      Right X27H385
    Peroneal
      Left X27U385
      Right X27T385
    Popliteal
      Left Distal X27N385
      Left Proximal X27L385
      Right Distal X27M385
      Right Proximal X27K385
    Posterior Tibial
      Left X27S385
      Right X27R385
  Four or More
    Anterior Tibial
      Left X27Q3C5
      Right X27P3C5
    Femoral
      Left X27J3C5
      Right X27H3C5
    Peroneal
      Left X27U3C5
      Right X27T3C5
    Popliteal
      Left Distal X27N3C5
      Left Proximal X27L3C5
      Right Distal X27M3C5
      Right Proximal X27K3C5
    Posterior Tibial
      Left X27S3C5
      Right X27R3C5
  Three
    Anterior Tibial
      Left X27Q3B5
      Right X27P3B5
    Femoral
      Left X27J3B5
      Right X27H3B5
    Peroneal
      Left X27U3B5
      Right X27T3B5
    Popliteal
      Left Distal X27N3B5
      Left Proximal X27L3B5

Subterms under main terms may continue to next column or page

Sustained Release Drug-eluting Intraluminal Device
— *continued*
Three — *continued*
Popliteal — *continued*
Right Distal X27M3B5
Right Proximal X27K3B5
Posterior Tibial
Left X27S3B5
Right X27R3B5
Two
Anterior Tibial
Left X27Q395
Right X27P395
Femoral
Left X27J395
Right X27H395
Peroneal
Left X27U395
Right X27T395
Popliteal
Left Distal X27N395
Left Proximal X27L395
Right Distal X27M395
Right Proximal X27K395
Posterior Tibial
Left X27S395
Right X27R395
Suture
Laceration repair *see* Repair
Ligation *see* Occlusion
Suture Removal
Extremity
Lower 8E0YXY8
Upper 8E0XXY8
Head and Neck Region 8E09XY8
Trunk Region 8E0WXY8
Sutureless valve, Perceval (rapid deployment technique) *see* Replacement, Valve, Aortic 02RF
Sweat gland *use* Skin
Sympathectomy *see* Excision, Peripheral Nervous System 01B
SynCardia (temporary) total artificial heart (TAH) *use* Synthetic Substitute, Pneumatic in 02R
SynCardia Total Artificial Heart *use* Synthetic Substitute
Synchra CRT-P *use* Cardiac Resynchronization Pacemaker Pulse Generator in 0JH
SynchroMed pump *use* Infusion Device, Pump in Subcutaneous Tissue and Fascia
Synechiotomy, iris *see* Release, Eye 08N
Synovectomy
Lower joint *see* Excision, Lower Joints 0SB
Upper joint *see* Excision, Upper Joints 0RB
Synthetic Human Angiotensin II XW0
Systemic Nuclear Medicine Therapy
Abdomen CW70
Anatomical Regions, Multiple CW7YYZZ
Chest CW73
Thyroid CW7G
Whole Body CW7N

T

tab-cel® *use* Tabelecleucel Immunotherapy
Tabelecleucel Immunotherapy XW0
Tagraxofusp-erzs Antineoplastic XW0
Takedown
Arteriovenous shunt *see* Removal of device from, Upper Arteries 03P
Arteriovenous shunt, with creation of new shunt *see* Bypass, Upper Arteries 031
Stoma
see Excision
see Reposition
Talent® Converter *use* Intraluminal Device
Talent® Occluder *use* Intraluminal Device
Talent® Stent Graft (abdominal) (thoracic) *use* Intraluminal Device
Talocalcaneal (subtalar) joint
use Tarsal Joint, Left
use Tarsal Joint, Right
Talocalcaneal ligament
use Foot Bursa and Ligament, Left
use Foot Bursa and Ligament, Right
Talocalcaneonavicular joint
use Tarsal Joint, Left
use Tarsal Joint, Right

Talocalcaneonavicular ligament
use Foot Bursa and Ligament, Left
use Foot Bursa and Ligament, Right
Talocrural joint
use Ankle Joint, Left
use Joint, Ankle, Right
Talofibular ligament
use Ankle Bursa and Ligament, Left
use Ankle Bursa and Ligament, Right
Talus bone
use Tarsal, Left
use Tarsal, Right
TandemHeart® System *use* Short-term External Heart Assist System in Heart and Great Vessels
Tarsectomy
see Excision, Lower Bones 0QB
see Resection, Lower Bones 0QT
Tarsometatarsal ligament
use Foot Bursa and Ligament, Left
use Foot Bursa and Ligament, Right
Tarsorrhaphy *see* Repair, Eye 08Q
Tattooing
Cornea 3E0CXMZ
Skin *see* Introduction of substance in or on, Skin 3E00
Taurolidine Anti-infective and Heparin Anticoagulant XY0YX28
TAXUS® Liberte® Paclitaxel-eluting Coronary Stent System *use* Intraluminal Device, Drug-eluting in Heart and Great Vessels
TBNA (transbronchial needle aspiration)
Fluid or gas *see* Drainage, Respiratory System 0B9
Tissue biopsy *see* Extraction, Respiratory System 0BD
Tecartus™ *use* Brexucabtagene Autoleucel Immunotherapy
TECENTRIQ® *use* Atezolizumab Antineoplastic
Teclistamab Antineoplastic XW01348
Telemetry 4A12X4Z
Ambulatory 4A12X45
Temperature gradient study 4A0ZXKZ
Temporal lobe *use* Cerebral Hemisphere
Temporalis muscle *use* Head Muscle
Temporoparietalis muscle *use* Head Muscle
Tendolysis *see* Release, Tendons 0LN
Tendonectomy
see Excision, Tendons 0LB
see Resection, Tendons 0LT
Tendonoplasty, tenoplasty
see Repair, Tendons 0LQ
see Replacement, Tendons 0LR
see Supplement, Tendons 0LU
Tendorrhaphy *see* Repair, Tendons 0LQ
Tendototomy
see Division, Tendons 0L8
see Drainage, Tendons 0L9
Tenectomy, tenonectomy
see Excision, Tendons 0LB
see Resection, Tendons 0LT
Tenolysis *see* Release, Tendons 0LN
Tenontorrhaphy *see* Repair, Tendons 0LQ
Tenontotomy
see Division, Tendons 0L8
see Drainage, Tendons 0L9
Tenorrhaphy *see* Repair, Tendons 0LQ
Tenosynovectomy
see Excision, Tendons 0LB
see Resection, Tendons 0LT
Tenotomy
see Division, Tendons 0L8
see Drainage, Tendons 0L9
Tensor fasciae latae muscle
use Hip Muscle, Left
use Hip Muscle, Right
Tensor veli palatini muscle *use* Tongue, Palate, Pharynx Muscle
Tenth cranial nerve *use* Vagus Nerve
Tentorium cerebelli *use* Dura Mater
Teres major muscle
use Shoulder Muscle, Left
use Shoulder Muscle, Right
Teres minor muscle
use Shoulder Muscle, Left
use Shoulder Muscle, Right
Terlipressin XW0
TERLIVAZ® *use* Terlipressin

Termination of pregnancy
Aspiration curettage 10A07ZZ
Dilation and curettage 10A07ZZ
Hysterotomy 10A00ZZ
Intra-amniotic injection 10A03ZZ
Laminaria 10A07ZW
Vacuum 10A07Z6
Testectomy
see Excision, Male Reproductive System 0VB
see Resection, Male Reproductive System 0VT
Testicular artery *use* Abdominal Aorta
Testing
Glaucoma 4A07XBZ
Hearing *see* Hearing Assessment, Diagnostic Audiology F13
Mental health *see* Psychological Tests
Muscle function, electromyography (EMG) *see* Measurement, Musculoskeletal 4A0F
Muscle function, manual *see* Motor Function Assessment, Rehabilitation F01
Neurophysiologic monitoring, intra-operative *see* Monitoring, Physiological Systems 4A1
Range of motion *see* Motor Function Assessment, Rehabilitation F01
Vestibular function *see* Vestibular Assessment, Diagnostic Audiology F15
Thalamectomy *see* Excision, Thalamus 00B9
Thalamotomy *see* Drainage, Thalamus 0099
Thenar muscle
use Hand Muscle, Left
use Hand Muscle, Right
Therapeutic Massage
Musculoskeletal System 8E0KX1Z
Reproductive System
Prostate 8E0VX1C
Rectum 8E0VX1D
Therapeutic occlusion coil(s) *use* Intraluminal Device
Thermography 4A0ZXKZ
Thermotherapy, prostate *see* Destruction, Prostate 0V50
Third cranial nerve *use* Oculomotor Nerve
Third occipital nerve *use* Cervical Nerve
Third ventricle *use* Cerebral Ventricle
Thoracectomy *see* Excision, Anatomical Regions, General 0WB
Thoracentesis *see* Drainage, Anatomical Regions, General 0W9
Thoracic aortic plexus *use* Thoracic Sympathetic Nerve
Thoracic esophagus *use* Esophagus, Middle
Thoracic facet joint *use* Thoracic Vertebral Joint
Thoracic ganglion *use* Thoracic Sympathetic Nerve
Thoracoacromial artery
use Axillary Artery, Left
use Axillary Artery, Right
Thoracocentesis *see* Drainage, Anatomical Regions, General 0W9
Thoracolumbar facet joint *use* Thoracolumbar Vertebral Joint
Thoracoplasty
see Repair, Anatomical Regions, General 0WQ
see Supplement, Anatomical Regions, General 0WU
Thoracostomy, for lung collapse *see* Drainage, Respiratory System 0B9
Thoracostomy tube *use* Drainage Device
Thoracotomy *see* Drainage, Anatomical Regions, General 0W9
Thoraflex™ Hybrid device *use* Branched Synthetic Substitute with Intraluminal Device in New Technology
Thoratec IVAD (Implantable Ventricular Assist Device) *use* Implantable Heart Assist System in Heart and Great Vessels
Thoratec Paracorporeal Ventricular Assist Device *use* Short-term External Heart Assist System in Heart and Great Vessels
Thrombectomy *see* Extirpation
Thrombolysis, Ultrasound assisted *see* Fragmentation, Artery
Thymectomy
see Excision, Lymphatic and Hemic Systems 07B
see Resection, Lymphatic and Hemic Systems 07T
Thymopexy
see Repair, Lymphatic and Hemic Systems 07Q
see Reposition, Lymphatic and Hemic Systems 07S
Thymus gland *use* Thymus
Thyroarytenoid muscle
use Neck Muscle, Left

Thyroarytenoid muscle — *continued*
  use Neck Muscle, Right
Thyrocervical trunk
  use Thyroid Artery, Left
  use Thyroid Artery, Right
Thyroid cartilage *use* Larynx
Thyroidectomy
  see Excision, Endocrine System ØGB
  see Resection, Endocrine System ØGT
Thyroidorrhaphy *see* Repair, Endocrine System ØGQ
Thyroidoscopy ØGJK4ZZ
Thyroidotomy *see* Drainage, Endocrine System ØG9
Tibial insert *use* Liner in Lower Joints
Tibial sesamoid
  use Metatarsal, Left
  use Metatarsal, Right
Tibialis anterior muscle
  use Lower Leg Muscle, Left
  use Lower Leg Muscle, Right
Tibialis posterior muscle
  use Lower Leg Muscle, Left
  use Lower Leg Muscle, Right
Tibiofemoral joint
  use Knee Joint, Left
  use Knee Joint, Right
  use Knee Joint, Tibial Surface, Left
  use Knee Joint, Tibial Surface, Right
Tibioperoneal trunk
  use Popliteal Artery, Left
  use Popliteal Artery, Right
Tisagenlecleucel *use* Tisagenlecleucel Immunotherapy
Tisagenlecleucel Immunotherapy XWØ
Tissue bank graft *use* Nonautologous Tissue Substitute
Tissue expander (inflatable) (injectable)
  use Tissue Expander in Skin and Breast
  use Tissue Expander in Subcutaneous Tissue and Fascia
Tissue Expander
  Insertion of device in
    Breast
      Bilateral ØHHV
      Left ØHHU
      Right ØHHT
    Nipple
      Left ØHHX
      Right ØHHW
    Subcutaneous Tissue and Fascia
      Abdomen ØJH8
      Back ØJH7
      Buttock ØJH9
      Chest ØJH6
      Face ØJH1
      Foot
        Left ØJHR
        Right ØJHQ
      Hand
        Left ØJHK
        Right ØJHJ
      Lower Arm
        Left ØJHH
        Right ØJHG
      Lower Leg
        Left ØJHP
        Right ØJHN
      Neck
        Left ØJH5
        Right ØJH4
      Pelvic Region ØJHC
      Perineum ØJHB
      Scalp ØJHØ
      Upper Arm
        Left ØJHF
        Right ØJHD
      Upper Leg
        Left ØJHM
        Right ØJHL
  Removal of device from
    Breast
      Left ØHPU
      Right ØHPT
    Subcutaneous Tissue and Fascia
      Head and Neck ØJPS
      Lower Extremity ØJPW
      Trunk ØJPT
      Upper Extremity ØJPV
  Revision of device in
    Breast
      Left ØHWU

Tissue Expander — *continued*
  Revision of device in — *continued*
    Breast — *continued*
      Right ØHWT
    Subcutaneous Tissue and Fascia
      Head and Neck ØJWS
      Lower Extremity ØJWW
      Trunk ØJWT
      Upper Extremity ØJWV
Tissue Plasminogen Activator (tPA) (r-tPA) *use* Other Thrombolytic
Titan Endoskeleton™
  use Interbody Fusion Device in Lower Joints
  use Interbody Fusion Device in Upper Joints
Titanium Sternal Fixation System (TSFS)
  use Internal Fixation Device, Rigid Plate in ØPS
  use Internal Fixation Device, Rigid Plate in ØPH
Tixagevimab and Cilgavimab Monoclonal Antibody XWØ23X7
Tocilizumab XWØ
Tomographic (Tomo) Nuclear Medicine Imaging
  Abdomen CW2Ø
  Abdomen and Chest CW24
  Abdomen and Pelvis CW21
  Anatomical Regions, Multiple CW2YYZZ
  Bladder, Kidneys and Ureters CT23
  Brain CØ2Ø
  Breast CH2YYZZ
    Bilateral CH22
    Left CH21
    Right CH2Ø
  Bronchi and Lungs CB22
  Central Nervous System CØ2YYZZ
  Cerebrospinal Fluid CØ25
  Chest CW23
  Chest and Abdomen CW24
  Chest and Neck CW26
  Digestive System CD2YYZZ
  Endocrine System CG2YYZZ
  Extremity
    Lower CW2D
      Bilateral CP2F
      Left CP2D
      Right CP2C
    Upper CW2M
      Bilateral CP2B
      Left CP29
      Right CP28
  Gallbladder CF24
  Gastrointestinal Tract CD27
  Gland, Parathyroid CG21
  Head and Neck CW2B
  Heart C22YYZZ
    Right and Left C226
  Hepatobiliary System and Pancreas CF2YYZZ
  Kidneys, Ureters and Bladder CT23
  Liver CF25
  Liver and Spleen CF26
  Lungs and Bronchi CB22
  Lymphatics and Hematologic System C72YYZZ
  Musculoskeletal System, Other CP2YYZZ
  Myocardium C22G
  Neck and Chest CW26
  Neck and Head CW2B
  Pancreas and Hepatobiliary System CF2YYZZ
  Pelvic Region CW2J
  Pelvis CP26
  Pelvis and Abdomen CW21
  Pelvis and Spine CP27
  Respiratory System CB2YYZZ
  Skin CH2YYZZ
  Skull CP21
  Skull and Cervical Spine CP23
  Spine
    Cervical CP22
    Cervical and Skull CP23
    Lumbar CP2H
    Thoracic CP2G
    Thoracolumbar CP2J
  Spine and Pelvis CP27
  Spleen C722
  Spleen and Liver CF26
  Subcutaneous Tissue CH2YYZZ
  Thorax CP24
  Ureters, Kidneys and Bladder CT23
  Urinary System CT2YYZZ
Tomography, computerized *see* Computerized Tomography (CT Scan)

Tongue, base of *use* Pharynx
Tonometry 4AØ7XBZ
Tonsillectomy
  see Excision, Mouth and Throat ØCB
  see Resection, Mouth and Throat ØCT
Tonsillotomy *see* Drainage, Mouth and Throat ØC9
TOPS™ System *use* Posterior Spinal Motion Preservation Device in New Technology
Total Anomalous Pulmonary Venous Return (TAPVR) repair
  see Bypass, Atrium, Left Ø217
  see Bypass, Vena Cava, Superior Ø21V
Total artificial (replacement) heart *use* Synthetic Substitute
Total parenteral nutrition (TPN) *see* Introduction of Nutritional Substance
Tourniquet, External *see* Compression, Anatomical Regions 2W1
Trachectomy
  see Excision, Trachea ØBB1
  see Resection, Trachea ØBT1
Trachelectomy
  see Excision, Cervix ØUBC
  see Resection, Cervix ØUTC
Trachelopexy
  see Repair, Cervix ØUQC
  see Reposition, Cervix ØUSC
Tracheloplasty *see* Repair, Cervix ØUQC
Trachelorrhaphy *see* Repair, Cervix ØUQC
Trachelotomy *see* Drainage, Cervix ØU9C
Tracheobronchial lymph node *use* Lymphatic, Thorax
Tracheoesophageal fistulization ØB11ØD6
Tracheolysis *see* Release, Respiratory System ØBN
Tracheoplasty
  see Repair, Respiratory System ØBQ
  see Supplement, Respiratory System ØBU
Tracheorrhaphy *see* Repair, Respiratory System ØBQ
Tracheoscopy ØBJ18ZZ
Tracheostomy *see* Bypass, Respiratory System ØB1
Tracheostomy Device
  Bypass, Trachea ØB11
  Change device in, Trachea ØB21XFZ
  Removal of device from, Trachea ØBP1
  Revision of device in, Trachea ØBW1
Tracheostomy tube *use* Tracheostomy Device in Respiratory System
Tracheotomy *see* Drainage, Respiratory System ØB9
Traction
  Abdominal Wall 2W63X
  Arm
    Lower
      Left 2W6DX
      Right 2W6CX
    Upper
      Left 2W6BX
      Right 2W6AX
  Back 2W65X
  Chest Wall 2W64X
  Extremity
    Lower
      Left 2W6MX
      Right 2W6LX
    Upper
      Left 2W69X
      Right 2W68X
  Face 2W61X
  Finger
    Left 2W6KX
    Right 2W6JX
  Foot
    Left 2W6TX
    Right 2W6SX
  Hand
    Left 2W6FX
    Right 2W6EX
  Head 2W60X
  Inguinal Region
    Left 2W67X
    Right 2W66X
  Leg
    Lower
      Left 2W6RX
      Right 2W6QX
    Upper
      Left 2W6PX
      Right 2W6NX
  Neck 2W62X

Traction — *continued*
  Thumb
    Left 2W6HX
    Right 2W6GX
  Toe
    Left 2W6VX
    Right 2W6UX
Tractotomy *see* Division, Central Nervous System and Cranial Nerves 008
Tragus
  use External Ear, Bilateral
  use External Ear, Left
  use External Ear, Right
Training, caregiver *see* Caregiver Training
TRAM (transverse rectus abdominis myocuta-neous) flap reconstruction
  Free *see* Replacement, Skin and Breast 0HR
  Pedicled *see* Transfer, Muscles 0KX
Transcatheter Pulmonary Valve (TPV) placement
  In conduit 02RH38L
  Native site 02RH38M
Transdermal Glomerular Filtration Rate (GFR) Measurement System XT25XE5
Transection *see* Division
Transfer
  Buccal Mucosa 0CX4
  Bursa and Ligament
    Abdomen
      Left 0MXJ
      Right 0MXH
    Ankle
      Left 0MXR
      Right 0MXQ
    Elbow
      Left 0MX4
      Right 0MX3
    Foot
      Left 0MXT
      Right 0MXS
    Hand
      Left 0MX8
      Right 0MX7
    Head and Neck 0MX0
    Hip
      Left 0MXM
      Right 0MXL
    Knee
      Left 0MXP
      Right 0MXN
    Lower Extremity
      Left 0MXW
      Right 0MXV
    Perineum 0MXK
    Rib(s) 0MXG
    Shoulder
      Left 0MX2
      Right 0MX1
    Spine
      Lower 0MXD
      Upper 0MXC
    Sternum 0MXF
    Upper Extremity
      Left 0MXB
      Right 0MX9
    Wrist
      Left 0MX6
      Right 0MX5
  Finger
    Left 0XXP0ZM
    Right 0XXN0ZL
  Gingiva
    Lower 0CX6
    Upper 0CX5
  Intestine
    Large 0DXE
    Small 0DX8
  Lip
    Lower 0CX1
    Upper 0CX0
  Muscle
    Abdomen
      Left 0KXL
      Right 0KXK
    Extraocular
      Left 08XM
      Right 08XL
    Facial 0KX1

Transfer — *continued*
  Muscle — *continued*
    Foot
      Left 0KXW
      Right 0KXV
    Hand
      Left 0KXD
      Right 0KXC
    Head 0KX0
    Hip
      Left 0KXP
      Right 0KXN
    Lower Arm and Wrist
      Left 0KXB
      Right 0KX9
    Lower Leg
      Left 0KXT
      Right 0KXS
    Neck
      Left 0KX3
      Right 0KX2
    Perineum 0KXM
    Shoulder
      Left 0KX6
      Right 0KX5
    Thorax
      Left 0KXJ
      Right 0KXH
    Tongue, Palate, Pharynx 0KX4
    Trunk
      Left 0KXG
      Right 0KXF
    Upper Arm
      Left 0KX8
      Right 0KX7
    Upper Leg
      Left 0KXR
      Right 0KXQ
  Nerve
    Abducens 00XL
    Accessory 00XR
    Acoustic 00XN
    Cervical 01X1
    Facial 00XM
    Femoral 01XD
    Glossopharyngeal 00XP
    Hypoglossal 00XS
    Lumbar 01XB
    Median 01X5
    Oculomotor 00XH
    Olfactory 00XF
    Optic 00XG
    Peroneal 01XH
    Phrenic 01X2
    Pudendal 01XC
    Radial 01X6
    Sciatic 01XF
    Thoracic 01X8
    Tibial 01XG
    Trigeminal 00XK
    Trochlear 00XJ
    Ulnar 01X4
    Vagus 00XQ
  Palate, Soft 0CX3
  Prepuce 0VXT
  Skin
    Abdomen 0HX7XZZ
    Back 0HX6XZZ
    Buttock 0HX8XZZ
    Chest 0HX5XZZ
    Ear
      Left 0HX3XZZ
      Right 0HX2XZZ
    Face 0HX1XZZ
    Foot
      Left 0HXNXZZ
      Right 0HXMXZZ
    Hand
      Left 0HXGXZZ
      Right 0HXFXZZ
    Inguinal 0HXAXZZ
    Lower Arm
      Left 0HXEXZZ
      Right 0HXDXZZ
    Lower Leg
      Left 0HXLXZZ
      Right 0HXKXZZ
    Neck 0HX4XZZ
    Perineum 0HX9XZZ

Transfer — *continued*
  Skin — *continued*
    Scalp 0HX0XZZ
    Upper Arm
      Left 0HXCXZZ
      Right 0HXBXZZ
    Upper Leg
      Left 0HXJXZZ
      Right 0HXHXZZ
  Stomach 0DX6
  Subcutaneous Tissue and Fascia
    Abdomen 0JX8
    Back 0JX7
    Buttock 0JX9
    Chest 0JX6
    Face 0JX1
    Foot
      Left 0JXR
      Right 0JXQ
    Hand
      Left 0JXK
      Right 0JXJ
    Lower Arm
      Left 0JXH
      Right 0JXG
    Lower Leg
      Left 0JXP
      Right 0JXN
    Neck
      Left 0JX5
      Right 0JX4
    Pelvic Region 0JXC
    Perineum 0JXB
    Scalp 0JX0
    Upper Arm
      Left 0JXF
      Right 0JXD
    Upper Leg
      Left 0JXM
      Right 0JXL
  Tendon
    Abdomen
      Left 0LXG
      Right 0LXF
    Ankle
      Left 0LXT
      Right 0LXS
    Foot
      Left 0LXW
      Right 0LXV
    Hand
      Left 0LX8
      Right 0LX7
    Head and Neck 0LX0
    Hip
      Left 0LXK
      Right 0LXJ
    Knee
      Left 0LXR
      Right 0LXQ
    Lower Arm and Wrist
      Left 0LX6
      Right 0LX5
    Lower Leg
      Left 0LXP
      Right 0LXN
    Perineum 0LXH
    Shoulder
      Left 0LX2
      Right 0LX1
    Thorax
      Left 0LXD
      Right 0LXC
    Trunk
      Left 0LXB
      Right 0LX9
    Upper Arm
      Left 0LX4
      Right 0LX3
    Upper Leg
      Left 0LXM
      Right 0LXL
  Tongue 0CX7
Transfusion
  Immunotherapy *see* New Technology, Anatomical Regions XW2
  Products of Conception
    Antihemophilic Factors 3027

Transfusion — *continued*
  Products of Conception — *continued*
    Blood
      Platelets 3027
      Red Cells 3027
        Frozen 3027
      White Cells 3027
      Whole 3027
    Factor IX 3027
    Fibrinogen 3027
    Globulin 3027
    Plasma
      Fresh 3027
      Frozen 3027
    Plasma Cryoprecipitate 3027
    Serum Albumin 3027
  Vein
    4-Factor Prothrombin Complex Concentrate 30283B1
    Central
      Antihemophilic Factors 30243V
      Blood
        Platelets 30243R
        Red Cells 30243N
          Frozen 30243P
        White Cells 30243Q
        Whole 30243H
      Bone Marrow 30243G
      Factor IX 30243W
      Fibrinogen 30243T
      Globulin 30243S
      Hematopoietic Stem/Progenitor Cells (HSPC), Genetically Modified 30243C0
      Pathogen Reduced Cryoprecipitated Fibrinogen Complex 30243D1
      Plasma
        Fresh 30243L
        Frozen 30243K
      Plasma Cryoprecipitate 30243M
      Serum Albumin 30243J
      Stem Cells
        Cord Blood 30243X
        Embryonic 30243AZ
        Hematopoietic 30243Y
        T-cell Depleted Hematopoietic 30243U
    Peripheral
      Antihemophilic Factors 30233V
      Blood
        Platelets 30233R
        Red Cells 30233N
          Frozen 30233P
        White Cells 30233Q
        Whole 30233H
      Bone Marrow 30233G
      Factor IX 30233W
      Fibrinogen 30233T
      Globulin 30233S
      Hematopoietic Stem/Progenitor Cells (HSPC), Genetically Modified 30233C0
      Pathogen Reduced Cryoprecipitated Fibrinogen Complex 30233D1
      Plasma
        Fresh 30233L
        Frozen 30233K
      Plasma Cryoprecipitate 30233M
      Serum Albumin 30233J
      Stem Cells
        Cord Blood 30233X
        Embryonic 30233AZ
        Hematopoietic 30233Y
        T-cell Depleted Hematopoietic 30233U
Transplant *see* Transplantation
Transplantation
  Bone marrow *see* Transfusion, Circulatory 302
  Esophagus 0DY50Z
  Face 0WY20Z
  Hand
    Left 0XYK0Z
    Right 0XYJ0Z
  Heart 02YA0Z
  Hematopoietic cell *see* Transfusion, Circulatory 302
  Intestine
    Large 0DYE0Z
    Small 0DY80Z

Transplantation — *continued*
  Kidney
    Left 0TY10Z
    Right 0TY00Z
  Liver 0FY00Z
  Lung
    Bilateral 0BYM0Z
    Left 0BYL0Z
    Lower Lobe
      Left 0BYJ0Z
      Right 0BYF0Z
    Middle Lobe, Right 0BYD0Z
    Right 0BYK0Z
    Upper Lobe
      Left 0BYG0Z
      Right 0BYC0Z
  Lung Lingula 0BYH0Z
  Ovary
    Left 0UY10Z
    Right 0UY00Z
  Pancreas 0FYG0Z
  Penis 0VYS0Z
  Products of Conception 10Y0
  Scrotum 0VY50Z
  Spleen 07YP0Z
  Stem cell *see* Transfusion, Circulatory 302
  Stomach 0DY60Z
  Thymus 07YM0Z
  Uterus 0UY90Z
Transposition
  see Bypass
  see Reposition
  see Transfer
Transversalis fascia *use* Subcutaneous Tissue and Fascia, Trunk
Transverse acetabular ligament
  use Hip Bursa and Ligament, Left
  use Hip Bursa and Ligament, Right
Transverse (cutaneous) cervical nerve *use* Cervical Plexus
Transverse facial artery
  use Temporal Artery, Left
  use Temporal Artery, Right
Transverse foramen *use* Cervical Vertebra
Transverse humeral ligament
  use Shoulder Bursa and Ligament, Left
  use Shoulder Bursa and Ligament, Right
Transverse ligament of atlas *use* Head and Neck Bursa and Ligament
Transverse process
  use Cervical Vertebra
  use Lumbar Vertebra
  use Thoracic Vertebra
Transverse Rectus Abdominis Myocutaneous Flap
  Replacement
    Bilateral 0HRV076
    Left 0HRU076
    Right 0HRT076
  Transfer
    Left 0KXL
    Right 0KXK
Transverse scapular ligament
  use Shoulder Bursa and Ligament, Left
  use Shoulder Bursa and Ligament, Right
Transverse thoracis muscle
  use Thorax Muscle, Left
  use Thorax Muscle, Right
Transversospinalis muscle
  use Trunk Muscle, Left
  use Trunk Muscle, Right
Transversus abdominis muscle
  use Abdomen Muscle, Left
  use Abdomen Muscle, Right
Trapezium bone
  use Carpal, Left
  use Carpal, Right
Trapezius muscle
  use Trunk Muscle, Left
  use Trunk Muscle, Right
Trapezoid bone
  use Carpal, Left
  use Carpal, Right
Treosulfan XW0
Triceps brachii muscle
  use Upper Arm Muscle, Left
  use Upper Arm Muscle, Right
Tricuspid annulus *use* Tricuspid Valve

Trifacial nerve *use* Trigeminal Nerve
Trifecta™ Valve (aortic) *use* Zooplastic Tissue in Heart and Great Vessels
Trigone of bladder *use* Bladder
TriGuard 3™ CEPD (cerebral embolic protection device) X2A6325
Trilaciclib XW0
Trimming, excisional *see* Excision
Triquetral bone
  use Carpal, Left
  use Carpal, Right
Trochanteric bursa
  use Hip Bursa and Ligament, Left
  use Hip Bursa and Ligament, Right
TUMT (transurethral microwave thermotherapy of prostate) 0V507ZZ
TUNA (transurethral needle ablation of prostate) 0V507ZZ
Tunneled central venous catheter *use* Vascular Access Device, Tunneled in Subcutaneous Tissue and Fascia
Tunneled spinal (intrathecal) catheter *use* Infusion Device
Turbinectomy
  see Excision, Ear, Nose, Sinus 09B
  see Resection, Ear, Nose, Sinus 09T
Turbinoplasty
  see Repair, Ear, Nose, Sinus 09Q
  see Replacement, Ear, Nose, Sinus 09R
  see Supplement, Ear, Nose, Sinus 09U
Turbinotomy
  see Division, Ear, Nose, Sinus 098
  see Drainage, Ear, Nose, Sinus 099
TURP (transurethral resection of prostate) 0VB07ZZ
  see Excision, Prostate 0VB0
  see Resection, Prostate 0VT0
Twelfth cranial nerve *use* Hypoglossal Nerve
Two lead pacemaker *use* Pacemaker, Dual Chamber in 0JH
Tympanic cavity
  use Middle Ear, Left
  use Middle Ear, Right
Tympanic nerve *use* Glossopharyngeal Nerve
Tympanic part of temoporal bone
  use Temporal Bone, Left
  use Temporal Bone, Right
Tympanogram *see* Hearing Assessment, Diagnostic Audiology F13
Tympanoplasty
  see Repair, Ear, Nose, Sinus 09Q
  see Replacement, Ear, Nose, Sinus 09R
  see Supplement, Ear, Nose, Sinus 09U
Tympanosympathectomy *see* Excision, Nerve, Head and Neck Sympathetic 01BK
Tympanotomy *see* Drainage, Ear, Nose, Sinus 099
TYRX Antibacterial Envelope *use* Anti-Infective Envelope

U

Ulnar collateral carpal ligament
  use Wrist Bursa and Ligament, Left
  use Wrist Bursa and Ligament, Right
Ulnar collateral ligament
  use Elbow Bursa and Ligament, Left
  use Elbow Bursa and Ligament, Right
Ulnar notch
  use Radius, Left
  use Radius, Right
Ulnar vein
  use Brachial Vein, Left
  use Brachial Vein, Right
Ultrafiltration
  Hemodialysis *see* Performance, Urinary 5A1D
  Therapeutic plasmapheresis *see* Pheresis, Circulatory 6A55
Ultraflex™ Precision Colonic Stent System *use* Intraluminal Device
ULTRAPRO Hernia System (UHS) *use* Synthetic Substitute
ULTRAPRO Partially Absorbable Lightweight Mesh *use* Synthetic Substitute
ULTRAPRO Plug *use* Synthetic Substitute
Ultrasonic osteogenic stimulator
  use Bone Growth Stimulator in Head and Facial Bones

Subterms under main terms may continue to next column or page

Ultrasonic osteogenic stimulator — *continued*
use Bone Growth Stimulator in Lower Bones
use Bone Growth Stimulator in Upper Bones
Ultrasonography
Abdomen BW40ZZZ
Abdomen and Pelvis BW41ZZZ
Abdominal Wall BH49ZZZ
Aorta
Abdominal, Intravascular B440ZZ3
Thoracic, Intravascular B340ZZ3
Appendix BD48ZZZ
Artery
Brachiocephalic-Subclavian, Right, Intravascular B341ZZ3
Celiac and Mesenteric, Intravascular B44KZZ3
Common Carotid
Bilateral, Intravascular B345ZZ3
Left, Intravascular B344ZZ3
Right, Intravascular B343ZZ3
Coronary
Multiple B241YZZ
Intravascular B241ZZ3
Transesophageal B241ZZ4
Single B240YZZ
Intravascular B240ZZ3
Transesophageal B240ZZ4
Femoral, Intravascular B44LZZ3
Inferior Mesenteric, Intravascular B445ZZ3
Internal Carotid
Bilateral, Intravascular B348ZZ3
Left, Intravascular B347ZZ3
Right, Intravascular B346ZZ3
Intra-Abdominal, Other, Intravascular B44BZZ3
Intracranial, Intravascular B34RZZ3
Lower Extremity
Bilateral, Intravascular B44HZZ3
Left, Intravascular B44GZZ3
Right, Intravascular B44FZZ3
Mesenteric and Celiac, Intravascular B44KZZ3
Ophthalmic, Intravascular B34VZZ3
Penile, Intravascular B44NZZ3
Pulmonary
Left, Intravascular B34TZZ3
Right, Intravascular B34SZZ3
Renal
Bilateral, Intravascular B448ZZ3
Left, Intravascular B447ZZ3
Right, Intravascular B446ZZ3
Subclavian, Left, Intravascular B342ZZ3
Superior Mesenteric, Intravascular B444ZZ3
Upper Extremity
Bilateral, Intravascular B34KZZ3
Left, Intravascular B34JZZ3
Right, Intravascular B34HZZ3
Bile Duct BF40ZZZ
Bile Duct and Gallbladder BF43ZZZ
Bladder BT40ZZZ
and Kidney BT4JZZZ
Brain B040ZZZ
Breast
Bilateral BH42ZZZ
Left BH41ZZZ
Right BH40ZZZ
Chest Wall BH4BZZZ
Coccyx BR4FZZZ
Connective Tissue
Lower Extremity BL41ZZZ
Upper Extremity BL40ZZZ
Duodenum BD49ZZZ
Elbow
Left, Densitometry BP4HZZ1
Right, Densitometry BP4GZZ1
Esophagus BD41ZZZ
Extremity
Lower BH48ZZZ
Upper BH47ZZZ
Eye
Bilateral B847ZZZ
Left B846ZZZ
Right B845ZZZ
Fallopian Tube
Bilateral BU42
Left BU41
Right BU40
Fetal Umbilical Cord BY47ZZZ
Fetus
First Trimester, Multiple Gestation BY4BZZZ

Ultrasonography — *continued*
Fetus — *continued*
Second Trimester, Multiple Gestation BY4DZZZ
Single
First Trimester BY49ZZZ
Second Trimester BY4CZZZ
Third Trimester BY4FZZZ
Third Trimester, Multiple Gestation BY4GZZZ
Gallbladder BF42ZZZ
Gallbladder and Bile Duct BF43ZZZ
Gastrointestinal Tract BD47ZZZ
Gland
Adrenal
Bilateral BG42ZZZ
Left BG41ZZZ
Right BG40ZZZ
Parathyroid BG43ZZZ
Thyroid BG44ZZZ
Hand
Left, Densitometry BP4PZZ1
Right, Densitometry BP4NZZ1
Head and Neck BH4CZZZ
Heart
Left B245YZZ
Intravascular B245ZZ3
Transesophageal B245ZZ4
Pediatric B24DYZZ
Intravascular B24DZZ3
Transesophageal B24DZZ4
Right B244YZZ
Intravascular B244ZZ3
Transesophageal B244ZZ4
Right and Left B246YZZ
Intravascular B246ZZ3
Transesophageal B246ZZ4
Heart with Aorta B24BYZZ
Intravascular B24BZZ3
Transesophageal B24BZZ4
Hepatobiliary System, All BF4CZZZ
Hip
Bilateral BQ42ZZZ
Left BQ41ZZZ
Right BQ40ZZZ
Kidney
and Bladder BT4JZZZ
Bilateral BT43ZZZ
Left BT42ZZZ
Right BT41ZZZ
Transplant BT49ZZZ
Knee
Bilateral BQ49ZZZ
Left BQ48ZZZ
Right BQ47ZZZ
Liver BF45ZZZ
Liver and Spleen BF46ZZZ
Mediastinum BB4CZZZ
Neck BW4FZZZ
Ovary
Bilateral BU45
Left BU44
Right BU43
Ovary and Uterus BU4C
Pancreas BF47ZZZ
Pelvic Region BW4GZZZ
Pelvis and Abdomen BW41ZZZ
Penis BV4BZZZ
Pericardium B24CYZZ
Intravascular B24CZZ3
Transesophageal B24CZZ4
Placenta BY48ZZZ
Pleura BB4BZZZ
Prostate and Seminal Vesicle BV49ZZZ
Rectum BD4CZZZ
Sacrum BR4FZZZ
Scrotum BV44ZZZ
Seminal Vesicle and Prostate BV49ZZZ
Shoulder
Left, Densitometry BP49ZZ1
Right, Densitometry BP48ZZ1
Spinal Cord B04BZZZ
Spine
Cervical BR40ZZZ
Lumbar BR49ZZZ
Thoracic BR47ZZZ
Spleen and Liver BF46ZZZ
Stomach BD42ZZZ
Tendon
Lower Extremity BL43ZZZ

Ultrasonography — *continued*
Tendon — *continued*
Upper Extremity BL42ZZZ
Ureter
Bilateral BT48ZZZ
Left BT47ZZZ
Right BT46ZZZ
Urethra BT45ZZZ
Uterus BU46
Uterus and Ovary BU4C
Vein
Jugular
Left, Intravascular B544ZZ3
Right, Intravascular B543ZZ3
Lower Extremity
Bilateral, Intravascular B54DZZ3
Left, Intravascular B54CZZ3
Right, Intravascular B54BZZ3
Portal, Intravascular B54TZZ3
Renal
Bilateral, Intravascular B54LZZ3
Left, Intravascular B54KZZ3
Right, Intravascular B54JZZ3
Spanchnic, Intravascular B54TZZ3
Subclavian
Left, Intravascular B547ZZ3
Right, Intravascular B546ZZ3
Upper Extremity
Bilateral, Intravascular B54PZZ3
Left, Intravascular B54NZZ3
Right, Intravascular B54MZZ3
Vena Cava
Inferior, Intravascular B549ZZ3
Superior, Intravascular B548ZZ3
Wrist
Left, Densitometry BP4MZZ1
Right, Densitometry BP4LZZ1
Ultrasound bone healing system
use Bone Growth Stimulator in Head and Facial Bones
use Bone Growth Stimulator in Lower Bones
use Bone Growth Stimulator in Upper Bones
Ultrasound Therapy
Heart 6A75
No Qualifier 6A75
Vessels
Head and Neck 6A75
Other 6A75
Peripheral 6A75
Ultraviolet Light Therapy, Skin 6A80
Umbilical artery
use Internal Iliac Artery, Left
use Internal Iliac Artery, Right
use Lower Artery
Uniplanar external fixator
use External Fixation Device, Monoplanar in 0PH
use External Fixation Device, Monoplanar in 0PS
use External Fixation Device, Monoplanar in 0QH
use External Fixation Device, Monoplanar in 0QS
UPLIZNA® use Inebilizumab-cdon
Upper GI series see Fluoroscopy, Gastrointestinal, Upper BD15
Ureteral orifice
use Ureter
use Ureter, Left
use Ureter, Right
use Ureters, Bilateral
Ureterectomy
see Excision, Urinary System 0TB
see Resection, Urinary System 0TT
Ureterocolostomy see Bypass, Urinary System 0T1
Ureterocystostomy see Bypass, Urinary System 0T1
Ureteroenterostomy see Bypass, Urinary System 0T1
Ureteroileostomy see Bypass, Urinary System 0T1
Ureterolithotomy see Extirpation, Urinary System 0TC
Ureterolysis see Release, Urinary System 0TN
Ureteroneocystostomy
see Bypass, Urinary System 0T1
see Reposition, Urinary System 0TS
Ureteropelvic junction (UPJ)
use Kidney Pelvis, Left
use Kidney Pelvis, Right
Ureteropexy
see Repair, Urinary System 0TQ
see Reposition, Urinary System 0TS
Ureteroplasty
see Repair, Urinary System 0TQ

Ureteroplasty — *continued*
  see Replacement, Urinary System ØTR
  see Supplement, Urinary System ØTU
Ureteroplication *see* Restriction, Urinary System ØTV
Ureteropyelography *see* Fluoroscopy, Urinary System BT1
Ureterorrhaphy *see* Repair, Urinary System ØTQ
Ureteroscopy ØTJ98ZZ
Ureterostomy
  see Bypass, Urinary System ØT1
  see Drainage, Urinary System ØT9
Ureterotomy *see* Drainage, Urinary System ØT9
Ureteroureterostomy *see* Bypass, Urinary System ØT1
Ureterovesical orifice
  use Ureter
  use Ureter, Left
  use Ureter, Right
  use Ureters, Bilateral
Urethral catheterization, indwelling ØT9B70Z
Urethrectomy
  see Excision, Urethra ØTBD
  see Resection, Urethra ØTTD
Urethrolithotomy *see* Extirpation, Urethra ØTCD
Urethrolysis *see* Release, Urethra ØTND
Urethropexy
  see Repair, Urethra ØTQD
  see Reposition, Urethra ØTSD
Urethroplasty
  see Repair, Urethra ØTQD
  see Replacement, Urethra ØTRD
  see Supplement, Urethra ØTUD
Urethrorrhaphy *see* Repair, Urethra ØTQD
Urethroscopy ØTJD8ZZ
Urethrotomy *see* Drainage, Urethra ØT9D
Urinary incontinence stimulator lead *use* Stimulator Lead in Urinary System
Urography *see* Fluoroscopy, Urinary System BT1
Ustekinumab *use* Other New Technology Therapeutic Substance
Uterine Artery
  use Internal Iliac Artery, Left
  use Internal Iliac Artery, Right
Uterine artery embolization (UAE) *see* Occlusion, Lower Arteries Ø4L
Uterine cornu *use* Uterus
Uterine tube
  use Fallopian Tube, Left
  use Fallopian Tube, Right
Uterine vein
  use Hypogastric Vein, Left
  use Hypogastric Vein, Right
Uvulectomy
  see Excision, Uvula ØCBN
  see Resection, Uvula ØCTN
Uvulorrhaphy *see* Repair, Uvula ØCQN
Uvulotomy *see* Drainage, Uvula ØC9N

V

Vabomere™ *use* Meropenem-vaborbactam Anti-infective
Vaccination *see* Introduction of Serum, Toxoid, and Vaccine
Vacuum extraction, obstetric 1ØD07Z6
Vaginal artery
  use Internal Iliac Artery, Left
  use Internal Iliac Artery, Right
Vaginal pessary *use* Intraluminal Device, Pessary in Female Reproductive System
Vaginal vein
  use Hypogastric Vein, Left
  use Hypogastric Vein, Right
Vaginectomy
  see Excision, Vagina ØUBG
  see Resection, Vagina ØUTG
Vaginofixation
  see Repair, Vagina ØUQG
  see Reposition, Vagina ØUSG
Vaginoplasty
  see Repair, Vagina ØUQG
  see Supplement, Vagina ØUUG
Vaginorrhaphy *see* Repair, Vagina ØUQG
Vaginoscopy ØUJH8ZZ
Vaginotomy *see* Drainage, Female Reproductive System ØU9

Vagotomy *see* Division, Nerve, Vagus ØØ8Q
Valiant Thoracic Stent Graft *use* Intraluminal Device
Valvotomy, valvulotomy
  see Division, Heart and Great Vessels Ø28
  see Release, Heart and Great Vessels Ø2N
Valvuloplasty
  see Repair, Heart and Great Vessels Ø2Q
  see Replacement, Heart and Great Vessels Ø2R
  see Supplement, Heart and Great Vessels Ø2U
Valvuloplasty, Alfieri Stitch *see* Restriction, Valve, Mitral Ø2VG
Vascular Access Device
  Totally Implantable
    Insertion of device in
      Abdomen ØJH8
      Chest ØJH6
      Lower Arm
        Left ØJHH
        Right ØJHG
      Lower Leg
        Left ØJHP
        Right ØJHN
      Upper Arm
        Left ØJHF
        Right ØJHD
      Upper Leg
        Left ØJHM
        Right ØJHL
    Removal of device from
      Lower Extremity ØJPW
      Trunk ØJPT
      Upper Extremity ØJPV
    Revision of device in
      Lower Extremity ØJWW
      Trunk ØJWT
      Upper Extremity ØJWV
  Tunneled
    Insertion of device in
      Abdomen ØJH8
      Chest ØJH6
      Lower Arm
        Left ØJHH
        Right ØJHG
      Lower Leg
        Left ØJHP
        Right ØJHN
      Upper Arm
        Left ØJHF
        Right ØJHD
      Upper Leg
        Left ØJHM
        Right ØJHL
    Removal of device from
      Lower Extremity ØJPW
      Trunk ØJPT
      Upper Extremity ØJPV
    Revision of device in
      Lower Extremity ØJWW
      Trunk ØJWT
      Upper Extremity ØJWV
Vasectomy *see* Excision, Male Reproductive System ØVB
Vasography
  see Fluoroscopy, Male Reproductive System BV1
  see Plain Radiography, Male Reproductive System BVØ
Vasoligation *see* Occlusion, Male Reproductive System ØVL
Vasorrhaphy *see* Repair, Male Reproductive System ØVQ
Vasostomy *see* Bypass, Male Reproductive System ØV1
Vasotomy
  Drainage *see* Drainage, Male Reproductive System ØV9
  With ligation *see* Occlusion, Male Reproductive System ØVL
Vasovasostomy *see* Repair, Male Reproductive System ØVQ
Vastus intermedius muscle
  use Upper Leg Muscle, Left
  use Upper Leg Muscle, Right
Vastus lateralis muscle
  use Upper Leg Muscle, Left
  use Upper Leg Muscle, Right
Vastus medialis muscle
  use Upper Leg Muscle, Left
  use Upper Leg Muscle, Right

VCG (vectorcardiogram) *see* Measurement, Cardiac 4AØ2
Vectra® Vascular Access Graft *use* Vascular Access Device, Tunneled in Subcutaneous Tissue and Fascia
Veklury *use* Remdesivir Anti-infective
Venclexta® *use* Venetoclax Antineoplastic
Venectomy
  see Excision, Lower Veins Ø6B
  see Excision, Upper Veins Ø5B
Venetoclax Antineoplastic XWØDXR5
Venography
  see Fluoroscopy, Veins B51
  see Plain Radiography, Veins B5Ø
Venorrhaphy
  see Repair, Lower Veins Ø6Q
  see Repair, Upper Veins Ø5Q
Venotripsy
  see Occlusion, Lower Veins Ø6L
  see Occlusion, Upper Veins Ø5L
Ventricular fold *use* Larynx
Ventriculoatriostomy *see* Bypass, Central Nervous System and Cranial Nerves ØØ1
Ventriculocisternostomy *see* Bypass, Central Nervous System and Cranial Nerves ØØ1
Ventriculogram, cardiac
  Combined left and right heart *see* Fluoroscopy, Heart, Right and Left B216
  Left ventricle *see* Fluoroscopy, Heart, Left B215
  Right ventricle *see* Fluoroscopy, Heart, Right B214
Ventriculopuncture, through previously implanted catheter 8C01X6J
Ventriculoscopy ØØJØ4ZZ
Ventriculostomy
  External drainage *see* Drainage, Cerebral Ventricle ØØ96
  Internal shunt *see* Bypass, Cerebral Ventricle ØØ16
Ventriculovenostomy *see* Bypass, Cerebral Ventricle ØØ16
Ventrio™ Hernia Patch *use* Synthetic Substitute
VEP (visual evoked potential) 4AØ7XØZ
Vermiform appendix *use* Appendix
Vermilion border
  use Lower Lip
  use Upper Lip
Versa *use* Pacemaker, Dual Chamber in ØJH
Version, obstetric
  External 1ØS0XZZ
  Internal 1ØS07ZZ
Vertebral arch
  use Cervical Vertebra
  use Lumbar Vertebra
  use Thoracic Vertebra
Vertebral body
  use Cervical Vertebra
  use Lumbar Vertebra
  use Thoracic Vertebra
Vertebral canal *use* Spinal Canal
Vertebral foramen
  use Cervical Vertebra
  use Lumbar Vertebra
  use Thoracic Vertebra
Vertebral lamina
  use Cervical Vertebra
  use Lumbar Vertebra
  use Thoracic Vertebra
Vertebral pedicle
  use Cervical Vertebra
  use Lumbar Vertebra
  use Thoracic Vertebra
Vesical vein
  use Hypogastric Vein, Left
  use Hypogastric Vein, Right
Vesicotomy *see* Drainage, Urinary System ØT9
Vesiculectomy
  see Excision, Male Reproductive System ØVB
  see Resection, Male Reproductive System ØVT
Vesiculogram, seminal *see* Plain Radiography, Male Reproductive System BVØ
Vesiculotomy *see* Drainage, Male Reproductive System ØV9
Vestibular Assessment F15Z
Vestibular (Scarpa's) ganglion *use* Acoustic Nerve
Vestibular nerve *use* Acoustic Nerve
Vestibular Treatment FØC
Vestibulocochlear nerve *use* Acoustic Nerve

VH-IVUS (virtual histology intravascular ultrasound) see Ultrasonography, Heart B24
Virchow's (supraclavicular) lymph node
    use Lymphatic, Left Neck
    use Lymphatic, Right Neck
Virtuoso (II) (DR) (VR) use Defibrillator Generator in ØJH
Vistogard® use Uridine Triacetate
Visualase™ MRI-Guided Laser Ablation System see Destruction
Vitrectomy
    see Excision, Eye Ø8B
    see Resection, Eye Ø8T
Vitreous body
    use Vitreous, Left
    use Vitreous, Right
Viva (XT) (S) use Cardiac Resynchronization Defibrillator Pulse Generator in ØJH
Vivistim® Paired VNS System Lead use Neurostimulator Lead with Paired Stimulation System in New Technology
Vocal fold
    use Vocal Cord, Left
    use Vocal Cord, Right
Vocational
    Assessment see Activities of Daily Living Assessment, Rehabilitation FØ2
    Retraining see Activities of Daily Living Treatment, Rehabilitation FØ8
Volar (palmar) digital vein
    use Hand Vein, Left
    use Hand Vein, Right
Volar (palmar) metacarpal vein
    use Hand Vein, Left
    use Hand Vein, Right
Vomer bone use Nasal Septum
Vomer of nasal septum use Nasal Bone
Voraxaze use Glucarpidase
Vulvectomy
    see Excision, Female Reproductive System ØUB
    see Resection, Female Reproductive System ØUT
V-Wave Interatrial Shunt System use Synthetic Substitute
VYXEOS™ use Cytarabine and Daunorubicin Liposome Antineoplastic

W

WALLSTENT® Endoprosthesis use Intraluminal Device
Washing see Irrigation
WavelinQ EndoAVF system
    Radial Artery, Left Ø31C3ZF
    Radial Artery, Right Ø31B3ZF
    Ulnar Artery, Left Ø31A3ZF
    Ulnar Artery, Right Ø3193ZF
Wedge resection, pulmonary see Excision, Respiratory System ØBB
Whole Blood Nucleic Acid-base Microbial Detection XXE5XM5
Whole Blood Reverse Transcription and Quantitative Real-time Polymerase Chain Reaction XXE5X38
Window see Drainage
Wiring, dental 2W31X9Z

X

Xact Carotid Stent System use Intraluminal Device
XENLETA™ use Lefamulin Anti-infective
Xenograft use Zooplastic Tissue in Heart and Great Vessels
XENOVIEW™ BB34Z3Z
XIENCE Everolimus Eluting Coronary Stent System use Intraluminal Device, Drug-eluting in Heart and Great Vessels
Xiphoid process use Sternum
XLIF® System use Interbody Fusion Device in Lower Joints
XOSPATA® use Gilteritinib Antineoplastic
X-ray see Plain Radiography
X-Spine Axle Cage
    use Spinal Stabilization Device, Interspinous Process in ØRH
    use Spinal Stabilization Device, Interspinous Process in ØSH
X-STOP® Spacer
    use Spinal Stabilization Device, Interspinous Process in ØRH
    use Spinal Stabilization Device, Interspinous Process in ØSH

Y

Yescarta® use Axicabtagene Ciloleucel Immunotherapy
Yoga Therapy 8EØZXY4

Z

Zenith AAA Endovascular Graft use Intraluminal Device
Zenith Flex® AAA Endovascular Graft use Intraluminal Device
Zenith TX2® TAA Endovascular Graft use Intraluminal Device
Zenith® Fenestrated AAA Endovascular Graft
    use Intraluminal Device, Branched or Fenestrated, One or Two Arteries in Ø4V
    use Intraluminal Device, Branched or Fenestrated, Three or More Arteries in Ø4V
Zenith® Renu™ AAA Ancillary Graft use Intraluminal Device
ZEPZELCA™ use Lurbinectedin
ZERBAXA® use Ceftolozane/Tazobactam Anti-infective
Zilver® PTX® (paclitaxel) Drug-Eluting Peripheral Stent
    use Intraluminal Device, Drug-eluting in Lower Arteries
    use Intraluminal Device, Drug-eluting in Upper Arteries
Zimmer® NexGen® LPS Mobile Bearing Knee use Synthetic Substitute
Zimmer® NexGen® LPS-Flex Mobile Knee use Synthetic Substitute
ZINPLAVA™ infusion see Introduction with qualifier Other Therapeutic Monoclonal Antibody
Zonule of Zinn
    use Lens, Left
    use Lens, Right
Zotarolimus-eluting Coronary Stent use Intraluminal Device, Drug-eluting in Heart and Great Vessels
Z-plasty, skin for scar contracture see Release, Skin and Breast ØHN
ZULRESSO™ use Brexanolone
Zygomatic process of frontal bone use Frontal Bone
Zygomatic process of temporal bone
    use Temporal Bone, Left
    use Temporal Bone, Right
Zygomaticus muscle use Facial Muscle
Zyvox use Oxazolidinones

ICD-10-PCS Tables

Central Nervous System and Cranial Nerves 001–00X

Character Meanings

This Character Meaning table is provided as a guide to assist the user in the identification of character members that may be found in this section of code tables. It **SHOULD NOT** be used to build a PCS code.

Operation–Character 3		Body Part–Character 4		Approach–Character 5		Device–Character 6		Qualifier–Character 7	
1	Bypass	0	Brain	0	Open	0	Drainage Device	0	Nasopharynx
2	Change	1	Cerebral Meninges	3	Percutaneous	1	Radioactive Element	1	Mastoid Sinus
5	Destruction	2	Dura Mater	4	Percutaneous Endoscopic	2	Monitoring Device	2	Atrium
7	Dilation	3	Epidural Space, Intracranial	X	External	3	Infusion Device	3	Blood Vessel OR Laser Interstitial Thermal Therapy
8	Division	4	Subdural Space, Intracranial			4	Radioactive Element, Cesium-131 Collagen Implant	4	Pleural Cavity
9	Drainage	5	Subarachnoid Space, Intracranial			7	Autologous Tissue Substitute	5	Intestine
B	Excision	6	Cerebral Ventricle			J	Synthetic Substitute	6	Peritoneal Cavity
C	Extirpation	7	Cerebral Hemisphere			K	Nonautologous Tissue Substitute	7	Urinary Tract
D	Extraction	8	Basal Ganglia			M	Neurostimulator Lead	8	Bone Marrow
F	Fragmentation	9	Thalamus			Y	Other Device	9	Fallopian Tube
H	Insertion	A	Hypothalamus			Z	No Device	A	Subgaleal Space
J	Inspection	B	Pons					B	Cerebral Cisterns
K	Map	C	Cerebellum					F	Olfactory Nerve
N	Release	D	Medulla Oblongata					G	Optic Nerve
P	Removal	E	Cranial Nerve					H	Oculomotor Nerve
Q	Repair	F	Olfactory Nerve					J	Trochlear Nerve
R	Replacement	G	Optic Nerve					K	Trigeminal Nerve
S	Reposition	H	Oculomotor Nerve					L	Abducens Nerve
T	Resection	J	Trochlear Nerve					M	Facial Nerve
U	Supplement	K	Trigeminal Nerve					N	Acoustic Nerve
W	Revision	L	Abducens Nerve					P	Glossopharyngeal Nerve
X	Transfer	M	Facial Nerve					Q	Vagus Nerve
		N	Acoustic Nerve					R	Accessory Nerve
		P	Glossopharyngeal Nerve					S	Hypoglossal Nerve
		Q	Vagus Nerve					X	Diagnostic
		R	Accessory Nerve					Z	No Qualifier
		S	Hypoglossal Nerve						
		T	Spinal Meninges						
		U	Spinal Canal						
		V	Spinal Cord						
		W	Cervical Spinal Cord						
		X	Thoracic Spinal Cord						
		Y	Lumbar Spinal Cord						

AHA Coding Clinic for table 001

2021, 2Q, 19	Electromagnetic stealth guided ventriculoperitoneal shunt insertion with endoscopy
2019, 4Q, 21-22	Cerebral ventricle bypass Qualifier
2018, 4Q, 86	Placement of lumboatrial shunt
2017, 4Q, 39-41	Dilation and bypass of cerebral ventricle
2015, 2Q, 9	Revision of ventriculoperitoneal (VP) shunt
2013, 2Q, 36	Insertion of ventriculoperitoneal shunt with laparoscopic assistance

AHA Coding Clinic for table 005

2022, 1Q, 50	Percutaneous ganglion balloon compression
2021, 3Q, 16	Decompression of Chiari malformation by excision
2021, 2Q, 17	Dorsal root entry zone procedure

AHA Coding Clinic for table 007

2017, 4Q, 39-41	Dilation and bypass of cerebral ventricle

AHA Coding Clinic for table 009

2018, 4Q, 85	Externalization of lumboatrial shunt
2017, 1Q, 50	Failed lumbar puncture
2015, 3Q, 10	Open evacuation of subdural hematoma
2015, 3Q, 11	Percutaneous drainage of subdural hematoma
2015, 3Q, 12	Subdural evacuation portal system (SEPS) placement
2015, 3Q, 12	Placement of ventriculostomy catheter via burr hole
2015, 2Q, 30	Drainage of syrinx
2015, 1Q, 31	Intrathecal chemotherapy
2014, 1Q, 8	Diagnostic lumbar tap
2014, 1Q, 8	Lumbar drainage port aspiration

AHA Coding Clinic for table 00B

2021, 3Q, 16	Decompression of Chiari malformation by excision
2017, 3Q, 17	Resection of schwannoma and placement of DuraGen and Lorenz cranial plating system
2016, 2Q, 12	Resection of malignant neoplasm of infratemporal fossa
2016, 2Q, 18	Amygdalohippocampectomy
2014, 4Q, 34	Resection of brain malignancy with implantation of chemotherapeutic wafer
2014, 3Q, 24	Repair of lipomyelomeningocele and tethered cord

AHA Coding Clinic for table 00C

2019, 3Q, 4	Evacuation of subdural hematoma and control of bleeding artery
2019, 2Q, 36	Evacuation of hematoma using NICO Brainpath® technology
2017, 4Q, 48	New and revised body part values - Extirpation spinal canal
2016, 2Q, 29	Decompressive craniectomy with cryopreservation and storage of bone flap
2015, 3Q, 10	Open evacuation of subdural hematoma
2015, 3Q, 11	Percutaneous drainage of subdural hematoma
2015, 3Q, 13	Evacuation of intracerebral hematoma

AHA Coding Clinic for table 00D

2021, 4Q, 38-40	Ultrasonic surgical aspiration of brain
2015, 3Q, 13	Nonexcisional debridement of cranial wound with removal and replacement of hardware

AHA Coding Clinic for table 00H

2020, 4Q, 43-44	Insertion of radioactive element
2020, 2Q, 15	Ommaya reservoir with ventricular catheter placement
2020, 2Q, 16	Ommaya reservoir placement for cerebrospinal fluid infusion therapy
2017, 4Q, 30-31	Radiotherapeutic brain implant
2017, 3Q, 13	Implantation of bilateral neurostimulator electrodes
2014, 3Q, 19	End of life replacement of Baclofen pump

AHA Coding Clinic for table 00J

2021, 2Q, 19	Electromagnetic stealth guided ventriculoperitoneal shunt insertion with endoscopy
2019, 2Q, 36	Evacuation of hematoma using NICO Brainpath® technology
2017, 1Q, 50	Failed lumbar puncture

AHA Coding Clinic for table 00N

2019, 2Q, 19	Cervical spinal fusion, decompression and placement of interfacet stabilization device
2019, 1Q, 28	Decompressive laminectomy of both spinal cord and nerve roots
2018, 3Q, 30	Decompressive laminectomy (release of spinal cord versus release of spinal meninges)
2017, 3Q, 10	Repair of Chiari malformation
2017, 2Q, 23	Decompression of spinal cord and placement of instrumentation
2016, 2Q, 29	Decompressive craniectomy with cryopreservation and storage of bone flap
2015, 2Q, 20	Cervical laminoplasty
2015, 2Q, 21	Multiple decompressive cervical laminectomies
2015, 2Q, 34	Decompressive laminectomy
2014, 3Q, 24	Repair of lipomyelomeningocele and tethered cord

AHA Coding Clinic for table 00P

2014, 3Q, 19	End of life replacement of Baclofen pump

AHA Coding Clinic for table 00Q

2014, 3Q, 7	Hemi-cranioplasty for repair of cranial defect
2013, 3Q, 25	Fracture of frontal bone with repair and coagulation for hemostasis

AHA Coding Clinic for table 00S

2014, 4Q, 35	Reimplantation of buccal nerve

AHA Coding Clinic for table 00U

2021, 3Q, 16	Decompression of Chiari malformation by excision
2018, 1Q, 9	Craniectomy with DuraGaurd placement
2017, 4Q, 62	Added and revised device values - Nerve substitutes
2017, 3Q, 10	Repair of Chiari malformation
2017, 3Q, 17	Resection of schwannoma and placement of DuraGen and Lorenz cranial plating system
2015, 4Q, 39	Dural patch graft
2014, 3Q, 24	Repair of lipomyelomeningocele and tethered cord

AHA Coding Clinic for table 00W

2018, 4Q, 86	Placement of lumboatrial shunt

Brain

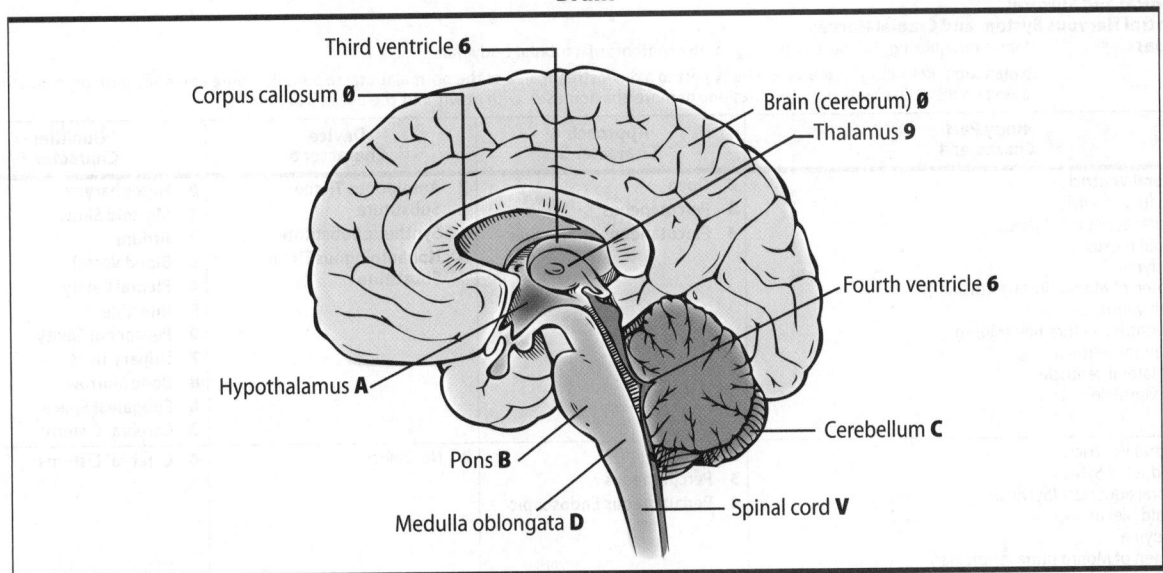

Third ventricle **6**

Corpus callosum **Ø**

Brain (cerebrum) **Ø**

Thalamus **9**

Fourth ventricle **6**

Hypothalamus **A**

Cerebellum **C**

Pons **B**

Spinal cord **V**

Medulla oblongata **D**

Cranial Nerves

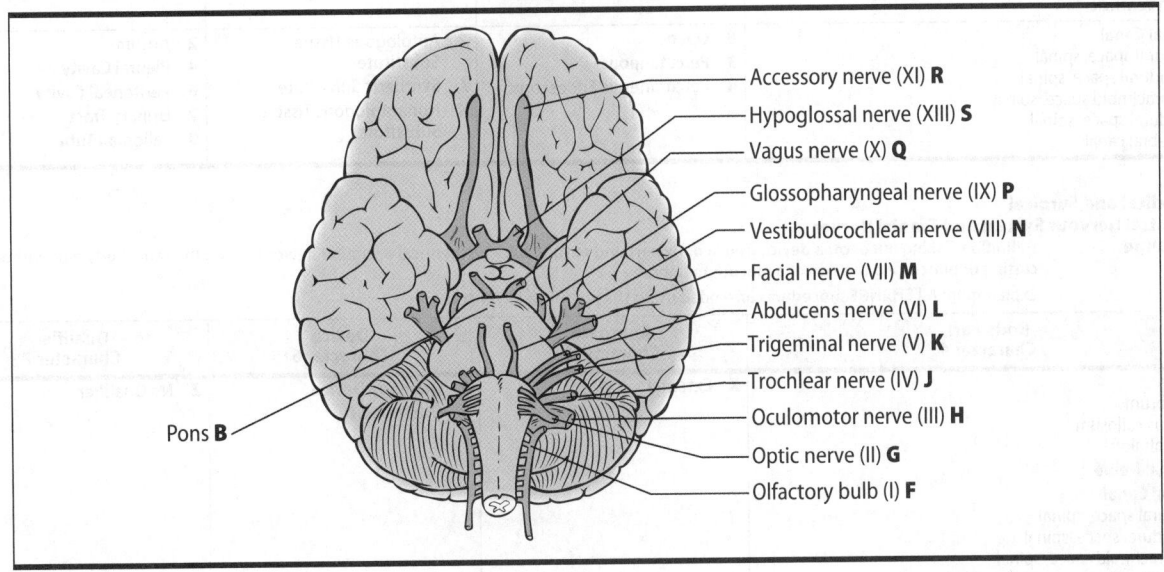

Accessory nerve (XI) **R**

Hypoglossal nerve (XIII) **S**

Vagus nerve (X) **Q**

Glossopharyngeal nerve (IX) **P**

Vestibulocochlear nerve (VIII) **N**

Facial nerve (VII) **M**

Abducens nerve (VI) **L**

Trigeminal nerve (V) **K**

Trochlear nerve (IV) **J**

Oculomotor nerve (III) **H**

Optic nerve (II) **G**

Olfactory bulb (I) **F**

Pons **B**

Ø   **Medical and Surgical**
Ø   **Central Nervous System and Cranial Nerves**
1   **Bypass**   Definition: Altering the route of passage of the contents of a tubular body part

Explanation: Rerouting contents of a body part to a downstream area of the normal route, to a similar route and body part, or to an abnormal route and dissimilar body part. Includes one or more anastomoses, with or without the use of a device.

Body Part Character 4	Approach Character 5	Device Character 6	Qualifier Character 7

6 Cerebral Ventricle
Aqueduct of Sylvius
Cerebral aqueduct (Sylvius)
Choroid plexus
Ependyma
Foramen of Monro (intraventricular)
Fourth ventricle
Interventricular foramen (Monro)
Left lateral ventricle
Right lateral ventricle
Third ventricle
	Ø Open
	3 Percutaneous
	4 Percutaneous Endoscopic
		7 Autologous Tissue
		   Substitute
		J Synthetic Substitute
		K Nonautologous Tissue
		   Substitute
			Ø Nasopharynx
			1 Mastoid Sinus
			2 Atrium
			3 Blood Vessel
			4 Pleural Cavity
			5 Intestine
			6 Peritoneal Cavity
			7 Urinary Tract
			8 Bone Marrow
			A Subgaleal Space
			B Cerebral Cisterns

6 Cerebral Ventricle Aqueduct of Sylvius Cerebral aqueduct (Sylvius) Choroid plexus Ependyma Foramen of Monro (intraventricular) Fourth ventricle Interventricular foramen (Monro) Left lateral ventricle Right lateral ventricle Third ventricle	Ø Open 3 Percutaneous 4 Percutaneous Endoscopic	Z No Device	B Cerebral Cisterns

U Spinal Canal
Epidural space, spinal
Extradural space, spinal
Subarachnoid space, spinal
Subdural space, spinal
Vertebral canal
	Ø Open
	3 Percutaneous
	4 Percutaneous Endoscopic
		7 Autologous Tissue
		   Substitute
		J Synthetic Substitute
		K Nonautologous Tissue
		   Substitute
			2 Atrium
			4 Pleural Cavity
			6 Peritoneal Cavity
			7 Urinary Tract
			9 Fallopian Tube

Ø   **Medical and Surgical**
Ø   **Central Nervous System and Cranial Nerves**
2   **Change**   Definition: Taking out or off a device from a body part and putting back an identical or similar device in or on the same body part without cutting or puncturing the skin or a mucous membrane

Explanation: All CHANGE procedures are coded using the approach EXTERNAL

Body Part Character 4	Approach Character 5	Device Character 6	Qualifier Character 7

Ø Brain
   Cerebrum
   Corpus callosum
   Encephalon
E Cranial Nerve
U Spinal Canal
   Epidural space, spinal
   Extradural space, spinal
   Subarachnoid space, spinal
   Subdural space, spinal
   Vertebral canal
	X External	Ø Drainage Device
		Y Other Device
			Z No Qualifier

Non-OR   All body part, approach, device, and qualifier values

Non-OR Procedure   DRG Non-OR Procedure   Valid OR Procedure   HAC Associated Procedure   Combination Only   New/Revised April   New/Revised October

134

ICD-10-PCS 2023

001–002

0   **Medical and Surgical**
0   **Central Nervous System and Cranial Nerves**
5   **Destruction**   Definition: Physical eradication of all or a portion of a body part by the direct use of energy, force, or a destructive agent

                             Explanation: None of the body part is physically taken out

Body Part Character 4		Approach Character 5	Device Character 6	Qualifier Character 7
0 Brain Cerebrum Corpus callosum Encephalon **W Cervical Spinal Cord** Dorsal root ganglion	**X Thoracic Spinal Cord** Dorsal root ganglion **Y Lumbar Spinal Cord** Cauda equina Conus medullaris Dorsal root ganglion	**0 Open** **3 Percutaneous** **4 Percutaneous Endoscopic**	**Z No Device**	**3 Laser Interstitial Thermal Therapy** **Z No Qualifier**

1 Cerebral Meninges
Arachnoid mater,
  intracranial
Leptomeninges,
  intracranial
Pia mater, intracranial
2 Dura Mater
Diaphragma sellae
Dura mater, intracranial
Falx cerebri
Tentorium cerebelli
6 Cerebral Ventricle
Aqueduct of Sylvius
Cerebral aqueduct
  (Sylvius)
Choroid plexus
Ependyma
Foramen of Monro
  (intraventricular)
Fourth ventricle
Interventricular foramen
  (Monro)
Left lateral ventricle
Right lateral ventricle
Third ventricle
7 Cerebral Hemisphere
Frontal lobe
Occipital lobe
Parietal lobe
Temporal lobe
8 Basal Ganglia
Basal nuclei
Claustrum
Corpus striatum
Globus pallidus
Substantia nigra
Subthalamic nucleus
9 Thalamus
Epithalamus
Geniculate nucleus
Metathalamus
Pulvinar
A Hypothalamus
Mammillary body
B Pons
Apneustic center
Basis pontis
Locus ceruleus
Pneumotaxic center
Pontine tegmentum
Superior olivary nucleus
C Cerebellum
Culmen
D Medulla Oblongata
Myelencephalon
F Olfactory Nerve
First cranial nerve
Olfactory bulb
G Optic Nerve
Optic chiasma
Second cranial nerve
	H Oculomotor Nerve
	Third cranial nerve
	J Trochlear Nerve
	Fourth cranial nerve
	K Trigeminal Nerve
	Fifth cranial nerve
	Gasserian ganglion
	Mandibular nerve
	Maxillary nerve
	Ophthalmic nerve
	Trifacial nerve
	L Abducens Nerve
	Sixth cranial nerve
	M Facial Nerve
	Chorda tympani
	Geniculate ganglion
	Greater superficial petrosal
	  nerve
	Nerve to the stapedius
	Parotid plexus
	Posterior auricular nerve
	Seventh cranial nerve
	Submandibular ganglion
	N Acoustic Nerve
	Cochlear nerve
	Eighth cranial nerve
	Scarpa's (vestibular)
	  ganglion
	Spiral ganglion
	Vestibular (Scarpa's)
	  ganglion
	Vestibular nerve
	Vestibulocochlear nerve
	P Glossopharyngeal Nerve
	Carotid sinus nerve
	Ninth cranial nerve
	Tympanic nerve
	Q Vagus Nerve
	Anterior vagal trunk
	Pharyngeal plexus
	Pneumogastric nerve
	Posterior vagal trunk
	Pulmonary plexus
	Recurrent laryngeal nerve
	Superior laryngeal nerve
	Tenth cranial nerve
	R Accessory Nerve
	Eleventh cranial nerve
	S Hypoglossal Nerve
	Twelfth cranial nerve
	T Spinal Meninges
	Arachnoid mater, spinal
	Denticulate (dentate)
	  ligament
	Dura mater, spinal
	Filum terminale
	Leptomeninges, spinal
	Pia mater, spinal
		0 Open
		3 Percutaneous
		4 Percutaneous Endoscopic
			Z No Device	**Z No Qualifier**

Non-OR	005[F,G,H,J,K,L,M,N,P,Q,R,S][0,3,4]ZZ

NC Noncovered Procedure   **LC** Limited Coverage   **QA** Questionable OB Admit   **NT** New Tech Add-on   ⊞ Combination Member   ♂ Male   ♀ Female

ICD-10-PCS 2023   135

Ø   **Medical and Surgical**
Ø   **Central Nervous System and Cranial Nerves**
7   **Dilation**   Definition: Expanding an orifice or the lumen of a tubular body part

Explanation: The orifice can be a natural orifice or an artificially created orifice. Accomplished by stretching a tubular body part using intraluminal pressure or by cutting part of the orifice or wall of the tubular body part.

Body Part Character 4	Approach Character 5	Device Character 6	Qualifier Character 7

6   Cerebral Ventricle
    Aqueduct of Sylvius
    Cerebral aqueduct (Sylvius)
    Choroid plexus
    Ependyma
    Foramen of Monro (intraventricular)
    Fourth ventricle
    Interventricular foramen (Monro)
    Left lateral ventricle
    Right lateral ventricle
    Third ventricle
	Ø Open
	3 Percutaneous
	4 Percutaneous Endoscopic
		Z No Device	Z No Qualifier

Ø   **Medical and Surgical**
Ø   **Central Nervous System and Cranial Nerves**
8   **Division**   Definition: Cutting into a body part, without draining fluids and/or gases from the body part, in order to separate or transect a body part

Explanation: All or a portion of the body part is separated into two or more portions

Body Part Character 4		Approach Character 5	Device Character 6	Qualifier Character 7

Ø   Brain
    Cerebrum
    Corpus callosum
    Encephalon
7   Cerebral Hemisphere
    Frontal lobe
    Occipital lobe
    Parietal lobe
    Temporal lobe
8   Basal Ganglia
    Basal nuclei
    Claustrum
    Corpus striatum
    Globus pallidus
    Substantia nigra
    Subthalamic nucleus
F   Olfactory Nerve
    First cranial nerve
    Olfactory bulb
G   Optic Nerve
    Optic chiasma
    Second cranial nerve
H   Oculomotor Nerve
    Third cranial nerve
J   Trochlear Nerve
    Fourth cranial nerve
K   Trigeminal Nerve
    Fifth cranial nerve
    Gasserian ganglion
    Mandibular nerve
    Maxillary nerve
    Ophthalmic nerve
    Trifacial nerve
L   Abducens Nerve
    Sixth cranial nerve
M   Facial Nerve
    Chorda tympani
    Geniculate ganglion
    Greater superficial petrosal
      nerve
    Nerve to the stapedius
    Parotid plexus
    Posterior auricular nerve
    Seventh cranial nerve
    Submandibular ganglion
	N Acoustic Nerve
	    Cochlear nerve
	    Eighth cranial nerve
	    Scarpa's (vestibular)
	      ganglion
	    Spiral ganglion
	    Vestibular (Scarpa's)
	      ganglion
	    Vestibular nerve
	    Vestibulocochlear nerve
	P Glossopharyngeal Nerve
	    Carotid sinus nerve
	    Ninth cranial nerve
	    Tympanic nerve
	Q Vagus Nerve
	    Anterior vagal trunk
	    Pharyngeal plexus
	    Pneumogastric nerve
	    Posterior vagal trunk
	    Pulmonary plexus
	    Recurrent laryngeal nerve
	    Superior laryngeal nerve
	    Tenth cranial nerve
	R Accessory Nerve
	    Eleventh cranial nerve
	S Hypoglossal Nerve
	    Twelfth cranial nerve
	W Cervical Spinal Cord
	    Dorsal root ganglion
	X Thoracic Spinal Cord
	    Dorsal root ganglion
	Y Lumbar Spinal Cord
	    Cauda equina
	    Conus medullaris
	    Dorsal root ganglion
		Ø Open
		3 Percutaneous
		4 Percutaneous Endoscopic
			Z No Device	Z No Qualifier

Non-OR Procedure   DRG Non-OR Procedure   Valid OR Procedure   HAC Associated Procedure   Combination Only   New/Revised April   New/Revised October

136   ICD-10-PCS 2023

Ø   Medical and Surgical
Ø   Central Nervous System and Cranial Nerves
9   Drainage   Definition: Taking or letting out fluids and/or gases from a body part

Explanation: The qualifier DIAGNOSTIC is used to identify drainage procedures that are biopsies

Body Part Character 4	Approach Character 5	Device Character 6	Qualifier Character 7
Ø Brain Cerebrum Corpus callosum Encephalon **1 Cerebral Meninges** Arachnoid mater, intracranial Leptomeninges, intracranial Pia mater, intracranial **2 Dura Mater** Diaphragma sellae Dura mater, intracranial Falx cerebri Tentorium cerebelli **3 Epidural Space, Intracranial** Extradural space, intracranial **4 Subdural Space, Intracranial** **5 Subarachnoid Space, Intracranial** **6 Cerebral Ventricle** Aqueduct of Sylvius Cerebral aqueduct (Sylvius) Choroid plexus Ependyma Foramen of Monro (intraventricular) Fourth ventricle Interventricular foramen (Monro) Left lateral ventricle Right lateral ventricle Third ventricle **7 Cerebral Hemisphere** Frontal lobe Occipital lobe Parietal lobe Temporal lobe **8 Basal Ganglia** Basal nuclei Claustrum Corpus striatum Globus pallidus Substantia nigra Subthalamic nucleus **9 Thalamus** Epithalamus Geniculate nucleus Metathalamus Pulvinar **A Hypothalamus** Mammillary body **B Pons** Apneustic center Basis pontis Locus ceruleus Pneumotaxic center Pontine tegmentum Superior olivary nucleus **C Cerebellum** Culmen **D Medulla Oblongata** Myelencephalon **F Olfactory Nerve** First cranial nerve Olfactory bulb	**G Optic Nerve** Optic chiasma Second cranial nerve **H Oculomotor Nerve** Third cranial nerve **J Trochlear Nerve** Fourth cranial nerve **K Trigeminal Nerve** Fifth cranial nerve Gasserian ganglion Mandibular nerve Maxillary nerve Ophthalmic nerve Trifacial nerve **L Abducens Nerve** Sixth cranial nerve **M Facial Nerve** Chorda tympani Geniculate ganglion Greater superficial petrosal nerve Nerve to the stapedius Parotid plexus Posterior auricular nerve Seventh cranial nerve Submandibular ganglion **N Acoustic Nerve** Cochlear nerve Eighth cranial nerve Scarpa's (vestibular) ganglion Spiral ganglion Vestibular (Scarpa's) ganglion Vestibular nerve Vestibulocochlear nerve **P Glossopharyngeal Nerve** Carotid sinus nerve Ninth cranial nerve Tympanic nerve **Q Vagus Nerve** Anterior vagal trunk Pharyngeal plexus Pneumogastric nerve Posterior vagal trunk Pulmonary plexus Recurrent laryngeal nerve Superior laryngeal nerve Tenth cranial nerve **R Accessory Nerve** Eleventh cranial nerve **S Hypoglossal Nerve** Twelfth cranial nerve **T Spinal Meninges** Arachnoid mater, spinal Denticulate (dentate) ligament Dura mater, spinal Filum terminale Leptomeninges, spinal Pia mater, spinal **U Spinal Canal** Epidural space, spinal Extradural space, spinal Subarachnoid space, spinal Subdural space, spinal Vertebral canal **W Cervical Spinal Cord** Dorsal root ganglion **X Thoracic Spinal Cord** Dorsal root ganglion **Y Lumbar Spinal Cord** Cauda equina Conus medullaris Dorsal root ganglion	**Ø Open** **3 Percutaneous** **4 Percutaneous Endoscopic**	**Ø Drainage Device**	**Z No Qualifier**

Non-OR	009[T,W,X,Y]30Z
Non-OR	009U[3,4]0Z

009 Continued on next page

NC Noncovered Procedure   **LC** Limited Coverage   **QA** Questionable OB Admit   **NT** New Tech Add-on   ⊞ Combination Member   ♂ Male   ♀ Female

ICD-10-PCS 2023   137

Ø   **Medical and Surgical**   ***Ø09 Continued***
Ø   **Central Nervous System and Cranial Nerves**
9   **Drainage**   Definition: Taking or letting out fluids and/or gases from a body part
                     Explanation: The qualifier DIAGNOSTIC is used to identify drainage procedures that are biopsies

Body Part Character 4		Approach Character 5	Device Character 6	Qualifier Character 7
Ø **Brain** Cerebrum Corpus callosum Encephalon	**G** **Optic Nerve** Optic chiasma Second cranial nerve	**Ø** Open **3** Percutaneous **4** Percutaneous Endoscopic	**Z** No Device	**X** Diagnostic **Z** No Qualifier

1 **Cerebral Meninges**
 Arachnoid mater,
     intracranial
 Leptomeninges,
     intracranial
 Pia mater, intracranial
	H **Oculomotor Nerve**
	 Third cranial nerve
	 J **Trochlear Nerve**
	 Fourth cranial nerve			

2 **Dura Mater** Diaphragma sellae Dura mater, intracranial Falx cerebri Tentorium cerebelli	**K** **Trigeminal Nerve** Fifth cranial nerve Gasserian ganglion Mandibular nerve Maxillary nerve Ophthalmic nerve Trifacial nerve			
3 **Epidural Space, Intracranial** Extradural space, intracranial	**L** **Abducens Nerve** Sixth cranial nerve			
4 **Subdural Space, Intracranial**	**M** **Facial Nerve** Chorda tympani Geniculate ganglion Greater superficial petrosal nerve Nerve to the stapedius Parotid plexus Posterior auricular nerve Seventh cranial nerve Submandibular ganglion			
5 **Subarachnoid Space, Intracranial**				

6 **Cerebral Ventricle**
 Aqueduct of Sylvius
 Cerebral aqueduct
     (Sylvius)
 Choroid plexus
 Ependyma
 Foramen of Monro
     (intraventricular)
 Fourth ventricle
 Interventricular foramen
     (Monro)
 Left lateral ventricle
 Right lateral ventricle
 Third ventricle
	N **Acoustic Nerve**
	 Cochlear nerve
	 Eighth cranial nerve
	 Scarpa's (vestibular) ganglion
	 Spiral ganglion
	 Vestibular (Scarpa's) ganglion
	 Vestibular nerve
	 Vestibulocochlear nerve			

7 **Cerebral Hemisphere** Frontal lobe Occipital lobe Parietal lobe Temporal lobe	**P** **Glossopharyngeal Nerve** Carotid sinus nerve Ninth cranial nerve Tympanic nerve **Q** **Vagus Nerve** Anterior vagal trunk			
8 **Basal Ganglia** Basal nuclei Claustrum Corpus striatum Globus pallidus Substantia nigra Subthalamic nucleus	Pharyngeal plexus Pneumogastric nerve Posterior vagal trunk Pulmonary plexus Recurrent laryngeal nerve Superior laryngeal nerve Tenth cranial nerve			
9 **Thalamus** Epithalamus Geniculate nucleus Metathalamus Pulvinar	**R** **Accessory Nerve** Eleventh cranial nerve **S** **Hypoglossal Nerve** Twelfth cranial nerve			
A **Hypothalamus** Mammillary body	**T** **Spinal Meninges** Arachnoid mater, spinal Denticulate (dentate) ligament Dura mater, spinal Filum terminale Leptomeninges, spinal Pia mater, spinal			
B **Pons** Apneustic center Basis pontis Locus ceruleus Pneumotaxic center Pontine tegmentum Superior olivary nucleus	**U** **Spinal Canal** Epidural space, spinal Extradural space, spinal Subarachnoid space, spinal Subdural space, spinal Vertebral canal			
C **Cerebellum** Culmen				
D **Medulla Oblongata** Myelencephalon	**W** **Cervical Spinal Cord** Dorsal root ganglion			
F **Olfactory Nerve** First cranial nerve Olfactory bulb	**X** **Thoracic Spinal Cord** Dorsal root ganglion **Y** **Lumbar Spinal Cord** Cauda equina Conus medullaris Dorsal root ganglion			

Non-OR   Ø09[Ø,1,2,3,4,5,6,7,8,9,A,B,C,D,F,G,H,J,K,L,M,N,P,Q,R,S][3,4]ZX
Non-OR   Ø09[T,W,X,Y]3Z[X,Z]
Non-OR   Ø09U[3,4]Z[X,Z]

Non-OR Procedure   DRG Non-OR Procedure   Valid OR Procedure   HAC Associated Procedure   Combination Only   New/Revised April   New/Revised October

0   **Medical and Surgical**
0   **Central Nervous System and Cranial Nerves**
B   **Excision**   Definition: Cutting out or off, without replacement, a portion of a body part
                   Explanation: The qualifier DIAGNOSTIC is used to identify excision procedures that are biopsies

Body Part Character 4		Approach Character 5	Device Character 6	Qualifier Character 7
0 Brain Cerebrum Corpus callosum Encephalon **1 Cerebral Meninges** Arachnoid mater, intracranial Leptomeninges, intracranial Pia mater, intracranial **2 Dura Mater** Diaphragma sellae Dura mater, intracranial Falx cerebri Tentorium cerebelli **6 Cerebral Ventricle** Aqueduct of Sylvius Cerebral aqueduct (Sylvius) Choroid plexus Ependyma Foramen of Monro (intraventricular) Fourth ventricle Interventricular foramen (Monro) Left lateral ventricle Right lateral ventricle Third ventricle **7 Cerebral Hemisphere** Frontal lobe Occipital lobe Parietal lobe Temporal lobe **8 Basal Ganglia** Basal nuclei Claustrum Corpus striatum Globus pallidus Substantia nigra Subthalamic nucleus **9 Thalamus** Epithalamus Geniculate nucleus Metathalamus Pulvinar **A Hypothalamus** Mammillary body **B Pons** Apneustic center Basis pontis Locus ceruleus Pneumotaxic center Pontine tegmentum Superior olivary nucleus **C Cerebellum** Culmen **D Medulla Oblongata** Myelencephalon **F Olfactory Nerve** First cranial nerve Olfactory bulb **G Optic Nerve** Optic chiasma Second cranial nerve	**H Oculomotor Nerve** Third cranial nerve **J Trochlear Nerve** Fourth cranial nerve **K Trigeminal Nerve** Fifth cranial nerve Gasserian ganglion Mandibular nerve Maxillary nerve Ophthalmic nerve Trifacial nerve **L Abducens Nerve** Sixth cranial nerve **M Facial Nerve** Chorda tympani Geniculate ganglion Greater superficial petrosal nerve Nerve to the stapedius Parotid plexus Posterior auricular nerve Seventh cranial nerve Submandibular ganglion **N Acoustic Nerve** Cochlear nerve Eighth cranial nerve Scarpa's (vestibular) ganglion Spiral ganglion Vestibular (Scarpa's) ganglion Vestibular nerve Vestibulocochlear nerve **P Glossopharyngeal Nerve** Carotid sinus nerve Ninth cranial nerve Tympanic nerve **Q Vagus Nerve** Anterior vagal trunk Pharyngeal plexus Pneumogastric nerve Posterior vagal trunk Pulmonary plexus Recurrent laryngeal nerve Superior laryngeal nerve Tenth cranial nerve **R Accessory Nerve** Eleventh cranial nerve **S Hypoglossal Nerve** Twelfth cranial nerve **T Spinal Meninges** Arachnoid mater, spinal Denticulate (dentate) ligament Dura mater, spinal Filum terminale Leptomeninges, spinal Pia mater, spinal **W Cervical Spinal Cord** Dorsal root ganglion **X Thoracic Spinal Cord** Dorsal root ganglion **Y Lumbar Spinal Cord** Cauda equina Conus medullaris Dorsal root ganglion	**0 Open** **3 Percutaneous** **4 Percutaneous Endoscopic**	**Z No Device**	**X Diagnostic** **Z No Qualifier**

Non-OR   00B[F,G,H,J,K,L,M,N,P,Q,R,S][3,4]ZX

NC Noncovered Procedure   **LC** Limited Coverage   **QA** Questionable OB Admit   **NT** New Tech Add-on   ⊞ Combination Member   ♂ Male   ♀ Female

ICD-10-PCS 2023   **139**

Central Nervous System and Cranial Nerves

Ø   **Medical and Surgical**
Ø   **Central Nervous System and Cranial Nerves**
C   **Extirpation**   Definition: Taking or cutting out solid matter from a body part

Explanation: The solid matter may be an abnormal byproduct of a biological function or a foreign body; it may be imbedded in a body part or in the lumen of a tubular body part. The solid matter may or may not have been previously broken into pieces.

Body Part Character 4		Approach Character 5	Device Character 6	Qualifier Character 7

Ø **Brain**
  Cerebrum
  Corpus callosum
  Encephalon
1 **Cerebral Meninges**
  Arachnoid mater,
    intracranial
  Leptomeninges,
    intracranial
  Pia mater, intracranial
2 **Dura Mater**
  Diaphragma sellae
  Dura mater, intracranial
  Falx cerebri
  Tentorium cerebelli
3 **Epidural Space,**
Intracranial
  Extradural space,
    intracranial
4 **Subdural Space,**
Intracranial
5 **Subarachnoid Space,**
Intracranial
6 **Cerebral Ventricle**
  Aqueduct of Sylvius
  Cerebral aqueduct
    (Sylvius)
  Choroid plexus
  Ependyma
  Foramen of Monro
    (intraventricular)
  Fourth ventricle
  Interventricular foramen
    (Monro)
  Left lateral ventricle
  Right lateral ventricle
  Third ventricle
7 **Cerebral Hemisphere**
  Frontal lobe
  Occipital lobe
  Parietal lobe
  Temporal lobe
8 **Basal Ganglia**
  Basal nuclei
  Claustrum
  Corpus striatum
  Globus pallidus
  Substantia nigra
  Subthalamic nucleus
9 **Thalamus**
  Epithalamus
  Geniculate nucleus
  Metathalamus
  Pulvinar
A **Hypothalamus**
  Mammillary body
B **Pons**
  Apneustic center
  Basis pontis
  Locus ceruleus
  Pneumotaxic center
  Pontine tegmentum
  Superior olivary nucleus
C **Cerebellum**
  Culmen
D **Medulla Oblongata**
  Myelencephalon
F **Olfactory Nerve**
  First cranial nerve
  Olfactory bulb
	G **Optic Nerve**
	  Optic chiasma
	  Second cranial nerve
	H **Oculomotor Nerve**
	  Third cranial nerve
	J **Trochlear Nerve**
	  Fourth cranial nerve
	K **Trigeminal Nerve**
	  Fifth cranial nerve
	  Gasserian ganglion
	  Mandibular nerve
	  Maxillary nerve
	  Ophthalmic nerve
	  Trifacial nerve
	L **Abducens Nerve**
	  Sixth cranial nerve
	M **Facial Nerve**
	  Chorda tympani
	  Geniculate ganglion
	  Greater superficial petrosal
	    nerve
	  Nerve to the stapedius
	  Parotid plexus
	  Posterior auricular nerve
	  Seventh cranial nerve
	  Submandibular ganglion
	N **Acoustic Nerve**
	  Cochlear nerve
	  Eighth cranial nerve
	  Scarpa's (vestibular)
	    ganglion
	  Spiral ganglion
	  Vestibular (Scarpa's)
	    ganglion
	  Vestibular nerve
	  Vestibulocochlear nerve
	P **Glossopharyngeal Nerve**
	  Carotid sinus nerve
	  Ninth cranial nerve
	  Tympanic nerve
	Q **Vagus Nerve**
	  Anterior vagal trunk
	  Pharyngeal plexus
	  Pneumogastric nerve
	  Posterior vagal trunk
	  Pulmonary plexus
	  Recurrent laryngeal nerve
	  Superior laryngeal nerve
	  Tenth cranial nerve
	R **Accessory Nerve**
	  Eleventh cranial nerve
	S **Hypoglossal Nerve**
	  Twelfth cranial nerve
	T **Spinal Meninges**
	  Arachnoid mater, spinal
	  Denticulate (dentate)
	    ligament
	  Dura mater, spinal
	  Filum terminale
	  Leptomeninges, spinal
	  Pia mater, spinal
	U **Spinal Canal**
	W **Cervical Spinal Cord**
	  Dorsal root ganglion
	X **Thoracic Spinal Cord**
	  Dorsal root ganglion
	Y **Lumbar Spinal Cord**
	  Cauda equina
	  Conus medullaris
	  Dorsal root ganglion
		Ø Open
		3 Percutaneous
		4 Percutaneous Endoscopic
			Z No Device	**Z** No Qualifier

Non-OR Procedure   DRG Non-OR Procedure   Valid OR Procedure   HAC Associated Procedure   Combination Only   New/Revised April   New/Revised October

140

ICD-10-PCS 2023

Ø **Medical and Surgical**
Ø **Central Nervous System and Cranial Nerves**
D **Extraction** Definition: Pulling or stripping out or off all or a portion of a body part by the use of force
Explanation: The qualifier DIAGNOSTIC is used to identify extraction procedures that are biopsies

Body Part Character 4		Approach Character 5	Device Character 6	Qualifier Character 7
Ø Brain Cerebrum Corpus callosum Encephalon **1 Cerebral Meninges** Arachnoid mater, intracranial Leptomeninges, intracranial Pia mater, intracranial **2 Dura Mater** Diaphragma sellae Dura mater, intracranial Falx cerebri Tentorium cerebelli **7 Cerebral Hemisphere** Frontal lobe Occipital lobe Parietal lobe Temporal lobe **C Cerebellum** Culmen **F Olfactory Nerve** First cranial nerve Olfactory bulb **G Optic Nerve** Optic chiasma Second cranial nerve **H Oculomotor Nerve** Third cranial nerve **J Trochlear Nerve** Fourth cranial nerve **K Trigeminal Nerve** Fifth cranial nerve Gasserian ganglion Mandibular nerve Maxillary nerve Ophthalmic nerve Trifacial nerve **L Abducens Nerve** Sixth cranial nerve	**M Facial Nerve** Chorda tympani Geniculate ganglion Greater superficial petrosal nerve Nerve to the stapedius Parotid plexus Posterior auricular nerve Seventh cranial nerve Submandibular ganglion **N Acoustic Nerve** Cochlear nerve Eighth cranial nerve Scarpa's (vestibular) ganglion Spiral ganglion Vestibular (Scarpa's) ganglion Vestibular nerve Vestibulocochlear nerve **P Glossopharyngeal Nerve** Carotid sinus nerve Ninth cranial nerve Tympanic nerve **Q Vagus Nerve** Anterior vagal trunk Pharyngeal plexus Pneumogastric nerve Posterior vagal trunk Pulmonary plexus Recurrent laryngeal nerve Superior laryngeal nerve Tenth cranial nerve **R Accessory Nerve** Eleventh cranial nerve **S Hypoglossal Nerve** Twelfth cranial nerve **T Spinal Meninges** Arachnoid mater, spinal Denticulate (dentate) ligament Dura mater, spinal Filum terminale Leptomeninges, spinal Pia mater, spinal	**Ø Open** **3 Percutaneous** **4 Percutaneous Endoscopic**	**Z No Device**	**Z No Qualifier**

0   **Medical and Surgical**
0   **Central Nervous System and Cranial Nerves**
F   **Fragmentation**   Definition: Breaking solid matter in a body part into pieces

             Explanation: Physical force (e.g., manual, ultrasonic) applied directly or indirectly is used to break the solid matter into pieces. The solid matter may be an abnormal byproduct of a biological function or a foreign body. The pieces of solid matter are not taken out.

Body Part Character 4	Approach Character 5	Device Character 6	Qualifier Character 7

3 Epidural Space, Intracranial   NC
    Extradural space, intracranial
4 Subdural Space, Intracranial   NC
5 Subarachnoid Space, Intracranial   NC
6 Cerebral Ventricle   NC
    Aqueduct of Sylvius
    Cerebral aqueduct (Sylvius)
    Choroid plexus
    Ependyma
    Foramen of Monro (intraventricular)
    Fourth ventricle
    Interventricular foramen (Monro)
    Left lateral ventricle
    Right lateral ventricle
    Third ventricle
U Spinal Canal
    Epidural space, spinal
    Extradural space, spinal
    Subarachnoid space, spinal
    Subdural space, spinal
    Vertebral canal
	0 Open
	3 Percutaneous
	4 Percutaneous Endoscopic
	X External
		Z No Device	**Z** No Qualifier

Non-OR   00F[3,4,5,6]XZZ
NC   00F[3,4,5,6]XZZ

0   **Medical and Surgical**
0   **Central Nervous System and Cranial Nerves**
H   **Insertion**   Definition: Putting in a nonbiological appliance that monitors, assists, performs, or prevents a physiological function but does not physically take the place of a body part

             Explanation: None

Body Part Character 4	Approach Character 5	Device Character 6	Qualifier Character 7

0 Brain ⊞
    Cerebrum
    Corpus callosum
    Encephalon
	0 Open	**1** Radioactive Element
		2 Monitoring Device
		3 Infusion Device
		4 Radioactive Element, Cesium-131
		    Collagen Implant
		M Neurostimulator Lead
		Y Other Device
			Z No Qualifier

0 Brain ⊞
    Cerebrum
    Corpus callosum
    Encephalon
	3 Percutaneous
	4 Percutaneous Endoscopic
		1 Radioactive Element
		2 Monitoring Device
		3 Infusion Device
		M Neurostimulator Lead
		Y Other Device
			Z No Qualifier

6 Cerebral Ventricle ⊞
    Aqueduct of Sylvius
    Cerebral aqueduct (Sylvius)
    Choroid plexus
    Ependyma
    Foramen of Monro (intraventricular)
    Fourth ventricle Interventricular foramen
    (Monro)
    Left lateral ventricle
    Right lateral ventricle
    Third ventricle
E Cranial Nerve ⊞
U Spinal Canal ⊞
    Epidural space, spinal
    Extradural space, spinal
    Subarachnoid space, spinal
    Subdural space, spinal
    Vertebral canal
V Spinal Cord ⊞
    Dorsal root ganglion
	0 Open
	3 Percutaneous
	4 Percutaneous Endoscopic
		1 Radioactive Element
		2 Monitoring Device
		3 Infusion Device
		M Neurostimulator Lead
		Y Other Device
			Z No Qualifier

DRG Non-OR 00H004Z		
Non-OR 00H[E,U,V]32Z	**See Appendix L for Procedure Combinations**	
Non-OR 00H[E,U][3,4]YZ	⊞ 00H00MZ	
Non-OR 00H[U,V][0,3,4]3Z	⊞ 00H0[3,4]MZ	
	⊞ 00H[6,E,U,V][0,3,4]MZ	

Non-OR Procedure   DRG Non-OR Procedure   Valid OR Procedure   HAC Associated Procedure   Combination Only   New/Revised April   New/Revised October

142   ICD-10-PCS 2023

00F–00H

Ø   **Medical and Surgical**
Ø   **Central Nervous System and Cranial Nerves**
J   **Inspection**   Definition: Visually and/or manually exploring a body part

Explanation: Visual exploration may be performed with or without optical instrumentation. Manual exploration may be performed directly or through intervening body layers.

Body Part Character 4	Approach Character 5	Device Character 6	Qualifier Character 7

Ø   **Brain**
    Cerebrum
    Corpus callosum
    Encephalon
E   **Cranial Nerve**
U   **Spinal Canal**
    Epidural space, spinal
    Extradural space, spinal
    Subarachnoid space, spinal
    Subdural space, spinal
    Vertebral canal
V   **Spinal Cord**
    Dorsal root ganglion
	Ø Open
	3 Percutaneous
	4 Percutaneous Endoscopic
		Z No Device	**Z** No Qualifier

Non-OR   ØØJ[Ø,E,U,V]3ZZ

Ø   **Medical and Surgical**
Ø   **Central Nervous System and Cranial Nerves**
K   **Map**   Definition: Locating the route of passage of electrical impulses and/or locating functional areas in a body part

Explanation: Applicable only to the cardiac conduction mechanism and the central nervous system

Body Part Character 4	Approach Character 5	Device Character 6	Qualifier Character 7

Ø   **Brain**
    Cerebrum
    Corpus callosum
    Encephalon
7   **Cerebral Hemisphere**
    Frontal lobe
    Occipital lobe
    Parietal lobe
    Temporal lobe
8   **Basal Ganglia**
    Basal nuclei
    Claustrum
    Corpus striatum
    Globus pallidus
    Substantia nigra
    Subthalamic nucleus
9   **Thalamus**
    Epithalamus
    Geniculate nucleus
    Metathalamus
    Pulvinar
A   **Hypothalamus**
    Mammillary body
B   **Pons**
    Apneustic center
    Basis pontis
    Locus ceruleus
    Pneumotaxic center
    Pontine tegmentum
    Superior olivary nucleus
C   **Cerebellum**
    Culmen
D   **Medulla Oblongata**
    Myelencephalon
	Ø Open
	3 Percutaneous
	4 Percutaneous Endoscopic
		Z No Device	**Z** No Qualifier

NC Noncovered Procedure   **LC** Limited Coverage   **QA** Questionable OB Admit   **NT** New Tech Add-on   ⊞ Combination Member   ♂ Male   ♀ Female

ICD-10-PCS 2023   **143**

Central Nervous System and Cranial Nerves

Ø   **Medical and Surgical**
Ø   **Central Nervous System and Cranial Nerves**
N   **Release**   Definition: Freeing a body part from an abnormal physical constraint by cutting or by the use of force
                       Explanation: Some of the restraining tissue may be taken out but none of the body part is taken out

Body Part Character 4		Approach Character 5	Device Character 6	Qualifier Character 7

Ø **Brain**
  Cerebrum
  Corpus callosum
  Encephalon
1 **Cerebral Meninges**
  Arachnoid mater,
    intracranial
  Leptomeninges,
    intracranial
  Pia mater, intracranial
2 **Dura Mater**
  Diaphragma sellae
  Dura mater, intracranial
  Falx cerebri
  Tentorium cerebelli
6 **Cerebral Ventricle**
  Aqueduct of Sylvius
  Cerebral aqueduct
    (Sylvius)
  Choroid plexus
  Ependyma
  Foramen of Monro
    (intraventricular)
  Fourth ventricle
  Interventricular foramen
    (Monro)
  Left lateral ventricle
  Right lateral ventricle
  Third ventricle
7 **Cerebral Hemisphere**
  Frontal lobe
  Occipital lobe
  Parietal lobe
  Temporal lobe
8 **Basal Ganglia**
  Basal nuclei
  Claustrum
  Corpus striatum
  Globus pallidus
  Substantia nigra
  Subthalamic nucleus
9 **Thalamus**
  Epithalamus
  Geniculate nucleus
  Metathalamus
  Pulvinar
A **Hypothalamus**
  Mammillary body
B **Pons**
  Apneustic center
  Basis pontis
  Locus ceruleus
  Pneumotaxic center
  Pontine tegmentum
  Superior olivary nucleus
C **Cerebellum**
  Culmen
D **Medulla Oblongata**
  Myelencephalon
F **Olfactory Nerve**
  First cranial nerve
  Olfactory bulb
G **Optic Nerve**
  Optic chiasma
  Second cranial nerve
	H **Oculomotor Nerve**
	  Third cranial nerve
	J **Trochlear Nerve**
	  Fourth cranial nerve
	K **Trigeminal Nerve**
	  Fifth cranial nerve
	  Gasserian ganglion
	  Mandibular nerve
	  Maxillary nerve
	  Ophthalmic nerve
	  Trifacial nerve
	L **Abducens Nerve**
	  Sixth cranial nerve
	M **Facial Nerve**
	  Chorda tympani
	  Geniculate ganglion
	  Greater superficial petrosal
	    nerve
	  Nerve to the stapedius
	  Parotid plexus
	  Posterior auricular nerve
	  Seventh cranial nerve
	  Submandibular ganglion
	N **Acoustic Nerve**
	  Cochlear nerve
	  Eighth cranial nerve
	  Scarpa's (vestibular)
	    ganglion
	  Spiral ganglion
	  Vestibular (Scarpa's)
	    ganglion
	  Vestibular nerve
	  Vestibulocochlear nerve
	P **Glossopharyngeal Nerve**
	  Carotid sinus nerve
	  Ninth cranial nerve
	  Tympanic nerve
	Q **Vagus Nerve**
	  Anterior vagal trunk
	  Pharyngeal plexus
	  Pneumogastric nerve
	  Posterior vagal trunk
	  Pulmonary plexus
	  Recurrent laryngeal nerve
	  Superior laryngeal nerve
	  Tenth cranial nerve
	R **Accessory Nerve**
	  Eleventh cranial nerve
	S **Hypoglossal Nerve**
	  Twelfth cranial nerve
	T **Spinal Meninges**
	  Arachnoid mater, spinal
	  Denticulate (dentate)
	    ligament
	  Dura mater, spinal
	  Filum terminale
	  Leptomeninges, spinal
	  Pia mater, spinal
	W **Cervical Spinal Cord**
	  Dorsal root ganglion
	X **Thoracic Spinal Cord**
	  Dorsal root ganglion
	Y **Lumbar Spinal Cord**
	  Cauda equina
	  Conus medullaris
	  Dorsal root ganglion
		Ø Open
		3 Percutaneous
		4 Percutaneous Endoscopic
			Z No Device	Z No Qualifier

Ø   **Medical and Surgical**
Ø   **Central Nervous System and Cranial Nerves**
P   **Removal**   Definition: Taking out or off a device from a body part

                       Explanation: If a device is taken out and a similar device put in without cutting or puncturing the skin or mucous membrane, the procedure is coded to the root operation CHANGE. Otherwise, the procedure for taking out a device is coded to the root operation REMOVAL.

Body Part Character 4	Approach Character 5	Device Character 6	Qualifier Character 7
Ø **Brain** Cerebrum Corpus callosum Encephalon V **Spinal Cord** Dorsal root ganglion	Ø Open 3 Percutaneous 4 Percutaneous Endoscopic	Ø Drainage Device 2 Monitoring Device 3 Infusion Device 7 Autologous Tissue Substitute J Synthetic Substitute K Nonautologous Tissue Substitute M Neurostimulator Lead Y Other Device	Z No Qualifier
Ø **Brain** Cerebrum Corpus callosum Encephalon V **Spinal Cord** Dorsal root ganglion	X External	Ø Drainage Device 2 Monitoring Device 3 Infusion Device M Neurostimulator Lead	Z No Qualifier
6 **Cerebral Ventricle** Aqueduct of Sylvius Cerebral aqueduct (Sylvius) Choroid plexus Ependyma Foramen of Monro (intraventricular) Fourth ventricle Interventricular foramen (Monro) Left lateral ventricle Right lateral ventricle Third ventricle U **Spinal Canal** Epidural space, spinal Extradural space, spinal Subarachnoid space, spinal Subdural space, spinal Vertebral canal	Ø Open 3 Percutaneous 4 Percutaneous Endoscopic	Ø Drainage Device 2 Monitoring Device 3 Infusion Device J Synthetic Substitute M Neurostimulator Lead Y Other Device	Z No Qualifier
6 **Cerebral Ventricle** Aqueduct of Sylvius Cerebral aqueduct (Sylvius) Choroid plexus Ependyma Foramen of Monro (intraventricular) Fourth ventricle Interventricular foramen (Monro) Left lateral ventricle Right lateral ventricle Third ventricle U **Spinal Canal** Epidural space, spinal Extradural space, spinal Subarachnoid space, spinal Subdural space, spinal Vertebral canal	X External	Ø Drainage Device 2 Monitoring Device 3 Infusion Device M Neurostimulator Lead	Z No Qualifier
E **Cranial Nerve**	Ø Open 3 Percutaneous 4 Percutaneous Endoscopic	Ø Drainage Device 2 Monitoring Device 3 Infusion Device 7 Autologous Tissue Substitute M Neurostimulator Lead Y Other Device	Z No Qualifier
E **Cranial Nerve**	X External	Ø Drainage Device 2 Monitoring Device 3 Infusion Device M Neurostimulator Lead	Z No Qualifier

Non-OR	ØØP[Ø,V]3[Ø,2,3]Z
Non-OR	ØØP[Ø,V][3,4]YZ
Non-OR	ØØP[Ø,V]X[Ø,2,3,M]Z
Non-OR	ØØP[6,U]3[Ø,2,3]Z
Non-OR	ØØP[6,U][3,4]YZ
Non-OR	ØØP[6,U]X[Ø,2,3,M]Z
Non-OR	ØØPE3[Ø,2,3]Z
Non-OR	ØØPE[3,4]YZ
Non-OR	ØØPEX[Ø,2,3,M]Z

NC Noncovered Procedure   LC Limited Coverage   QA Questionable OB Admit   NT New Tech Add-on   ⊞ Combination Member   ♂ Male   ♀ Female

ICD-10-PCS 2023   **145**

Central Nervous System and Cranial Nerves

Ø   **Medical and Surgical**
Ø   **Central Nervous System and Cranial Nerves**
Q   **Repair**   Definition: Restoring, to the extent possible, a body part to its normal anatomic structure and function
                       Explanation: Used only when the method to accomplish the repair is not one of the other root operations

Body Part Character 4		Approach Character 5	Device Character 6	Qualifier Character 7
Ø **Brain**	H **Oculomotor Nerve**	Ø Open	Z No Device	Z No Qualifier
Cerebrum	Third cranial nerve	3 Percutaneous		
Corpus callosum	J **Trochlear Nerve**	4 Percutaneous Endoscopic		
Encephalon	Fourth cranial nerve			
1 **Cerebral Meninges**	K **Trigeminal Nerve**			
Arachnoid mater,	Fifth cranial nerve			
intracranial	Gasserian ganglion			
Leptomeninges,	Mandibular nerve			
intracranial	Maxillary nerve			
Pia mater, intracranial	Ophthalmic nerve			
2 **Dura Mater**	Trifacial nerve			
Diaphragma sellae	L **Abducens Nerve**			
Dura mater, intracranial	Sixth cranial nerve			
Falx cerebri	M **Facial Nerve**			
Tentorium cerebelli	Chorda tympani			
6 **Cerebral Ventricle**	Geniculate ganglion			
Aqueduct of Sylvius	Greater superficial petrosal			
Cerebral aqueduct	nerve			
(Sylvius)	Nerve to the stapedius			
Choroid plexus	Parotid plexus			
Ependyma	Posterior auricular nerve			
Foramen of Monro	Seventh cranial nerve			
(intraventricular)	Submandibular ganglion			
Fourth ventricle	N **Acoustic Nerve**			
Interventricular foramen	Cochlear nerve			
(Monro)	Eighth cranial nerve			
Left lateral ventricle	Scarpa's (vestibular)			
Right lateral ventricle	ganglion			
Third ventricle	Spiral ganglion			
7 **Cerebral Hemisphere**	Vestibular (Scarpa's)			
Frontal lobe	ganglion			
Occipital lobe	Vestibular nerve			
Parietal lobe	Vestibulocochlear nerve			
Temporal lobe	P **Glossopharyngeal Nerve**			
8 **Basal Ganglia**	Carotid sinus nerve			
Basal nuclei	Ninth cranial nerve			
Claustrum	Tympanic nerve			
Corpus striatum	Q **Vagus Nerve**			
Globus pallidus	Anterior vagal trunk			
Substantia nigra	Pharyngeal plexus			
Subthalamic nucleus	Pneumogastric nerve			
9 **Thalamus**	Posterior vagal trunk			
Epithalamus	Pulmonary plexus			
Geniculate nucleus	Recurrent laryngeal nerve			
Metathalamus	Superior laryngeal nerve			
Pulvinar	Tenth cranial nerve			
A **Hypothalamus**	R **Accessory Nerve**			
Mammillary body	Eleventh cranial nerve			
B **Pons**	S **Hypoglossal Nerve**			
Apneustic center	Twelfth cranial nerve			
Basis pontis	T **Spinal Meninges**			
Locus ceruleus	Arachnoid mater, spinal			
Pneumotaxic center	Denticulate (dentate)			
Pontine tegmentum	ligament			
Superior olivary nucleus	Dura mater, spinal			
C **Cerebellum**	Filum terminale			
Culmen	Leptomeninges, spinal			
D **Medulla Oblongata**	Pia mater, spinal			
Myelencephalon	W **Cervical Spinal Cord**			
F **Olfactory Nerve**	Dorsal root ganglion			
First cranial nerve	X **Thoracic Spinal Cord**			
Olfactory bulb	Dorsal root ganglion			
G **Optic Nerve**	Y **Lumbar Spinal Cord**			
Optic chiasma	Cauda equina			
Second cranial nerve	Conus medullaris			
	Dorsal root ganglion			

Non-OR Procedure   DRG Non-OR Procedure   Valid OR Procedure   HAC Associated Procedure   Combination Only   New/Revised April   New/Revised October

146   ICD-10-PCS 2023

0   **Medical and Surgical**
0   **Central Nervous System and Cranial Nerves**
R   **Replacement**   Definition: Putting in or on biological or synthetic material that physically takes the place and/or function of all or a portion of a body part

Explanation: The body part may have been taken out or replaced, or may be taken out, physically eradicated, or rendered nonfunctional during the REPLACEMENT procedure. A REMOVAL procedure is coded for taking out the device used in a previous replacement procedure.

Body Part Character 4		Approach Character 5	Device Character 6	Qualifier Character 7

1 Cerebral Meninges
Arachnoid mater,
  intracranial
Leptomeninges,
  intracranial
Pia mater, intracranial
2 Dura Mater
Diaphragma sellae
Dura mater, intracranial
Falx cerebri
Tentorium cerebelli
6 Cerebral Ventricle
Aqueduct of Sylvius
Cerebral aqueduct
  (Sylvius)
Choroid plexus
Ependyma
Foramen of Monro
  (intraventricular)
Fourth ventricle
Interventricular foramen
  (Monro)
Left lateral ventricle
Right lateral ventricle
Third ventricle
F Olfactory Nerve
First cranial nerve
Olfactory bulb
G Optic Nerve
Optic chiasma
Second cranial nerve
H Oculomotor Nerve
Third cranial nerve
J Trochlear Nerve
Fourth cranial nerve
K Trigeminal Nerve
Fifth cranial nerve
Gasserian ganglion
Mandibular nerve
Maxillary nerve
Ophthalmic nerve
Trifacial nerve
L Abducens Nerve
Sixth cranial nerve
	M Facial Nerve
	Chorda tympani
	Geniculate ganglion
	Greater superficial petrosal
	  nerve
	Nerve to the stapedius
	Parotid plexus
	Posterior auricular nerve
	Seventh cranial nerve
	Submandibular ganglion
	N Acoustic Nerve
	Cochlear nerve
	Eighth cranial nerve
	Scarpa's (vestibular)
	  ganglion
	Spiral ganglion
	Vestibular (Scarpa's)
	  ganglion
	Vestibular nerve
	Vestibulocochlear nerve
	P Glossopharyngeal Nerve
	Carotid sinus nerve
	Ninth cranial nerve
	Tympanic nerve
	Q Vagus Nerve
	Anterior vagal trunk
	Pharyngeal plexus
	Pneumogastric nerve
	Posterior vagal trunk
	Pulmonary plexus
	Recurrent laryngeal nerve
	Superior laryngeal nerve
	Tenth cranial nerve
	R Accessory Nerve
	Eleventh cranial nerve
	S Hypoglossal Nerve
	Twelfth cranial nerve
	T Spinal Meninges
	Arachnoid mater, spinal
	Denticulate (dentate)
	  ligament
	Dura mater, spinal
	Filum terminale
	Leptomeninges, spinal
	Pia mater, spinal
		0 Open
		4 Percutaneous Endoscopic
			7 Autologous Tissue
			  Substitute
			J Synthetic Substitute
			K Nonautologous Tissue
			  Substitute
				Z No Qualifier

NC Noncovered Procedure   **LC** Limited Coverage   **OA** Questionable OB Admit   **NT** New Tech Add-on   ✛ Combination Member   ♂ Male   ♀ Female

ICD-10-PCS 2023   **147**

Central Nervous System and Cranial Nerves

Ø   Medical and Surgical
Ø   Central Nervous System and Cranial Nerves
S   Reposition   Definition: Moving to its normal location, or other suitable location, all or a portion of a body part

Explanation: The body part is moved to a new location from an abnormal location, or from a normal location where it is not functioning correctly. The body part may or may not be cut out or off to be moved to the new location.

Body Part Character 4		Approach Character 5	Device Character 6	Qualifier Character 7

F Olfactory Nerve
First cranial nerve
Olfactory bulb
G Optic Nerve
Optic chiasma
Second cranial nerve
H Oculomotor Nerve
Third cranial nerve
J Trochlear Nerve
Fourth cranial nerve
K Trigeminal Nerve
Fifth cranial nerve
Gasserian ganglion
Mandibular nerve
Maxillary nerve
Ophthalmic nerve
Trifacial nerve
L Abducens Nerve
Sixth cranial nerve
M Facial Nerve
Chorda tympani
Geniculate ganglion
Greater superficial petrosal
   nerve
Nerve to the stapedius
Parotid plexus
Posterior auricular nerve
Seventh cranial nerve
Submandibular ganglion
	N Acoustic Nerve
	Cochlear nerve
	Eighth cranial nerve
	Scarpa's (vestibular)
	   ganglion
	Spiral ganglion
	Vestibular (Scarpa's)
	   ganglion
	Vestibular nerve
	Vestibulocochlear nerve
	P Glossopharyngeal Nerve
	Carotid sinus nerve
	Ninth cranial nerve
	Tympanic nerve
	Q Vagus Nerve
	Anterior vagal trunk
	Pharyngeal plexus
	Pneumogastric nerve
	Posterior vagal trunk
	Pulmonary plexus
	Recurrent laryngeal nerve
	Superior laryngeal nerve
	Tenth cranial nerve
	R Accessory Nerve
	Eleventh cranial nerve
	S Hypoglossal Nerve
	Twelfth cranial nerve
	W Cervical Spinal Cord
	Dorsal root ganglion
	X Thoracic Spinal Cord
	Dorsal root ganglion
	Y Lumbar Spinal Cord
	Cauda equina
	Conus medullaris
	Dorsal root ganglion
		Ø Open
		3 Percutaneous
		4 Percutaneous Endoscopic
			Z No Device	**Z No Qualifier**

Ø   Medical and Surgical
Ø   Central Nervous System and Cranial Nerves
T   Resection   Definition: Cutting out or off, without replacement, all of a body part

Explanation: None

Body Part Character 4	Approach Character 5	Device Character 6	Qualifier Character 7
7 Cerebral Hemisphere Frontal lobe Occipital lobe Parietal lobe Temporal lobe	**Ø Open** **3 Percutaneous** **4 Percutaneous Endoscopic**	**Z No Device**	**Z No Qualifier**

0   Medical and Surgical
0   Central Nervous System and Cranial Nerves
U   Supplement   Definition: Putting in or on biological or synthetic material that physically reinforces and/or augments the function of a portion of a body part

Explanation: The biological material is non-living, or is living and from the same individual. The body part may have been previously replaced, and the SUPPLEMENT procedure is performed to physically reinforce and/or augment the function of the replaced body part.

Body Part Character 4		Approach Character 5	Device Character 6	Qualifier Character 7

1 Cerebral Meninges
  Arachnoid mater,
    intracranial
  Leptomeninges,
    intracranial
  Pia mater, intracranial
2 Dura Mater
  Diaphragma sellae
  Dura mater, intracranial
  Falx cerebri
  Tentorium cerebelli
6 Cerebral Ventricle
  Aqueduct of Sylvius
  Cerebral aqueduct
    (Sylvius)
  Choroid plexus
  Ependyma
  Foramen of Monro
    (intraventricular)
  Fourth ventricle
  Interventricular foramen
    (Monro)
  Left lateral ventricle
  Right lateral ventricle
  Third ventricle
F Olfactory Nerve
  First cranial nerve
  Olfactory bulb
G Optic Nerve
  Optic chiasma
  Second cranial nerve
H Oculomotor Nerve
  Third cranial nerve
J Trochlear Nerve
  Fourth cranial nerve
K Trigeminal Nerve
  Fifth cranial nerve
  Gasserian ganglion
  Mandibular nerve
  Maxillary nerve
  Ophthalmic nerve
  Trifacial nerve
L Abducens Nerve
  Sixth cranial nerve
	M Facial Nerve
	  Chorda tympani
	  Geniculate ganglion
	  Greater superficial petrosal
	    nerve
	  Nerve to the stapedius
	  Parotid plexus
	  Posterior auricular nerve
	  Seventh cranial nerve
	  Submandibular ganglion
	N Acoustic Nerve
	  Cochlear nerve
	  Eighth cranial nerve
	  Scarpa's (vestibular)
	    ganglion
	  Spiral ganglion
	  Vestibular (Scarpa's)
	    ganglion
	  Vestibular nerve
	  Vestibulocochlear nerve
	P Glossopharyngeal Nerve
	  Carotid sinus nerve
	  Ninth cranial nerve
	  Tympanic nerve
	Q Vagus Nerve
	  Anterior vagal trunk
	  Pharyngeal plexus
	  Pneumogastric nerve
	  Posterior vagal trunk
	  Pulmonary plexus
	  Recurrent laryngeal nerve
	  Superior laryngeal nerve
	  Tenth cranial nerve
	R Accessory Nerve
	  Eleventh cranial nerve
	S Hypoglossal Nerve
	  Twelfth cranial nerve
	T Spinal Meninges
	  Arachnoid mater, spinal
	  Denticulate (dentate)
	    ligament
	  Dura mater, spinal
	  Filum terminale
	  Leptomeninges, spinal
	  Pia mater, spinal
		0 Open
		3 Percutaneous
		4 Percutaneous Endoscopic
			7 Autologous Tissue
			  Substitute
			J Synthetic Substitute
			K Nonautologous Tissue
			  Substitute
				Z No Qualifier

NC Noncovered Procedure   LC Limited Coverage   QA Questionable OB Admit   NT New Tech Add-on   ⊞ Combination Member   ♂ Male   ♀ Female

ICD-10-PCS 2023   149

0   **Medical and Surgical**
0   **Central Nervous System and Cranial Nerves**
W   **Revision**   Definition: Correcting, to the extent possible, a portion of a malfunctioning device or the position of a displaced device

                   Explanation: Revision can include correcting a malfunctioning or displaced device by taking out or putting in components of the device such as a screw or pin

Body Part Character 4	Approach Character 5	Device Character 6	Qualifier Character 7

0 **Brain**
    Cerebrum
    Corpus callosum
    Encephalon
V **Spinal Cord**
    Dorsal root ganglion
	0 Open
	3 Percutaneous
	4 Percutaneous Endoscopic
		0 Drainage Device
		2 Monitoring Device
		3 Infusion Device
		7 Autologous Tissue Substitute
		J Synthetic Substitute
		K Nonautologous Tissue Substitute
		M Neurostimulator Lead
		Y Other Device
			Z No Qualifier

0 **Brain**
    Cerebrum
    Corpus callosum
    Encephalon
V **Spinal Cord**
    Dorsal root ganglion
	X External	**0** Drainage Device
		2 Monitoring Device
		3 Infusion Device
		7 Autologous Tissue Substitute
		J Synthetic Substitute
		K Nonautologous Tissue Substitute
		M Neurostimulator Lead
			Z No Qualifier

6 **Cerebral Ventricle**
    Aqueduct of Sylvius
    Cerebral aqueduct (Sylvius)
    Choroid plexus
    Ependyma
    Foramen of Monro (intraventricular)
    Fourth ventricle
    Interventricular foramen (Monro)
    Left lateral ventricle
    Right lateral ventricle
    Third ventricle
U **Spinal Canal**
    Epidural space, spinal
    Extradural space, spinal
    Subarachnoid space, spinal
    Subdural space, spinal
    Vertebral canal
	0 Open
	3 Percutaneous
	4 Percutaneous Endoscopic
		0 Drainage Device
		2 Monitoring Device
		3 Infusion Device
		J Synthetic Substitute
		M Neurostimulator Lead
		Y Other Device
			Z No Qualifier

6 **Cerebral Ventricle**
    Aqueduct of Sylvius
    Cerebral aqueduct (Sylvius)
    Choroid plexus
    Ependyma
    Foramen of Monro (intraventricular)
    Fourth ventricle
    Interventricular foramen (Monro)
    Left lateral ventricle
    Right lateral ventricle
    Third ventricle
U **Spinal Canal**
    Epidural space, spinal
    Extradural space, spinal
    Subarachnoid space, spinal
    Subdural space, spinal
    Vertebral canal
	X External	**0** Drainage Device
		2 Monitoring Device
		3 Infusion Device
		J Synthetic Substitute
		M Neurostimulator Lead
			Z No Qualifier

E **Cranial Nerve**	**0** Open **3** Percutaneous **4** Percutaneous Endoscopic	**0** Drainage Device **2** Monitoring Device **3** Infusion Device **7** Autologous Tissue Substitute **M** Neurostimulator Lead **Y** Other Device	**Z** No Qualifier
E **Cranial Nerve**	**X** External	**0** Drainage Device **2** Monitoring Device **3** Infusion Device **7** Autologous Tissue Substitute **M** Neurostimulator Lead	**Z** No Qualifier

Non-OR	00W[0,V][3,4]YZ
Non-OR	00W[0,V]X[0,2,3,7,J,K,M]Z
Non-OR	00W[6,U][3,4]YZ
Non-OR	00W[6,U]X[0,2,3,J,M]Z
Non-OR	00WE[3,4]YZ
Non-OR	00WEX[0,2,3,7,M]Z

Non-OR Procedure   DRG Non-OR Procedure   Valid OR Procedure   HAC Associated Procedure   Combination Only   New/Revised April   New/Revised October

150   ICD-10-PCS 2023

0 Medical and Surgical
0 Central Nervous System and Cranial Nerves
X Transfer Definition: Moving, without taking out, all or a portion of a body part to another location to take over the function of all or a portion of a body part
Explanation: The body part transferred remains connected to its vascular and nervous supply

Body Part Character 4	Approach Character 5	Device Character 6	Qualifier Character 7
F Olfactory Nerve First cranial nerve Olfactory bulb **G Optic Nerve** Optic chiasma Second cranial nerve **H Oculomotor Nerve** Third cranial nerve **J Trochlear Nerve** Fourth cranial nerve **K Trigeminal Nerve** Fifth cranial nerve Gasserian ganglion Mandibular nerve Maxillary nerve Ophthalmic nerve Trifacial nerve **L Abducens Nerve** Sixth cranial nerve **M Facial Nerve** Chorda tympani Geniculate ganglion Greater superficial petrosal nerve Nerve to the stapedius Parotid plexus Posterior auricular nerve Seventh cranial nerve Submandibular ganglion **N Acoustic Nerve** Cochlear nerve Eighth cranial nerve Scarpa's (vestibular) ganglion Spiral ganglion Vestibular (Scarpa's) ganglion Vestibular nerve Vestibulocochlear nerve **P Glossopharyngeal Nerve** Carotid sinus nerve Ninth cranial nerve Tympanic nerve **Q Vagus Nerve** Anterior vagal trunk Pharyngeal plexus Pneumogastric nerve Posterior vagal trunk Pulmonary plexus Recurrent laryngeal nerve Superior laryngeal nerve Tenth cranial nerve **R Accessory Nerve** Eleventh cranial nerve **S Hypoglossal Nerve** Twelfth cranial nerve	**0 Open** **4 Percutaneous Endoscopic**	**Z No Device**	**F Olfactory Nerve** **G Optic Nerve** **H Oculomotor Nerve** **J Trochlear Nerve** **K Trigeminal Nerve** **L Abducens Nerve** **M Facial Nerve** **N Acoustic Nerve** **P Glossopharyngeal Nerve** **Q Vagus Nerve** **R Accessory Nerve** **S Hypoglossal Nerve**

0   Medical and Surgical
0   Central Nervous System and Cranial Nerves
X   Transfer   Definition: Moving, without taking out, all or a portion of a body part to another location to take over the function of all or a portion of a body part
       Explanation: The body part transferred remains connected to its vascular and nervous supply

Body Part (Character 4)	Approach (Character 5)	Device (Character 6)	Qualifier (Character 7)

8   Olfactory Nerve
    First cranial nerve
    Olfactory bulb
9   Optic Nerve
    Optic chiasma
    Second cranial nerve
H   Oculomotor Nerve
    Third cranial nerve
J   Trochlear Nerve
    Fourth cranial nerve
K   Trigeminal Nerve
    Gasserian ganglion
    Mandibular nerve
    Maxillary nerve
    Ophthalmic nerve
    Trifacial nerve
L   Abducens Nerve
    Sixth cranial nerve
M   Facial Nerve
    Chorda tympani
    Geniculate ganglion
    Greater superficial petrosal nerve
    Nerve to the stapedius
    Parotid plexus
    Posterior auricular nerve
    Seventh cranial nerve
    Submandibular ganglion
N   Acoustic Nerve
    Cochlear nerve
    Eighth cranial nerve
    Scarpa's (vestibular) ganglion
    Spiral ganglion
    Vestibular (Scarpa's) ganglion
    Vestibular nerve
    Vestibulocochlear nerve
P   Glossopharyngeal Nerve
    Carotid sinus nerve
    Ninth cranial nerve
    Tympanic nerve
Q   Vagus Nerve
    Anterior vagal trunk
    Pharyngeal plexus
    Pneumogastric nerve
    Posterior vagal trunk
    Pulmonary plexus
    Recurrent laryngeal nerve
    Superior laryngeal nerve
    Tenth cranial nerve
R   Accessory Nerve
    Eleventh cranial nerve
S   Hypoglossal Nerve
    Twelfth cranial nerve
	0 Open
	4 Percutaneous Endoscopic
		Z No Device	F Olfactory Nerve
			G Optic Nerve
			H Oculomotor Nerve
			J Trochlear Nerve
			K Trigeminal Nerve
			L Abducens Nerve
			M Facial Nerve
			N Acoustic Nerve
			P Glossopharyngeal Nerve
			Q Vagus Nerve
			R Accessory Nerve
			S Hypoglossal Nerve

Peripheral Nervous System 012–01X

Character Meanings

This Character Meaning table is provided as a guide to assist the user in the identification of character members that may be found in this section of code tables. It **SHOULD NOT** be used to build a PCS code.

Operation–Character 3	Body Part–Character 4	Approach–Character 5	Device–Character 6	Qualifier–Character 7
2 Change	0 Cervical Plexus	0 Open	0 Drainage Device	1 Cervical Nerve
5 Destruction	1 Cervical Nerve	3 Percutaneous	1 Radioactive Element	2 Phrenic Nerve
8 Division	2 Phrenic Nerve	4 Percutaneous Endoscopic	2 Monitoring Device	4 Ulnar Nerve
9 Drainage	3 Brachial Plexus	X External	7 Autologous Tissue Substitute	5 Median Nerve
B Excision	4 Ulnar Nerve		J Synthetic Substitute	6 Radial Nerve
C Extirpation	5 Median Nerve		K Nonautologous Tissue Substitute	8 Thoracic Nerve
D Extraction	6 Radial Nerve		M Neurostimulator Lead	B Lumbar Nerve
H Insertion	8 Thoracic Nerve		Y Other Device	C Perineal Nerve
J Inspection	9 Lumbar Plexus		Z No Device	D Femoral Nerve
N Release	A Lumbosacral Plexus			F Sciatic Nerve
P Removal	B Lumbar Nerve			G Tibial Nerve
Q Repair	C Pudendal Nerve			H Peroneal Nerve
R Replacement	D Femoral Nerve			X Diagnostic
S Reposition	F Sciatic Nerve			Z No Qualifier
U Supplement	G Tibial Nerve			
W Revision	H Peroneal Nerve			
X Transfer	K Head and Neck Sympathetic Nerve			
	L Thoracic Sympathetic Nerve			
	M Abdominal Sympathetic Nerve			
	N Lumbar Sympathetic Nerve			
	P Sacral Sympathetic Nerve			
	Q Sacral Plexus			
	R Sacral Nerve			
	Y Peripheral Nerve			

AHA Coding Clinic for table 01B
2018, 2Q, 22   Excision of synovial cyst
2017, 2Q, 19   Thoracic outlet decompression with sympathectomy

AHA Coding Clinic for table 01H
2020, 4Q, 43-44   Insertion of radioactive element

AHA Coding Clinic for table 01N
2019, 1Q, 28   Decompressive laminectomy of both spinal cord and nerve roots
2018, 2Q, 22   Excision of synovial cyst
2017, 2Q, 19   Thoracic outlet decompression with sympathectomy
2016, 2Q, 16   Decompressive laminectomy/foraminotomy and lumbar discectomy
2016, 2Q, 17   Removal of longitudinal ligament to decompress cervical nerve root
2016, 2Q, 23   Thoracic outlet syndrome and release of brachial plexus
2015, 2Q, 34   Decompressive laminectomy
2014, 3Q, 33   Radial fracture treatment with open reduction internal fixation, and release of carpal ligament

AHA Coding Clinic for table 01Q
2019, 3Q, 32   Breast reconstruction with neurotization

AHA Coding Clinic for table 01S
2021, 3Q, 19   Elbow amputation and targeted muscle reinnervation

AHA Coding Clinic for table 01U
2019, 3Q, 32   Breast reconstruction with neurotization
2017, 4Q, 62   Added and revised device values - Nerve substitutes

Median and Ulnar Nerves

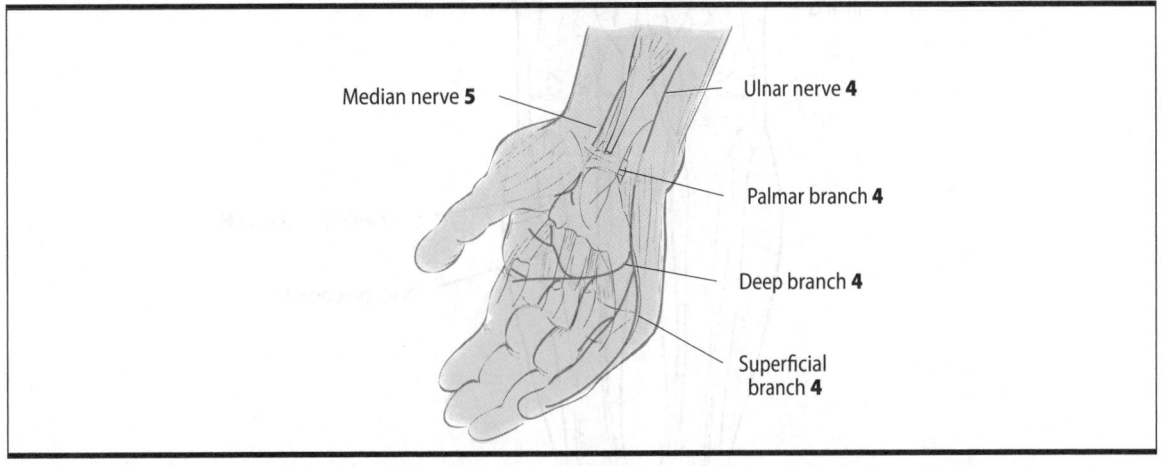

Median nerve **5**
Ulnar nerve **4**
Palmar branch **4**
Deep branch **4**
Superficial branch **4**

Peripheral Nervous System

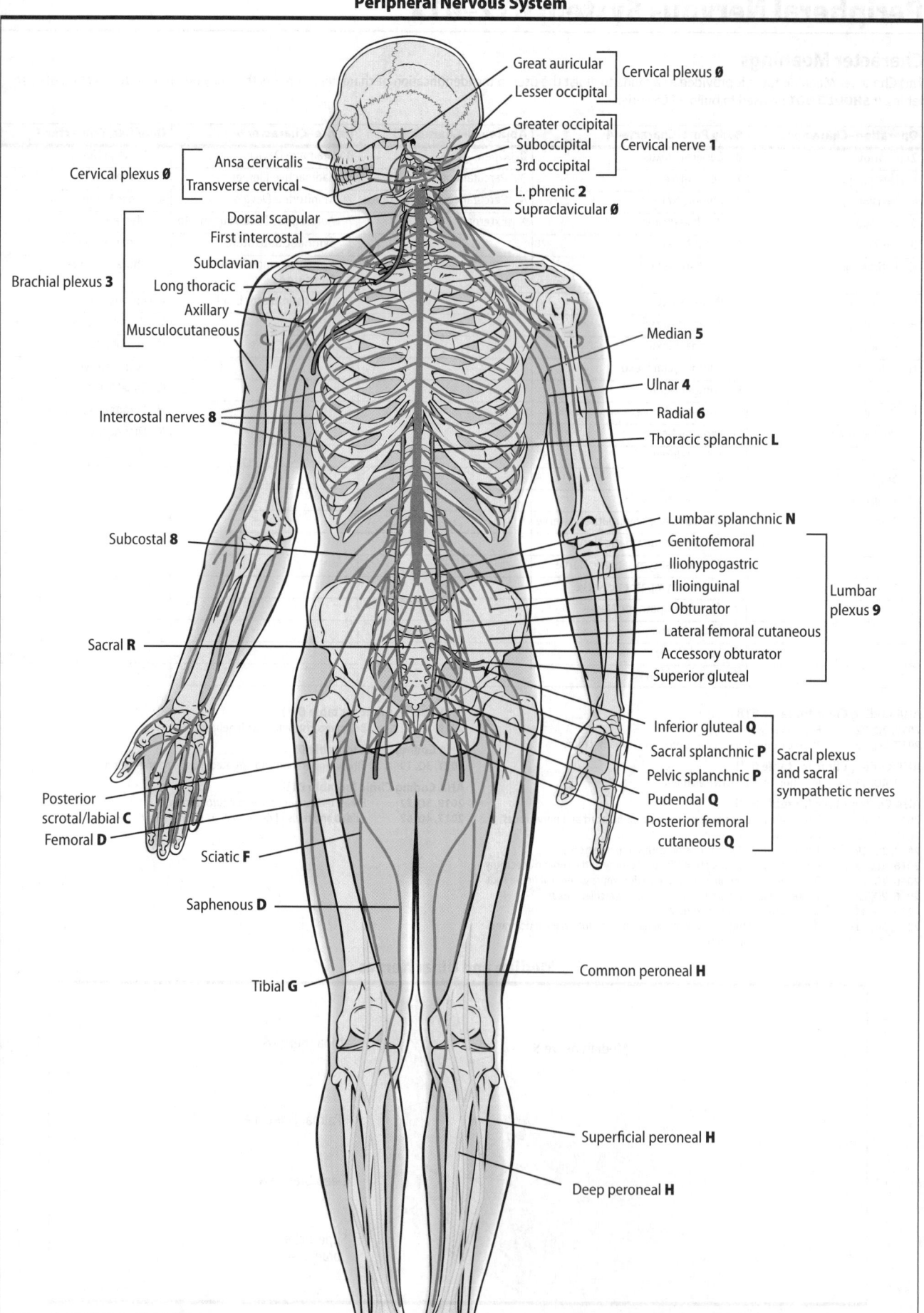

Great auricular — Cervical plexus Ø
Lesser occipital

Greater occipital
Suboccipital — Cervical nerve 1
3rd occipital

Cervical plexus Ø

Ansa cervicalis
Transverse cervical

L. phrenic 2
Supraclavicular Ø

Dorsal scapular
First intercostal
Subclavian
Long thoracic — Brachial plexus 3
Axillary
Musculocutaneous

Median 5
Ulnar 4
Radial 6
Thoracic splanchnic L

Intercostal nerves 8

Subcostal 8

Lumbar splanchnic N
Genitofemoral
Iliohypogastric
Ilioinguinal
Obturator — Lumbar plexus 9
Lateral femoral cutaneous
Accessory obturator
Superior gluteal

Sacral R

Inferior gluteal Q
Sacral splanchnic P
Pelvic splanchnic P — Sacral plexus and sacral sympathetic nerves
Pudendal Q
Posterior femoral cutaneous Q

Posterior scrotal/labial C
Femoral D

Sciatic F

Saphenous D

Common peroneal H

Tibial G

Superficial peroneal H

Deep peroneal H

Ø   Medical and Surgical
1   Peripheral Nervous System
2   Change   Definition: Taking out or off a device from a body part and putting back an identical or similar device in or on the same body part without cutting or puncturing the skin or a mucous membrane

          Explanation: All CHANGE procedures are coded using the approach EXTERNAL

Body Part Character 4	Approach Character 5	Device Character 6	Qualifier Character 7
Y Peripheral Nerve	X External	Ø Drainage Device Y Other Device	Z No Qualifier

Non-OR	All body part, approach, device, and qualifier values

Ø   Medical and Surgical
1   Peripheral Nervous System
5   Destruction   Definition: Physical eradication of all or a portion of a body part by the direct use of energy, force, or a destructive agent

          Explanation: None of the body part is physically taken out

Body Part Character 4		Approach Character 5	Device Character 6	Qualifier Character 7

Ø   **Cervical Plexus**
    Ansa cervicalis
    Cutaneous (transverse) cervical nerve
    Great auricular nerve
    Lesser occipital nerve
    Supraclavicular nerve
    Transverse (cutaneous) cervical nerve
1   **Cervical Nerve**
    Greater occipital nerve
    Spinal nerve, cervical
    Suboccipital nerve
    Third occipital nerve
2   **Phrenic Nerve**
    Accessory phrenic nerve
3   **Brachial Plexus**
    Axillary nerve
    Dorsal scapular nerve
    First intercostal nerve
    Long thoracic nerve
    Musculocutaneous nerve
    Subclavius nerve
    Suprascapular nerve
4   **Ulnar Nerve**
    Cubital nerve
5   **Median Nerve**
    Anterior interosseous nerve
    Palmar cutaneous nerve
6   **Radial Nerve**
    Dorsal digital nerve
    Musculospiral nerve
    Palmar cutaneous nerve
    Posterior interosseous nerve
8   **Thoracic Nerve**
    Intercostal nerve
    Intercostobrachial nerve
    Spinal nerve, thoracic
    Subcostal nerve
9   **Lumbar Plexus**
    Accessory obturator nerve
    Genitofemoral nerve
    Iliohypogastric nerve
    Ilioinguinal nerve
    Lateral femoral cutaneous nerve
    Obturator nerve
    Superior gluteal nerve
A   **Lumbosacral Plexus**
B   **Lumbar Nerve**
    Lumbosacral trunk
    Spinal nerve, lumbar
    Superior clunic (cluneal) nerve
C   **Pudendal Nerve**
    Posterior labial nerve
    Posterior scrotal nerve
D   **Femoral Nerve**
    Anterior crural nerve
    Saphenous nerve
F   **Sciatic Nerve**
    Ischiatic nerve
G   **Tibial Nerve**
    Lateral plantar nerve
    Medial plantar nerve
    Medial popliteal nerve
    Medial sural cutaneous nerve
	H **Peroneal Nerve**
	    Common fibular nerve
	    Common peroneal nerve
	    External popliteal nerve
	    Lateral sural cutaneous nerve
	K **Head and Neck Sympathetic Nerve**
	    Cavernous plexus
	    Cervical ganglion
	    Ciliary ganglion
	    Internal carotid plexus
	    Otic ganglion
	    Pterygopalatine (sphenopalatine)
	      ganglion
	    Sphenopalatine (pterygopalatine)
	      ganglion
	    Stellate ganglion
	    Submandibular ganglion
	    Submaxillary ganglion
	L **Thoracic Sympathetic Nerve**
	    Cardiac plexus
	    Esophageal plexus
	    Greater splanchnic nerve
	    Inferior cardiac nerve
	    Least splanchnic nerve
	    Lesser splanchnic nerve
	    Middle cardiac nerve
	    Pulmonary plexus
	    Superior cardiac nerve
	    Thoracic aortic plexus
	    Thoracic ganglion
	M **Abdominal Sympathetic Nerve**
	    Abdominal aortic plexus
	    Auerbach's (myenteric) plexus
	    Celiac (solar) plexus
	    Celiac ganglion
	    Gastric plexus
	    Hepatic plexus
	    Inferior hypogastric plexus
	    Inferior mesenteric ganglion
	    Inferior mesenteric plexus
	    Meissner's (submucous) plexus
	    Myenteric (Auerbach's) plexus
	    Pancreatic plexus
	    Pelvic splanchnic nerve
	    Renal nerve
	    Renal plexus
	    Solar (celiac) plexus
	    Splenic plexus
	    Submucous (Meissner's) plexus
	    Superior hypogastric plexus
	    Superior mesenteric ganglion
	    Superior mesenteric plexus
	    Suprarenal plexus
	N **Lumbar Sympathetic Nerve**
	    Lumbar ganglion
	    Lumbar splanchnic nerve
	P **Sacral Sympathetic Nerve**
	    Ganglion impar (ganglion of
	      Walther)
	    Pelvic splanchnic nerve
	    Sacral ganglion
	    Sacral splanchnic nerve
	Q **Sacral Plexus**
	    Inferior gluteal nerve
	    Posterior femoral cutaneous nerve
	    Pudendal nerve
	R **Sacral Nerve**
	    Spinal nerve, sacral
		Ø Open
		3 Percutaneous
		4 Percutaneous
		    Endoscopic
			Z No Device	Z No Qualifier

Non-OR	Ø15[Ø,2,3,4,5,6,9,A,C,D,F,G,H,Q][Ø,3,4]ZZ	Non-OR	Ø15[1,8,B,R]3ZZ

NC Noncovered Procedure   LC Limited Coverage   QA Questionable OB Admit   NT New Tech Add-on   ⊞ Combination Member   ♂ Male   ♀ Female

ICD-10-PCS 2023   **155**

Ø12–Ø15

Peripheral Nervous System

Ø   **Medical and Surgical**
1   **Peripheral Nervous System**
8   **Division**   Definition: Cutting into a body part, without draining fluids and/or gases from the body part, in order to separate or transect a body part
                   Explanation: All or a portion of the body part is separated into two or more portions

Body Part Character 4		Approach Character 5	Device Character 6	Qualifier Character 7

Ø Cervical Plexus
Ansa cervicalis
Cutaneous (transverse) cervical
   nerve
Great auricular nerve
Lesser occipital nerve
Supraclavicular nerve
Transverse (cutaneous) cervical
   nerve
1 Cervical Nerve
Greater occipital nerve
Spinal nerve, cervical
Suboccipital nerve
Third occipital nerve
2 Phrenic Nerve
Accessory phrenic nerve
3 Brachial Plexus
Axillary nerve
Dorsal scapular nerve
First intercostal nerve
Long thoracic nerve
Musculocutaneous nerve
Subclavius nerve
Suprascapular nerve
4 Ulnar Nerve
Cubital nerve
5 Median Nerve
Anterior interosseous nerve
Palmar cutaneous nerve
6 Radial Nerve
Dorsal digital nerve
Musculospiral nerve
Palmar cutaneous nerve
Posterior interosseous nerve
8 Thoracic Nerve
Intercostal nerve
Intercostobrachial nerve
Spinal nerve, thoracic
Subcostal nerve
9 Lumbar Plexus
Accessory obturator nerve
Genitofemoral nerve
Iliohypogastric nerve
Ilioinguinal nerve
Lateral femoral cutaneous
   nerve
Obturator nerve
Superior gluteal nerve
A Lumbosacral Plexus
B Lumbar Nerve
Lumbosacral trunk
Spinal nerve, lumbar
Superior clunic (cluneal) nerve
C Pudendal Nerve
Posterior labial nerve
Posterior scrotal nerve
D Femoral Nerve
Anterior crural nerve
Saphenous nerve
F Sciatic Nerve
Ischiatic nerve
G Tibial Nerve
Lateral plantar nerve
Medial plantar nerve
Medial popliteal nerve
Medial sural cutaneous nerve
	H Peroneal Nerve
	Common fibular nerve
	Common peroneal nerve
	External popliteal nerve
	Lateral sural cutaneous nerve
	K Head and Neck Sympathetic
	Nerve
	Cavernous plexus
	Cervical ganglion
	Ciliary ganglion
	Internal carotid plexus
	Otic ganglion
	Pterygopalatine
	   (sphenopalatine) ganglion
	Sphenopalatine
	   (pterygopalatine) ganglion
	Stellate ganglion
	Submandibular ganglion
	Submaxillary ganglion
	L Thoracic Sympathetic Nerve
	Cardiac plexus
	Esophageal plexus
	Greater splanchnic nerve
	Inferior cardiac nerve
	Least splanchnic nerve
	Lesser splanchnic nerve
	Middle cardiac nerve
	Pulmonary plexus
	Superior cardiac nerve
	Thoracic aortic plexus
	Thoracic ganglion
	M Abdominal Sympathetic
	Nerve
	Abdominal aortic plexus
	Auerbach's (myenteric) plexus
	Celiac (solar) plexus
	Celiac ganglion
	Gastric plexus
	Hepatic plexus
	Inferior hypogastric plexus
	Inferior mesenteric ganglion
	Inferior mesenteric plexus
	Meissner's (submucous) plexus
	Myenteric (Auerbach's) plexus
	Pancreatic plexus
	Pelvic splanchnic nerve
	Renal nerve
	Renal plexus
	Solar (celiac) plexus
	Splenic plexus
	Submucous (Meissner's) plexus
	Superior hypogastric plexus
	Superior mesenteric ganglion
	Superior mesenteric plexus
	Suprarenal plexus
	N Lumbar Sympathetic Nerve
	Lumbar ganglion
	Lumbar splanchnic nerve
	P Sacral Sympathetic Nerve
	Ganglion impar (ganglion of
	   Walther)
	Pelvic splanchnic nerve
	Sacral ganglion
	Sacral splanchnic nerve
	Q Sacral Plexus
	Inferior gluteal nerve
	Posterior femoral cutaneous
	   nerve
	Pudendal nerve
	R Sacral Nerve
	Spinal nerve, sacral
		Ø Open
		3 Percutaneous
		4 Percutaneous Endoscopic
			Z No Device	**Z No Qualifier**

Non-OR Procedure   DRG Non-OR Procedure   Valid OR Procedure   HAC Associated Procedure   Combination Only   New/Revised April   New/Revised October

156

ICD-10-PCS 2023

Ø18–Ø18

Ø   Medical and Surgical
1   Peripheral Nervous System
9   Drainage   Definition: Taking or letting out fluids and/or gases from a body part
                     Explanation: The qualifier DIAGNOSTIC is used to identify drainage procedures that are biopsies

Body Part Character 4		Approach Character 5	Device Character 6	Qualifier Character 7

Ø Cervical Plexus
  Ansa cervicalis
  Cutaneous (transverse) cervical
    nerve
  Great auricular nerve
  Lesser occipital nerve
  Supraclavicular nerve
  Transverse (cutaneous) cervical
    nerve
1 Cervical Nerve
  Greater occipital nerve
  Spinal nerve, cervical
  Suboccipital nerve
  Third occipital nerve
2 Phrenic Nerve
  Accessory phrenic nerve
3 Brachial Plexus
  Axillary nerve
  Dorsal scapular nerve
  First intercostal nerve
  Long thoracic nerve
  Musculocutaneous nerve
  Subclavius nerve
  Suprascapular nerve
4 Ulnar Nerve
  Cubital nerve
5 Median Nerve
  Anterior interosseous nerve
  Palmar cutaneous nerve
6 Radial Nerve
  Dorsal digital nerve
  Musculospiral nerve
  Palmar cutaneous nerve
  Posterior interosseous nerve
8 Thoracic Nerve
  Intercostal nerve
  Intercostobrachial nerve
  Spinal nerve, thoracic
  Subcostal nerve
9 Lumbar Plexus
  Accessory obturator nerve
  Genitofemoral nerve
  Iliohypogastric nerve
  Ilioinguinal nerve
  Lateral femoral cutaneous
    nerve
  Obturator nerve
  Superior gluteal nerve
A Lumbosacral Plexus
B Lumbar Nerve
  Lumbosacral trunk
  Spinal nerve, lumbar
  Superior clunic (cluneal) nerve
C Pudendal Nerve
  Posterior labial nerve
  Posterior scrotal nerve
D Femoral Nerve
  Anterior crural nerve
  Saphenous nerve
F Sciatic Nerve
  Ischiatic nerve
G Tibial Nerve
  Lateral plantar nerve
  Medial plantar nerve
  Medial popliteal nerve
  Medial sural cutaneous nerve
	H Peroneal Nerve
	  Common fibular nerve
	  Common peroneal nerve
	  External popliteal nerve
	  Lateral sural cutaneous nerve
	K Head and Neck Sympathetic
	** Nerve**
	  Cavernous plexus
	  Cervical ganglion
	  Ciliary ganglion
	  Internal carotid plexus
	  Otic ganglion
	  Pterygopalatine
	    (sphenopalatine) ganglion
	  Sphenopalatine
	    (pterygopalatine) ganglion
	  Stellate ganglion
	  Submandibular ganglion
	  Submaxillary ganglion
	L Thoracic Sympathetic Nerve
	  Cardiac plexus
	  Esophageal plexus
	  Greater splanchnic nerve
	  Inferior cardiac nerve
	  Least splanchnic nerve
	  Lesser splanchnic nerve
	  Middle cardiac nerve
	  Pulmonary plexus
	  Superior cardiac nerve
	  Thoracic aortic plexus
	  Thoracic ganglion
	M Abdominal Sympathetic
	** Nerve**
	  Abdominal aortic plexus
	  Auerbach's (myenteric) plexus
	  Celiac (solar) plexus
	  Celiac ganglion
	  Gastric plexus
	  Hepatic plexus
	  Inferior hypogastric plexus
	  Inferior mesenteric ganglion
	  Inferior mesenteric plexus
	  Meissner's (submucous) plexus
	  Myenteric (Auerbach's) plexus
	  Pancreatic plexus
	  Pelvic splanchnic nerve
	  Renal nerve
	  Renal plexus
	  Solar (celiac) plexus
	  Splenic plexus
	  Submucous (Meissner's) plexus
	  Superior hypogastric plexus
	  Superior mesenteric ganglion
	  Superior mesenteric plexus
	  Suprarenal plexus
	N Lumbar Sympathetic Nerve
	  Lumbar ganglion
	  Lumbar splanchnic nerve
	P Sacral Sympathetic Nerve
	  Ganglion impar (ganglion of
	    Walther)
	  Pelvic splanchnic nerve
	  Sacral ganglion
	  Sacral splanchnic nerve
	Q Sacral Plexus
	  Inferior gluteal nerve
	  Posterior femoral cutaneous
	    nerve
	  Pudendal nerve
	R Sacral Nerve
	  Spinal nerve, sacral
		Ø Open
		3 Percutaneous
		4 Percutaneous Endoscopic
			Ø Drainage Device	**Z No Qualifier**

Non-OR   Ø19[Ø,1,2,3,4,5,6,8,9,A,B,C,D,F,G,H,K,L,M,N,P,Q,R]3ØZ

Ø19 Continued on next page

Peripheral Nervous System

Ø   **Medical and Surgical**
1   **Peripheral Nervous System**
9   **Drainage**   Definition: Taking or letting out fluids and/or gases from a body part

Ø19 Continued

Explanation: The qualifier DIAGNOSTIC is used to identify drainage procedures that are biopsies

Body Part Character 4		Approach Character 5	Device Character 6	Qualifier Character 7
Ø **Cervical Plexus** Ansa cervicalis Cutaneous (transverse) cervical nerve Great auricular nerve Lesser occipital nerve Supraclavicular nerve Transverse (cutaneous) cervical nerve 1 **Cervical Nerve** Greater occipital nerve Spinal nerve, cervical Suboccipital nerve Third occipital nerve 2 **Phrenic Nerve** Accessory phrenic nerve 3 **Brachial Plexus** Axillary nerve Dorsal scapular nerve First intercostal nerve Long thoracic nerve Musculocutaneous nerve Subclavius nerve Suprascapular nerve 4 **Ulnar Nerve** Cubital nerve 5 **Median Nerve** Anterior interosseous nerve Palmar cutaneous nerve 6 **Radial Nerve** Dorsal digital nerve Musculospiral nerve Palmar cutaneous nerve Posterior interosseous nerve 8 **Thoracic Nerve** Intercostal nerve Intercostobrachial nerve Spinal nerve, thoracic Subcostal nerve 9 **Lumbar Plexus** Accessory obturator nerve Genitofemoral nerve Iliohypogastric nerve Ilioinguinal nerve Lateral femoral cutaneous nerve Obturator nerve Superior gluteal nerve A **Lumbosacral Plexus** B **Lumbar Nerve** Lumbosacral trunk Spinal nerve, lumbar Superior clunic (cluneal) nerve C **Pudendal Nerve** Posterior labial nerve Posterior scrotal nerve D **Femoral Nerve** Anterior crural nerve Saphenous nerve F **Sciatic Nerve** Ischiatic nerve G **Tibial Nerve** Lateral plantar nerve Medial plantar nerve Medial popliteal nerve Medial sural cutaneous nerve	H **Peroneal Nerve** Common fibular nerve Common peroneal nerve External popliteal nerve Lateral sural cutaneous nerve K **Head and Neck Sympathetic Nerve** Cavernous plexus Cervical ganglion Ciliary ganglion Internal carotid plexus Otic ganglion Pterygopalatine (sphenopalatine) ganglion Sphenopalatine (pterygopalatine) ganglion Stellate ganglion Submandibular ganglion Submaxillary ganglion L **Thoracic Sympathetic Nerve** Cardiac plexus Esophageal plexus Greater splanchnic nerve Inferior cardiac nerve Least splanchnic nerve Lesser splanchnic nerve Middle cardiac nerve Pulmonary plexus Superior cardiac nerve Thoracic aortic plexus Thoracic ganglion M **Abdominal Sympathetic Nerve** Abdominal aortic plexus Auerbach's (myenteric) plexus Celiac (solar) plexus Celiac ganglion Gastric plexus Hepatic plexus Inferior hypogastric plexus Inferior mesenteric ganglion Inferior mesenteric plexus Meissner's (submucous) plexus Myenteric (Auerbach's) plexus Pancreatic plexus Pelvic splanchnic nerve Renal nerve Renal plexus Solar (celiac) plexus Splenic plexus Submucous (Meissner's) plexus Superior hypogastric plexus Superior mesenteric ganglion Superior mesenteric plexus Suprarenal plexus N **Lumbar Sympathetic Nerve** Lumbar ganglion Lumbar splanchnic nerve P **Sacral Sympathetic Nerve** Ganglion impar (ganglion of Walther) Pelvic splanchnic nerve Sacral ganglion Sacral splanchnic nerve Q **Sacral Plexus** Inferior gluteal nerve Posterior femoral cutaneous nerve Pudendal nerve R **Sacral Nerve** Spinal nerve, sacral	Ø **Open** 3 **Percutaneous** 4 **Percutaneous Endoscopic**	Z **No Device**	X **Diagnostic** Z **No Qualifier**

Non-OR	Ø19[Ø,1,2,3,4,5,6,8,9,A,B,C,D,F,G,H,Q,R][3,4]ZX
Non-OR	Ø19[Ø,1,2,3,4,5,6,8,9,A,B,C,D,F,G,H,K,L,M,N,P,Q,R]3ZZ

Non-OR Procedure   DRG Non-OR Procedure   Valid OR Procedure   HAC Associated Procedure   Combination Only   New/Revised April   New/Revised October

0   Medical and Surgical
1   Peripheral Nervous System
B   Excision   Definition: Cutting out or off, without replacement, a portion of a body part
                   Explanation: The qualifier DIAGNOSTIC is used to identify excision procedures that are biopsies

Body Part Character 4		Approach Character 5	Device Character 6	Qualifier Character 7

0 Cervical Plexus
Ansa cervicalis
Cutaneous (transverse) cervical
   nerve
Great auricular nerve
Lesser occipital nerve
Supraclavicular nerve
Transverse (cutaneous) cervical
   nerve
1 Cervical Nerve
Greater occipital nerve
Spinal nerve, cervical
Suboccipital nerve
Third occipital nerve
2 Phrenic Nerve
Accessory phrenic nerve
3 Brachial Plexus
Axillary nerve
Dorsal scapular nerve
First intercostal nerve
Long thoracic nerve
Musculocutaneous nerve
Subclavius nerve
Suprascapular nerve
4 Ulnar Nerve
Cubital nerve
5 Median Nerve
Anterior interosseous nerve
Palmar cutaneous nerve
6 Radial Nerve
Dorsal digital nerve
Musculospiral nerve
Palmar cutaneous nerve
Posterior interosseous nerve
8 Thoracic Nerve
Intercostal nerve
Intercostobrachial nerve
Spinal nerve, thoracic
Subcostal nerve
9 Lumbar Plexus
Accessory obturator nerve
Genitofemoral nerve
Iliohypogastric nerve
Ilioinguinal nerve
Lateral femoral cutaneous
   nerve
Obturator nerve
Superior gluteal nerve
A Lumbosacral Plexus
B Lumbar Nerve
Lumbosacral trunk
Spinal nerve, lumbar
Superior clunic (cluneal) nerve
C Pudendal Nerve
Posterior labial nerve
Posterior scrotal nerve
D Femoral Nerve
Anterior crural nerve
Saphenous nerve
F Sciatic Nerve
Ischiatic nerve
G Tibial Nerve
Lateral plantar nerve
Medial plantar nerve
Medial popliteal nerve
Medial sural cutaneous nerve
	H Peroneal Nerve
	Common fibular nerve
	Common peroneal nerve
	External popliteal nerve
	Lateral sural cutaneous nerve
	K Head and Neck Sympathetic
	   Nerve
	Cavernous plexus
	Cervical ganglion
	Ciliary ganglion
	Internal carotid plexus
	Otic ganglion
	Pterygopalatine
	   (sphenopalatine) ganglion
	Sphenopalatine
	   (pterygopalatine) ganglion
	Stellate ganglion
	Submandibular ganglion
	Submaxillary ganglion
	L Thoracic Sympathetic
	   Nerve
	Cardiac plexus
	Esophageal plexus
	Greater splanchnic nerve
	Inferior cardiac nerve
	Least splanchnic nerve
	Lesser splanchnic nerve
	Middle cardiac nerve
	Pulmonary plexus
	Superior cardiac nerve
	Thoracic aortic plexus
	Thoracic ganglion
	M Abdominal Sympathetic
	   Nerve
	Abdominal aortic plexus
	Auerbach's (myenteric) plexus
	Celiac (solar) plexus
	Celiac ganglion
	Gastric plexus
	Hepatic plexus
	Inferior hypogastric plexus
	Inferior mesenteric ganglion
	Inferior mesenteric plexus
	Meissner's (submucous) plexus
	Myenteric (Auerbach's) plexus
	Pancreatic plexus
	Pelvic splanchnic nerve
	Renal nerve
	Renal plexus
	Solar (celiac) plexus
	Splenic plexus
	Submucous (Meissner's) plexus
	Superior hypogastric plexus
	Superior mesenteric ganglion
	Superior mesenteric plexus
	Suprarenal plexus
	N Lumbar Sympathetic Nerve
	Lumbar ganglion
	Lumbar splanchnic nerve
	P Sacral Sympathetic Nerve
	Ganglion impar (ganglion of
	   Walther)
	Pelvic splanchnic nerve
	Sacral ganglion
	Sacral splanchnic nerve
	Q Sacral Plexus
	Inferior gluteal nerve
	Posterior femoral cutaneous
	   nerve
	Pudendal nerve
	R Sacral Nerve
	Spinal nerve, sacral
		0 Open
		3 Percutaneous
		4 Percutaneous Endoscopic
			Z No Device	**X** Diagnostic
				Z No Qualifier

Non-OR   01B[0,1,2,3,4,5,6,8,9,A,B,C,D,F,G,H,Q,R][3,4]ZX

NC Noncovered Procedure   **LC** Limited Coverage   **QA** Questionable OB Admit   **NT** New Tech Add-on   ⊞ Combination Member   ♂ Male   ♀ Female

ICD-10-PCS 2023   159

Peripheral Nervous System

Ø   **Medical and Surgical**
1   **Peripheral Nervous System**
C   **Extirpation**   Definition: Taking or cutting out solid matter from a body part

Explanation: The solid matter may be an abnormal byproduct of a biological function or a foreign body; it may be imbedded in a body part or in the lumen of a tubular body part. The solid matter may or may not have been previously broken into pieces.

Body Part Character 4		Approach Character 5	Device Character 6	Qualifier Character 7

Ø Cervical Plexus
  Ansa cervicalis
  Cutaneous (transverse) cervical
    nerve
  Great auricular nerve
  Lesser occipital nerve
  Supraclavicular nerve
  Transverse (cutaneous) cervical
    nerve
1 Cervical Nerve
  Greater occipital nerve
  Spinal nerve, cervical
  Suboccipital nerve
  Third occipital nerve
2 Phrenic Nerve
  Accessory phrenic nerve
3 Brachial Plexus
  Axillary nerve
  Dorsal scapular nerve
  First intercostal nerve
  Long thoracic nerve
  Musculocutaneous nerve
  Subclavius nerve
  Suprascapular nerve
4 Ulnar Nerve
  Cubital nerve
5 Median Nerve
  Anterior interosseous nerve
  Palmar cutaneous nerve
6 Radial Nerve
  Dorsal digital nerve
  Musculospiral nerve
  Palmar cutaneous nerve
  Posterior interosseous nerve
8 Thoracic Nerve
  Intercostal nerve
  Intercostobrachial nerve
  Spinal nerve, thoracic
  Subcostal nerve
9 Lumbar Plexus
  Accessory obturator nerve
  Genitofemoral nerve
  Iliohypogastric nerve
  Ilioinguinal nerve
  Lateral femoral cutaneous
    nerve
  Obturator nerve
  Superior gluteal nerve
A Lumbosacral Plexus
B Lumbar Nerve
  Lumbosacral trunk
  Spinal nerve, lumbar
  Superior clunic (cluneal) nerve
C Pudendal Nerve
  Posterior labial nerve
  Posterior scrotal nerve
D Femoral Nerve
  Anterior crural nerve
  Saphenous nerve
F Sciatic Nerve
  Ischiatic nerve
G Tibial Nerve
  Lateral plantar nerve
  Medial plantar nerve
  Medial popliteal nerve
  Medial sural cutaneous nerve
	H Peroneal Nerve
	  Common fibular nerve
	  Common peroneal nerve
	  External popliteal nerve
	  Lateral sural cutaneous nerve
	K Head and Neck Sympathetic
	  Nerve
	  Cavernous plexus
	  Cervical ganglion
	  Ciliary ganglion
	  Internal carotid plexus
	  Otic ganglion
	  Pterygopalatine
	    (sphenopalatine) ganglion
	  Sphenopalatine
	    (pterygopalatine) ganglion
	  Stellate ganglion
	  Submandibular ganglion
	  Submaxillary ganglion
	L Thoracic Sympathetic Nerve
	  Cardiac plexus
	  Esophageal plexus
	  Greater splanchnic nerve
	  Inferior cardiac nerve
	  Least splanchnic nerve
	  Lesser splanchnic nerve
	  Middle cardiac nerve
	  Pulmonary plexus
	  Superior cardiac nerve
	  Thoracic aortic plexus
	  Thoracic ganglion
	M Abdominal Sympathetic
	  Nerve
	  Abdominal aortic plexus
	  Auerbach's (myenteric) plexus
	  Celiac (solar) plexus
	  Celiac ganglion
	  Gastric plexus
	  Hepatic plexus
	  Inferior hypogastric plexus
	  Inferior mesenteric ganglion
	  Inferior mesenteric plexus
	  Meissner's (submucous) plexus
	  Myenteric (Auerbach's) plexus
	  Pancreatic plexus
	  Pelvic splanchnic nerve
	  Renal nerve
	  Renal plexus
	  Solar (celiac) plexus
	  Splenic plexus
	  Submucous (Meissner's) plexus
	  Superior hypogastric plexus
	  Superior mesenteric ganglion
	  Superior mesenteric plexus
	  Suprarenal plexus
	N Lumbar Sympathetic Nerve
	  Lumbar ganglion
	  Lumbar splanchnic nerve
	P Sacral Sympathetic Nerve
	  Ganglion impar (ganglion of
	    Walther)
	  Pelvic splanchnic nerve
	  Sacral ganglion
	  Sacral splanchnic nerve
	Q Sacral Plexus
	  Inferior gluteal nerve
	  Posterior femoral cutaneous
	    nerve
	  Pudendal nerve
	R Sacral Nerve
	  Spinal nerve, sacral
		Ø Open
		3 Percutaneous
		4 Percutaneous Endoscopic
			Z No Device	**Z No Qualifier**

Non-OR Procedure   DRG Non-OR Procedure   Valid OR Procedure   HAC Associated Procedure   Combination Only   New/Revised April   New/Revised October

160   ICD-10-PCS 2023

Ø   **Medical and Surgical**
1   **Peripheral Nervous System**
D   **Extraction**   Definition: Pulling or stripping out or off all or a portion of a body part by the use of force
                      Explanation: The qualifier DIAGNOSTIC is used to identify extraction procedures that are biopsies

Body Part Character 4		Approach Character 5	Device Character 6	Qualifier Character 7

Ø Cervical Plexus
Ansa cervicalis
Cutaneous (transverse) cervical
   nerve
Great auricular nerve
Lesser occipital nerve
Supraclavicular nerve
Transverse (cutaneous) cervical
   nerve
1 Cervical Nerve
Greater occipital nerve
Spinal nerve, cervical
Suboccipital nerve
Third occipital nerve
2 Phrenic Nerve
Accessory phrenic nerve
3 Brachial Plexus
Axillary nerve
Dorsal scapular nerve
First intercostal nerve
Long thoracic nerve
Musculocutaneous nerve
Subclavius nerve
Suprascapular nerve
4 Ulnar Nerve
Cubital nerve
5 Median Nerve
Anterior interosseous nerve
Palmar cutaneous nerve
6 Radial Nerve
Dorsal digital nerve
Musculospiral nerve
Palmar cutaneous nerve
Posterior interosseous nerve
8 Thoracic Nerve
Intercostal nerve
Intercostobrachial nerve
Spinal nerve, thoracic
Subcostal nerve
9 Lumbar Plexus
Accessory obturator nerve
Genitofemoral nerve
Iliohypogastric nerve
Ilioinguinal nerve
Lateral femoral cutaneous nerve
Obturator nerve
Superior gluteal nerve
A Lumbosacral Plexus
B Lumbar Nerve
Lumbosacral trunk
Spinal nerve, lumbar
Superior clunic (cluneal) nerve
C Pudendal Nerve]
Posterior labial nerve
Posterior scrotal nerve
D Femoral Nerve
Anterior crural nerve
Saphenous nerve
F Sciatic Nerve
Ischiatic nerve
G Tibial Nerve
Lateral plantar nerve
Medial plantar nerve
Medial popliteal nerve
Medial sural cutaneous nerve
	H Peroneal Nerve
	Common fibular nerve
	Common peroneal nerve
	External popliteal nerve
	Lateral sural cutaneous nerve
	K Head and Neck Sympathetic
	Nerve
	Cavernous plexus
	Cervical ganglion
	Ciliary ganglion
	Internal carotid plexus
	Otic ganglion
	Pterygopalatine
	   (sphenopalatine) ganglion
	Sphenopalatine
	   (pterygopalatine) ganglion
	Stellate ganglion
	Submandibular ganglion
	Submaxillary ganglion
	L Thoracic Sympathetic Nerve
	Cardiac plexus
	Esophageal plexus
	Greater splanchnic nerve
	Inferior cardiac nerve
	Least splanchnic nerve
	Lesser splanchnic nerve
	Middle cardiac nerve
	Pulmonary plexus
	Superior cardiac nerve
	Thoracic aortic plexus
	Thoracic ganglion
	M Abdominal Sympathetic Nerve
	Abdominal aortic plexus
	Auerbach's (myenteric) plexus
	Celiac (solar) plexus
	Celiac ganglion
	Gastric plexus
	Hepatic plexus
	Inferior hypogastric plexus
	Inferior mesenteric ganglion
	Inferior mesenteric plexus
	Meissner's (submucous) plexus
	Myenteric (Auerbach's) plexus
	Pancreatic plexus
	Pelvic splanchnic nerve
	Renal nerve
	Renal plexus
	Solar (celiac) plexus
	Splenic plexus
	Submucous (Meissner's) plexus
	Superior hypogastric plexus
	Superior mesenteric ganglion
	Superior mesenteric plexus
	Suprarenal plexus
	N Lumbar Sympathetic Nerve
	Lumbar ganglion
	Lumbar splanchnic nerve
	P Sacral Sympathetic Nerve
	Ganglion impar (ganglion of
	   Walther)
	Pelvic splanchnic nerve
	Sacral ganglion
	Sacral splanchnic nerve
	Q Sacral Plexus
	Inferior gluteal nerve
	Posterior femoral cutaneous
	   nerve
	Pudendal nerve
	R Sacral Nerve
	Spinal nerve, sacral
		Ø Open
		3 Percutaneous
		4 Percutaneous Endoscopic
			Z No Device	**Z No Qualifier**

NC Noncovered Procedure   **LC** Limited Coverage   **QA** Questionable OB Admit   **NT** New Tech Add-on   ⊞ Combination Member   ♂ Male   ♀ Female

ICD-10-PCS 2023   161

01D–01D

Peripheral Nervous System

Ø **Medical and Surgical**
1 **Peripheral Nervous System**
H **Insertion** Definition: Putting in a nonbiological appliance that monitors, assists, performs, or prevents a physiological function but does not physically take the place of a body part
Explanation: None

Body Part Character 4		Approach Character 5	Device Character 6	Qualifier Character 7
Y Peripheral Nerve ⊞		**Ø** Open **3** Percutaneous **4** Percutaneous Endoscopic	**1** Radioactive Element **2** Monitoring Device **M** Neurostimulator Lead **Y** Other Device	**Z** No Qualifier

Non-OR   Ø1HY31Z
Non-OR   Ø1HY[3,4]YZ

See Appendix L for Procedure Combinations
⊞   Ø1HY[Ø,3,4]MZ

Ø **Medical and Surgical**
1 **Peripheral Nervous System**
J **Inspection** Definition: Visually and/or manually exploring a body part
Explanation: Visual exploration may be performed with or without optical instrumentation. Manual exploration may be performed directly or through intervening body layers.

Body Part Character 4		Approach Character 5	Device Character 6	Qualifier Character 7
Y Peripheral Nerve		**Ø** Open **3** Percutaneous **4** Percutaneous Endoscopic	**Z** No Device	**Z** No Qualifier

Non-OR   Ø1JY3ZZ

Non-OR Procedure   DRG Non-OR Procedure   Valid OR Procedure   HAC Associated Procedure   Combination Only   New/Revised April   New/Revised October

162

ICD-10-PCS 2023

Ø Medical and Surgical
1 Peripheral Nervous System
N Release   Definition: Freeing a body part from an abnormal physical constraint by cutting or by the use of force
                Explanation: Some of the restraining tissue may be taken out but none of the body part is taken out

Body Part Character 4	Approach Character 5	Device Character 6	Qualifier Character 7

Ø Cervical Plexus
Ansa cervicalis
Cutaneous (transverse) cervical
  nerve
Great auricular nerve
Lesser occipital nerve
Supraclavicular nerve
Transverse (cutaneous) cervical
  nerve
1 Cervical Nerve
Greater occipital nerve
Spinal nerve, cervical
Suboccipital nerve
Third occipital nerve
2 Phrenic Nerve
Accessory phrenic nerve
3 Brachial Plexus
Axillary nerve
Dorsal scapular nerve
First intercostal nerve
Long thoracic nerve
Musculocutaneous nerve
Subclavius nerve
Suprascapular nerve
4 Ulnar Nerve
Cubital nerve
5 Median Nerve
Anterior interosseous nerve
Palmar cutaneous nerve
6 Radial Nerve
Dorsal digital nerve
Musculospiral nerve
Palmar cutaneous nerve
Posterior interosseous nerve
8 Thoracic Nerve
Intercostal nerve
Intercostobrachial nerve
Spinal nerve, thoracic
Subcostal nerve
9 Lumbar Plexus
Accessory obturator nerve
Genitofemoral nerve
Iliohypogastric nerve
Ilioinguinal nerve
Lateral femoral cutaneous nerve
Obturator nerve
Superior gluteal nerve
A Lumbosacral Plexus
B Lumbar Nerve
Lumbosacral trunk
Spinal nerve, lumbar
Superior clunic (cluneal) nerve
C Pudendal Nerve
Posterior labial nerve
Posterior scrotal nerve
D Femoral Nerve
Anterior crural nerve
Saphenous nerve
F Sciatic Nerve
Ischiatic nerve
G Tibial Nerve
Lateral plantar nerve
Medial plantar nerve
Medial popliteal nerve
Medial sural cutaneous nerve
	H Peroneal Nerve
	Common fibular nerve
	Common peroneal nerve
	External popliteal nerve
	Lateral sural cutaneous nerve
	K Head and Neck Sympathetic
	   Nerve
	Cavernous plexus
	Cervical ganglion
	Ciliary ganglion
	Internal carotid plexus
	Otic ganglion
	Pterygopalatine
	    (sphenopalatine) ganglion
	Sphenopalatine
	    (pterygopalatine) ganglion
	Stellate ganglion
	Submandibular ganglion
	Submaxillary ganglion
	L Thoracic Sympathetic Nerve
	Cardiac plexus
	Esophageal plexus
	Greater splanchnic nerve
	Inferior cardiac nerve
	Least splanchnic nerve
	Lesser splanchnic nerve
	Middle cardiac nerve
	Pulmonary plexus
	Superior cardiac nerve
	Thoracic aortic plexus
	Thoracic ganglion
	M Abdominal Sympathetic
	   Nerve
	Abdominal aortic plexus
	Auerbach's (myenteric) plexus
	Celiac (solar) plexus
	Celiac ganglion
	Gastric plexus
	Hepatic plexus
	Inferior hypogastric plexus
	Inferior mesenteric ganglion
	Inferior mesenteric plexus
	Meissner's (submucous) plexus
	Myenteric (Auerbach's) plexus
	Pancreatic plexus
	Pelvic splanchnic nerve
	Renal nerve
	Renal plexus
	Solar (celiac) plexus
	Splenic plexus
	Submucous (Meissner's) plexus
	Superior hypogastric plexus
	Superior mesenteric ganglion
	Superior mesenteric plexus
	Suprarenal plexus
	N Lumbar Sympathetic Nerve
	Lumbar ganglion
	Lumbar splanchnic nerve
	P Sacral Sympathetic Nerve
	Ganglion impar (ganglion of
	   Walther)
	Pelvic splanchnic nerve
	Sacral ganglion
	Sacral splanchnic nerve
	Q Sacral Plexus
	Inferior gluteal nerve
	Posterior femoral cutaneous
	   nerve
	Pudendal nerve
	R Sacral Nerve
	Spinal nerve, sacral
		Ø Open
		3 Percutaneous
		4 Percutaneous Endoscopic
			Z No Device	**Z** No Qualifier

Ø   Medical and Surgical
1   Peripheral Nervous System
P   Removal   Definition: Taking out or off a device from a body part

Explanation: If a device is taken out and a similar device put in without cutting or puncturing the skin or mucous membrane, the procedure is coded to the root operation CHANGE. Otherwise, the procedure for taking out a device is coded to the root operation REMOVAL.

Body Part Character 4	Approach Character 5	Device Character 6	Qualifier Character 7
Y Peripheral Nerve	Ø Open 3 Percutaneous 4 Percutaneous Endoscopic	Ø Drainage Device 2 Monitoring Device 7 Autologous Tissue Substitute M Neurostimulator Lead Y Other Device	Z No Qualifier
Y Peripheral Nerve	X External	Ø Drainage Device 2 Monitoring Device M Neurostimulator Lead	Z No Qualifier

Non-OR   Ø1PY3[Ø,2]Z
Non-OR   Ø1PY[3,4]YZ
Non-OR   Ø1PYX[Ø,2,M]Z

0   Medical and Surgical
1   Peripheral Nervous System
Q   Repair   Definition: Restoring, to the extent possible, a body part to its normal anatomic structure and function
                    Explanation: Used only when the method to accomplish the repair is not one of the other root operations

Body Part Character 4		Approach Character 5	Device Character 6	Qualifier Character 7

0   Cervical Plexus
   Ansa cervicalis
   Cutaneous (transverse) cervical
        nerve
   Great auricular nerve
   Lesser occipital nerve
   Supraclavicular nerve
   Transverse (cutaneous) cervical
        nerve
1   Cervical Nerve
   Greater occipital nerve
   Spinal nerve, cervical
   Suboccipital nerve
   Third occipital nerve
2   Phrenic Nerve
   Accessory phrenic nerve
3   Brachial Plexus
   Axillary nerve
   Dorsal scapular nerve
   First intercostal nerve
   Long thoracic nerve
   Musculocutaneous nerve
   Subclavius nerve
   Suprascapular nerve
4   Ulnar Nerve
   Cubital nerve
5   Median Nerve
   Anterior interosseous nerve
   Palmar cutaneous nerve
6   Radial Nerve
   Dorsal digital nerve
   Musculospiral nerve
   Palmar cutaneous nerve
   Posterior interosseous nerve
8   Thoracic Nerve
   Intercostal nerve
   Intercostobrachial nerve
   Spinal nerve, thoracic
   Subcostal nerve
9   Lumbar Plexus
   Accessory obturator nerve
   Genitofemoral nerve
   Iliohypogastric nerve
   Ilioinguinal nerve
   Lateral femoral cutaneous
        nerve
   Obturator nerve
   Superior gluteal nerve
A   Lumbosacral Plexus
B   Lumbar Nerve
   Lumbosacral trunk
   Spinal nerve, lumbar
   Superior clunic (cluneal) nerve
C   Pudendal Nerve
   Posterior labial nerve
   Posterior scrotal nerve
D   Femoral Nerve
   Anterior crural nerve
   Saphenous nerve
F   Sciatic Nerve
   Ischiatic nerve
G   Tibial Nerve
   Lateral plantar nerve
   Medial plantar nerve
   Medial popliteal nerve
   Medial sural cutaneous nerve
	H Peroneal Nerve
	   Common fibular nerve
	   Common peroneal nerve
	   External popliteal nerve
	   Lateral sural cutaneous nerve
	**K Head and Neck Sympathetic
	     Nerve**
	   Cavernous plexus
	   Cervical ganglion
	   Ciliary ganglion
	   Internal carotid plexus
	   Otic ganglion
	   Pterygopalatine
	        (sphenopalatine) ganglion
	   Sphenopalatine
	        (pterygopalatine) ganglion
	   Stellate ganglion
	   Submandibular ganglion
	   Submaxillary ganglion
	L Thoracic Sympathetic Nerve
	   Cardiac plexus
	   Esophageal plexus
	   Greater splanchnic nerve
	   Inferior cardiac nerve
	   Least splanchnic nerve
	   Lesser splanchnic nerve
	   Middle cardiac nerve
	   Pulmonary plexus
	   Superior cardiac nerve
	   Thoracic aortic plexus
	   Thoracic ganglion
	**M Abdominal Sympathetic
	     Nerve**
	   Abdominal aortic plexus
	   Auerbach's (myenteric) plexus
	   Celiac (solar) plexus
	   Celiac ganglion
	   Gastric plexus
	   Hepatic plexus
	   Inferior hypogastric plexus
	   Inferior mesenteric ganglion
	   Inferior mesenteric plexus
	   Meissner's (submucous) plexus
	   Myenteric (Auerbach's) plexus
	   Pancreatic plexus
	   Pelvic splanchnic nerve
	   Renal nerve
	   Renal plexus
	   Solar (celiac) plexus
	   Splenic plexus
	   Submucous (Meissner's) plexus
	   Superior hypogastric plexus
	   Superior mesenteric ganglion
	   Superior mesenteric plexus
	   Suprarenal plexus
	N Lumbar Sympathetic Nerve
	   Lumbar ganglion
	   Lumbar splanchnic nerve
	P Sacral Sympathetic Nerve
	   Ganglion impar (ganglion of
	        Walther)
	   Pelvic splanchnic nerve
	   Sacral ganglion
	   Sacral splanchnic nerve
	Q Sacral Plexus
	   Inferior gluteal nerve
	   Posterior femoral cutaneous
	        nerve
	   Pudendal nerve
	R Sacral Nerve
	   Spinal nerve, sacral
		0 Open
		3 Percutaneous
		4 Percutaneous Endoscopic
			Z No Device	**Z No Qualifier**

NC Noncovered Procedure   **LC** Limited Coverage   **QA** Questionable OB Admit   **NT** New Tech Add-on   ✛ Combination Member   ♂Male   ♀Female

ICD-10-PCS 2023   **165**

Ø   **Medical and Surgical**
1   **Peripheral Nervous System**
R   **Replacement**   Definition: Putting in or on biological or synthetic material that physically takes the place and/or function of all or a portion of a body part
                            Explanation: The body part may have been taken out or replaced, or may be taken out, physically eradicated, or rendered nonfunctional during
                            the REPLACEMENT procedure. A REMOVAL procedure is coded for taking out the device used in a previous replacement procedure.

Body Part Character 4	Approach Character 5	Device Character 6	Qualifier Character 7
1 Cervical Nerve Greater occipital nerve Spinal nerve, cervical Suboccipital nerve Third occipital nerve **2 Phrenic Nerve** Accessory phrenic nerve **4 Ulnar Nerve** Cubital nerve **5 Median Nerve** Anterior interosseous nerve Palmar cutaneous nerve **6 Radial Nerve** Dorsal digital nerve Musculospiral nerve Palmar cutaneous nerve Posterior interosseous nerve **8 Thoracic Nerve** Intercostal nerve Intercostobrachial nerve Spinal nerve, thoracic Subcostal nerve **B Lumbar Nerve** Lumbosacral trunk Spinal nerve, lumbar Superior clunic (cluneal) nerve **C Pudendal Nerve** Posterior labial nerve Posterior scrotal nerve **D Femoral Nerve** Anterior crural nerve Saphenous nerve **F Sciatic Nerve** Ischiatic nerve **G Tibial Nerve** Lateral plantar nerve Medial plantar nerve Medial popliteal nerve Medial sural cutaneous nerve **H Peroneal Nerve** Common fibular nerve Common peroneal nerve External popliteal nerve Lateral sural cutaneous nerve **R Sacral Nerve** Spinal nerve, sacral	**Ø Open** **4 Percutaneous Endoscopic**	**7 Autologous Tissue Substitute** **J Synthetic Substitute** **K Nonautologous Tissue Substitute**	**Z No Qualifier**

Ø   **Medical and Surgical**
1   **Peripheral Nervous System**
S   **Reposition**   Definition: Moving to its normal location, or other suitable location, all or a portion of a body part

                           Explanation: The body part is moved to a new location from an abnormal location, or from a normal location where it is not functioning correctly. The body part may or may not be cut out or off to be moved to the new location.

Body Part Character 4	Approach Character 5	Device Character 6	Qualifier Character 7

Ø **Cervical Plexus**
   Ansa cervicalis
   Cutaneous (transverse) cervical nerve
   Great auricular nerve
   Lesser occipital nerve
   Supraclavicular nerve
   Transverse (cutaneous) cervical nerve
	Ø Open
	3 Percutaneous
	4 Percutaneous Endoscopic
		Z No Device	**Z** No Qualifier

1 **Cervical Nerve**
   Greater occipital nerve
   Spinal nerve, cervical
   Suboccipital nerve
   Third occipital nerve			

2 **Phrenic Nerve** Accessory phrenic nerve			

3 **Brachial Plexus**
   Axillary nerve
   Dorsal scapular nerve
   First intercostal nerve
   Long thoracic nerve
   Musculocutaneous nerve
   Subclavius nerve
   Suprascapular nerve			

4 **Ulnar Nerve** Cubital nerve			

5 **Median Nerve**
   Anterior interosseous nerve
   Palmar cutaneous nerve			

6 **Radial Nerve**
   Dorsal digital nerve
   Musculospiral nerve
   Palmar cutaneous nerve
   Posterior interosseous nerve			

8 **Thoracic Nerve**
   Intercostal nerve
   Intercostobrachial nerve
   Spinal nerve, thoracic
   Subcostal nerve			

9 **Lumbar Plexus**
   Accessory obturator nerve
   Genitofemoral nerve
   Iliohypogastric nerve
   Ilioinguinal nerve
   Lateral femoral cutaneous nerve
   Obturator nerve
   Superior gluteal nerve			

A **Lumbosacral Plexus**			

B **Lumbar Nerve**
   Lumbosacral trunk
   Spinal nerve, lumbar
   Superior clunic (cluneal) nerve			

C **Pudendal Nerve**
   Posterior labial nerve
   Posterior scrotal nerve			

D **Femoral Nerve**
   Anterior crural nerve
   Saphenous nerve			

F **Sciatic Nerve** Ischiatic nerve			

G **Tibial Nerve**
   Lateral plantar nerve
   Medial plantar nerve
   Medial popliteal nerve
   Medial sural cutaneous nerve			

H **Peroneal Nerve**
   Common fibular nerve
   Common peroneal nerve
   External popliteal nerve
   Lateral sural cutaneous nerve			

Q **Sacral Plexus**
   Inferior gluteal nerve
   Posterior femoral cutaneous nerve
   Pudendal nerve			

R **Sacral Nerve** Spinal nerve, sacral			

NC Noncovered Procedure   **LC** Limited Coverage   **QA** Questionable OB Admit   **NT** New Tech Add-on   ⊞ Combination Member   ♂ Male   ♀ Female

ICD-10-PCS 2023   **167**

Peripheral Nervous System

0   Medical and Surgical
1   Peripheral Nervous System
U   Supplement   Definition: Putting in or on biological or synthetic material that physically reinforces and/or augments the function of a portion of a body part

Explanation: The biological material is non-living, or is living and from the same individual. The body part may have been previously replaced, and the SUPPLEMENT procedure is performed to physically reinforce and/or augment the function of the replaced body part.

Body Part Character 4	Approach Character 5	Device Character 6	Qualifier Character 7

1   Cervical Nerve
    Greater occipital nerve
    Spinal nerve, cervical
    Suboccipital nerve
    Third occipital nerve
2   Phrenic Nerve
    Accessory phrenic nerve
4   Ulnar Nerve
    Cubital nerve
5   Median Nerve
    Anterior interosseous nerve
    Palmar cutaneous nerve
6   Radial Nerve
    Dorsal digital nerve
    Musculospiral nerve
    Palmar cutaneous nerve
    Posterior interosseous nerve
8   Thoracic Nerve
    Intercostal nerve
    Intercostobrachial nerve
    Spinal nerve, thoracic
    Subcostal nerve
B   Lumbar Nerve
    Lumbosacral trunk
    Spinal nerve, lumbar
    Superior clunic (cluneal) nerve
C   Pudendal Nerve
    Posterior labial nerve
    Posterior scrotal nerve
D   Femoral Nerve
    Anterior crural nerve
    Saphenous nerve
F   Sciatic Nerve
    Ischiatic nerve
G   Tibial Nerve
    Lateral plantar nerve
    Medial plantar nerve
    Medial popliteal nerve
    Medial sural cutaneous nerve
H   Peroneal Nerve
    Common fibular nerve
    Common peroneal nerve
    External popliteal nerve
    Lateral sural cutaneous nerve
R   Sacral Nerve
    Spinal nerve, sacral
	0 Open
	3 Percutaneous
	4 Percutaneous Endoscopic
		7 Autologous Tissue Substitute
		J Synthetic Substitute
		K Nonautologous Tissue Substitute
			Z No Qualifier

0   Medical and Surgical
1   Peripheral Nervous System
W   Revision   Definition: Correcting, to the extent possible, a portion of a malfunctioning device or the position of a displaced device

Explanation: Revision can include correcting a malfunctioning or displaced device by taking out or putting in components of the device such as a screw or pin

Body Part Character 4	Approach Character 5	Device Character 6	Qualifier Character 7
Y Peripheral Nerve	**0 Open** **3 Percutaneous** **4 Percutaneous Endoscopic**	**0 Drainage Device** **2 Monitoring Device** **7 Autologous Tissue Substitute** **M Neurostimulator Lead** **Y Other Device**	**Z No Qualifier**
Y Peripheral Nerve	**X External**	**0 Drainage Device** **2 Monitoring Device** **7 Autologous Tissue Substitute** **M Neurostimulator Lead**	**Z No Qualifier**

Non-OR	01WY[3,4]YZ
Non-OR	01WYX[0,2,7,M]Z

Ø   **Medical and Surgical**
1   **Peripheral Nervous System**
X   **Transfer**   Definition: Moving, without taking out, all or a portion of a body part to another location to take over the function of all or a portion of a body part
                   Explanation: The body part transferred remains connected to its vascular and nervous supply

Body Part Character 4	Approach Character 5	Device Character 6	Qualifier Character 7
1 Cervical Nerve Greater occipital nerve Spinal nerve, cervical Suboccipital nerve Third occipital nerve **2 Phrenic Nerve** Accessory phrenic nerve	Ø Open 4 Percutaneous Endoscopic	Z No Device	1 Cervical Nerve 2 Phrenic Nerve
4 Ulnar Nerve Cubital nerve **5 Median Nerve** Anterior interosseous nerve Palmar cutaneous nerve **6 Radial Nerve** Dorsal digital nerve Musculospiral nerve Palmar cutaneous nerve Posterior interosseous nerve	Ø Open 4 Percutaneous Endoscopic	Z No Device	4 Ulnar Nerve 5 Median Nerve 6 Radial Nerve
8 Thoracic Nerve Intercostal nerve Intercostobrachial nerve Spinal nerve, thoracic Subcostal nerve	Ø Open 4 Percutaneous Endoscopic	Z No Device	8 Thoracic Nerve
B Lumbar Nerve Lumbosacral trunk Spinal nerve, lumbar Superior clunic (cluneal) nerve **C Pudendal Nerve** Posterior labial nerve Posterior scrotal nerve	Ø Open 4 Percutaneous Endoscopic	Z No Device	B Lumbar Nerve C Perineal Nerve
D Femoral Nerve Anterior crural nerve Saphenous nerve **F Sciatic Nerve** Ischiatic nerve **G Tibial Nerve** Lateral plantar nerve Medial plantar nerve Medial popliteal nerve Medial sural cutaneous nerve **H Peroneal Nerve** Common fibular nerve Common peroneal nerve External popliteal nerve Lateral sural cutaneous nerve	Ø Open 4 Percutaneous Endoscopic	Z No Device	D Femoral Nerve F Sciatic Nerve G Tibial Nerve H Peroneal Nerve

NC Noncovered Procedure   LC Limited Coverage   QA Questionable OB Admit   NT New Tech Add-on   ⊞ Combination Member   ♂ Male   ♀ Female

ICD-10-PCS 2023   **169**

0 Medical and Surgical
1 Peripheral Nervous System
X Transfer: Moving, without taking out, all or a portion of a body part to another location to take over the function of all or a portion of a body part

Explanation: The body part transferred remains connected to its scalp and nerve supply

Body Part – Character 4	Approach – Character 5	Device – Character 6	Qualifier – Character 7
1 Cervical Nerve Greater occipital nerve Spinal accessory nerve Suboccipital nerve Third occipital nerve **2 Phrenic Nerve** Accessory phrenic nerve	**0 Open** **4 Percutaneous Endoscopic**	**Z No Device**	**1 Cervical Nerve** **2 Phrenic Nerve**
4 Ulnar Nerve Cubital nerve **5 Median Nerve** Anterior interosseous nerve Palmar cutaneous nerve **6 Radial Nerve** Dorsal digital nerve Musculospiral nerve Palmar cutaneous nerve Posterior interosseous nerve	**0 Open** **4 Percutaneous Endoscopic**	**Z No Device**	**4 Ulnar Nerve** **5 Median Nerve** **6 Radial Nerve**
7 Thoracic Nerve Intercostal nerve Intercostobrachial nerve Spinal nerve, thoracic Subcostal nerve	**0 Open** **4 Percutaneous Endoscopic**	**Z No Device**	**8 Thoracic Nerve**
8 Lumbar Nerve Lumbosacral trunk Spinal nerve, lumbar **C Perineal Nerve** Posterior scrotal nerve	**0 Open** **4 Percutaneous Endoscopic**	**Z No Device**	**A Lumbar Nerve** **C Perineal Nerve**
D Femoral Nerve Anterior crural nerve Saphenous nerve **F Sciatic Nerve** Ischiatic nerve **G Tibial Nerve** Lateral plantar nerve Medial plantar nerve Medial popliteal nerve Medial sural cutaneous nerve **H Peroneal Nerve** Common fibular nerve Common peroneal nerve External popliteal nerve Lateral sural cutaneous nerve	**0 Open** **4 Percutaneous Endoscopic**	**Z No Device**	**D Femoral Nerve** **F Sciatic Nerve** **G Tibial Nerve** **H Peroneal Nerve**

Heart and Great Vessels Ø21–Ø2Y

Character Meanings

This Character Meaning table is provided as a guide to assist the user in the identification of character members that may be found in this section of code tables. It **SHOULD NOT** be used to build a PCS code.

Operation–Character 3	Body Part–Character 4	Approach–Character 5	Device–Character 6	Qualifier–Character 7
1 Bypass	Ø Coronary Artery, One Artery	Ø Open	Ø Monitoring Device, Pressure Sensor	Ø Allogeneic OR Ultrasonic
4 Creation	1 Coronary Artery, Two Arteries	3 Percutaneous	2 Monitoring Device	1 Syngeneic
5 Destruction	2 Coronary Artery, Three Arteries	4 Percutaneous Endoscopic	3 Infusion Device	2 Zooplastic OR Common Atrioventricular Valve
7 Dilation	3 Coronary Artery, Four or More Arteries	X External	4 Intraluminal Device, Drug-eluting	3 Coronary Artery
8 Division	4 Coronary Vein		5 Intraluminal Device, Drug-eluting, Two	4 Coronary Vein
B Excision	5 Atrial Septum		6 Intraluminal Device, Drug-eluting, Three	5 Coronary Circulation
C Extirpation	6 Atrium, Right		7 Intraluminal Device, Drug-eluting, Four or More OR Autologous Tissue Substitute	6 Bifurcation OR Atrium, Right
F Fragmentation	7 Atrium, Left		8 Zooplastic Tissue	7 Atrium, Left OR Orbital Atherectomy Technique
H Insertion	8 Conduction Mechanism		9 Autologous Venous Tissue	8 Internal Mammary, Right
J Inspection	9 Chordae Tendineae		A Autologous Arterial Tissue	9 Internal Mammary, Left
K Map	A Heart		C Extraluminal Device	A Innominate Artery
L Occlusion	B Heart, Right		D Intraluminal Device	B Subclavian
N Release	C Heart, Left		E Intraluminal Device, Two OR Intraluminal Device, Branched or Fenestrated, One or Two Arteries	C Thoracic Artery
P Removal	D Papillary Muscle		F Intraluminal Device, Three OR Intraluminal Device, Branched or Fenestrated, Three or More Arteries	D Carotid
Q Repair	F Aortic Valve		G Intraluminal Device, Four or More	E Atrioventricular Valve, Left
R Replacement	G Mitral Valve		J Synthetic Substitute OR Cardiac Lead, Pacemaker	F Abdominal Artery
S Reposition	H Pulmonary Valve		K Nonautologous Tissue Substitute OR Cardiac Lead, Defibrillator	G Atrioventricular Valve, Right OR Axillary Artery
T Resection	J Tricuspid Valve		L Biologic with Synthetic Substitute, Autoregulated Electrohydraulic	H Transapical OR Brachial Artery
U Supplement	K Ventricle, Right		M Cardiac Lead OR Synthetic Substitute, Pneumatic	J Truncal Valve OR Temporary OR Intraoperative
V Restriction	L Ventricle, Left		N Intracardiac Pacemaker	K Left Atrial Appendage
			Q Implantable Heart Assist System	L In Existing Conduit
			R Short-term External Heart Assist System	M Native Site
W Revision	M Ventricular Septum		T Intraluminal Device, Radioactive	N Rapid Deployment Technique
Y Transplantation	N Pericardium		Y Other Device	P Pulmonary Trunk
	P Pulmonary Trunk		Z No Device	Q Pulmonary Artery, Right
	Q Pulmonary Artery, Right			R Pulmonary Artery, Left
	R Pulmonary Artery, Left			S Pulmonary Vein, Right OR Biventricular
	S Pulmonary Vein, Right			T Pulmonary Vein, Left OR Ductus Arteriosus
	T Pulmonary Vein, Left			U Pulmonary Vein, Confluence
	V Superior Vena Cava			V Lower Extremity Artery
	W Thoracic Aorta, Descending			W Aorta
	X Thoracic Aorta, Ascending/Arch			X Diagnostic
	Y Great Vessel			Z No Qualifier

AHA Coding Clinic for Heart and Great Vessels

2022, 1Q, 10-13	Procedures performed on a continuous vessel, ICD-10-PCS Guideline B4.1c

AHA Coding Clinic for table Ø21

2022, 1Q, 54	Coronary artery bypass graft surgery
2021, 3Q, 22	Left internal mammary artery free graft between obtuse marginal saphenous vein graft and left anterior descending artery
2020, 4Q, 44-45	Atrium bypass qualifier
2020, 1Q, 24	Pulmonary artery unifocalization
2020, 1Q, 37	Bypass of ascending aorta to brachiocephalic artery
2019, 4Q, 23	Bypass thoracic aorta to innominate artery
2019, 3Q, 30	Aortic aneurysm repair with debranching of common carotid and brachiocephalic arteries
2018, 4Q, 45-46	Descending thoracic aorta bypass
2018, 3Q, 8	Coronary artery bypass graft surgery (revision versus total redo)
2018, 3Q, 26	Coronary artery bypass graft surgery with endarterectomy
2017, 4Q, 56	Added approach values - Percutaneous heart valve procedures
2017, 1Q, 19	Norwood Sano procedure
2016, 4Q, 80-81	Thoracic aorta, ascending/arch and descending
2016, 4Q, 82-83	Coronary artery, number of arteries
2016, 4Q, 102-109	Correction of congenital heart defects
2016, 4Q, 144	Repair of atrial septal defect and anomalous pulmonary venous return
2016, 4Q, 145	Modified Warden procedure for repair of septal defect and right partial anomalous pulmonary venous return
2016, 1Q, 27	Aortocoronary bypass graft utilizing Y-graft
2015, 4Q, 22, 24	Congenital heart corrective procedures
2015, 3Q, 16	Revision of previous truncus arteriosus surgery with ventricle to pulmonary artery conduit
2014, 3Q, 3	Blalock-Taussig shunt procedure
2014, 3Q, 8	Coronary artery bypass graft utilizing internal mammary as pedicle graft
2014, 3Q, 20	MAZE procedure performed with coronary artery bypass graft
2014, 3Q, 29	Fontan completion procedure stage II
2014, 3Q, 30	Creation of conduit from right ventricle to pulmonary artery
2014, 1Q, 10	Repair of thoracic aortic aneurysm & coronary artery bypass graft
2013, 2Q, 37	Coronary artery release performed during coronary artery bypass graft

AHA Coding Clinic for table Ø24

2016, 4Q, 101	Root operation Creation
2016, 4Q, 102-109	Correction of congenital heart defects

AHA Coding Clinic for table Ø25

2020, 1Q, 32	Ablation convergent procedure (catheter-based and thoracoscopic ablations)
2018, 3Q, 27	Alcohol septal ablation
2016, 4Q, 80-81	Thoracic aorta, ascending/arch and descending
2016, 3Q, 43-44	Peri-pulmonary catheter ablation
2016, 3Q, 44-45	Maze procedure
2016, 2Q, 17	Photodynamic therapy for treatment of malignant mesothelioma
2014, 4Q, 47	Catheter ablation of peripulmonary veins
2014, 3Q, 19	Ablation of ventricular tachycardia with Impella® support
2014, 3Q, 20	MAZE procedure performed with coronary artery bypass graft
2013, 2Q, 38	Catheter ablation to treat atrial fibrillation

AHA Coding Clinic for table Ø27

2018, 3Q, 7	Coronary brachytherapy with angioplasty
2018, 3Q, 10	Disruption of perma-catheter fibrin sheath via angioplasty of superior vena cava
2018, 2Q, 24	Coronary artery bifurcation
2017, 4Q, 32-33	Corrective surgery of left ventricular outflow tract obstruction
2016, 4Q, 80-81	Thoracic aorta, ascending/arch and descending
2016, 4Q, 82-83	Coronary artery, number of arteries
2016, 4Q, 84-85	Coronary artery, number of stents
2016, 4Q, 86-88	Coronary and peripheral artery bifurcation
2016, 1Q, 16	Pulmonary valvotomy and dilation of annulus
2015, 4Q, 13	New Section X codes—New Technology procedures
2015, 3Q, 9	Failed attempt to treat coronary artery occlusion
2015, 3Q, 10	Coronary angioplasty with unsuccessful stent insertion
2015, 3Q, 16	Revision of previous truncus arteriosus surgery with ventricle to pulmonary artery conduit
2015, 2Q, 3-5	Coronary artery intervention site
2014, 2Q, 4	Coronary angioplasty of bypassed vessel

AHA Coding Clinic for table Ø2B

2019, 3Q, 32	Endomyocardial biopsy and right heart catheterization
2019, 2Q, 20	Pericardiectomy for constrictive pericarditis
2017, 1Q, 38	Mitral valve repair and chordae tendineae transfer
2016, 4Q, 80-81	Thoracic aorta, ascending/arch and descending
2015, 2Q, 23	Annuloplasty ring

AHA Coding Clinic for table Ø2C

2021, 4Q, 41	Coronary orbital atherectomy
2019, 4Q, 25	Coronary artery to root operation Supplement
2018, 3Q, 26	Coronary artery bypass graft surgery with endarterectomy
2018, 2Q, 24	Coronary artery bifurcation
2017, 2Q, 23	Thrombectomy via Fogarty catheter
2016, 4Q, 80-81	Thoracic aorta, ascending/arch and descending
2016, 4Q, 82-83	Coronary artery, number of arteries
2016, 4Q, 86-87	Coronary and peripheral artery bifurcation
2016, 2Q, 24	Repair/decalcification of mitral valve
2016, 2Q, 25	Aortic valve surgery with excision of calcium deposits

AHA Coding Clinic for table Ø2F

2021, 4Q, 41-42	Coronary intravascular lithotripsy
2020, 4Q, 45-49	New fragmentation tables
2020, 4Q, 49-50	Intravascular ultrasound assisted thrombolysis
2020, 4Q, 50	Intravascular lithotripsy

AHA Coding Clinic for table Ø2H

2022, 2Q, 25	Temporary-permanent pacemaker placement
2021, 2Q, 23	Clarification of lead placement in bundle of HIS
2019, 4Q, 23-24	Coronary artery Body Part to root operation Insertion
2019, 3Q, 19	Insertion of left ventricular catheter
2019, 3Q, 23	Placement of pacemaker lead in Bundle of HIS
2019, 1Q, 24	Replacement of left ventricular assist device with retention of outflow graft
2018, 4Q, 94	Insertion and removal of failed Watchman™ device
2018, 2Q, 3-5	Intra-aortic balloon pump
2018, 2Q, 19	Pacing lead attached to automatic implantable cardioverter defibrillator
2017, 4Q, 42-45	Insertion of external heart assist devices
2017, 4Q, 63-64	Added and revised device values - Vascular access reservoir
2017, 4Q, 104	Placement of Watchman™ left atrial appendage device
2017, 3Q, 11	Placement of peripherally inserted central catheter using 3CG ECG technology
2017, 2Q, 24	Tunneled catheter versus totally implantable catheter
2017, 2Q, 26	Exchange of tunneled catheter
2017, 1Q, 10-11	External heart assist device
2016, 4Q, 80-81	Thoracic aorta, ascending/arch and descending
2016, 4Q, 95	Intracardiac pacemaker
2016, 4Q, 137-138	Heart assist device systems
2016, 2Q, 15	Removal and replacement of tunneled internal jugular catheter
2015, 4Q, 14	New Section X codes—New Technology procedures
2015, 4Q, 26-31	Vascular access devices
2015, 3Q, 35	Swan Ganz catheterization
2015, 2Q, 31	Leadless pacemaker insertion
2015, 2Q, 33	Totally implantable central venous access device (Port-a-Cath)
2013, 3Q, 18	Placement of peripherally inserted central catheter (PICC)

AHA Coding Clinic for table Ø2J

2015, 3Q, 9	Failed attempt to treat coronary artery occlusion

AHA Coding Clinic for table Ø2K

2020, 1Q, 32	Ablation convergent procedure (catheter-based and thoracoscopic ablations)

AHA Coding Clinic for table Ø2L

2018, 4Q, 94	Insertion and removal of failed Watchman™ device
2017, 4Q, 31	Resuscitative endovascular balloon occlusion of the aorta
2017, 4Q, 33-34	Occlusion/ligation of pulmonary trunk & right pulmonary artery
2016, 4Q, 102-109	Correction of congenital heart defects
2016, 2Q, 26	Embolization of pulmonary arteriovenous fistula
2015, 4Q, 23	Congenital heart corrective procedures
2014, 3Q, 20	MAZE procedure performed with coronary artery bypass graft

AHA Coding Clinic for table Ø2N

2021, 3Q, 26	Cavoatrial junction tear with repair and relief of cardiac tamponade
2019, 2Q, 13	Unroofing of anomalous coronary artery
2019, 2Q, 20	Pericardiectomy for constrictive pericarditis
2017, 4Q, 35	Release of myocardial bridge
2016, 4Q, 80-81	Thoracic aorta, ascending/arch and descending
2014, 3Q, 16	Repair of Tetralogy of Fallot

AHA Coding Clinic for table Ø2P

2022, 2Q, 25	Temporary-permanent pacemaker placement
2019, 1Q, 24	Replacement of left ventricular assist device with retention of outflow graft
2018, 4Q, 52-54	Percutaneous extracorporeal membrane oxygenation
2018, 4Q, 85	Externalization of lumboatrial shunt
2018, 4Q, 94	Insertion and removal of failed Watchman™ device
2018, 2Q, 3-5	Intra-aortic balloon pump
2017, 4Q, 42-45	Insertion of external heart assist devices
2017, 4Q, 104	Placement of Watchman™ left atrial appendage device
2017, 3Q, 18	Intra-aortic balloon pump removal
2017, 2Q, 24	Tunneled catheter versus totally implantable catheter
2017, 2Q, 26	Exchange of tunneled catheter
2017, 1Q, 11	External heart assist device
2017, 1Q, 13	SynCardia total artificial heart
2016, 4Q, 95-96	Intracardiac pacemaker
2016, 4Q, 137-139	Heart assist device systems
2016, 3Q, 19	Nonoperative removal of peripherally inserted central catheter
2016, 2Q, 15	Removal and replacement of tunneled internal jugular catheter
2015, 4Q, 31	Vascular access devices
2015, 3Q, 33	Approach values for repositioning and removal of cardiac lead

AHA Coding Clinic for table 02Q

2022, 1Q, 40	Repair of common atrioventricular valve using Alfieri stitch
2022, 1Q, 41	Common atrioventricular valve repair with commissuroplasty sutures
2021, 3Q, 26	Cavoatrial junction tear with repair and relief of cardiac tamponade
2018, 1Q, 12	Percutaneous balloon valvuloplasty & cardiac catheterization with ventriculogram
2017, 1Q, 18	Sutureless repair of pulmonary vein stenosis
2016, 4Q, 80-81	Thoracic aorta, ascending/arch and descending
2016, 4Q, 82-83	Coronary artery, number of arteries
2016, 4Q, 101	Root operation Creation
2016, 4Q, 102-109	Correction of congenital heart defects
2015, 4Q, 23	Congenital heart corrective procedures
2015, 3Q, 16	Vascular ring surgery and double aortic arch
2015, 2Q, 23	Annuloplasty ring
2013, 3Q, 26	Transcatheter replacement of heart valve (TAVR) with measurements

AHA Coding Clinic for table 02R

2021, 4Q, 42-43	Total artificial heart systems
2021, 4Q, 43	Transcatheter replacement of pulmonary valve
2020, 1Q, 25	Elephant trunk repair of aortic dissection
2019, 4Q, 24	Coronary artery Body Part to root operation Insertion
2019, 4Q, 46	Cerebral embolic filtration
2019, 3Q, 23	Replacement of atrioventricular valve
2019, 3Q, 24	Valve sparing aortic root replacement with modified Gleason Vascutek® graft to ascending aorta
2019, 1Q, 31	Transcatheter aortic valve in valve replacement
2018, 3Q, 11	Transcatheter aortic valve replacement via transaortic approach
2018, 1Q, 12	Percutaneous balloon valvuloplasty & cardiac catheterization with ventriculogram
2017, 4Q, 55-56	Added approach values - Percutaneous heart valve procedures
2017, 1Q, 13	SynCardia total artificial heart
2016, 4Q, 80-81	Thoracic aorta, ascending/arch and descending
2016, 3Q, 32	Transcatheter tricuspid valve replacement
2014, 1Q, 10	Repair of thoracic aortic aneurysm & coronary artery bypass graft

AHA Coding Clinic for table 02S

2016, 4Q, 80-81	Thoracic aorta, ascending/arch and descending
2016, 4Q, 82-83	Coronary artery, number of arteries
2016, 4Q, 102-109	Correction of congenital heart defects
2015, 4Q, 23	Congenital heart corrective procedures

AHA Coding Clinic for table 02U

2022, 1Q, 37	Insertion of amplatzer occluder device into atrium
2022, 1Q, 38	Reconstruction of aorto-mitral curtain using bovine pericardium
2021, 3Q, 28	Repair mitral valve with Pascal® system
2020, 4Q, 52	Transapical mitral valve repair with device
2020, 1Q, 24	Pulmonary artery unifocalization
2019, 4Q, 25	Coronary artery to root operation Supplement
2018, 1Q, 12	Percutaneous balloon valvuloplasty & cardiac catheterization with ventriculogram
2017, 4Q, 36	Alfieri stitch procedure
2017, 3Q, 7	Senning procedure (arterial switch)
2017, 1Q, 19	Norwood Sano procedure
2016, 4Q, 80-81	Thoracic aorta, ascending/arch and descending
2016, 4Q, 101	Root operation Creation
2016, 4Q, 102-109	Correction of congenital heart defects
2016, 2Q, 23	Repair of tetralogy of Fallot with autologous pericardial patch graft
2016, 2Q, 26	Aortic valve replacement with aortic root enlargement
2015, 4Q, 22-24	Congenital heart corrective procedures
2015, 3Q, 16	Revision of previous truncus arteriosus surgery with ventricle to pulmonary artery conduit
2015, 2Q, 23	Annuloplasty ring
2014, 3Q, 16	Repair of tetralogy of Fallot

AHA Coding Clinic for table 02V

2022, 1Q, 40	Repair of common atrioventricular valve using Alfieri stitch
2021, 4Q, 44	Restriction of left ventricle
2020, 1Q, 25	Elephant trunk repair of aortic dissection
2017, 4Q, 35-36	Alfieri stitch procedure
2016, 4Q, 80-81	Thoracic aorta, ascending/arch and descending
2016, 4Q, 89-92	Branched and fenestrated endograft repair of aneurysms

AHA Coding Clinic for table 02W

2019, 1Q, 24	Replacement of left ventricular assist device with retention of outflow graft
2018, 3Q, 8	Coronary artery bypass graft surgery (revision versus total redo)
2018, 3Q, 9	Fibrin sheath stripping of malfunctioning port-a-cath
2018, 1Q, 17	Repositioning of Impella short-term external heart assist device
2017, 4Q, 42-45	Insertion of external heart assist devices
2017, 4Q, 55-56	Added approach values - Percutaneous heart valve procedures
2016, 4Q, 85	Coronary artery, number of stents
2016, 4Q, 95-96	Intracardiac pacemaker
2015, 3Q, 32	Approach values for repositioning and removal of cardiac lead
2014, 3Q, 31	Closure of paravalvular leak using Amplatzer® vascular plug

AHA Coding Clinic for table 02Y

2013, 3Q, 18	Heart transplant surgery

Coronary Arteries

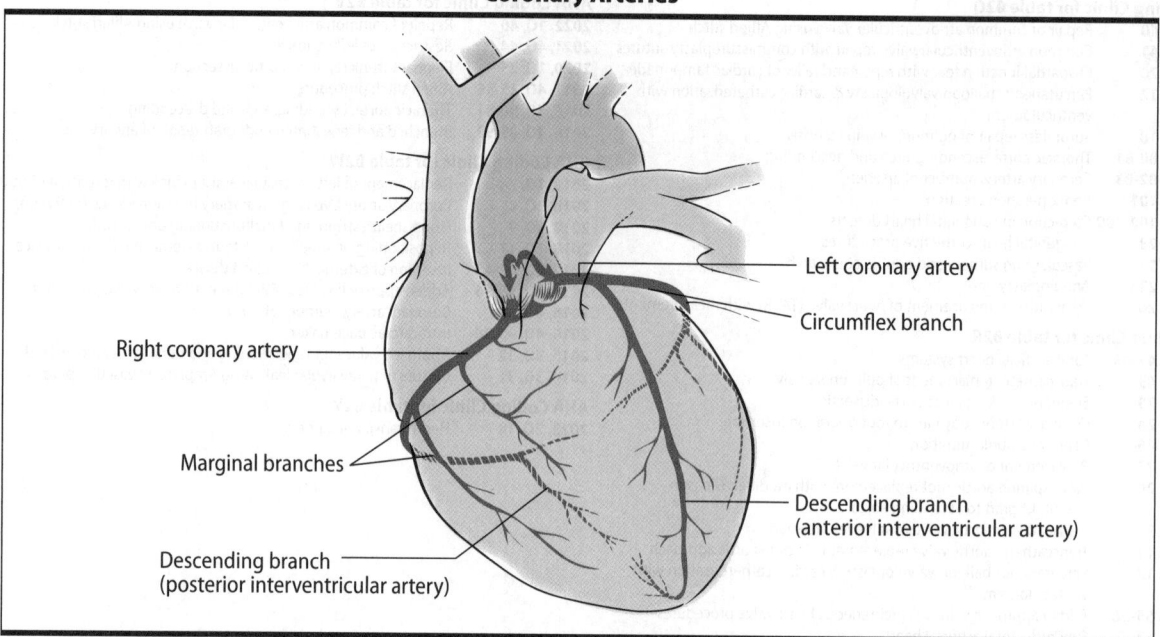

- Left coronary artery
- Circumflex branch
- Right coronary artery
- Marginal branches
- Descending branch (anterior interventricular artery)
- Descending branch (posterior interventricular artery)

Heart Anatomy

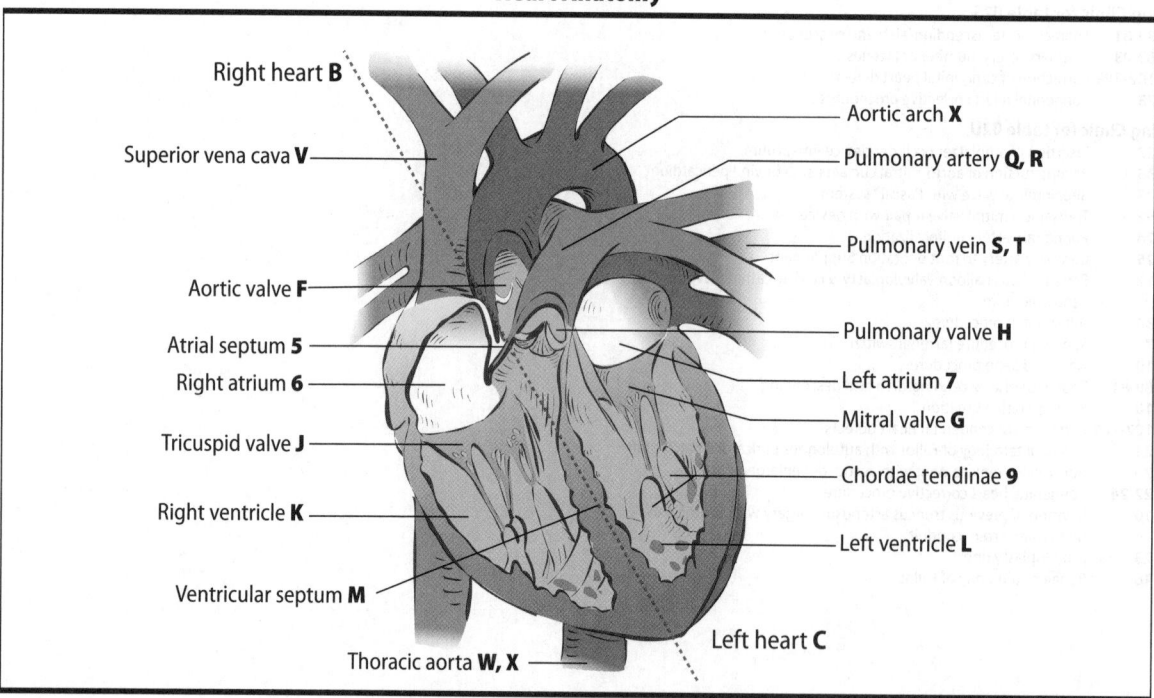

- Right heart **B**
- Superior vena cava **V**
- Aortic valve **F**
- Atrial septum **5**
- Right atrium **6**
- Tricuspid valve **J**
- Right ventricle **K**
- Ventricular septum **M**
- Thoracic aorta **W, X**
- Aortic arch **X**
- Pulmonary artery **Q, R**
- Pulmonary vein **S, T**
- Pulmonary valve **H**
- Left atrium **7**
- Mitral valve **G**
- Chordae tendinae **9**
- Left ventricle **L**
- Left heart **C**

Ø **Medical and Surgical**
2 **Heart and Great Vessels**
1 **Bypass**　　　Definition: Altering the route of passage of the contents of a tubular body part

Explanation: Rerouting contents of a body part to a downstream area of the normal route, to a similar route and body part, or to an abnormal route and dissimilar body part. Includes one or more anastomoses, with or without the use of a device.

Body Part Character 4	Approach Character 5	Device Character 6	Qualifier Character 7
Ø Coronary Artery, One Artery 1 Coronary Artery, Two Arteries 2 Coronary Artery, Three Arteries 3 Coronary Artery, Four or More Arteries	Ø Open	8 Zooplastic Tissue 9 Autologous Venous Tissue A Autologous Arterial Tissue J Synthetic Substitute K Nonautologous Tissue Substitute	3 Coronary Artery 8 Internal Mammary, Right 9 Internal Mammary, Left C Thoracic Artery F Abdominal Artery W Aorta
Ø Coronary Artery, One Artery 1 Coronary Artery, Two Arteries 2 Coronary Artery, Three Arteries 3 Coronary Artery, Four or More Arteries	Ø Open	Z No Device	3 Coronary Artery 8 Internal Mammary, Right 9 Internal Mammary, Left C Thoracic Artery F Abdominal Artery
Ø Coronary Artery, One Artery 1 Coronary Artery, Two Arteries 2 Coronary Artery, Three Arteries 3 Coronary Artery, Four or More Arteries	3 Percutaneous	4 Intraluminal Device, Drug-eluting D Intraluminal Device	4 Coronary Vein
Ø Coronary Artery, One Artery 1 Coronary Artery, Two Arteries 2 Coronary Artery, Three Arteries 3 Coronary Artery, Four or More Arteries	4 Percutaneous Endoscopic	4 Intraluminal Device, Drug-eluting D Intraluminal Device	4 Coronary Vein
Ø Coronary Artery, One Artery 1 Coronary Artery, Two Arteries 2 Coronary Artery, Three Arteries 3 Coronary Artery, Four or More Arteries	4 Percutaneous Endoscopic	8 Zooplastic Tissue 9 Autologous Venous Tissue A Autologous Arterial Tissue J Synthetic Substitute K Nonautologous Tissue Substitute	3 Coronary Artery 8 Internal Mammary, Right 9 Internal Mammary, Left C Thoracic Artery F Abdominal Artery W Aorta
Ø Coronary Artery, One Artery 1 Coronary Artery, Two Arteries 2 Coronary Artery, Three Arteries 3 Coronary Artery, Four or More Arteries	4 Percutaneous Endoscopic	Z No Device	3 Coronary Artery 8 Internal Mammary, Right 9 Internal Mammary, Left C Thoracic Artery F Abdominal Artery
6 Atrium, Right Atrium dextrum cordis Right auricular appendix Sinus venosus	Ø Open 4 Percutaneous Endoscopic	8 Zooplastic Tissue 9 Autologous Venous Tissue A Autologous Arterial Tissue J Synthetic Substitute K Nonautologous Tissue Substitute	P Pulmonary Trunk Q Pulmonary Artery, Right R Pulmonary Artery, Left
6 Atrium, Right Atrium dextrum cordis Right auricular appendix Sinus venosus	Ø Open 4 Percutaneous Endoscopic	Z No Device	7 Atrium, Left P Pulmonary Trunk Q Pulmonary Artery, Right R Pulmonary Artery, Left
6 Atrium, Right Atrium dextrum cordis Right auricular appendix Sinus venosus	3 Percutaneous	Z No Device	7 Atrium, Left
7 Atrium, Left Atrium pulmonale Left auricular appendix	Ø Open 4 Percutaneous Endoscopic	8 Zooplastic Tissue 9 Autologous Venous Tissue A Autologous Arterial Tissue J Synthetic Substitute K Nonautologous Tissue Substitute Z No Device	P Pulmonary Trunk Q Pulmonary Artery, Right R Pulmonary Artery, Left S Pulmonary Vein, Right T Pulmonary Vein, Left U Pulmonary Vein, Confluence
7 Atrium, Left Atrium pulmonale Left auricular appendix	3 Percutaneous	J Synthetic Substitute	6 Atrium, Right
K Ventricle, Right Conus arteriosus L Ventricle, Left	Ø Open 4 Percutaneous Endoscopic	8 Zooplastic Tissue 9 Autologous Venous Tissue A Autologous Arterial Tissue J Synthetic Substitute K Nonautologous Tissue Substitute	P Pulmonary Trunk Q Pulmonary Artery, Right R Pulmonary Artery, Left

HAC　Ø21[Ø,1,2,3]Ø[8,9,A,J,K][3,8,9,C,F,W] when reported with SDx J98.51 or J98.59
HAC　Ø21[Ø,1,2,3]ØZ[3,8,9,C,F] when reported with SDx J98.51 or J98.59
HAC　Ø21[Ø,1,2,3]4[8,9,A,J,K][3,8,9,C,F,W] when reported with SDx J98.51 or J98.59
HAC　Ø21[Ø,1,2,3]4Z[3,8,9,C,F] when reported with SDx J98.51 or J98.59

Ø21 Continued on next page

NC Noncovered Procedure　**LC** Limited Coverage　**QA** Questionable OB Admit　**NT** New Tech Add-on　⊞ Combination Member　♂ Male　♀ Female

Ø **Medical and Surgical**
2 **Heart and Great Vessels**
1 **Bypass**　　Definition: Altering the route of passage of the contents of a tubular body part

Explanation: Rerouting contents of a body part to a downstream area of the normal route, to a similar route and body part, or to an abnormal route and dissimilar body part. Includes one or more anastomoses, with or without the use of a device.

Body Part Character 4	Approach Character 5	Device Character 6	Qualifier Character 7
K Ventricle, Right 　Conus arteriosus **L** Ventricle, Left	**Ø** Open **4** Percutaneous Endoscopic	**Z** No Device	**5** Coronary Circulation **8** Internal Mammary, Right **9** Internal Mammary, Left **C** Thoracic Artery **F** Abdominal Artery **P** Pulmonary Trunk **Q** Pulmonary Artery, Right **R** Pulmonary Artery, Left **W** Aorta
P Pulmonary Trunk **Q** Pulmonary Artery, Right **R** Pulmonary Artery, Left 　Arterial canal (duct) 　Botallo's duct 　Pulmoaortic canal	**Ø** Open **4** Percutaneous Endoscopic	**8** Zooplastic Tissue **9** Autologous Venous Tissue **A** Autologous Arterial Tissue **J** Synthetic Substitute **K** Nonautologous Tissue Substitute **Z** No Device	**A** Innominate Artery **B** Subclavian **D** Carotid
V Superior Vena Cava 　Cavoatrial junction 　Precava	**Ø** Open **4** Percutaneous Endoscopic	**8** Zooplastic Tissue **9** Autologous Venous Tissue **A** Autologous Arterial Tissue **J** Synthetic Substitute **K** Nonautologous Tissue Substitute **Z** No Device	**P** Pulmonary Trunk **Q** Pulmonary Artery, Right **R** Pulmonary Artery, Left **S** Pulmonary Vein, Right **T** Pulmonary Vein, Left **U** Pulmonary Vein, Confluence
W Thoracic Aorta, Descending	**Ø** Open	**8** Zooplastic Tissue **9** Autologous Venous Tissue **A** Autologous Arterial Tissue **J** Synthetic Substitute **K** Nonautologous Tissue Substitute	**A** Innominate Artery **B** Subclavian **D** Carotid **F** Abdominal Artery **G** Axillary Artery **H** Brachial Artery **P** Pulmonary Trunk **Q** Pulmonary Artery, Right **R** Pulmonary Artery, Left **V** Lower Extremity Artery
W Thoracic Aorta, Descending	**Ø** Open	**Z** No Device	**A** Innominate Artery **B** Subclavian **D** Carotid **P** Pulmonary Trunk **Q** Pulmonary Artery, Right **R** Pulmonary Artery, Left
W Thoracic Aorta, Descending	**4** Percutaneous Endoscopic	**8** Zooplastic Tissue **9** Autologous Venous Tissue **A** Autologous Arterial Tissue **J** Synthetic Substitute **K** Nonautologous Tissue Substitute **Z** No Device	**A** Innominate Artery **B** Subclavian **D** Carotid **P** Pulmonary Trunk **Q** Pulmonary Artery, Right **R** Pulmonary Artery, Left
X Thoracic Aorta, Ascending/Arch 　Aortic arch 　Ascending aorta	**Ø** Open **4** Percutaneous Endoscopic	**8** Zooplastic Tissue **9** Autologous Venous Tissue **A** Autologous Arterial Tissue **J** Synthetic Substitute **K** Nonautologous Tissue Substitute **Z** No Device	**A** Innominate Artery **B** Subclavian **D** Carotid **P** Pulmonary Trunk **Q** Pulmonary Artery, Right **R** Pulmonary Artery, Left

Ø **Medical and Surgical**
2 **Heart and Great Vessels**
4 **Creation**　　Definition: Putting in or on biological or synthetic material to form a new body part that to the extent possible replicates the anatomic structure or function of an absent body part

Explanation: Used for gender reassignment surgery and corrective procedures in individuals with congenital anomalies

Body Part Character 4	Approach Character 5	Device Character 6	Qualifier Character 7
F Aortic Valve 　Aortic annulus	**Ø** Open	**7** Autologous Tissue **8** Zooplastic Tissue **J** Synthetic Substitute **K** Nonautologous Tissue Substitute	**J** Truncal Valve
G Mitral Valve 　Bicuspid valve 　Left atrioventricular valve 　Mitral annulus **J** Tricuspid Valve 　Right atrioventricular valve 　Tricuspid annulus	**Ø** Open	**7** Autologous Tissue **8** Zooplastic Tissue **J** Synthetic Substitute **K** Nonautologous Tissue Substitute	**2** Common Atrioventricular Valve

Non-OR Procedure　　DRG Non-OR Procedure　　Valid OR Procedure　　HAC Associated Procedure　　Combination Only　　New/Revised April　　New/Revised October

Ø   **Medical and Surgical**
2   **Heart and Great Vessels**
5   **Destruction**   Definition: Physical eradication of all or a portion of a body part by the direct use of energy, force, or a destructive agent
                 Explanation: None of the body part is physically taken out

Body Part Character 4	Approach Character 5	Device Character 6	Qualifier Character 7
4 **Coronary Vein**	Ø Open	Z No Device	Z No Qualifier
5 **Atrial Septum**	3 Percutaneous		
Interatrial septum	4 Percutaneous Endoscopic		
6 **Atrium, Right**			
Atrium dextrum cordis			
Right auricular appendix			
Sinus venosus			
8 **Conduction Mechanism**			
Atrioventricular node			
Bundle of His			
Bundle of Kent			
Sinoatrial node			
9 **Chordae Tendineae**			
D **Papillary Muscle**			
F **Aortic Valve**			
Aortic annulus			
G **Mitral Valve**			
Bicuspid valve			
Left atrioventricular valve			
Mitral annulus			
H **Pulmonary Valve**			
Pulmonary annulus			
Pulmonic valve			
J **Tricuspid Valve**			
Right atrioventricular valve			
Tricuspid annulus			
K **Ventricle, Right**			
Conus arteriosus			
L **Ventricle, Left**			
M **Ventricular Septum**			
Interventricular septum			
N **Pericardium**			
P **Pulmonary Trunk**			
Q **Pulmonary Artery, Right**			
R **Pulmonary Artery, Left**			
Arterial canal (duct)			
Botallo's duct			
Pulmoaortic canal			
S **Pulmonary Vein, Right**			
Right inferior pulmonary vein			
Right superior pulmonary vein			
T **Pulmonary Vein, Left**			
Left inferior pulmonary vein			
Left superior pulmonary vein			
V **Superior Vena Cava**			
Cavoatrial junction			
Precava			
W **Thoracic Aorta, Descending**			
X **Thoracic Aorta, Ascending/Arch**			
Aortic arch			
Ascending aorta			
7 **Atrium, Left**	Ø Open	Z No Device	K Left Atrial Appendage
Atrium pulmonale	3 Percutaneous		Z No Qualifier
Left auricular appendix	4 Percutaneous Endoscopic		

DRG Non-OR   Ø257[Ø,3,4]ZK

NC Noncovered Procedure   LC Limited Coverage   QA Questionable OB Admit   NT New Tech Add-on   ⊞ Combination Member   ♂ Male   ♀ Female

ICD-10-PCS 2023   177

Ø25–Ø25

Heart and Great Vessels

Ø   **Medical and Surgical**
2   **Heart and Great Vessels**
7   **Dilation**   Definition: Expanding an orifice or the lumen of a tubular body part

                     Explanation: The orifice can be a natural orifice or an artificially created orifice. Accomplished by stretching a tubular body part using intraluminal pressure or by cutting part of the orifice or wall of the tubular body part.

Body Part Character 4	Approach Character 5	Device Character 6	Qualifier Character 7
Ø Coronary Artery, One Artery 1 Coronary Artery, Two Arteries 2 Coronary Artery, Three Arteries 3 Coronary Artery, Four or More Arteries	Ø Open 3 Percutaneous 4 Percutaneous Endoscopic	4 Intraluminal Device, Drug-eluting 5 Intraluminal Device, Drug-eluting, Two 6 Intraluminal Device, Drug-eluting, Three 7 Intraluminal Device, Drug-eluting, Four or More D Intraluminal Device E Intraluminal Device, Two F Intraluminal Device, Three G Intraluminal Device, Four or More T Intraluminal Device, Radioactive Z No Device	6 Bifurcation Z No Qualifier

F   Aortic Valve
     Aortic annulus
G   Mitral Valve
     Bicuspid valve
     Left atrioventricular valve
     Mitral annulus
H   Pulmonary Valve
     Pulmonary annulus
     Pulmonic valve
J   Tricuspid Valve
     Right atrioventricular valve
     Tricuspid annulus
K   Ventricle, Right
     Conus arteriosus
L   Ventricle, Left
P   Pulmonary Trunk
Q   Pulmonary Artery, Right
S   Pulmonary Vein, Right
     Right inferior pulmonary vein
     Right superior pulmonary vein
T   Pulmonary Vein, Left
     Left inferior pulmonary vein
     Left superior pulmonary vein
V   Superior Vena Cava
     Cavoatrial junction
     Precava
W   Thoracic Aorta, Descending
X   Thoracic Aorta, Ascending/Arch
     Aortic arch
     Ascending aorta
	Ø Open
	3 Percutaneous
	4 Percutaneous Endoscopic
		4 Intraluminal Device, Drug-eluting
		D Intraluminal Device
		Z No Device
			Z No Qualifier

R   Pulmonary Artery, Left
     Arterial canal (duct)
     Botallo's duct
     Pulmoaortic canal
	Ø Open
	3 Percutaneous
	4 Percutaneous Endoscopic
		4 Intraluminal Device, Drug-eluting
		D Intraluminal Device
		Z No Device
			T Ductus Arteriosus
			Z No Qualifier

Ø   **Medical and Surgical**
2   **Heart and Great Vessels**
8   **Division**   Definition: Cutting into a body part, without draining fluids and/or gases from the body part, in order to separate or transect a body part

                     Explanation: All or a portion of the body part is separated into two or more portions

Body Part Character 4	Approach Character 5	Device Character 6	Qualifier Character 7

8   Conduction Mechanism
     Atrioventricular node
     Bundle of His
     Bundle of Kent
     Sinoatrial node
9   Chordae Tendineae
D   Papillary Muscle
	Ø Open
	3 Percutaneous
	4 Percutaneous Endoscopic
		Z No Device	Z No Qualifier

Non-OR Procedure   DRG Non-OR Procedure   Valid OR Procedure   HAC Associated Procedure   Combination Only   New/Revised April   New/Revised October

178   ICD-10-PCS 2023

Ø   **Medical and Surgical**
2   **Heart and Great Vessels**
B   **Excision**   Definition: Cutting out or off, without replacement, a portion of a body part

                         Explanation: The qualifier DIAGNOSTIC is used to identify excision procedures that are biopsies

Body Part Character 4	Approach Character 5	Device Character 6	Qualifier Character 7
4 **Coronary Vein**	**Ø** Open	**Z** No Device	**X** Diagnostic
5 **Atrial Septum**	**3** Percutaneous		**Z** No Qualifier
Interatrial septum	**4** Percutaneous Endoscopic		
6 **Atrium, Right**			
Atrium dextrum cordis			
Right auricular appendix			
Sinus venosus			
8 **Conduction Mechanism**			
Atrioventricular node			
Bundle of His			
Bundle of Kent			
Sinoatrial node			
9 **Chordae Tendineae**			
D **Papillary Muscle**			
F **Aortic Valve**			
Aortic annulus			
G **Mitral Valve**			
Bicuspid valve			
Left atrioventricular valve			
Mitral annulus			
H **Pulmonary Valve**			
Pulmonary annulus			
Pulmonic valve			
J **Tricuspid Valve**			
Right atrioventricular valve			
Tricuspid annulus			
K **Ventricle, Right** `NC`			
Conus arteriosus			
L **Ventricle, Left** `NC`			
M **Ventricular Septum**			
Interventricular septum			
N **Pericardium**			
P **Pulmonary Trunk**			
Q **Pulmonary Artery, Right**			
R **Pulmonary Artery, Left**			
Arterial canal (duct)			
Botallo's duct			
Pulmoaortic canal			
S **Pulmonary Vein, Right**			
Right inferior pulmonary vein			
Right superior pulmonary vein			
T **Pulmonary Vein, Left**			
Left inferior pulmonary vein			
Left superior pulmonary vein			
V **Superior Vena Cava**			
Cavoatrial junction			
Precava			
W **Thoracic Aorta, Descending**			
X **Thoracic Aorta, Ascending/Arch**			
Aortic arch			
Ascending aorta			
7 **Atrium, Left**	**Ø** Open	**Z** No Device	**K** Left Atrial Appendage
Atrium pulmonale	**3** Percutaneous		**X** Diagnostic
Left auricular appendix	**4** Percutaneous Endoscopic		**Z** No Qualifier

DRG Non-OR   02B7[Ø,3,4]ZK
Non-OR   02B[4,5,6,8,9,D,F,G,H,J,K,L,M][Ø,3,4]ZX
`NC`   02B[K,L][Ø,3,4]ZZ

0 **Medical and Surgical**
2 **Heart and Great Vessels**
C **Extirpation**   Definition: Taking or cutting out solid matter from a body part

Explanation: The solid matter may be an abnormal byproduct of a biological function or a foreign body; it may be imbedded in a body part or in the lumen of a tubular body part. The solid matter may or may not have been previously broken into pieces.

Body Part Character 4	Approach Character 5	Device Character 6	Qualifier Character 7
0 **Coronary Artery, One Artery** **1** **Coronary Artery, Two Arteries** **2** **Coronary Artery, Three Arteries** **3** **Coronary Artery, Four or More Arteries**	**0** Open **4** Percutaneous Endoscopic	**Z** No Device	**6** Bifurcation **Z** No Qualifier
0 **Coronary Artery, One Artery** **1** **Coronary Artery, Two Arteries** **2** **Coronary Artery, Three Arteries** **3** **Coronary Artery, Four or More Arteries**	**3** Percutaneous	**Z** No Device	**6** Bifurcation **7** Orbital Atherectomy Technique **Z** No Qualifier

4 **Coronary Vein**
5 **Atrial Septum**
   Interatrial septum
6 **Atrium, Right**
   Atrium dextrum cordis
   Right auricular appendix
   Sinus venosus
7 **Atrium, Left**
   Atrium pulmonale
   Left auricular appendix
8 **Conduction Mechanism**
   Atrioventricular node
   Bundle of His
   Bundle of Kent
   Sinoatrial node
9 **Chordae Tendineae**
D **Papillary Muscle**
F **Aortic Valve**
   Aortic annulus
G **Mitral Valve**
   Bicuspid valve
   Left atrioventricular valve
   Mitral annulus
H **Pulmonary Valve**
   Pulmonary annulus
   Pulmonic valve
J **Tricuspid Valve**
   Right atrioventricular valve
   Tricuspid annulus
K **Ventricle, Right**
   Conus arteriosus
L **Ventricle, Left**
M **Ventricular Septum**
   Interventricular septum
N **Pericardium**
P **Pulmonary Trunk**
Q **Pulmonary Artery, Right**
R **Pulmonary Artery, Left**
   Arterial canal (duct)
   Botallo's duct
   Pulmoaortic canal
S **Pulmonary Vein, Right**
   Right inferior pulmonary vein
   Right superior pulmonary vein
T **Pulmonary Vein, Left**
   Left inferior pulmonary vein
   Left superior pulmonary vein
V **Superior Vena Cava**
   Cavoatrial junction
   Precava
W **Thoracic Aorta, Descending**
X **Thoracic Aorta, Ascending/Arch**
   Aortic arch
   Ascending aorta
	0 Open
	3 Percutaneous
	4 Percutaneous Endoscopic
		Z No Device	**Z** No Qualifier

Non-OR Procedure   DRG Non-OR Procedure   Valid OR Procedure   HAC Associated Procedure   Combination Only   New/Revised April   New/Revised October

180

ICD-10-PCS 2023

0　**Medical and Surgical**
2　**Heart and Great Vessels**
F　**Fragmentation**　　Definition: Breaking solid matter in a body part into pieces
　　　　　　　　　　　　Explanation: Physical force (e.g., manual, ultrasonic) applied directly or indirectly is used to break the solid matter into pieces. The solid matter may be an abnormal byproduct of a biological function or a foreign body. The pieces of solid matter are not taken out.

Body Part Character 4	Approach Character 5	Device Character 6	Qualifier Character 7
0 Coronary Artery, One Artery **1 Coronary Artery, Two Arteries** **2 Coronary Artery, Three Arteries** **3 Coronary Artery, Four or More Arteries**	**3 Percutaneous**	**Z No Device** [NT]	**Z No Qualifier**
N Pericardium [NC]	**0 Open** **3 Percutaneous** **4 Percutaneous Endoscopic** **X External**	**Z No Device**	**Z No Qualifier**
P Pulmonary Trunk **Q Pulmonary Artery, Right** **R Pulmonary Artery, Left** 　Arterial canal (duct) 　Botallo's duct 　Pulmoaortic canal **S Pulmonary Vein, Right** 　Right inferior pulmonary vein 　Right superior pulmonary vein **T Pulmonary Vein, Left** 　Left inferior pulmonary vein 　Left superior pulmonary vein	**3 Percutaneous**	**Z No Device**	**0 Ultrasonic** **Z No Qualifier**

Non-OR　02FNXZZ
[NC]　02FNXZZ
[NT]　02F[0,1,2,3]3ZZ for Shockwave C2 Intravascular Lithotripsy (IVL) System

Heart and Great Vessels

0   **Medical and Surgical**
2   **Heart and Great Vessels**
H   **Insertion**   Definition: Putting in a nonbiological appliance that monitors, assists, performs, or prevents a physiological function but does not physically take the place of a body part
            Explanation: None

Body Part Character 4	Approach Character 5	Device Character 6	Qualifier Character 7
0 Coronary Artery, One Artery **1** Coronary Artery, Two Arteries **2** Coronary Artery, Three Arteries **3** Coronary Artery, Four or More Arteries	**0** Open **3** Percutaneous **4** Percutaneous Endoscopic	**D** Intraluminal Device **Y** Other Device	**Z** No Qualifier

4 Coronary Vein ⊞
6 Atrium, Right ⊞
    Atrium dextrum cordis
    Right auricular appendix
    Sinus venosus
7 Atrium, Left ⊞
    Atrium pulmonale
    Left auricular appendix
K Ventricle, Right ⊞
    Conus arteriosus
L Ventricle, Left ⊞
	0 Open
	3 Percutaneous
	4 Percutaneous Endoscopic
		0 Monitoring Device, Pressure Sensor
		2 Monitoring Device
		3 Infusion Device
		D Intraluminal Device
		J Cardiac Lead, Pacemaker
		K Cardiac Lead, Defibrillator
		M Cardiac Lead
		N Intracardiac Pacemaker
		Y Other Device
			Z No Qualifier

A Heart NC	**0** Open **3** Percutaneous **4** Percutaneous Endoscopic	**Q** Implantable Heart Assist System **Y** Other Device	**Z** No Qualifier
A Heart ⊞	**0** Open **3** Percutaneous **4** Percutaneous Endoscopic	**R** Short-term External Heart Assist System	**J** Intraoperative **S** Biventricular **Z** No Qualifier
N Pericardium ⊞	**0** Open **3** Percutaneous **4** Percutaneous Endoscopic	**0** Monitoring Device, Pressure Sensor **2** Monitoring Device **J** Cardiac Lead, Pacemaker **K** Cardiac Lead, Defibrillator **M** Cardiac Lead **Y** Other Device	**Z** No Qualifier

P Pulmonary Trunk
Q Pulmonary Artery, Right
R Pulmonary Artery, Left
    Arterial canal (duct)
    Botallo's duct
    Pulmoaortic canal
S Pulmonary Vein, Right
    Right inferior pulmonary vein
    Right superior pulmonary vein
T Pulmonary Vein, Left
    Left inferior pulmonary vein
    Left superior pulmonary vein
V Superior Vena Cava
    Cavoatrial junction
    Precava
W Thoracic Aorta, Descending
	0 Open
	3 Percutaneous
	4 Percutaneous Endoscopic
		0 Monitoring Device, Pressure Sensor
		2 Monitoring Device
		3 Infusion Device
		D Intraluminal Device
		Y Other Device
			Z No Qualifier

X Thoracic Aorta, Ascending/Arch
    Aortic arch
    Ascending aorta
	0 Open
	3 Percutaneous
	4 Percutaneous Endoscopic
		0 Monitoring Device, Pressure Sensor
		2 Monitoring Device
		3 Infusion Device
		D Intraluminal Device
			Z No Qualifier

DRG Non-OR	02H[4,6,7,K,L][0,3,4][J,M]Z	**HAC**	02H43[J,K,M]Z when reported with SDx K68.11 or T81.40-T81.49, T82.7 with 7th character A
DRG Non-OR	02HK32Z		
DRG Non-OR	02HN[0,3,4][J,M]Z	**HAC**	02H[6,K]33Z when reported with SDx J95.811
Non-OR	02H[4,6,7,L]3[2,3]Z	**HAC**	02H[6,7]3[J,M]Z when reported with SDx K68.11 or T81.40-T81.49, T82.7 with 7th character A
Non-OR	02H[6,7]3MZ		
Non-OR	02HK3[0,3]Z	**HAC**	02H[K,L]3JZ when reported with SDx K68.11 or T81.40-T81.49, T82.7 with 7th character A
Non-OR	02HN32Z		
Non-OR	02HP[0,3,4][0,2,3]Z	**HAC**	02HN[0,3,4][J,M]Z when reported with SDx K68.11 or T81.40-T81.49, T82.7 with 7th character A
Non-OR	02H[Q,R][0,3,4][2,3]Z		
Non-OR	02H[S,T,V,W][0,3,4]3Z	**HAC**	02H[S,T,V][3,4]3Z when reported with SDx J95.811
Non-OR	02H[S,T,V,W]32Z	**NC**	02HA[3,4]QZ
Non-OR	02HW[0,3]0Z		
Non-OR	02HX[0,3,4][0,3]Z	**See Appendix L for Procedure Combinations**	
		⊞	02H[4,6,7,K,L][0,3,4][J,K,M]Z
		⊞	02HA[0,4]R[S,Z]
		⊞	02HA3RS
		⊞	02HN[0,3,4][J,K,M]Z

0   Medical and Surgical
2   Heart and Great Vessels
J   Inspection   Definition: Visually and/or manually exploring a body part

Explanation: Visual exploration may be performed with or without optical instrumentation. Manual exploration may be performed directly or through intervening body layers.

Body Part Character 4	Approach Character 5	Device Character 6	Qualifier Character 7
A Heart Y Great Vessel	0 Open 3 Percutaneous 4 Percutaneous Endoscopic	Z No Device	Z No Qualifier

Non-OR   02J[A,Y]3ZZ

---

0   Medical and Surgical
2   Heart and Great Vessels
K   Map   Definition: Locating the route of passage of electrical impulses and/or locating functional areas in a body part

Explanation: Applicable only to the cardiac conduction mechanism and the central nervous system

Body Part Character 4	Approach Character 5	Device Character 6	Qualifier Character 7

8   Conduction Mechanism
    Atrioventricular node
    Bundle of His
    Bundle of Kent
    Sinoatrial node
	0 Open
	3 Percutaneous
	4 Percutaneous Endoscopic
		Z No Device	Z No Qualifier

DRG Non-OR   02K8[0,3,4]ZZ

---

0   Medical and Surgical
2   Heart and Great Vessels
L   Occlusion   Definition: Completely closing an orifice or the lumen of a tubular body part

Explanation: The orifice can be a natural orifice or an artificially created orifice

Body Part Character 4	Approach Character 5	Device Character 6	Qualifier Character 7

7   Atrium, Left
    Atrium pulmonale
    Left auricular appendix
	0 Open
	3 Percutaneous
	4 Percutaneous Endoscopic
		C Extraluminal Device
		D Intraluminal Device
		Z No Device
			K Left Atrial Appendage

H   Pulmonary Valve
    Pulmonary annulus
    Pulmonic valve
P   Pulmonary Trunk
Q   Pulmonary Artery, Right
S   Pulmonary Vein, Right
    Right inferior pulmonary vein
    Right superior pulmonary vein
T   Pulmonary Vein, Left
    Left inferior pulmonary vein
    Left superior pulmonary vein
V   Superior Vena Cava
    Cavoatrial junction
    Precava
	0 Open
	3 Percutaneous
	4 Percutaneous Endoscopic
		C Extraluminal Device
		D Intraluminal Device
		Z No Device
			Z No Qualifier

R   Pulmonary Artery, Left
    Arterial canal (duct)
    Botallo's duct
    Pulmoaortic canal
	0 Open
	3 Percutaneous
	4 Percutaneous Endoscopic
		C Extraluminal Device
		D Intraluminal Device
		Z No Device
			T Ductus Arteriosus
			Z No Qualifier

W Thoracic Aorta, Descending	3 Percutaneous	D Intraluminal Device	J Temporary

DRG Non-OR   02L7[0,3,4][C,D,Z]K

NC Noncovered Procedure   LC Limited Coverage   QA Questionable OB Admit   NT New Tech Add-on   ⊞ Combination Member   ♂ Male   ♀ Female

ICD-10-PCS 2023   183

Heart and Great Vessels

Ø   **Medical and Surgical**
2   **Heart and Great Vessels**
N   **Release**   Definition: Freeing a body part from an abnormal physical constraint by cutting or by the use of force
                      Explanation: Some of the restraining tissue may be taken out but none of the body part is taken out

Body Part Character 4	Approach Character 5	Device Character 6	Qualifier Character 7

Ø   **Coronary Artery, One Artery**
1   **Coronary Artery, Two Arteries**
2   **Coronary Artery, Three Arteries**
3   **Coronary Artery, Four or More Arteries**
4   **Coronary Vein**
5   **Atrial Septum**
     Interatrial septum
6   **Atrium, Right**
     Atrium dextrum cordis
     Right auricular appendix
     Sinus venosus
7   **Atrium, Left**
     Atrium pulmonale
     Left auricular appendix
8   **Conduction Mechanism**
     Atrioventricular node
     Bundle of His
     Bundle of Kent
     Sinoatrial node
9   **Chordae Tendineae**
D   **Papillary Muscle**
F   **Aortic Valve**
     Aortic annulus
G   **Mitral Valve**
     Bicuspid valve
     Left atrioventricular valve
     Mitral annulus
H   **Pulmonary Valve**
     Pulmonary annulus
     Pulmonic valve
J   **Tricuspid Valve**
     Right atrioventricular valve
     Tricuspid annulus
K   **Ventricle, Right**
     Conus arteriosus
L   **Ventricle, Left**
M   **Ventricular Septum**
     Interventricular septum
N   **Pericardium**
P   **Pulmonary Trunk**
Q   **Pulmonary Artery, Right**
R   **Pulmonary Artery, Left**
     Arterial canal (duct)
     Botallo's duct
     Pulmoaortic canal
S   **Pulmonary Vein, Right**
     Right inferior pulmonary vein
     Right superior pulmonary vein
T   **Pulmonary Vein, Left**
     Left inferior pulmonary vein
     Left superior pulmonary vein
V   **Superior Vena Cava**
     Cavoatrial junction
     Precava
W   **Thoracic Aorta, Descending**
X   **Thoracic Aorta, Ascending/Arch**
     Aortic arch
     Ascending aorta
	Ø Open
	3 Percutaneous
	4 Percutaneous Endoscopic
		Z No Device	Z No Qualifier

Non-OR Procedure   DRG Non-OR Procedure   Valid OR Procedure   HAC Associated Procedure   Combination Only   New/Revised April   New/Revised October

184   ICD-10-PCS 2023

Ø   Medical and Surgical
2   Heart and Great Vessels
P   Removal   Definition: Taking out or off a device from a body part

                      Explanation: If a device is taken out and a similar device put in without cutting or puncturing the skin or mucous membrane, the procedure is coded to the root operation CHANGE. Otherwise, the procedure for taking out a device is coded to the root operation REMOVAL.

Body Part Character 4	Approach Character 5	Device Character 6	Qualifier Character 7
A Heart	Ø Open 3 Percutaneous 4 Percutaneous Endoscopic	2 Monitoring Device 3 Infusion Device 7 Autologous Tissue Substitute 8 Zooplastic Tissue C Extraluminal Device D Intraluminal Device J Synthetic Substitute K Nonautologous Tissue Substitute M Cardiac Lead N Intracardiac Pacemaker Q Implantable Heart Assist System Y Other Device	Z No Qualifier
A Heart ⊞	Ø Open 3 Percutaneous 4 Percutaneous Endoscopic	R Short-term External Heart Assist System	S Biventricular Z No Qualifier
A Heart	X External	2 Monitoring Device 3 Infusion Device D Intraluminal Device M Cardiac Lead	Z No Qualifier
Y Great Vessel	Ø Open 3 Percutaneous 4 Percutaneous Endoscopic	2 Monitoring Device 3 Infusion Device 7 Autologous Tissue Substitute 8 Zooplastic Tissue C Extraluminal Device D Intraluminal Device J Synthetic Substitute K Nonautologous Tissue Substitute Y Other Device	Z No Qualifier
Y Great Vessel	X External	2 Monitoring Device 3 Infusion Device D Intraluminal Device	Z No Qualifier

Non-OR   Ø2PA3[2,3,D]Z
Non-OR   Ø2PA[3,4]YZ
Non-OR   Ø2PAX[2,3,D,M]Z
Non-OR   Ø2PY3[2,3,D]Z
Non-OR   Ø2PY[3,4]YZ
Non-OR   Ø2PYX[2,3,D]Z
HAC   Ø2PA[Ø,3,4]MZ when reported with SDx K68.11 or T81.4Ø-T81.49, T82.7 with 7th character A
HAC   Ø2PAXMZ when reported with SDx K68.11 or T81.4Ø-T81.49, T82.7 with 7th character A

See Appendix L for Procedure Combinations
⊞   Ø2PA[Ø,3,4]RZ

NC Noncovered Procedure   LC Limited Coverage   QA Questionable OB Admit   NT New Tech Add-on   ⊞ Combination Member   ♂ Male   ♀ Female

ICD-10-PCS 2023   185

0 Medical and Surgical
2 Heart and Great Vessels
Q Repair   Definition: Restoring, to the extent possible, a body part to its normal anatomic structure and function
          Explanation: Used only when the method to accomplish the repair is not one of the other root operations

Body Part Character 4	Approach Character 5	Device Character 6	Qualifier Character 7
0 **Coronary Artery, One Artery**	**0** **Open**	**Z** **No Device**	**Z** **No Qualifier**
1 **Coronary Artery, Two Arteries**	**3** **Percutaneous**		
2 **Coronary Artery, Three Arteries**	**4** **Percutaneous Endoscopic**		
3 **Coronary Artery, Four or More** Arteries			
4 **Coronary Vein**			
5 **Atrial Septum** Interatrial septum			
6 **Atrium, Right** Atrium dextrum cordis Right auricular appendix Sinus venosus			
7 **Atrium, Left** Atrium pulmonale Left auricular appendix			
8 **Conduction Mechanism** Atrioventricular node Bundle of His Bundle of Kent Sinoatrial node			
9 **Chordae Tendineae**			
A **Heart**			
B **Heart, Right** Right coronary sulcus			
C **Heart, Left** Left coronary sulcus Obtuse margin			
D **Papillary Muscle**			
H **Pulmonary Valve** Pulmonary annulus Pulmonic valve			
K **Ventricle, Right** Conus arteriosus			
L **Ventricle, Left**			
M **Ventricular Septum** Interventricular septum			
N **Pericardium**			
P **Pulmonary Trunk**			
Q **Pulmonary Artery, Right**			
R **Pulmonary Artery, Left** Arterial canal (duct) Botallo's duct Pulmoaortic canal			
S **Pulmonary Vein, Right** Right inferior pulmonary vein Right superior pulmonary vein			
T **Pulmonary Vein, Left** Left inferior pulmonary vein Left superior pulmonary vein			
V **Superior Vena Cava** Cavoatrial junction Precava			
W **Thoracic Aorta, Descending**			
X **Thoracic Aorta, Ascending/Arch** Aortic arch Ascending aorta			
F **Aortic Valve** Aortic annulus	**0** **Open** **3** **Percutaneous** **4** **Percutaneous Endoscopic**	**Z** **No Device**	**J** **Truncal Valve** **Z** **No Qualifier**
G **Mitral Valve** Bicuspid valve Left atrioventricular valve Mitral annulus	**0** **Open** **3** **Percutaneous** **4** **Percutaneous Endoscopic**	**Z** **No Device**	**E** **Atrioventricular Valve, Left** **Z** **No Qualifier**
J **Tricuspid Valve** Right atrioventricular valve Tricuspid annulus	**0** **Open** **3** **Percutaneous** **4** **Percutaneous Endoscopic**	**Z** **No Device**	**G** **Atrioventricular Valve, Right** **Z** **No Qualifier**

Non-OR Procedure   DRG Non-OR Procedure   Valid OR Procedure   HAC Associated Procedure   Combination Only   New/Revised April   New/Revised October

186

ICD-10-PCS 2023

0   Medical and Surgical
2   Heart and Great Vessels
R   Replacement   Definition: Putting in or on biological or synthetic material that physically takes the place and/or function of all or a portion of a body part

Explanation: The body part may have been taken out or replaced, or may be taken out, physically eradicated, or rendered nonfunctional during the REPLACEMENT procedure. A REMOVAL procedure is coded for taking out the device used in a previous replacement procedure.

Body Part Character 4	Approach Character 5	Device Character 6	Qualifier Character 7
5 Atrial Septum Interatrial septum **6 Atrium, Right** Atrium dextrum cordis Right auricular appendix Sinus venosus **7 Atrium, Left** Atrium pulmonale Left auricular appendix **9 Chordae Tendineae** **D Papillary Muscle** **K Ventricle, Right** ⊞ Conus arteriosus **L Ventricle, Left** ⊞ **M Ventricular Septum** Interventricular septum **N Pericardium** **P Pulmonary Trunk** **Q Pulmonary Artery, Right** **R Pulmonary Artery, Left** Arterial canal (duct) Botallo's duct Pulmoaortic canal **S Pulmonary Vein, Right** Right inferior pulmonary vein Right superior pulmonary vein **T Pulmonary Vein, Left** Left inferior pulmonary vein Left superior pulmonary vein **V Superior Vena Cava** Cavoatrial junction Precava **W Thoracic Aorta, Descending** **X Thoracic Aorta, Ascending/Arch** Aortic arch Ascending aorta	**0** Open **4** Percutaneous Endoscopic	**7** Autologous Tissue Substitute **8** Zooplastic Tissue **J** Synthetic Substitute **K** Nonautologous Tissue Substitute	**Z** No Qualifier
A Heart	**0** Open	**L** Biologic with Synthetic Substitute, Autoregulated Electrohydraulic **M** Synthetic Substitute, Pneumatic	**Z** No Qualifier
F Aortic Valve Aortic annulus	**0** Open **4** Percutaneous Endoscopic	**7** Autologous Tissue Substitute **J** Synthetic Substitute **K** Nonautologous Tissue Substitute	**Z** No Qualifier
F Aortic Valve Aortic annulus	**0** Open **4** Percutaneous Endoscopic	**8** Zooplastic Tissue	**N** Rapid Deployment Technique **Z** No Qualifier
F Aortic Valve Aortic annulus	**3** Percutaneous	**7** Autologous Tissue Substitute **J** Synthetic Substitute **K** Nonautologous Tissue Substitute	**H** Transapical **Z** No Qualifier
F Aortic Valve Aortic annulus	**3** Percutaneous	**8** Zooplastic Tissue	**H** Transapical **N** Rapid Deployment Technique **Z** No Qualifier
G Mitral Valve Bicuspid valve Left atrioventricular valve Mitral annulus **J Tricuspid Valve** Right atrioventricular valve Tricuspid annulus	**0** Open **4** Percutaneous Endoscopic	**7** Autologous Tissue Substitute **8** Zooplastic Tissue **J** Synthetic Substitute **K** Nonautologous Tissue Substitute	**Z** No Qualifier
G Mitral Valve Bicuspid valve Left atrioventricular valve Mitral annulus **J Tricuspid Valve** Right atrioventricular valve Tricuspid annulus	**3** Percutaneous	**7** Autologous Tissue Substitute **8** Zooplastic Tissue **J** Synthetic Substitute **K** Nonautologous Tissue Substitute	**H** Transapical **Z** No Qualifier
H Pulmonary Valve Pulmonary annulus Pulmonic valve	**0** Open **4** Percutaneous Endoscopic	**7** Autologous Tissue Substitute **8** Zooplastic Tissue **J** Synthetic Substitute **K** Nonautologous Tissue Substitute	**Z** No Qualifier
H Pulmonary Valve Pulmonary annulus Pulmonic valve	**3** Percutaneous	**7** Autologous Tissue Substitute **J** Synthetic Substitute **K** Nonautologous Tissue Substitute	**H** Transapical **Z** No Qualifier
H Pulmonary Valve Pulmonary annulus Pulmonic valve	**3** Percutaneous	**8** Zooplastic Tissue NT	**H** Transapical **L** In Existing Conduit **M** Native Site **Z** No Qualifier

NT   02RH38M for Harmony™ Transcatheter Pulmonary Valve (TPV) System   **See Appendix L for Procedure Combinations**
⊞   02R[K,L]0JZ

NC Noncovered Procedure   LC Limited Coverage   QA Questionable OB Admit   NT New Tech Add-on   ⊞ Combination Member   ♂ Male   ♀ Female

Heart and Great Vessels

0   **Medical and Surgical**
2   **Heart and Great Vessels**
S   **Reposition**   Definition: Moving to its normal location, or other suitable location, all or a portion of a body part

Explanation: The body part is moved to a new location from an abnormal location, or from a normal location where it is not functioning correctly. The body part may or may not be cut out or off to be moved to the new location.

Body Part Character 4	Approach Character 5	Device Character 6	Qualifier Character 7
0 **Coronary Artery, One Artery**	**0** Open	**Z** No Device	**Z** No Qualifier
1 **Coronary Artery, Two Arteries**			
P **Pulmonary Trunk**			
Q **Pulmonary Artery, Right**			
R **Pulmonary Artery, Left**			
Arterial canal (duct)			
Botallo's duct			
Pulmoaortic canal			
S **Pulmonary Vein, Right**			
Right inferior pulmonary vein			
Right superior pulmonary vein			
T **Pulmonary Vein, Left**			
Left inferior pulmonary vein			
Left superior pulmonary vein			
V **Superior Vena Cava**			
Cavoatrial junction			
Precava			
W **Thoracic Aorta, Descending**			
X **Thoracic Aorta, Ascending/Arch**			
Aortic arch			
Ascending aorta			

0   **Medical and Surgical**
2   **Heart and Great Vessels**
T   **Resection**   Definition: Cutting out or off, without replacement, all of a body part

Explanation: None

Body Part Character 4	Approach Character 5	Device Character 6	Qualifier Character 7
5 **Atrial Septum**	**0** Open	**Z** No Device	**Z** No Qualifier
Interatrial septum	**3** Percutaneous		
8 **Conduction Mechanism**	**4** Percutaneous Endoscopic		
Atrioventricular node			
Bundle of His			
Bundle of Kent			
Sinoatrial node			
9 **Chordae Tendineae**			
D **Papillary Muscle**			
H **Pulmonary Valve**			
Pulmonary annulus			
Pulmonic valve			
M **Ventricular Septum**			
Interventricular septum			
N **Pericardium**			

Non-OR Procedure   DRG Non-OR Procedure   Valid OR Procedure   HAC Associated Procedure   Combination Only   New/Revised April   New/Revised October

188

ICD-10-PCS 2023

0   **Medical and Surgical**
2   **Heart and Great Vessels**
U   **Supplement**   Definition: Putting in or on biological or synthetic material that physically reinforces and/or augments the function of a portion of a body part
                            Explanation: The biological material is non-living, or is living and from the same individual. The body part may have been previously replaced, and the SUPPLEMENT procedure is performed to physically reinforce and/or augment the function of the replaced body part.

Body Part Character 4	Approach Character 5	Device Character 6	Qualifier Character 7

0   **Coronary Artery, One Artery**
1   **Coronary Artery, Two Arteries**
2   **Coronary Artery, Three Arteries**
3   **Coronary Artery, Four or More**
     Arteries
5   **Atrial Septum**
     Interatrial septum
6   **Atrium, Right**
     Atrium dextrum cordis
     Right auricular appendix
     Sinus venosus
7   **Atrium, Left**
     Atrium pulmonale
     Left auricular appendix
9   **Chordae Tendineae**
A   **Heart**
D   **Papillary Muscle**
H   **Pulmonary Valve**
     Pulmonary annulus
     Pulmonic valve
K   **Ventricle, Right**
     Conus arteriosus
L   **Ventricle, Left**
M   **Ventricular Septum**
     Interventricular septum
N   **Pericardium**
P   **Pulmonary Trunk**
Q   **Pulmonary Artery, Right**
R   **Pulmonary Artery, Left**
     Arterial canal (duct)
     Botallo's duct
     Pulmoaortic canal
S   **Pulmonary Vein, Right**
     Right inferior pulmonary vein
     Right superior pulmonary vein
T   **Pulmonary Vein, Left**
     Left inferior pulmonary vein
     Left superior pulmonary vein
V   **Superior Vena Cava**
     Cavoatrial junction
     Precava
W   **Thoracic Aorta, Descending**
X   **Thoracic Aorta, Ascending/Arch**
     Aortic arch
     Ascending aorta
	0 **Open**
	3 **Percutaneous**
	4 **Percutaneous Endoscopic**
		7 **Autologous Tissue Substitute**
		8 **Zooplastic Tissue**
		J **Synthetic Substitute**
		K **Nonautologous Tissue Substitute**
			Z **No Qualifier**

F **Aortic Valve** Aortic annulus	**0** **Open** **3** **Percutaneous** **4** **Percutaneous Endoscopic**	**7** **Autologous Tissue Substitute** **8** **Zooplastic Tissue** **J** **Synthetic Substitute** **K** **Nonautologous Tissue Substitute**	**J** **Truncal Valve** **Z** **No Qualifier**

G   **Mitral Valve**
     Bicuspid valve
     Left atrioventricular valve
     Mitral annulus
	0 **Open**
	4 **Percutaneous Endoscopic**
		7 **Autologous Tissue Substitute**
		8 **Zooplastic Tissue**
		J **Synthetic Substitute**
		K **Nonautologous Tissue Substitute**
			E **Atrioventricular Valve, Left**
			Z **No Qualifier**

G   **Mitral Valve**
     Bicuspid valve
     Left atrioventricular valve
     Mitral annulus
	3 **Percutaneous**	**7** **Autologous Tissue Substitute**
		8 **Zooplastic Tissue**
		K **Nonautologous Tissue Substitute**
			E **Atrioventricular Valve, Left**
			Z **No Qualifier**

G   **Mitral Valve**
     Bicuspid valve
     Left atrioventricular valve
     Mitral annulus
	3 **Percutaneous**	**J** **Synthetic Substitute**	**E** **Atrioventricular Valve, Left**
			H **Transapical**
			Z **No Qualifier**

J   **Tricuspid Valve**
     Right atrioventricular valve
     Tricuspid annulus
	0 **Open**
	3 **Percutaneous**
	4 **Percutaneous Endoscopic**
		7 **Autologous Tissue Substitute**
		8 **Zooplastic Tissue**
		J **Synthetic Substitute**
		K **Nonautologous Tissue Substitute**
			G **Atrioventricular Valve, Right**
			Z **No Qualifier**

     DRG Non-OR   02U7[3,4]JZ

0 Medical and Surgical
2 Heart and Great Vessels
V Restriction Definition: Partially closing an orifice or the lumen of a tubular body part
Explanation: The orifice can be a natural orifice or an artificially created orifice

Body Part Character 4	Approach Character 5	Device Character 6	Qualifier Character 7
A Heart	**Ø** Open **3** Percutaneous **4** Percutaneous Endoscopic	**C** Extraluminal Device **Z** No Device	**Z** No Qualifier
G Mitral Valve Bicuspid valve Left atrioventricular valve Mitral annulus	**Ø** Open **3** Percutaneous **4** Percutaneous Endoscopic	**Z** No Device	**Z** No Qualifier
L Ventricle, Left **P** Pulmonary Trunk **Q** Pulmonary Artery, Right **S** Pulmonary Vein, Right Right inferior pulmonary vein Right superior pulmonary vein **T** Pulmonary Vein, Left Left inferior pulmonary vein Left superior pulmonary vein **V** Superior Vena Cava Cavoatrial junction Precava	**Ø** Open **3** Percutaneous **4** Percutaneous Endoscopic	**C** Extraluminal Device **D** Intraluminal Device **Z** No Device	**Z** No Qualifier
R Pulmonary Artery, Left Arterial canal (duct) Botallo's duct Pulmoaortic canal	**Ø** Open **3** Percutaneous **4** Percutaneous Endoscopic	**C** Extraluminal Device **D** Intraluminal Device **Z** No Device	**T** Ductus Arteriosus **Z** No Qualifier
W Thoracic Aorta, Descending **X** Thoracic Aorta, Ascending/Arch Aortic arch Ascending aorta	**Ø** Open **3** Percutaneous **4** Percutaneous Endoscopic	**C** Extraluminal Device **D** Intraluminal Device **E** Intraluminal Device, Branched or Fenestrated, One or Two Arteries **F** Intraluminal Device, Branched or Fenestrated, Three or More Arteries **Z** No Device	**Z** No Qualifier

0   **Medical and Surgical**
2   **Heart and Great Vessels**
W   **Revision**   Definition: Correcting, to the extent possible, a portion of a malfunctioning device or the position of a displaced device

Explanation: Revision can include correcting a malfunctioning or displaced device by taking out or putting in components of the device such as a screw or pin

Body Part Character 4	Approach Character 5	Device Character 6	Qualifier Character 7
5 Atrial Septum Interatrial septum **M Ventricular Septum** Interventricular septum	**0** Open **4** Percutaneous Endoscopic	**J** Synthetic Substitute	**Z** No Qualifier
A Heart LC ✚	**0** Open **3** Percutaneous **4** Percutaneous Endoscopic	**2** Monitoring Device **3** Infusion Device **7** Autologous Tissue Substitute **8** Zooplastic Tissue **C** Extraluminal Device **D** Intraluminal Device **J** Synthetic Substitute **K** Nonautologous Tissue Substitute **M** Cardiac Lead **N** Intracardiac Pacemaker **Q** Implantable Heart Assist System **Y** Other Device	**Z** No Qualifier
A Heart ✚	**0** Open **3** Percutaneous **4** Percutaneous Endoscopic	**R** Short-term External Heart Assist System	**S** Biventricular **Z** No Qualifier
A Heart	**X** External	**2** Monitoring Device **3** Infusion Device **7** Autologous Tissue Substitute **8** Zooplastic Tissue **C** Extraluminal Device **D** Intraluminal Device **J** Synthetic Substitute **K** Nonautologous Tissue Substitute **M** Cardiac Lead **N** Intracardiac Pacemaker **Q** Implantable Heart Assist System	**Z** No Qualifier
A Heart	**X** External	**R** Short-term External Heart Assist System	**S** Biventricular **Z** No Qualifier
F Aortic Valve Aortic annulus **G Mitral Valve** Bicuspid valve Left atrioventricular valve Mitral annulus **H Pulmonary Valve** Pulmonary annulus Pulmonic valve **J Tricuspid Valve** Right atrioventricular valve Tricuspid annulus	**0** Open **3** Percutaneous **4** Percutaneous Endoscopic	**7** Autologous Tissue Substitute **8** Zooplastic Tissue **J** Synthetic Substitute **K** Nonautologous Tissue Substitute	**Z** No Qualifier
Y Great Vessel	**0** Open **3** Percutaneous **4** Percutaneous Endoscopic	**2** Monitoring Device **3** Infusion Device **7** Autologous Tissue Substitute **8** Zooplastic Tissue **C** Extraluminal Device **D** Intraluminal Device **J** Synthetic Substitute **K** Nonautologous Tissue Substitute **Y** Other Device	**Z** No Qualifier
Y Great Vessel	**X** External	**2** Monitoring Device **3** Infusion Device **7** Autologous Tissue Substitute **8** Zooplastic Tissue **C** Extraluminal Device **D** Intraluminal Device **J** Synthetic Substitute **K** Nonautologous Tissue Substitute	**Z** No Qualifier

Non-OR 02WA3[2,3,D]Z	**HAC** 02WA[0,3,4]MZ when reported with T81.40–T81.49, T82.7 with 7th character A
Non-OR 02WA[3,4]YZ	**LC** 02WA[3,4]QZ
Non-OR 02WAX[2,3,7,8,C,D,J,K,M,N,Q]Z	
Non-OR 02WAXRZ	**See Appendix L for Procedure Combinations**
Non-OR 02WY3[2,3]Z	✚ 02WA[0,3,4]QZ
Non-OR 02WY[3,4]YZ	✚ 02WA[0,3,4]RZ
Non-OR 02WYX[2,3,7,8,C,D,J,K]Z	

NC Noncovered Procedure   LC Limited Coverage   QA Questionable OB Admit   NT New Tech Add-on   ✚ Combination Member   ♂ Male   ♀ Female

Heart and Great Vessels

Ø **Medical and Surgical**
2 **Heart and Great Vessels**
Y **Transplantation** Definition: Putting in or on all or a portion of a living body part taken from another individual or animal to physically take the place and/or function of all or a portion of a similar body part

Explanation: The native body part may or may not be taken out, and the transplanted body part may take over all or a portion of its function

Body Part Character 4	Approach Character 5	Device Character 6	Qualifier Character 7
A Heart LC	Ø Open	Z No Device	Ø Allogeneic 1 Syngeneic 2 Zooplastic

LC	Ø2YAØZ[Ø,1,2]

Upper Arteries Ø31–Ø3W

Character Meanings

This Character Meaning table is provided as a guide to assist the user in the identification of character members that may be found in this section of code tables. It **SHOULD NOT** be used to build a PCS code.

Operation–Character 3	Body Part–Character 4	Approach–Character 5	Device–Character 6	Qualifier–Character 7
1 Bypass	Ø Internal Mammary Artery, Right	Ø Open	Ø Drainage Device	Ø Upper Arm Artery, Right OR Ultrasonic
5 Destruction	1 Internal Mammary Artery, Left	3 Percutaneous	2 Monitoring Device	1 Upper Arm Artery, Left OR Drug-Coated Balloon
7 Dilation	2 Innominate Artery	4 Percutaneous Endoscopic	3 Infusion Device	2 Upper Arm Artery, Bilateral
9 Drainage	3 Subclavian Artery, Right	X External	4 Intraluminal Device, Drug-eluting	3 Lower Arm Artery, Right
B Excision	4 Subclavian Artery, Left		5 Intraluminal Device, Drug-eluting, Two	4 Lower Arm Artery, Left
C Extirpation	5 Axillary Artery, Right		6 Intraluminal Device, Drug-eluting, Three	5 Lower Arm Artery, Bilateral
F Fragmentation	6 Axillary Artery, Left		7 Intraluminal Device, Drug-eluting, Four or More OR Autologous Tissue Substitute	6 Upper Leg Artery, Right
H Insertion	7 Brachial Artery, Right		9 Autologous Venous Tissue	7 Upper Leg Artery, Left OR Stent Retriever
J Inspection	8 Brachial Artery, Left		A Autologous Arterial Tissue	8 Upper Leg Artery, Bilateral
L Occlusion	9 Ulnar Artery, Right		B Intraluminal Device, Bioactive	9 Lower Leg Artery, Right
N Release	A Ulnar Artery, Left		C Extraluminal Device	B Lower Leg Artery, Left
P Removal	B Radial Artery, Right		D Intraluminal Device	C Lower Leg Artery, Bilateral
Q Repair	C Radial Artery, Left		E Intraluminal Device, Two	D Upper Arm Vein
R Replacement	D Hand Artery, Right		F Intraluminal Device, Three	F Lower Arm Vein
S Reposition	F Hand Artery, Left		G Intraluminal Device, Four or More	G Intracranial Artery
U Supplement	G Intracranial Artery		H Intraluminal Device, Flow Diverter	J Extracranial Artery, Right
V Restriction	H Common Carotid Artery, Right		J Synthetic Substitute	K Extracranial Artery, Left
W Revision	J Common Carotid Artery, Left		K Nonautologous Tissue Substitute	M Pulmonary Artery, Right
	K Internal Carotid Artery, Right		M Stimulator Lead	N Pulmonary Artery, Left
	L Internal Carotid Artery, Left		Y Other Device	T Abdominal Artery
	M External Carotid Artery, Right		Z No Device	V Superior Vena Cava
	N External Carotid Artery, Left			W Lower Extremity Vein
	P Vertebral Artery, Right			X Diagnostic
	Q Vertebral Artery, Left			Y Upper Artery
	R Face Artery			Z No Qualifier
	S Temporal Artery, Right			
	T Temporal Artery, Left			
	U Thyroid Artery, Right			
	V Thyroid Artery, Left			
	Y Upper Artery			

AHA Coding Clinic for Upper Arteries

2022, 1Q, 10-13   Procedures performed on a continuous vessel, ICD-10-PCS Guideline B4.1c

AHA Coding Clinic for table 031

2021, 4Q, 45-46   Percutaneous bypass of brachial artery for arteriovenous fistula creation
2021, 3Q, 14   Arteriovenous fistula revision with graft to cephalic vein stump
2019, 4Q, 26   Upper artery bypass Qualifier
2019, 4Q, 26   Percutaneous approach upper artery bypass
2017, 4Q, 64-65   New qualifier values - Left to right carotid bypass
2017, 2Q, 22   Carotid artery to subclavian artery transposition
2017, 1Q, 31   Left to right common carotid artery bypass
2016, 3Q, 37   Insertion of arteriovenous graft using HeRO device
2016, 3Q, 39   Revision of arteriovenous graft
2013, 4Q, 125   Stage II cephalic vein transposition (superficialization) of arteriovenous fistula
2013, 1Q, 27   Creation of radial artery fistula

AHA Coding Clinic for table 037

2020, 4Q, 70-71   Cerebral embolic filtration extracorporeal flow reversal circuit
2019, 4Q, 27   Bifurcation Qualifier
2019, 3Q, 29   Transcarotid arterial catheterization
2018, 2Q, 24   Coronary artery bifurcation
2016, 4Q, 86   Peripheral artery, number of stents
2016, 4Q, 86-87   Coronary and peripheral artery bifurcation
2015, 1Q, 32   Deployment of stent for herniated/migrated coil in basilar artery

AHA Coding Clinic for table 03B

2016, 2Q, 12   Resection of malignant neoplasm of infratemporal fossa

AHA Coding Clinic for table 03C

2022, 1Q, 43   Cerebral thrombectomy with failed stent retriever deployment and aspiration of thrombus
2021, 2Q, 13   Thromboendarterectomy with deconstruction of internal carotid artery
2020, 3Q, 38   Thrombectomy of arteriovenous fistula with angioplasty and stent placement
2019, 4Q, 27   Bifurcation Qualifier
2018, 4Q, 47-48   Endovascular thrombectomy with stent retriever
2018, 2Q, 24   Coronary artery bifurcation
2017, 4Q, 64-65   New qualifier values - Left to right carotid bypass
2017, 2Q, 23   Thrombectomy via Fogarty catheter
2016, 4Q, 86-87   Coronary and peripheral artery bifurcation
2016, 2Q, 11   Carotid endarterectomy with patch angioplasty
2015, 1Q, 29   Discontinued carotid endarterectomy

AHA Coding Clinic for table 03F

2021, 4Q, 46   Fragmentation of intracranial artery
2020, 4Q, 45-49   New fragmentation tables
2020, 4Q, 49-50   Intravascular ultrasound assisted thrombolysis
2020, 4Q, 50   Intravascular lithotripsy

AHA Coding Clinic for table 03H

2020, 1Q, 25   Elephant trunk repair of aortic dissection
2016, 2Q, 32   Arterial catheter placement

AHA Coding Clinic for table 03J

2021, 1Q, 16   Placement of Sentinel™ embolic protection device with deployment of single filter
2015, 1Q, 29   Discontinued carotid endarterectomy

AHA Coding Clinic for table 03L

2021, 2Q, 13   Thromboendarterectomy with deconstruction of internal carotid artery
2016, 2Q, 30   Clipping (occlusion) of cerebral artery, decompressive craniectomy and storage of bone flap in abdominal wall
2014, 4Q, 20   Control of epistaxis
2014, 4Q, 37   Endovascular embolization of arteriovenous malformation using Onyx-18 liquid

AHA Coding Clinic for table 03Q

2017, 1Q, 31   Left to right common carotid artery bypass

AHA Coding Clinic for table 03S

2017, 2Q, 22   Carotid artery to subclavian artery transposition
2015, 3Q, 27   Moyamoya disease and hemispheric pial synangiosis with craniotomy

AHA Coding Clinic for table 03U

2019, 1Q, 22   Cerebral artery fusiform aneurysm repair via wrapping
2016, 2Q, 11   Carotid endarterectomy with patch angioplasty

AHA Coding Clinic for table 03V

2019, 4Q, 27-28   Aneurysm treatment using flow diverter stent
2019, 1Q, 22   Cerebral artery fusiform aneurysm repair via wrapping
2016, 1Q, 19   Embolization of superior hypophyseal aneurysm using stent-assisted coil

AHA Coding Clinic for table 03W

2016, 3Q, 39   Revision of arteriovenous graft
2015, 1Q, 32   Deployment of stent for herniated/migrated coil in basilar artery

Upper Arteries

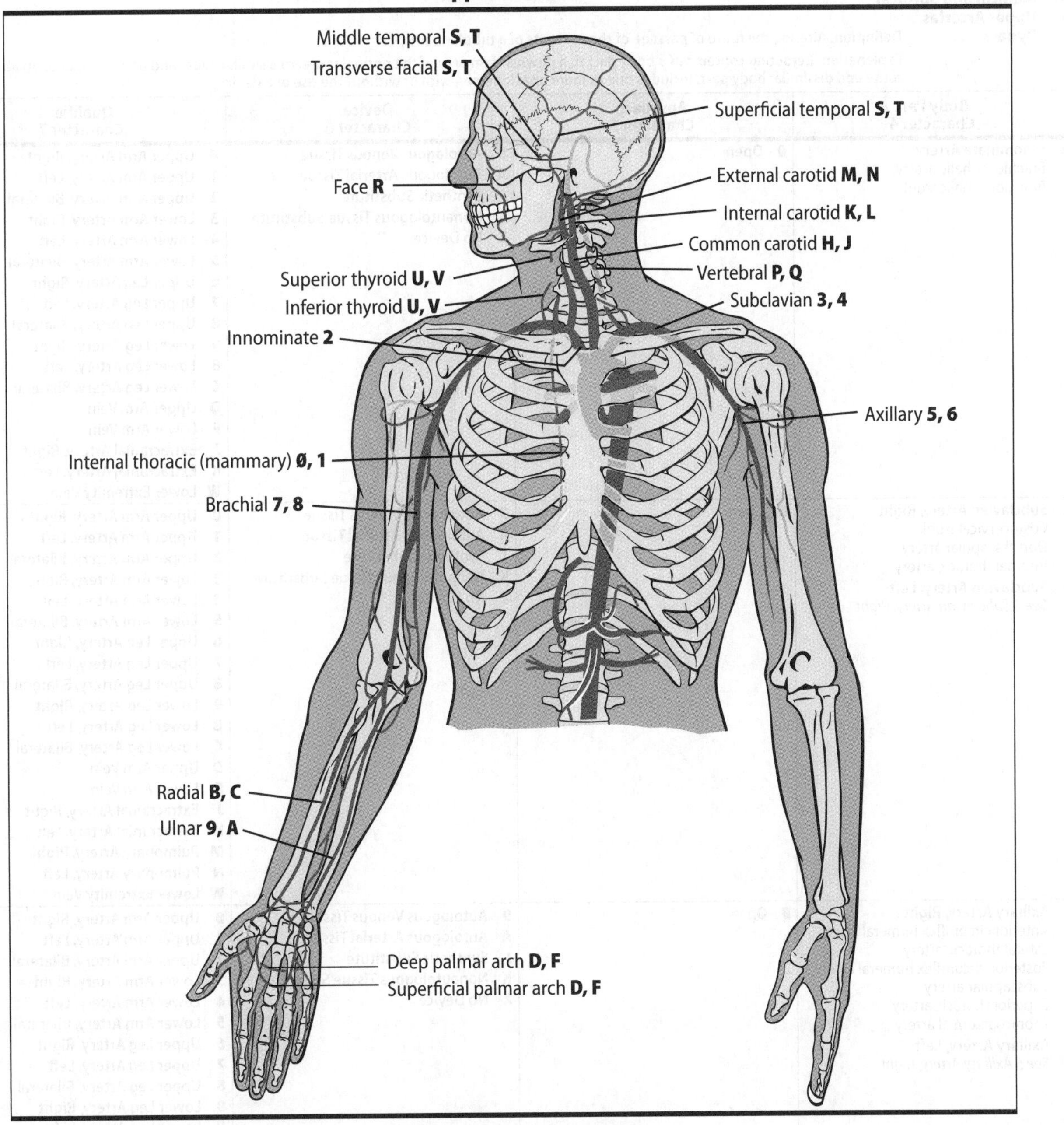

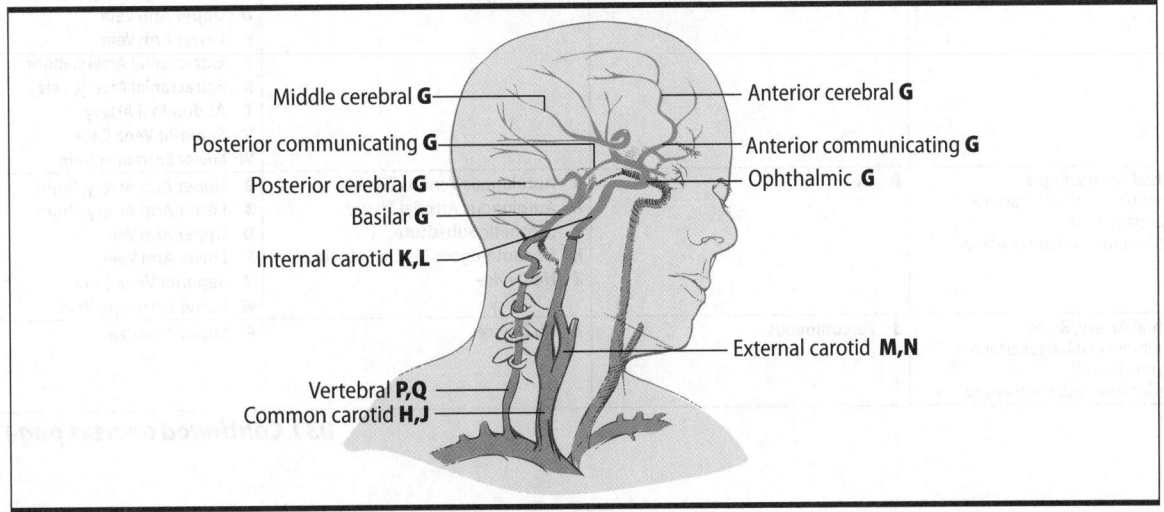

Middle temporal **S, T**
Transverse facial **S, T**
Superficial temporal **S, T**
Face **R**
External carotid **M, N**
Internal carotid **K, L**
Common carotid **H, J**
Superior thyroid **U, V**
Vertebral **P, Q**
Inferior thyroid **U, V**
Subclavian **3, 4**
Innominate **2**
Axillary **5, 6**
Internal thoracic (mammary) **Ø, 1**
Brachial **7, 8**
Radial **B, C**
Ulnar **9, A**
Deep palmar arch **D, F**
Superficial palmar arch **D, F**

Head and Neck Arteries

Middle cerebral **G**
Anterior cerebral **G**
Posterior communicating **G**
Anterior communicating **G**
Posterior cerebral **G**
Ophthalmic **G**
Basilar **G**
Internal carotid **K,L**
External carotid **M,N**
Vertebral **P,Q**
Common carotid **H,J**

Ø   Medical and Surgical
3   Upper Arteries
1   Bypass   Definition: Altering the route of passage of the contents of a tubular body part

Explanation: Rerouting contents of a body part to a downstream area of the normal route, to a similar route and body part, or to an abnormal route and dissimilar body part. Includes one or more anastomoses, with or without the use of a device.

Body Part Character 4	Approach Character 5	Device Character 6	Qualifier Character 7
2 Innominate Artery Brachiocephalic artery Brachiocephalic trunk	Ø Open	9 Autologous Venous Tissue A Autologous Arterial Tissue J Synthetic Substitute K Nonautologous Tissue Substitute Z No Device	Ø Upper Arm Artery, Right 1 Upper Arm Artery, Left 2 Upper Arm Artery, Bilateral 3 Lower Arm Artery, Right 4 Lower Arm Artery, Left 5 Lower Arm Artery, Bilateral 6 Upper Leg Artery, Right 7 Upper Leg Artery, Left 8 Upper Leg Artery, Bilateral 9 Lower Leg Artery, Right B Lower Leg Artery, Left C Lower Leg Artery, Bilateral D Upper Arm Vein F Lower Arm Vein J Extracranial Artery, Right K Extracranial Artery, Left W Lower Extremity Vein
3 Subclavian Artery, Right Costocervical trunk Dorsal scapular artery Internal thoracic artery **4 Subclavian Artery, Left** *See 3 Subclavian Artery, Right*	Ø Open	9 Autologous Venous Tissue A Autologous Arterial Tissue J Synthetic Substitute K Nonautologous Tissue Substitute Z No Device	Ø Upper Arm Artery, Right 1 Upper Arm Artery, Left 2 Upper Arm Artery, Bilateral 3 Lower Arm Artery, Right 4 Lower Arm Artery, Left 5 Lower Arm Artery, Bilateral 6 Upper Leg Artery, Right 7 Upper Leg Artery, Left 8 Upper Leg Artery, Bilateral 9 Lower Leg Artery, Right B Lower Leg Artery, Left C Lower Leg Artery, Bilateral D Upper Arm Vein F Lower Arm Vein J Extracranial Artery, Right K Extracranial Artery, Left M Pulmonary Artery, Right N Pulmonary Artery, Left W Lower Extremity Vein
5 Axillary Artery, Right Anterior circumflex humeral artery Lateral thoracic artery Posterior circumflex humeral artery Subscapular artery Superior thoracic artery Thoracoacromial artery **6 Axillary Artery, Left** *See 5 Axillary Artery, Right*	Ø Open	9 Autologous Venous Tissue A Autologous Arterial Tissue J Synthetic Substitute K Nonautologous Tissue Substitute Z No Device	Ø Upper Arm Artery, Right 1 Upper Arm Artery, Left 2 Upper Arm Artery, Bilateral 3 Lower Arm Artery, Right 4 Lower Arm Artery, Left 5 Lower Arm Artery, Bilateral 6 Upper Leg Artery, Right 7 Upper Leg Artery, Left 8 Upper Leg Artery, Bilateral 9 Lower Leg Artery, Right B Lower Leg Artery, Left C Lower Leg Artery, Bilateral D Upper Arm Vein F Lower Arm Vein J Extracranial Artery, Right K Extracranial Artery, Left T Abdominal Artery V Superior Vena Cava W Lower Extremity Vein
7 Brachial Artery, Right Inferior ulnar collateral artery Profunda brachii Superior ulnar collateral artery	Ø Open	9 Autologous Venous Tissue A Autologous Arterial Tissue J Synthetic Substitute K Nonautologous Tissue Substitute Z No Device	Ø Upper Arm Artery, Right 3 Lower Arm Artery, Right D Upper Arm Vein F Lower Arm Vein V Superior Vena Cava W Lower Extremity Vein
7 Brachial Artery, Right Inferior ulnar collateral artery Profunda brachii Superior ulnar collateral artery	3 Percutaneous	Z No Device	F Lower Arm Vein

Ø31 Continued on next page

Non-OR Procedure   DRG Non-OR Procedure   Valid OR Procedure   HAC Associated Procedure   Combination Only   New/Revised April   New/Revised October

196   ICD-10-PCS 2023

Ø31–Ø31

Ø   **Medical and Surgical**   *Ø31 Continued*
3   **Upper Arteries**
1   **Bypass**   Definition: Altering the route of passage of the contents of a tubular body part

Explanation: Rerouting contents of a body part to a downstream area of the normal route, to a similar route and body part, or to an abnormal route and dissimilar body part. Includes one or more anastomoses, with or without the use of a device.

Body Part Character 4	Approach Character 5	Device Character 6	Qualifier Character 7
8 **Brachial Artery, Left** Inferior ulnar collateral artery Profunda brachii Superior ulnar collateral artery	**Ø** Open	**9** Autologous Venous Tissue **A** Autologous Arterial Tissue **J** Synthetic Substitute **K** Nonautologous Tissue Substitute **Z** No Device	**1** Upper Arm Artery, Left **4** Lower Arm Artery, Left **D** Upper Arm Vein **F** Lower Arm Vein **V** Superior Vena Cava **W** Lower Extremity Vein
8 **Brachial Artery, Left** Inferior ulnar collateral artery Profunda brachii Superior ulnar collateral artery	**3** Percutaneous	**Z** No Device	**F** Lower Arm Vein
9 **Ulnar Artery, Right** Anterior ulnar recurrent artery Common interosseous artery Posterior ulnar recurrent artery **B** **Radial Artery, Right** Radial recurrent artery	**Ø** Open	**9** Autologous Venous Tissue **A** Autologous Arterial Tissue **J** Synthetic Substitute **K** Nonautologous Tissue Substitute **Z** No Device	**3** Lower Arm Artery, Right **F** Lower Arm Vein
9 **Ulnar Artery, Right** Anterior ulnar recurrent artery Common interosseous artery Posterior ulnar recurrent artery **B** **Radial Artery, Right** Radial recurrent artery	**3** Percutaneous	**Z** No Device	**F** Lower Arm Vein
A **Ulnar Artery, Left** Anterior ulnar recurrent artery Common interosseous artery Posterior ulnar recurrent artery **C** **Radial Artery, Left** Radial recurrent artery	**Ø** Open	**9** Autologous Venous Tissue **A** Autologous Arterial Tissue **J** Synthetic Substitute **K** Nonautologous Tissue Substitute **Z** No Device	**4** Lower Arm Artery, Left **F** Lower Arm Vein
A **Ulnar Artery, Left** Anterior ulnar recurrent artery Common interosseous artery Posterior ulnar recurrent artery **C** **Radial Artery, Left** Radial recurrent artery	**3** Percutaneous	**Z** No Device	**F** Lower Arm Vein

G **Intracranial Artery**
Anterior cerebral artery
Anterior choroidal artery
Anterior communicating artery
Basilar artery
Circle of Willis
Internal carotid artery, intracranial
   portion
Middle cerebral artery
Ophthalmic artery
Posterior cerebral artery
Posterior communicating artery
Posterior inferior cerebellar artery
   (PICA)
S **Temporal Artery, Right**
Middle temporal artery
Superficial temporal artery
Transverse facial artery
T **Temporal Artery, Left**
See S Temporal Artery, Right
	Ø Open	**9** Autologous Venous Tissue
		A Autologous Arterial Tissue
		J Synthetic Substitute
		K Nonautologous Tissue Substitute
		Z No Device
			G Intracranial Artery

H **Common Carotid Artery, Right** **J** **Common Carotid Artery, Left**	**Ø** Open	**9** Autologous Venous Tissue **A** Autologous Arterial Tissue **J** Synthetic Substitute **K** Nonautologous Tissue Substitute **Z** No Device	**G** Intracranial Artery **J** Extracranial Artery, Right **K** Extracranial Artery, Left **Y** Upper Artery

Ø31 Continued on next page

NC Noncovered Procedure   **LC** Limited Coverage   **QA** Questionable OB Admit   **NT** New Tech Add-on   ⊞ Combination Member   ♂ Male   ♀ Female

Ø Medical and Surgical
3 Upper Arteries
1 Bypass

Ø31 Continued

Definition: Altering the route of passage of the contents of a tubular body part

Explanation: Rerouting contents of a body part to a downstream area of the normal route, to a similar route and body part, or to an abnormal route and dissimilar body part. Includes one or more anastomoses, with or without the use of a device.

Body Part Character 4	Approach Character 5	Device Character 6	Qualifier Character 7

K Internal Carotid Artery, Right
  Caroticotympanic artery
  Carotid sinus
L Internal Carotid Artery, Left
  Caroticotympanic artery
  Carotid sinus
M External Carotid Artery, Right
  Ascending pharyngeal artery
  Internal maxillary artery
  Lingual artery
  Maxillary artery
  Occipital artery
  Posterior auricular artery
  Superior thyroid artery
N External Carotid Artery, Left
  Ascending pharyngeal artery
  Internal maxillary artery
  Lingual artery
  Maxillary artery
  Occipital artery
  Posterior auricular artery
  Superior thyroid artery
	Ø Open	**9 Autologous Venous Tissue**
		A Autologous Arterial Tissue
		J Synthetic Substitute
		K Nonautologous Tissue Substitute
		Z No Device
			J Extracranial Artery, Right
			K Extracranial Artery, Left

Non-OR Procedure   DRG Non-OR Procedure   Valid OR Procedure   HAC Associated Procedure   Combination Only   New/Revised April   New/Revised October

198

ICD-10-PCS 2023

Ø31–Ø31

Ø   **Medical and Surgical**
3   **Upper Arteries**
5   **Destruction**   Definition: Physical eradication of all or a portion of a body part by the direct use of energy, force, or a destructive agent
                          Explanation: None of the body part is physically taken out

Body Part Character 4		Approach Character 5	Device Character 6	Qualifier Character 7
Ø Internal Mammary Artery, Right Anterior intercostal artery Internal thoracic artery Musculophrenic artery Pericardiophrenic artery Superior epigastric artery **1 Internal Mammary Artery, Left** *See Ø Internal Mammary Artery, Right* **2 Innominate Artery** Brachiocephalic artery Brachiocephalic trunk **3 Subclavian Artery, Right** Costocervical trunk Dorsal scapular artery Internal thoracic artery **4 Subclavian Artery, Left** *See 3 Subclavian Artery, Right* **5 Axillary Artery, Right** Anterior circumflex humeral artery Lateral thoracic artery Posterior circumflex humeral artery Subscapular artery Superior thoracic artery Thoracoacromial artery **6 Axillary Artery, Left** *See 5 Axillary Artery, Right* **7 Brachial Artery, Right** Inferior ulnar collateral artery Profunda brachii Superior ulnar collateral artery **8 Brachial Artery, Left** *See 7 Brachial Artery, Right* **9 Ulnar Artery, Right** Anterior ulnar recurrent artery Common interosseous artery Posterior ulnar recurrent artery **A Ulnar Artery, Left** *See 9 Ulnar Artery, Right* **B Radial Artery, Right** Radial recurrent artery **C Radial Artery, Left** *See B Radial Artery, Right* **D Hand Artery, Right** Deep palmar arch Princeps pollicis artery Radialis indicis Superficial palmar arch **F Hand Artery, Left** *See D Hand Artery, Right* **G Intracranial Artery** Anterior cerebral artery Anterior choroidal artery Anterior communicating artery Basilar artery Circle of Willis Internal carotid artery, intracranial portion Middle cerebral artery Ophthalmic artery Posterior cerebral artery Posterior communicating artery Posterior inferior cerebellar artery (PICA)	**H Common Carotid Artery, Right** **J Common Carotid Artery, Left** **K Internal Carotid Artery, Right** Caroticotympanic artery Carotid sinus **L Internal Carotid Artery, Left** *See K Internal Carotid Artery, Right* **M External Carotid Artery, Right** Ascending pharyngeal artery Internal maxillary artery Lingual artery Maxillary artery Occipital artery Posterior auricular artery Superior thyroid artery **N External Carotid Artery, Left** *See M External Carotid Artery, Right* **P Vertebral Artery, Right** Anterior spinal artery Posterior spinal artery **Q Vertebral Artery, Left** *See P Vertebral Artery, Right* **R Face Artery** Angular artery Ascending palatine artery External maxillary artery Facial artery Inferior labial artery Submental artery Superior labial artery **S Temporal Artery, Right** Middle temporal artery Superficial temporal artery Transverse facial artery **T Temporal Artery, Left** *See S Temporal Artery, Right* **U Thyroid Artery, Right** Cricothyroid artery Hyoid artery Sternocleidomastoid artery Superior laryngeal artery Superior thyroid artery Thyrocervical trunk **V Thyroid Artery, Left** *See U Thyroid Artery, Right* **Y Upper Artery** Aortic intercostal artery Bronchial artery Esophageal artery Subcostal artery	**Ø Open** **3 Percutaneous** **4 Percutaneous Endoscopic**	**Z No Device**	**Z No Qualifier**

NC Noncovered Procedure   **LC** Limited Coverage   **QA** Questionable OB Admit   **NT** New Tech Add-on   ⊞ Combination Member   ♂ Male   ♀ Female

ICD-10-PCS 2023   **199**

035–035

Upper Arteries

Ø	Medical and Surgical
3	Upper Arteries
7	Dilation

Definition: Expanding an orifice or the lumen of a tubular body part

Explanation: The orifice can be a natural orifice or an artificially created orifice. Accomplished by stretching a tubular body part using intraluminal pressure or by cutting part of the orifice or wall of the tubular body part.

Body Part Character 4		Approach Character 5	Device Character 6	Qualifier Character 7
Ø Internal Mammary Artery, Right Anterior intercostal artery Internal thoracic artery Musculophrenic artery Pericardiophrenic artery Superior epigastric artery **1 Internal Mammary Artery, Left** *See Ø Internal Mammary Artery, Right* **2 Innominate Artery** Brachiocephalic artery Brachiocephalic trunk **3 Subclavian Artery, Right** Costocervical trunk Dorsal scapular artery Internal thoracic artery **4 Subclavian Artery, Left** *See 3 Subclavian Artery, Right* **5 Axillary Artery, Right** Anterior circumflex humeral artery Lateral thoracic artery Posterior circumflex humeral artery Subscapular artery Superior thoracic artery Thoracoacromial artery	**6 Axillary Artery, Left** *See 5 Axillary Artery, Right* **7 Brachial Artery, Right** Inferior ulnar collateral artery Profunda brachii Superior ulnar collateral artery **8 Brachial Artery, Left** *See 7 Brachial Artery, Right* **9 Ulnar Artery, Right** Anterior ulnar recurrent artery Common interosseous artery Posterior ulnar recurrent artery **A Ulnar Artery, Left** *See 9 Ulnar Artery, Right* **B Radial Artery, Right** Radial recurrent artery **C Radial Artery, Left** *See B Radial Artery, Right*	**Ø Open** **3 Percutaneous** **4 Percutaneous Endoscopic**	**4 Intraluminal Device, Drug-eluting** **5 Intraluminal Device, Drug-eluting, Two** **6 Intraluminal Device, Drug-eluting, Three** **7 Intraluminal Device, Drug-eluting, Four or More** **E Intraluminal Device, Two** **F Intraluminal Device, Three** **G Intraluminal Device, Four or More**	**Z No Qualifier**
Ø Internal Mammary Artery, Right Anterior intercostal artery Internal thoracic artery Musculophrenic artery Pericardiophrenic artery Superior epigastric artery **1 Internal Mammary Artery, Left** *See Ø Internal Mammary Artery, Right* **2 Innominate Artery** Brachiocephalic artery Brachiocephalic trunk **3 Subclavian Artery, Right** Costocervical trunk Dorsal scapular artery Internal thoracic artery **4 Subclavian Artery, Left** *See 3 Subclavian Artery, Right* **5 Axillary Artery, Right** Anterior circumflex humeral artery Lateral thoracic artery Posterior circumflex humeral artery Subscapular artery Superior thoracic artery Thoracoacromial artery	**6 Axillary Artery, Left** *See 5 Axillary Artery, Right* **7 Brachial Artery, Right** Inferior ulnar collateral artery Profunda brachii Superior ulnar collateral artery **8 Brachial Artery, Left** *See 7 Brachial Artery, Right* **9 Ulnar Artery, Right** Anterior ulnar recurrent artery Common interosseous artery Posterior ulnar recurrent artery **A Ulnar Artery, Left** *See 9 Ulnar Artery, Right* **B Radial Artery, Right** Radial recurrent artery **C Radial Artery, Left** *See B Radial Artery, Right*	**Ø Open** **3 Percutaneous** **4 Percutaneous Endoscopic**	**D Intraluminal Device** **Z No Device**	**1 Drug-Coated Balloon** **Z No Qualifier**

Ø37 Continued on next page

Non-OR Procedure   DRG Non-OR Procedure   Valid OR Procedure   HAC Associated Procedure   Combination Only   New/Revised April   New/Revised October

Ø   **Medical and Surgical**   *Ø37 Continued*
3   **Upper Arteries**
7   **Dilation**   Definition: Expanding an orifice or the lumen of a tubular body part

Explanation: The orifice can be a natural orifice or an artificially created orifice. Accomplished by stretching a tubular body part using intraluminal pressure or by cutting part of the orifice or wall of the tubular body part.

Body Part Character 4		Approach Character 5	Device Character 6	Qualifier Character 7

D Hand Artery, Right
Deep palmar arch
Princeps pollicis artery
Radialis indicis
Superficial palmar arch
F Hand Artery, Left
See D Hand Artery, Right
G Intracranial Artery [NC]
Anterior cerebral artery
Anterior choroidal artery
Anterior communicating artery
Basilar artery
Circle of Willis
Internal carotid artery,
   intracranial portion
Middle cerebral artery
Ophthalmic artery
Posterior cerebral artery
Posterior communicating
   artery
Posterior inferior cerebellar
   artery (PICA)
**H Common Carotid Artery,
   Right**
J Common Carotid Artery, Left
K Internal Carotid Artery, Right
Caroticotympanic artery
Carotid sinus
L Internal Carotid Artery, Left
*See K Internal Carotid Artery,
   Right*
M External Carotid Artery, Right
Ascending pharyngeal artery
Internal maxillary artery
Lingual artery
Maxillary artery
Occipital artery
Posterior auricular artery
Superior thyroid artery
	N External Carotid Artery, Left
	*See M External Carotid Artery,
	   Right*
	P Vertebral Artery, Right
	Anterior spinal artery
	Posterior spinal artery
	Q Vertebral Artery, Left
	See P Vertebral Artery, Right
	R Face Artery
	Angular artery
	Ascending palatine artery
	External maxillary artery
	Facial artery
	Inferior labial artery
	Submental artery
	Superior labial artery
	S Temporal Artery, Right
	Middle temporal artery
	Superficial temporal artery
	Transverse facial artery
	T Temporal Artery, Left
	See S Temporal Artery, Right
	U Thyroid Artery, Right
	Cricothyroid artery
	Hyoid artery
	Sternocleidomastoid artery
	Superior laryngeal artery
	Superior thyroid artery
	Thyrocervical trunk
	V Thyroid Artery, Left
	See U Thyroid Artery, Right
	Y Upper Artery
	Aortic intercostal artery
	Bronchial artery
	Esophageal artery
	Subcostal artery
		Ø Open
		3 Percutaneous
		4 Percutaneous Endoscopic
			**4 Intraluminal Device,
			   Drug-eluting**
			**5 Intraluminal Device, Drug-
			   eluting, Two**
			**6 Intraluminal Device, Drug-
			   eluting, Three**
			**7 Intraluminal Device, Drug-
			   eluting, Four or More**
			D Intraluminal Device
			E Intraluminal Device, Two
			F Intraluminal Device, Three
			**G Intraluminal Device, Four
			   or More**
			Z No Device
				Z No Qualifier

[NC]   Ø37G[3,4]ZZ

[NC] Noncovered Procedure   [LC] Limited Coverage   [QA] Questionable OB Admit   [NT] New Tech Add-on   ⊞ Combination Member   ♂ Male   ♀ Female

ICD-10-PCS 2023   201

Ø37–Ø37

Ø   Medical and Surgical
3   Upper Arteries
9   Drainage   Definition: Taking or letting out fluids and/or gases from a body part

Explanation: The qualifier DIAGNOSTIC is used to identify drainage procedures that are biopsies

Body Part Character 4		Approach Character 5	Device Character 6	Qualifier Character 7
Ø Internal Mammary Artery, Right Anterior intercostal artery Internal thoracic artery Musculophrenic artery Pericardiophrenic artery Superior epigastric artery	**H Common Carotid Artery, Right** **J Common Carotid Artery, Left** **K Internal Carotid Artery, Right** Caroticotympanic artery Carotid sinus	**Ø Open** **3 Percutaneous** **4 Percutaneous Endoscopic**	**Ø Drainage Device**	**Z No Qualifier**
1 Internal Mammary Artery, Left *See Ø Internal Mammary Artery, Right above*	**L Internal Carotid Artery, Left** *See K Internal Carotid Artery, Right*			
2 Innominate Artery Brachiocephalic artery Brachiocephalic trunk	**M External Carotid Artery, Right** Ascending pharyngeal artery Internal maxillary artery Lingual artery Maxillary artery Occipital artery Posterior auricular artery Superior thyroid artery			
3 Subclavian Artery, Right Costocervical trunk Dorsal scapular artery Internal thoracic artery				
4 Subclavian Artery, Left *See 3 Subclavian Artery, Right*	**N External Carotid Artery, Left** *See M External Carotid Artery, Right*			
5 Axillary Artery, Right Anterior circumflex humeral artery Lateral thoracic artery Posterior circumflex humeral artery Subscapular artery Superior thoracic artery Thoracoacromial artery	**P Vertebral Artery, Right** Anterior spinal artery Posterior spinal artery **Q Vertebral Artery, Left** *See P Vertebral Artery, Right* **R Face Artery** Angular artery Ascending palatine artery External maxillary artery Facial artery Inferior labial artery Submental artery Superior labial artery			
6 Axillary Artery, Left *See 5 Axillary Artery, Right*				
7 Brachial Artery, Right Inferior ulnar collateral artery Profunda brachii Superior ulnar collateral artery	**S Temporal Artery, Right** Middle temporal artery Superficial temporal artery Transverse facial artery			
8 Brachial Artery, Left *See 7 Brachial Artery, Right*				
9 Ulnar Artery, Right Anterior ulnar recurrent artery Common interosseous artery Posterior ulnar recurrent artery	**T Temporal Artery, Left** *See S Temporal Artery, Right* **U Thyroid Artery, Right** Cricothyroid artery Hyoid artery Sternocleidomastoid artery Superior laryngeal artery Superior thyroid artery Thyrocervical trunk			
A Ulnar Artery, Left *See 9 Ulnar Artery, Right*				
B Radial Artery, Right Radial recurrent artery				
C Radial Artery, Left *See B Radial Artery, Right*	**V Thyroid Artery, Left** *See U Thyroid Artery, Right*			
D Hand Artery, Right Deep palmar arch Princeps pollicis artery Radialis indicis Superficial palmar arch	**Y Upper Artery** Aortic intercostal artery Bronchial artery Esophageal artery Subcostal artery			
F Hand Artery, Left *See D Hand Artery, Right*				
G Intracranial Artery Anterior cerebral artery Anterior choroidal artery Anterior communicating artery Basilar artery Circle of Willis Internal carotid artery, intracranial portion Middle cerebral artery Ophthalmic artery Posterior cerebral artery Posterior communicating artery Posterior inferior cerebellar artery (PICA)				

Non-OR   Ø39[Ø,1,2,3,4,5,6,7,8,9,A,B,C,D,F,G,H,J,K,L,M,N,P,Q,R,S,T,U,V,Y][Ø,3,4]ØZ

Ø39 Continued on next page

Non-OR Procedure   DRG Non-OR Procedure   Valid OR Procedure   HAC Associated Procedure   Combination Only   New/Revised April   New/Revised October

202   ICD-10-PCS 2023

Ø39–Ø39

Ø   **Medical and Surgical**   *039 Continued*
3   **Upper Arteries**
9   **Drainage**   Definition: Taking or letting out fluids and/or gases from a body part

                       Explanation: The qualifier DIAGNOSTIC is used to identify drainage procedures that are biopsies

Body Part Character 4		Approach Character 5	Device Character 6	Qualifier Character 7
Ø Internal Mammary Artery, Right Anterior intercostal artery Internal thoracic artery Musculophrenic artery Pericardiophrenic artery Superior epigastric artery	**H Common Carotid Artery, Right** **J Common Carotid Artery, Left** **K Internal Carotid Artery, Right** Caroticotympanic artery Carotid sinus	**Ø Open** **3 Percutaneous** **4 Percutaneous Endoscopic**	**Z No Device**	**X Diagnostic** **Z No Qualifier**
1 Internal Mammary Artery, Left *See Ø Internal Mammary Artery, Right*	**L Internal Carotid Artery, Left** *See K Internal Carotid Artery, Right*			
2 Innominate Artery Brachiocephalic artery Brachiocephalic trunk	**M External Carotid Artery, Right** Ascending pharyngeal artery Internal maxillary artery Lingual artery			
3 Subclavian Artery, Right Costocervical trunk Dorsal scapular artery Internal thoracic artery	Maxillary artery Occipital artery Posterior auricular artery Superior thyroid artery			
4 Subclavian Artery, Left *See 3 Subclavian Artery, Right*	**N External Carotid Artery, Left** *See M External Carotid Artery, Right*			
5 Axillary Artery, Right Anterior circumflex humeral artery Lateral thoracic artery Posterior circumflex humeral artery Subscapular artery Superior thoracic artery Thoracoacromial artery	**P Vertebral Artery, Right** Anterior spinal artery Posterior spinal artery **Q Vertebral Artery, Left** *See P Vertebral Artery, Right* **R Face Artery** Angular artery Ascending palatine artery External maxillary artery			
6 Axillary Artery, Left *See 5 Axillary Artery, Right*	Facial artery Inferior labial artery			
7 Brachial Artery, Right Inferior ulnar collateral artery Profunda brachii Superior ulnar collateral artery	Submental artery Superior labial artery **S Temporal Artery, Right** Middle temporal artery			
8 Brachial Artery, Left *See 7 Brachial Artery, Right*	Superficial temporal artery Transverse facial artery			
9 Ulnar Artery, Right Anterior ulnar recurrent artery Common interosseous artery Posterior ulnar recurrent artery	**T Temporal Artery, Left** *See S Temporal Artery, Right* **U Thyroid Artery, Right** Cricothyroid artery			
A Ulnar Artery, Left *See 9 Ulnar Artery, Right*	Hyoid artery Sternocleidomastoid artery Superior laryngeal artery			
B Radial Artery, Right Radial recurrent artery	Superior thyroid artery Thyrocervical trunk			
C Radial Artery, Left *See B Radial Artery, Right*	**V Thyroid Artery, Left** *See U Thyroid Artery, Right*			
D Hand Artery, Right Deep palmar arch Princeps pollicis artery Radialis indicis Superficial palmar arch	**Y Upper Artery** Aortic intercostal artery Bronchial artery Esophageal artery Subcostal artery			
F Hand Artery, Left *See D Hand Artery, Right*				
G Intracranial Artery Anterior cerebral artery Anterior choroidal artery Anterior communicating artery Basilar artery Circle of Willis Internal carotid artery, intracranial portion Middle cerebral artery Ophthalmic artery Posterior cerebral artery Posterior communicating artery Posterior inferior cerebellar artery (PICA)				

Non-OR   Ø39[Ø,1,2,3,4,5,6,7,8,9,A,B,C,D,F,G,H,J,K,L,M,N,P,Q,R,S,T,U,V,Y]3ZX
Non-OR   Ø39[Ø,1,2,3,4,5,6,7,8,9,A,B,C,D,F,G,H,J,K,L,M,N,P,Q,R,S,T,U,V,Y][Ø,3,4]ZZ

NC Noncovered Procedure   **LC** Limited Coverage   **QA** Questionable OB Admit   **NT** New Tech Add-on   ⊞ Combination Member   ♂ Male   ♀ Female

ICD-10-PCS 2023   **203**

Ø39–Ø39

Ø   Medical and Surgical
3   Upper Arteries
B   Excision   Definition: Cutting out or off, without replacement, a portion of a body part

                   Explanation: The qualifier DIAGNOSTIC is used to identify excision procedures that are biopsies

Body Part Character 4		Approach Character 5	Device Character 6	Qualifier Character 7
Ø Internal Mammary Artery, Right Anterior intercostal artery Internal thoracic artery Musculophrenic artery Pericardiophrenic artery Superior epigastric artery	**H Common Carotid Artery, Right**	**Ø Open** **3 Percutaneous** **4 Percutaneous Endoscopic**	**Z No Device**	**X Diagnostic** **Z No Qualifier**
	J Common Carotid Artery, Left			
	K Internal Carotid Artery, Right Caroticotympanic artery Carotid sinus			
1 Internal Mammary Artery, Left *See Ø Internal Mammary Artery, Right*	**L Internal Carotid Artery, Left** *See K Internal Carotid Artery, Right*			
2 Innominate Artery Brachiocephalic artery Brachiocephalic trunk	**M External Carotid Artery, Right** Ascending pharyngeal artery Internal maxillary artery Lingual artery Maxillary artery Occipital artery Posterior auricular artery Superior thyroid artery			
3 Subclavian Artery, Right Costocervical trunk Dorsal scapular artery Internal thoracic artery				
4 Subclavian Artery, Left *See 3 Subclavian Artery, Right*	**N External Carotid Artery, Left** *See M External Carotid Artery, Right*			
5 Axillary Artery, Right Anterior circumflex humeral artery Lateral thoracic artery Posterior circumflex humeral artery Subscapular artery Superior thoracic artery Thoracoacromial artery	**P Vertebral Artery, Right** Anterior spinal artery Posterior spinal artery			
	Q Vertebral Artery, Left *See P Vertebral Artery, Right*			
	R Face Artery Angular artery Ascending palatine artery External maxillary artery Facial artery Inferior labial artery Submental artery Superior labial artery			
6 Axillary Artery, Left *See 5 Axillary Artery, Right*				
7 Brachial Artery, Right Inferior ulnar collateral artery Profunda brachii Superior ulnar collateral artery	**S Temporal Artery, Right** Middle temporal artery Superficial temporal artery Transverse facial artery			
8 Brachial Artery, Left *See 7 Brachial Artery, Right*	**T Temporal Artery, Left** *See S Temporal Artery, Right*			
9 Ulnar Artery, Right Anterior ulnar recurrent artery Common interosseous artery Posterior ulnar recurrent artery	**U Thyroid Artery, Right** Cricothyroid artery Hyoid artery Sternocleidomastoid artery Superior laryngeal artery Superior thyroid artery Thyrocervical trunk			
A Ulnar Artery, Left *See 9 Ulnar Artery, Right*				
B Radial Artery, Right Radial recurrent artery				
C Radial Artery, Left *See B Radial Artery, Right*	**V Thyroid Artery, Left** *See U Thyroid Artery, Right*			
D Hand Artery, Right Deep palmar arch Princeps pollicis artery Radialis indicis Superficial palmar arch	**Y Upper Artery** Aortic intercostal artery Bronchial artery Esophageal artery Subcostal artery			
F Hand Artery, Left *See D Hand Artery, Right*				
G Intracranial Artery Anterior cerebral artery Anterior choroidal artery Anterior communicating artery Basilar artery Circle of Willis Internal carotid artery, intracranial portion Middle cerebral artery Ophthalmic artery Posterior cerebral artery Posterior communicating artery Posterior inferior cerebellar artery (PICA)				

Non-OR Procedure   DRG Non-OR Procedure   Valid OR Procedure   HAC Associated Procedure   Combination Only   New/Revised April   New/Revised October

0   **Medical and Surgical**
3   **Upper Arteries**
C   **Extirpation**   Definition: Taking or cutting out solid matter from a body part

Explanation: The solid matter may be an abnormal byproduct of a biological function or a foreign body; it may be imbedded in a body part or in the lumen of a tubular body part. The solid matter may or may not have been previously broken into pieces.

Body Part Character 4		Approach Character 5	Device Character 6	Qualifier Character 7
0 Internal Mammary Artery, Right Anterior intercostal artery Internal thoracic artery Musculophrenic artery Pericardiophrenic artery Superior epigastric artery **1 Internal Mammary Artery, Left** *See 0 Internal Mammary Artery, Right* **2 Innominate Artery** Brachiocephalic artery Brachiocephalic trunk **3 Subclavian Artery, Right** Costocervical trunk Dorsal scapular artery Internal thoracic artery **4 Subclavian Artery, Left** *See 3 Subclavian Artery, Right* **5 Axillary Artery, Right** Anterior circumflex humeral artery Lateral thoracic artery Posterior circumflex humeral artery Subscapular artery Superior thoracic artery Thoracoacromial artery **6 Axillary Artery, Left** *See 5 Axillary Artery, Right* **7 Brachial Artery, Right** Inferior ulnar collateral artery Profunda brachii Superior ulnar collateral artery **8 Brachial Artery, Left** *See 7 Brachial Artery, Right* **9 Ulnar Artery, Right** Anterior ulnar recurrent artery Common interosseous artery Posterior ulnar recurrent artery	**A Ulnar Artery, Left** *See 9 Ulnar Artery, Right* **B Radial Artery, Right** Radial recurrent artery **C Radial Artery, Left** *See B Radial Artery, Right* **D Hand Artery, Right** Deep palmar arch Princeps pollicis artery Radialis indicis Superficial palmar arch **F Hand Artery, Left** *See D Hand Artery, Right* **R Face Artery** Angular artery Ascending palatine artery External maxillary artery Facial artery Inferior labial artery Submental artery Superior labial artery **S Temporal Artery, Right** Middle temporal artery Superficial temporal artery Transverse facial artery **T Temporal Artery, Left** *See S Temporal Artery, Right* **U Thyroid Artery, Right** Cricothyroid artery Hyoid artery Sternocleidomastoid artery Superior laryngeal artery Superior thyroid artery Thyrocervical trunk **V Thyroid Artery, Left** *See U Thyroid Artery, Right* **Y Upper Artery** Aortic intercostal artery Bronchial artery Esophageal artery Subcostal artery	**0** Open **3** Percutaneous **4** Percutaneous Endoscopic	**Z** No Device	**Z** No Qualifier
G Intracranial Artery Anterior cerebral artery Anterior choroidal artery Anterior communicating artery Basilar artery Circle of Willis Internal carotid artery, intracranial portion Middle cerebral artery Ophthalmic artery Posterior cerebral artery Posterior communicating artery Posterior inferior cerebellar artery (PICA) **H Common Carotid Artery, Right** **J Common Carotid Artery, Left** **K Internal Carotid Artery, Right** Caroticotympanic artery Carotid sinus	**L Internal Carotid Artery, Left** *See K Internal Carotid Artery, Right* **M External Carotid Artery, Right** Ascending pharyngeal artery Internal maxillary artery Lingual artery Maxillary artery Occipital artery Posterior auricular artery Superior thyroid artery **N External Carotid Artery, Left** *See M External Carotid Artery, Right* **P Vertebral Artery, Right** Anterior spinal artery Posterior spinal artery **Q Vertebral Artery, Left** *See P Vertebral Artery, Right*	**0** Open **4** Percutaneous Endoscopic	**Z** No Device	**Z** No Qualifier

03C Continued on next page

NC Noncovered Procedure   **LC** Limited Coverage   **QA** Questionable OB Admit   **NT** New Tech Add-on   ⊞ Combination Member   ♂ Male   ♀ Female

ICD-10-PCS 2023   205

03C–03C

Ø Medical and Surgical
3 Upper Arteries
C Extirpation

Definition: Taking or cutting out solid matter from a body part

Explanation: The solid matter may be an abnormal byproduct of a biological function or a foreign body; it may be imbedded in a body part or in the lumen of a tubular body part. The solid matter may or may not have been previously broken into pieces.

Body Part Character 4		Approach Character 5	Device Character 6	Qualifier Character 7
G Intracranial Artery Anterior cerebral artery Anterior choroidal artery Anterior communicating artery Basilar artery Circle of Willis Internal carotid artery, intracranial portion Middle cerebral artery Ophthalmic artery Posterior cerebral artery Posterior communicating artery Posterior inferior cerebellar artery (PICA) **H Common Carotid Artery, Right** **J Common Carotid Artery, Left** **K Internal Carotid Artery, Right** Caroticotympanic artery Carotid sinus	**L Internal Carotid Artery, Left** *See K Internal Carotid Artery, Right* **M External Carotid Artery, Right** Ascending pharyngeal artery Internal maxillary artery Lingual artery Maxillary artery Occipital artery Posterior auricular artery Superior thyroid artery **N External Carotid Artery, Left** *See M External Carotid Artery, Right* **P Vertebral Artery, Right** Anterior spinal artery Posterior spinal artery **Q Vertebral Artery, Left** *See P Vertebral Artery, Right*	**3 Percutaneous**	**Z No Device**	**7 Stent Retriever** **Z No Qualifier**

Ø Medical and Surgical
3 Upper Arteries
F Fragmentation

Definition: Breaking solid matter in a body part into pieces

Explanation: Physical force (e.g., manual, ultrasonic) applied directly or indirectly is used to break the solid matter into pieces. The solid matter may be an abnormal byproduct of a biological function or a foreign body. The pieces of solid matter are not taken out.

Body Part Character 4		Approach Character 5	Device Character 6	Qualifier Character 7
2 Innominate Artery Brachiocephalic artery Brachiocephalic trunk **3 Subclavian Artery, Right** Costocervical trunk Dorsal scapular artery Internal thoracic artery **4 Subclavian Artery, Left** *See 3 Subclavian Artery, Right* **5 Axillary Artery, Right** Anterior circumflex humeral artery Lateral thoracic artery Posterior circumflex humeral artery Subscapular artery Superior thoracic artery Thoracoacromial artery **6 Axillary Artery, Left** *See 5 Axillary Artery, Right* **7 Brachial Artery, Right** Inferior ulnar collateral artery Profunda brachii Superior ulnar collateral artery **8 Brachial Artery, Left** *See 7 Brachial Artery, Right*	**9 Ulnar Artery, Right** Anterior ulnar recurrent artery Common interosseous artery Posterior ulnar recurrent artery **A Ulnar Artery, Left** *See 9 Ulnar Artery, Right* **B Radial Artery, Right** Radial recurrent artery **C Radial Artery, Left** *See B Radial Artery, Right* **G Intracranial Artery** Anterior cerebral artery Anterior choroidal artery Anterior communicating artery Basilar artery Circle of Willis Internal carotid artery, intracranial portion Middle cerebral artery Ophthalmic artery Posterior cerebral artery Posterior communicating artery Posterior inferior cerebellar artery (PICA) **Y Upper Artery** Aortic intercostal artery Bronchial artery Esophageal artery Subcostal artery	**3 Percutaneous**	**Z No Device**	**Ø Ultrasonic** **Z No Qualifier**

03C Continued on next page

Ø **Medical and Surgical**
3 **Upper Arteries**
H **Insertion**   Definition: Putting in a nonbiological appliance that monitors, assists, performs, or prevents a physiological function but does not physically take the place of a body part
          Explanation: None

Body Part Character 4		Approach Character 5	Device Character 6	Qualifier Character 7
Ø **Internal Mammary Artery, Right** Anterior intercostal artery Internal thoracic artery Musculophrenic artery Pericardiophrenic artery Superior epigastric artery **1** **Internal Mammary Artery, Left** *See* Ø *Internal Mammary Artery, Right* **2** **Innominate Artery** Brachiocephalic artery Brachiocephalic trunk **3** **Subclavian Artery, Right** Costocervical trunk Dorsal scapular artery Internal thoracic artery **4** **Subclavian Artery, Left** *See* 3 *Subclavian Artery, Right* **5** **Axillary Artery, Right** Anterior circumflex humeral artery Lateral thoracic artery Posterior circumflex humeral artery Subscapular artery Superior thoracic artery Thoracoacromial artery **6** **Axillary Artery, Left** *See* 5 *Axillary Artery, Right* **7** **Brachial Artery, Right** Inferior ulnar collateral artery Profunda brachii Superior ulnar collateral artery **8** **Brachial Artery, Left** *See* 7 *Brachial Artery, Right* **9** **Ulnar Artery, Right** Anterior ulnar recurrent artery Common interosseous artery Posterior ulnar recurrent artery **A** **Ulnar Artery, Left** *See* 9 *Ulnar Artery, Right* **B** **Radial Artery, Right** Radial recurrent artery **C** **Radial Artery, Left** *See* B *Radial Artery, Right* **D** **Hand Artery, Right** Deep palmar arch Princeps pollicis artery Radialis indicis Superficial palmar arch **F** **Hand Artery, Left** *See* D *Hand Artery, Right*	**G** **Intracranial Artery** Anterior cerebral artery Anterior choroidal artery Anterior communicating artery Basilar artery Circle of Willis Internal carotid artery, intracranial portion Middle cerebral artery Ophthalmic artery Posterior cerebral artery Posterior communicating artery Posterior inferior cerebellar artery (PICA) **H** **Common Carotid Artery, Right** **J** **Common Carotid Artery, Left** **M** **External Carotid Artery, Right** Ascending pharyngeal artery Internal maxillary artery Lingual artery Maxillary artery Occipital artery Posterior auricular artery Superior thyroid artery **N** **External Carotid Artery, Left** *See* M *External Carotid Artery, Right* **P** **Vertebral Artery, Right** Anterior spinal artery Posterior spinal artery **Q** **Vertebral Artery, Left** *See* P *Vertebral Artery, Right* **R** **Face Artery** Angular artery Ascending palatine artery External maxillary artery Facial artery Inferior labial artery Submental artery Superior labial artery **S** **Temporal Artery, Right** Middle temporal artery Superficial temporal artery Transverse facial artery **T** **Temporal Artery, Left** *See* S *Temporal Artery, Right* **U** **Thyroid Artery, Right** Cricothyroid artery Hyoid artery Sternocleidomastoid artery Superior laryngeal artery Superior thyroid artery Thyrocervical trunk **V** **Thyroid Artery, Left** *See* U *Thyroid Artery, Right*	**Ø** Open **3** Percutaneous **4** Percutaneous Endoscopic	**3** Infusion Device **D** Intraluminal Device	**Z** No Qualifier
K **Internal Carotid Artery, Right** Caroticotympanic artery Carotid sinus **L** **Internal Carotid Artery, Left** *See* K *Internal Carotid Artery, Right*		**Ø** Open **3** Percutaneous **4** Percutaneous Endoscope	**3** Infusion Device **D** Intraluminal Device **M** Stimulator Lead	**Z** No Qualifier
Y **Upper Artery** Aortic intercostal artery Bronchial artery Esophageal artery Subcostal artery		**Ø** Open **3** Percutaneous **4** Percutaneous Endoscopic	**2** Monitoring Device **3** Infusion Device **D** Intraluminal Device **Y** Other Device	**Z** No Qualifier

Non-OR	Ø3H[Ø,1,2,3,4,5,6,7,8,9,A,B,C,D,F,G,H,J,M,N,P,Q,R,S,T,U,V][Ø,3,4]3Z
Non-OR	Ø3H[K,L][Ø,3,4]3Z
Non-OR	Ø3HY[Ø,3,4]3Z
Non-OR	Ø3HY32Z
Non-OR	Ø3HY[3,4]YZ

NC Noncovered Procedure   LC Limited Coverage   QA Questionable OB Admit   NT New Tech Add-on   ⊞ Combination Member   ♂Male   ♀Female

0 Medical and Surgical
3 Upper Arteries
J Inspection   Definition: Visually and/or manually exploring a body part

Explanation: Visual exploration may be performed with or without optical instrumentation. Manual exploration may be performed directly or through intervening body layers.

Body Part Character 4	Approach Character 5	Device Character 6	Qualifier Character 7

Y Upper Artery
   Aortic intercostal artery
   Bronchial artery
   Esophageal artery
   Subcostal artery
	0 Open
	3 Percutaneous
	4 Percutaneous Endoscopic
	X External
		Z No Device	Z No Qualifier

Non-OR   03JY[3,4,X]ZZ

Non-OR Procedure   DRG Non-OR Procedure   Valid OR Procedure   HAC Associated Procedure   Combination Only   New/Revised April   New/Revised October

208   ICD-10-PCS 2023

03J–03J

Ø   Medical and Surgical
3   Upper Arteries
L   Occlusion   Definition: Completely closing an orifice or the lumen of a tubular body part
                          Explanation: The orifice can be a natural orifice or an artificially created orifice

Body Part Character 4		Approach Character 5	Device Character 6	Qualifier Character 7
Ø Internal Mammary Artery, Right Anterior intercostal artery Internal thoracic artery Musculophrenic artery Pericardiophrenic artery Superior epigastric artery **1 Internal Mammary Artery, Left** *See Ø Internal Mammary Artery, Left* **2 Innominate Artery** Brachiocephalic artery Brachiocephalic trunk **3 Subclavian Artery, Right** Costocervical trunk Dorsal scapular artery Internal thoracic artery **4 Subclavian Artery, Left** *See 3 Subclavian Artery, Right* **5 Axillary Artery, Right** Anterior circumflex humeral artery Lateral thoracic artery Posterior circumflex humeral artery Subscapular artery Superior thoracic artery Thoracoacromial artery **6 Axillary Artery, Left** *See 5 Axillary Artery, Right* **7 Brachial Artery, Right** Inferior ulnar collateral artery Profunda brachii Superior ulnar collateral artery **8 Brachial Artery, Left** *See 7 Brachial Artery, Right* **9 Ulnar Artery, Right** Anterior ulnar recurrent artery Common interosseous artery Posterior ulnar recurrent artery	**A Ulnar Artery, Left** *See 9 Ulnar Artery, Right* **B Radial Artery, Right** Radial recurrent artery **C Radial Artery, Left** *See B Radial Artery, Right* **D Hand Artery, Right** Deep palmar arch Princeps pollicis artery Radialis indicis Superficial palmar arch **F Hand Artery, Left** *See D Hand Artery, Right* **R Face Artery** Angular artery Ascending palatine artery External maxillary artery Facial artery Inferior labial artery Submental artery Superior labial artery **S Temporal Artery, Right** Middle temporal artery Superficial temporal artery Transverse facial artery **T Temporal Artery, Left** *See S Temporal Artery, Right* **U Thyroid Artery, Right** Cricothyroid artery Hyoid artery Sternocleidomastoid artery Superior laryngeal artery Superior thyroid artery Thyrocervical trunk **V Thyroid Artery, Left** *See U Thyroid Artery, Right* **Y Upper Artery** Aortic intercostal artery Bronchial artery Esophageal artery Subcostal artery	**Ø Open** **3 Percutaneous** **4 Percutaneous Endoscopic**	**C Extraluminal Device** **D Intraluminal Device** **Z No Device**	**Z No Qualifier**
G Intracranial Artery Anterior cerebral artery Anterior choroidal artery Anterior communicating artery Basilar artery Circle of Willis Internal carotid artery, intracranial portion Middle cerebral artery Ophthalmic artery Posterior cerebral artery Posterior communicating artery Posterior inferior cerebellar artery (PICA) **H Common Carotid Artery, Right** **J Common Carotid Artery, Left** **K Internal Carotid Artery, Right** Caroticotympanic artery Carotid sinus	**L Internal Carotid Artery, Left** *See K Internal Carotid Artery, Right* **M External Carotid Artery, Right** Ascending pharyngeal artery Internal maxillary artery Lingual artery Maxillary artery Occipital artery Posterior auricular artery Superior thyroid artery **N External Carotid Artery, Left** *See M External Carotid Artery, Right* **P Vertebral Artery, Right** Anterior spinal artery Posterior spinal artery **Q Vertebral Artery, Left** *See P Vertebral Artery, Right*	**Ø Open** **3 Percutaneous** **4 Percutaneous Endoscopic**	**B Intraluminal Device, Bioactive** **C Extraluminal Device** **D Intraluminal Device** **Z No Device**	**Z No Qualifier**

NC Noncovered Procedure   LC Limited Coverage   QA Questionable OB Admit   NT New Tech Add-on   ⊞ Combination Member   ♂ Male   ♀ Female

ICD-10-PCS 2023   **209**

Ø3L–Ø3L

Upper Arteries

Ø Medical and Surgical
3 Upper Arteries
N Release   Definition: Freeing a body part from an abnormal physical constraint by cutting or by the use of force
              Explanation: Some of the restraining tissue may be taken out but none of the body part is taken out

Body Part Character 4		Approach Character 5	Device Character 6	Qualifier Character 7
Ø Internal Mammary Artery, Right	**H Common Carotid Artery, Right**	**Ø Open**	**Z No Device**	**Z No Qualifier**
Anterior intercostal artery	**J Common Carotid Artery, Left**	**3 Percutaneous**		
Internal thoracic artery	**K Internal Carotid Artery, Right**	**4 Percutaneous Endoscopic**		
Musculophrenic artery	Caroticotympanic artery			
Pericardiophrenic artery	Carotid sinus			
Superior epigastric artery	**L Internal Carotid Artery, Left**			
1 Internal Mammary Artery, Left	*See K Internal Carotid Artery, Right*			
See Ø Internal Mammary Artery, Right	**M External Carotid Artery, Right**			
2 Innominate Artery	Ascending pharyngeal artery			
Brachiocephalic artery	Internal maxillary artery			
Brachiocephalic trunk	Lingual artery			
3 Subclavian Artery, Right	Maxillary artery			
Costocervical trunk	Occipital artery			
Dorsal scapular artery	Posterior auricular artery			
Internal thoracic artery	Superior thyroid artery			
4 Subclavian Artery, Left	**N External Carotid Artery, Left**			
See 3 Subclavian Artery, Right	*See M External Carotid Artery, Right*			
5 Axillary Artery, Right	**P Vertebral Artery, Right**			
Anterior circumflex humeral artery	Anterior spinal artery			
Lateral thoracic artery	Posterior spinal artery			
Posterior circumflex humeral artery	**Q Vertebral Artery, Left**			
Subscapular artery	*See P Vertebral Artery, Right*			
Superior thoracic artery	**R Face Artery**			
Thoracoacromial artery	Angular artery			
6 Axillary Artery, Left	Ascending palatine artery			
See 5 Axillary Artery, Right	External maxillary artery			
7 Brachial Artery, Right	Facial artery			
Inferior ulnar collateral artery	Inferior labial artery			
Profunda brachii	Submental artery			
Superior ulnar collateral artery	Superior labial artery			
8 Brachial Artery, Left	**S Temporal Artery, Right**			
See 7 Brachial Artery, Right	Middle temporal artery			
9 Ulnar Artery, Right	Superficial temporal artery			
Anterior ulnar recurrent artery	Transverse facial artery			
Common interosseous artery	**T Temporal Artery, Left**			
Posterior ulnar recurrent artery	*See S Temporal Artery, Right*			
A Ulnar Artery, Left	**U Thyroid Artery, Right**			
See 9 Ulnar Artery, Right	Cricothyroid artery			
B Radial Artery, Right	Hyoid artery			
Radial recurrent artery	Sternocleidomastoid artery			
C Radial Artery, Left	Superior laryngeal artery			
See B Radial Artery, Right	Superior thyroid artery			
D Hand Artery, Right	Thyrocervical trunk			
Deep palmar arch	**V Thyroid Artery, Left**			
Princeps pollicis artery	*See U Thyroid Artery, Right*			
Radialis indicis	**Y Upper Artery**			
Superficial palmar arch	Aortic intercostal artery			
F Hand Artery, Left	Bronchial artery			
See D Hand Artery, Right	Esophageal artery			
G Intracranial Artery	Subcostal artery			
Anterior cerebral artery				
Anterior choroidal artery				
Anterior communicating artery				
Basilar artery				
Circle of Willis				
Internal carotid artery, intracranial portion				
Middle cerebral artery				
Ophthalmic artery				
Posterior cerebral artery				
Posterior communicating artery				
Posterior inferior cerebellar artery (PICA)				

0   **Medical and Surgical**
3   **Upper Arteries**
P   **Removal**   Definition: Taking out or off a device from a body part

Explanation: If a device is taken out and a similar device put in without cutting or puncturing the skin or mucous membrane, the procedure is coded to the root operation CHANGE. Otherwise, the procedure for taking out a device is coded to the root operation REMOVAL.

Body Part Character 4	Approach Character 5	Device Character 6	Qualifier Character 7

Y   Upper Artery
   Aortic intercostal artery
   Bronchial artery
   Esophageal artery
   Subcostal artery
	0 Open
	3 Percutaneous
	4 Percutaneous Endoscopic
		0 Drainage Device
		2 Monitoring Device
		3 Infusion Device
		7 Autologous Tissue Substitute
		C Extraluminal Device
		D Intraluminal Device
		J Synthetic Substitute
		K Nonautologous Tissue Substitute
		M Stimulator Lead
		Y Other Device
			Z No Qualifier

Y   Upper Artery
   Aortic intercostal artery
   Bronchial artery
   Esophageal artery
   Subcostal artery
	X External	**0** Drainage Device
		2 Monitoring Device
		3 Infusion Device
		D Intraluminal Device
		M Stimulator Lead
			Z No Qualifier

Non-OR	03PY3[0,2,3,D]Z
Non-OR	03PY[3,4]YZ
Non-OR	03PYX[0,2,3,D,M]Z

Upper Arteries

Ø   **Medical and Surgical**
3   **Upper Arteries**
Q   **Repair**   Definition: Restoring, to the extent possible, a body part to its normal anatomic structure and function

Explanation: Used only when the method to accomplish the repair is not one of the other root operations

Body Part Character 4		Approach Character 5	Device Character 6	Qualifier Character 7
Ø Internal Mammary Artery, Right Anterior intercostal artery Internal thoracic artery Musculophrenic artery Pericardiophrenic artery Superior epigastric artery **1 Internal Mammary Artery, Left** *See Ø Internal Mammary Artery, Right* **2 Innominate Artery** Brachiocephalic artery Brachiocephalic trunk **3 Subclavian Artery, Right** Costocervical trunk Dorsal scapular artery Internal thoracic artery **4 Subclavian Artery, Left** *See 3 Subclavian Artery, Right* **5 Axillary Artery, Right** Anterior circumflex humeral artery Lateral thoracic artery Posterior circumflex humeral artery Subscapular artery Superior thoracic artery Thoracoacromial artery **6 Axillary Artery, Left** *See 5 Axillary Artery, Right* **7 Brachial Artery, Right** Inferior ulnar collateral artery Profunda brachii Superior ulnar collateral artery **8 Brachial Artery, Left** *See 7 Brachial Artery, Right* **9 Ulnar Artery, Right** Anterior ulnar recurrent artery Common interosseous artery Posterior ulnar recurrent artery **A Ulnar Artery, Left** *See 9 Ulnar Artery, Right* **B Radial Artery, Right** Radial recurrent artery **C Radial Artery, Left** *See B Radial Artery, Right* **D Hand Artery, Right** Deep palmar arch Princeps pollicis artery Radialis indicis Superficial palmar arch **F Hand Artery, Left** *See D Hand Artery, Right* **G Intracranial Artery** Anterior cerebral artery Anterior choroidal artery Anterior communicating artery Basilar artery Circle of Willis Internal carotid artery, intracranial portion Middle cerebral artery Ophthalmic artery Posterior cerebral artery Posterior communicating artery Posterior inferior cerebellar artery (PICA)	**H Common Carotid Artery, Right** **J Common Carotid Artery, Left** **K Internal Carotid Artery, Right** Caroticotympanic artery Carotid sinus **L Internal Carotid Artery, Left** *See K Internal Carotid Artery, Right* **M External Carotid Artery, Right** Ascending pharyngeal artery Internal maxillary artery Lingual artery Maxillary artery Occipital artery Posterior auricular artery Superior thyroid artery **N External Carotid Artery, Left** *See M External Carotid Artery, Right* **P Vertebral Artery, Right** Anterior spinal artery Posterior spinal artery **Q Vertebral Artery, Left** *See P Vertebral Artery, Right* **R Face Artery** Angular artery Ascending palatine artery External maxillary artery Facial artery Inferior labial artery Submental artery Superior labial artery **S Temporal Artery, Right** Middle temporal artery Superficial temporal artery Transverse facial artery **T Temporal Artery, Left** *See S Temporal Artery, Right* **U Thyroid Artery, Right** Cricothyroid artery Hyoid artery Sternocleidomastoid artery Superior laryngeal artery Superior thyroid artery Thyrocervical trunk **V Thyroid Artery, Left** *See U Thyroid Artery, Right* **Y Upper Artery** Aortic intercostal artery Bronchial artery Esophageal artery Subcostal artery	**Ø Open** **3 Percutaneous** **4 Percutaneous Endoscopic**	**Z No Device**	**Z No Qualifier**

Non-OR Procedure   DRG Non-OR Procedure   Valid OR Procedure   HAC Associated Procedure   Combination Only   New/Revised April   New/Revised October

212   ICD-10-PCS 2023

Ø   **Medical and Surgical**
3   **Upper Arteries**
R   **Replacement**   Definition: Putting in or on biological or synthetic material that physically takes the place and/or function of all or a portion of a body part
                     Explanation: The body part may have been taken out or replaced, or may be taken out, physically eradicated, or rendered nonfunctional during the REPLACEMENT procedure. A REMOVAL procedure is coded for taking out the device used in a previous replacement procedure.

Body Part Character 4		Approach Character 5	Device Character 6	Qualifier Character 7

Ø **Internal Mammary Artery, Right**
   Anterior intercostal artery
   Internal thoracic artery
   Musculophrenic artery
   Pericardiophrenic artery
   Superior epigastric artery
1 **Internal Mammary Artery, Left**
   See Ø Internal Mammary Artery, Right
2 **Innominate Artery**
   Brachiocephalic artery
   Brachiocephalic trunk
3 **Subclavian Artery, Right**
   Costocervical trunk
   Dorsal scapular artery
   Internal thoracic artery
4 **Subclavian Artery, Left**
   See 3 Subclavian Artery, Right
5 **Axillary Artery, Right**
   Anterior circumflex humeral artery
   Lateral thoracic artery
   Posterior circumflex humeral artery
   Subscapular artery
   Superior thoracic artery
   Thoracoacromial artery
6 **Axillary Artery, Left**
   See 5 Axillary Artery, Right
7 **Brachial Artery, Right**
   Inferior ulnar collateral artery
   Profunda brachii
   Superior ulnar collateral artery
8 **Brachial Artery, Left**
   See 7 Brachial Artery, Right
9 **Ulnar Artery, Right**
   Anterior ulnar recurrent artery
   Common interosseous artery
   Posterior ulnar recurrent artery
A **Ulnar Artery, Left**
   See 9 Ulnar Artery, Right
B **Radial Artery, Right**
   Radial recurrent artery
C **Radial Artery, Left**
   See B Radial Artery, Right
D **Hand Artery, Right**
   Deep palmar arch
   Princeps pollicis artery
   Radialis indicis
   Superficial palmar arch
F **Hand Artery, Left**
   See D Hand Artery, Right
G **Intracranial Artery**
   Anterior cerebral artery
   Anterior choroidal artery
   Anterior communicating artery
   Basilar artery
   Circle of Willis
   Internal carotid artery, intracranial portion
   Middle cerebral artery
   Ophthalmic artery
   Posterior cerebral artery
   Posterior communicating artery
   Posterior inferior cerebellar artery (PICA)
	H **Common Carotid Artery, Right**
	J **Common Carotid Artery, Left**
	K **Internal Carotid Artery, Right**
	   Caroticotympanic artery
	   Carotid sinus
	L **Internal Carotid Artery, Left**
	   See K Internal Carotid Artery, Right
	M **External Carotid Artery, Right**
	   Ascending pharyngeal artery
	   Internal maxillary artery
	   Lingual artery
	   Maxillary artery
	   Occipital artery
	   Posterior auricular artery
	   Superior thyroid artery
	N **External Carotid Artery, Left**
	   See M External Carotid Artery, Right
	P **Vertebral Artery, Right**
	   Anterior spinal artery
	   Posterior spinal artery
	Q **Vertebral Artery, Left**
	   See P Vertebral Artery, Right
	R **Face Artery**
	   Angular artery
	   Ascending palatine artery
	   External maxillary artery
	   Facial artery
	   Inferior labial artery
	   Submental artery
	   Superior labial artery
	S **Temporal Artery, Right**
	   Middle temporal artery
	   Superficial temporal artery
	   Transverse facial artery
	T **Temporal Artery, Left**
	   See S Temporal Artery, Right
	U **Thyroid Artery, Right**
	   Cricothyroid artery
	   Hyoid artery
	   Sternocleidomastoid artery
	   Superior laryngeal artery
	   Superior thyroid artery
	   Thyrocervical trunk
	V **Thyroid Artery, Left**
	   See U Thyroid Artery, Right
	Y **Upper Artery**
	   Aortic intercostal artery
	   Bronchial artery
	   Esophageal artery
	   Subcostal artery
		Ø Open
		4 Percutaneous Endoscopic
			7 Autologous Tissue Substitute
			J Synthetic Substitute
			K Nonautologous Tissue Substitute
				Z No Qualifier

NC Noncovered Procedure   LC Limited Coverage   QA Questionable OB Admit   NT New Tech Add-on   ⊞ Combination Member   ♂ Male   ♀ Female

ICD-10-PCS 2023   213

Upper Arteries

Ø   **Medical and Surgical**
3   **Upper Arteries**
S   **Reposition**   Definition: Moving to its normal location, or other suitable location, all or a portion of a body part

Explanation: The body part is moved to a new location from an abnormal location, or from a normal location where it is not functioning correctly. The body part may or may not be cut out or off to be moved to the new location.

Body Part Character 4		Approach Character 5	Device Character 6	Qualifier Character 7
Ø Internal Mammary Artery, Right Anterior intercostal artery Internal thoracic artery Musculophrenic artery Pericardiophrenic artery Superior epigastric artery **1 Internal Mammary Artery, Left** *See Ø Internal Mammary Artery, Right* **2 Innominate Artery** Brachiocephalic artery Brachiocephalic trunk **3 Subclavian Artery, Right** Costocervical trunk Dorsal scapular artery Internal thoracic artery **4 Subclavian Artery, Left** *See 3 Subclavian Artery, Right* **5 Axillary Artery, Right** Anterior circumflex humeral artery Lateral thoracic artery Posterior circumflex humeral artery Subscapular artery Superior thoracic artery Thoracoacromial artery **6 Axillary Artery, Left** *See 5 Axillary Artery, Right* **7 Brachial Artery, Right** Inferior ulnar collateral artery Profunda brachii Superior ulnar collateral artery **8 Brachial Artery, Left** *See 7 Brachial Artery, Right* **9 Ulnar Artery, Right** Anterior ulnar recurrent artery Common interosseous artery Posterior ulnar recurrent artery **A Ulnar Artery, Left** *See 9 Ulnar Artery, Right* **B Radial Artery, Right** Radial recurrent artery **C Radial Artery, Left** *See B Radial Artery, Right* **D Hand Artery, Right** Deep palmar arch Princeps pollicis artery Radialis indicis Superficial palmar arch **F Hand Artery, Left** *See D Hand Artery, Right* **G Intracranial Artery** Anterior cerebral artery Anterior choroidal artery Anterior communicating artery Basilar artery Circle of Willis Internal carotid artery, intracranial portion Middle cerebral artery Ophthalmic artery Posterior cerebral artery Posterior communicating artery Posterior inferior cerebellar artery (PICA)	**H Common Carotid Artery, Right** **J Common Carotid Artery, Left** **K Internal Carotid Artery, Right** Caroticotympanic artery Carotid sinus **L Internal Carotid Artery, Left** *See K Internal Carotid Artery, Right* **M External Carotid Artery, Right** Ascending pharyngeal artery Internal maxillary artery Lingual artery Maxillary artery Occipital artery Posterior auricular artery Superior thyroid artery **N External Carotid Artery, Left** *See M External Carotid Artery, Right* **P Vertebral Artery, Right** Anterior spinal artery Posterior spinal artery **Q Vertebral Artery, Left** *See P Vertebral Artery, Right* **R Face Artery** Angular artery Ascending palatine artery External maxillary artery Facial artery Inferior labial artery Submental artery Superior labial artery **S Temporal Artery, Right** Middle temporal artery Superficial temporal artery Transverse facial artery **T Temporal Artery, Left** *See S Temporal Artery, Right* **U Thyroid Artery, Right** Cricothyroid artery Hyoid artery Sternocleidomastoid artery Superior laryngeal artery Superior thyroid artery Thyrocervical trunk **V Thyroid Artery, Left** *See U Thyroid Artery, Right* **Y Upper Artery** Aortic intercostal artery Bronchial artery Esophageal artery Subcostal artery	**Ø Open** **3 Percutaneous** **4 Percutaneous Endoscopic**	**Z No Device**	**Z No Qualifier**

Non-OR Procedure   DRG Non-OR Procedure   Valid OR Procedure   HAC Associated Procedure   Combination Only   New/Revised April   New/Revised October

214   ICD-10-PCS 2023

Ø   **Medical and Surgical**
3   **Upper Arteries**
U   **Supplement**   Definition: Putting in or on biological or synthetic material that physically reinforces and/or augments the function of a portion of a body part
Explanation: The biological material is non-living, or is living and from the same individual. The body part may have been previously replaced, and the SUPPLEMENT procedure is performed to physically reinforce and/or augment the function of the replaced body part.

Body Part Character 4		Approach Character 5	Device Character 6	Qualifier Character 7
Ø Internal Mammary Artery, Right Anterior intercostal artery Internal thoracic artery Musculophrenic artery Pericardiophrenic artery Superior epigastric artery **1 Internal Mammary Artery, Left** *See Ø Internal Mammary Artery, Right* **2 Innominate Artery** Brachiocephalic artery Brachiocephalic trunk **3 Subclavian Artery, Right** Costocervical trunk Dorsal scapular artery Internal thoracic artery **4 Subclavian Artery, Left** *See 3 Subclavian Artery, Right* **5 Axillary Artery, Right** Anterior circumflex humeral artery Lateral thoracic artery Posterior circumflex humeral artery Subscapular artery Superior thoracic artery Thoracoacromial artery **6 Axillary Artery, Left** *See 5 Axillary Artery, Right* **7 Brachial Artery, Right** Inferior ulnar collateral artery Profunda brachii Superior ulnar collateral artery **8 Brachial Artery, Left** *See 7 Brachial Artery, Right* **9 Ulnar Artery, Right** Anterior ulnar recurrent artery Common interosseous artery Posterior ulnar recurrent artery **A Ulnar Artery, Left** *See 9 Ulnar Artery, Right* **B Radial Artery, Right** Radial recurrent artery **C Radial Artery, Left** *See B Radial Artery, Right* **D Hand Artery, Right** Deep palmar arch Princeps pollicis artery Radialis indicis Superficial palmar arch **F Hand Artery, Left** *See D Hand Artery, Right* **G Intracranial Artery** Anterior cerebral artery Anterior choroidal artery Anterior communicating artery Basilar artery Circle of Willis Internal carotid artery, intracranial portion Middle cerebral artery Ophthalmic artery Posterior cerebral artery Posterior communicating artery Posterior inferior cerebellar artery (PICA)	**H Common Carotid Artery, Right** **J Common Carotid Artery, Left** **K Internal Carotid Artery, Right** Caroticotympanic artery Carotid sinus **L Internal Carotid Artery, Left** *See K Internal Carotid Artery, Right* **M External Carotid Artery, Right** Ascending pharyngeal artery Internal maxillary artery Lingual artery Maxillary artery Occipital artery Posterior auricular artery Superior thyroid artery **N External Carotid Artery, Left** *See M External Carotid Artery, Right* **P Vertebral Artery, Right** Anterior spinal artery Posterior spinal artery **Q Vertebral Artery, Left** *See P Vertebral Artery, Right* **R Face Artery** Angular artery Ascending palatine artery External maxillary artery Facial artery Inferior labial artery Submental artery Superior labial artery **S Temporal Artery, Right** Middle temporal artery Superficial temporal artery Transverse facial artery **T Temporal Artery, Left** *See S Temporal Artery, Right* **U Thyroid Artery, Right** Cricothyroid artery Hyoid artery Sternocleidomastoid artery Superior laryngeal artery Superior thyroid artery Thyrocervical trunk **V Thyroid Artery, Left** *See U Thyroid Artery, Right* **Y Upper Artery** Aortic intercostal artery Bronchial artery Esophageal artery Subcostal artery	**Ø Open** **3 Percutaneous** **4 Percutaneous Endoscopic**	**7 Autologous Tissue Substitute** **J Synthetic Substitute** **K Nonautologous Tissue Substitute**	**Z No Qualifier**

NC Noncovered Procedure   LC Limited Coverage   QA Questionable OB Admit   NT New Tech Add-on   ⊞ Combination Member   ♂ Male   ♀ Female

ICD-10-PCS 2023   **215**

Ø3U–Ø3U

Upper Arteries

Ø   Medical and Surgical
3   Upper Arteries
V   Restriction   Definition: Partially closing an orifice or the lumen of a tubular body part
                   Explanation: The orifice can be a natural orifice or an artificially created orifice

Body Part Character 4	Approach Character 5	Device Character 6	Qualifier Character 7

Ø Internal Mammary Artery, Right
  Anterior intercostal artery
  Internal thoracic artery
  Musculophrenic artery
  Pericardiophrenic artery
  Superior epigastric artery
1 Internal Mammary Artery, Left
  See Ø Internal Mammary Artery,
    Right
2 Innominate Artery
  Brachiocephalic artery
  Brachiocephalic trunk
3 Subclavian Artery, Right
  Costocervical trunk
  Dorsal scapular artery
  Internal thoracic artery
4 Subclavian Artery, Left
  See 3 Subclavian Artery, Right
5 Axillary Artery, Right
  Anterior circumflex humeral artery
  Lateral thoracic artery
  Posterior circumflex humeral artery
  Subscapular artery
  Superior thoracic artery
  Thoracoacromial artery
6 Axillary Artery, Left
  See 5 Axillary Artery, Right
7 Brachial Artery, Right
  Inferior ulnar collateral artery
  Profunda brachii
  Superior ulnar collateral artery
8 Brachial Artery, Left
  See 7 Brachial Artery, Right
9 Ulnar Artery, Right
  Anterior ulnar recurrent artery
  Common interosseous artery
  Posterior ulnar recurrent artery
A Ulnar Artery, Left
  See 9 Ulnar Artery, Right
	B Radial Artery, Right
	  Radial recurrent artery
	C Radial Artery, Left
	  See B Radial Artery, Right
	D Hand Artery, Right
	  Deep palmar arch
	  Princeps pollicis artery
	  Radialis indicis
	  Superficial palmar arch
	F Hand Artery, Left
	  See D Hand Artery, Right
	R Face Artery
	  Angular artery
	  Ascending palatine artery
	  External maxillary artery
	  Facial artery
	  Inferior labial artery
	  Submental artery
	  Superior labial artery
	S Temporal Artery, Right
	  Middle temporal artery
	  Superficial temporal artery
	  Transverse facial artery
	T Temporal Artery, Left
	  See S Temporal Artery, Right
	U Thyroid Artery, Right
	  Cricothyroid artery
	  Hyoid artery
	  Sternocleidomastoid artery
	  Superior laryngeal artery
	  Superior thyroid artery
	  Thyrocervical trunk
	V Thyroid Artery, Left
	  See U Thyroid Artery, Right
	Y Upper Artery
	  Aortic intercostal artery
	  Bronchial artery
	  Esophageal artery
	  Subcostal artery
		Ø Open
		3 Percutaneous
		4 Percutaneous
		  Endoscopic
			C Extraluminal Device
			D Intraluminal Device
			Z No Device
				Z No Qualifier

G Intracranial Artery
  Anterior cerebral artery
  Anterior choroidal artery
  Anterior communicating artery
  Basilar artery
  Circle of Willis
  Internal carotid artery,
    intracranial portion
  Middle cerebral artery
  Ophthalmic artery
  Posterior cerebral artery
  Posterior communicating artery
  Posterior inferior cerebellar artery
    (PICA)
H Common Carotid Artery, Right
J Common Carotid Artery, Left
K Internal Carotid Artery, Right
  Caroticotympanic artery
  Carotid sinus
	L Internal Carotid Artery, Left
	  See K Internal Carotid Artery, Right
	M External Carotid Artery, Right
	  Ascending pharyngeal artery
	  Internal maxillary artery
	  Lingual artery
	  Maxillary artery
	  Occipital artery
	  Posterior auricular artery
	  Superior thyroid artery
	N External Carotid Artery, Left
	  See M External Carotid Artery, Right
	P Vertebral Artery, Right
	  Anterior spinal artery
	  Posterior spinal artery
	Q Vertebral Artery, Left
	  See P Vertebral Artery, Right
		Ø Open
		3 Percutaneous
		4 Percutaneous
		  Endoscopic
			B Intraluminal Device,
			  Bioactive
			C Extraluminal Device
			D Intraluminal Device
			H Intraluminal Device,
			  Flow Diverter
			Z No Device
				Z No Qualifier

Non-OR Procedure   DRG Non-OR Procedure   Valid OR Procedure   HAC Associated Procedure   Combination Only   New/Revised April   New/Revised October
216   ICD-10-PCS 2023
Ø3V–Ø3V

Ø   **Medical and Surgical**
3   **Upper Arteries**
W   **Revision**   Definition: Correcting, to the extent possible, a portion of a malfunctioning device or the position of a displaced device

                            Explanation: Revision can include correcting a malfunctioning or displaced device by taking out or putting in components of the device such as a screw or pin

Body Part Character 4	Approach Character 5	Device Character 6	Qualifier Character 7

Y **Upper Artery**
    Aortic intercostal artery
    Bronchial artery
    Esophageal artery
    Subcostal artery
	Ø Open
	3 Percutaneous
	4 Percutaneous Endoscopic
		Ø Drainage Device
		2 Monitoring Device
		3 Infusion Device
		7 Autologous Tissue Substitute
		C Extraluminal Device
		D Intraluminal Device
		J Synthetic Substitute
		K Nonautologous Tissue Substitute
		M Stimulator Lead
		Y Other Device
			Z No Qualifier

Y **Upper Artery**
    Aortic intercostal artery
    Bronchial artery
    Esophageal artery
    Subcostal artery
	X External	**Ø** Drainage Device
		2 Monitoring Device
		3 Infusion Device
		7 Autologous Tissue Substitute
		C Extraluminal Device
		D Intraluminal Device
		J Synthetic Substitute
		K Nonautologous Tissue Substitute
		M Stimulator Lead
			Z No Qualifier

Non-OR   Ø3WY3[Ø,2,3]Z
Non-OR   Ø3WY[3,4]YZ
Non-OR   Ø3WYX[Ø,2,3,7,C,D,J,K,M]Z

Lower Arteries Ø41–Ø4W

Character Meanings

This Character Meaning table is provided as a guide to assist the user in the identification of character members that may be found in this section of code tables. It **SHOULD NOT** be used to build a PCS code.

Operation–Character 3	Body Part–Character 4	Approach–Character 5	Device–Character 6	Qualifier–Character 7
1 Bypass	Ø Abdominal Aorta	Ø Open	Ø Drainage Device	Ø Abdominal Aorta OR Ultrasonic
5 Destruction	1 Celiac Artery	3 Percutaneous	1 Radioactive Element	1 Celiac Artery OR Drug-Coated Balloon
7 Dilation	2 Gastric Artery	4 Percutaneous Endoscopic	2 Monitoring Device	2 Mesenteric Artery
9 Drainage	3 Hepatic Artery	X External	3 Infusion Device	3 Renal Artery, Right
B Excision	4 Splenic Artery		4 Intraluminal Device, Drug-eluting	4 Renal Artery, Left
C Extirpation	5 Superior Mesenteric Artery		5 Intraluminal Device, Drug-eluting, Two	5 Renal Artery, Bilateral
F Fragmentation	6 Colic Artery, Right		6 Intraluminal Device, Drug-eluting, Three	6 Common Iliac Artery, Right
H Insertion	7 Colic Artery, Left		7 Intraluminal Device, Drug-eluting, Four or More OR Autologous Tissue Substitute	7 Common Iliac Artery, Left
J Inspection	8 Colic Artery, Middle		9 Autologous Venous Tissue	8 Common Iliac Arteries, Bilateral
L Occlusion	9 Renal Artery, Right		A Autologous Arterial Tissue	9 Internal Iliac Artery, Right
N Release	A Renal Artery, Left		C Extraluminal Device	B Internal Iliac Artery, Left
P Removal	B Inferior Mesenteric Artery		D Intraluminal Device	C Internal Iliac Arteries, Bilateral
Q Repair	C Common Iliac Artery, Right		E Intraluminal Device, Two OR Intraluminal Device, Branched or Fenestrated, One or Two Arteries	D External Iliac Artery, Right
R Replacement	D Common Iliac Artery, Left		F Intraluminal Device, Three OR Intraluminal Device, Branched or Fenestrated, Three or More Arteries	F External Iliac Artery, Left
S Reposition	E Internal Iliac Artery, Right		G Intraluminal Device, Four or More	G External Iliac Arteries, Bilateral
U Supplement	F Internal Iliac Artery, Left		J Synthetic Substitute	H Femoral Artery, Right
V Restriction	H External Iliac Artery, Right		K Nonautologous Tissue Substitute	J Femoral Artery, Left OR Temporary
W Revision	J External Iliac Artery, Left		Y Other Device	K Femoral Arteries, Bilateral
	K Femoral Artery, Right		Z No Device	L Popliteal Artery
	L Femoral Artery, Left			M Peroneal Artery
	M Popliteal Artery, Right			N Posterior Tibial Artery
	N Popliteal Artery, Left			P Foot Artery
	P Anterior Tibial Artery, Right			Q Lower Extremity Artery
	Q Anterior Tibial Artery, Left			R Lower Artery
	R Posterior Tibial Artery, Right			S Lower Extremity Vein
	S Posterior Tibial Artery, Left			T Uterine Artery, Right
	T Peroneal Artery, Right			U Uterine Artery, Left
	U Peroneal Artery, Left			V Prostatic Artery, Right
	V Foot Artery, Right			W Prostatic Artery, Left
	W Foot Artery, Left			X Diagnostic
	Y Lower Artery			Z No Qualifier

AHA Coding Clinic for Lower Arteries

2022, 1Q, 10-13	Procedures performed on a continuous vessel, ICD-10-PCS Guideline B4.1c

AHA Coding Clinic for table 041

2019, 1Q, 23	Endovascular repair of shaggy aorta and deployment of chimney stent grafts
2018, 3Q, 25	Femoral artery to tibioperoneal trunk bypass
2017, 4Q, 46-47	New and revised body part values - Bypass hepatic artery to renal artery
2017, 3Q, 5	Femoral artery to posterior tibial artery bypass using autologous and synthetic grafts
2017, 3Q, 16	Abdominal aortic debranching with bypass of external iliac artery to bilateral renal arteries and superior mesenteric artery
2017, 1Q, 32	Peroneal artery to dorsalis pedis artery bypass using saphenous vein graft
2016, 2Q, 18	Femoral-tibial artery bypass and saphenous vein graft
2015, 3Q, 28	Bilateral renal artery bypass

AHA Coding Clinic for table 047

2020, 4Q, 50	Intravascular lithotripsy
2019, 4Q, 27	Bifurcation Qualifier
2019, 2Q, 14	Revision of occluded femoral-popliteal bypass graft
2018, 2Q, 24	Coronary artery bifurcation
2016, 4Q, 86	Peripheral artery, number of stents
2016, 4Q, 86-88	Coronary and peripheral artery bifurcation
2016, 3Q, 39	Infrarenal abdominal aortic aneurysm repair with iliac graft extension
2015, 4Q, 4-7, 15	Drug-coated balloon angioplasty in peripheral vessels
2015, 3Q, 9	Aborted endovascular stenting of superficial femoral artery

AHA Coding Clinic for table 04C

2021, 1Q, 15	Iliofemoral endarterectomy and furthest point of entry
2019, 4Q, 27	Bifurcation Qualifier
2019, 1Q, 23	Endovascular repair of shaggy aorta and deployment of chimney stent grafts
2018, 2Q, 24	Coronary artery bifurcation
2017, 2Q, 23	Thrombectomy via Fogarty catheter
2016, 4Q, 86-88	Coronary and peripheral artery bifurcation
2016, 1Q, 31	Iliofemoral endarterectomy with patch repair
2015, 1Q, 29	Discontinued carotid endarterectomy
2015, 1Q, 36	Percutaneous mechanical thrombectomy of femoropopliteal bypass graft

AHA Coding Clinic for table 04F

2020, 4Q, 45-49	New fragmentation tables
2020, 4Q, 49-50	Intravascular ultrasound assisted thrombolysis
2020, 4Q, 50-51	Intravascular lithotripsy

AHA Coding Clinic for table 04H

2019, 3Q, 20	Removal and revision of ECMO component
2019, 1Q, 23	Endovascular repair of shaggy aorta and deployment of chimney stent grafts
2017, 1Q, 30	Insertion of umbilical artery catheter

AHA Coding Clinic for table 04L

2020, 3Q, 43	Staged laparoscopic gastric conduit and placement of feeding tube
2018, 2Q, 18	Transverse rectus abdominis myocutaneous (TRAM) delay
2017, 4Q, 31	Resuscitative endovascular balloon occlusion of the aorta
2015, 2Q, 27	Uterine artery embolization using Gelfoam
2014, 3Q, 26	Coil embolization of gastroduodenal artery with chemoembolization of hepatic artery
2014, 1Q, 24	Endovascular embolization for gastrointestinal bleeding

AHA Coding Clinic for table 04N

2015, 2Q, 28	Release and replacement of celiac artery

AHA Coding Clinic for table 04P

2019, 3Q, 20	Removal and revision of ECMO component

AHA Coding Clinic for table 04Q

2014, 1Q, 21	Repair of femoral artery pseudoaneurysm

AHA Coding Clinic for table 04R

2019, 1Q, 22	Abdominal aortic aneurysm repair using tube graft
2015, 2Q, 28	Release and replacement of celiac artery

AHA Coding Clinic for table 04U

2019, 1Q, 22	Abdominal aortic aneurysm repair using tube graft
2016, 2Q, 18	Femoral-tibial artery bypass and saphenous vein graft
2016, 1Q, 31	Iliofemoral endarterectomy with patch repair
2014, 4Q, 37	Bovine patch arterioplasty
2014, 1Q, 22	Repair of pseudoaneurysm of femoral-popliteal bypass graft

AHA Coding Clinic for table 04V

2021, 3Q, 23	Transcatheter embolization of splenic artery
2019, 4Q, 27	Bifurcation Qualifier
2019, 1Q, 22	Abdominal aortic aneurysm repair using tube graft
2018, 2Q, 24	Coronary artery bifurcation
2016, 4Q, 86-87	Coronary and peripheral artery bifurcation
2016, 4Q, 89-93	Branched and fenestrated endograft repair of aneurysms
2016, 3Q, 39	Infrarenal abdominal aortic aneurysm repair with iliac graft extension
2014, 1Q, 9	Endovascular repair of abdominal aortic aneurysm

AHA Coding Clinic for table 04W

2020, 3Q, 5	Types of endoleaks following endovascular aneurysm repair
2019, 2Q, 14	Revision of occluded femoral-popliteal bypass graft
2015, 1Q, 36	Revision of femoropopliteal bypass graft
2014, 1Q, 9	Endovascular repair of endoleak
2014, 1Q, 22	Repair of pseudoaneurysm of femoral-popliteal bypass graft

Lower Arteries

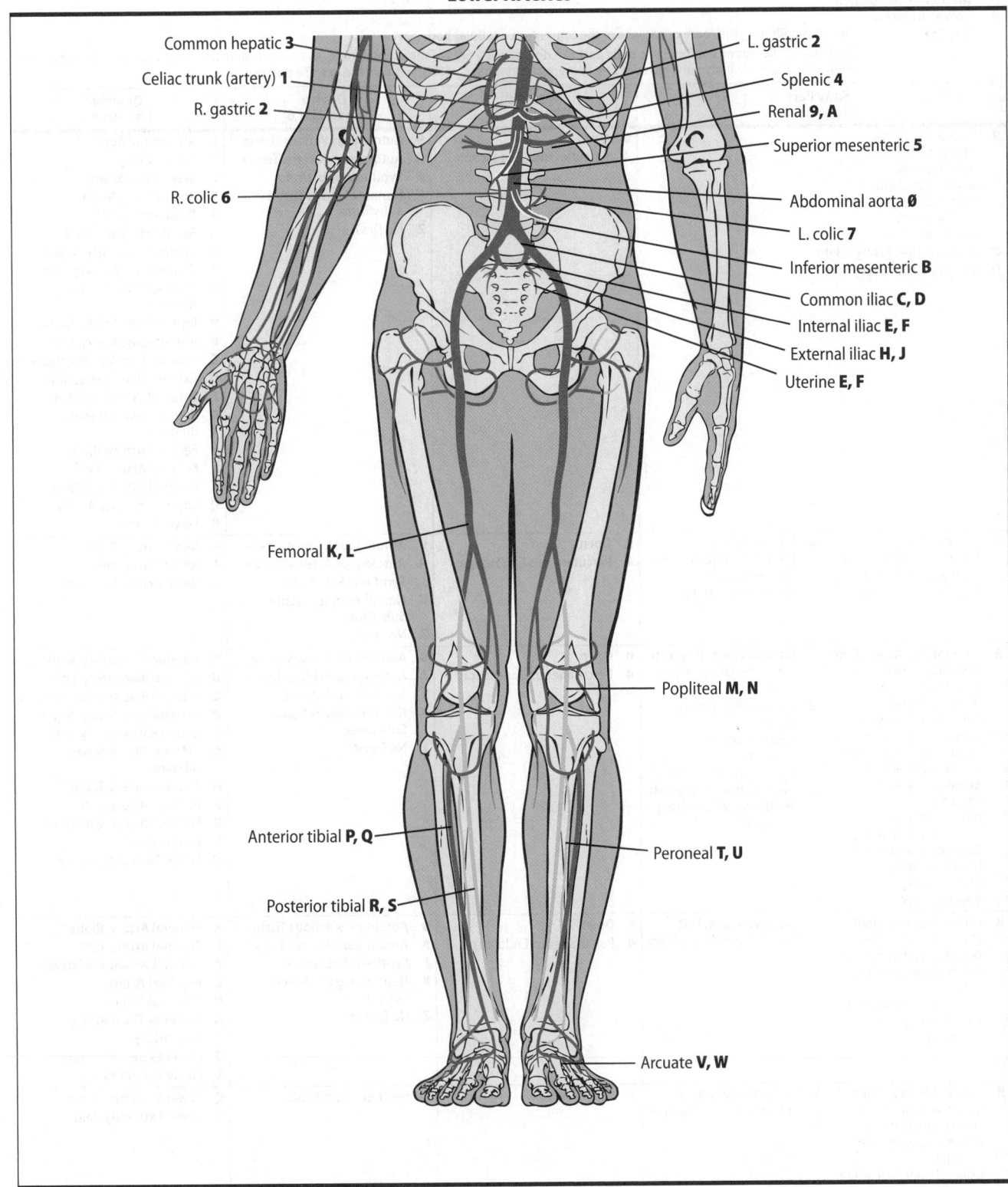

Common hepatic **3**
Celiac trunk (artery) **1**
R. gastric **2**
R. colic **6**

L. gastric **2**
Splenic **4**
Renal **9, A**
Superior mesenteric **5**
Abdominal aorta **Ø**
L. colic **7**
Inferior mesenteric **B**
Common iliac **C, D**
Internal iliac **E, F**
External iliac **H, J**
Uterine **E, F**

Femoral **K, L**

Popliteal **M, N**

Anterior tibial **P, Q**

Peroneal **T, U**

Posterior tibial **R, S**

Arcuate **V, W**

Ø   Medical and Surgical
4   Lower Arteries
1   Bypass   Definition: Altering the route of passage of the contents of a tubular body part

Explanation: Rerouting contents of a body part to a downstream area of the normal route, to a similar route and body part, or to an abnormal route and dissimilar body part. Includes one or more anastomoses, with or without the use of a device.

Body Part — Character 4		Approach — Character 5	Device — Character 6	Qualifier — Character 7
Ø **Abdominal Aorta** Inferior phrenic artery Lumbar artery Median sacral artery Middle suprarenal artery Ovarian artery Testicular artery C **Common Iliac Artery, Right** D **Common Iliac Artery, Left**		Ø Open 4 Percutaneous Endoscopic	9 Autologous Venous Tissue A Autologous Arterial Tissue J Synthetic Substitute K Nonautologous Tissue Substitute Z No Device	Ø Abdominal Aorta 1 Celiac Artery 2 Mesenteric Artery 3 Renal Artery, Right 4 Renal Artery, Left 5 Renal Artery, Bilateral 6 Common Iliac Artery, Right 7 Common Iliac Artery, Left 8 Common Iliac Arteries, Bilateral 9 Internal Iliac Artery, Right B Internal Iliac Artery, Left C Internal Iliac Arteries, Bilateral D External Iliac Artery, Right F External Iliac Artery, Left G External Iliac Arteries, Bilateral H Femoral Artery, Right J Femoral Artery, Left K Femoral Arteries, Bilateral Q Lower Extremity Artery R Lower Artery
3 **Hepatic Artery** Common hepatic artery Gastroduodenal artery Hepatic artery proper	4 **Splenic Artery** Left gastroepiploic artery Pancreatic artery Short gastric artery	Ø Open 4 Percutaneous Endoscopic	9 Autologous Venous Tissue A Autologous Arterial Tissue J Synthetic Substitute K Nonautologous Tissue Substitute Z No Device	3 Renal Artery, Right 4 Renal Artery, Left 5 Renal Artery, Bilateral
E **Internal Iliac Artery, Right** Deferential artery Hypogastric artery Iliolumbar artery Inferior gluteal artery Inferior vesical artery Internal pudendal artery Lateral sacral artery Middle rectal artery Obturator artery Prostatic artery Superior gluteal artery Superior vesical artery Umbilical artery Uterine artery Vaginal artery	F **Internal Iliac Artery, Left** *See E Internal Iliac Artery, Right* H **External Iliac Artery, Right** Deep circumflex iliac artery Inferior epigastric artery J **External Iliac Artery, Left** *See H External Iliac Artery, Right*	Ø Open 4 Percutaneous Endoscopic	9 Autologous Venous Tissue A Autologous Arterial Tissue J Synthetic Substitute K Nonautologous Tissue Substitute Z No Device	9 Internal Iliac Artery, Right B Internal Iliac Artery, Left C Internal Iliac Arteries, Bilateral D External Iliac Artery, Right F External Iliac Artery, Left G External Iliac Arteries, Bilateral H Femoral Artery, Right J Femoral Artery, Left K Femoral Arteries, Bilateral P Foot Artery Q Lower Extremity Artery
K **Femoral Artery, Right** Circumflex iliac artery Deep femoral artery Descending genicular artery External pudendal artery Superficial epigastric artery	L **Femoral Artery, Left** *See K Femoral Artery, Right*	Ø Open 4 Percutaneous Endoscopic	9 Autologous Venous Tissue A Autologous Arterial Tissue J Synthetic Substitute K Nonautologous Tissue Substitute Z No Device	H Femoral Artery, Right J Femoral Artery, Left K Femoral Arteries, Bilateral L Popliteal Artery M Peroneal Artery N Posterior Tibial Artery P Foot Artery Q Lower Extremity Artery S Lower Extremity Vein
K **Femoral Artery, Right** Circumflex iliac artery Deep femoral artery Descending genicular artery External pudendal artery Superficial epigastric artery	L **Femoral Artery, Left** *See K Femoral Artery, Right*	3 Percutaneous	J Synthetic Substitute	Q Lower Extremity Artery S Lower Extremity Vein
M **Popliteal Artery, Right** Inferior genicular artery Middle genicular artery Superior genicular artery Sural artery Tibioperoneal trunk	N **Popliteal Artery, Left** *See M Popliteal Artery, Right*	Ø Open 4 Percutaneous Endoscopic	9 Autologous Venous Tissue A Autologous Arterial Tissue J Synthetic Substitute K Nonautologous Tissue Substitute Z No Device	L Popliteal Artery M Peroneal Artery P Foot Artery Q Lower Extremity Artery S Lower Extremity Vein

Ø41 Continued on next page

Non-OR Procedure   DRG Non-OR Procedure   Valid OR Procedure   HAC Associated Procedure   Combination Only   New/Revised April   New/Revised October

222   ICD-10-PCS 2023

Ø　**Medical and Surgical**
4　**Lower Arteries**
1　**Bypass**

041 Continued

Definition: Altering the route of passage of the contents of a tubular body part

Explanation: Rerouting contents of a body part to a downstream area of the normal route, to a similar route and body part, or to an abnormal route and dissimilar body part. Includes one or more anastomoses, with or without the use of a device.

Body Part Character 4		Approach Character 5	Device Character 6	Qualifier Character 7
M **Popliteal Artery, Right** Inferior genicular artery Middle genicular artery Superior genicular artery Sural artery Tibioperoneal trunk	**N** **Popliteal Artery, Left** *See* M Popliteal Artery, *Right*	**3** Percutaneous	**J** Synthetic Substitute	**Q** Lower Extremity Artery **S** Lower Extremity Vein
P **Anterior Tibial Artery, Right** Anterior lateral malleolar artery Anterior medial malleolar artery Anterior tibial recurrent artery Dorsalis pedis artery Posterior tibial recurrent artery	**Q** **Anterior Tibial Artery, Left** *See* P Anterior Tibial Artery, *Right* **R** **Posterior Tibial Artery, Right** **S** **Posterior Tibial Artery, Left**	**Ø** Open **3** Percutaneous **4** Percutaneous Endoscopic	**J** Synthetic Substitute	**Q** Lower Extremity Artery **S** Lower Extremity Vein
T **Peroneal Artery, Right** Fibular artery **U** **Peroneal Artery, Left** *See* T Peroneal Artery, *Right*	**V** **Foot Artery, Right** Arcuate artery Dorsal metatarsal artery Lateral plantar artery Lateral tarsal artery Medial plantar artery **W** **Foot Artery, Left** *See* V Foot Artery, *Right*	**Ø** Open **4** Percutaneous Endoscopic	**9** Autologous Venous Tissue **A** Autologous Arterial Tissue **J** Synthetic Substitute **K** Nonautologous Tissue Substitute **Z** No Device	**P** Foot Artery **Q** Lower Extremity Artery **S** Lower Extremity Vein
T **Peroneal Artery, Right** Fibular artery **U** **Peroneal Artery, Left** *See* T Peroneal Artery, *Right*	**V** **Foot Artery, Right** Arcuate artery Dorsal metatarsal artery Lateral plantar artery Lateral tarsal artery Medial plantar artery **W** **Foot Artery, Left** *See* V Foot Artery, *Right*	**3** Percutaneous	**J** Synthetic Substitute	**Q** Lower Extremity Artery **S** Lower Extremity Vein

NC Noncovered Procedure　　**LC** Limited Coverage　　**QA** Questionable OB Admit　　**NT** New Tech Add-on　　⊞ Combination Member　　♂ Male　　♀ Female

ICD-10-PCS 2023　　　　　　　　　　　　　　　　　　　　　　　　　　　　　　　　　　　　　223

041–041

Lower Arteries

Ø   Medical and Surgical
4   Lower Arteries
5   Destruction   Definition: Physical eradication of all or a portion of a body part by the direct use of energy, force, or a destructive agent
                 Explanation: None of the body part is physically taken out

Body Part — Character 4	Approach — Character 5	Device — Character 6	Qualifier — Character 7
Ø Abdominal Aorta Inferior phrenic artery Lumbar artery Median sacral artery Middle suprarenal artery Ovarian artery Testicular artery **1 Celiac Artery** Celiac trunk **2 Gastric Artery** Left gastric artery Right gastric artery **3 Hepatic Artery** Common hepatic artery Gastroduodenal artery Hepatic artery proper **4 Splenic Artery** Left gastroepiploic artery Pancreatic artery Short gastric artery **5 Superior Mesenteric Artery** Ileal artery Ileocolic artery Inferior pancreaticoduodenal artery Jejunal artery **6 Colic Artery, Right** **7 Colic Artery, Left** **8 Colic Artery, Middle** **9 Renal Artery, Right** Inferior suprarenal artery Renal segmental artery **A Renal Artery, Left** *See 9 Renal Artery, Right* **B Inferior Mesenteric Artery** Sigmoid artery Superior rectal artery **C Common Iliac Artery, Right** **D Common Iliac Artery, Left** **E Internal Iliac Artery, Right** Deferential artery Hypogastric artery Iliolumbar artery Inferior gluteal artery Inferior vesical artery Internal pudendal artery Lateral sacral artery Middle rectal artery Obturator artery Prostatic artery Superior gluteal artery Superior vesical artery Umbilical artery Uterine artery Vaginal artery	**F Internal Iliac Artery, Left** *See E Internal Iliac Artery, Right* **H External Iliac Artery, Right** Deep circumflex iliac artery Inferior epigastric artery **J External Iliac Artery, Left** *See H External Iliac Artery, Right* **K Femoral Artery, Right** Circumflex iliac artery Deep femoral artery Descending genicular artery External pudendal artery Superficial epigastric artery **L Femoral Artery, Left** *See K Femoral Artery, Right* **M Popliteal Artery, Right** Inferior genicular artery Middle genicular artery Superior genicular artery Sural artery Tibioperoneal trunk **N Popliteal Artery, Left** *See M Popliteal Artery, Right* **P Anterior Tibial Artery, Right** Anterior lateral malleolar artery Anterior medial malleolar artery Anterior tibial recurrent artery Dorsalis pedis artery Posterior tibial recurrent artery **Q Anterior Tibial Artery, Left** *See P Anterior Tibial Artery, Right* **R Posterior Tibial Artery, Right** **S Posterior Tibial Artery, Left** **T Peroneal Artery, Right** Fibular artery **U Peroneal Artery, Left** *See T Peroneal Artery, Right* **V Foot Artery, Right** Arcuate artery Dorsal metatarsal artery Lateral plantar artery Lateral tarsal artery Medial plantar artery **W Foot Artery, Left** *See V Foot Artery, Right* **Y Lower Artery** Umbilical artery	**Ø Open** **3 Percutaneous** **4 Percutaneous Endoscopic**	**Z No Device**	**Z No Qualifier**

Ø   **Medical and Surgical**
4   **Lower Arteries**
7   **Dilation**   Definition: Expanding an orifice or the lumen of a tubular body part

                       Explanation: The orifice can be a natural orifice or an artificially created orifice. Accomplished by stretching a tubular body part using intraluminal pressure or by cutting part of the orifice or wall of the tubular body part.

Body Part — Character 4		Approach — Character 5	Device — Character 6	Qualifier — Character 7
Ø **Abdominal Aorta**	**F** **Internal Iliac Artery, Left**	**Ø** Open	**4** Intraluminal Device, Drug-eluting	**1** Drug-Coated Balloon
Inferior phrenic artery	*See E Internal Iliac Artery, Right*	**3** Percutaneous	**D** Intraluminal Device	**Z** No Qualifier
Lumbar artery	**H** **External Iliac Artery, Right**	**4** Percutaneous Endoscopic	**Z** No Device	
Median sacral artery	Deep circumflex iliac artery			
Middle suprarenal artery	Inferior epigastric artery			
Ovarian artery	**J** **External Iliac Artery, Left**			
Testicular artery	*See H External Iliac Artery, Right*			
1 **Celiac Artery**	**K** **Femoral Artery, Right**			
Celiac trunk	Circumflex iliac artery			
2 **Gastric Artery**	Deep femoral artery			
Left gastric artery	Descending genicular artery			
Right gastric artery	External pudendal artery			
3 **Hepatic Artery**	Superficial epigastric artery			
Common hepatic artery	**L** **Femoral Artery, Left**			
Gastroduodenal artery	*See K Femoral Artery, Right*			
Hepatic artery proper	**M** **Popliteal Artery, Right**			
4 **Splenic Artery**	Inferior genicular artery			
Left gastroepiploic artery	Middle genicular artery			
Pancreatic artery	Superior genicular artery			
Short gastric artery	Sural artery			
5 **Superior Mesenteric Artery**	Tibioperoneal trunk			
Ileal artery	**N** **Popliteal Artery, Left**			
Ileocolic artery	*See M Popliteal Artery, Right*			
Inferior pancreaticoduodenal artery	**P** **Anterior Tibial Artery, Right**			
Jejunal artery	Anterior lateral malleolar artery			
6 **Colic Artery, Right**	Anterior medial malleolar artery			
7 **Colic Artery, Left**	Anterior tibial recurrent artery			
8 **Colic Artery, Middle**	Dorsalis pedis artery			
9 **Renal Artery, Right**	Posterior tibial recurrent artery			
Inferior suprarenal artery	**Q** **Anterior Tibial Artery, Left**			
Renal segmental artery	*See P Anterior Tibial Artery, Right*			
A **Renal Artery, Left**	**R** **Posterior Tibial Artery, Right**			
See 9 Renal Artery, Right	**S** **Posterior Tibial Artery, Left**			
B **Inferior Mesenteric Artery**	**T** **Peroneal Artery, Right**			
Sigmoid artery	Fibular artery			
Superior rectal artery	**U** **Peroneal Artery, Left**			
C **Common Iliac Artery, Right**	*See T Peroneal Artery, Right*			
D **Common Iliac Artery, Left**	**V** **Foot Artery, Right**			
E **Internal Iliac Artery, Right**	Arcuate artery			
Deferential artery	Dorsal metatarsal artery			
Hypogastric artery	Lateral plantar artery			
Iliolumbar artery	Lateral tarsal artery			
Inferior gluteal artery	Medial plantar artery			
Inferior vesical artery	**W** **Foot Artery, Left**			
Internal pudendal artery	*See V Foot Artery, Right*			
Lateral sacral artery	**Y** **Lower Artery**			
Middle rectal artery	Umbilical artery			
Obturator artery				
Prostatic artery				
Superior gluteal artery				
Superior vesical artery				
Umbilical artery				
Uterine artery				
Vaginal artery				

Ø47 Continued on next page

NC Noncovered Procedure   **LC** Limited Coverage   **QA** Questionable OB Admit   **NT** New Tech Add-on   ⊞ Combination Member   ♂ Male   ♀ Female

ICD-10-PCS 2023   225

047–047

Lower Arteries

Ø   **Medical and Surgical**
4   **Lower Arteries**
7   **Dilation**   Definition: Expanding an orifice or the lumen of a tubular body part

Ø47 Continued

Explanation: The orifice can be a natural orifice or an artificially created orifice. Accomplished by stretching a tubular body part using intraluminal pressure or by cutting part of the orifice or wall of the tubular body part.

Body Part Character 4		Approach Character 5	Device Character 6	Qualifier Character 7

Ø Abdominal Aorta
Inferior phrenic artery
Lumbar artery
Median sacral artery
Middle suprarenal artery
Ovarian artery
Testicular artery
1 Celiac Artery
Celiac trunk
2 Gastric Artery
Left gastric artery
Right gastric artery
3 Hepatic Artery
Common hepatic artery
Gastroduodenal artery
Hepatic artery proper
4 Splenic Artery
Left gastroepiploic artery
Pancreatic artery
Short gastric artery
5 Superior Mesenteric Artery
Ileal artery
Ileocolic artery
Inferior pancreaticoduodenal
  artery
Jejunal artery
6 Colic Artery, Right
7 Colic Artery, Left
8 Colic Artery, Middle
9 Renal Artery, Right
Inferior suprarenal artery
Renal segmental artery
A Renal Artery, Left
See 9 Renal Artery, Right
B Inferior Mesenteric Artery
Sigmoid artery
Superior rectal artery
C Common Iliac Artery, Right
D Common Iliac Artery, Left
E Internal Iliac Artery, Right
Deferential artery
Hypogastric artery
Iliolumbar artery
Inferior gluteal artery
Inferior vesical artery
Internal pudendal artery
Lateral sacral artery
Middle rectal artery
Obturator artery
Prostatic artery
Superior gluteal artery
Superior vesical artery
Umbilical artery
Uterine artery
Vaginal artery
	F Internal Iliac Artery, Left
	See E Internal Iliac Artery, Right
	H External Iliac Artery, Right
	Deep circumflex iliac artery
	Inferior epigastric artery
	J External Iliac Artery, Left
	See H External Iliac Artery, Right
	K Femoral Artery, Right
	Circumflex iliac artery
	Deep femoral artery
	Descending genicular artery
	External pudendal artery
	Superficial epigastric artery
	L Femoral Artery, Left
	See K Femoral Artery, Right
	M Popliteal Artery, Right
	Inferior genicular artery
	Middle genicular artery
	Superior genicular artery
	Sural artery
	Tibioperoneal trunk
	N Popliteal Artery, Left
	See M Popliteal Artery, Right
	P Anterior Tibial Artery, Right
	Anterior lateral malleolar
	  artery
	Anterior medial malleolar
	  artery
	Anterior tibial recurrent artery
	Dorsalis pedis artery
	Posterior tibial recurrent artery
	Q Anterior Tibial Artery, Left
	See P Anterior Tibial Artery,
	Right
	R Posterior Tibial Artery, Right
	S Posterior Tibial Artery, Left
	T Peroneal Artery, Right
	Fibular artery
	U Peroneal Artery, Left
	See T Peroneal Artery, Right
	V Foot Artery, Right
	Arcuate artery
	Dorsal metatarsal artery
	Lateral plantar artery
	Lateral tarsal artery
	Medial plantar artery
	W Foot Artery, Left
	See V Foot Artery, Right
	Y Lower Artery
	Umbilical artery
		Ø Open
		3 Percutaneous
		4 Percutaneous Endoscopic
			**5 Intraluminal Device, Drug-
			eluting, Two**
			**6 Intraluminal Device, Drug-
			eluting, Three**
			**7 Intraluminal Device, Drug-
			eluting, Four or More**
			E Intraluminal Device, Two
			F Intraluminal Device, Three
			**G Intraluminal Device, Four
			or More**
				Z No Qualifier

Non-OR Procedure   DRG Non-OR Procedure   Valid OR Procedure   HAC Associated Procedure   Combination Only   New/Revised April   New/Revised October

226   ICD-10-PCS 2023

Ø47–Ø47

Ø   Medical and Surgical
4   Lower Arteries
9   Drainage   Definition: Taking or letting out fluids and/or gases from a body part

Explanation: The qualifier DIAGNOSTIC is used to identify drainage procedures that are biopsies

Body Part Character 4		Approach Character 5	Device Character 6	Qualifier Character 7

Ø Abdominal Aorta
Inferior phrenic artery
Lumbar artery
Median sacral artery
Middle suprarenal artery
Ovarian artery
Testicular artery
1 Celiac Artery
Celiac trunk
2 Gastric Artery
Left gastric artery
Right gastric artery
3 Hepatic Artery
Common hepatic artery
Gastroduodenal artery
Hepatic artery proper
4 Splenic Artery
Left gastroepiploic artery
Pancreatic artery
Short gastric artery
5 Superior Mesenteric Artery
Ileal artery
Ileocolic artery
Inferior pancreaticoduodenal
   artery
Jejunal artery
6 Colic Artery, Right
7 Colic Artery, Left
8 Colic Artery, Middle
9 Renal Artery, Right
Inferior suprarenal artery
Renal segmental artery
A Renal Artery, Left
See 9 Renal Artery, Right
B Inferior Mesenteric Artery
Sigmoid artery
Superior rectal artery
C Common Iliac Artery, Right
D Common Iliac Artery, Left
E Internal Iliac Artery, Right
Deferential artery
Hypogastric artery
Iliolumbar artery
Inferior gluteal artery
Inferior vesical artery
Internal pudendal artery
Lateral sacral artery
Middle rectal artery
Obturator artery
Prostatic artery
Superior gluteal artery
Superior vesical artery
Umbilical artery
Uterine artery
Vaginal artery
	F Internal Iliac Artery, Left
	See E Internal Iliac Artery, Right
	H External Iliac Artery, Right
	Deep circumflex iliac artery
	Inferior epigastric artery
	J External Iliac Artery, Left
	See H External Iliac Artery, Right
	K Femoral Artery, Right
	Circumflex iliac artery
	Deep femoral artery
	Descending genicular artery
	External pudendal artery
	Superficial epigastric artery
	L Femoral Artery, Left
	See K Femoral Artery, Right
	M Popliteal Artery, Right
	Inferior genicular artery
	Middle genicular artery
	Superior genicular artery
	Sural artery
	Tibioperoneal trunk
	N Popliteal Artery, Left
	See M Popliteal Artery, Right
	P Anterior Tibial Artery, Right
	Anterior lateral malleolar
	   artery
	Anterior medial malleolar
	   artery
	Anterior tibial recurrent artery
	Dorsalis pedis artery
	Posterior tibial recurrent artery
	Q Anterior Tibial Artery, Left
	See P Anterior Tibial Artery,
	* Right*
	R Posterior Tibial Artery, Right
	S Posterior Tibial Artery, Left
	T Peroneal Artery, Right
	Fibular artery
	U Peroneal Artery, Left
	See T Peroneal Artery, Right
	V Foot Artery, Right
	Arcuate artery
	Dorsal metatarsal artery
	Lateral plantar artery
	Lateral tarsal artery
	Medial plantar artery
	W Foot Artery, Left
	See V Foot Artery, Right
	Y Lower Artery
	Umbilical artery
		Ø Open
		3 Percutaneous
		4 Percutaneous Endoscopic
			Ø Drainage Device	**Z No Qualifier**

Non-OR   Ø49[Ø,1,2,3,4,5,6,7,8,9,A,B,C,D,E,F,H,J,K,L,M,N,P,Q,R,S,T,U,V,W,Y][Ø,3,4]ØZ

Ø49 Continued on next page

NC Noncovered Procedure   LC Limited Coverage   OA Questionable OB Admit   NT New Tech Add-on   ⊞ Combination Member   ♂ Male   ♀ Female

ICD-10-PCS 2023   227

Ø49–Ø49

Lower Arteries

Ø	Medical and Surgical	
4	Lower Arteries	
9	Drainage	

049 Continued

Definition: Taking or letting out fluids and/or gases from a body part

Explanation: The qualifier DIAGNOSTIC is used to identify drainage procedures that are biopsies

Body Part — Character 4		Approach — Character 5	Device — Character 6	Qualifier — Character 7
Ø Abdominal Aorta Inferior phrenic artery Lumbar artery Median sacral artery Middle suprarenal artery Ovarian artery Testicular artery **1 Celiac Artery** Celiac trunk **2 Gastric Artery** Left gastric artery Right gastric artery **3 Hepatic Artery** Common hepatic artery Gastroduodenal artery Hepatic artery proper **4 Splenic Artery** Left gastroepiploic artery Pancreatic artery Short gastric artery **5 Superior Mesenteric Artery** Ileal artery Ileocolic artery Inferior pancreaticoduodenal artery Jejunal artery **6 Colic Artery, Right** **7 Colic Artery, Left** **8 Colic Artery, Middle** **9 Renal Artery, Right** Inferior suprarenal artery Renal segmental artery **A Renal Artery, Left** *See 9 Renal Artery, Right* **B Inferior Mesenteric Artery** Sigmoid artery Superior rectal artery **C Common Iliac Artery, Right** **D Common Iliac Artery, Left** **E Internal Iliac Artery, Right** Deferential artery Hypogastric artery Iliolumbar artery Inferior gluteal artery Inferior vesical artery Internal pudendal artery Lateral sacral artery Middle rectal artery Obturator artery Prostatic artery Superior gluteal artery Superior vesical artery Umbilical artery Uterine artery Vaginal artery	**F Internal Iliac Artery, Left** *See E Internal Iliac Artery, Right* **H External Iliac Artery, Right** Deep circumflex iliac artery Inferior epigastric artery **J External Iliac Artery, Left** *See H External Iliac Artery, Right* **K Femoral Artery, Right** Circumflex iliac artery Deep femoral artery Descending genicular artery External pudendal artery Superficial epigastric artery **L Femoral Artery, Left** *See K Femoral Artery, Right* **M Popliteal Artery, Right** Inferior genicular artery Middle genicular artery Superior genicular artery Sural artery Tibioperoneal trunk **N Popliteal Artery, Left** *See M Popliteal Artery, Right* **P Anterior Tibial Artery, Right** Anterior lateral malleolar artery Anterior medial malleolar artery Anterior tibial recurrent artery Dorsalis pedis artery Posterior tibial recurrent artery **Q Anterior Tibial Artery, Left** *See P Anterior Tibial Artery, Right* **R Posterior Tibial Artery, Right** **S Posterior Tibial Artery, Left** **T Peroneal Artery, Right** Fibular artery **U Peroneal Artery, Left** *See T Peroneal Artery, Right* **V Foot Artery, Right** Arcuate artery Dorsal metatarsal artery Lateral plantar artery Lateral tarsal artery Medial plantar artery **W Foot Artery, Left** *See V Foot Artery, Right* **Y Lower Artery** Umbilical artery	**Ø** Open **3** Percutaneous **4** Percutaneous Endoscopic	**Z** No Device	**X** Diagnostic **Z** No Qualifier

Non-OR   049[Ø,1,2,3,4,5,6,7,8,9,A,B,C,D,E,F,H,J,K,L,M,N,P,Q,R,S,T,U,V,W,Y]3ZX

Non-OR   049[Ø,1,2,3,4,5,6,7,8,9,A,B,C,D,E,F,H,J,K,L,M,N,P,Q,R,S,T,U,V,W,Y][Ø,3,4]ZZ

Non-OR Procedure   DRG Non-OR Procedure   Valid OR Procedure   HAC Associated Procedure   Combination Only   New/Revised April   New/Revised October

228   ICD-10-PCS 2023

0   **Medical and Surgical**
4   **Lower Arteries**
B   **Excision**   Definition: Cutting out or off, without replacement, a portion of a body part
                          Explanation: The qualifier DIAGNOSTIC is used to identify excision procedures that are biopsies

Body Part Character 4		Approach Character 5	Device Character 6	Qualifier Character 7

0 **Abdominal Aorta**
 Inferior phrenic artery
 Lumbar artery
 Median sacral artery
 Middle suprarenal artery
 Ovarian artery
 Testicular artery
 1 **Celiac Artery**
 Celiac trunk
 2 **Gastric Artery**
 Left gastric artery
 Right gastric artery
 3 **Hepatic Artery**
 Common hepatic artery
 Gastroduodenal artery
 Hepatic artery proper
 4 **Splenic Artery**
 Left gastroepiploic artery
 Pancreatic artery
 Short gastric artery
 5 **Superior Mesenteric Artery**
 Ileal artery
 Ileocolic artery
 Inferior pancreaticoduodenal
    artery
 Jejunal artery
 6 **Colic Artery, Right**
 7 **Colic Artery, Left**
 8 **Colic Artery, Middle**
 9 **Renal Artery, Right**
 Inferior suprarenal artery
 Renal segmental artery
 A **Renal Artery, Left**
 See 9 Renal Artery, Right
 B **Inferior Mesenteric Artery**
 Sigmoid artery
 Superior rectal artery
 C **Common Iliac Artery, Right**
 D **Common Iliac Artery, Left**
 E **Internal Iliac Artery, Right**
 Deferential artery
 Hypogastric artery
 Iliolumbar artery
 Inferior gluteal artery
 Inferior vesical artery
 Internal pudendal artery
 Lateral sacral artery
 Middle rectal artery
 Obturator artery
 Prostatic artery
 Superior gluteal artery
 Superior vesical artery
 Umbilical artery
 Uterine artery
 Vaginal artery
	F **Internal Iliac Artery, Left**
	 See E Internal Iliac Artery, Right
	 H **External Iliac Artery, Right**
	 Deep circumflex iliac artery
	 Inferior epigastric artery
	 J **External Iliac Artery, Left**
	 See H External Iliac Artery, Right
	 K **Femoral Artery, Right**
	 Circumflex iliac artery
	 Deep femoral artery
	 Descending genicular artery
	 External pudendal artery
	 Superficial epigastric artery
	 L **Femoral Artery, Left**
	 See K Femoral Artery, Right
	 M **Popliteal Artery, Right**
	 Inferior genicular artery
	 Middle genicular artery
	 Superior genicular artery
	 Sural artery
	 Tibioperoneal trunk
	 N **Popliteal Artery, Left**
	 See M Popliteal Artery, Right
	 P **Anterior Tibial Artery, Right**
	 Anterior lateral malleolar
	    artery
	 Anterior medial malleolar
	    artery
	 Anterior tibial recurrent artery
	 Dorsalis pedis artery
	 Posterior tibial recurrent artery
	 Q **Anterior Tibial Artery, Left**
	 See P Anterior Tibial Artery,
	    Right
	 R **Posterior Tibial Artery, Right**
	 S **Posterior Tibial Artery, Left**
	 T **Peroneal Artery, Right**
	 Fibular artery
	 U **Peroneal Artery, Left**
	 See T Peroneal Artery, Right
	 V **Foot Artery, Right**
	 Arcuate artery
	 Dorsal metatarsal artery
	 Lateral plantar artery
	 Lateral tarsal artery
	 Medial plantar artery
	 W **Foot Artery, Left**
	 See V Foot Artery, Right
	 Y **Lower Artery**
	 Umbilical artery
		0 Open
		 3 Percutaneous
		 4 Percutaneous Endoscopic
			Z No Device	**X** Diagnostic
				 Z No Qualifier

Lower Arteries

0   Medical and Surgical
4   Lower Arteries
C   Extirpation   Definition: Taking or cutting out solid matter from a body part

Explanation: The solid matter may be an abnormal byproduct of a biological function or a foreign body; it may be imbedded in a body part or in the lumen of a tubular body part. The solid matter may or may not have been previously broken into pieces.

Body Part Character 4		Approach Character 5	Device Character 6	Qualifier Character 7

0 Abdominal Aorta
Inferior phrenic artery
Lumbar artery
Median sacral artery
Middle suprarenal artery
Ovarian artery
Testicular artery
1 Celiac Artery
Celiac trunk
2 Gastric Artery
Left gastric artery
Right gastric artery
3 Hepatic Artery
Common hepatic artery
Gastroduodenal artery
Hepatic artery proper
4 Splenic Artery
Left gastroepiploic artery
Pancreatic artery
Short gastric artery
5 Superior Mesenteric Artery
Ileal artery
Ileocolic artery
Inferior pancreaticoduodenal
   artery
Jejunal artery
6 Colic Artery, Right
7 Colic Artery, Left
8 Colic Artery, Middle
9 Renal Artery, Right
Inferior suprarenal artery
Renal segmental artery
A Renal Artery, Left
See 9 Renal Artery, Right
B Inferior Mesenteric Artery
Sigmoid artery
Superior rectal artery
C Common Iliac Artery, Right
D Common Iliac Artery, Left
E Internal Iliac Artery, Right
Deferential artery
Hypogastric artery
Iliolumbar artery
Inferior gluteal artery
Inferior vesical artery
Internal pudendal artery
Lateral sacral artery
Middle rectal artery
Obturator artery
Prostatic artery
Superior gluteal artery
Superior vesical artery
Umbilical artery
Uterine artery
Vaginal artery
	F Internal Iliac Artery, Left
	See E Internal Iliac Artery, Right
	H External Iliac Artery, Right
	Deep circumflex iliac artery
	Inferior epigastric artery
	J External Iliac Artery, Left
	See H External Iliac Artery, Right
	K Femoral Artery, Right
	Circumflex iliac artery
	Deep femoral artery
	Descending genicular artery
	External pudendal artery
	Superficial epigastric artery
	L Femoral Artery, Left
	See K Femoral Artery, Right
	M Popliteal Artery, Right
	Inferior genicular artery
	Middle genicular artery
	Superior genicular artery
	Sural artery
	Tibioperoneal trunk
	N Popliteal Artery, Left
	See M Popliteal Artery, Right
	P Anterior Tibial Artery, Right
	Anterior lateral malleolar artery
	Anterior medial malleolar artery
	Anterior tibial recurrent artery
	Dorsalis pedis artery
	Posterior tibial recurrent artery
	Q Anterior Tibial Artery, Left
	See P Anterior Tibial Artery,
	   Right
	R Posterior Tibial Artery, Right
	S Posterior Tibial Artery, Left
	T Peroneal Artery, Right
	Fibular artery
	U Peroneal Artery, Left
	See T Peroneal Artery, Right
	V Foot Artery, Right
	Arcuate artery
	Dorsal metatarsal artery
	Lateral plantar artery
	Lateral tarsal artery
	Medial plantar artery
	W Foot Artery, Left
	See V Foot Artery, Right
	Y Lower Artery
	Umbilical artery
		0 Open
		3 Percutaneous
		4 Percutaneous Endoscopic
			Z No Device	**Z No Qualifier**

Non-OR Procedure   DRG Non-OR Procedure   Valid OR Procedure   HAC Associated Procedure   Combination Only   New/Revised April   New/Revised October

230   ICD-10-PCS 2023

04C–04C

Ø   **Medical and Surgical**
4   **Lower Arteries**
F   **Fragmentation**   Definition: Breaking solid matter in a body part into pieces
           Explanation: Physical force (e.g., manual, ultrasonic) applied directly or indirectly is used to break the solid matter into pieces. The solid matter may be an abnormal byproduct of a biological function or a foreign body. The pieces of solid matter are not taken out.

Body Part Character 4	Approach Character 5	Device Character 6	Qualifier Character 7

C **Common Iliac Artery, Right**
D **Common Iliac Artery, Left**
E **Internal Iliac Artery, Right**
   Deferential artery
   Hypogastric artery
   Iliolumbar artery
   Inferior gluteal artery
   Inferior vesical artery
   Internal pudendal artery
   Lateral sacral artery
   Middle rectal artery
   Obturator artery
   Prostatic artery
   Superior gluteal artery
   Superior vesical artery
   Umbilical artery
   Uterine artery
   Vaginal artery
F **Internal Iliac Artery, Left**
   See E Internal Iliac Artery, Right
H **External Iliac Artery, Right**
   Deep circumflex iliac artery
   Inferior epigastric artery
J **External Iliac Artery, Left**
   See H External Iliac Artery, Right
K **Femoral Artery, Right**
   Circumflex iliac artery
   Deep femoral artery
   Descending genicular artery
   External pudendal artery
   Superficial epigastric artery
L **Femoral Artery, Left**
   See K Femoral Artery, Right
M **Popliteal Artery, Right**
   Inferior genicular artery
   Middle genicular artery
   Superior genicular artery
   Sural artery
   Tibioperoneal trunk
N **Popliteal Artery, Left**
   See M Popliteal Artery, Right
P **Anterior Tibial Artery, Right**
   Anterior lateral malleolar artery
   Anterior medial malleolar artery
   Anterior tibial recurrent artery
   Dorsalis pedis artery
   Posterior tibial recurrent artery
Q **Anterior Tibial Artery, Left**
   See P Anterior Tibial Artery, Right
R **Posterior Tibial Artery, Right**
S **Posterior Tibial Artery, Left**
T **Peroneal Artery, Right**
   Fibular artery
U **Peroneal Artery, Left**
   See T Peroneal Artery, Right
Y **Lower Artery**
   Umbilical artery
	3 Percutaneous	**Z** No Device	**Ø** Ultrasonic
			Z No Qualifier

NC Noncovered Procedure   **LC** Limited Coverage   **QA** Questionable OB Admit   **NT** New Tech Add-on   ⊞ Combination Member   ♂ Male   ♀ Female

ICD-10-PCS 2023   231

Lower Arteries

0 Medical and Surgical
4 Lower Arteries
H Insertion Definition: Putting in a nonbiological appliance that monitors, assists, performs, or prevents a physiological function but does not physically take the place of a body part

Explanation: None

Body Part Character 4		Approach Character 5	Device Character 6	Qualifier Character 7
0 Abdominal Aorta Inferior phrenic artery Lumbar artery Median sacral artery Middle suprarenal artery Ovarian artery Testicular artery		**0** Open **3** Percutaneous **4** Percutaneous Endoscopic	**2** Monitoring Device **3** Infusion Device **D** Intraluminal Device	**Z** No Qualifier
1 Celiac Artery Celiac trunk **2 Gastric Artery** Left gastric artery Right gastric artery **3 Hepatic Artery** Common hepatic artery Gastroduodenal artery Hepatic artery proper **4 Splenic Artery** Left gastroepiploic artery Pancreatic artery Short gastric artery **5 Superior Mesenteric Artery** Ileal artery Ileocolic artery Inferior pancreaticoduodenal artery Jejunal artery **6 Colic Artery, Right** **7 Colic Artery, Left** **8 Colic Artery, Middle** **9 Renal Artery, Right** Inferior suprarenal artery Renal segmental artery **A Renal Artery, Left** *See 9 Renal Artery, Right* **B Inferior Mesenteric Artery** Sigmoid artery Superior rectal artery **C Common Iliac Artery, Right** **D Common Iliac Artery, Left** **E Internal Iliac Artery, Right** Deferential artery Hypogastric artery Iliolumbar artery Inferior gluteal artery Inferior vesical artery Internal pudendal artery Lateral sacral artery Middle rectal artery Obturator artery Prostatic artery Superior gluteal artery Superior vesical artery Umbilical artery Uterine artery Vaginal artery	**F Internal Iliac Artery, Left** *See E Internal Iliac Artery, Right* **H External Iliac Artery, Right** Deep circumflex iliac artery Inferior epigastric artery **J External Iliac Artery, Left** *See H External Iliac Artery, Right* **K Femoral Artery, Right** Circumflex iliac artery Deep femoral artery Descending genicular artery External pudendal artery Superficial epigastric artery **L Femoral Artery, Left** *See K Femoral Artery, Right* **M Popliteal Artery, Right** Inferior genicular artery Middle genicular artery Superior genicular artery Sural artery Tibioperoneal trunk **N Popliteal Artery, Left** *See M Popliteal Artery, Right* **P Anterior Tibial Artery, Right** Anterior lateral malleolar artery Anterior medial malleolar artery Anterior tibial recurrent artery Dorsalis pedis artery Posterior tibial recurrent artery **Q Anterior Tibial Artery, Left** *See P Anterior Tibial Artery, Right* **R Posterior Tibial Artery, Right** **S Posterior Tibial Artery, Left** **T Peroneal Artery, Right** Fibular artery **U Peroneal Artery, Left** *See T Peroneal Artery, Right* **V Foot Artery, Right** Arcuate artery Dorsal metatarsal artery Lateral plantar artery Lateral tarsal artery Medial plantar artery **W Foot Artery, Left** *See V Foot Artery, Right*	**0** Open **3** Percutaneous **4** Percutaneous Endoscopic	**3** Infusion Device **D** Intraluminal Device	**Z** No Qualifier
Y Lower Artery Umbilical artery		**0** Open **3** Percutaneous **4** Percutaneous Endoscopic	**2** Monitoring Device **3** Infusion Device **D** Intraluminal Device **Y** Other Device	**Z** No Qualifier

Non-OR	04H0[0,3,4][2,3]Z
Non-OR	04H[1,2,3,4,5,6,7,8,9,A,B,C,D,E,F,H,J,K,L,M,N,P,Q,R,S,T,U,V,W][0,3,4]3Z
Non-OR	04HY32Z
Non-OR	04HY[0,3,4]3Z
Non-OR	04HY[3,4]YZ

Non-OR Procedure   DRG Non-OR Procedure   Valid OR Procedure   HAC Associated Procedure   Combination Only   New/Revised April   New/Revised October

232

ICD-10-PCS 2023

Ø   **Medical and Surgical**
4   **Lower Arteries**
J   **Inspection**   Definition: Visually and/or manually exploring a body part

Explanation: Visual exploration may be performed with or without optical instrumentation. Manual exploration may be performed directly or through intervening body layers.

Body Part Character 4	Approach Character 5	Device Character 6	Qualifier Character 7
Y Lower Artery Umbilical artery	**Ø** Open **3** Percutaneous **4** Percutaneous Endoscopic **X** External	**Z** No Device	**Z** No Qualifier

Non-OR   04JY[3,4,X]ZZ

Ø   **Medical and Surgical**
4   **Lower Arteries**
L   **Occlusion**   Definition: Completely closing an orifice or the lumen of a tubular body part

Explanation: The orifice can be a natural orifice or an artificially created orifice

Body Part Character 4	Approach Character 5	Device Character 6	Qualifier Character 7

Ø Abdominal Aorta
   Inferior phrenic artery
   Lumbar artery
   Median sacral artery
   Middle suprarenal artery
   Ovarian artery
   Testicular artery
	Ø Open
	4 Percutaneous Endoscopic
		C Extraluminal Device
		D Intraluminal Device
		Z No Device
			Z No Qualifier

Ø Abdominal Aorta
   Inferior phrenic artery
   Lumbar artery
   Median sacral artery
   Middle suprarenal artery
   Ovarian artery
   Testicular artery
	3 Percutaneous	**C** Extraluminal Device
		Z No Device
			Z No Qualifier

Ø Abdominal Aorta
   Inferior phrenic artery
   Lumbar artery
   Median sacral artery
   Middle suprarenal artery
   Ovarian artery
   Testicular artery
	3 Percutaneous	**D** Intraluminal Device	**J** Temporary
			Z No Qualifier

04L Continued on next page

Lower Arteries

0   **Medical and Surgical**
4   **Lower Arteries**
L   **Occlusion**

04L Continued

Definition: Completely closing an orifice or the lumen of a tubular body part
Explanation: The orifice can be a natural orifice or an artificially created orifice

Body Part — Character 4	Approach — Character 5	Device — Character 6	Qualifier — Character 7
1 **Celiac Artery** — Celiac trunk 2 **Gastric Artery** — Left gastric artery, Right gastric artery 3 **Hepatic Artery** — Common hepatic artery, Gastroduodenal artery, Hepatic artery proper 4 **Splenic Artery** — Left gastroepiploic artery, Pancreatic artery, Short gastric artery 5 **Superior Mesenteric Artery** — Ileal artery, Ileocolic artery, Inferior pancreaticoduodenal artery, Jejunal artery 6 **Colic Artery, Right** 7 **Colic Artery, Left** 8 **Colic Artery, Middle** 9 **Renal Artery, Right** — Inferior suprarenal artery, Renal segmental artery A **Renal Artery, Left** *See 9 Renal Artery, Right* B **Inferior Mesenteric Artery** — Sigmoid artery, Superior rectal artery C **Common Iliac Artery, Right** D **Common Iliac Artery, Left** H **External Iliac Artery, Right** — Deep circumflex iliac artery, Inferior epigastric artery J **External Iliac Artery, Left** *See H External Iliac Artery, Right* K **Femoral Artery, Right** — Circumflex iliac artery, Deep femoral artery, Descending genicular artery, External pudendal artery, Superficial epigastric artery L **Femoral Artery, Left** *See K Femoral Artery, Right* M **Popliteal Artery, Right** — Inferior genicular artery, Middle genicular artery, Superior genicular artery, Sural artery, Tibioperoneal trunk N **Popliteal Artery, Left** *See M Popliteal Artery, Right* P **Anterior Tibial Artery, Right** — Anterior lateral malleolar artery, Anterior medial malleolar artery, Anterior tibial recurrent artery, Dorsalis pedis artery, Posterior tibial recurrent artery Q **Anterior Tibial Artery, Left** *See P Anterior Tibial Artery, Right* R **Posterior Tibial Artery, Right** S **Posterior Tibial Artery, Left** T **Peroneal Artery, Right** — Fibular artery U **Peroneal Artery, Left** *See T Peroneal Artery, Right* V **Foot Artery, Right** — Arcuate artery, Dorsal metatarsal artery, Lateral plantar artery, Lateral tarsal artery, Medial plantar artery W **Foot Artery, Left** *See V Foot Artery, Right* Y **Lower Artery** — Umbilical artery	0 Open 3 Percutaneous 4 Percutaneous Endoscopic	C Extraluminal Device D Intraluminal Device Z No Device	Z No Qualifier
E **Internal Iliac Artery, Right** — Deferential artery, Hypogastric artery, Iliolumbar artery, Inferior gluteal artery, Inferior vesical artery, Internal pudendal artery, Lateral sacral artery, Middle rectal artery, Obturator artery, Prostatic artery, Superior gluteal artery, Superior vesical artery, Umbilical artery, Uterine artery, Vaginal artery	0 Open 3 Percutaneous 4 Percutaneous Endoscopic	C Extraluminal Device D Intraluminal Device Z No Device	T Uterine Artery, Right ♀ V Prostatic Artery, Right ♂ Z No Qualifier
F **Internal Iliac Artery, Left** — Deferential artery, Hypogastric artery, Iliolumbar artery, Inferior gluteal artery, Inferior vesical artery, Internal pudendal artery, Lateral sacral artery, Middle rectal artery, Obturator artery, Prostatic artery, Superior gluteal artery, Superior vesical artery, Umbilical artery, Uterine artery, Vaginal artery	0 Open 3 Percutaneous 4 Percutaneous Endoscopic	C Extraluminal Device D Intraluminal Device Z No Device	U Uterine Artery, Left ♀ W Prostatic Artery, Left ♂ Z No Qualifier

♀   04LE[0,3,4][C,D,Z]T
♀   04LF[0,3,4][C,D,Z]U
♂   04LE[0,3,4][C,D,Z]V
♂   04LF[0,3,4][C,D,Z]W

0   **Medical and Surgical**
4   **Lower Arteries**
N   **Release**   Definition: Freeing a body part from an abnormal physical constraint by cutting or by the use of force
                  Explanation: Some of the restraining tissue may be taken out but none of the body part is taken out

Body Part Character 4		Approach Character 5	Device Character 6	Qualifier Character 7

0 **Abdominal Aorta**
  Inferior phrenic artery
  Lumbar artery
  Median sacral artery
  Middle suprarenal artery
  Ovarian artery
  Testicular artery
1 **Celiac Artery**
  Celiac trunk
2 **Gastric Artery**
  Left gastric artery
  Right gastric artery
3 **Hepatic Artery**
  Common hepatic artery
  Gastroduodenal artery
  Hepatic artery proper
4 **Splenic Artery**
  Left gastroepiploic artery
  Pancreatic artery
  Short gastric artery
5 **Superior Mesenteric Artery**
  Ileal artery
  Ileocolic artery
  Inferior pancreaticoduodenal artery
  Jejunal artery
6 **Colic Artery, Right**
7 **Colic Artery, Left**
8 **Colic Artery, Middle**
9 **Renal Artery, Right**
  Inferior suprarenal artery
  Renal segmental artery
A **Renal Artery, Left**
  See 9 Renal Artery, Right
B **Inferior Mesenteric Artery**
  Sigmoid artery
  Superior rectal artery
C **Common Iliac Artery, Right**
D **Common Iliac Artery, Left**
E **Internal Iliac Artery, Right**
  Deferential artery
  Hypogastric artery
  Iliolumbar artery
  Inferior gluteal artery
  Inferior vesical artery
  Internal pudendal artery
  Lateral sacral artery
  Middle rectal artery
  Obturator artery
  Prostatic artery
  Superior gluteal artery
  Superior vesical artery
  Umbilical artery
  Uterine artery
  Vaginal artery
	F **Internal Iliac Artery, Left**
	  See E Internal Iliac Artery, Right
	H **External Iliac Artery, Right**
	  Deep circumflex iliac artery
	  Inferior epigastric artery
	J **External Iliac Artery, Left**
	  See H External Iliac Artery, Right
	K **Femoral Artery, Right**
	  Circumflex iliac artery
	  Deep femoral artery
	  Descending genicular artery
	  External pudendal artery
	  Superficial epigastric artery
	L **Femoral Artery, Left**
	  See K Femoral Artery, Right
	M **Popliteal Artery, Right**
	  Inferior genicular artery
	  Middle genicular artery
	  Superior genicular artery
	  Sural artery
	  Tibioperoneal trunk
	N **Popliteal Artery, Left**
	  See M Popliteal Artery, Right
	P **Anterior Tibial Artery, Right**
	  Anterior lateral malleolar artery
	  Anterior medial malleolar artery
	  Anterior tibial recurrent artery
	  Dorsalis pedis artery
	  Posterior tibial recurrent artery
	Q **Anterior Tibial Artery, Left**
	  See P Anterior Tibial Artery, Right
	R **Posterior Tibial Artery, Right**
	S **Posterior Tibial Artery, Left**
	T **Peroneal Artery, Right**
	  Fibular artery
	U **Peroneal Artery, Left**
	  See T Peroneal Artery, Right
	V **Foot Artery, Right**
	  Arcuate artery
	  Dorsal metatarsal artery
	  Lateral plantar artery
	  Lateral tarsal artery
	  Medial plantar artery
	W **Foot Artery, Left**
	  See V Foot Artery, Right
	Y **Lower Artery**
	  Umbilical artery
		0 Open
		3 Percutaneous
		4 Percutaneous Endoscopic
			Z No Device	**Z** No Qualifier

NC Noncovered Procedure   **LC** Limited Coverage   **QA** Questionable OB Admit   **NT** New Tech Add-on   ⊞ Combination Member   ♂ Male   ♀ Female

ICD-10-PCS 2023   235

04N–04N

Lower Arteries

Ø	**Medical and Surgical**
4	**Lower Arteries**
P	**Removal**

Definition: Taking out or off a device from a body part

Explanation: If a device is taken out and a similar device put in without cutting or puncturing the skin or mucous membrane, the procedure is coded to the root operation CHANGE. Otherwise, the procedure for taking out a device is coded to the root operation REMOVAL.

Body Part Character 4	Approach Character 5	Device Character 6	Qualifier Character 7
Y Lower Artery Umbilical artery	Ø Open 3 Percutaneous 4 Percutaneous Endoscopic	Ø Drainage Device 2 Monitoring Device 3 Infusion Device 7 Autologous Tissue Substitute C Extraluminal Device D Intraluminal Device J Synthetic Substitute K Nonautologous Tissue Substitute Y Other Device	Z No Qualifier
Y Lower Artery Umbilical artery	X External	Ø Drainage Device 1 Radioactive Element 2 Monitoring Device 3 Infusion Device D Intraluminal Device	Z No Qualifier

Non-OR	Ø4PY3[Ø,2,3,D]Z
Non-OR	Ø4PY[3,4]YZ
Non-OR	Ø4PYX[Ø,1,2,3,D]Z

Non-OR Procedure   DRG Non-OR Procedure   Valid OR Procedure   HAC Associated Procedure   Combination Only   New/Revised April   New/Revised October

236   ICD-10-PCS 2023

Ø   Medical and Surgical
4   Lower Arteries
Q   Repair   Definition: Restoring, to the extent possible, a body part to its normal anatomic structure and function

Explanation: Used only when the method to accomplish the repair is not one of the other root operations

Body Part Character 4		Approach Character 5	Device Character 6	Qualifier Character 7

Ø Abdominal Aorta
  Inferior phrenic artery
  Lumbar artery
  Median sacral artery
  Middle suprarenal artery
  Ovarian artery
  Testicular artery
1 Celiac Artery
  Celiac trunk
2 Gastric Artery
  Left gastric artery
  Right gastric artery
3 Hepatic Artery
  Common hepatic artery
  Gastroduodenal artery
  Hepatic artery proper
4 Splenic Artery
  Left gastroepiploic artery
  Pancreatic artery
  Short gastric artery
5 Superior Mesenteric Artery
  Ileal artery
  Ileocolic artery
  Inferior pancreaticoduodenal
    artery
  Jejunal artery
6 Colic Artery, Right
7 Colic Artery, Left
8 Colic Artery, Middle
9 Renal Artery, Right
  Inferior suprarenal artery
  Renal segmental artery
A Renal Artery, Left
  See 9 Renal Artery, Right
B Inferior Mesenteric Artery
  Sigmoid artery
  Superior rectal artery
C Common Iliac Artery, Right
D Common Iliac Artery, Left
E Internal Iliac Artery, Right
  Deferential artery
  Hypogastric artery
  Iliolumbar artery
  Inferior gluteal artery
  Inferior vesical artery
  Internal pudendal artery
  Lateral sacral artery
  Middle rectal artery
  Obturator artery
  Prostatic artery
  Superior gluteal artery
  Superior vesical artery
  Umbilical artery
  Uterine artery
  Vaginal artery
	F Internal Iliac Artery, Left
	  *See E Internal Iliac Artery,
	    Right*
	H External Iliac Artery, Right
	  Deep circumflex iliac artery
	  Inferior epigastric artery
	J External Iliac Artery, Left
	  *See H External Iliac Artery,
	    Right*
	K Femoral Artery, Right
	  Circumflex iliac artery
	  Deep femoral artery
	  Descending genicular artery
	  External pudendal artery
	  Superficial epigastric artery
	L Femoral Artery, Left
	  See K Femoral Artery, Right
	M Popliteal Artery, Right
	  Inferior genicular artery
	  Middle genicular artery
	  Superior genicular artery
	  Sural artery
	  Tibioperoneal trunk
	N Popliteal Artery, Left
	  See M Popliteal Artery, Right
	P Anterior Tibial Artery, Right
	  Anterior lateral malleolar
	    artery
	  Anterior medial malleolar
	    artery
	  Anterior tibial recurrent
	    artery
	  Dorsalis pedis artery
	  Posterior tibial recurrent
	    artery
	Q Anterior Tibial Artery, Left
	  *See P Anterior Tibial Artery,
	    Right*
	**R Posterior Tibial Artery,
	  Right**
	S Posterior Tibial Artery, Left
	T Peroneal Artery, Right
	  Fibular artery
	U Peroneal Artery, Left
	  See T Peroneal Artery, Right
	V Foot Artery, Right
	  Arcuate artery
	  Dorsal metatarsal artery
	  Lateral plantar artery
	  Lateral tarsal artery
	  Medial plantar artery
	W Foot Artery, Left
	  See V Foot Artery, Right
	Y Lower Artery
	  Umbilical artery
		Ø Open
		3 Percutaneous
		4 Percutaneous Endoscopic
			Z No Device	**Z No Qualifier**

NC Noncovered Procedure   **LC** Limited Coverage   **QA** Questionable OB Admit   **NT** New Tech Add-on   ⊞ Combination Member   ♂ Male   ♀ Female

ICD-10-PCS 2023   237

04Q–04Q

Ø **Medical and Surgical**
4 **Lower Arteries**
R **Replacement** Definition: Putting in or on biological or synthetic material that physically takes the place and/or function of all or a portion of a body part
Explanation: The body part may have been taken out or replaced, or may be taken out, physically eradicated, or rendered nonfunctional during the REPLACEMENT procedure. A REMOVAL procedure is coded for taking out the device used in a previous replacement procedure.

Body Part Character 4		Approach Character 5	Device Character 6	Qualifier Character 7

Ø **Abdominal Aorta**
 Inferior phrenic artery
 Lumbar artery
 Median sacral artery
 Middle suprarenal artery
 Ovarian artery
 Testicular artery
1 **Celiac Artery**
 Celiac trunk
2 **Gastric Artery**
 Left gastric artery
 Right gastric artery
3 **Hepatic Artery**
 Common hepatic artery
 Gastroduodenal artery
 Hepatic artery proper
4 **Splenic Artery**
 Left gastroepiploic artery
 Pancreatic artery
 Short gastric artery
5 **Superior Mesenteric Artery**
 Ileal artery
 Ileocolic artery
 Inferior pancreaticoduodenal
  artery
 Jejunal artery
6 **Colic Artery, Right**
7 **Colic Artery, Left**
8 **Colic Artery, Middle**
9 **Renal Artery, Right**
 Inferior suprarenal artery
 Renal segmental artery
A **Renal Artery, Left**
 See 9 Renal Artery, Right
B **Inferior Mesenteric Artery**
 Sigmoid artery
 Superior rectal artery
C **Common Iliac Artery, Right**
D **Common Iliac Artery, Left**
E **Internal Iliac Artery, Right**
 Deferential artery
 Hypogastric artery
 Iliolumbar artery
 Inferior gluteal artery
 Inferior vesical artery
 Internal pudendal artery
 Lateral sacral artery
 Middle rectal artery
 Obturator artery
 Prostatic artery
 Superior gluteal artery
 Superior vesical artery
 Umbilical artery
 Uterine artery
 Vaginal artery
	F **Internal Iliac Artery, Left**
	 See E Internal Iliac Artery, Right
	H **External Iliac Artery, Right**
	 Deep circumflex iliac artery
	 Inferior epigastric artery
	J **External Iliac Artery, Left**
	 See H External Iliac Artery, Right
	K **Femoral Artery, Right**
	 Circumflex iliac artery
	 Deep femoral artery
	 Descending genicular artery
	 External pudendal artery
	 Superficial epigastric artery
	L **Femoral Artery, Left**
	 See K Femoral Artery, Right
	M **Popliteal Artery, Right**
	 Inferior genicular artery
	 Middle genicular artery
	 Superior genicular artery
	 Sural artery
	 Tibioperoneal trunk
	N **Popliteal Artery, Left**
	 See M Popliteal Artery, Right
	P **Anterior Tibial Artery, Right**
	 Anterior lateral malleolar
	  artery
	 Anterior medial malleolar
	  artery
	 Anterior tibial recurrent artery
	 Dorsalis pedis artery
	 Posterior tibial recurrent artery
	Q **Anterior Tibial Artery, Left**
	 See P Anterior Tibial Artery,
	 Right
	R **Posterior Tibial Artery, Right**
	S **Posterior Tibial Artery, Left**
	T **Peroneal Artery, Right**
	 Fibular artery
	U **Peroneal Artery, Left**
	 See T Peroneal Artery, Right
	V **Foot Artery, Right**
	 Arcuate artery
	 Dorsal metatarsal artery
	 Lateral plantar artery
	 Lateral tarsal artery
	 Medial plantar artery
	W **Foot Artery, Left**
	 See V Foot Artery, Right
	Y **Lower Artery**
	 Umbilical artery
		Ø **Open**
		4 **Percutaneous Endoscopic**
			7 **Autologous Tissue**
			 Substitute
			J **Synthetic Substitute**
			K **Nonautologous Tissue**
			 Substitute
				Z **No Qualifier**

Non-OR Procedure   DRG Non-OR Procedure   Valid OR Procedure   HAC Associated Procedure   Combination Only   New/Revised April   New/Revised October

238

ICD-10-PCS 2023

Ø Medical and Surgical
4 Lower Arteries
S Reposition   Definition: Moving to its normal location, or other suitable location, all or a portion of a body part

Explanation: The body part is moved to a new location from an abnormal location, or from a normal location where it is not functioning correctly. The body part may or may not be cut out or off to be moved to the new location.

Body Part Character 4		Approach Character 5	Device Character 6	Qualifier Character 7

Ø Abdominal Aorta
Inferior phrenic artery
Lumbar artery
Median sacral artery
Middle suprarenal artery
Ovarian artery
Testicular artery
1 Celiac Artery
Celiac trunk
2 Gastric Artery
Left gastric artery
Right gastric artery
3 Hepatic Artery
Common hepatic artery
Gastroduodenal artery
Hepatic artery proper
4 Splenic Artery
Left gastroepiploic artery
Pancreatic artery
Short gastric artery
5 Superior Mesenteric Artery
Ileal artery
Ileocolic artery
Inferior pancreaticoduodenal
   artery
Jejunal artery
6 Colic Artery, Right
7 Colic Artery, Left
8 Colic Artery, Middle
9 Renal Artery, Right
Inferior suprarenal artery
Renal segmental artery
A Renal Artery, Left
See 9 Renal Artery, Right
B Inferior Mesenteric Artery
Sigmoid artery
Superior rectal artery
C Common Iliac Artery, Right
D Common Iliac Artery, Left
E Internal Iliac Artery, Right
Deferential artery
Hypogastric artery
Iliolumbar artery
Inferior gluteal artery
Inferior vesical artery
Internal pudendal artery
Lateral sacral artery
Middle rectal artery
Obturator artery
Prostatic artery
Superior gluteal artery
Superior vesical artery
Umbilical artery
Uterine artery
Vaginal artery
	F Internal Iliac Artery, Left
	See E Internal Iliac Artery, Right
	H External Iliac Artery, Right
	Deep circumflex iliac artery
	Inferior epigastric artery
	J External Iliac Artery, Left
	See H External Iliac Artery, Right
	K Femoral Artery, Right
	Circumflex iliac artery
	Deep femoral artery
	Descending genicular artery
	External pudendal artery
	Superficial epigastric artery
	L Femoral Artery, Left
	See K Femoral Artery, Right
	M Popliteal Artery, Right
	Inferior genicular artery
	Middle genicular artery
	Superior genicular artery
	Sural artery
	Tibioperoneal trunk
	N Popliteal Artery, Left
	See M Popliteal Artery, Right
	P Anterior Tibial Artery, Right
	Anterior lateral malleolar
	   artery
	Anterior medial malleolar
	   artery
	Anterior tibial recurrent artery
	Dorsalis pedis artery
	Posterior tibial recurrent artery
	Q Anterior Tibial Artery, Left
	See P Anterior Tibial Artery,
	Right
	R Posterior Tibial Artery, Right
	S Posterior Tibial Artery, Left
	T Peroneal Artery, Right
	Fibular artery
	U Peroneal Artery, Left
	See T Peroneal Artery, Right
	V Foot Artery, Right
	Arcuate artery
	Dorsal metatarsal artery
	Lateral plantar artery
	Lateral tarsal artery
	Medial plantar artery
	W Foot Artery, Left
	See V Foot Artery, Right
	Y Lower Artery
	Umbilical artery
		Ø Open
		3 Percutaneous
		4 Percutaneous Endoscopic
			Z No Device	**Z No Qualifier**

NC Noncovered Procedure   LC Limited Coverage   QA Questionable OB Admit   NT New Tech Add-on   ⊞ Combination Member   ♂ Male   ♀ Female

ICD-10-PCS 2023

239

04S–04S

Lower Arteries

0   **Medical and Surgical**
4   **Lower Arteries**
U   **Supplement**   Definition: Putting in or on biological or synthetic material that physically reinforces and/or augments the function of a portion of a body part

Explanation: The biological material is non-living, or is living and from the same individual. The body part may have been previously replaced, and the SUPPLEMENT procedure is performed to physically reinforce and/or augment the function of the replaced body part.

Body Part Character 4		Approach Character 5	Device Character 6	Qualifier Character 7
0 **Abdominal Aorta** Inferior phrenic artery Lumbar artery Median sacral artery Middle suprarenal artery Ovarian artery Testicular artery **1** **Celiac Artery** Celiac trunk **2** **Gastric Artery** Left gastric artery Right gastric artery **3** **Hepatic Artery** Common hepatic artery Gastroduodenal artery Hepatic artery proper **4** **Splenic Artery** Left gastroepiploic artery Pancreatic artery Short gastric artery **5** **Superior Mesenteric Artery** Ileal artery Ileocolic artery Inferior pancreaticoduodenal artery Jejunal artery **6** **Colic Artery, Right** **7** **Colic Artery, Left** **8** **Colic Artery, Middle** **9** **Renal Artery, Right** Inferior suprarenal artery Renal segmental artery **A** **Renal Artery, Left** *See 9 Renal Artery, Right* **B** **Inferior Mesenteric Artery** Sigmoid artery Superior rectal artery **C** **Common Iliac Artery, Right** **D** **Common Iliac Artery, Left** **E** **Internal Iliac Artery, Right** Deferential artery Hypogastric artery Iliolumbar artery Inferior gluteal artery Inferior vesical artery Internal pudendal artery Lateral sacral artery Middle rectal artery Obturator artery Prostatic artery Superior gluteal artery Superior vesical artery Umbilical artery Uterine artery Vaginal artery	**F** **Internal Iliac Artery, Left** *See E Internal Iliac Artery, Right* **H** **External Iliac Artery, Right** Deep circumflex iliac artery Inferior epigastric artery **J** **External Iliac Artery, Left** *See H External Iliac Artery, Right* **K** **Femoral Artery, Right** Circumflex iliac artery Deep femoral artery Descending genicular artery External pudendal artery Superficial epigastric artery **L** **Femoral Artery, Left** *See K Femoral Artery, Right* **M** **Popliteal Artery, Right** Inferior genicular artery Middle genicular artery Superior genicular artery Sural artery Tibioperoneal trunk **N** **Popliteal Artery, Left** *See M Popliteal Artery, Right* **P** **Anterior Tibial Artery, Right** Anterior lateral malleolar artery Anterior medial malleolar artery Anterior tibial recurrent artery Dorsalis pedis artery Posterior tibial recurrent artery **Q** **Anterior Tibial Artery, Left** *See P Anterior Tibial Artery, Right* **R** **Posterior Tibial Artery, Right** **S** **Posterior Tibial Artery, Left** **T** **Peroneal Artery, Right** Fibular artery **U** **Peroneal Artery, Left** *See T Peroneal Artery, Right* **V** **Foot Artery, Right** Arcuate artery Dorsal metatarsal artery Lateral plantar artery Lateral tarsal artery Medial plantar artery **W** **Foot Artery, Left** *See V Foot Artery, Right* **Y** **Lower Artery** Umbilical artery	**0** Open **3** Percutaneous **4** Percutaneous Endoscopic	**7** Autologous Tissue Substitute **J** Synthetic Substitute **K** Nonautologous Tissue Substitute	**Z** No Qualifier

Non-OR Procedure   DRG Non-OR Procedure   Valid OR Procedure   HAC Associated Procedure   Combination Only   New/Revised April   New/Revised October

240   ICD-10-PCS 2023

Ø   Medical and Surgical
4   Lower Arteries
V   Restriction   Definition: Partially closing an orifice or the lumen of a tubular body part
                        Explanation: The orifice can be a natural orifice or an artificially created orifice

Body Part Character 4		Approach Character 5	Device Character 6	Qualifier Character 7
Ø Abdominal Aorta Inferior phrenic artery Lumbar artery Median sacral artery Middle suprarenal artery Ovarian artery Testicular artery		**Ø** Open **3** Percutaneous **4** Percutaneous Endoscopic	**C** Extraluminal Device **E** Intraluminal Device, Branched or Fenestrated, One or Two Arteries **F** Intraluminal Device, Branched or Fenestrated, Three or More Arteries **Z** No Device	**Z** No Qualifier
Ø Abdominal Aorta Inferior phrenic artery Lumbar artery Median sacral artery Middle suprarenal artery Ovarian artery Testicular artery		**Ø** Open **3** Percutaneous **4** Percutaneous Endoscopic	**D** Intraluminal Device	**J** Temporary **Z** No Qualifier
1 Celiac Artery Celiac trunk **2 Gastric Artery** Left gastric artery Right gastric artery **3 Hepatic Artery** Common hepatic artery Gastroduodenal artery Hepatic artery proper **4 Splenic Artery** Left gastroepiploic artery Pancreatic artery Short gastric artery **5 Superior Mesenteric Artery** Ileal artery Ileocolic artery Inferior pancreaticoduodenal artery Jejunal artery **6 Colic Artery, Right** **7 Colic Artery, Left** **8 Colic Artery, Middle** **9 Renal Artery, Right** Inferior suprarenal artery Renal segmental artery **A Renal Artery, Left** *See 9 Renal Artery, Right* **B Inferior Mesenteric Artery** Sigmoid artery Superior rectal artery **E Internal Iliac Artery, Right** Deferential artery Hypogastric artery Iliolumbar artery Inferior gluteal artery Inferior vesical artery Internal pudendal artery Lateral sacral artery Middle rectal artery Obturator artery Prostatic artery Superior gluteal artery Superior vesical artery Umbilical artery Uterine artery Vaginal artery **F Internal Iliac Artery, Left** *See E Internal Iliac Artery, Right*	**H External Iliac Artery, Right** Deep circumflex iliac artery Inferior epigastric artery **J External Iliac Artery, Left** *See H External Iliac Artery, Right* **K Femoral Artery, Right** Circumflex iliac artery Deep femoral artery Descending genicular artery External pudendal artery Superficial epigastric artery **L Femoral Artery, Left** *See K Femoral Artery, Right* **M Popliteal Artery, Right** Inferior genicular artery Middle genicular artery Superior genicular artery Sural artery Tibioperoneal trunk **N Popliteal Artery, Left** *See M Popliteal Artery, Right* **P Anterior Tibial Artery, Right** Anterior lateral malleolar artery Anterior medial malleolar artery Anterior tibial recurrent artery Dorsalis pedis artery Posterior tibial recurrent artery **Q Anterior Tibial Artery, Left** *See P Anterior Tibial Artery, Right* **R Posterior Tibial Artery, Right** **S Posterior Tibial Artery, Left** **T Peroneal Artery, Right** Fibular artery **U Peroneal Artery, Left** *See T Peroneal Artery, Right* **V Foot Artery, Right** Arcuate artery Dorsal metatarsal artery Lateral plantar artery Lateral tarsal artery Medial plantar artery **W Foot Artery, Left** *See V Foot Artery, Right* **Y Lower Artery** Umbilical artery	**Ø** Open **3** Percutaneous **4** Percutaneous Endoscopic	**C** Extraluminal Device **D** Intraluminal Device **Z** No Device	**Z** No Qualifier
C Common Iliac Artery, Right **D Common Iliac Artery, Left**		**Ø** Open **3** Percutaneous **4** Percutaneous Endoscopic	**C** Extraluminal Device **D** Intraluminal Device **E** Intraluminal Device, Branched or Fenestrated, One or Two Arteries **Z** No Device	**Z** No Qualifier

NC Noncovered Procedure   **LC** Limited Coverage   **QA** Questionable OB Admit   **NT** New Tech Add-on   ⊞ Combination Member   ♂ Male   ♀ Female

ICD-10-PCS 2023   241

Lower Arteries

Ø　**Medical and Surgical**
4　**Lower Arteries**
W　**Revision**　　Definition: Correcting, to the extent possible, a portion of a malfunctioning device or the position of a displaced device
　　　　　　　　　Explanation: Revision can include correcting a malfunctioning or displaced device by taking out or putting in components of the device such as a screw or pin

Body Part Character 4	Approach Character 5	Device Character 6	Qualifier Character 7
Y　Lower Artery 　　Umbilical artery	Ø　Open 3　Percutaneous 4　Percutaneous Endoscopic	Ø　Drainage Device 2　Monitoring Device 3　Infusion Device 7　Autologous Tissue 　　Substitute C　Extraluminal Device D　Intraluminal Device J　Synthetic Substitute K　Nonautologous Tissue 　　Substitute Y　Other Device	Z　No Qualifier
Y　Lower Artery 　　Umbilical artery	X　External	Ø　Drainage Device 2　Monitoring Device 3　Infusion Device 7　Autologous Tissue 　　Substitute C　Extraluminal Device D　Intraluminal Device J　Synthetic Substitute K　Nonautologous Tissue 　　Substitute	Z　No Qualifier

Non-OR　Ø4WY3[Ø,2,3]Z
Non-OR　Ø4WY[3,4]YZ
Non-OR　Ø4WYX[Ø,2,3,7,C,D,J,K]Z

Upper Veins Ø51–Ø5W

Character Meanings

This Character Meaning table is provided as a guide to assist the user in the identification of character members that may be found in this section of code tables. It **SHOULD NOT** be used to build a PCS code.

Operation–Character 3		Body Part–Character 4		Approach–Character 5		Device–Character 6		Qualifier–Character 7	
1	Bypass	Ø	Azygos Vein	Ø	Open	Ø	Drainage Device	Ø	Ultrasonic
5	Destruction	1	Hemiazygos Vein	3	Percutaneous	2	Monitoring Device	1	Drug-Coated Balloon
7	Dilation	3	Innominate Vein, Right	4	Percutaneous Endoscopic	3	Infusion Device	X	Diagnostic
9	Drainage	4	Innominate Vein, Left	X	External	7	Autologous Tissue Substitute	Y	Upper Vein
B	Excision	5	Subclavian Vein, Right			9	Autologous Venous Tissue	Z	No Qualifier
C	Extirpation	6	Subclavian Vein, Left			A	Autologous Arterial Tissue		
D	Extraction	7	Axillary Vein, Right			C	Extraluminal Device		
F	Fragmentation	8	Axillary Vein, Left			D	Intraluminal Device		
H	Insertion	9	Brachial Vein, Right			J	Synthetic Substitute		
J	Inspection	A	Brachial Vein, Left			K	Nonautologous Tissue Substitute		
L	Occlusion	B	Basilic Vein, Right			M	Neurostimulator Lead		
N	Release	C	Basilic Vein, Left			Y	Other Device		
P	Removal	D	Cephalic Vein, Right			Z	No Device		
Q	Repair	F	Cephalic Vein, Left						
R	Replacement	G	Hand Vein, Right						
S	Reposition	H	Hand Vein, Left						
U	Supplement	L	Intracranial Vein						
V	Restriction	M	Internal Jugular Vein, Right						
W	Revision	N	Internal Jugular Vein, Left						
		P	External Jugular Vein, Right						
		Q	External Jugular Vein, Left						
		R	Vertebral Vein, Right						
		S	Vertebral Vein, Left						
		T	Face Vein, Right						
		V	Face Vein, Left						
		Y	Upper Vein						

AHA Coding Clinic for Upper Veins
2022, 1Q, 10-13   Procedures performed on a continuous vessel, ICD-10-PCS Guideline B4.1c

AHA Coding Clinic for table Ø51
2020, 1Q, 28   Free flap microvascular breast reconstruction
2017, 3Q, 15   Bypass of innominate vein to atrial appendage

AHA Coding Clinic for table Ø57
2020, 3Q, 38   Thrombectomy of arteriovenous fistula with angioplasty and stent placement

AHA Coding Clinic for table Ø59
2018, 3Q, 7   Catheter placement for treatment of congestive heart failure

AHA Coding Clinic for table Ø5B
2021, 2Q, 15   Excision of pituitary macroadenoma within cavernous sinus
2020, 3Q, 40   Excision of ulceration of arteriovenous fistula
2020, 1Q, 24   Resection of vascular malformation, likely cavernoma
2016, 2Q, 12   Resection of malignant neoplasm of infratemporal fossa

AHA Coding Clinic for table Ø5C
2020, 3Q, 37   Repair of aneurysm of arteriovenous fistula with endovenectomy
2020, 3Q, 38   Thrombectomy of arteriovenous fistula with angioplasty and stent placement

AHA Coding Clinic for table Ø5F
2020, 4Q, 45-49   New fragmentation tables
2020, 4Q, 49-50   Intravascular ultrasound assisted thrombolysis
2020, 4Q, 50   Intravascular lithotripsy

AHA Coding Clinic for table Ø5H
2016, 4Q, 97-98   Phrenic neurostimulator

AHA Coding Clinic for table Ø5P
2016, 4Q, 97-98   Phrenic neurostimulator

AHA Coding Clinic for table Ø5Q
2017, 3Q, 15   Bypass of innominate vein to atrial appendage

AHA Coding Clinic for table Ø5S
2013, 4Q, 125   Stage II cephalic vein transposition (superficialization) of arteriovenous fistula

AHA Coding Clinic for table Ø5V
2020, 3Q, 37   Repair of aneurysm of arteriovenous fistula with endovenectomy

AHA Coding Clinic for table Ø5W
2016, 4Q, 97-98   Phrenic neurostimulator

Head and Neck Veins

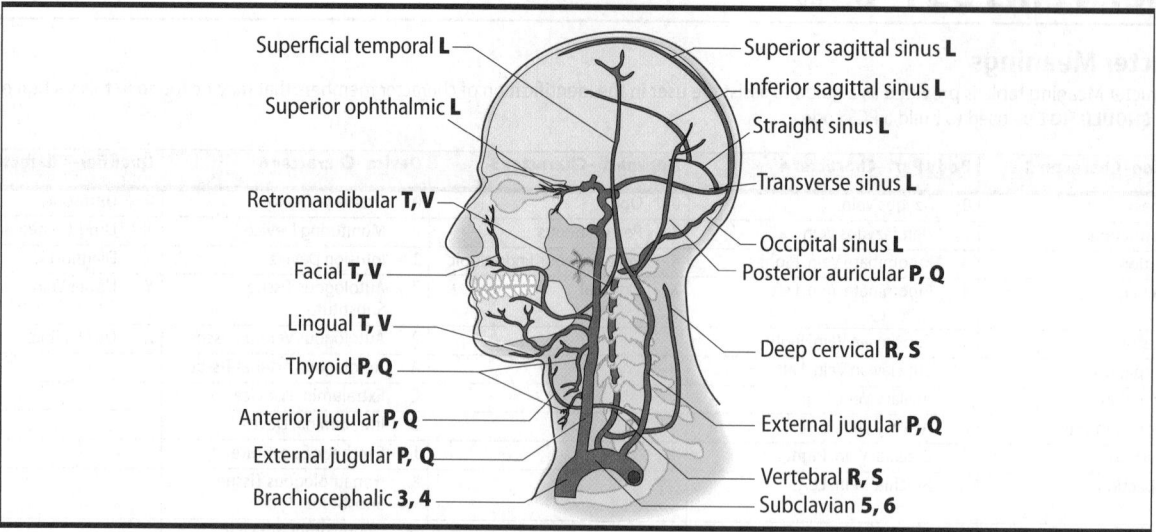

Superficial temporal **L**
Superior ophthalmic **L**
Retromandibular **T, V**
Facial **T, V**
Lingual **T, V**
Thyroid **P, Q**
Anterior jugular **P, Q**
External jugular **P, Q**
Brachiocephalic **3, 4**

Superior sagittal sinus **L**
Inferior sagittal sinus **L**
Straight sinus **L**
Transverse sinus **L**
Occipital sinus **L**
Posterior auricular **P, Q**
Deep cervical **R, S**
External jugular **P, Q**
Vertebral **R, S**
Subclavian **5, 6**

Upper Veins

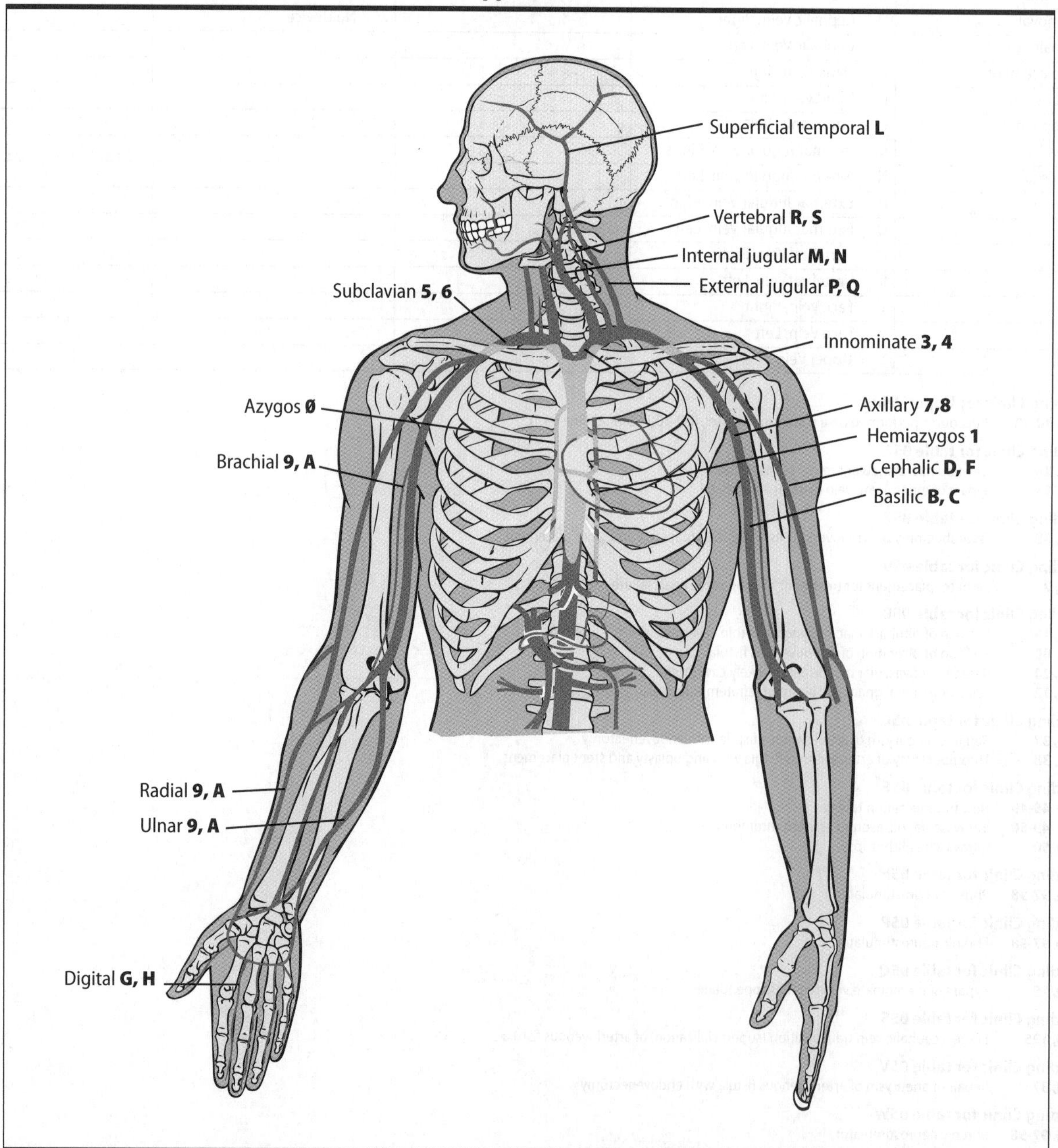

Superficial temporal **L**
Vertebral **R, S**
Internal jugular **M, N**
External jugular **P, Q**
Subclavian **5, 6**
Innominate **3, 4**
Azygos **Ø**
Axillary **7, 8**
Brachial **9, A**
Hemiazygos **1**
Cephalic **D, F**
Basilic **B, C**
Radial **9, A**
Ulnar **9, A**
Digital **G, H**

Upper Veins *(margin)*

Ø   **Medical and Surgical**
5   **Upper Veins**
1   **Bypass**   **Definition:** Altering the route of passage of the contents of a tubular body part

                                   Explanation: Rerouting contents of a body part to a downstream area of the normal route, to a similar route and body part, or to an abnormal route and dissimilar body part. Includes one or more anastomoses, with or without the use of a device.

Body Part Character 4	Approach Character 5	Device Character 6	Qualifier Character 7

Ø **Azygos Vein**
   Right ascending lumbar vein
   Right subcostal vein
	Ø Open
	4 Percutaneous Endoscopic
		7 Autologous Tissue Substitute
		9 Autologous Venous Tissue
		A Autologous Arterial Tissue
		J Synthetic Substitute
		K Nonautologous Tissue Substitute
		Z No Device
			Y Upper Vein

1 **Hemiazygos Vein**
   Left ascending lumbar vein
   Left subcostal vein			

3 **Innominate Vein, Right**
   Brachiocephalic vein
   Inferior thyroid vein			

4 **Innominate Vein, Left** *See 3 Innominate Vein, Right*			
5 **Subclavian Vein, Right**			
6 **Subclavian Vein, Left**			
7 **Axillary Vein, Right**			
8 **Axillary Vein, Left**			

9 **Brachial Vein, Right**
   Radial vein
   Ulnar vein			

A **Brachial Vein, Left** *See 9 Brachial Vein, Right*			

B **Basilic Vein, Right**
   Median antebrachial vein
   Median cubital vein			

C **Basilic Vein, Left** *See B Basilic Vein, Right*			
D **Cephalic Vein, Right** Accessory cephalic vein			
F **Cephalic Vein, Left** *See D Cephalic Vein, Right*			

G **Hand Vein, Right**
   Dorsal metacarpal vein
   Palmar (volar) digital vein
   Palmar (volar) metacarpal vein
   Superficial palmar venous arch
   Volar (palmar) digital vein
   Volar (palmar) metacarpal vein			

H **Hand Vein, Left** *See G Hand Vein, Right*			

L **Intracranial Vein**
   Anterior cerebral vein
   Basal (internal) cerebral vein
   Dural venous sinus
   Great cerebral vein
   Inferior cerebellar vein
   Inferior cerebral vein
   Internal (basal) cerebral vein
   Middle cerebral vein
   Ophthalmic vein
   Superior cerebellar vein
   Superior cerebral vein			

M **Internal Jugular Vein, Right**			
N **Internal Jugular Vein, Left**			
P **External Jugular Vein, Right** Posterior auricular vein			
Q **External Jugular Vein, Left** *See P External Jugular Vein, Right*			

R **Vertebral Vein, Right**
   Deep cervical vein
   Suboccipital venous plexus			

S **Vertebral Vein, Left** *See R Vertebral Vein, Right*			

T **Face Vein, Right**
   Angular vein
   Anterior facial vein
   Common facial vein
   Deep facial vein
   Frontal vein
   Posterior facial (retromandibular) vein
   Supraorbital vein			

V **Face Vein, Left** *See T Face Vein, Right*			

NC Noncovered Procedure   **LC** Limited Coverage   **QA** Questionable OB Admit   **NT** New Tech Add-on   ⊞ Combination Member   ♂ Male   ♀ Female

ICD-10-PCS 2023   **245**

Ø51-Ø51 *(margin)*

Ø Medical and Surgical
5 Upper Veins
5 Destruction   Definition: Physical eradication of all or a portion of a body part by the direct use of energy, force, or a destructive agent
                        Explanation: None of the body part is physically taken out

Body Part Character 4	Approach Character 5	Device Character 6	Qualifier Character 7
Ø Azygos Vein Right ascending lumbar vein Right subcostal vein **1 Hemiazygos Vein** Left ascending lumbar vein Left subcostal vein **3 Innominate Vein, Right** Brachiocephalic vein Inferior thyroid vein **4 Innominate Vein, Left** *See 3 Innominate Vein, Right* **5 Subclavian Vein, Right** **6 Subclavian Vein, Left** **7 Axillary Vein, Right** **8 Axillary Vein, Left** **9 Brachial Vein, Right** Radial vein Ulnar vein **A Brachial Vein, Left** *See 9 Brachial Vein, Right* **B Basilic Vein, Right** Median antebrachial vein Median cubital vein **C Basilic Vein, Left** *See B Basilic Vein, Right* **D Cephalic Vein, Right** Accessory cephalic vein **F Cephalic Vein, Left** *See D Cephalic Vein, Right* **G Hand Vein, Right** Dorsal metacarpal vein Palmar (volar) digital vein Palmar (volar) metacarpal vein Superficial palmar venous arch Volar (palmar) digital vein Volar (palmar) metacarpal vein **H Hand Vein, Left** *See G Hand Vein, Right* **L Intracranial Vein** Anterior cerebral vein Basal (internal) cerebral vein Dural venous sinus Great cerebral vein Inferior cerebellar vein Inferior cerebral vein Internal (basal) cerebral vein Middle cerebral vein Ophthalmic vein Superior cerebellar vein Superior cerebral vein **M Internal Jugular Vein, Right** **N Internal Jugular Vein, Left** **P External Jugular Vein, Right** Posterior auricular vein **Q External Jugular Vein, Left** *See P External Jugular Vein, Right* **R Vertebral Vein, Right** Deep cervical vein Suboccipital venous plexus **S Vertebral Vein, Left** *See R Vertebral Vein, Right* **T Face Vein, Right** Angular vein Anterior facial vein Common facial vein Deep facial vein Frontal vein Posterior facial (retromandibular) vein Supraorbital vein **V Face Vein, Left** *See T Face Vein, Right* **Y Upper Vein**	**Ø Open** **3 Percutaneous** **4 Percutaneous Endoscopic**	**Z No Device**	**Z No Qualifier**

Ø Medical and Surgical
5 Upper Veins
7 Dilation Definition: Expanding an orifice or the lumen of a tubular body part

Explanation: The orifice can be a natural orifice or an artificially created orifice. Accomplished by stretching a tubular body part using intraluminal pressure or by cutting part of the orifice or wall of the tubular body part.

Body Part Character 4	Approach Character 5	Device Character 6	Qualifier Character 7
Ø Azygos Vein Right ascending lumbar vein Right subcostal vein **1 Hemiazygos Vein** Left ascending lumbar vein Left subcostal vein **G Hand Vein, Right** Dorsal metacarpal vein Palmar (volar) digital vein Palmar (volar) metacarpal vein Superficial palmar venous arch Volar (palmar) digital vein Volar (palmar) metacarpal vein **H Hand Vein, Left** *See G Hand Vein, Right* **L Intracranial Vein** `NC` Anterior cerebral vein Basal (internal) cerebral vein Dural venous sinus Great cerebral vein Inferior cerebellar vein Inferior cerebral vein Internal (basal) cerebral vein Middle cerebral vein Ophthalmic vein Superior cerebellar vein Superior cerebral vein **M Internal Jugular Vein, Right** **N Internal Jugular Vein, Left** **P External Jugular Vein, Right** Posterior auricular vein **Q External Jugular Vein, Left** *See P External Jugular Vein, Right* **R Vertebral Vein, Right** Deep cervical vein Suboccipital venous plexus **S Vertebral Vein, Left** *See R Vertebral Vein, Right* **T Face Vein, Right** Angular vein Anterior facial vein Common facial vein Deep facial vein Frontal vein Posterior facial (retromandibular) vein Supraorbital vein **V Face Vein, Left** *See T Face Vein, Right* **Y Upper Vein**	**Ø Open** **3 Percutaneous** **4 Percutaneous Endoscopic**	**D Intraluminal Device** **Z No Device**	**Z No Qualifier**
3 Innominate Vein, Right Brachiocephalic vein Inferior thyroid vein **4 Innominate Vein, Left** *See 3 Innominate Vein, Right* **5 Subclavian Vein, Right** **6 Subclavian Vein, Left** **7 Axillary Vein, Right** **8 Axillary Vein, Left** **9 Brachial Vein, Right** Radial vein Ulnar vein **A Brachial Vein, Left** *See 9 Brachial Vein, Right* **B Basilic Vein, Right** Median antebrachial vein Median cubital vein **C Basilic Vein, Left** *See B Basilic Vein, Right* **D Cephalic Vein, Right** Accessory cephalic vein **F Cephalic Vein, Left** *See D Cephalic Vein, Right*	**Ø Open** **3 Percutaneous** **4 Percutaneous Endoscopic**	**D Intraluminal Device** **Z No Device**	**1 Drug-Coated Balloon** **Z No Qualifier**

`NC` Ø57L[3,4]ZZ

`NC` Noncovered Procedure `LC` Limited Coverage `QA` Questionable OB Admit `NT` New Tech Add-on ⊞ Combination Member ♂ Male ♀ Female

ICD-10-PCS 2023 247

Upper Veins

Ø   **Medical and Surgical**
5   **Upper Veins**
9   **Drainage**   Definition: Taking or letting out fluids and/or gases from a body part

                     Explanation: The qualifier DIAGNOSTIC is used to identify drainage procedures that are biopsies

Body Part Character 4		Approach Character 5	Device Character 6	Qualifier Character 7

Ø Azygos Vein
  Right ascending lumbar vein
  Right subcostal vein
1 Hemiazygos Vein
  Left ascending lumbar vein
  Left subcostal vein
3 Innominate Vein, Right
  Brachiocephalic vein
  Inferior thyroid vein
4 Innominate Vein, Left
  See 3 Innominate Vein, Right
5 Subclavian Vein, Right
6 Subclavian Vein, Left
7 Axillary Vein, Right
8 Axillary Vein, Left
9 Brachial Vein, Right
  Radial vein
  Ulnar vein
A Brachial Vein, Left
  See 9 Brachial Vein, Right
B Basilic Vein, Right
  Median antebrachial vein
  Median cubital vein
C Basilic Vein, Left
  See B Basilic Vein, Right
D Cephalic Vein, Right
  Accessory cephalic vein
F Cephalic Vein, Left
  See D Cephalic Vein, Right
G Hand Vein, Right
  Dorsal metacarpal vein
  Palmar (volar) digital vein
  Palmar (volar) metacarpal vein
  Superficial palmar venous arch
  Volar (palmar) digital vein
  Volar (palmar) metacarpal vein
	H Hand Vein, Left
	  See G Hand Vein, Right
	L Intracranial Vein
	  Anterior cerebral vein
	  Basal (internal) cerebral vein
	  Dural venous sinus
	  Great cerebral vein
	  Inferior cerebellar vein
	  Inferior cerebral vein
	  Internal (basal) cerebral vein
	  Middle cerebral vein
	  Ophthalmic vein
	  Superior cerebellar vein
	  Superior cerebral vein
	M Internal Jugular Vein, Right
	N Internal Jugular Vein, Left
	P External Jugular Vein, Right
	  Posterior auricular vein
	Q External Jugular Vein, Left
	  See P External Jugular Vein, Right
	R Vertebral Vein, Right
	  Deep cervical vein
	  Suboccipital venous plexus
	S Vertebral Vein, Left
	  See R Vertebral Vein, Right
	T Face Vein, Right
	  Angular vein
	  Anterior facial vein
	  Common facial vein
	  Deep facial vein
	  Frontal vein
	  Posterior facial
	    (retromandibular) vein
	  Supraorbital vein
	V Face Vein, Left
	  See T Face Vein, Right
	Y Upper Vein
		Ø Open
		3 Percutaneous
		4 Percutaneous Endoscopic
			Ø Drainage Device	**Z No Qualifier**

Ø Azygos Vein
  Right ascending lumbar vein
  Right subcostal vein
1 Hemiazygos Vein
  Left ascending lumbar vein
  Left subcostal vein
3 Innominate Vein, Right
  Brachiocephalic vein
  Inferior thyroid vein
4 Innominate Vein, Left
  See 3 Innominate Vein, Right
5 Subclavian Vein, Right
6 Subclavian Vein, Left
7 Axillary Vein, Right
8 Axillary Vein, Left
9 Brachial Vein, Right
  Radial vein
  Ulnar vein
A Brachial Vein, Left
  See 9 Brachial Vein, Right
B Basilic Vein, Right
  Median antebrachial vein
  Median cubital vein
C Basilic Vein, Left
  See B Basilic Vein, Right
D Cephalic Vein, Right
  Accessory cephalic vein
F Cephalic Vein, Left
  See D Cephalic Vein, Right
G Hand Vein, Right
  Dorsal metacarpal vein
  Palmar (volar) digital vein
  Palmar (volar) metacarpal vein
  Superficial palmar venous arch
  Volar (palmar) digital vein
  Volar (palmar) metacarpal vein
	H Hand Vein, Left
	  See G Hand Vein, Right
	L Intracranial Vein
	  Anterior cerebral vein
	  Basal (internal) cerebral vein
	  Dural venous sinus
	  Great cerebral vein
	  Inferior cerebellar vein
	  Inferior cerebral vein
	  Internal (basal) cerebral vein
	  Middle cerebral vein
	  Ophthalmic vein
	  Superior cerebellar vein
	  Superior cerebral vein
	M Internal Jugular Vein, Right
	N Internal Jugular Vein, Left
	P External Jugular Vein, Right
	  Posterior auricular vein
	Q External Jugular Vein, Left
	  See P External Jugular Vein, Right
	R Vertebral Vein, Right
	  Deep cervical vein
	  Suboccipital venous plexus
	S Vertebral Vein, Left
	  See R Vertebral Vein, Right
	T Face Vein, Right
	  Angular vein
	  Anterior facial vein
	  Common facial vein
	  Deep facial vein
	  Frontal vein
	  Posterior facial
	    (retromandibular) vein
	  Supraorbital vein
	V Face Vein, Left
	  See T Face Vein, Right
	Y Upper Vein
		Ø Open
		3 Percutaneous
		4 Percutaneous Endoscopic
			Z No Device	**X Diagnostic**
				Z No Qualifier

Non-OR   Ø59[Ø,1,3,4,5,6,7,8,9,A,B,C,D,F,G,H,L,M,N,P,Q,R,S,T,V,Y][Ø,3,4]ØZ
Non-OR   Ø59[Ø,1,3,4,5,6,7,8,9,A,B,C,D,F,G,H,L,M,N,P,Q,R,S,T,V,Y]3ZX
Non-OR   Ø59[Ø,1,3,4,5,6,7,8,9,A,B,C,D,F,G,H,L,M,N,P,Q,R,S,T,V,Y][Ø,3,4]ZZ

Non-OR Procedure   DRG Non-OR Procedure   Valid OR Procedure   HAC Associated Procedure   Combination Only   New/Revised April   New/Revised October

248   ICD-10-PCS 2023

Ø **Medical and Surgical**
5 **Upper Veins**
B **Excision**   Definition: Cutting out or off, without replacement, a portion of a body part
          Explanation: The qualifier DIAGNOSTIC is used to identify excision procedures that are biopsies

Body Part Character 4	Approach Character 5	Device Character 6	Qualifier Character 7
Ø **Azygos Vein** Right ascending lumbar vein Right subcostal vein	**Ø** Open **3** Percutaneous **4** Percutaneous Endoscopic	**Z** No Device	**X** Diagnostic **Z** No Qualifier
1 **Hemiazygos Vein** Left ascending lumbar vein Left subcostal vein			
3 **Innominate Vein, Right** Brachiocephalic vein Inferior thyroid vein			
4 **Innominate Vein, Left** *See 3 Innominate Vein, Right*			
5 **Subclavian Vein, Right**			
6 **Subclavian Vein, Left**			
7 **Axillary Vein, Right**			
8 **Axillary Vein, Left**			
9 **Brachial Vein, Right** Radial vein Ulnar vein			
A **Brachial Vein, Left** *See 9 Brachial Vein, Right*			
B **Basilic Vein, Right** Median antebrachial vein Median cubital vein			
C **Basilic Vein, Left** *See B Basilic Vein, Right*			
D **Cephalic Vein, Right** Accessory cephalic vein			
F **Cephalic Vein, Left** *See D Cephalic Vein, Right*			
G **Hand Vein, Right** Dorsal metacarpal vein Palmar (volar) digital vein Palmar (volar) metacarpal vein Superficial palmar venous arch Volar (palmar) digital vein Volar (palmar) metacarpal vein			
H **Hand Vein, Left** *See G Hand Vein, Right*			
L **Intracranial Vein** Anterior cerebral vein Basal (internal) cerebral vein Dural venous sinus Great cerebral vein Inferior cerebellar vein Inferior cerebral vein Internal (basal) cerebral vein Middle cerebral vein Ophthalmic vein Superior cerebellar vein Superior cerebral vein			
M **Internal Jugular Vein, Right**			
N **Internal Jugular Vein, Left**			
P **External Jugular Vein, Right** Posterior auricular vein			
Q **External Jugular Vein, Left** *See P External Jugular Vein, Right*			
R **Vertebral Vein, Right** Deep cervical vein Suboccipital venous plexus			
S **Vertebral Vein, Left** *See R Vertebral Vein, Right*			
T **Face Vein, Right** Angular vein Anterior facial vein Common facial vein Deep facial vein Frontal vein Posterior facial (retromandibular) vein Supraorbital vein			
V **Face Vein, Left** *See T Face Vein, Right*			
Y **Upper Vein**			

NC Noncovered Procedure   **LC** Limited Coverage   **QA** Questionable OB Admit   **NT** New Tech Add-on   ⊞ Combination Member   ♂ Male   ♀ Female

ICD-10-PCS 2023   249

Ø5B–Ø5B

Ø Medical and Surgical
5 Upper Veins
C Extirpation   Definition: Taking or cutting out solid matter from a body part

Explanation: The solid matter may be an abnormal byproduct of a biological function or a foreign body; it may be imbedded in a body part or in the lumen of a tubular body part. The solid matter may or may not have been previously broken into pieces.

Body Part Character 4	Approach Character 5	Device Character 6	Qualifier Character 7
Ø Azygos Vein Right ascending lumbar vein Right subcostal vein **1 Hemiazygos Vein** Left ascending lumbar vein Left subcostal vein **3 Innominate Vein, Right** Brachiocephalic vein Inferior thyroid vein **4 Innominate Vein, Left** *See 3 Innominate Vein, Right* **5 Subclavian Vein, Right** **6 Subclavian Vein, Left** **7 Axillary Vein, Right** **8 Axillary Vein, Left** **9 Brachial Vein, Right** Radial vein Ulnar vein **A Brachial Vein, Left** *See 9 Brachial Vein, Right* **B Basilic Vein, Right** Median antebrachial vein Median cubital vein **C Basilic Vein, Left** *See B Basilic Vein, Right* **D Cephalic Vein, Right** Accessory cephalic vein **F Cephalic Vein, Left** *See D Cephalic Vein, Right* **G Hand Vein, Right** Dorsal metacarpal vein Palmar (volar) digital vein Palmar (volar) metacarpal vein Superficial palmar venous arch Volar (palmar) digital vein Volar (palmar) metacarpal vein **H Hand Vein, Left** *See G Hand Vein, Right* **L Intracranial Vein** Anterior cerebral vein Basal (internal) cerebral vein Dural venous sinus Great cerebral vein Inferior cerebellar vein Inferior cerebral vein Internal (basal) cerebral vein Middle cerebral vein Ophthalmic vein Superior cerebellar vein Superior cerebral vein **M Internal Jugular Vein, Right** **N Internal Jugular Vein, Left** **P External Jugular Vein, Right** Posterior auricular vein **Q External Jugular Vein, Left** *See P External Jugular Vein, Right* **R Vertebral Vein, Right** Deep cervical vein Suboccipital venous plexus **S Vertebral Vein, Left** *See R Vertebral Vein, Right* **T Face Vein, Right** Angular vein Anterior facial vein Common facial vein Deep facial vein Frontal vein Posterior facial (retromandibular) vein Supraorbital vein **V Face Vein, Left** *See T Face Vein, Right* **Y Upper Vein**	**Ø Open** **3 Percutaneous** **4 Percutaneous Endoscopic**	**Z No Device**	**Z No Qualifier**

Non-OR Procedure   DRG Non-OR Procedure   Valid OR Procedure   HAC Associated Procedure   Combination Only   New/Revised April   New/Revised October

250   ICD-10-PCS 2023

Ø   Medical and Surgical
5   Upper Veins
D   Extraction   Definition: Pulling or stripping out or off all or a portion of a body part by the use of force
                             Explanation: The qualifier DIAGNOSTIC is used to identify extraction procedures that are biopsies

Body Part Character 4	Approach Character 5	Device Character 6	Qualifier Character 7
9 Brachial Vein, Right Radial vein Ulnar vein	**Ø Open** **3 Percutaneous**	**Z No Device**	**Z No Qualifier**
A Brachial Vein, Left *See 9 Brachial Vein, Right*			
B Basilic Vein, Right Median antebrachial vein Median cubital vein			
C Basilic Vein, Left *See B Basilic Vein, Right*			
D Cephalic Vein, Right Accessory cephalic vein			
F Cephalic Vein, Left *See D Cephalic Vein, Right*			
G Hand Vein, Right Dorsal metacarpal vein Palmar (volar) digital vein Palmar (volar) metacarpal vein Superficial palmar venous arch Volar (palmar) digital vein Volar (palmar) metacarpal vein			
H Hand Vein, Left *See G Hand Vein, Right*			
Y Upper Vein			

Ø   Medical and Surgical
5   Upper Veins
F   Fragmentation   Definition: Breaking solid matter in a body part into pieces
                             Explanation: Physical force (e.g., manual, ultrasonic) applied directly or indirectly is used to break the solid matter into pieces. The solid matter may be an abnormal byproduct of a biological function or a foreign body. The pieces of solid matter are not taken out.

Body Part Character 4	Approach Character 5	Device Character 6	Qualifier Character 7
3 Innominate Vein, Right Brachiocephalic vein Inferior thyroid vein	**3 Percutaneous**	**Z No Device**	**Ø Ultrasonic** **Z No Qualifier**
4 Innominate Vein, Left *See 3 Innominate Vein, Right*			
5 Subclavian Vein, Right			
6 Subclavian Vein, Left			
7 Axillary Vein, Right			
8 Axillary Vein, Left			
9 Brachial Vein, Right Radial vein Ulnar vein			
A Brachial Vein, Left *See 9 Brachial Vein, Right*			
B Basilic Vein, Right Median antebrachial vein Median cubital vein			
C Basilic Vein, Left *See B Basilic Vein, Right*			
D Cephalic Vein, Right Accessory cephalic vein			
F Cephalic Vein, Left *See D Cephalic Vein, Right*			
Y Upper Vein			

Upper Veins

Ø   **Medical and Surgical**
5   **Upper Veins**
H   **Insertion**   Definition: Putting in a nonbiological appliance that monitors, assists, performs, or prevents a physiological function but does not physically take the place of a body part

Explanation: None

Body Part Character 4		Approach Character 5	Device Character 6	Qualifier Character 7
Ø **Azygos Vein** ⊞ Right ascending lumbar vein Right subcostal vein		Ø Open 3 Percutaneous 4 Percutaneous Endoscopic	2 Monitoring Device 3 Infusion Device D Intraluminal Device M Neurostimulator Lead	Z No Qualifier
1 **Hemiazygos Vein** Left ascending lumbar vein Left subcostal vein 5 **Subclavian Vein, Right** 6 **Subclavian Vein, Left** 7 **Axillary Vein, Right** 8 **Axillary Vein, Left** 9 **Brachial Vein, Right** Radial vein Ulnar vein A **Brachial Vein, Left** *See 9 Brachial Vein, Right* B **Basilic Vein, Right** Median antebrachial vein Median cubital vein C **Basilic Vein, Left** *See B Basilic Vein, Right* D **Cephalic Vein, Right** Accessory cephalic vein F **Cephalic Vein, Left** *See D Cephalic Vein, Right* G **Hand Vein, Right** Dorsal metacarpal vein Palmar (volar) digital vein Palmar (volar) metacarpal vein Superficial palmar venous arch Volar (palmar) digital vein Volar (palmar) metacarpal vein H **Hand Vein, Left** *See G Hand Vein, Right*	L **Intracranial Vein** Anterior cerebral vein Basal (internal) cerebral vein Dural venous sinus Great cerebral vein Inferior cerebellar vein Inferior cerebral vein Internal (basal) cerebral vein Middle cerebral vein Ophthalmic vein Superior cerebellar vein Superior cerebral vein M **Internal Jugular Vein, Right** N **Internal Jugular Vein, Left** P **External Jugular Vein, Right** Posterior auricular vein Q **External Jugular Vein, Left** *See P External Jugular Vein, Right* R **Vertebral Vein, Right** Deep cervical vein Suboccipital venous plexus S **Vertebral Vein, Left** *See R Vertebral Vein, Right* T **Face Vein, Right** Angular vein Anterior facial vein Common facial vein Deep facial vein Frontal vein Posterior facial (retromandibular) vein Supraorbital vein V **Face Vein, Left** *See T Face Vein, Right*	Ø Open 3 Percutaneous 4 Percutaneous Endoscopic	3 Infusion Device D Intraluminal Device	Z No Qualifier
3 **Innominate Vein, Right** ⊞ Brachiocephalic vein Inferior thyroid vein 4 **Innominate Vein, Left** ⊞ *See 3 Innominate Vein, Right*		Ø Open 3 Percutaneous 4 Percutaneous Endoscopic	3 Infusion Device D Intraluminal Device M Neurostimulator Lead	Z No Qualifier
Y **Upper Vein**		Ø Open 3 Percutaneous 4 Percutaneous Endoscopic	2 Monitoring Device 3 Infusion Device D Intraluminal Device Y Other Device	Z No Qualifier

Non-OR	Ø5HØ[Ø,3,4]3Z			
Non-OR	Ø5H[1,5,6,7,8,9,A,B,C,D,F,G,H,L,M,N,P,Q,R,S,T,V][Ø,3,4]3Z			
Non-OR	Ø5H[3,4][Ø,3,4]3Z			
Non-OR	Ø5HY[Ø,3,4]3Z			
Non-OR	Ø5HY32Z			
Non-OR	Ø5HY[3,4]YZ			
HAC	Ø5HØ[3,4]3Z when reported with SDx J95.811			
HAC	Ø5H[1,5,6][3,4]3Z when reported with SDx J95.811			
HAC	Ø5H[M,N,P,Q]33Z when reported with SDx J95.811			
HAC	Ø5H[3,4][3,4]3Z when reported with SDx J95.811			

See Appendix L for Procedure Combinations
⊞   Ø5HØ[Ø,3,4]MZ
⊞   Ø5H[3,4][Ø,3,4]MZ

Ø   **Medical and Surgical**
5   **Upper Veins**
J   **Inspection**   Definition: Visually and/or manually exploring a body part

Explanation: Visual exploration may be performed with or without optical instrumentation. Manual exploration may be performed directly or through intervening body layers.

Body Part Character 4	Approach Character 5	Device Character 6	Qualifier Character 7
Y **Upper Vein**	Ø Open 3 Percutaneous 4 Percutaneous Endoscopic X External	Z No Device	Z No Qualifier

Non-OR	Ø5JY[3,X]ZZ

Non-OR Procedure   DRG Non-OR Procedure   Valid OR Procedure   HAC Associated Procedure   Combination Only   New/Revised April   New/Revised October

Ø5H–Ø5J

0   **Medical and Surgical**
5   **Upper Veins**
L   **Occlusion**   Definition: Completely closing an orifice or the lumen of a tubular body part
                         Explanation: The orifice can be a natural orifice or an artificially created orifice

Body Part Character 4	Approach Character 5	Device Character 6	Qualifier Character 7

0   **Azygos Vein**
    Right ascending lumbar vein
    Right subcostal vein
1   **Hemiazygos Vein**
    Left ascending lumbar vein
    Left subcostal vein
3   **Innominate Vein, Right**
    Brachiocephalic vein
    Inferior thyroid vein
4   **Innominate Vein, Left**
    See 3 Innominate Vein, Right
5   **Subclavian Vein, Right**
6   **Subclavian Vein, Left**
7   **Axillary Vein, Right**
8   **Axillary Vein, Left**
9   **Brachial Vein, Right**
    Radial vein
    Ulnar vein
A   **Brachial Vein, Left**
    See 9 Brachial Vein, Right
B   **Basilic Vein, Right**
    Median antebrachial vein
    Median cubital vein
C   **Basilic Vein, Left**
    See B Basilic Vein, Right
D   **Cephalic Vein, Right**
    Accessory cephalic vein
F   **Cephalic Vein, Left**
    See D Cephalic Vein, Right
G   **Hand Vein, Right**
    Dorsal metacarpal vein
    Palmar (volar) digital vein
    Palmar (volar) metacarpal vein
    Superficial palmar venous arch
    Volar (palmar) digital vein
    Volar (palmar) metacarpal vein
H   **Hand Vein, Left**
    See G Hand Vein, Right
L   **Intracranial Vein**
    Anterior cerebral vein
    Basal (internal) cerebral vein
    Dural venous sinus
    Great cerebral vein
    Inferior cerebellar vein
    Inferior cerebral vein
    Internal (basal) cerebral vein
    Middle cerebral vein
    Ophthalmic vein
    Superior cerebellar vein
    Superior cerebral vein
M   **Internal Jugular Vein, Right**
N   **Internal Jugular Vein, Left**
P   **External Jugular Vein, Right**
    Posterior auricular vein
Q   **External Jugular Vein, Left**
    See P External Jugular Vein, Right
R   **Vertebral Vein, Right**
    Deep cervical vein
    Suboccipital venous plexus
S   **Vertebral Vein, Left**
    See R Vertebral Vein, Right
T   **Face Vein, Right**
    Angular vein
    Anterior facial vein
    Common facial vein
    Deep facial vein
    Frontal vein
    Posterior facial (retromandibular) vein
    Supraorbital vein
V   **Face Vein, Left**
    See T Face Vein, Right
Y   **Upper Vein**
	0 Open
	3 Percutaneous
	4 Percutaneous Endoscopic
		C Extraluminal Device
		D Intraluminal Device
		Z No Device
			Z No Qualifier

NC Noncovered Procedure   LC Limited Coverage   QA Questionable OB Admit   NT New Tech Add-on   ⊞ Combination Member   ♂ Male   ♀ Female

ICD-10-PCS 2023   253

05L–05L

Upper Veins

0 Medical and Surgical
5 Upper Veins
N Release

Definition: Freeing a body part from an abnormal physical constraint by cutting or by the use of force

Explanation: Some of the restraining tissue may be taken out but none of the body part is taken out

Body Part Character 4	Approach Character 5	Device Character 6	Qualifier Character 7
0 Azygos Vein Right ascending lumbar vein Right subcostal vein	**0 Open** **3 Percutaneous** **4 Percutaneous Endoscopic**	**Z No Device**	**Z No Qualifier**
1 Hemiazygos Vein Left ascending lumbar vein Left subcostal vein			
3 Innominate Vein, Right Brachiocephalic vein Inferior thyroid vein			
4 Innominate Vein, Left *See 3 Innominate Vein, Right*			
5 Subclavian Vein, Right			
6 Subclavian Vein, Left			
7 Axillary Vein, Right			
8 Axillary Vein, Left			
9 Brachial Vein, Right Radial vein Ulnar vein			
A Brachial Vein, Left *See 9 Brachial Vein, Right*			
B Basilic Vein, Right Median antebrachial vein Median cubital vein			
C Basilic Vein, Left *See B Basilic Vein, Right*			
D Cephalic Vein, Right Accessory cephalic vein			
F Cephalic Vein, Left *See D Cephalic Vein, Right*			
G Hand Vein, Right Dorsal metacarpal vein Palmar (volar) digital vein Palmar (volar) metacarpal vein Superficial palmar venous arch Volar (palmar) digital vein Volar (palmar) metacarpal vein			
H Hand Vein, Left *See G Hand Vein, Right*			
L Intracranial Vein Anterior cerebral vein Basal (internal) cerebral vein Dural venous sinus Great cerebral vein Inferior cerebellar vein Inferior cerebral vein Internal (basal) cerebral vein Middle cerebral vein Ophthalmic vein Superior cerebellar vein Superior cerebral vein			
M Internal Jugular Vein, Right			
N Internal Jugular Vein, Left			
P External Jugular Vein, Right Posterior auricular vein			
Q External Jugular Vein, Left *See P External Jugular Vein, Right*			
R Vertebral Vein, Right Deep cervical vein Suboccipital venous plexus			
S Vertebral Vein, Left *See R Vertebral Vein, Right*			
T Face Vein, Right Angular vein Anterior facial vein Common facial vein Deep facial vein Frontal vein Posterior facial (retromandibular) vein Supraorbital vein			
V Face Vein, Left *See T Face Vein, Right*			
Y Upper Vein			

Non-OR Procedure   DRG Non-OR Procedure   Valid OR Procedure   HAC Associated Procedure   Combination Only   New/Revised April   New/Revised October

254

ICD-10-PCS 2023

Ø   **Medical and Surgical**
5   **Upper Veins**
P   **Removal**   Definition: Taking out or off a device from a body part

Explanation: If a device is taken out and a similar device put in without cutting or puncturing the skin or mucous membrane, the procedure is coded to the root operation CHANGE. Otherwise, the procedure for taking out a device is coded to the root operation REMOVAL.

Body Part Character 4		Approach Character 5		Device Character 6		Qualifier Character 7	
Ø	**Azygos Vein** Right ascending lumbar vein Right subcostal vein	Ø 3 4 X	Open Percutaneous Percutaneous Endoscopic External	2 M	Monitoring Device Neurostimulator Lead	Z	No Qualifier
3 4	**Innominate Vein, Right** Brachiocephalic vein Inferior thyroid vein **Innominate Vein, Left** *See 3 Innominate Vein, Right*	Ø 3 4 X	Open Percutaneous Percutaneous Endoscopic External	M	Neurostimulator Lead	Z	No Qualifier
Y	**Upper Vein**	Ø 3 4	Open Percutaneous Percutaneous Endoscopic	Ø 2 3 7 C D J K Y	Drainage Device Monitoring Device Infusion Device Autologous Tissue Substitute Extraluminal Device Intraluminal Device Synthetic Substitute Nonautologous Tissue Substitute Other Device	Z	No Qualifier
Y	**Upper Vein**	X	External	Ø 2 3 D	Drainage Device Monitoring Device Infusion Device Intraluminal Device	Z	No Qualifier

Non-OR   Ø5PØ[Ø,3,4,X]2Z
Non-OR   Ø5PY3[Ø,2,3]Z
Non-OR   Ø5PY[3,4]YZ
Non-OR   Ø5PYX[Ø,2,3,D]Z

Ø   **Medical and Surgical**
5   **Upper Veins**
Q   **Repair**   Definition: Restoring, to the extent possible, a body part to its normal anatomic structure and function

Explanation: Used only when the method to accomplish the repair is not one of the other root operations

Body Part Character 4	Approach Character 5	Device Character 6	Qualifier Character 7

Ø   **Azygos Vein**
    Right ascending lumbar vein
    Right subcostal vein
 1   **Hemiazygos Vein**
    Left ascending lumbar vein
    Left subcostal vein
 3   **Innominate Vein, Right**
    Brachiocephalic vein
    Inferior thyroid vein
 4   **Innominate Vein, Left**
    See 3 Innominate Vein, Right
 5   **Subclavian Vein, Right**
 6   **Subclavian Vein, Left**
 7   **Axillary Vein, Right**
 8   **Axillary Vein, Left**
 9   **Brachial Vein, Right**
    Radial vein
    Ulnar vein
 A   **Brachial Vein, Left**
    See 9 Brachial Vein, Right
 B   **Basilic Vein, Right**
    Median antebrachial vein
    Median cubital vein
 C   **Basilic Vein, Left**
    See B Basilic Vein, Right
 D   **Cephalic Vein, Right**
    Accessory cephalic vein
 F   **Cephalic Vein, Left**
    See D Cephalic Vein, Right
 G   **Hand Vein, Right**
    Dorsal metacarpal vein
    Palmar (volar) digital vein
    Palmar (volar) metacarpal vein
    Superficial palmar venous arch
    Volar (palmar) digital vein
    Volar (palmar) metacarpal vein
 H   **Hand Vein, Left**
    See G Hand Vein, Right
 L   **Intracranial Vein**
    Anterior cerebral vein
    Basal (internal) cerebral vein
    Dural venous sinus
    Great cerebral vein
    Inferior cerebellar vein
    Inferior cerebral vein
    Internal (basal) cerebral vein
    Middle cerebral vein
    Ophthalmic vein
    Superior cerebellar vein
    Superior cerebral vein
 M   **Internal Jugular Vein, Right**
 N   **Internal Jugular Vein, Left**
 P   **External Jugular Vein, Right**
    Posterior auricular vein
 Q   **External Jugular Vein, Left**
    See P External Jugular Vein, Right
 R   **Vertebral Vein, Right**
    Deep cervical vein
    Suboccipital venous plexus
 S   **Vertebral Vein, Left**
    See R Vertebral Vein, Right
 T   **Face Vein, Right**
    Angular vein
    Anterior facial vein
    Common facial vein
    Deep facial vein
    Frontal vein
    Posterior facial (retromandibular) vein
    Supraorbital vein
 V   **Face Vein, Left**
    See T Face Vein, Right
 Y   **Upper Vein**
	Ø Open
	 3 Percutaneous
	 4 Percutaneous Endoscopic
		Z No Device	**Z** No Qualifier

Non-OR Procedure   DRG Non-OR Procedure   Valid OR Procedure   HAC Associated Procedure   Combination Only   New/Revised April   New/Revised October

256   ICD-10-PCS 2023

Ø	**Medical and Surgical**		
5	**Upper Veins**		
R	**Replacement**	Definition: Putting in or on biological or synthetic material that physically takes the place and/or function of all or a portion of a body part	

Explanation: The body part may have been taken out or replaced, or may be taken out, physically eradicated, or rendered nonfunctional during the REPLACEMENT procedure. A REMOVAL procedure is coded for taking out the device used in a previous replacement procedure.

Body Part Character 4	Approach Character 5	Device Character 6	Qualifier Character 7
Ø Azygos Vein Right ascending lumbar vein Right subcostal vein **1 Hemiazygos Vein** Left ascending lumbar vein Left subcostal vein **3 Innominate Vein, Right** Brachiocephalic vein Inferior thyroid vein **4 Innominate Vein, Left** *See 3 Innominate Vein, Right* **5 Subclavian Vein, Right** **6 Subclavian Vein, Left** **7 Axillary Vein, Right** **8 Axillary Vein, Left** **9 Brachial Vein, Right** Radial vein Ulnar vein **A Brachial Vein, Left** *See 9 Brachial Vein, Right* **B Basilic Vein, Right** Median antebrachial vein Median cubital vein **C Basilic Vein, Left** *See B Basilic Vein, Right* **D Cephalic Vein, Right** Accessory cephalic vein **F Cephalic Vein, Left** *See D Cephalic Vein, Right* **G Hand Vein, Right** Dorsal metacarpal vein Palmar (volar) digital vein Palmar (volar) metacarpal vein Superficial palmar venous arch Volar (palmar) digital vein Volar (palmar) metacarpal vein **H Hand Vein, Left** *See G Hand Vein, Right* **L Intracranial Vein** Anterior cerebral vein Basal (internal) cerebral vein Dural venous sinus Great cerebral vein Inferior cerebellar vein Inferior cerebral vein Internal (basal) cerebral vein Middle cerebral vein Ophthalmic vein Superior cerebellar vein Superior cerebral vein **M Internal Jugular Vein, Right** **N Internal Jugular Vein, Left** **P External Jugular Vein, Right** Posterior auricular vein **Q External Jugular Vein, Left** *See P External Jugular Vein, Right* **R Vertebral Vein, Right** Deep cervical vein Suboccipital venous plexus **S Vertebral Vein, Left** *See R Vertebral Vein, Right* **T Face Vein, Right** Angular vein Anterior facial vein Common facial vein Deep facial vein Frontal vein Posterior facial (retromandibular) vein Supraorbital vein **V Face Vein, Left** *See T Face Vein, Right* **Y Upper Vein**	**Ø Open** **4 Percutaneous Endoscopic**	**7 Autologous Tissue Substitute** **J Synthetic Substitute** **K Nonautologous Tissue Substitute**	**Z No Qualifier**

NC Noncovered Procedure   **LC** Limited Coverage   **QA** Questionable OB Admit   **NT** New Tech Add-on   ⊞ Combination Member   ♂ Male   ♀ Female

ICD-10-PCS 2023   257

Ø5R–Ø5R

Ø   **Medical and Surgical**
5   **Upper Veins**
S   **Reposition**   Definition: Moving to its normal location, or other suitable location, all or a portion of a body part

Explanation: The body part is moved to a new location from an abnormal location, or from a normal location where it is not functioning correctly. The body part may or may not be cut out or off to be moved to the new location.

Body Part Character 4	Approach Character 5	Device Character 6	Qualifier Character 7

Ø   **Azygos Vein**
    Right ascending lumbar vein
    Right subcostal vein
1   **Hemiazygos Vein**
    Left ascending lumbar vein
    Left subcostal vein
3   **Innominate Vein, Right**
    Brachiocephalic vein
    Inferior thyroid vein
4   **Innominate Vein, Left**
    See 3 Innominate Vein, Right
5   **Subclavian Vein, Right**
6   **Subclavian Vein, Left**
7   **Axillary Vein, Right**
8   **Axillary Vein, Left**
9   **Brachial Vein, Right**
    Radial vein
    Ulnar vein
A   **Brachial Vein, Left**
    See 9 Brachial Vein, Right
B   **Basilic Vein, Right**
    Median antebrachial vein
    Median cubital vein
C   **Basilic Vein, Left**
    See B Basilic Vein, Right
D   **Cephalic Vein, Right**
    Accessory cephalic vein
F   **Cephalic Vein, Left**
    See D Cephalic Vein, Right
G   **Hand Vein, Right**
    Dorsal metacarpal vein
    Palmar (volar) digital vein
    Palmar (volar) metacarpal vein
    Superficial palmar venous arch
    Volar (palmar) digital vein
    Volar (palmar) metacarpal vein
H   **Hand Vein, Left**
    See G Hand Vein, Right
L   **Intracranial Vein**
    Anterior cerebral vein
    Basal (internal) cerebral vein
    Dural venous sinus
    Great cerebral vein
    Inferior cerebellar vein
    Inferior cerebral vein
    Internal (basal) cerebral vein
    Middle cerebral vein
    Ophthalmic vein
    Superior cerebellar vein
    Superior cerebral vein
M   **Internal Jugular Vein, Right**
N   **Internal Jugular Vein, Left**
P   **External Jugular Vein, Right**
    Posterior auricular vein
Q   **External Jugular Vein, Left**
    See P External Jugular Vein, Right
R   **Vertebral Vein, Right**
    Deep cervical vein
    Suboccipital venous plexus
S   **Vertebral Vein, Left**
    See R Vertebral Vein, Right
T   **Face Vein, Right**
    Angular vein
    Anterior facial vein
    Common facial vein
    Deep facial vein
    Frontal vein
    Posterior facial (retromandibular) vein
    Supraorbital vein
V   **Face Vein, Left**
    See T Face Vein, Right
Y   **Upper Vein**
	Ø Open
	3 Percutaneous
	4 Percutaneous Endoscopic
		Z No Device	**Z** No Qualifier

Ø   Medical and Surgical
5   Upper Veins
U   Supplement   Definition: Putting in or on biological or synthetic material that physically reinforces and/or augments the function of a portion of a body part
                         Explanation: The biological material is non-living, or is living and from the same individual. The body part may have been previously replaced, and the SUPPLEMENT procedure is performed to physically reinforce and/or augment the function of the replaced body part.

Body Part Character 4	Approach Character 5	Device Character 6	Qualifier Character 7

Ø   **Azygos Vein**
    Right ascending lumbar vein
    Right subcostal vein
	Ø Open
	3 Percutaneous
	4 Percutaneous Endoscopic
		7 Autologous Tissue Substitute
		J Synthetic Substitute
		K Nonautologous Tissue Substitute
			Z No Qualifier

1   **Hemiazygos Vein**
    Left ascending lumbar vein
    Left subcostal vein			

3   **Innominate Vein, Right**
    Brachiocephalic vein
    Inferior thyroid vein			

4 **Innominate Vein, Left** *See 3 Innominate Vein, Right*			
5 **Subclavian Vein, Right**			
6 **Subclavian Vein, Left**			
7 **Axillary Vein, Right**			
8 **Axillary Vein, Left**			

9   **Brachial Vein, Right**
    Radial vein
    Ulnar vein			

A **Brachial Vein, Left** *See 9 Brachial Vein, Right*			

B   **Basilic Vein, Right**
    Median antebrachial vein
    Median cubital vein			

C **Basilic Vein, Left** *See B Basilic Vein, Right*			
D **Cephalic Vein, Right** Accessory cephalic vein			
F **Cephalic Vein, Left** *See D Cephalic Vein, Right*			

G   **Hand Vein, Right**
    Dorsal metacarpal vein
    Palmar (volar) digital vein
    Palmar (volar) metacarpal vein
    Superficial palmar venous arch
    Volar (palmar) digital vein
    Volar (palmar) metacarpal vein			

H **Hand Vein, Left** *See G Hand Vein, Right*			

L   **Intracranial Vein**
    Anterior cerebral vein
    Basal (internal) cerebral vein
    Dural venous sinus
    Great cerebral vein
    Inferior cerebellar vein
    Inferior cerebral vein
    Internal (basal) cerebral vein
    Middle cerebral vein
    Ophthalmic vein
    Superior cerebellar vein
    Superior cerebral vein			

M **Internal Jugular Vein, Right**			
N **Internal Jugular Vein, Left**			
P **External Jugular Vein, Right** Posterior auricular vein			
Q **External Jugular Vein, Left** *See P External Jugular Vein, Right*			

R   **Vertebral Vein, Right**
    Deep cervical vein
    Suboccipital venous plexus			

S **Vertebral Vein, Left** *See R Vertebral Vein, Right*			

T   **Face Vein, Right**
    Angular vein
    Anterior facial vein
    Common facial vein
    Deep facial vein
    Frontal vein
    Posterior facial (retromandibular) vein
    Supraorbital vein			

V **Face Vein, Left** *See T Face Vein, Right*			
Y **Upper Vein**			

NC Noncovered Procedure   **LC** Limited Coverage   **QA** Questionable OB Admit   **NT** New Tech Add-on   ✛ Combination Member   ♂ Male   ♀ Female

Upper Veins

Ø   **Medical and Surgical**
5   **Upper Veins**
V   **Restriction**   Definition: Partially closing an orifice or the lumen of a tubular body part
                   Explanation: The orifice can be a natural orifice or an artificially created orifice

Body Part Character 4	Approach Character 5	Device Character 6	Qualifier Character 7

Ø **Azygos Vein**
  Right ascending lumbar vein
  Right subcostal vein
1 **Hemiazygos Vein**
  Left ascending lumbar vein
  Left subcostal vein
3 **Innominate Vein, Right**
  Brachiocephalic vein
  Inferior thyroid vein
4 **Innominate Vein, Left**
  See 3 Innominate Vein, Right
5 **Subclavian Vein, Right**
6 **Subclavian Vein, Left**
7 **Axillary Vein, Right**
8 **Axillary Vein, Left**
9 **Brachial Vein, Right**
  Radial vein
  Ulnar vein
A **Brachial Vein, Left**
  See 9 Brachial Vein, Right
B **Basilic Vein, Right**
  Median antebrachial vein
  Median cubital vein
C **Basilic Vein, Left**
  See B Basilic Vein, Right
D **Cephalic Vein, Right**
  Accessory cephalic vein
F **Cephalic Vein, Left**
  See D Cephalic Vein, Right
G **Hand Vein, Right**
  Dorsal metacarpal vein
  Palmar (volar) digital vein
  Palmar (volar) metacarpal vein
  Superficial palmar venous arch
  Volar (palmar) digital vein
  Volar (palmar) metacarpal vein
H **Hand Vein, Left**
  See G Hand Vein, Right
L **Intracranial Vein**
  Anterior cerebral vein
  Basal (internal) cerebral vein
  Dural venous sinus
  Great cerebral vein
  Inferior cerebellar vein
  Inferior cerebral vein
  Internal (basal) cerebral vein
  Middle cerebral vein
  Ophthalmic vein
  Superior cerebellar vein
  Superior cerebral vein
M **Internal Jugular Vein, Right**
N **Internal Jugular Vein, Left**
P **External Jugular Vein, Right**
  Posterior auricular vein
Q **External Jugular Vein, Left**
  See P External Jugular Vein, Right
R **Vertebral Vein, Right**
  Deep cervical vein
  Suboccipital venous plexus
S **Vertebral Vein, Left**
  See R Vertebral Vein, Right
T **Face Vein, Right**
  Angular vein
  Anterior facial vein
  Common facial vein
  Deep facial vein
  Frontal vein
  Posterior facial (retromandibular) vein
  Supraorbital vein
V **Face Vein, Left**
  See T Face Vein, Right
Y **Upper Vein**
	Ø **Open**
	3 **Percutaneous**
	4 **Percutaneous Endoscopic**
		C **Extraluminal Device**
		D **Intraluminal Device**
		Z **No Device**
			Z **No Qualifier**

0   Medical and Surgical
5   Upper Veins
W   Revision   Definition: Correcting, to the extent possible, a portion of a malfunctioning device or the position of a displaced device

Explanation: Revision can include correcting a malfunctioning or displaced device by taking out or putting in components of the device such as a screw or pin

Body Part Character 4	Approach Character 5	Device Character 6	Qualifier Character 7
0 Azygos Vein Right ascending lumbar vein Right subcostal vein	**0 Open** **3 Percutaneous** **4 Percutaneous Endoscopic** **X External**	**2 Monitoring Device** **M Neurostimulator Lead**	**Z No Qualifier**
3 Innominate Vein, Right Brachiocephalic vein Inferior thyroid vein **4 Innominate Vein, Left** *See 3 Innominate Vein, Right*	**0 Open** **3 Percutaneous** **4 Percutaneous Endoscopic** **X External**	**M Neurostimulator Lead**	**Z No Qualifier**
Y Upper Vein	**0 Open** **3 Percutaneous** **4 Percutaneous Endoscopic**	**0 Drainage Device** **2 Monitoring Device** **3 Infusion Device** **7 Autologous Tissue Substitute** **C Extraluminal Device** **D Intraluminal Device** **J Synthetic Substitute** **K Nonautologous Tissue Substitute** **Y Other Device**	**Z No Qualifier**
Y Upper Vein	**X External**	**0 Drainage Device** **2 Monitoring Device** **3 Infusion Device** **7 Autologous Tissue Substitute** **C Extraluminal Device** **D Intraluminal Device** **J Synthetic Substitute** **K Nonautologous Tissue Substitute**	**Z No Qualifier**

Non-OR	05W0XMZ
Non-OR	05W[3,4]XMZ
Non-OR	05WY3[0,2,3]Z
Non-OR	05WY[3,4]YZ
Non-OR	05WYX[0,2,3,7,C,D,J,K]Z

NC Noncovered Procedure   LC Limited Coverage   QA Questionable OB Admit   NT New Tech Add-on   ⊞ Combination Member   ♂ Male   ♀ Female

ICD-10-PCS 2023   261

05W–05W

Lower Veins Ø61–Ø6W

Character Meanings

This Character Meaning table is provided as a guide to assist the user in the identification of character members that may be found in this section of code tables. It **SHOULD NOT** be used to build a PCS code.

Operation–Character 3		Body Part–Character 4		Approach–Character 5		Device–Character 6		Qualifier–Character 7	
1	Bypass	Ø	Inferior Vena Cava	Ø	Open	Ø	Drainage Device	Ø	Ultrasonic
5	Destruction	1	Splenic Vein	3	Percutaneous	2	Monitoring Device	4	Hepatic Vein
7	Dilation	2	Gastric Vein	4	Percutaneous Endoscopic	3	Infusion Device	5	Superior Mesenteric Vein
9	Drainage	3	Esophageal Vein	7	Via Natural or Artificial Opening	7	Autologous Tissue Substitute	6	Inferior Mesenteric Vein
B	Excision	4	Hepatic Vein	8	Via Natural or Artificial Opening Endoscopic	9	Autologous Venous Tissue	9	Renal Vein, Right
C	Extirpation	5	Superior Mesenteric Vein	X	External	A	Autologous Arterial Tissue	B	Renal Vein, Left
D	Extraction	6	Inferior Mesenteric Vein			C	Extraluminal Device	C	Hemorrhoidal Plexus
F	Fragmentation	7	Colic Vein			D	Intraluminal Device	P	Pulmonary Trunk
H	Insertion	8	Portal Vein			J	Synthetic Substitute	Q	Pulmonary Artery, Right
J	Inspection	9	Renal Vein, Right			K	Nonautologous Tissue Substitute	R	Pulmonary Artery, Left
L	Occlusion	B	Renal Vein, Left			Y	Other Device	T	Via Umbilical Vein
N	Release	C	Common Iliac Vein, Right			Z	No Device	X	Diagnostic
P	Removal	D	Common Iliac Vein, Left					Y	Lower Vein
Q	Repair	F	External Iliac Vein, Right					Z	No Qualifier
R	Replacement	G	External Iliac Vein, Left						
S	Reposition	H	Hypogastric Vein, Right						
U	Supplement	J	Hypogastric Vein, Left						
V	Restriction	M	Femoral Vein, Right						
W	Revision	N	Femoral Vein, Left						
		P	Saphenous Vein, Right						
		Q	Saphenous Vein, Left						
		T	Foot Vein, Right						
		V	Foot Vein, Left						
		Y	Lower Vein						

AHA Coding Clinic for Lower Veins
2022, 1Q, 10-13 Procedures performed on a continuous vessel, ICD-10-PCS Guideline B4.1c

AHA Coding Clinic for table Ø61
2017, 4Q, 36-38 Fontan completion procedure
2017, 4Q, 66-67 New qualifier values - Portal to hepatic shunt

AHA Coding Clinic for table Ø6B
2020, 1Q, 28 Free flap microvascular breast reconstruction
2017, 3Q, 5 Femoral artery to posterior tibial artery bypass using autologous and synthetic grafts
2017, 1Q, 31 Left to right common carotid artery bypass
2017, 1Q, 32 Peroneal artery to dorsalis pedis artery bypass using saphenous vein graft
2016, 3Q, 31 Femoral to peroneal artery bypass with in-situ saphenous vein graft and lysis of valves
2016, 2Q, 18 Femoral-tibial artery bypass and saphenous vein graft
2016, 1Q, 27 Aortocoronary bypass graft utilizing Y-graft
2014, 3Q, 8 Excision of saphenous vein for coronary artery bypass graft
2014, 3Q, 20 MAZE procedure performed with coronary artery bypass graft
2014, 1Q, 10 Repair of thoracic aortic aneurysm & coronary artery bypass graft

AHA Coding Clinic for table Ø6F
2020, 4Q, 45-49 New fragmentation tables
2020, 4Q, 49-50 Intravascular ultrasound assisted thrombolysis
2020, 4Q, 50 Intravascular lithotripsy

AHA Coding Clinic for table Ø6H
2021, 3Q, 18 Placement and removal of cannulas for extracorporeal membrane oxygenation
2017, 3Q, 11 Placement of peripherally inserted central catheter using 3CG ECG technology
2017, 1Q, 31 Umbilical vein catheterization
2017, 1Q, 31 Central catheter placement in femoral vein
2013, 3Q, 18 Heart transplant surgery

AHA Coding Clinic for table Ø6L
2021, 4Q, 47 Endoscopic banding of hemorrhoidal plexus
2021, 4Q, 49 Division of liver for staged hepatectomy
2020, 3Q, 44 Cardiophrenic vein embolization
2019, 4Q, 28 Transorifice occlusion of gastric varices
2018, 2Q, 18 Transverse rectus abdominis myocutaneous (TRAM) delay
2017, 4Q, 57-58 Added approach values - Transorifice esophageal vein banding
2013, 4Q, 112 Endoscopic banding of esophageal varices

AHA Coding Clinic for table Ø6P
2021, 3Q, 18 Placement and removal of cannulas for extracorporeal membrane oxygenation

AHA Coding Clinic for table Ø6V
2018, 3Q, 11 Transvenous transcatheter placement of valve in inferior vena cava
2018, 1Q, 10 Revision of transjugular intrahepatic portosystemic shunt

AHA Coding Clinic for table Ø6W
2019, 2Q, 39 Transjugular intrahepatic portosystemic shunt revision
2018, 1Q, 10 Revision of transjugular intrahepatic portosystemic shunt
2014, 3Q, 25 Revision of transjugular intrahepatic portosystemic shunt (TIPS)

Lower Veins

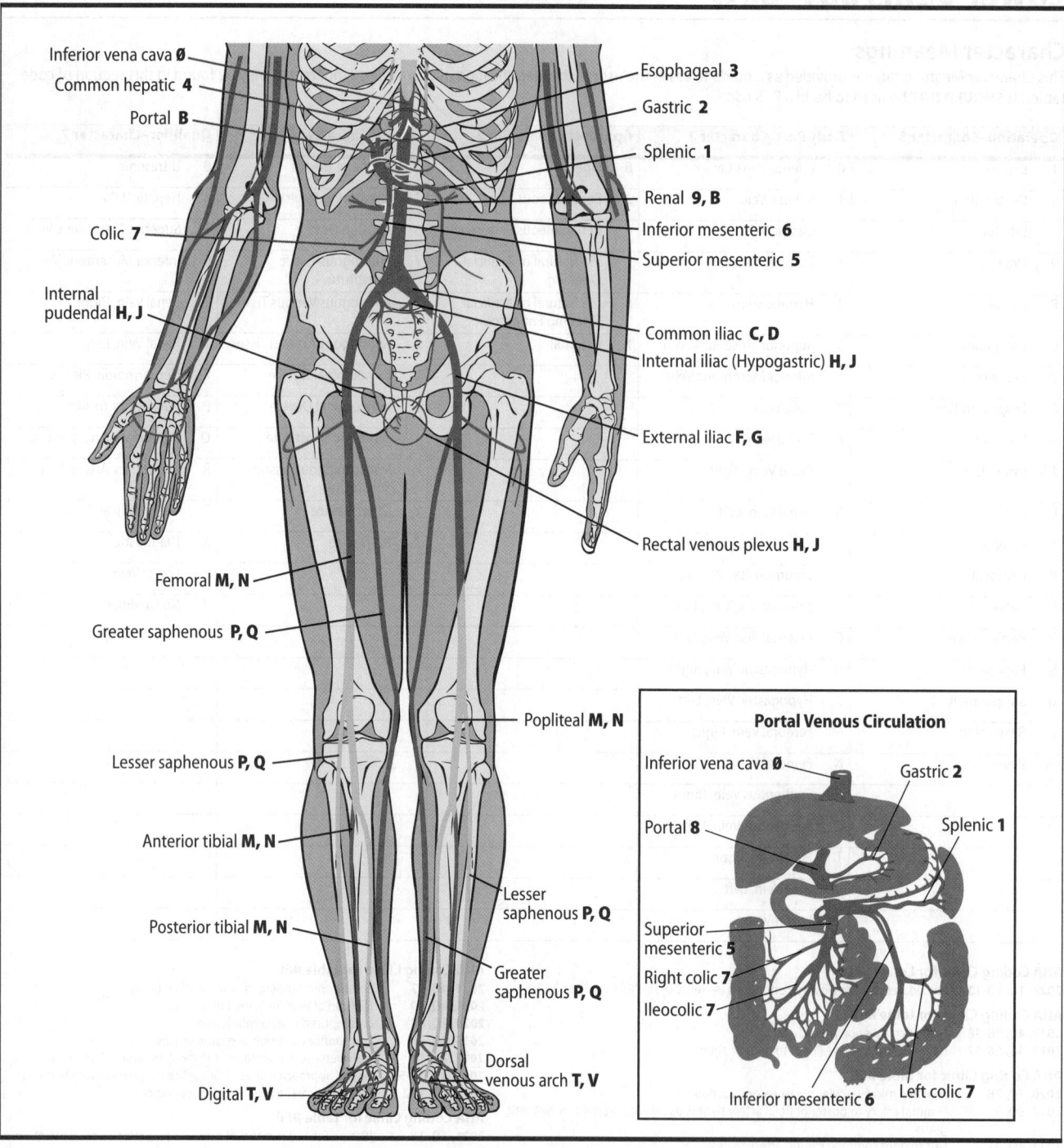

Inferior vena cava **Ø**
Common hepatic **4**
Portal **B**
Colic **7**
Internal pudendal **H, J**
Femoral **M, N**
Greater saphenous **P, Q**
Lesser saphenous **P, Q**
Anterior tibial **M, N**
Posterior tibial **M, N**
Digital **T, V**

Esophageal **3**
Gastric **2**
Splenic **1**
Renal **9, B**
Inferior mesenteric **6**
Superior mesenteric **5**
Common iliac **C, D**
Internal iliac (Hypogastric) **H, J**
External iliac **F, G**
Rectal venous plexus **H, J**
Popliteal **M, N**
Lesser saphenous **P, Q**
Greater saphenous **P, Q**
Dorsal venous arch **T, V**

Portal Venous Circulation

Inferior vena cava **Ø**
Portal **8**
Superior mesenteric **5**
Right colic **7**
Ileocolic **7**
Gastric **2**
Splenic **1**
Inferior mesenteric **6**
Left colic **7**

Ø Medical and Surgical
6 Lower Veins
1 Bypass   Definition: Altering the route of passage of the contents of a tubular body part

Explanation: Rerouting contents of a body part to a downstream area of the normal route, to a similar route and body part, or to an abnormal route and dissimilar body part. Includes one or more anastomoses, with or without the use of a device.

Body Part — Character 4		Approach — Character 5	Device — Character 6	Qualifier — Character 7
Ø Inferior Vena Cava Postcava Right inferior phrenic vein Right ovarian vein Right second lumbar vein Right suprarenal vein Right testicular vein		**Ø Open** **4 Percutaneous Endoscopic**	**7 Autologous Tissue Substitute** **9 Autologous Venous Tissue** **A Autologous Arterial Tissue** **J Synthetic Substitute** **K Nonautologous Tissue Substitute** **Z No Device**	**5 Superior Mesenteric Vein** **6 Inferior Mesenteric Vein** **P Pulmonary Trunk** **Q Pulmonary Artery, Right** **R Pulmonary Artery, Left** **Y Lower Vein**
1 Splenic Vein Left gastroepiploic vein Pancreatic vein		**Ø Open** **4 Percutaneous Endoscopic**	**7 Autologous Tissue Substitute** **9 Autologous Venous Tissue** **A Autologous Arterial Tissue** **J Synthetic Substitute** **K Nonautologous Tissue Substitute** **Z No Device**	**9 Renal Vein, Right** **B Renal Vein, Left** **Y Lower Vein**
2 Gastric Vein **3 Esophageal Vein** **4 Hepatic Vein** **5 Superior Mesenteric Vein** Right gastroepiploic vein **6 Inferior Mesenteric Vein** Sigmoid vein Superior rectal vein **7 Colic Vein** Ileocolic vein Left colic vein Middle colic vein Right colic vein **9 Renal Vein, Right** **B Renal Vein, Left** Left inferior phrenic vein Left ovarian vein Left second lumbar vein Left suprarenal vein Left testicular vein **C Common Iliac Vein, Right** **D Common Iliac Vein, Left** **F External Iliac Vein, Right** **G External Iliac Vein, Left** **H Hypogastric Vein, Right** Gluteal vein Internal iliac vein Internal pudendal vein Lateral sacral vein Middle hemorrhoidal vein Obturator vein Uterine vein Vaginal vein Vesical vein	**J Hypogastric Vein, Left** *See H Hypogastric Vein, Right* **M Femoral Vein, Right** Deep femoral (profunda femoris) vein Popliteal vein Profunda femoris (deep femoral) vein **N Femoral Vein, Left** *See M Femoral Vein, Right* **P Saphenous Vein, Right** External pudendal vein Great(er) saphenous vein Lesser saphenous vein Small saphenous vein Superficial circumflex iliac vein Superficial epigastric vein **Q Saphenous Vein, Left** *See P Saphenous Vein, Right* **T Foot Vein, Right** Common digital vein Dorsal metatarsal vein Dorsal venous arch Plantar digital vein Plantar metatarsal vein Plantar venous arch **V Foot Vein, Left** *See T Foot Vein, Right*	**Ø Open** **4 Percutaneous Endoscopic**	**7 Autologous Tissue Substitute** **9 Autologous Venous Tissue** **A Autologous Arterial Tissue** **J Synthetic Substitute** **K Nonautologous Tissue Substitute** **Z No Device**	**Y Lower Vein**
8 Portal Vein Hepatic portal vein		**Ø Open**	**7 Autologous Tissue Substitute** **9 Autologous Venous Tissue** **A Autologous Arterial Tissue** **J Synthetic Substitute** **K Nonautologous Tissue Substitute** **Z No Device**	**9 Renal Vein, Right** **B Renal Vein, Left** **Y Lower Vein**
8 Portal Vein Hepatic portal vein		**3 Percutaneous**	**J Synthetic Substitute**	**4 Hepatic Vein** **Y Lower Vein**
8 Portal Vein Hepatic portal vein		**4 Percutaneous Endoscopic**	**7 Autologous Tissue Substitute** **9 Autologous Venous Tissue** **A Autologous Arterial Tissue** **K Nonautologous Tissue Substitute** **Z No Device**	**9 Renal Vein, Right** **B Renal Vein, Left** **Y Lower Vein**
8 Portal Vein Hepatic portal vein		**4 Percutaneous Endoscopic**	**J Synthetic Substitute**	**4 Hepatic Vein** **9 Renal Vein, Right** **B Renal Vein, Left** **Y Lower Vein**

NC Noncovered Procedure   **LC** Limited Coverage   **QA** Questionable OB Admit   **NT** New Tech Add-on   ⊞ Combination Member   ♂ Male   ♀ Female

ICD-10-PCS 2023   265

Ø61–Ø61

Lower Veins

Ø **Medical and Surgical**
6 **Lower Veins**
5 **Destruction**　　Definition: Physical eradication of all or a portion of a body part by the direct use of energy, force, or a destructive agent
　　　　　　　　　　　Explanation: None of the body part is physically taken out

Body Part Character 4	Approach Character 5	Device Character 6	Qualifier Character 7
Ø **Inferior Vena Cava** 　Postcava 　Right inferior phrenic vein 　Right ovarian vein 　Right second lumbar vein 　Right suprarenal vein 　Right testicular vein 1 **Splenic Vein** 　Left gastroepiploic vein 　Pancreatic vein 2 **Gastric Vein** 3 **Esophageal Vein** 4 **Hepatic Vein** 5 **Superior Mesenteric Vein** 　Right gastroepiploic vein 6 **Inferior Mesenteric Vein** 　Sigmoid vein 　Superior rectal vein 7 **Colic Vein** 　Ileocolic vein 　Left colic vein 　Middle colic vein 　Right colic vein 8 **Portal Vein** 　Hepatic portal vein 9 **Renal Vein, Right** B **Renal Vein, Left** 　Left inferior phrenic vein 　Left ovarian vein 　Left second lumbar vein 　Left suprarenal vein 　Left testicular vein C **Common Iliac Vein, Right** D **Common Iliac Vein, Left** F **External Iliac Vein, Right** G **External Iliac Vein, Left** H **Hypogastric Vein, Right** 　Gluteal vein 　Internal iliac vein 　Internal pudendal vein 　Lateral sacral vein 　Middle hemorrhoidal vein 　Obturator vein 　Uterine vein 　Vaginal vein 　Vesical vein J **Hypogastric Vein, Left** 　*See H Hypogastric Vein, Right* M **Femoral Vein, Right** 　Deep femoral (profunda femoris) vein 　Popliteal vein 　Profunda femoris (deep femoral) vein N **Femoral Vein, Left** 　*See M Femoral Vein, Right* P **Saphenous Vein, Right** 　External pudendal vein 　Great(er) saphenous vein 　Lesser saphenous vein 　Small saphenous vein 　Superficial circumflex iliac vein 　Superficial epigastric vein Q **Saphenous Vein, Left** 　*See P Saphenous Vein, Right* T **Foot Vein, Right** 　Common digital vein 　Dorsal metatarsal vein 　Dorsal venous arch 　Plantar digital vein 　Plantar metatarsal vein 　Plantar venous arch V **Foot Vein, Left** 　*See T Foot Vein, Right*	Ø **Open** 3 **Percutaneous** 4 **Percutaneous Endoscopic**	Z **No Device**	Z **No Qualifier**
Y **Lower Vein**	Ø **Open** 3 **Percutaneous** 4 **Percutaneous Endoscopic**	Z **No Device**	C **Hemorrhoidal Plexus** Z **No Qualifier**

Non-OR Procedure　　DRG Non-OR Procedure　　Valid OR Procedure　　HAC Associated Procedure　　Combination Only　　New/Revised April　　New/Revised October

266　　ICD-10-PCS 2023

Ø   Medical and Surgical
6   Lower Veins
7   Dilation   Definition: Expanding an orifice or the lumen of a tubular body part

Explanation: The orifice can be a natural orifice or an artificially created orifice. Accomplished by stretching a tubular body part using intraluminal pressure or by cutting part of the orifice or wall of the tubular body part.

Body Part Character 4	Approach Character 5	Device Character 6	Qualifier Character 7
Ø **Inferior Vena Cava** Postcava Right inferior phrenic vein Right ovarian vein Right second lumbar vein Right suprarenal vein Right testicular vein	**Ø** Open **3** Percutaneous **4** Percutaneous Endoscopic	**D** Intraluminal Device **Z** No Device	**Z** No Qualifier
1 **Splenic Vein** Left gastroepiploic vein Pancreatic vein			
2 **Gastric Vein**			
3 **Esophageal Vein**			
4 **Hepatic Vein**			
5 **Superior Mesenteric Vein** Right gastroepiploic vein			
6 **Inferior Mesenteric Vein** Sigmoid vein Superior rectal vein			
7 **Colic Vein** Ileocolic vein Left colic vein Middle colic vein Right colic vein			
8 **Portal Vein** Hepatic portal vein			
9 **Renal Vein, Right**			
B **Renal Vein, Left** Left inferior phrenic vein Left ovarian vein Left second lumbar vein Left suprarenal vein Left testicular vein			
C **Common Iliac Vein, Right**			
D **Common Iliac Vein, Left**			
F **External Iliac Vein, Right**			
G **External Iliac Vein, Left**			
H **Hypogastric Vein, Right** Gluteal vein Internal iliac vein Internal pudendal vein Lateral sacral vein Middle hemorrhoidal vein Obturator vein Uterine vein Vaginal vein Vesical vein			
J **Hypogastric Vein, Left** *See* H Hypogastric Vein, Right			
M **Femoral Vein, Right** Deep femoral (profunda femoris) vein Popliteal vein Profunda femoris (deep femoral) vein			
N **Femoral Vein, Left** *See* M Femoral Vein, Right			
P **Saphenous Vein, Right** External pudendal vein Great(er) saphenous vein Lesser saphenous vein Small saphenous vein Superficial circumflex iliac vein Superficial epigastric vein			
Q **Saphenous Vein, Left** *See* P Saphenous Vein, Right			
T **Foot Vein, Right** Common digital vein Dorsal metatarsal vein Dorsal venous arch Plantar digital vein Plantar metatarsal vein Plantar venous arch			
V **Foot Vein, Left** *See* T Foot Vein, Right			
Y **Lower Vein**			

NC Noncovered Procedure   **LC** Limited Coverage   **QA** Questionable OB Admit   **NT** New Tech Add-on   ⊞ Combination Member   ♂ Male   ♀ Female

ICD-10-PCS 2023   267

Lower Veins

Ø **Medical and Surgical**
6 **Lower Veins**
9 **Drainage**   Definition: Taking or letting out fluids and/or gases from a body part

                       Explanation: The qualifier DIAGNOSTIC is used to identify drainage procedures that are biopsies

Body Part Character 4	Approach Character 5	Device Character 6	Qualifier Character 7

Ø **Inferior Vena Cava**
  Postcava
  Right inferior phrenic vein
  Right ovarian vein
  Right second lumbar vein
  Right suprarenal vein
  Right testicular vein
1 **Splenic Vein**
  Left gastroepiploic vein
  Pancreatic vein
2 **Gastric Vein**
3 **Esophageal Vein**
4 **Hepatic Vein**
5 **Superior Mesenteric Vein**
  Right gastroepiploic vein
6 **Inferior Mesenteric Vein**
  Sigmoid vein
  Superior rectal vein
7 **Colic Vein**
  Ileocolic vein
  Left colic vein
  Middle colic vein
  Right colic vein
8 **Portal Vein**
  Hepatic portal vein
9 **Renal Vein, Right**
B **Renal Vein, Left**
  Left inferior phrenic vein
  Left ovarian vein
  Left second lumbar vein
  Left suprarenal vein
  Left testicular vein
C **Common Iliac Vein, Right**
D **Common Iliac Vein, Left**
F **External Iliac Vein, Right**
G **External Iliac Vein, Left**
H **Hypogastric Vein, Right**
  Gluteal vein
  Internal iliac vein
  Internal pudendal vein
  Lateral sacral vein
  Middle hemorrhoidal vein
  Obturator vein
  Uterine vein
  Vaginal vein
  Vesical vein
J **Hypogastric Vein, Left**
  See H Hypogastric Vein, Right
M **Femoral Vein, Right**
  Deep femoral (profunda femoris) vein
  Popliteal vein
  Profunda femoris (deep femoral) vein
N **Femoral Vein, Left**
  See M Femoral Vein, Right
P **Saphenous Vein, Right**
  External pudendal vein
  Great(er) saphenous vein
  Lesser saphenous vein
  Small saphenous vein
  Superficial circumflex iliac vein
  Superficial epigastric vein
Q **Saphenous Vein, Left**
  See P Saphenous Vein, Right
T **Foot Vein, Right**
  Common digital vein
  Dorsal metatarsal vein
  Dorsal venous arch
  Plantar digital vein
  Plantar metatarsal vein
  Plantar venous arch
V **Foot Vein, Left**
  See T Foot Vein, Right
Y **Lower Vein**
	Ø **Open**
	3 **Percutaneous**
	4 **Percutaneous Endoscopic**
		Ø **Drainage Device**	Z **No Qualifier**

Non-OR	Ø69[Ø,1,2,4,5,6,7,8,9,B,C,D,F,G,H,J,M,N,P,Q,T,V,Y][Ø,3,4]ØZ
Non-OR	Ø69330Z

Ø69 Continued on next page

Non-OR Procedure   DRG Non-OR Procedure   Valid OR Procedure   HAC Associated Procedure   Combination Only   New/Revised April   New/Revised October

Ø **Medical and Surgical**   *Ø69 Continued*
6 **Lower Veins**
9 **Drainage**   Definition: Taking or letting out fluids and/or gases from a body part
                       Explanation: The qualifier DIAGNOSTIC is used to identify drainage procedures that are biopsies

Body Part Character 4	Approach Character 5	Device Character 6	Qualifier Character 7
Ø **Inferior Vena Cava** 　Postcava 　Right inferior phrenic vein 　Right ovarian vein 　Right second lumbar vein 　Right suprarenal vein 　Right testicular vein	**Ø** Open **3** Percutaneous **4** Percutaneous Endoscopic	**Z** No Device	**X** Diagnostic **Z** No Qualifier
1 **Splenic Vein** 　Left gastroepiploic vein 　Pancreatic vein			
2 **Gastric Vein**			
3 **Esophageal Vein**			
4 **Hepatic Vein**			
5 **Superior Mesenteric Vein** 　Right gastroepiploic vein			
6 **Inferior Mesenteric Vein** 　Sigmoid vein 　Superior rectal vein			
7 **Colic Vein** 　Ileocolic vein 　Left colic vein 　Middle colic vein 　Right colic vein			
8 **Portal Vein** 　Hepatic portal vein			
9 **Renal Vein, Right**			
B **Renal Vein, Left** 　Left inferior phrenic vein 　Left ovarian vein 　Left second lumbar vein 　Left suprarenal vein 　Left testicular vein			
C **Common Iliac Vein, Right**			
D **Common Iliac Vein, Left**			
F **External Iliac Vein, Right**			
G **External Iliac Vein, Left**			
H **Hypogastric Vein, Right** 　Gluteal vein 　Internal iliac vein 　Internal pudendal vein 　Lateral sacral vein 　Middle hemorrhoidal vein 　Obturator vein 　Uterine vein 　Vaginal vein 　Vesical vein			
J **Hypogastric Vein, Left** 　*See H Hypogastric Vein, Right*			
M **Femoral Vein, Right** 　Deep femoral (profunda femoris) vein 　Popliteal vein 　Profunda femoris (deep femoral) vein			
N **Femoral Vein, Left** 　*See M Femoral Vein, Right*			
P **Saphenous Vein, Right** 　External pudendal vein 　Great(er) saphenous vein 　Lesser saphenous vein 　Small saphenous vein 　Superficial circumflex iliac vein 　Superficial epigastric vein			
Q **Saphenous Vein, Left** 　*See P Saphenous Vein, Right*			
T **Foot Vein, Right** 　Common digital vein 　Dorsal metatarsal vein 　Dorsal venous arch 　Plantar digital vein 　Plantar metatarsal vein 　Plantar venous arch			
V **Foot Vein, Left** 　*See T Foot Vein, Right*			
Y **Lower Vein**			

Non-OR	Ø69[Ø,1,2,3,4,5,6,7,8,9,B,C,D,F,G,H,J,M,N,P,Q,T,V,Y]3ZX
Non-OR	Ø69[Ø,1,2,4,5,6,7,8,9,B,C,D,F,G,H,J,M,N,P,Q,T,V,Y][Ø,3,4]ZZ
Non-OR	Ø6933ZZ

 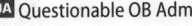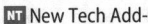

0   Medical and Surgical
6   Lower Veins
B   Excision   Definition: Cutting out or off, without replacement, a portion of a body part

Explanation: The qualifier DIAGNOSTIC is used to identify excision procedures that are biopsies

Body Part Character 4	Approach Character 5	Device Character 6	Qualifier Character 7
0 Inferior Vena Cava Postcava Right inferior phrenic vein Right ovarian vein Right second lumbar vein Right suprarenal vein Right testicular vein **1 Splenic Vein** Left gastroepiploic vein Pancreatic vein **2 Gastric Vein** **3 Esophageal Vein** **4 Hepatic Vein** **5 Superior Mesenteric Vein** Right gastroepiploic vein **6 Inferior Mesenteric Vein** Sigmoid vein Superior rectal vein **7 Colic Vein** Ileocolic vein Left colic vein Middle colic vein Right colic vein **8 Portal Vein** Hepatic portal vein **9 Renal Vein, Right** **B Renal Vein, Left** Left inferior phrenic vein Left ovarian vein Left second lumbar vein Left suprarenal vein Left testicular vein **C Common Iliac Vein, Right** **D Common Iliac Vein, Left** **F External Iliac Vein, Right** **G External Iliac Vein, Left** **H Hypogastric Vein, Right** Gluteal vein Internal iliac vein Internal pudendal vein Lateral sacral vein Middle hemorrhoidal vein Obturator vein Uterine vein Vaginal vein Vesical vein **J Hypogastric Vein, Left** *See H Hypogastric Vein, Right* **M Femoral Vein, Right** Deep femoral (profunda femoris) vein Popliteal vein Profunda femoris (deep femoral) vein **N Femoral Vein, Left** *See M Femoral Vein, Right* **P Saphenous Vein, Right** External pudendal vein Great(er) saphenous vein Lesser saphenous vein Small saphenous vein Superficial circumflex iliac vein Superficial epigastric vein **Q Saphenous Vein, Left** *See P Saphenous Vein, Right* **T Foot Vein, Right** Common digital vein Dorsal metatarsal vein Dorsal venous arch Plantar digital vein Plantar metatarsal vein Plantar venous arch **V Foot Vein, Left** *See T Foot Vein, Right*	**0 Open** **3 Percutaneous** **4 Percutaneous Endoscopic**	**Z No Device**	**X Diagnostic** **Z No Qualifier**
Y Lower Vein	**0 Open** **3 Percutaneous** **4 Percutaneous Endoscopic**	**Z No Device**	**C Hemorrhoidal Plexus** **X Diagnostic** **Z No Qualifier**

Non-OR Procedure   DRG Non-OR Procedure   Valid OR Procedure   HAC Associated Procedure   Combination Only   New/Revised April   New/Revised October

Ø   **Medical and Surgical**
6   **Lower Veins**
C   **Extirpation**   Definition: Taking or cutting out solid matter from a body part
                           Explanation: The solid matter may be an abnormal byproduct of a biological function or a foreign body; it may be imbedded in a body part or in
                           the lumen of a tubular body part. The solid matter may or may not have been previously broken into pieces.

Body Part Character 4	Approach Character 5	Device Character 6	Qualifier Character 7
Ø Inferior Vena Cava Postcava Right inferior phrenic vein Right ovarian vein Right second lumbar vein Right suprarenal vein Right testicular vein	**Ø Open** **3 Percutaneous** **4 Percutaneous Endoscopic**	**Z No Device**	**Z No Qualifier**
1 Splenic Vein Left gastroepiploic vein Pancreatic vein			
2 Gastric Vein			
3 Esophageal Vein			
4 Hepatic Vein			
5 Superior Mesenteric Vein Right gastroepiploic vein			
6 Inferior Mesenteric Vein Sigmoid vein Superior rectal vein			
7 Colic Vein Ileocolic vein Left colic vein Middle colic vein Right colic vein			
8 Portal Vein Hepatic portal vein			
9 Renal Vein, Right			
B Renal Vein, Left Left inferior phrenic vein Left ovarian vein Left second lumbar vein Left suprarenal vein Left testicular vein			
C Common Iliac Vein, Right			
D Common Iliac Vein, Left			
F External Iliac Vein, Right			
G External Iliac Vein, Left			
H Hypogastric Vein, Right Gluteal vein Internal iliac vein Internal pudendal vein Lateral sacral vein Middle hemorrhoidal vein Obturator vein Uterine vein Vaginal vein Vesical vein			
J Hypogastric Vein, Left *See H Hypogastric Vein, Right*			
M Femoral Vein, Right Deep femoral (profunda femoris) vein Popliteal vein Profunda femoris (deep femoral) vein			
N Femoral Vein, Left *See M Femoral Vein, Right*			
P Saphenous Vein, Right External pudendal vein Great(er) saphenous vein Lesser saphenous vein Small saphenous vein Superficial circumflex iliac vein Superficial epigastric vein			
Q Saphenous Vein, Left *See P Saphenous Vein, Right*			
T Foot Vein, Right Common digital vein Dorsal metatarsal vein Dorsal venous arch Plantar digital vein Plantar metatarsal vein Plantar venous arch			
V Foot Vein, Left *See T Foot Vein, Right*			
Y Lower Vein			

NC Noncovered Procedure   **LC** Limited Coverage   **QA** Questionable OB Admit   **NT** New Tech Add-on   ⊞ Combination Member   ♂ Male   ♀ Female

Lower Veins

0   **Medical and Surgical**
6   **Lower Veins**
D   **Extraction**   Definition: Pulling or stripping out or off all or a portion of a body part by the use of force
                           Explanation: The qualifier DIAGNOSTIC is used to identify extraction procedures that are biopsies

Body Part Character 4	Approach Character 5	Device Character 6	Qualifier Character 7

M   **Femoral Vein, Right**
    Deep femoral (profunda femoris) vein
    Popliteal vein
    Profunda femoris (deep femoral) vein
N   **Femoral Vein, Left**
    See M Femoral Vein, Right
P   **Saphenous Vein, Right**
    External pudendal vein
    Great(er) saphenous vein
    Lesser saphenous vein
    Small saphenous vein
    Superficial circumflex iliac vein
    Superficial epigastric vein
Q   **Saphenous Vein, Left**
    See P Saphenous Vein, Right
T   **Foot Vein, Right**
    Common digital vein
    Dorsal metatarsal vein
    Dorsal venous arch
    Plantar digital vein
    Plantar metatarsal vein
    Plantar venous arch
V   **Foot Vein, Left**
    See T Foot Vein, Right
Y   **Lower Vein**
	0 Open
	3 Percutaneous
	4 Percutaneous Endoscopic
		Z No Device	**Z** No Qualifier

0   **Medical and Surgical**
6   **Lower Veins**
F   **Fragmentation**   Definition: Breaking solid matter in a body part into pieces
                           Explanation: Physical force (e.g., manual, ultrasonic) applied directly or indirectly is used to break the solid matter into pieces. The solid matter may be an abnormal byproduct of a biological function or a foreign body. The pieces of solid matter are not taken out.

Body Part Character 4	Approach Character 5	Device Character 6	Qualifier Character 7

C   **Common Iliac Vein, Right**
D   **Common Iliac Vein, Left**
F   **External Iliac Vein, Right**
G   **External Iliac Vein, Left**
H   **Hypogastric Vein, Right**
    Gluteal vein
    Internal iliac vein
    Internal pudendal vein
    Lateral sacral vein
    Middle hemorrhoidal vein
    Obturator vein
    Uterine vein
    Vaginal vein
    Vesical vein
J   **Hypogastric Vein, Left**
    See H Hypogastric Vein, Right
M   **Femoral Vein, Right**
    Deep femoral (profunda femoris) vein
    Popliteal vein
    Profunda femoris (deep femoral) vein
N   **Femoral Vein, Left**
    See M Femoral Vein, Right
P   **Saphenous Vein, Right**
    External pudendal vein
    Great(er) saphenous vein
    Lesser saphenous vein
    Small saphenous vein
    Superficial circumflex iliac vein
    Superficial epigastric vein
Q   **Saphenous Vein, Left**
    See P Saphenous Vein, Right
Y   **Lower Vein**
	3 Percutaneous	**Z** No Device	**0** Ultrasonic
			Z No Qualifier

Non-OR Procedure   DRG Non-OR Procedure   Valid OR Procedure   HAC Associated Procedure   Combination Only   New/Revised April   New/Revised October

272

ICD-10-PCS 2023

06D–06F

Ø Medical and Surgical
6 Lower Veins
H Insertion
    Definition: Putting in a nonbiological appliance that monitors, assists, performs, or prevents a physiological function but does not physically take the place of a body part
    Explanation: None

Body Part Character 4		Approach Character 5	Device Character 6	Qualifier Character 7
Ø **Inferior Vena Cava** Postcava Right inferior phrenic vein Right ovarian vein Right second lumbar vein Right suprarenal vein Right testicular vein		Ø Open 3 Percutaneous	3 Infusion Device	T Via Umbilical Vein Z No Qualifier
Ø **Inferior Vena Cava** Postcava Right inferior phrenic vein Right ovarian vein Right second lumbar vein Right suprarenal vein Right testicular vein		Ø Open 3 Percutaneous	D Intraluminal Device	Z No Qualifier
Ø **Inferior Vena Cava** Postcava Right inferior phrenic vein Right ovarian vein Right second lumbar vein Right suprarenal vein Right testicular vein		4 Percutaneous Endoscopic	3 Infusion Device D Intraluminal Device	Z No Qualifier

1 **Splenic Vein**
  Left gastroepiploic vein
  Pancreatic vein
2 **Gastric Vein**
3 **Esophageal Vein**
4 **Hepatic Vein**
5 **Superior Mesenteric Vein**
  Right gastroepiploic vein
6 **Inferior Mesenteric Vein**
  Sigmoid vein
  Superior rectal vein
7 **Colic Vein**
  Ileocolic vein
  Left colic vein
  Middle colic vein
  Right colic vein
8 **Portal Vein**
  Hepatic portal vein
9 **Renal Vein, Right**
B **Renal Vein, Left**
  Left inferior phrenic vein
  Left ovarian vein
  Left second lumbar vein
  Left suprarenal vein
  Left testicular vein
C **Common Iliac Vein, Right**
D **Common Iliac Vein, Left**
F **External Iliac Vein, Right**
G **External Iliac Vein, Left**
	H **Hypogastric Vein, Right**
	  Gluteal vein
	  Internal iliac vein
	  Internal pudendal vein
	  Lateral sacral vein
	  Middle hemorrhoidal vein
	  Obturator vein
	  Uterine vein
	  Vaginal vein
	  Vesical vein
	J **Hypogastric Vein, Left**
	  See H Hypogastric Vein, Right
	M **Femoral Vein, Right**
	  Deep femoral (profunda femoris) vein
	  Popliteal vein
	  Profunda femoris (deep femoral) vein
	N **Femoral Vein, Left**
	  See M Femoral Vein, Right
	P **Saphenous Vein, Right**
	  External pudendal vein
	  Great(er) saphenous vein
	  Lesser saphenous vein
	  Small saphenous vein
	  Superficial circumflex iliac vein
	  Superficial epigastric vein
	Q **Saphenous Vein, Left**
	  See P Saphenous Vein, Right
	T **Foot Vein, Right**
	  Common digital vein
	  Dorsal metatarsal vein
	  Dorsal venous arch
	  Plantar digital vein
	  Plantar metatarsal vein
	  Plantar venous arch
	V **Foot Vein, Left**
	  See T Foot Vein, Right
		Ø Open
		3 Percutaneous
		4 Percutaneous Endoscopic
			3 Infusion Device
			D Intraluminal Device
				Z No Qualifier

Y **Lower Vein**		Ø Open 3 Percutaneous 4 Percutaneous Endoscopic	2 Monitoring Device 3 Infusion Device D Intraluminal Device Y Other Device	Z No Qualifier

Non-OR	06H0[Ø,3]3[T,Z]
Non-OR	06H03DZ
Non-OR	06H043Z
Non-OR	06H[1,2,3,4,5,6,7,8,9,B,C,D,F,G,H,J,M,N,P,Q,T,V][Ø,3,4]3Z
Non-OR	06HY[Ø,3,4]3Z
Non-OR	06HY32Z
Non-OR	06HY[3,4]YZ

NC Noncovered Procedure   **LC** Limited Coverage   **QA** Questionable OB Admit   **NT** New Tech Add-on   ⊞ Combination Member   ♂ Male   ♀ Female

ICD-10-PCS 2023   273

06H–06H

Ø Medical and Surgical
6 Lower Veins
J Inspection Definition: Visually and/or manually exploring a body part

Explanation: Visual exploration may be performed with or without optical instrumentation. Manual exploration may be performed directly or through intervening body layers.

Body Part Character 4	Approach Character 5	Device Character 6	Qualifier Character 7
Y Lower Vein	Ø Open 3 Percutaneous 4 Percutaneous Endoscopic X External	Z No Device	Z No Qualifier

Non-OR 06JY[3,X]ZZ

Ø Medical and Surgical
6 Lower Veins
L Occlusion Definition: Completely closing an orifice or the lumen of a tubular body part

Explanation: The orifice can be a natural orifice or an artificially created orifice

Body Part Character 4	Approach Character 5	Device Character 6	Qualifier Character 7
Ø Inferior Vena Cava Postcava Right inferior phrenic vein Right ovarian vein Right second lumbar vein Right suprarenal vein Right testicular vein 1 Splenic Vein Left gastroepiploic vein Pancreatic vein 4 Hepatic Vein 5 Superior Mesenteric Vein Right gastroepiploic vein 6 Inferior Mesenteric Vein Sigmoid vein Superior rectal vein 7 Colic Vein Ileocolic vein Left colic vein Middle colic vein Right colic vein 8 Portal Vein Hepatic portal vein 9 Renal Vein, Right B Renal Vein, Left Left inferior phrenic vein Left ovarian vein Left second lumbar vein Left suprarenal vein Left testicular vein C Common Iliac Vein, Right D Common Iliac Vein, Left F External Iliac Vein, Right G External Iliac Vein, Left	H Hypogastric Vein, Right Gluteal vein Internal iliac vein Internal pudendal vein Lateral sacral vein Middle hemorrhoidal vein Obturator vein Uterine vein Vaginal vein Vesical vein J Hypogastric Vein, Left *See H Hypogastric Vein, Right* M Femoral Vein, Right Deep femoral (profunda femoris) vein Popliteal vein Profunda femoris (deep femoral) vein N Femoral Vein, Left *See M Femoral Vein, Right* P Saphenous Vein, Right External pudendal vein Great(er) saphenous vein Lesser saphenous vein Small saphenous vein Superficial circumflex iliac vein Superficial epigastric vein Q Saphenous Vein, Left *See P Saphenous Vein, Right* T Foot Vein, Right Common digital vein Dorsal metatarsal vein Dorsal venous arch Plantar digital vein Plantar metatarsal vein Plantar venous arch V Foot Vein, Left *See T Foot Vein, Right*	Ø Open 3 Percutaneous 4 Percutaneous Endoscopic	C Extraluminal Device D Intraluminal Device Z No Device	Z No Qualifier
2 Gastric Vein 3 Esophageal Vein	Ø Open 3 Percutaneous 4 Percutaneous Endoscopic 7 Via Natural or Artificial Opening 8 Via Natural or Artificial Opening Endoscopic	C Extraluminal Device D Intraluminal Device Z No Device	Z No Qualifier
Y Lower Vein	Ø Open 3 Percutaneous 4 Percutaneous Endoscopic 7 Via Natural or Artificial Opening 8 Via Natural or Artificial Opening Endoscopic	C Extraluminal Device D Intraluminal Device Z No Device	C Hemorrhoidal Plexus Z No Qualifier

Non-OR 06L2[7,8][C,D,Z]Z
Non-OR 06L3[3,4,7,8][C,D,Z]Z

Non-OR Procedure   DRG Non-OR Procedure   Valid OR Procedure   HAC Associated Procedure   Combination Only   New/Revised April   New/Revised October

274 ICD-10-PCS 2023

06J–06L

0   **Medical and Surgical**
6   **Lower Veins**
N   **Release**   Definition: Freeing a body part from an abnormal physical constraint by cutting or by the use of force
                      Explanation: Some of the restraining tissue may be taken out but none of the body part is taken out

Body Part Character 4		Approach Character 5	Device Character 6	Qualifier Character 7

0 **Inferior Vena Cava**
    Postcava
    Right inferior phrenic vein
    Right ovarian vein
    Right second lumbar vein
    Right suprarenal vein
    Right testicular vein
1 **Splenic Vein**
    Left gastroepiploic vein
    Pancreatic vein
2 **Gastric Vein**
3 **Esophageal Vein**
4 **Hepatic Vein**
5 **Superior Mesenteric Vein**
    Right gastroepiploic vein
6 **Inferior Mesenteric Vein**
    Sigmoid vein
    Superior rectal vein
7 **Colic Vein**
    Ileocolic vein
    Left colic vein
    Middle colic vein
    Right colic vein
8 **Portal Vein**
    Hepatic portal vein
9 **Renal Vein, Right**
B **Renal Vein, Left**
    Left inferior phrenic vein
    Left ovarian vein
    Left second lumbar vein
    Left suprarenal vein
    Left testicular vein
C **Common Iliac Vein, Right**
D **Common Iliac Vein, Left**
F **External Iliac Vein, Right**
G **External Iliac Vein, Left**
	H **Hypogastric Vein, Right**
	    Gluteal vein
	    Internal iliac vein
	    Internal pudendal vein
	    Lateral sacral vein
	    Middle hemorrhoidal vein
	    Obturator vein
	    Uterine vein
	    Vaginal vein
	    Vesical vein
	J **Hypogastric Vein, Left**
	    See H Hypogastric Vein, Right
	M **Femoral Vein, Right**
	    Deep femoral (profunda
	       femoris) vein
	    Popliteal vein
	    Profunda femoris (deep
	       femoral) vein
	N **Femoral Vein, Left**
	    See M Femoral Vein, Right
	P **Saphenous Vein, Right**
	    External pudendal vein
	    Great(er) saphenous vein
	    Lesser saphenous vein
	    Small saphenous vein
	    Superficial circumflex iliac vein
	    Superficial epigastric vein
	Q **Saphenous Vein, Left**
	    See P Saphenous Vein, Right
	T **Foot Vein, Right**
	    Common digital vein
	    Dorsal metatarsal vein
	    Dorsal venous arch
	    Plantar digital vein
	    Plantar metatarsal vein
	    Plantar venous arch
	V **Foot Vein, Left**
	    See T Foot Vein, Right
	Y **Lower Vein**
		0 **Open**
		3 **Percutaneous**
		4 **Percutaneous Endoscopic**
			Z **No Device**	**Z** **No Qualifier**

0   **Medical and Surgical**
6   **Lower Veins**
P   **Removal**   Definition: Taking out or off a device from a body part
                      Explanation: If a device is taken out and a similar device put in without cutting or puncturing the skin or mucous membrane, the procedure is coded to the root operation CHANGE. Otherwise, the procedure for taking out a device is coded to the root operation REMOVAL.

Body Part Character 4	Approach Character 5	Device Character 6	Qualifier Character 7

Y Lower Vein	**0** **Open**
	3 **Percutaneous**
	4 **Percutaneous Endoscopic**
		0 **Drainage Device**
		2 **Monitoring Device**
		3 **Infusion Device**
		7 **Autologous Tissue**
		    Substitute
		C **Extraluminal Device**
		D **Intraluminal Device**
		J **Synthetic Substitute**
		K **Nonautologous Tissue**
		    Substitute
		Y **Other Device**
			Z **No Qualifier**

Y Lower Vein	**X** **External**	**0** **Drainage Device** **2** **Monitoring Device** **3** **Infusion Device** **D** **Intraluminal Device**	**Z** **No Qualifier**

Non-OR	06PY3[0,2,3]Z
Non-OR	06PY[3,4]YZ
Non-OR	06PYX[0,2,3,D]Z

NC Noncovered Procedure   LC Limited Coverage   QA Questionable OB Admit   NT New Tech Add-on   ⊞ Combination Member   ♂ Male   ♀ Female

Lower Veins

0 Medical and Surgical
6 Lower Veins
Q Repair

Definition: Restoring, to the extent possible, a body part to its normal anatomic structure and function
Explanation: Used only when the method to accomplish the repair is not one of the other root operations

Body Part Character 4	Approach Character 5	Device Character 6	Qualifier Character 7
0 Inferior Vena Cava Postcava Right inferior phrenic vein Right ovarian vein Right second lumbar vein Right suprarenal vein Right testicular vein	**0 Open** **3 Percutaneous** **4 Percutaneous Endoscopic**	**Z No Device**	**Z No Qualifier**
1 Splenic Vein Left gastroepiploic vein Pancreatic vein			
2 Gastric Vein			
3 Esophageal Vein			
4 Hepatic Vein			
5 Superior Mesenteric Vein Right gastroepiploic vein			
6 Inferior Mesenteric Vein Sigmoid vein Superior rectal vein			
7 Colic Vein Ileocolic vein Left colic vein Middle colic vein Right colic vein			
8 Portal Vein Hepatic portal vein			
9 Renal Vein, Right			
B Renal Vein, Left Left inferior phrenic vein Left ovarian vein Left second lumbar vein Left suprarenal vein Left testicular vein			
C Common Iliac Vein, Right			
D Common Iliac Vein, Left			
F External Iliac Vein, Right			
G External Iliac Vein, Left			
H Hypogastric Vein, Right Gluteal vein Internal iliac vein Internal pudendal vein Lateral sacral vein Middle hemorrhoidal vein Obturator vein Uterine vein Vaginal vein Vesical vein			
J Hypogastric Vein, Left *See H Hypogastric Vein, Right*			
M Femoral Vein, Right Deep femoral (profunda femoris) vein Popliteal vein Profunda femoris (deep femoral) vein			
N Femoral Vein, Left *See M Femoral Vein, Right*			
P Saphenous Vein, Right External pudendal vein Great(er) saphenous vein Lesser saphenous vein Small saphenous vein Superficial circumflex iliac vein Superficial epigastric vein			
Q Saphenous Vein, Left *See P Saphenous Vein, Right*			
T Foot Vein, Right Common digital vein Dorsal metatarsal vein Dorsal venous arch Plantar digital vein Plantar metatarsal vein Plantar venous arch			
V Foot Vein, Left *See T Foot Vein, Right*			
Y Lower Vein			

Ø   **Medical and Surgical**
6   **Lower Veins**
R   **Replacement**   Definition: Putting in or on biological or synthetic material that physically takes the place and/or function of all or a portion of a body part

Explanation: The body part may have been taken out or replaced, or may be taken out, physically eradicated, or rendered nonfunctional during the REPLACEMENT procedure. A REMOVAL procedure is coded for taking out the device used in a previous replacement procedure.

Body Part Character 4	Approach Character 5	Device Character 6	Qualifier Character 7
Ø Inferior Vena Cava Postcava Right inferior phrenic vein Right ovarian vein Right second lumbar vein Right suprarenal vein Right testicular vein **1 Splenic Vein** Left gastroepiploic vein Pancreatic vein **2 Gastric Vein** **3 Esophageal Vein** **4 Hepatic Vein** **5 Superior Mesenteric Vein** Right gastroepiploic vein **6 Inferior Mesenteric Vein** Sigmoid vein Superior rectal vein **7 Colic Vein** Ileocolic vein Left colic vein Middle colic vein Right colic vein **8 Portal Vein** Hepatic portal vein **9 Renal Vein, Right** **B Renal Vein, Left** Left inferior phrenic vein Left ovarian vein Left second lumbar vein Left suprarenal vein Left testicular vein **C Common Iliac Vein, Right** **D Common Iliac Vein, Left** **F External Iliac Vein, Right** **G External Iliac Vein, Left** **H Hypogastric Vein, Right** Gluteal vein Internal iliac vein Internal pudendal vein Lateral sacral vein Middle hemorrhoidal vein Obturator vein Uterine vein Vaginal vein Vesical vein **J Hypogastric Vein, Left** *See* H Hypogastric Vein, Right **M Femoral Vein, Right** Deep femoral (profunda femoris) vein Popliteal vein Profunda femoris (deep femoral) vein **N Femoral Vein, Left** *See* M Femoral Vein, Right **P Saphenous Vein, Right** External pudendal vein Great(er) saphenous vein Lesser saphenous vein Small saphenous vein Superficial circumflex iliac vein Superficial epigastric vein **Q Saphenous Vein, Left** *See* P Saphenous Vein, Right **T Foot Vein, Right** Common digital vein Dorsal metatarsal vein Dorsal venous arch Plantar digital vein Plantar metatarsal vein Plantar venous arch **V Foot Vein, Left** *See* T Foot Vein, Right **Y Lower Vein**	**Ø Open** **4 Percutaneous Endoscopic**	**7 Autologous Tissue Substitute** **J Synthetic Substitute** **K Nonautologous Tissue Substitute**	**Z No Qualifier**

0   **Medical and Surgical**
6   **Lower Veins**
S   **Reposition**   Definition: Moving to its normal location, or other suitable location, all or a portion of a body part

Explanation: The body part is moved to a new location from an abnormal location, or from a normal location where it is not functioning correctly. The body part may or may not be cut out or off to be moved to the new location.

Body Part Character 4	Approach Character 5	Device Character 6	Qualifier Character 7

0 **Inferior Vena Cava**
   Postcava
   Right inferior phrenic vein
   Right ovarian vein
   Right second lumbar vein
   Right suprarenal vein
   Right testicular vein
1 **Splenic Vein**
   Left gastroepiploic vein
   Pancreatic vein
2 **Gastric Vein**
3 **Esophageal Vein**
4 **Hepatic Vein**
5 **Superior Mesenteric Vein**
   Right gastroepiploic vein
6 **Inferior Mesenteric Vein**
   Sigmoid vein
   Superior rectal vein
7 **Colic Vein**
   Ileocolic vein
   Left colic vein
   Middle colic vein
   Right colic vein
8 **Portal Vein**
   Hepatic portal vein
9 **Renal Vein, Right**
B **Renal Vein, Left**
   Left inferior phrenic vein
   Left ovarian vein
   Left second lumbar vein
   Left suprarenal vein
   Left testicular vein
C **Common Iliac Vein, Right**
D **Common Iliac Vein, Left**
F **External Iliac Vein, Right**
G **External Iliac Vein, Left**
H **Hypogastric Vein, Right**
   Gluteal vein
   Internal iliac vein
   Internal pudendal vein
   Lateral sacral vein
   Middle hemorrhoidal vein
   Obturator vein
   Uterine vein
   Vaginal vein
   Vesical vein
J **Hypogastric Vein, Left**
   See H Hypogastric Vein, Right
M **Femoral Vein, Right**
   Deep femoral (profunda femoris) vein
   Popliteal vein
   Profunda femoris (deep femoral) vein
N **Femoral Vein, Left**
   See M Femoral Vein, Right
P **Saphenous Vein, Right**
   External pudendal vein
   Great(er) saphenous vein
   Lesser saphenous vein
   Small saphenous vein
   Superficial circumflex iliac vein
   Superficial epigastric vein
Q **Saphenous Vein, Left**
   See P Saphenous Vein, Right
T **Foot Vein, Right**
   Common digital vein
   Dorsal metatarsal vein
   Dorsal venous arch
   Plantar digital vein
   Plantar metatarsal vein
   Plantar venous arch
V **Foot Vein, Left**
   See T Foot Vein, Right
Y **Lower Vein**
	0 Open
	3 Percutaneous
	4 Percutaneous Endoscopic
		Z No Device	**Z** No Qualifier

Non-OR Procedure   DRG Non-OR Procedure   Valid OR Procedure   HAC Associated Procedure   Combination Only   New/Revised April   New/Revised October

278   ICD-10-PCS 2023

Ø   **Medical and Surgical**
6   **Lower Veins**
U   **Supplement**   Definition: Putting in or on biological or synthetic material that physically reinforces and/or augments the function of a portion of a body part
                    Explanation: The biological material is non-living, or is living and from the same individual. The body part may have been previously replaced, and the SUPPLEMENT procedure is performed to physically reinforce and/or augment the function of the replaced body part.

Body Part Character 4	Approach Character 5	Device Character 6	Qualifier Character 7

Ø   **Inferior Vena Cava**
    Postcava
    Right inferior phrenic vein
    Right ovarian vein
    Right second lumbar vein
    Right suprarenal vein
    Right testicular vein
1   **Splenic Vein**
    Left gastroepiploic vein
    Pancreatic vein
2   **Gastric Vein**
3   **Esophageal Vein**
4   **Hepatic Vein**
5   **Superior Mesenteric Vein**
    Right gastroepiploic vein
6   **Inferior Mesenteric Vein**
    Sigmoid vein
    Superior rectal vein
7   **Colic Vein**
    Ileocolic vein
    Left colic vein
    Middle colic vein
    Right colic vein
8   **Portal Vein**
    Hepatic portal vein
9   **Renal Vein, Right**
B   **Renal Vein, Left**
    Left inferior phrenic vein
    Left ovarian vein
    Left second lumbar vein
    Left suprarenal vein
    Left testicular vein
C   **Common Iliac Vein, Right**
D   **Common Iliac Vein, Left**
F   **External Iliac Vein, Right**
G   **External Iliac Vein, Left**
H   **Hypogastric Vein, Right**
    Gluteal vein
    Internal iliac vein
    Internal pudendal vein
    Lateral sacral vein
    Middle hemorrhoidal vein
    Obturator vein
    Uterine vein
    Vaginal vein
    Vesical vein
J   **Hypogastric Vein, Left**
    See H Hypogastric Vein, Right
M   **Femoral Vein, Right**
    Deep femoral (profunda femoris) vein
    Popliteal vein
    Profunda femoris (deep femoral) vein
N   **Femoral Vein, Left**
    See M Femoral Vein, Right
P   **Saphenous Vein, Right**
    External pudendal vein
    Great(er) saphenous vein
    Lesser saphenous vein
    Small saphenous vein
    Superficial circumflex iliac vein
    Superficial epigastric vein
Q   **Saphenous Vein, Left**
    See P Saphenous Vein, Right
T   **Foot Vein, Right**
    Common digital vein
    Dorsal metatarsal vein
    Dorsal venous arch
    Plantar digital vein
    Plantar metatarsal vein
    Plantar venous arch
V   **Foot Vein, Left**
    See T Foot Vein, Right
Y   **Lower Vein**
	Ø Open
	3 Percutaneous
	4 Percutaneous Endoscopic
		7 Autologous Tissue Substitute
		J Synthetic Substitute
		K Nonautologous Tissue Substitute
			Z No Qualifier

NC Noncovered Procedure   **LC** Limited Coverage   **QA** Questionable OB Admit   **NT** New Tech Add-on   ⊞ Combination Member   ♂ Male   ♀ Female

ICD-10-PCS 2023   **279**

Ø6U–Ø6U

Lower Veins

Ø   **Medical and Surgical**
6   **Lower Veins**
V   **Restriction**   Definition: Partially closing an orifice or the lumen of a tubular body part
                           Explanation: The orifice can be a natural orifice or an artificially created orifice

Body Part Character 4	Approach Character 5	Device Character 6	Qualifier Character 7
Ø Inferior Vena Cava Postcava Right inferior phrenic vein Right ovarian vein Right second lumbar vein Right suprarenal vein Right testicular vein **1 Splenic Vein** Left gastroepiploic vein Pancreatic vein **2 Gastric Vein** **3 Esophageal Vein** **4 Hepatic Vein** **5 Superior Mesenteric Vein** Right gastroepiploic vein **6 Inferior Mesenteric Vein** Sigmoid vein Superior rectal vein **7 Colic Vein** Ileocolic vein Left colic vein Middle colic vein Right colic vein **8 Portal Vein** Hepatic portal vein **9 Renal Vein, Right** **B Renal Vein, Left** Left inferior phrenic vein Left ovarian vein Left second lumbar vein Left suprarenal vein Left testicular vein **C Common Iliac Vein, Right** **D Common Iliac Vein, Left** **F External Iliac Vein, Right** **G External Iliac Vein, Left** **H Hypogastric Vein, Right** Gluteal vein Internal iliac vein Internal pudendal vein Lateral sacral vein Middle hemorrhoidal vein Obturator vein Uterine vein Vaginal vein Vesical vein **J Hypogastric Vein, Left** *See H Hypogastric Vein, Right* **M Femoral Vein, Right** Deep femoral (profunda femoris) vein Popliteal vein Profunda femoris (deep femoral) vein **N Femoral Vein, Left** *See M Femoral Vein, Right* **P Saphenous Vein, Right** External pudendal vein Great(er) saphenous vein Lesser saphenous vein Small saphenous vein Superficial circumflex iliac vein Superficial epigastric vein **Q Saphenous Vein, Left** *See P Saphenous Vein, Right* **T Foot Vein, Right** Common digital vein Dorsal metatarsal vein Dorsal venous arch Plantar digital vein Plantar metatarsal vein Plantar venous arch **V Foot Vein, Left** *See T Foot Vein, Right* **Y Lower Vein**	**Ø Open** **3 Percutaneous** **4 Percutaneous Endoscopic**	**C Extraluminal Device** **D Intraluminal Device** **Z No Device**	**Z No Qualifier**

Non-OR Procedure   DRG Non-OR Procedure   Valid OR Procedure   HAC Associated Procedure   Combination Only   New/Revised April   New/Revised October

280   ICD-10-PCS 2023

Ø   Medical and Surgical
6   Lower Veins
W   Revision   Definition: Correcting, to the extent possible, a portion of a malfunctioning device or the position of a displaced device

Explanation: Revision can include correcting a malfunctioning or displaced device by taking out or putting in components of the device such as a screw or pin

Body Part Character 4	Approach Character 5	Device Character 6	Qualifier Character 7
Y Lower Vein	**Ø** Open **3** Percutaneous **4** Percutaneous Endoscopic	**Ø** Drainage Device **2** Monitoring Device **3** Infusion Device **7** Autologous Tissue Substitute **C** Extraluminal Device **D** Intraluminal Device **J** Synthetic Substitute **K** Nonautologous Tissue Substitute **Y** Other Device	**Z** No Qualifier
Y Lower Vein	**X** External	**Ø** Drainage Device **2** Monitoring Device **3** Infusion Device **7** Autologous Tissue Substitute **C** Extraluminal Device **D** Intraluminal Device **J** Synthetic Substitute **K** Nonautologous Tissue Substitute	**Z** No Qualifier

Non-OR	Ø6WY3[Ø,2,3]Z
Non-OR	Ø6WY[3,4]YZ
Non-OR	Ø6WYX[Ø,2,3,7,C,D,J,K]Z

NC Noncovered Procedure   LC Limited Coverage   QA Questionable OB Admit   NT New Tech Add-on   ⊞ Combination Member   ♂ Male   ♀ Female

ICD-10-PCS 2023   281

Lymphatic and Hemic Systems Ø72–Ø7Y

Character Meanings*

This Character Meaning table is provided as a guide to assist the user in the identification of character members that may be found in this section of code tables. It **SHOULD NOT** be used to build a PCS code.

Operation–Character 3	Body Part–Character 4	Approach–Character 5	Device–Character 6	Qualifier–Character 7
2 Change	Ø Lymphatic, Head	Ø Open	Ø Drainage Device	Ø Allogeneic
5 Destruction	1 Lymphatic, Right Neck	3 Percutaneous	1 Radioactive Element	1 Syngeneic
9 Drainage	2 Lymphatic, Left Neck	4 Percutaneous Endoscopic	3 Infusion Device	2 Zooplastic
B Excision	3 Lymphatic, Right Upper Extremity	8 Via Natural or Artificial Opening Endoscopic	7 Autologous Tissue Substitute	X Diagnostic
C Extirpation	4 Lymphatic, Left Upper Extremity	X External	C Extraluminal Device	Z No Qualifier
D Extraction	5 Lymphatic, Right Axillary		D Intraluminal Device	
H Insertion	6 Lymphatic, Left Axillary		J Synthetic Substitute	
J Inspection	7 Lymphatic, Thorax		K Nonautologous Tissue Substitute	
L Occlusion	8 Lymphatic, Internal Mammary, Right		Y Other Device	
N Release	9 Lymphatic, Internal Mammary, Left		Z No Device	
P Removal	B Lymphatic, Mesenteric			
Q Repair	C Lymphatic, Pelvis			
S Reposition	D Lymphatic, Aortic			
T Resection	F Lymphatic, Right Lower Extremity			
U Supplement	G Lymphatic, Left Lower Extremity			
V Restriction	H Lymphatic, Right Inguinal			
W Revision	J Lymphatic, Left Inguinal			
Y Transplantation	K Thoracic Duct			
	L Cisterna Chyli			
	M Thymus			
	N Lymphatic			
	P Spleen			
	Q Bone Marrow, Sternum			
	R Bone Marrow, Iliac			
	S Bone Marrow, Vertebral			
	T Bone Marrow			

* Includes lymph vessels and lymph nodes.

AHA Coding Clinic for table Ø79

2021, 4Q, 47	Extraction of bone marrow from other sites
2018, 4Q, 84	Fine needle aspiration biopsy of lymphatic tissue
2017, 1Q, 34	Lymphovenous bypass following mastectomy
2014, 1Q, 26	Transbronchial needle aspiration lymph node biopsy
2013, 4Q, 111	Transbronchial needle aspiration lymph node biopsy

AHA Coding Clinic for table Ø7B

2022, 1Q, 14	Reduction mammoplasty for breast symmetry
2019, 1Q, 3-8	Whipple procedure
2018, 4Q, 84	Fine needle aspiration biopsy of lymphatic tissue
2018, 1Q, 22	Resection of lymph node chains
2016, 1Q, 30	Axillary lymph node resection with modified radical mastectomy
2014, 3Q, 10	Selective excision of paratracheal lymph nodes
2014, 1Q, 20	Fiducial marker placement
2014, 1Q, 26	Transbronchial endoscopic lymph node aspiration biopsy

AHA Coding Clinic for table Ø7D

2022, 1Q, 54	Extraction of bone marrow from other sites
2021, 4Q, 47	Extraction of bone marrow from other sites
2018, 4Q, 84	Fine needle aspiration biopsy of lymphatic tissue
2013, 4Q, 111	Root operation for bone marrow biopsy

AHA Coding Clinic for table Ø7H

| 2020, 4Q, 43-44 | Insertion of radioactive element |
| 2020, 1Q, 53 | Bone marrow body part |

AHA Coding Clinic for table Ø7Q

| 2017, 1Q, 34 | Lymphovenous bypass following mastectomy |

AHA Coding Clinic for table Ø7S

| 2019, 3Q, 29 | Thymus transplant for T-Cell production |

AHA Coding Clinic for table Ø7T

2018, 1Q, 22	Resection of lymph node chains
2016, 2Q, 12	Resection of malignant neoplasm of infratemporal fossa
2016, 1Q, 30	Axillary lymph node resection with modified radical mastectomy
2015, 4Q, 13	New Section X codes—New Technology procedures
2014, 3Q, 9	Radical resection of level I lymph nodes
2014, 3Q, 16	Repair of Tetralogy of Fallot

AHA Coding Clinic for table Ø7Y

| 2019, 3Q, 29 | Thymus transplant for T-Cell production |

Lymphatic System

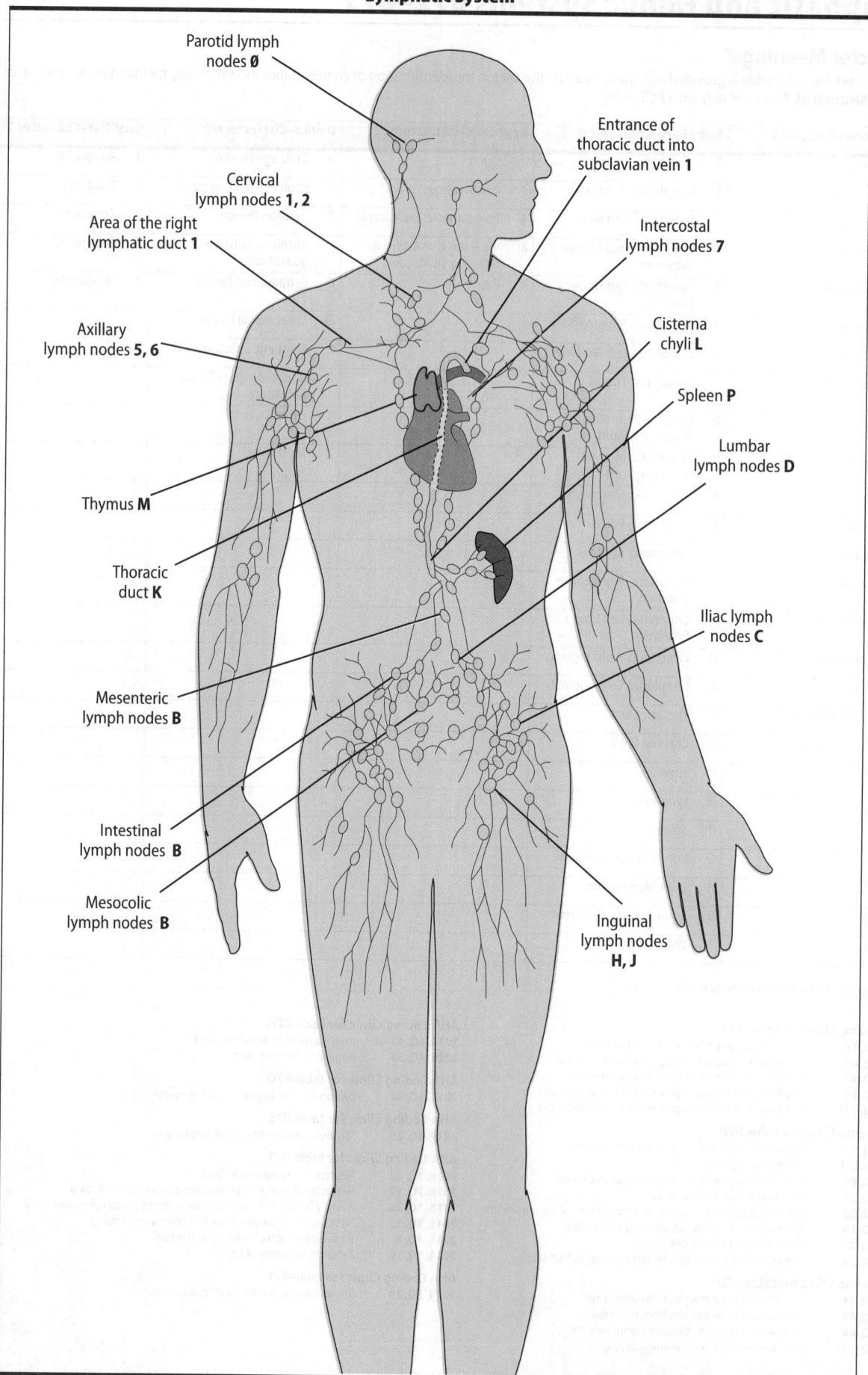

Parotid lymph nodes Ø

Entrance of thoracic duct into subclavian vein 1

Cervical lymph nodes 1, 2

Intercostal lymph nodes 7

Area of the right lymphatic duct 1

Cisterna chyli L

Axillary lymph nodes 5, 6

Spleen P

Lumbar lymph nodes D

Thymus M

Thoracic duct K

Mesenteric lymph nodes B

Iliac lymph nodes C

Intestinal lymph nodes B

Mesocolic lymph nodes B

Inguinal lymph nodes H, J

Ø Medical and Surgical
7 Lymphatic and Hemic Systems
2 Change   Definition: Taking out or off a device from a body part and putting back an identical or similar device in or on the same body part without cutting or puncturing the skin or a mucous membrane

Explanation: All CHANGE procedures are coded using the approach EXTERNAL

Body Part Character 4		Approach Character 5	Device Character 6	Qualifier Character 7
K Thoracic Duct Left jugular trunk Left subclavian trunk **L Cisterna Chyli** Intestinal lymphatic trunk Lumbar lymphatic trunk	**M Thymus** Thymus gland **N Lymphatic** **P Spleen** Accessory spleen **T Bone Marrow**	**X** External	**Ø** Drainage Device **Y** Other Device	**Z** No Qualifier

Non-OR   All body part, approach, device, and qualifier values

---

Ø Medical and Surgical
7 Lymphatic and Hemic Systems
5 Destruction   Definition: Physical eradication of all or a portion of a body part by the direct use of energy, force, or a destructive agent

Explanation: None of the body part is physically taken out

Body Part Character 4		Approach Character 5	Device Character 6	Qualifier Character 7
Ø Lymphatic, Head Buccinator lymph node Infraauricular lymph node Infraparotid lymph node Parotid lymph node Preauricular lymph node Submandibular lymph node Submaxillary lymph node Submental lymph node Subparotid lymph node Suprahyoid lymph node **1 Lymphatic, Right Neck** Cervical lymph node Jugular lymph node Mastoid (postauricular) lymph node Occipital lymph node Postauricular (mastoid) lymph node Retropharyngeal lymph node Right jugular trunk Right lymphatic duct Right subclavian trunk Supraclavicular (Virchow's) lymph node Virchow's (supraclavicular) lymph node **2 Lymphatic, Left Neck** Cervical lymph node Jugular lymph node Mastoid (postauricular) lymph node Occipital lymph node Postauricular (mastoid) lymph node Retropharyngeal lymph node Supraclavicular (Virchow's) lymph node Virchow's (supraclavicular) lymph node **3 Lymphatic, Right Upper Extremity** Cubital lymph node Deltopectoral (infraclavicular) lymph node Epitrochlear lymph node Infraclavicular (deltopectoral) lymph node Supratrochlear lymph node **4 Lymphatic, Left Upper Extremity** *See 3 Lymphatic, Right Upper Extremity* **5 Lymphatic, Right Axillary** Anterior (pectoral) lymph node Apical (subclavicular) lymph node Brachial (lateral) lymph node Central axillary lymph node Lateral (brachial) lymph node Pectoral (anterior) lymph node Posterior (subscapular) lymph node Subclavicular (apical) lymph node Subscapular (posterior) lymph node	**6 Lymphatic, Left Axillary** *See 5 Lymphatic, Right Axillary* **7 Lymphatic, Thorax** Intercostal lymph node Mediastinal lymph node Parasternal lymph node Paratracheal lymph node Tracheobronchial lymph node **8 Lymphatic, Internal Mammary, Right** **9 Lymphatic, Internal Mammary, Left** **B Lymphatic, Mesenteric** Inferior mesenteric lymph node Pararectal lymph node Superior mesenteric lymph node **C Lymphatic, Pelvis** Common iliac (subaortic) lymph node Gluteal lymph node Iliac lymph node Inferior epigastric lymph node Obturator lymph node Sacral lymph node Subaortic (common iliac) lymph node Suprainguinal lymph node **D Lymphatic, Aortic** Celiac lymph node Gastric lymph node Hepatic lymph node Lumbar lymph node Pancreaticosplenic lymph node Paraaortic lymph node Retroperitoneal lymph node **F Lymphatic, Right Lower Extremity** Femoral lymph node Popliteal lymph node **G Lymphatic, Left Lower Extremity** *See F Lymphatic, Right Lower Extremity* **H Lymphatic, Right Inguinal** **J Lymphatic, Left Inguinal** **K Thoracic Duct** Left jugular trunk Left subclavian trunk **L Cisterna Chyli** Intestinal lymphatic trunk Lumbar lymphatic trunk **M Thymus** Thymus gland **P Spleen** Accessory spleen	**Ø** Open **3** Percutaneous **4** Percutaneous Endoscopic	**Z** No Device	**Z** No Qualifier

---

NC Noncovered Procedure   **LC** Limited Coverage   **QA** Questionable OB Admit   **NT** New Tech Add-on   ⊞ Combination Member   ♂ Male   ♀ Female

ICD-10-PCS 2023   285

072–075

Lymphatic and Hemic Systems

Ø   **Medical and Surgical**
7   **Lymphatic and Hemic Systems**
9   **Drainage**   Definition: Taking or letting out fluids and/or gases from a body part
                       Explanation: The qualifier DIAGNOSTIC is used to identify drainage procedures that are biopsies

Body Part Character 4		Approach Character 5	Device Character 6	Qualifier Character 7
Ø Lymphatic, Head Buccinator lymph node Infraauricular lymph node Infraparotid lymph node Parotid lymph node Preauricular lymph node Submandibular lymph node Submaxillary lymph node Submental lymph node Subparotid lymph node Suprahyoid lymph node **1 Lymphatic, Right Neck** Cervical lymph node Jugular lymph node Mastoid (postauricular) lymph node Occipital lymph node Postauricular (mastoid) lymph node Retropharyngeal lymph node Right jugular trunk Right lymphatic duct Right subclavian trunk Supraclavicular (Virchow's) lymph node Virchow's (supraclavicular) lymph node **2 Lymphatic, Left Neck** Cervical lymph node Jugular lymph node Mastoid (postauricular) lymph node Occipital lymph node Postauricular (mastoid) lymph node Retropharyngeal lymph node Supraclavicular (Virchow's) lymph node Virchow's (supraclavicular) lymph node **3 Lymphatic, Right Upper Extremity** Cubital lymph node Deltopectoral (infraclavicular) lymph node Epitrochlear lymph node Infraclavicular (deltopectoral) lymph node Supratrochlear lymph node **4 Lymphatic, Left Upper Extremity** *See 3 Lymphatic, Right Upper Extremity* **5 Lymphatic, Right Axillary** Anterior (pectoral) lymph node Apical (subclavicular) lymph node Brachial (lateral) lymph node Central axillary lymph node Lateral (brachial) lymph node Pectoral (anterior) lymph node Posterior (subscapular) lymph node Subclavicular (apical) lymph node Subscapular (posterior) lymph node	**6 Lymphatic, Left Axillary** *See 5 Lymphatic, Right Axillary* **7 Lymphatic, Thorax** Intercostal lymph node Mediastinal lymph node Parasternal lymph node Paratracheal lymph node Tracheobronchial lymph node **8 Lymphatic, Internal Mammary, Right** **9 Lymphatic, Internal Mammary, Left** **B Lymphatic, Mesenteric** Inferior mesenteric lymph node Pararectal lymph node Superior mesenteric lymph node **C Lymphatic, Pelvis** Common iliac (subaortic) lymph node Gluteal lymph node Iliac lymph node Inferior epigastric lymph node Obturator lymph node Sacral lymph node Subaortic (common iliac) lymph node Suprainguinal lymph node **D Lymphatic, Aortic** Celiac lymph node Gastric lymph node Hepatic lymph node Lumbar lymph node Pancreaticosplenic lymph node Paraaortic lymph node Retroperitoneal lymph node **F Lymphatic, Right Lower Extremity** Femoral lymph node Popliteal lymph node **G Lymphatic, Left Lower Extremity** *See F Lymphatic, Right Lower Extremity* **H Lymphatic, Right Inguinal** **J Lymphatic, Left Inguinal** **K Thoracic Duct** Left jugular trunk Left subclavian trunk **L Cisterna Chyli** Intestinal lymphatic trunk Lumbar lymphatic trunk	**Ø Open** **3 Percutaneous** **4 Percutaneous Endoscopic** **8 Via Natural or Artificial Opening Endoscopic**	**Ø Drainage Device**	**Z No Qualifier**

Non-OR   Ø79[Ø,1,2,3,4,5,6,7,8,9,B,C,D,F,G,H,J,K,L][3,8]ØZ

Ø79 Continued on next page

Ø **Medical and Surgical**
7 **Lymphatic and Hemic Systems**
9 **Drainage**   Definition: Taking or letting out fluids and/or gases from a body part

Ø79 Continued

Explanation: The qualifier DIAGNOSTIC is used to identify drainage procedures that are biopsies

Body Part Character 4		Approach Character 5	Device Character 6	Qualifier Character 7

Ø Lymphatic, Head
Buccinator lymph node
Infraauricular lymph node
Infraparotid lymph node
Parotid lymph node
Preauricular lymph node
Submandibular lymph node
Submaxillary lymph node
Submental lymph node
Subparotid lymph node
Suprahyoid lymph node
1 Lymphatic, Right Neck
Cervical lymph node
Jugular lymph node
Mastoid (postauricular) lymph node
Occipital lymph node
Postauricular (mastoid) lymph node
Retropharyngeal lymph node
Right jugular trunk
Right lymphatic duct
Right subclavian trunk
Supraclavicular (Virchow's) lymph
  node
Virchow's (supraclavicular) lymph
  node
2 Lymphatic, Left Neck
Cervical lymph node
Jugular lymph node
Mastoid (postauricular) lymph node
Occipital lymph node
Postauricular (mastoid) lymph node
Retropharyngeal lymph node
Supraclavicular (Virchow's) lymph
  node
Virchow's (supraclavicular) lymph
  node
3 Lymphatic, Right Upper Extremity
Cubital lymph node
Deltopectoral (infraclavicular) lymph
  node
Epitrochlear lymph node
Infraclavicular (deltopectoral) lymph
  node
Supratrochlear lymph node
4 Lymphatic, Left Upper Extremity
See 3 Lymphatic, Right Upper Extremity
5 Lymphatic, Right Axillary
Anterior (pectoral) lymph node
Apical (subclavicular) lymph node
Brachial (lateral) lymph node
Central axillary lymph node
Lateral (brachial) lymph node
Pectoral (anterior) lymph node
Posterior (subscapular) lymph node
Subclavicular (apical) lymph node
Subscapular (posterior) lymph node
	6 Lymphatic, Left Axillary
	See 5 Lymphatic, Right Axillary
	7 Lymphatic, Thorax
	Intercostal lymph node
	Mediastinal lymph node
	Parasternal lymph node
	Paratracheal lymph node
	Tracheobronchial lymph node
	8 Lymphatic, Internal Mammary, Right
	9 Lymphatic, Internal Mammary, Left
	B Lymphatic, Mesenteric
	Inferior mesenteric lymph node
	Pararectal lymph node
	Superior mesenteric lymph node
	C Lymphatic, Pelvis
	Common iliac (subaortic) lymph node
	Gluteal lymph node
	Iliac lymph node
	Inferior epigastric lymph node
	Obturator lymph node
	Sacral lymph node
	Subaortic (common iliac) lymph node
	Suprainguinal lymph node
	D Lymphatic, Aortic
	Celiac lymph node
	Gastric lymph node
	Hepatic lymph node
	Lumbar lymph node
	Pancreaticosplenic lymph node
	Paraaortic lymph node
	Retroperitoneal lymph node
	F Lymphatic, Right Lower Extremity
	Femoral lymph node
	Popliteal lymph node
	G Lymphatic, Left Lower Extremity
	See F Lymphatic, Right Lower Extremity
	H Lymphatic, Right Inguinal
	J Lymphatic, Left Inguinal
	K Thoracic Duct
	Left jugular trunk
	Left subclavian trunk
	L Cisterna Chyli
	Intestinal lymphatic trunk
	Lumbar lymphatic trunk
		Ø Open
		3 Percutaneous
		**4 Percutaneous
		  Endoscopic**
		**8 Via Natural or
		  Artificial Opening
		  Endoscopic**
			Z No Device	**X Diagnostic**
				Z No Qualifier

M Thymus Thymus gland **P Spleen** Accessory spleen **T Bone Marrow**		**Ø Open** **3 Percutaneous** **4 Percutaneous Endoscopic**	**Ø Drainage Device**	**Z No Qualifier**
M Thymus Thymus gland **P Spleen** Accessory spleen **T Bone Marrow**		**Ø Open** **3 Percutaneous** **4 Percutaneous Endoscopic**	**Z No Device**	**X Diagnostic** **Z No Qualifier**

Non-OR	Ø79[Ø,1,2,3,4,5,6,7,8,9,B,C,D,F,G,H,J,K,L]8ZX
Non-OR	Ø79[Ø,1,2,3,4,5,6,7,8,9,B,C,D,F,G,H,J,K,L][3,8]ZZ
Non-OR	Ø79M3ØZ
Non-OR	Ø79P[3,4]ØZ
Non-OR	Ø79T[Ø,3,4]ØZ
Non-OR	Ø79M3ZZ
Non-OR	Ø79P[3,4]Z[X,Z]
Non-OR	Ø79T[Ø,3,4]Z[X,Z]

NC Noncovered Procedure **LC** Limited Coverage **QA** Questionable OB Admit **NT** New Tech Add-on ⊞ Combination Member ♂ Male ♀ Female

ICD-10-PCS 2023   287

Ø79–Ø79

Ø Medical and Surgical
7 Lymphatic and Hemic Systems
B Excision — Definition: Cutting out or off, without replacement, a portion of a body part
Explanation: The qualifier DIAGNOSTIC is used to identify excision procedures that are biopsies

Body Part Character 4		Approach Character 5	Device Character 6	Qualifier Character 7
Ø Lymphatic, Head	**6 Lymphatic, Left Axillary**	**Ø** Open	**Z** No Device	**X** Diagnostic
Buccinator lymph node	*See 5 Lymphatic, Right Axillary*	**3** Percutaneous		**Z** No Qualifier
Infraauricular lymph node	**7 Lymphatic, Thorax**	**4** Percutaneous Endoscopic		
Infraparotid lymph node	Intercostal lymph node			
Parotid lymph node	Mediastinal lymph node			
Preauricular lymph node	Parasternal lymph node			
Submandibular lymph node	Paratracheal lymph node			
Submaxillary lymph node	Tracheobronchial lymph node			
Submental lymph node	**8 Lymphatic, Internal Mammary, Right**			
Subparotid lymph node	**9 Lymphatic, Internal Mammary, Left**			
Suprahyoid lymph node	**B Lymphatic, Mesenteric**			
1 Lymphatic, Right Neck	Inferior mesenteric lymph node			
Cervical lymph node	Pararectal lymph node			
Jugular lymph node	Superior mesenteric lymph node			
Mastoid (postauricular) lymph node	**C Lymphatic, Pelvis**			
Occipital lymph node	Common iliac (subaortic) lymph node			
Postauricular (mastoid) lymph node	Gluteal lymph node			
Retropharyngeal lymph node	Iliac lymph node			
Right jugular trunk	Inferior epigastric lymph node			
Right lymphatic duct	Obturator lymph node			
Right subclavian trunk	Sacral lymph node			
Supraclavicular (Virchow's) lymph node	Subaortic (common iliac) lymph node			
Virchow's (supraclavicular) lymph node	Suprainguinal lymph node			
2 Lymphatic, Left Neck	**D Lymphatic, Aortic**			
Cervical lymph node	Celiac lymph node			
Jugular lymph node	Gastric lymph node			
Mastoid (postauricular) lymph node	Hepatic lymph node			
Occipital lymph node	Lumbar lymph node			
Postauricular (mastoid) lymph node	Pancreaticosplenic lymph node			
Retropharyngeal lymph node	Paraaortic lymph node			
Supraclavicular (Virchow's) lymph node	Retroperitoneal lymph node			
Virchow's (supraclavicular) lymph node	**F Lymphatic, Right Lower Extremity**			
3 Lymphatic, Right Upper Extremity	Femoral lymph node			
Cubital lymph node	Popliteal lymph node			
Deltopectoral (infraclavicular) lymph node	**G Lymphatic, Left Lower Extremity**			
Epitrochlear lymph node	*See F Lymphatic, Right Lower Extremity*			
Infraclavicular (deltopectoral) lymph node	**H Lymphatic, Right Inguinal** ⊞			
Supratrochlear lymph node	**J Lymphatic, Left Inguinal** ⊞			
4 Lymphatic, Left Upper Extremity	**K Thoracic Duct**			
See 3 Lymphatic, Right Upper Extremity	Left jugular trunk			
5 Lymphatic, Right Axillary	Left subclavian trunk			
Anterior (pectoral) lymph node	**L Cisterna Chyli**			
Apical (subclavicular) lymph node	Intestinal lymphatic trunk			
Brachial (lateral) lymph node	Lumbar lymphatic trunk			
Central axillary lymph node	**M Thymus**			
Lateral (brachial) lymph node	Thymus gland			
Pectoral (anterior) lymph node	**P Spleen**			
Posterior (subscapular) lymph node	Accessory spleen			
Subclavicular (apical) lymph node				
Subscapular (posterior) lymph node				

Non-OR Ø7BP[3,4]ZX

See Appendix L for Procedure Combinations
⊞ Ø7B[H,J][Ø,4]ZZ

Non-OR Procedure   DRG Non-OR Procedure   Valid OR Procedure   HAC Associated Procedure   Combination Only   New/Revised April   New/Revised October

288

ICD-10-PCS 2023

0   **Medical and Surgical**
7   **Lymphatic and Hemic Systems**
C   **Extirpation**   Definition: Taking or cutting out solid matter from a body part

                  Explanation: The solid matter may be an abnormal byproduct of a biological function or a foreign body; it may be imbedded in a body part or in the lumen of a tubular body part. The solid matter may or may not have been previously broken into pieces.

Body Part Character 4		Approach Character 5	Device Character 6	Qualifier Character 7

0   **Lymphatic, Head**
    Buccinator lymph node
    Infraauricular lymph node
    Infraparotid lymph node
    Parotid lymph node
    Preauricular lymph node
    Submandibular lymph node
    Submaxillary lymph node
    Submental lymph node
    Subparotid lymph node
    Suprahyoid lymph node
1   **Lymphatic, Right Neck**
    Cervical lymph node
    Jugular lymph node
    Mastoid (postauricular) lymph node
    Occipital lymph node
    Postauricular (mastoid) lymph node
    Retropharyngeal lymph node
    Right jugular trunk
    Right lymphatic duct
    Right subclavian trunk
    Supraclavicular (Virchow's) lymph
       node
    Virchow's (supraclavicular) lymph
       node
2   **Lymphatic, Left Neck**
    Cervical lymph node
    Jugular lymph node
    Mastoid (postauricular) lymph node
    Occipital lymph node
    Postauricular (mastoid) lymph node
    Retropharyngeal lymph node
    Supraclavicular (Virchow's) lymph
       node
    Virchow's (supraclavicular) lymph
       node
3   **Lymphatic, Right Upper Extremity**
    Cubital lymph node
    Deltopectoral (infraclavicular) lymph
       node
    Epitrochlear lymph node
    Infraclavicular (deltopectoral) lymph
       node
    Supratrochlear lymph node
4   **Lymphatic, Left Upper Extremity**
    See 3 Lymphatic, Right Upper Extremity
5   **Lymphatic, Right Axillary**
    Anterior (pectoral) lymph node
    Apical (subclavicular) lymph node
    Brachial (lateral) lymph node
    Central axillary lymph node
    Lateral (brachial) lymph node
    Pectoral (anterior) lymph node
    Posterior (subscapular) lymph node
    Subclavicular (apical) lymph node
    Subscapular (posterior) lymph node
	6 **Lymphatic, Left Axillary**
	    See 5 Lymphatic, Right Axillary
	7 **Lymphatic, Thorax**
	    Intercostal lymph node
	    Mediastinal lymph node
	    Parasternal lymph node
	    Paratracheal lymph node
	    Tracheobronchial lymph node
	8 **Lymphatic, Internal Mammary, Right**
	9 **Lymphatic, Internal Mammary, Left**
	B **Lymphatic, Mesenteric**
	    Inferior mesenteric lymph node
	    Pararectal lymph node
	    Superior mesenteric lymph node
	C **Lymphatic, Pelvis**
	    Common iliac (subaortic) lymph node
	    Gluteal lymph node
	    Iliac lymph node
	    Inferior epigastric lymph node
	    Obturator lymph node
	    Sacral lymph node
	    Subaortic (common iliac) lymph node
	    Suprainguinal lymph node
	D **Lymphatic, Aortic**
	    Celiac lymph node
	    Gastric lymph node
	    Hepatic lymph node
	    Lumbar lymph node
	    Pancreaticosplenic lymph node
	    Paraaortic lymph node
	    Retroperitoneal lymph node
	F **Lymphatic, Right Lower Extremity**
	    Femoral lymph node
	    Popliteal lymph node
	G **Lymphatic, Left Lower Extremity**
	    See F Lymphatic, Right Lower Extremity
	H **Lymphatic, Right Inguinal**
	J **Lymphatic, Left Inguinal**
	K **Thoracic Duct**
	    Left jugular trunk
	    Left subclavian trunk
	L **Cisterna Chyli**
	    Intestinal lymphatic trunk
	    Lumbar lymphatic trunk
	M **Thymus**
	    Thymus gland
	P **Spleen**
	    Accessory spleen
		0 Open
		3 Percutaneous
		4 Percutaneous
		    Endoscopic
			Z No Device	**Z** No Qualifier

Non-OR   07CP[3,4]ZZ

NC Noncovered Procedure   **LC** Limited Coverage   **QA** Questionable OB Admit   **NT** New Tech Add-on   ⊞ Combination Member   ♂ Male   ♀ Female

ICD-10-PCS 2023   289

Ø   Medical and Surgical
7   Lymphatic and Hemic Systems
D   Extraction   Definition: Pulling or stripping out or off all or a portion of a body part by the use of force
           Explanation: The qualifier DIAGNOSTIC is used to identify extraction procedures that are biopsies

Body Part Character 4		Approach Character 5	Device Character 6	Qualifier Character 7

Ø Lymphatic, Head
Buccinator lymph node
Infraauricular lymph node
Infraparotid lymph node
Parotid lymph node
Preauricular lymph node
Submandibular lymph node
Submaxillary lymph node
Submental lymph node
Subparotid lymph node
Suprahyoid lymph node
1 Lymphatic, Right Neck
Cervical lymph node
Jugular lymph node
Mastoid (postauricular) lymph
  node
Occipital lymph node
Postauricular (mastoid) lymph
  node
Retropharyngeal lymph node
Right jugular trunk
Right lymphatic duct
Right subclavian trunk
Supraclavicular (Virchow's)
  lymph node
Virchow's (supraclavicular)
  lymph node
2 Lymphatic, Left Neck
Cervical lymph node
Jugular lymph node
Mastoid (postauricular) lymph
  node
Occipital lymph node
Postauricular (mastoid) lymph
  node
Retropharyngeal lymph node
Supraclavicular (Virchow's)
  lymph node
Virchow's (supraclavicular)
  lymph node
**3 Lymphatic, Right Upper
  Extremity**
Cubital lymph node
Deltopectoral (infraclavicular)
  lymph node
Epitrochlear lymph node
Infraclavicular (deltopectoral)
  lymph node
Supratrochlear lymph node
**4 Lymphatic, Left Upper
  Extremity**
*See 3 Lymphatic, Right Upper
  Extremity*
5 Lymphatic, Right Axillary
Anterior (pectoral) lymph node
Apical (subclavicular) lymph
  node
Brachial (lateral) lymph node
Central axillary lymph node
Lateral (brachial) lymph node
Pectoral (anterior) lymph node
Posterior (subscapular) lymph
  node
Subclavicular (apical) lymph
  node
Subscapular (posterior) lymph
  node
	6 Lymphatic, Left Axillary
	See 5 Lymphatic, Right Axillary
	7 Lymphatic, Thorax
	Intercostal lymph node
	Mediastinal lymph node
	Parasternal lymph node
	Paratracheal lymph node
	Tracheobronchial lymph node
	**8 Lymphatic, Internal
	  Mammary, Right**
	**9 Lymphatic, Internal
	  Mammary, Left**
	B Lymphatic, Mesenteric
	Inferior mesenteric lymph
	  node
	Pararectal lymph node
	Superior mesenteric lymph
	  node
	C Lymphatic, Pelvis
	Common iliac (subaortic)
	  lymph node
	Gluteal lymph node
	Iliac lymph node
	Inferior epigastric lymph node
	Obturator lymph node
	Sacral lymph node
	Subaortic (common iliac)
	  lymph node
	Suprainguinal lymph node
	D Lymphatic, Aortic
	Celiac lymph node
	Gastric lymph node
	Hepatic lymph node
	Lumbar lymph node
	Pancreaticosplenic lymph
	  node
	Paraaortic lymph node
	Retroperitoneal lymph node
	**F Lymphatic, Right Lower
	  Extremity**
	Femoral lymph node
	Popliteal lymph node
	**G Lymphatic, Left Lower
	  Extremity**
	*See F Lymphatic, Right Lower
	  Extremity*
	H Lymphatic, Right Inguinal
	J Lymphatic, Left Inguinal
	K Thoracic Duct
	Left jugular trunk
	Left subclavian trunk
	L Cisterna Chyli
	Intestinal lymphatic trunk
	Lumbar lymphatic trunk
		3 Percutaneous
		4 Percutaneous Endoscopic
		**8 Via Natural or Artificial
		  Opening Endoscopic**
			Z No Device	**X Diagnostic**

M Thymus Thymus gland **P Spleen** Accessory spleen		**3 Percutaneous** **4 Percutaneous Endoscopic**	**Z No Device**	**X Diagnostic**
Q Bone Marrow, Sternum **R Bone Marrow, Iliac** **S Bone Marrow, Vertebral** **T Bone Marrow**		**Ø Open** **3 Percutaneous**	**Z No Device**	**X Diagnostic** **Z No Qualifier**

Non-OR   All body part, approach, device, and qualifier values

Non-OR Procedure   DRG Non-OR Procedure   Valid OR Procedure   HAC Associated Procedure   Combination Only   New/Revised April   New/Revised October

Ø   Medical and Surgical
7   Lymphatic and Hemic Systems
H   Insertion   Definition: Putting in a nonbiological appliance that monitors, assists, performs, or prevents a physiological function but does not physically take the place of a body part

Explanation: None

Body Part Character 4	Approach Character 5	Device Character 6	Qualifier Character 7

K   Thoracic Duct
     Left jugular trunk
     Left subclavian trunk
L   Cisterna Chyli
     Intestinal lymphatic trunk
     Lumbar lymphatic trunk
M   Thymus
     Thymus gland
N   Lymphatic
P   Spleen
     Accessory spleen
T   Bone Marrow
	Ø Open
	3 Percutaneous
	4 Percutaneous Endoscopic
		1 Radioactive Element
		3 Infusion Device
		Y Other Device
			Z No Qualifier

Non-OR	07H[K,L,M,N,P][Ø,4]3Z
Non-OR	07H[K,L,M,N,P,T]3[1,3,Y]Z
Non-OR	07H[N,P]4YZ
Non-OR	07HT[Ø,4][1,3,Y]Z

Ø   Medical and Surgical
7   Lymphatic and Hemic Systems
J   Inspection   Definition: Visually and/or manually exploring a body part

Explanation: Visual exploration may be performed with or without optical instrumentation. Manual exploration may be performed directly or through intervening body layers.

Body Part Character 4	Approach Character 5	Device Character 6	Qualifier Character 7

K   Thoracic Duct
     Left jugular trunk
     Left subclavian trunk
L   Cisterna Chyli
     Intestinal lymphatic trunk
     Lumbar lymphatic trunk
M   Thymus
     Thymus gland
T   Bone Marrow
	Ø Open
	3 Percutaneous
	4 Percutaneous Endoscopic
		Z No Device	Z No Qualifier

N Lymphatic	Ø Open 3 Percutaneous 4 Percutaneous Endoscopic 8 Via Natural or Artificial Opening Endoscopic X External	Z No Device	Z No Qualifier
P Spleen Accessory spleen	Ø Open 3 Percutaneous 4 Percutaneous Endoscopic X External	Z No Device	Z No Qualifier

Non-OR	07J[K,L,M]3ZZ
Non-OR	07JT[Ø,3,4]ZZ
Non-OR	07JN[3,8,X]ZZ
Non-OR	07JP[3,4,X]ZZ

NC Noncovered Procedure   LC Limited Coverage   QA Questionable OB Admit   NT New Tech Add-on   ⊞ Combination Member   ♂ Male   ♀ Female

ICD-10-PCS 2023   291

Ø Medical and Surgical
7 Lymphatic and Hemic Systems
L Occlusion   Definition: Completely closing an orifice or the lumen of a tubular body part
Explanation: The orifice can be a natural orifice or an artificially created orifice

Body Part Character 4		Approach Character 5	Device Character 6	Qualifier Character 7
Ø Lymphatic, Head Buccinator lymph node Infraauricular lymph node Infraparotid lymph node Parotid lymph node Preauricular lymph node Submandibular lymph node Submaxillary lymph node Submental lymph node Subparotid lymph node Suprahyoid lymph node **1 Lymphatic, Right Neck** Cervical lymph node Jugular lymph node Mastoid (postauricular) lymph node Occipital lymph node Postauricular (mastoid) lymph node Retropharyngeal lymph node Right jugular trunk Right lymphatic duct Right subclavian trunk Supraclavicular (Virchow's) lymph node Virchow's (supraclavicular) lymph node **2 Lymphatic, Left Neck** Cervical lymph node Jugular lymph node Mastoid (postauricular) lymph node Occipital lymph node Postauricular (mastoid) lymph node Retropharyngeal lymph node Supraclavicular (Virchow's) lymph node Virchow's (supraclavicular) lymph node **3 Lymphatic, Right Upper Extremity** Cubital lymph node Deltopectoral (infraclavicular) lymph node Epitrochlear lymph node Infraclavicular (deltopectoral) lymph node Supratrochlear lymph node **4 Lymphatic, Left Upper Extremity** *See 3 Lymphatic, Right Upper Extremity* **5 Lymphatic, Right Axillary** Anterior (pectoral) lymph node Apical (subclavicular) lymph node Brachial (lateral) lymph node Central axillary lymph node Lateral (brachial) lymph node Pectoral (anterior) lymph node Posterior (subscapular) lymph node Subclavicular (apical) lymph node Subscapular (posterior) lymph node	**6 Lymphatic, Left Axillary** *See 5 Lymphatic, Right Axillary* **7 Lymphatic, Thorax** Intercostal lymph node Mediastinal lymph node Parasternal lymph node Paratracheal lymph node Tracheobronchial lymph node **8 Lymphatic, Internal Mammary, Right** **9 Lymphatic, Internal Mammary, Left** **B Lymphatic, Mesenteric** Inferior mesenteric lymph node Pararectal lymph node Superior mesenteric lymph node **C Lymphatic, Pelvis** Common iliac (subaortic) lymph node Gluteal lymph node Iliac lymph node Inferior epigastric lymph node Obturator lymph node Sacral lymph node Subaortic (common iliac) lymph node Suprainguinal lymph node **D Lymphatic, Aortic** Celiac lymph node Gastric lymph node Hepatic lymph node Lumbar lymph node Pancreaticosplenic lymph node Paraaortic lymph node Retroperitoneal lymph node **F Lymphatic, Right Lower Extremity** Femoral lymph node Popliteal lymph node **G Lymphatic, Left Lower Extremity** *See F Lymphatic, Right Lower Extremity* **H Lymphatic, Right Inguinal** **J Lymphatic, Left Inguinal** **K Thoracic Duct** Left jugular trunk Left subclavian trunk **L Cisterna Chyli** Intestinal lymphatic trunk Lumbar lymphatic trunk	**Ø Open** **3 Percutaneous** **4 Percutaneous Endoscopic**	**C Extraluminal Device** **D Intraluminal Device** **Z No Device**	**Z No Qualifier**

Non-OR Procedure   DRG Non-OR Procedure   Valid OR Procedure   HAC Associated Procedure   Combination Only   New/Revised April   New/Revised October

292
ICD-10-PCS 2023

Ø Medical and Surgical
7 Lymphatic and Hemic Systems
N Release   Definition: Freeing a body part from an abnormal physical constraint by cutting or by the use of force
                 Explanation: Some of the restraining tissue may be taken out but none of the body part is taken out

Body Part Character 4		Approach Character 5	Device Character 6	Qualifier Character 7

Ø Lymphatic, Head
 Buccinator lymph node
 Infraauricular lymph node
 Infraparotid lymph node
 Parotid lymph node
 Preauricular lymph node
 Submandibular lymph node
 Submaxillary lymph node
 Submental lymph node
 Subparotid lymph node
 Suprahyoid lymph node
 1 Lymphatic, Right Neck
 Cervical lymph node
 Jugular lymph node
 Mastoid (postauricular) lymph node
 Occipital lymph node
 Postauricular (mastoid) lymph node
 Retropharyngeal lymph node
 Right jugular trunk
 Right lymphatic duct
 Right subclavian trunk
 Supraclavicular (Virchow's) lymph
    node
 Virchow's (supraclavicular) lymph
    node
 2 Lymphatic, Left Neck
 Cervical lymph node
 Jugular lymph node
 Mastoid (postauricular) lymph node
 Occipital lymph node
 Postauricular (mastoid) lymph node
 Retropharyngeal lymph node
 Supraclavicular (Virchow's) lymph
    node
 Virchow's (supraclavicular) lymph
    node
 3 Lymphatic, Right Upper Extremity
 Cubital lymph node
 Deltopectoral (infraclavicular) lymph
    node
 Epitrochlear lymph node
 Infraclavicular (deltopectoral) lymph
    node
 Supratrochlear lymph node
 4 Lymphatic, Left Upper Extremity
 See 3 Lymphatic, Right Upper Extremity
 5 Lymphatic, Right Axillary
 Anterior (pectoral) lymph node
 Apical (subclavicular) lymph node
 Brachial (lateral) lymph node
 Central axillary lymph node
 Lateral (brachial) lymph node
 Pectoral (anterior) lymph node
 Posterior (subscapular) lymph node
 Subclavicular (apical) lymph node
 Subscapular (posterior) lymph node
	6 Lymphatic, Left Axillary
	 See 5 Lymphatic, Right Axillary
	 7 Lymphatic, Thorax
	 Intercostal lymph node
	 Mediastinal lymph node
	 Parasternal lymph node
	 Paratracheal lymph node
	 Tracheobronchial lymph node
	 8 Lymphatic, Internal Mammary, Right
	 9 Lymphatic, Internal Mammary, Left
	 B Lymphatic, Mesenteric
	 Inferior mesenteric lymph node
	 Pararectal lymph node
	 Superior mesenteric lymph node
	 C Lymphatic, Pelvis
	 Common iliac (subaortic) lymph node
	 Gluteal lymph node
	 Iliac lymph node
	 Inferior epigastric lymph node
	 Obturator lymph node
	 Sacral lymph node
	 Subaortic (common iliac) lymph node
	 Suprainguinal lymph node
	 D Lymphatic, Aortic
	 Celiac lymph node
	 Gastric lymph node
	 Hepatic lymph node
	 Lumbar lymph node
	 Pancreaticosplenic lymph node
	 Paraaortic lymph node
	 Retroperitoneal lymph node
	 F Lymphatic, Right Lower Extremity
	 Femoral lymph node
	 Popliteal lymph node
	 G Lymphatic, Left Lower Extremity
	 See F Lymphatic, Right Lower Extremity
	 H Lymphatic, Right Inguinal
	 J Lymphatic, Left Inguinal
	 K Thoracic Duct
	 Left jugular trunk
	 Left subclavian trunk
	 L Cisterna Chyli
	 Intestinal lymphatic trunk
	 Lumbar lymphatic trunk
	 M Thymus
	 Thymus gland
	 P Spleen
	 Accessory spleen
		Ø Open
		 3 Percutaneous
		 4 Percutaneous Endoscopic
			Z No Device	**Z No Qualifier**

NC Noncovered Procedure   **LC** Limited Coverage   **QA** Questionable OB Admit   **NT** New Tech Add-on   ⊞ Combination Member   ♂ Male   ♀ Female

ICD-10-PCS 2023   293

Ø   Medical and Surgical
7   Lymphatic and Hemic Systems
P   Removal   Definition: Taking out or off a device from a body part

Explanation: If a device is taken out and a similar device put in without cutting or puncturing the skin or mucous membrane, the procedure is coded to the root operation CHANGE. Otherwise, the procedure for taking out a device is coded to the root operation REMOVAL.

Body Part Character 4	Approach Character 5	Device Character 6	Qualifier Character 7

K   Thoracic Duct
    Left jugular trunk
    Left subclavian trunk
L   Cisterna Chyli
    Intestinal lymphatic trunk
    Lumbar lymphatic trunk
N   Lymphatic
	Ø Open
	3 Percutaneous
	4 Percutaneous Endoscopic
		Ø Drainage Device
		3 Infusion Device
		7 Autologous Tissue
		    Substitute
		C Extraluminal Device
		D Intraluminal Device
		J Synthetic Substitute
		K Nonautologous Tissue
		    Substitute
		Y Other Device
			Z No Qualifier

K   Thoracic Duct
    Left jugular trunk
    Left subclavian trunk
L   Cisterna Chyli
    Intestinal lymphatic trunk
    Lumbar lymphatic trunk
N   Lymphatic
	X External	Ø Drainage Device
		3 Infusion Device
		D Intraluminal Device
			Z No Qualifier

M   Thymus
    Thymus gland
P   Spleen
    Accessory spleen
	Ø Open
	3 Percutaneous
	4 Percutaneous Endoscopic
		Ø Drainage Device
		3 Infusion Device
		Y Other Device
			Z No Qualifier

M   Thymus
    Thymus gland
P   Spleen
    Accessory spleen
	X External	Ø Drainage Device
		3 Infusion Device
			Z No Qualifier

T Bone Marrow	Ø Open 3 Percutaneous 4 Percutaneous Endoscopic X External	Ø Drainage Device	Z No Qualifier

Non-OR	07P[K,L,N][3,4]YZ
Non-OR	07P[K,L,N]X[Ø,3,D]Z
Non-OR	07P[M,P][3,4]YZ
Non-OR	07P[M,P]X[Ø,3]Z
Non-OR	07PT[Ø,3,4,X]ØZ

Non-OR Procedure   DRG Non-OR Procedure   Valid OR Procedure   HAC Associated Procedure   Combination Only   New/Revised April   New/Revised October

294

ICD-10-PCS 2023

Ø   **Medical and Surgical**
7   **Lymphatic and Hemic Systems**
Q   **Repair**   Definition: Restoring, to the extent possible, a body part to its normal anatomic structure and function
              Explanation: Used only when the method to accomplish the repair is not one of the other root operations

Body Part Character 4		Approach Character 5	Device Character 6	Qualifier Character 7

Ø **Lymphatic, Head**
   Buccinator lymph node
   Infraauricular lymph node
   Infraparotid lymph node
   Parotid lymph node
   Preauricular lymph node
   Submandibular lymph node
   Submaxillary lymph node
   Submental lymph node
   Subparotid lymph node
   Suprahyoid lymph node
1 **Lymphatic, Right Neck**
   Cervical lymph node
   Jugular lymph node
   Mastoid (postauricular) lymph node
   Occipital lymph node
   Postauricular (mastoid) lymph node
   Retropharyngeal lymph node
   Right jugular trunk
   Right lymphatic duct
   Right subclavian trunk
   Supraclavicular (Virchow's) lymph
     node
   Virchow's (supraclavicular) lymph
     node
2 **Lymphatic, Left Neck**
   Cervical lymph node
   Jugular lymph node
   Mastoid (postauricular) lymph node
   Occipital lymph node
   Postauricular (mastoid) lymph node
   Retropharyngeal lymph node
   Supraclavicular (Virchow's) lymph
     node
   Virchow's (supraclavicular) lymph
     node
3 **Lymphatic, Right Upper Extremity**
   Cubital lymph node
   Deltopectoral (infraclavicular) lymph
     node
   Epitrochlear lymph node
   Infraclavicular (deltopectoral) lymph
     node
   Supratrochlear lymph node
4 **Lymphatic, Left Upper Extremity**
   See 3 Lymphatic, Right Upper Extremity
5 **Lymphatic, Right Axillary**
   Anterior (pectoral) lymph node
   Apical (subclavicular) lymph node
   Brachial (lateral) lymph node
   Central axillary lymph node
   Lateral (brachial) lymph node
   Pectoral (anterior) lymph node
   Posterior (subscapular) lymph node
   Subclavicular (apical) lymph node
   Subscapular (posterior) lymph node
	6 **Lymphatic, Left Axillary**
	   See 5 Lymphatic, Right Axillary
	7 **Lymphatic, Thorax**
	   Intercostal lymph node
	   Mediastinal lymph node
	   Parasternal lymph node
	   Paratracheal lymph node
	   Tracheobronchial lymph node
	8 **Lymphatic, Internal Mammary, Right**
	9 **Lymphatic, Internal Mammary, Left**
	B **Lymphatic, Mesenteric**
	   Inferior mesenteric lymph node
	   Pararectal lymph node
	   Superior mesenteric lymph node
	C **Lymphatic, Pelvis**
	   Common iliac (subaortic) lymph node
	   Gluteal lymph node
	   Iliac lymph node
	   Inferior epigastric lymph node
	   Obturator lymph node
	   Sacral lymph node
	   Subaortic (common iliac) lymph node
	   Suprainguinal lymph node
	D **Lymphatic, Aortic**
	   Celiac lymph node
	   Gastric lymph node
	   Hepatic lymph node
	   Lumbar lymph node
	   Pancreaticosplenic lymph node
	   Paraaortic lymph node
	   Retroperitoneal lymph node
	F **Lymphatic, Right Lower Extremity**
	   Femoral lymph node
	   Popliteal lymph node
	G **Lymphatic, Left Lower Extremity**
	   See F Lymphatic, Right Lower Extremity
	H **Lymphatic, Right Inguinal**
	J **Lymphatic, Left Inguinal**
	K **Thoracic Duct**
	   Left jugular trunk
	   Left subclavian trunk
	L **Cisterna Chyli**
	   Intestinal lymphatic trunk
	   Lumbar lymphatic trunk
		Ø **Open**
		3 **Percutaneous**
		4 **Percutaneous
		   Endoscopic**
		8 **Via Natural or
		   Artificial Opening
		   Endoscopic**
			Z **No Device**	Z **No Qualifier**

M **Thymus**
   Thymus gland
P **Spleen**
   Accessory spleen
		Ø **Open**
		3 **Percutaneous**
		4 **Percutaneous
		   Endoscopic**
			Z **No Device**	Z **No Qualifier**

Lymphatic and Hemic Systems (side tab)

Ø **Medical and Surgical**
7 **Lymphatic and Hemic Systems**
S **Reposition** Definition: Moving to its normal location, or other suitable location, all or a portion of a body part

Explanation: The body part is moved to a new location from an abnormal location, or from a normal location where it is not functioning correctly. The body part may or may not be cut out or off to be moved to the new location.

Body Part Character 4	Approach Character 5	Device Character 6	Qualifier Character 7
M Thymus 　Thymus gland P Spleen 　Accessory spleen	Ø Open	Z No Device	Z No Qualifier

Ø **Medical and Surgical**
7 **Lymphatic and Hemic Systems**
T **Resection** Definition: Cutting out or off, without replacement, all of a body part

Explanation: None

Body Part Character 4	Approach Character 5	Device Character 6	Qualifier Character 7
Ø **Lymphatic, Head** 　Buccinator lymph node 　Infraauricular lymph node 　Infraparotid lymph node 　Parotid lymph node 　Preauricular lymph node 　Submandibular lymph node 　Submaxillary lymph node 　Submental lymph node 　Subparotid lymph node 　Suprahyoid lymph node 1 **Lymphatic, Right Neck** 　Cervical lymph node 　Jugular lymph node 　Mastoid (postauricular) lymph node 　Occipital lymph node 　Postauricular (mastoid) lymph node 　Retropharyngeal lymph node 　Right jugular trunk 　Right lymphatic duct 　Right subclavian trunk 　Supraclavicular (Virchow's) lymph node 　Virchow's (supraclavicular) lymph node 2 **Lymphatic, Left Neck** 　Cervical lymph node 　Jugular lymph node 　Mastoid (postauricular) lymph node 　Occipital lymph node 　Postauricular (mastoid) lymph node 　Retropharyngeal lymph node 　Supraclavicular (Virchow's) lymph node 　Virchow's (supraclavicular) lymph node 3 **Lymphatic, Right Upper Extremity** 　Cubital lymph node 　Deltopectoral (infraclavicular) lymph node 　Epitrochlear lymph node 　Infraclavicular (deltopectoral) lymph node 　Supratrochlear lymph node 4 **Lymphatic, Left Upper Extremity** 　*See 3 Lymphatic, Right Upper Extremity* 5 **Lymphatic, Right Axillary** ⊞ 　Anterior (pectoral) lymph node 　Apical (subclavicular) lymph node 　Brachial (lateral) lymph node 　Central axillary lymph node 　Lateral (brachial) lymph node 　Pectoral (anterior) lymph node 　Posterior (subscapular) lymph node 　Subclavicular (apical) lymph node 　Subscapular (posterior) lymph node 6 **Lymphatic, Left Axillary** ⊞ 　*See 5 Lymphatic, Right Axillary* 7 **Lymphatic, Thorax** ⊞ 　Intercostal lymph node 　Mediastinal lymph node 　Parasternal lymph node 　Paratracheal lymph node 　Tracheobronchial lymph node 8 **Lymphatic, Internal Mammary, Right** ⊞ 9 **Lymphatic, Internal Mammary, Left** ⊞ B **Lymphatic, Mesenteric** 　Inferior mesenteric lymph node 　Pararectal lymph node 　Superior mesenteric lymph node C **Lymphatic, Pelvis** 　Common iliac (subaortic) lymph node 　Gluteal lymph node 　Iliac lymph node 　Inferior epigastric lymph node 　Obturator lymph node 　Sacral lymph node 　Subaortic (common iliac) lymph node 　Suprainguinal lymph node D **Lymphatic, Aortic** 　Celiac lymph node 　Gastric lymph node 　Hepatic lymph node 　Lumbar lymph node 　Pancreaticosplenic lymph node 　Paraaortic lymph node 　Retroperitoneal lymph node F **Lymphatic, Right Lower Extremity** 　Femoral lymph node 　Popliteal lymph node G **Lymphatic, Left Lower Extremity** 　*See F Lymphatic, Right Lower Extremity* H **Lymphatic, Right Inguinal** J **Lymphatic, Left Inguinal** K **Thoracic Duct** 　Left jugular trunk 　Left subclavian trunk L **Cisterna Chyli** 　Intestinal lymphatic trunk 　Lumbar lymphatic trunk M **Thymus** 　Thymus gland P **Spleen** 　Accessory spleen	Ø Open 4 Percutaneous Endoscopic	Z No Device	Z No Qualifier

See Appendix L for Procedure Combinations
　⊞　07T[5,6,7,8,9]ØZZ

Ø   Medical and Surgical
7   Lymphatic and Hemic Systems
U   Supplement   Definition: Putting in or on biological or synthetic material that physically reinforces and/or augments the function of a portion of a body part
                     Explanation: The biological material is non-living, or is living and from the same individual. The body part may have been previously replaced, and the SUPPLEMENT procedure is performed to physically reinforce and/or augment the function of the replaced body part.

Body Part Character 4	Approach Character 5	Device Character 6	Qualifier Character 7

Ø Lymphatic, Head
  Buccinator lymph node
  Infraauricular lymph node
  Infraparotid lymph node
  Parotid lymph node
  Preauricular lymph node
  Submandibular lymph node
  Submaxillary lymph node
  Submental lymph node
  Subparotid lymph node
  Suprahyoid lymph node
1 Lymphatic, Right Neck
  Cervical lymph node
  Jugular lymph node
  Mastoid (postauricular) lymph node
  Occipital lymph node
  Postauricular (mastoid) lymph node
  Retropharyngeal lymph node
  Right jugular trunk
  Right lymphatic duct
  Right subclavian trunk
  Supraclavicular (Virchow's) lymph
    node
  Virchow's (supraclavicular) lymph
    node
2 Lymphatic, Left Neck
  Cervical lymph node
  Jugular lymph node
  Mastoid (postauricular) lymph node
  Occipital lymph node
  Postauricular (mastoid) lymph node
  Retropharyngeal lymph node
  Supraclavicular (Virchow's) lymph
    node
  Virchow's (supraclavicular) lymph
    node
3 Lymphatic, Right Upper Extremity
  Cubital lymph node
  Deltopectoral (infraclavicular) lymph
    node
  Epitrochlear lymph node
  Infraclavicular (deltopectoral) lymph
    node
  Supratrochlear lymph node
4 Lymphatic, Left Upper Extremity
  See 3 Lymphatic, Right Upper Extremity
5 Lymphatic, Right Axillary
  Anterior (pectoral) lymph node
  Apical (subclavicular) lymph node
  Brachial (lateral) lymph node
  Central axillary lymph node
  Lateral (brachial) lymph node
  Pectoral (anterior) lymph node
  Posterior (subscapular) lymph node
  Subclavicular (apical) lymph node
  Subscapular (posterior) lymph node
	Ø Open
	**4 Percutaneous
	   Endoscopic**
		**7 Autologous Tissue
		   Substitute**
		J Synthetic Substitute
		**K Nonautologous
		   Tissue Substitute**
			Z No Qualifier

(continued, Body Part column, second sub-column)

6 Lymphatic, Left Axillary
  See 5 Lymphatic, Right Axillary
7 Lymphatic, Thorax
  Intercostal lymph node
  Mediastinal lymph node
  Parasternal lymph node
  Paratracheal lymph node
  Tracheobronchial lymph node
8 Lymphatic, Internal Mammary, Right
9 Lymphatic, Internal Mammary, Left
B Lymphatic, Mesenteric
  Inferior mesenteric lymph node
  Pararectal lymph node
  Superior mesenteric lymph node
C Lymphatic, Pelvis
  Common iliac (subaortic) lymph node
  Gluteal lymph node
  Iliac lymph node
  Inferior epigastric lymph node
  Obturator lymph node
  Sacral lymph node
  Subaortic (common iliac) lymph node
  Suprainguinal lymph node
D Lymphatic, Aortic
  Celiac lymph node
  Gastric lymph node
  Hepatic lymph node
  Lumbar lymph node
  Pancreaticosplenic lymph node
  Paraaortic lymph node
  Retroperitoneal lymph node
F Lymphatic, Right Lower Extremity
  Femoral lymph node
  Popliteal lymph node
G Lymphatic, Left Lower Extremity
  See F Lymphatic, Right Lower Extremity
H Lymphatic, Right Inguinal
J Lymphatic, Left Inguinal
K Thoracic Duct
  Left jugular trunk
  Left subclavian trunk
L Cisterna Chyli
  Intestinal lymphatic trunk
  Lumbar lymphatic trunk

NC Noncovered Procedure   **LC** Limited Coverage   **QA** Questionable OB Admit   **NT** New Tech Add-on   ⊞ Combination Member   ♂ Male   ♀ Female

ICD-10-PCS 2023   **297**

Lymphatic and Hemic Systems *(side tab)*

Ø   Medical and Surgical
7   Lymphatic and Hemic Systems
V   Restriction   Definition: Partially closing an orifice or the lumen of a tubular body part

Explanation: The orifice can be a natural orifice or an artificially created orifice

Body Part Character 4		Approach Character 5	Device Character 6	Qualifier Character 7

Ø Lymphatic, Head
Buccinator lymph node
Infraauricular lymph node
Infraparotid lymph node
Parotid lymph node
Preauricular lymph node
Submandibular lymph node
Submaxillary lymph node
Submental lymph node
Subparotid lymph node
Suprahyoid lymph node
1 Lymphatic, Right Neck
Cervical lymph node
Jugular lymph node
Mastoid (postauricular) lymph node
Occipital lymph node
Postauricular (mastoid) lymph node
Retropharyngeal lymph node
Right jugular trunk
Right lymphatic duct
Right subclavian trunk
Supraclavicular (Virchow's) lymph
   node
Virchow's (supraclavicular) lymph
   node
2 Lymphatic, Left Neck
Cervical lymph node
Jugular lymph node
Mastoid (postauricular) lymph node
Occipital lymph node
Postauricular (mastoid) lymph node
Retropharyngeal lymph node
Supraclavicular (Virchow's) lymph
   node
Virchow's (supraclavicular) lymph
   node
3 Lymphatic, Right Upper Extremity
Cubital lymph node
Deltopectoral (infraclavicular) lymph
   node
Epitrochlear lymph node
Infraclavicular (deltopectoral) lymph
   node
Supratrochlear lymph node
4 Lymphatic, Left Upper Extremity
See 3 Lymphatic, Right Upper Extremity
5 Lymphatic, Right Axillary
Anterior (pectoral) lymph node
Apical (subclavicular) lymph node
Brachial (lateral) lymph node
Central axillary lymph node
Lateral (brachial) lymph node
Pectoral (anterior) lymph node
Posterior (subscapular) lymph node
Subclavicular (apical) lymph node
Subscapular (posterior) lymph node
	6 Lymphatic, Left Axillary
	See 5 Lymphatic, Right Axillary
	7 Lymphatic, Thorax
	Intercostal lymph node
	Mediastinal lymph node
	Parasternal lymph node
	Paratracheal lymph node
	Tracheobronchial lymph node
	8 Lymphatic, Internal Mammary, Right
	9 Lymphatic, Internal Mammary, Left
	B Lymphatic, Mesenteric
	Inferior mesenteric lymph node
	Pararectal lymph node
	Superior mesenteric lymph node
	C Lymphatic, Pelvis
	Common iliac (subaortic) lymph node
	Gluteal lymph node
	Iliac lymph node
	Inferior epigastric lymph node
	Obturator lymph node
	Sacral lymph node
	Subaortic (common iliac) lymph node
	Suprainguinal lymph node
	D Lymphatic, Aortic
	Celiac lymph node
	Gastric lymph node
	Hepatic lymph node
	Lumbar lymph node
	Pancreaticosplenic lymph node
	Paraaortic lymph node
	Retroperitoneal lymph node
	F Lymphatic, Right Lower Extremity
	Femoral lymph node
	Popliteal lymph node
	G Lymphatic, Left Lower Extremity
	See F Lymphatic, Right Lower Extremity
	H Lymphatic, Right Inguinal
	J Lymphatic, Left Inguinal
	K Thoracic Duct
	Left jugular trunk
	Left subclavian trunk
	L Cisterna Chyli
	Intestinal lymphatic trunk
	Lumbar lymphatic trunk
		Ø Open
		3 Percutaneous
		4 Percutaneous
		   Endoscopic
			C Extraluminal Device
			D Intraluminal Device
			Z No Device
				Z No Qualifier

Non-OR Procedure   DRG Non-OR Procedure   Valid OR Procedure   HAC Associated Procedure   Combination Only   New/Revised April   New/Revised October

298   ICD-10-PCS 2023

Ø7V–Ø7V *(side tab, bottom)*

Ø   Medical and Surgical
7   Lymphatic and Hemic Systems
W   Revision   Definition: Correcting, to the extent possible, a portion of a malfunctioning device or the position of a displaced device

                     Explanation: Revision can include correcting a malfunctioning or displaced device by taking out or putting in components of the device such as a screw or pin

Body Part Character 4	Approach Character 5	Device Character 6	Qualifier Character 7

K Thoracic Duct
     Left jugular trunk
     Left subclavian trunk
L Cisterna Chyli
     Intestinal lymphatic trunk
     Lumbar lymphatic trunk
N Lymphatic
	Ø Open
	3 Percutaneous
	4 Percutaneous Endoscopic
		Ø Drainage Device
		3 Infusion Device
		7 Autologous Tissue
		     Substitute
		C Extraluminal Device
		D Intraluminal Device
		J Synthetic Substitute
		K Nonautologous Tissue
		     Substitute
		Y Other Device
			Z No Qualifier

K Thoracic Duct
     Left jugular trunk
     Left subclavian trunk
L Cisterna Chyli
     Intestinal lymphatic trunk
     Lumbar lymphatic trunk
N Lymphatic
	X External	**Ø** Drainage Device
		3 Infusion Device
		7 Autologous Tissue
		     Substitute
		C Extraluminal Device
		D Intraluminal Device
		J Synthetic Substitute
		K Nonautologous Tissue
		     Substitute
			Z No Qualifier

M Thymus
     Thymus gland
P Spleen
     Accessory spleen
	Ø Open
	3 Percutaneous
	4 Percutaneous Endoscopic
		Ø Drainage Device
		3 Infusion Device
		Y Other Device
			Z No Qualifier

M Thymus
     Thymus gland
P Spleen
     Accessory spleen
	X External	**Ø** Drainage Device
		3 Infusion Device
			Z No Qualifier

T Bone Marrow	**Ø** Open **3** Percutaneous **4** Percutaneous Endoscopic **X** External	**Ø** Drainage Device	**Z** No Qualifier

Non-OR	Ø7W[K,L,N][3,4]YZ
Non-OR	Ø7W[K,L,N]X[Ø,3,7,C,D,J,K]Z
Non-OR	Ø7W[M,P][3,4]YZ
Non-OR	Ø7W[M,P]X[Ø,3]Z
Non-OR	Ø7WT[Ø,3,4,X]ØZ

Ø   Medical and Surgical
7   Lymphatic and Hemic Systems
Y   Transplantation   Definition: Putting in or on all or a portion of a living body part taken from another individual or animal to physically take the place and/or function of all or a portion of a similar body part

                     Explanation: The native body part may or may not be taken out, and the transplanted body part may take over all or a portion of its function

Body Part Character 4	Approach Character 5	Device Character 6	Qualifier Character 7

M Thymus
     Thymus gland
P Spleen
     Accessory spleen
	Ø Open	**Z** No Device	**Ø** Allogeneic
			1 Syngeneic
			2 Zooplastic

NC Noncovered Procedure   **LC** Limited Coverage   **QA** Questionable OB Admit   **NT** New Tech Add-on   ⊞ Combination Member   ♂ Male   ♀ Female

ICD-10-PCS 2023   **299**

Eye Ø8Ø–Ø8X

Character Meanings

This Character Meaning table is provided as a guide to assist the user in the identification of character members that may be found in this section of code tables. It **SHOULD NOT** be used to build a PCS code.

Operation–Character 3		Body Part–Character 4		Approach–Character 5		Device–Character 6		Qualifier–Character 7	
Ø	Alteration	Ø	Eye, Right	Ø	Open	Ø	Drainage Device OR Synthetic Substitute, Intraocular Telescope	3	Nasal Cavity
1	Bypass	1	Eye, Left	3	Percutaneous	1	Radioactive Element	4	Sclera
2	Change	2	Anterior Chamber, Right	7	Via Natural or Artificial Opening	3	Infusion Device	X	Diagnostic
5	Destruction	3	Anterior Chamber, Left	8	Via Natural or Artificial Opening Endoscopic	5	Epiretinal Visual Prosthesis	Z	No Qualifier
7	Dilation	4	Vitreous, Right	X	External	7	Autologous Tissue Substitute		
9	Drainage	5	Vitreous, Left			C	Extraluminal Device		
B	Excision	6	Sclera, Right			D	Intraluminal Device		
C	Extirpation	7	Sclera, Left			J	Synthetic Substitute		
D	Extraction	8	Cornea, Right			K	Nonautologous Tissue Substitute		
F	Fragmentation	9	Cornea, Left			Y	Other Device		
H	Insertion	A	Choroid, Right			Z	No Device		
J	Inspection	B	Choroid, Left						
L	Occlusion	C	Iris, Right						
M	Reattachment	D	Iris, Left						
N	Release	E	Retina, Right						
P	Removal	F	Retina, Left						
Q	Repair	G	Retinal Vessel, Right						
R	Replacement	H	Retinal Vessel, Left						
S	Reposition	J	Lens, Right						
T	Resection	K	Lens, Left						
U	Supplement	L	Extraocular Muscle, Right						
V	Restriction	M	Extraocular Muscle, Left						
W	Revision	N	Upper Eyelid, Right						
X	Transfer	P	Upper Eyelid, Left						
		Q	Lower Eyelid, Right						
		R	Lower Eyelid, Left						
		S	Conjunctiva, Right						
		T	Conjunctiva, Left						
		V	Lacrimal Gland, Right						
		W	Lacrimal Gland, Left						
		X	Lacrimal Duct, Right						
		Y	Lacrimal Duct, Left						

AHA Coding Clinic for table Ø81
2019, 1Q, 27   Glaucoma tube shunt

AHA Coding Clinic for table Ø89
2016, 2Q, 21   Laser trabeculoplasty

AHA Coding Clinic for table Ø8B
2014, 4Q, 35   Vitrectomy with air/fluid exchange
2014, 4Q, 36   Pars plans vitrectomy without mention of instillation of oil, air or fluid

AHA Coding Clinic for table Ø8J
2015, 1Q, 35   Attempted removal of foreign body from cornea

AHA Coding Clinic for table Ø8N
2015, 2Q, 24   Penetrating keratoplasty and anterior segment reconstruction

AHA Coding Clinic for table Ø8Q
2018, 3Q, 13   Repair of ruptured globe

AHA Coding Clinic for table Ø8R
2015, 2Q, 24   Penetrating keratoplasty and anterior segment reconstruction
2015, 2Q, 25   Penetrating keratoplasty and placement of viscoelastic eye with paracentesis

AHA Coding Clinic for table Ø8T
2015, 2Q, 12   Orbital exenteration

AHA Coding Clinic for table Ø8U
2014, 3Q, 31   Corneal amniotic membrane transplantation

Eye

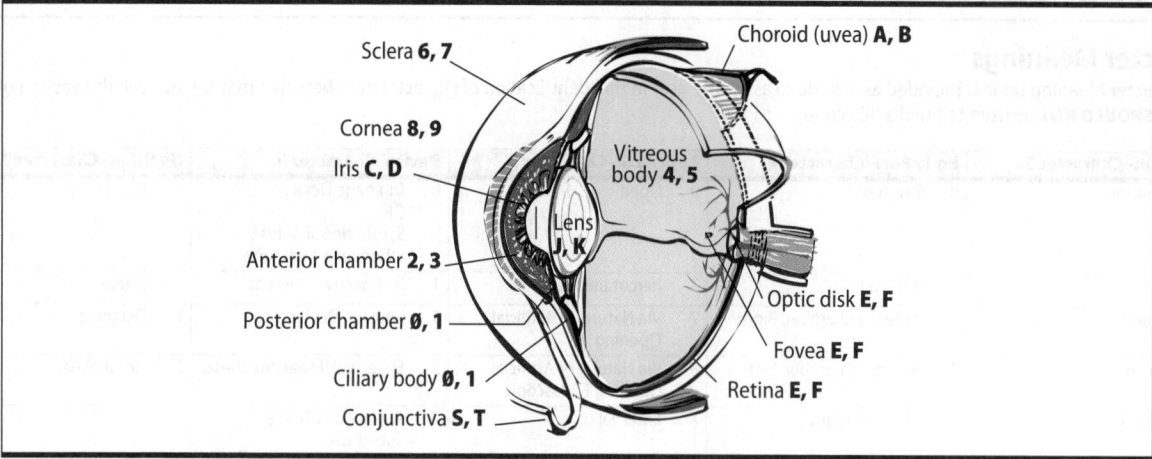

Choroid (uvea) **A, B**

Sclera **6, 7**

Cornea **8, 9**

Iris **C, D**

Vitreous body **4, 5**

Lens **J, K**

Anterior chamber **2, 3**

Posterior chamber **Ø, 1**

Ciliary body **Ø, 1**

Conjunctiva **S, T**

Optic disk **E, F**

Fovea **E, F**

Retina **E, F**

Eye Musculature

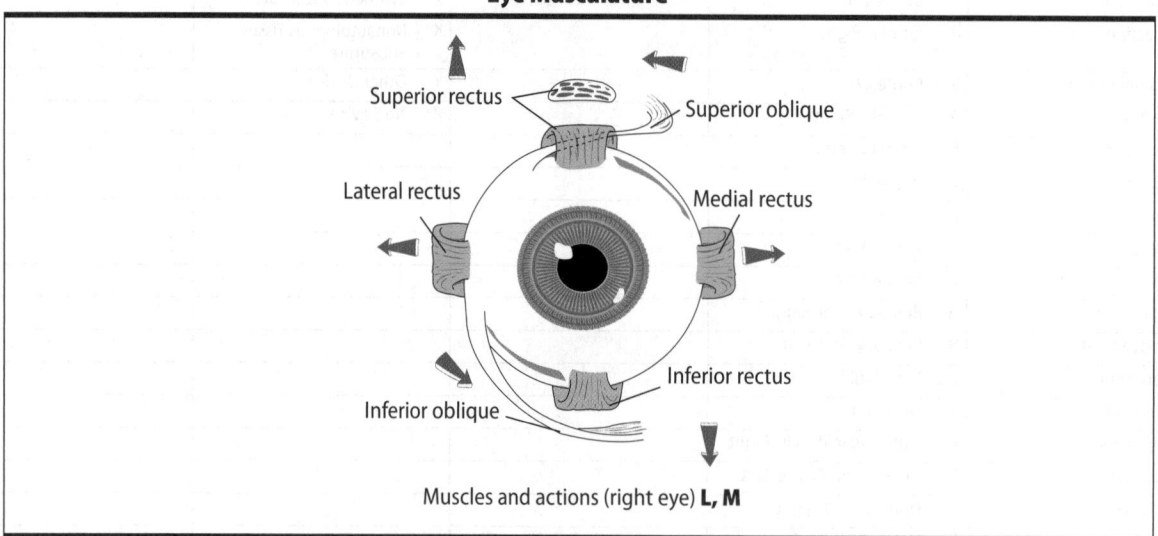

Superior rectus

Superior oblique

Lateral rectus

Medial rectus

Inferior oblique

Inferior rectus

Muscles and actions (right eye) **L, M**

Lacrimal System

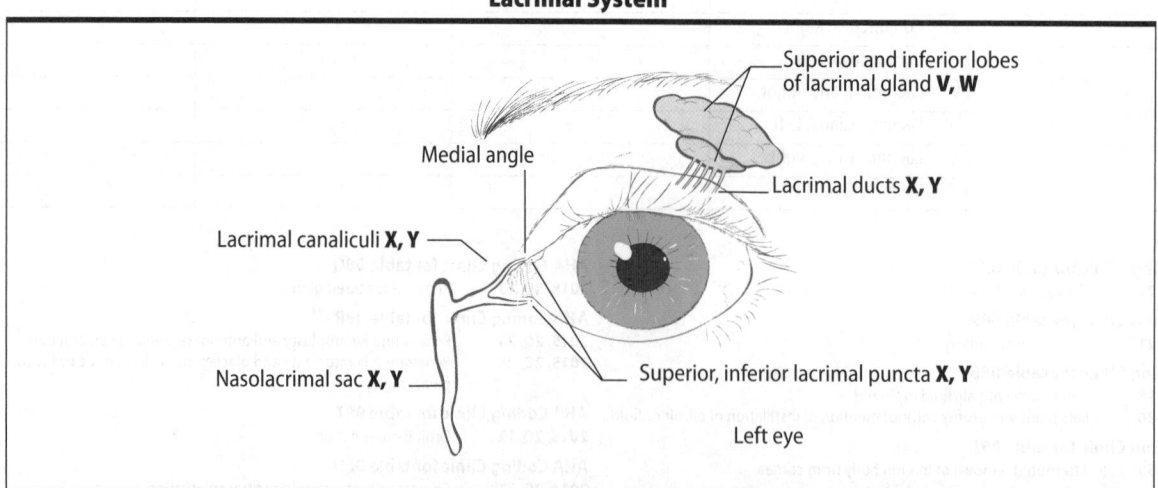

Superior and inferior lobes of lacrimal gland **V, W**

Medial angle

Lacrimal ducts **X, Y**

Lacrimal canaliculi **X, Y**

Nasolacrimal sac **X, Y**

Superior, inferior lacrimal puncta **X, Y**

Left eye

Ø   **Medical and Surgical**
8   **Eye**
Ø   **Alteration**   Definition: Modifying the anatomic structure of a body part without affecting the function of the body part

                                Explanation: Principal purpose is to improve appearance

Body Part Character 4	Approach Character 5	Device Character 6	Qualifier Character 7

N Upper Eyelid, Right
    Lateral canthus
    Levator palpebrae superioris muscle
    Orbicularis oculi muscle
    Superior tarsal plate
P Upper Eyelid, Left
    See N Upper Eyelid, Right
Q Lower Eyelid, Right
    Inferior tarsal plate
    Medial canthus
R Lower Eyelid, Left
    See Q Lower Eyelid, Right
	Ø Open
	3 Percutaneous
	X External
		7 Autologous Tissue Substitute
		J Synthetic Substitute
		K Nonautologous Tissue Substitute
		Z No Device
			Z No Qualifier

Non-OR   All body part, approach, device, and qualifier values

Ø   **Medical and Surgical**
8   **Eye**
1   **Bypass**   Definition: Altering the route of passage of the contents of a tubular body part

                                Explanation: Rerouting contents of a body part to a downstream area of the normal route, to a similar route and body part, or to an abnormal route and dissimilar body part. Includes one or more anastomoses, with or without the use of a device.

Body Part Character 4	Approach Character 5	Device Character 6	Qualifier Character 7

2 Anterior Chamber, Right
    Aqueous humour
3 Anterior Chamber, Left
    See 2 Anterior Chamber, Right
	3 Percutaneous	**J** Synthetic Substitute
		K Nonautologous Tissue Substitute
		Z No Device
			4 Sclera

X Lacrimal Duct, Right
    Lacrimal canaliculus
    Lacrimal punctum
    Lacrimal sac
    Nasolacrimal duct
Y Lacrimal Duct, Left
    See X Lacrimal Duct, Right
	Ø Open
	3 Percutaneous
		J Synthetic Substitute
		K Nonautologous Tissue Substitute
		Z No Device
			3 Nasal Cavity

Ø   **Medical and Surgical**
8   **Eye**
2   **Change**   Definition: Taking out or off a device from a body part and putting back an identical or similar device in or on the same body part without cutting or puncturing the skin or a mucous membrane

                                Explanation: All CHANGE procedures are coded using the approach EXTERNAL

Body Part Character 4	Approach Character 5	Device Character 6	Qualifier Character 7

Ø Eye, Right
    Ciliary body
    Posterior chamber
1 Eye, Left
    See Ø Eye, Right
	X External	**Ø** Drainage Device
		Y Other Device
			Z No Qualifier

Non-OR   All body part, approach, device, and qualifier values

NC Noncovered Procedure   **LC** Limited Coverage   **QA** Questionable OB Admit   **NT** New Tech Add-on   ⊞ Combination Member   ♂ Male   ♀ Female

ICD-10-PCS 2023   303

080–082

Ø Medical and Surgical
8 Eye
5 Destruction Definition: Physical eradication of all or a portion of a body part by the direct use of energy, force, or a destructive agent

Explanation: None of the body part is physically taken out

Body Part Character 4		Approach Character 5	Device Character 6	Qualifier Character 7
Ø Eye, Right Ciliary body Posterior chamber **1 Eye, Left** *See Ø Eye, Right* **6 Sclera, Right** **7 Sclera, Left**	**8 Cornea, Right** **9 Cornea, Left** **S Conjunctiva, Right** Plica semilunaris **T Conjunctiva, Left** *See S Conjunctiva, Right*	**X External**	**Z No Device**	**Z No Qualifier**
2 Anterior Chamber, Right Aqueous humour **3 Anterior Chamber, Left** *See 2 Anterior Chamber, Right* **4 Vitreous, Right** Vitreous body **5 Vitreous, Left** *See 4 Vitreous, Right* **C Iris, Right** **D Iris, Left**	**E Retina, Right** Fovea Macula Optic disc **F Retina, Left** *See E Retina, Right* **G Retinal Vessel, Right** **H Retinal Vessel, Left** **J Lens, Right** Zonule of Zinn **K Lens, Left** *See J Lens, Right*	**3 Percutaneous**	**Z No Device**	**Z No Qualifier**
A Choroid, Right **B Choroid, Left** **L Extraocular Muscle, Right** Inferior oblique muscle Inferior rectus muscle Lateral rectus muscle Medial rectus muscle Superior oblique muscle Superior rectus muscle	**M Extraocular Muscle, Left** *See L Extraocular Muscle, Right* **V Lacrimal Gland, Right** **W Lacrimal Gland, Left**	**Ø Open** **3 Percutaneous**	**Z No Device**	**Z No Qualifier**
N Upper Eyelid, Right Lateral canthus Levator palpebrae superioris muscle Orbicularis oculi muscle Superior tarsal plate **P Upper Eyelid, Left** *See N Upper Eyelid, Right*	**Q Lower Eyelid, Right** Inferior tarsal plate Medial canthus **R Lower Eyelid, Left** *See Q Lower Eyelid, Right*	**Ø Open** **3 Percutaneous** **X External**	**Z No Device**	**Z No Qualifier**
X Lacrimal Duct, Right Lacrimal canaliculus Lacrimal punctum Lacrimal sac Nasolacrimal duct	**Y Lacrimal Duct, Left** *See X Lacrimal Duct, Right*	**Ø Open** **3 Percutaneous** **7 Via Natural or Artificial Opening** **8 Via Natural or Artificial Opening Endoscopic**	**Z No Device**	**Z No Qualifier**

Non-OR	Ø85[E,F]3ZZ

Ø Medical and Surgical
8 Eye
7 Dilation Definition: Expanding an orifice or the lumen of a tubular body part

Explanation: The orifice can be a natural orifice or an artificially created orifice. Accomplished by stretching a tubular body part using intraluminal pressure or by cutting part of the orifice or wall of the tubular body part.

Body Part Character 4	Approach Character 5	Device Character 6	Qualifier Character 7
X Lacrimal Duct, Right Lacrimal canaliculus Lacrimal punctum Lacrimal sac Nasolacrimal duct **Y Lacrimal Duct, Left** *See X Lacrimal Duct, Right*	**Ø Open** **3 Percutaneous** **7 Via Natural or Artificial Opening** **8 Via Natural or Artificial Opening Endoscopic**	**D Intraluminal Device** **Z No Device**	**Z No Qualifier**

Non-OR Procedure   DRG Non-OR Procedure   Valid OR Procedure   HAC Associated Procedure   Combination Only   New/Revised April   New/Revised October

304   ICD-10-PCS 2023

Ø   **Medical and Surgical**
8   **Eye**
9   **Drainage**   Definition: Taking or letting out fluids and/or gases from a body part
                 Explanation: The qualifier DIAGNOSTIC is used to identify drainage procedures that are biopsies

Body Part Character 4		Approach Character 5	Device Character 6	Qualifier Character 7

Ø Eye, Right
  Ciliary body
  Posterior chamber
1 Eye, Left
  See Ø Eye, Right
6 Sclera, Right
7 Sclera, Left
	8 Cornea, Right
	9 Cornea, Left
	S Conjunctiva, Right
	  Plica semilunaris
	T Conjunctiva, Left
	  See S Conjunctiva, Right
		X External	Ø Drainage Device	Z No Qualifier

Ø Eye, Right
  Ciliary body
  Posterior chamber
1 Eye, Left
  See Ø Eye, Right
6 Sclera, Right
7 Sclera, Left
	8 Cornea, Right
	9 Cornea, Left
	S Conjunctiva, Right
	  Plica semilunaris
	T Conjunctiva, Left
	  See S Conjunctiva, Right
		X External	Z No Device	X Diagnostic
				Z No Qualifier

2 Anterior Chamber, Right
  Aqueous humour
3 Anterior Chamber, Left
  See 2 Anterior Chamber, Right
4 Vitreous, Right
  Vitreous body
5 Vitreous, Left
  See 4 Vitreous, Right
C Iris, Right
D Iris, Left
	E Retina, Right
	  Fovea
	  Macula
	  Optic disc
	F Retina, Left
	  See E Retina, Right
	G Retinal Vessel, Right
	H Retinal Vessel, Left
	J Lens, Right
	  Zonule of Zinn
	K Lens, Left
	  See J Lens, Right
		3 Percutaneous	Ø Drainage Device	Z No Qualifier

2 Anterior Chamber, Right
  Aqueous humour
3 Anterior Chamber, Left
  See 2 Anterior Chamber, Right
4 Vitreous, Right
  Vitreous body
5 Vitreous, Left
  See 4 Vitreous, Right
C Iris, Right
D Iris, Left
	E Retina, Right
	  Fovea
	  Macula
	  Optic disc
	F Retina, Left
	  See E Retina, Right
	G Retinal Vessel, Right
	H Retinal Vessel, Left
	J Lens, Right
	  Zonule of Zinn
	K Lens, Left
	  See J Lens, Right
		3 Percutaneous	Z No Device	X Diagnostic
				Z No Qualifier

A Choroid, Right
B Choroid, Left
L Extraocular Muscle, Right
  Inferior oblique muscle
  Inferior rectus muscle
  Lateral rectus muscle
  Medial rectus muscle
  Superior oblique muscle
  Superior rectus muscle
	M Extraocular Muscle, Left
	  See L Extraocular Muscle, Right
	V Lacrimal Gland, Right
	W Lacrimal Gland, Left
		Ø Open
		3 Percutaneous
			Ø Drainage Device	Z No Qualifier

A Choroid, Right
B Choroid, Left
L Extraocular Muscle, Right
  Inferior oblique muscle
  Inferior rectus muscle
  Lateral rectus muscle
  Medial rectus muscle
  Superior oblique muscle
  Superior rectus muscle
	M Extraocular Muscle, Left
	  See L Extraocular Muscle, Right
	V Lacrimal Gland, Right
	W Lacrimal Gland, Left
		Ø Open
		3 Percutaneous
			Z No Device	X Diagnostic
				Z No Qualifier

N Upper Eyelid, Right
  Lateral canthus
  Levator palpebrae superioris
    muscle
  Orbicularis oculi muscle
  Superior tarsal plate
P Upper Eyelid, Left
  See N Upper Eyelid, Right
	Q Lower Eyelid, Right
	  Inferior tarsal plate
	  Medial canthus
	R Lower Eyelid, Left
	  See Q Lower Eyelid, Right
		Ø Open
		3 Percutaneous
		X External
			Ø Drainage Device	Z No Qualifier

Non-OR   Ø89[Ø,1,6,7,8,9,S,T]XZ[X,Z]
Non-OR   Ø89[N,P,Q,R][Ø,3,X]ØZ

Ø89 Continued on next page

NC Noncovered Procedure   LC Limited Coverage   QA Questionable OB Admit   NT New Tech Add-on   ⊞ Combination Member   ♂ Male   ♀ Female

Ø   **Medical and Surgical**   *Ø89 Continued*
8   **Eye**
9   **Drainage**   Definition: Taking or letting out fluids and/or gases from a body part
                 Explanation: The qualifier DIAGNOSTIC is used to identify drainage procedures that are biopsies

Body Part Character 4		Approach Character 5	Device Character 6	Qualifier Character 7

N Upper Eyelid, Right
   Lateral canthus
   Levator palpebrae superioris
     muscle
   Orbicularis oculi muscle
   Superior tarsal plate
P Upper Eyelid, Left
   See N Upper Eyelid, Right
	Q Lower Eyelid, Right
	   Inferior tarsal plate
	   Medial canthus
	R Lower Eyelid, Left
	   See Q Lower Eyelid, Right
		Ø Open
		3 Percutaneous
		X External
			Z No Device	**X** Diagnostic
				Z No Qualifier

X Lacrimal Duct, Right
   Lacrimal canaliculus
   Lacrimal punctum
   Lacrimal sac
   Nasolacrimal duct
	Y Lacrimal Duct, Left
	   See X Lacrimal Duct, Right
		Ø Open
		3 Percutaneous
		7 Via Natural or Artificial
		   Opening
		8 Via Natural or Artificial
		   Opening Endoscopic
			Ø Drainage Device	**Z** No Qualifier

X Lacrimal Duct, Right
   Lacrimal canaliculus
   Lacrimal punctum
   Lacrimal sac
   Nasolacrimal duct
	Y Lacrimal Duct, Left
	   See X Lacrimal Duct, Right
		Ø Open
		3 Percutaneous
		7 Via Natural or Artificial
		   Opening
		8 Via Natural or Artificial
		   Opening Endoscopic
			Z No Device	**X** Diagnostic
				Z No Qualifier

Non-OR   Ø89[N,P,Q,R]ØZZ
Non-OR   Ø89[N,P,Q,R][3,X]Z[X,Z]

Ø   **Medical and Surgical**
8   **Eye**
B   **Excision**   Definition: Cutting out or off, without replacement, a portion of a body part
                 Explanation: The qualifier DIAGNOSTIC is used to identify excision procedures that are biopsies

Body Part Character 4		Approach Character 5	Device Character 6	Qualifier Character 7

Ø Eye, Right
   Ciliary body
   Posterior chamber
1 Eye, Left
   See Ø Eye, Right
N Upper Eyelid, Right
   Lateral canthus
   Levator palpebrae superioris
     muscle
   Orbicularis oculi muscle
   Superior tarsal plate
	P Upper Eyelid, Left
	   See N Upper Eyelid, Right
	Q Lower Eyelid, Right
	   Inferior tarsal plate
	   Medial canthus
	R Lower Eyelid, Left
	   See Q Lower Eyelid, Right
		Ø Open
		3 Percutaneous
		X External
			Z No Device	**X** Diagnostic
				Z No Qualifier

4 Vitreous, Right
   Vitreous body
5 Vitreous, Left
   See 4 Vitreous, Right
C Iris, Right
D Iris, Left
E Retina, Right
   Fovea
   Macula
   Optic disc
	F Retina, Left
	   See E Retina, Right
	J Lens, Right
	   Zonule of Zinn
	K Lens, Left
	   See J Lens, Right
		3 Percutaneous	**Z** No Device	**X** Diagnostic
				Z No Qualifier

6 Sclera, Right
7 Sclera, Left
8 Cornea, Right
9 Cornea, Left
	S Conjunctiva, Right
	   Plica semilunaris
	T Conjunctiva, Left
	   See S Conjunctiva, Right
		X External	**Z** No Device	**X** Diagnostic
				Z No Qualifier

A Choroid, Right
B Choroid, Left
L Extraocular Muscle, Right
   Inferior oblique muscle
   Inferior rectus muscle
   Lateral rectus muscle
   Medial rectus muscle
   Superior oblique muscle
   Superior rectus muscle
	M Extraocular Muscle, Left
	   See L Extraocular Muscle, Right
	V Lacrimal Gland, Right
	W Lacrimal Gland, Left
		Ø Open
		3 Percutaneous
			Z No Device	**X** Diagnostic
				Z No Qualifier

X Lacrimal Duct, Right
   Lacrimal canaliculus
   Lacrimal punctum
   Lacrimal sac
   Nasolacrimal duct
	Y Lacrimal Duct, Left
	   See X Lacrimal Duct, Right
		Ø Open
		3 Percutaneous
		7 Via Natural or Artificial
		   Opening
		8 Via Natural or Artificial
		   Opening Endoscopic
			Z No Device	**X** Diagnostic
				Z No Qualifier

Ø89–Ø8B

Non-OR Procedure   DRG Non-OR Procedure   Valid OR Procedure   HAC Associated Procedure   Combination Only   New/Revised April   New/Revised October

306   ICD-10-PCS 2023

Ø   **Medical and Surgical**
8   **Eye**
C   **Extirpation**   Definition: Taking or cutting out solid matter from a body part

Explanation: The solid matter may be an abnormal byproduct of a biological function or a foreign body; it may be imbedded in a body part or in the lumen of a tubular body part. The solid matter may or may not have been previously broken into pieces.

Body Part Character 4	Approach Character 5	Device Character 6	Qualifier Character 7
Ø Eye, Right Ciliary body Posterior chamber **1 Eye, Left** *See Ø Eye, Right* **6 Sclera, Right** **7 Sclera, Left** **8 Cornea, Right** **9 Cornea, Left** **S Conjunctiva, Right** Plica semilunaris **T Conjunctiva, Left** *See S Conjunctiva, Right*	**X** External	**Z** No Device	**Z** No Qualifier
2 Anterior Chamber, Right Aqueous humour **3 Anterior Chamber, Left** *See 2 Anterior Chamber, Right* **4 Vitreous, Right** Vitreous body **5 Vitreous, Left** *See 4 Vitreous, Right* **C Iris, Right** **D Iris, Left** **E Retina, Right** Fovea Macula Optic disc **F Retina, Left** *See E Retina, Right* **G Retinal Vessel, Right** **H Retinal Vessel, Left** **J Lens, Right** Zonule of Zinn **K Lens, Left** *See J Lens, Right*	**3** Percutaneous **X** External	**Z** No Device	**Z** No Qualifier
A Choroid, Right **B Choroid, Left** **L Extraocular Muscle, Right** Inferior oblique muscle Inferior rectus muscle Lateral rectus muscle Medial rectus muscle Superior oblique muscle Superior rectus muscle **M Extraocular Muscle, Left** *See L Extraocular Muscle, Right* **N Upper Eyelid, Right** Lateral canthus Levator palpebrae superioris muscle Orbicularis oculi muscle Superior tarsal plate **P Upper Eyelid, Left** *See N Upper Eyelid, Right* **Q Lower Eyelid, Right** Inferior tarsal plate Medial canthus **R Lower Eyelid, Left** *See Q Lower Eyelid, Right* **V Lacrimal Gland, Right** **W Lacrimal Gland, Left**	**Ø** Open **3** Percutaneous **X** External	**Z** No Device	**Z** No Qualifier
X Lacrimal Duct, Right Lacrimal canaliculus Lacrimal punctum Lacrimal sac Nasolacrimal duct **Y Lacrimal Duct, Left** *See X Lacrimal Duct, Right*	**Ø** Open **3** Percutaneous **7** Via Natural or Artificial Opening **8** Via Natural or Artificial Opening Endoscopic	**Z** No Device	**Z** No Qualifier

Non-OR	Ø8C[Ø,1,6,7,S,T]XZZ
Non-OR	Ø8C[2,3]XZZ
Non-OR	Ø8C[N,P,Q,R][Ø,3,X]ZZ

NC Noncovered Procedure   **LC** Limited Coverage   **QA** Questionable OB Admit   **NT** New Tech Add-on   ✚ Combination Member   ♂ Male   ♀ Female

ICD-10-PCS 2023   **307**

Ø8C–Ø8C

0   Medical and Surgical
8   Eye
D   Extraction   Definition: Pulling or stripping out or off all or a portion of a body part by the use of force

Explanation: The qualifier DIAGNOSTIC is used to identify extraction procedures that are biopsies

Body Part Character 4	Approach Character 5	Device Character 6	Qualifier Character 7
8 Cornea, Right 9 Cornea, Left	X External	Z No Device	X Diagnostic Z No Qualifier

J Lens, Right
   Zonule of Zinn
K Lens, Left
   See J Lens, Right
	3 Percutaneous	Z No Device	Z No Qualifier

0   Medical and Surgical
8   Eye
F   Fragmentation   Definition: Breaking solid matter in a body part into pieces

Explanation: Physical force (e.g., manual, ultrasonic) applied directly or indirectly is used to break the solid matter into pieces. The solid matter may be an abnormal byproduct of a biological function or a foreign body. The pieces of solid matter are not taken out.

Body Part Character 4	Approach Character 5	Device Character 6	Qualifier Character 7

4 Vitreous, Right **NC**
   Vitreous body
5 Vitreous, Left **NC**
   See 4 Vitreous, Right
	3 Percutaneous
	X External
		Z No Device	Z No Qualifier

Non-OR 08F[4,5]XZZ
NC   08F[4,5]XZZ

0   Medical and Surgical
8   Eye
H   Insertion   Definition: Putting in a nonbiological appliance that monitors, assists, performs, or prevents a physiological function but does not physically take the place of a body part

Explanation: None

Body Part Character 4	Approach Character 5	Device Character 6	Qualifier Character 7

0 Eye, Right
   Ciliary body
   Posterior chamber
1 Eye, Left
   See 0 Eye, Right
	0 Open	5 Epiretinal Visual Prosthesis
		Y Other Device
			Z No Qualifier

0 Eye, Right
   Ciliary body
   Posterior chamber
1 Eye, Left
   See 0 Eye, Right
	3 Percutaneous	1 Radioactive Element
		3 Infusion Device
		Y Other Device
			Z No Qualifier

0 Eye, Right
   Ciliary body
   Posterior chamber
1 Eye, Left
   See 0 Eye, Right
	7 Via Natural or Artificial Opening
	8 Via Natural or Artificial Opening Endoscopic
		Y Other Device	Z No Qualifier

0 Eye, Right
   Ciliary body
   Posterior chamber
1 Eye, Left
   See 0 Eye, Right
	X External	1 Radioactive Element
		3 Infusion Device
			Z No Qualifier

Non-OR 08H[0,1]3YZ
Non-OR 08H[0,1][7,8]YZ

Non-OR Procedure   DRG Non-OR Procedure   Valid OR Procedure   HAC Associated Procedure   Combination Only   New/Revised April   New/Revised October

308   ICD-10-PCS 2023

08D–08H

Ø   Medical and Surgical
8   Eye
J   Inspection   Definition: Visually and/or manually exploring a body part

Explanation: Visual exploration may be performed with or without optical instrumentation. Manual exploration may be performed directly or through intervening body layers.

Body Part Character 4	Approach Character 5	Device Character 6	Qualifier Character 7

Ø   Eye, Right
    Ciliary body
    Posterior chamber
1   Eye, Left
    See Ø Eye, Right
J   Lens, Right
    Zonule of Zinn
K   Lens, Left
    See J Lens, Right
	X External	Z No Device	Z No Qualifier

L   Extraocular Muscle, Right
    Inferior oblique muscle
    Inferior rectus muscle
    Lateral rectus muscle
    Medial rectus muscle
    Superior oblique muscle
    Superior rectus muscle
M   Extraocular Muscle, Left
    See L Extraocular Muscle, Right
	Ø Open
	X External
		Z No Device	Z No Qualifier

Non-OR   08J[0,1,J,K]XZZ
Non-OR   08J[L,M]XZZ

Ø   Medical and Surgical
8   Eye
L   Occlusion   Definition: Completely closing an orifice or the lumen of a tubular body part

Explanation: The orifice can be a natural orifice or an artificially created orifice

Body Part Character 4	Approach Character 5	Device Character 6	Qualifier Character 7

X   Lacrimal Duct, Right
    Lacrimal canaliculus
    Lacrimal punctum
    Lacrimal sac
    Nasolacrimal duct
Y   Lacrimal Duct, Left
    See X Lacrimal Duct, Right
	Ø Open
	3 Percutaneous
		C Extraluminal Device
		D Intraluminal Device
		Z No Device
			Z No Qualifier

X   Lacrimal Duct, Right
    Lacrimal canaliculus
    Lacrimal punctum
    Lacrimal sac
    Nasolacrimal duct
Y   Lacrimal Duct, Left
    See X Lacrimal Duct, Right
	7 Via Natural or Artificial Opening
	8 Via Natural or Artificial Opening
	    Endoscopic
		D Intraluminal Device
		Z No Device
			Z No Qualifier

Ø   Medical and Surgical
8   Eye
M   Reattachment   Definition: Putting back in or on all or a portion of a separated body part to its normal location or other suitable location

Explanation: Vascular circulation and nervous pathways may or may not be reestablished

Body Part Character 4	Approach Character 5	Device Character 6	Qualifier Character 7

N   Upper Eyelid, Right
    Lateral canthus
    Levator palpebrae superioris muscle
    Orbicularis oculi muscle
    Superior tarsal plate
P   Upper Eyelid, Left
    See N Upper Eyelid, Right
Q   Lower Eyelid, Right
    Inferior tarsal plate
    Medial canthus
R   Lower Eyelid, Left
    See Q Lower Eyelid, Right
	X External	Z No Device	Z No Qualifier

NC Noncovered Procedure   LC Limited Coverage   QA Questionable OB Admit   NT New Tech Add-on   ⊞ Combination Member   ♂ Male   ♀ Female

Ø   **Medical and Surgical**
8   **Eye**
N   **Release**   Definition: Freeing a body part from an abnormal physical constraint by cutting or by the use of force
                        Explanation: Some of the restraining tissue may be taken out but none of the body part is taken out

Body Part Character 4	Approach Character 5	Device Character 6	Qualifier Character 7

Ø   **Eye, Right**
    Ciliary body
    Posterior chamber
1   **Eye, Left**
    See Ø Eye, Right
6   **Sclera, Right**
7   **Sclera, Left**
8   **Cornea, Right**
9   **Cornea, Left**
S   **Conjunctiva, Right**
    Plica semilunaris
T   **Conjunctiva, Left**
    See S Conjunctiva, Right
	X External	**Z** No Device	**Z** No Qualifier

2   **Anterior Chamber, Right**
    Aqueous humour
3   **Anterior Chamber, Left**
    See 2 Anterior Chamber, Right
4   **Vitreous, Right**
    Vitreous body
5   **Vitreous, Left**
    See 4 Vitreous, Right
C   **Iris, Right**
D   **Iris, Left**
E   **Retina, Right**
    Fovea
    Macula
    Optic disc
F   **Retina, Left**
    See E Retina, Right
G   **Retinal Vessel, Right**
H   **Retinal Vessel, Left**
J   **Lens, Right**
    Zonule of Zinn
K   **Lens, Left**
    See J Lens, Right
	3 Percutaneous	**Z** No Device	**Z** No Qualifier

A   **Choroid, Right**
B   **Choroid, Left**
L   **Extraocular Muscle, Right**
    Inferior oblique muscle
    Inferior rectus muscle
    Lateral rectus muscle
    Medial rectus muscle
    Superior oblique muscle
    Superior rectus muscle
M   **Extraocular Muscle, Left**
    See L Extraocular Muscle, Right
V   **Lacrimal Gland, Right**
W   **Lacrimal Gland, Left**
	Ø Open
	3 Percutaneous
		Z No Device	**Z** No Qualifier

N   **Upper Eyelid, Right**
    Lateral canthus
    Levator palpebrae superioris muscle
    Orbicularis oculi muscle
    Superior tarsal plate
P   **Upper Eyelid, Left**
    See N Upper Eyelid, Right
Q   **Lower Eyelid, Right**
    Inferior tarsal plate
    Medial canthus
R   **Lower Eyelid, Left**
    See Q Lower Eyelid, Right
	Ø Open
	3 Percutaneous
	X External
		Z No Device	**Z** No Qualifier

X   **Lacrimal Duct, Right**
    Lacrimal canaliculus
    Lacrimal punctum
    Lacrimal sac
    Nasolacrimal duct
Y   **Lacrimal Duct, Left**
    See X Lacrimal Duct, Right
	Ø Open
	3 Percutaneous
	7 Via Natural or Artificial Opening
	8 Via Natural or Artificial Opening
	      Endoscopic
		Z No Device	**Z** No Qualifier

Non-OR Procedure   DRG Non-OR Procedure   Valid OR Procedure   HAC Associated Procedure   Combination Only   New/Revised April   New/Revised October

310   ICD-10-PCS 2023

Ø8N–Ø8N

0   **Medical and Surgical**
8   **Eye**
P   **Removal**   Definition: Taking out or off a device from a body part

                       Explanation: If a device is taken out and a similar device put in without cutting or puncturing the skin or mucous membrane, the procedure is coded to the root operation CHANGE. Otherwise, the procedure for taking out a device is coded to the root operation REMOVAL.

Body Part Character 4	Approach Character 5	Device Character 6	Qualifier Character 7

0   Eye, Right
     Ciliary body
     Posterior chamber
1   Eye, Left
     See 0 Eye, Right
	0 Open
	3 Percutaneous
	7 Via Natural or Artificial Opening
	8 Via Natural or Artificial Opening
	     Endoscopic
		0 Drainage Device
		1 Radioactive Element
		3 Infusion Device
		7 Autologous Tissue Substitute
		C Extraluminal Device
		D Intraluminal Device
		J Synthetic Substitute
		K Nonautologous Tissue Substitute
		Y Other Device
			Z No Qualifier

0   Eye, Right
     Ciliary body
     Posterior chamber
1   Eye, Left
     See 0 Eye, Right
	X External	**0** Drainage Device
		1 Radioactive Element
		3 Infusion Device
		7 Autologous Tissue Substitute
		C Extraluminal Device
		D Intraluminal Device
		J Synthetic Substitute
		K Nonautologous Tissue Substitute
			Z No Qualifier

J   Lens, Right
     Zonule of Zinn
K   Lens, Left
     See J Lens, Right
	3 Percutaneous	**J** Synthetic Substitute
		Y Other Device
			Z No Qualifier

L   Extraocular Muscle, Right
     Inferior oblique muscle
     Inferior rectus muscle
     Lateral rectus muscle
     Medial rectus muscle
     Superior oblique muscle
     Superior rectus muscle
M   Extraocular Muscle, Left
     See L Extraocular Muscle, Right
	0 Open
	3 Percutaneous
		0 Drainage Device
		7 Autologous Tissue Substitute
		J Synthetic Substitute
		K Nonautologous Tissue Substitute
		Y Other Device
			Z No Qualifier

Non-OR	08P[0,1]3YZ
Non-OR	08P[0,1][7,8][0,3,D,Y]Z
Non-OR	08P[0,1]X[0,1,3,C,D,J]Z
Non-OR	08P[J,K]3YZ
Non-OR	08P[L,M]3YZ

NC Noncovered Procedure   **LC** Limited Coverage   **QA** Questionable OB Admit   **NT** New Tech Add-on   ⊞ Combination Member   ♂ Male   ♀ Female

ICD-10-PCS 2023   311

08P–08P

Ø   Medical and Surgical
8   Eye
Q   Repair   Definition: Restoring, to the extent possible, a body part to its normal anatomic structure and function
Explanation: Used only when the method to accomplish the repair is not one of the other root operations

Body Part Character 4	Approach Character 5	Device Character 6	Qualifier Character 7

Ø Eye, Right
   Ciliary body
   Posterior chamber
1 Eye, Left
   See Ø Eye, Right
6 Sclera, Right
7 Sclera, Left
8 Cornea, Right ⬛NC
9 Cornea, Left ⬛NC
S Conjunctiva, Right
   Plica semilunaris
T Conjunctiva, Left
   See S Conjunctiva, Right
	X External	**Z** No Device	**Z** No Qualifier

2 Anterior Chamber, Right
   Aqueous humour
3 Anterior Chamber, Left
   See 2 Anterior Chamber, Right
4 Vitreous, Right
   Vitreous body
5 Vitreous, Left
   See 4 Vitreous, Right
C Iris, Right
D Iris, Left
E Retina, Right
   Fovea
   Macula
   Optic disc
F Retina, Left
   See E Retina, Right
G Retinal Vessel, Right
H Retinal Vessel, Left
J Lens, Right
   Zonule of Zinn
K Lens, Left
   See J Lens, Right
	3 Percutaneous	**Z** No Device	**Z** No Qualifier

A Choroid, Right
B Choroid, Left
L Extraocular Muscle, Right
   Inferior oblique muscle
   Inferior rectus muscle
   Lateral rectus muscle
   Medial rectus muscle
   Superior oblique muscle
   Superior rectus muscle
M Extraocular Muscle, Left
   See L Extraocular Muscle, Right
V Lacrimal Gland, Right
W Lacrimal Gland, Left
	Ø Open
	3 Percutaneous
		Z No Device	**Z** No Qualifier

N Upper Eyelid, Right
   Lateral canthus
   Levator palpebrae superioris muscle
   Orbicularis oculi muscle
   Superior tarsal plate
P Upper Eyelid, Left
   See N Upper Eyelid, Right
Q Lower Eyelid, Right
   Inferior tarsal plate
   Medial canthus
R Lower Eyelid, Left
   See Q Lower Eyelid, Right
	Ø Open
	3 Percutaneous
	X External
		Z No Device	**Z** No Qualifier

X Lacrimal Duct, Right
   Lacrimal canaliculus
   Lacrimal punctum
   Lacrimal sac
   Nasolacrimal duct
Y Lacrimal Duct, Left
   See X Lacrimal Duct, Right
	Ø Open
	3 Percutaneous
	7 Via Natural or Artificial Opening
	8 Via Natural or Artificial Opening
	   Endoscopic
		Z No Device	**Z** No Qualifier

Non-OR   Ø8Q[N,P,Q,R][Ø,3,X]ZZ
NC   Ø8Q[8,9]XZZ

Ø8Q–Ø8Q

Non-OR Procedure   DRG Non-OR Procedure   Valid OR Procedure   HAC Associated Procedure   Combination Only   New/Revised April   New/Revised October
312   ICD-10-PCS 2023

Ø   Medical and Surgical
8   Eye
R   Replacement   Definition: Putting in or on biological or synthetic material that physically takes the place and/or function of all or a portion of a body part

Explanation: The body part may have been taken out or replaced, or may be taken out, physically eradicated, or rendered nonfunctional during the REPLACEMENT procedure. A REMOVAL procedure is coded for taking out the device used in a previous replacement procedure.

Body Part Character 4	Approach Character 5	Device Character 6	Qualifier Character 7
Ø Eye, Right Ciliary body Posterior chamber **1 Eye, Left** *See Ø Eye, Right* **A Choroid, Right** **B Choroid, Left**	**Ø Open** **3 Percutaneous**	**7 Autologous Tissue Substitute** **J Synthetic Substitute** **K Nonautologous Tissue Substitute**	**Z No Qualifier**
4 Vitreous, Right Vitreous body **5 Vitreous, Left** *See 4 Vitreous, Right* **C Iris, Right** **D Iris, Left** **G Retinal Vessel, Right** **H Retinal Vessel, Left**	**3 Percutaneous**	**7 Autologous Tissue Substitute** **J Synthetic Substitute** **K Nonautologous Tissue Substitute**	**Z No Qualifier**
6 Sclera, Right **7 Sclera, Left** **S Conjunctiva, Right** Plica semilunaris **T Conjunctiva, Left** *See S Conjunctiva, Right*	**X External**	**7 Autologous Tissue Substitute** **J Synthetic Substitute** **K Nonautologous Tissue Substitute**	**Z No Qualifier**
8 Cornea, Right **9 Cornea, Left**	**3 Percutaneous** **X External**	**7 Autologous Tissue Substitute** **J Synthetic Substitute** **K Nonautologous Tissue Substitute**	**Z No Qualifier**
J Lens, Right Zonule of Zinn **K Lens, Left** *See J Lens, Right*	**3 Percutaneous**	**Ø Synthetic Substitute, Intraocular Telescope** **7 Autologous Tissue Substitute** **J Synthetic Substitute** **K Nonautologous Tissue Substitute**	**Z No Qualifier**
N Upper Eyelid, Right Lateral canthus Levator palpebrae superioris muscle Orbicularis oculi muscle Superior tarsal plate **P Upper Eyelid, Left** *See N Upper Eyelid, Right* **Q Lower Eyelid, Right** Inferior tarsal plate Medial canthus **R Lower Eyelid, Left** *See Q Lower Eyelid, Right*	**Ø Open** **3 Percutaneous** **X External**	**7 Autologous Tissue Substitute** **J Synthetic Substitute** **K Nonautologous Tissue Substitute**	**Z No Qualifier**
X Lacrimal Duct, Right Lacrimal canaliculus Lacrimal punctum Lacrimal sac Nasolacrimal duct **Y Lacrimal Duct, Left** *See X Lacrimal Duct, Right*	**Ø Open** **3 Percutaneous** **7 Via Natural or Artificial Opening** **8 Via Natural or Artificial Opening Endoscopic**	**7 Autologous Tissue Substitute** **J Synthetic Substitute** **K Nonautologous Tissue Substitute**	**Z No Qualifier**

NC Noncovered Procedure   **LC** Limited Coverage   **OA** Questionable OB Admit   **NT** New Tech Add-on   ⊞ Combination Member   ♂Male   ♀Female

ICD-10-PCS 2023   313

Ø8R–Ø8R

Ø   Medical and Surgical
8   Eye
S   Reposition   Definition: Moving to its normal location, or other suitable location, all or a portion of a body part

Explanation: The body part is moved to a new location from an abnormal location, or from a normal location where it is not functioning correctly. The body part may or may not be cut out or off to be moved to the new location.

Body Part Character 4	Approach Character 5	Device Character 6	Qualifier Character 7

C Iris, Right
D Iris, Left
G Retinal Vessel, Right
H Retinal Vessel, Left
J Lens, Right
    Zonule of Zinn
K Lens, Left
    See J Lens, Right
	3 Percutaneous	**Z** No Device	**Z** No Qualifier

L Extraocular Muscle, Right
    Inferior oblique muscle
    Inferior rectus muscle
    Lateral rectus muscle
    Medial rectus muscle
    Superior oblique muscle
    Superior rectus muscle
M Extraocular Muscle, Left
    See L Extraocular Muscle, Right
V Lacrimal Gland, Right
W Lacrimal Gland, Left
	Ø Open
	3 Percutaneous
		Z No Device	**Z** No Qualifier

N Upper Eyelid, Right
    Lateral canthus
    Levator palpebrae superioris muscle
    Orbicularis oculi muscle
    Superior tarsal plate
P Upper Eyelid, Left
    See N Upper Eyelid, Right
Q Lower Eyelid, Right
    Inferior tarsal plate
    Medial canthus
R Lower Eyelid, Left
    See Q Lower Eyelid, Right
	Ø Open
	3 Percutaneous
	X External
		Z No Device	**Z** No Qualifier

X Lacrimal Duct, Right
    Lacrimal canaliculus
    Lacrimal punctum
    Lacrimal sac
    Nasolacrimal duct
Y Lacrimal Duct, Left
    See X Lacrimal Duct, Right
	Ø Open
	3 Percutaneous
	7 Via Natural or Artificial Opening
	8 Via Natural or Artificial Opening Endoscopic
		Z No Device	**Z** No Qualifier

Non-OR Procedure   DRG Non-OR Procedure   Valid OR Procedure   HAC Associated Procedure   Combination Only   New/Revised April   New/Revised October

Ø   Medical and Surgical
8   Eye
T   Resection   Definition: Cutting out or off, without replacement, all of a body part
                  Explanation: None

Body Part Character 4	Approach Character 5	Device Character 6	Qualifier Character 7

Ø Eye, Right
  Ciliary body
  Posterior chamber
1 Eye, Left
  See Ø Eye, Right
8 Cornea, Right
9 Cornea, Left
	X External	**Z No Device**	**Z No Qualifier**

4 Vitreous, Right
  Vitreous body
5 Vitreous, Left
  See 4 Vitreous, Right
C Iris, Right
D Iris, Left
J Lens, Right
  Zonule of Zinn
K Lens, Left
  See J Lens, Right
	3 Percutaneous	**Z No Device**	**Z No Qualifier**

L Extraocular Muscle, Right
  Inferior oblique muscle
  Inferior rectus muscle
  Lateral rectus muscle
  Medial rectus muscle
  Superior oblique muscle
  Superior rectus muscle
M Extraocular Muscle, Left
  See L Extraocular Muscle, Right
V Lacrimal Gland, Right
W Lacrimal Gland, Left
	Ø Open
	3 Percutaneous
		Z No Device	**Z No Qualifier**

N Upper Eyelid, Right
  Lateral canthus
  Levator palpebrae superioris muscle
  Orbicularis oculi muscle
  Superior tarsal plate
P Upper Eyelid, Left
  See N Upper Eyelid, Right
Q Lower Eyelid, Right
  Inferior tarsal plate
  Medial canthus
R Lower Eyelid, Left
  See Q Lower Eyelid, Right
	Ø Open
	X External
		Z No Device	**Z No Qualifier**

X Lacrimal Duct, Right
  Lacrimal canaliculus
  Lacrimal punctum
  Lacrimal sac
  Nasolacrimal duct
Y Lacrimal Duct, Left
  See X Lacrimal Duct, Right
	Ø Open
	3 Percutaneous
	7 Via Natural or Artificial Opening
	**8 Via Natural or Artificial Opening
	   Endoscopic**
		Z No Device	**Z No Qualifier**

Ø   **Medical and Surgical**
8   **Eye**
U   **Supplement**   Definition: Putting in or on biological or synthetic material that physically reinforces and/or augments the function of a portion of a body part
                     Explanation: The biological material is non-living, or is living and from the same individual. The body part may have been previously replaced, and the SUPPLEMENT procedure is performed to physically reinforce and/or augment the function of the replaced body part.

Body Part Character 4	Approach Character 5	Device Character 6	Qualifier Character 7

Ø   Eye, Right
     Ciliary body
     Posterior chamber
1   Eye, Left
     See Ø Eye, Right
C   Iris, Right
D   Iris, Left
E   Retina, Right
     Fovea
     Macula
     Optic disc
F   Retina, Left
     See E Retina, Right
G   Retinal Vessel, Right
H   Retinal Vessel, Left
L   Extraocular Muscle, Right
     Inferior oblique muscle
     Inferior rectus muscle
     Lateral rectus muscle
     Medial rectus muscle
     Superior oblique muscle
     Superior rectus muscle
M   Extraocular Muscle, Left
     See L Extraocular Muscle, Right
	Ø Open
	3 Percutaneous
		7 Autologous Tissue Substitute
		J Synthetic Substitute
		K Nonautologous Tissue Substitute
			Z No Qualifier

8   Cornea, Right   **NC**
9   Cornea, Left   **NC**
N   Upper Eyelid, Right
     Lateral canthus
     Levator palpebrae superioris muscle
     Orbicularis oculi muscle
     Superior tarsal plate
P   Upper Eyelid, Left
     See N Upper Eyelid, Right
Q   Lower Eyelid, Right
     Inferior tarsal plate
     Medial canthus
R   Lower Eyelid, Left
     See Q Lower Eyelid, Right
	Ø Open
	3 Percutaneous
	X External
		7 Autologous Tissue Substitute
		J Synthetic Substitute
		K Nonautologous Tissue Substitute
			Z No Qualifier

X   Lacrimal Duct, Right
     Lacrimal canaliculus
     Lacrimal punctum
     Lacrimal sac
     Nasolacrimal duct
Y   Lacrimal Duct, Left
     See X Lacrimal Duct, Right
	Ø Open
	3 Percutaneous
	7 Via Natural or Artificial Opening
	8 Via Natural or Artificial Opening
	     Endoscopic
		7 Autologous Tissue Substitute
		J Synthetic Substitute
		K Nonautologous Tissue Substitute
			Z No Qualifier

NC   Ø8U[8,9][Ø,3,X]KZ

Ø   **Medical and Surgical**
8   **Eye**
V   **Restriction**   Definition: Partially closing an orifice or the lumen of a tubular body part
                Explanation: The orifice can be a natural orifice or an artificially created orifice

Body Part Character 4	Approach Character 5	Device Character 6	Qualifier Character 7

X   Lacrimal Duct, Right
     Lacrimal canaliculus
     Lacrimal punctum
     Lacrimal sac
     Nasolacrimal duct
Y   Lacrimal Duct, Left
     See X Lacrimal Duct, Right
	Ø Open
	3 Percutaneous
		C Extraluminal Device
		D Intraluminal Device
		Z No Device
			Z No Qualifier

X   Lacrimal Duct, Right
     Lacrimal canaliculus
     Lacrimal punctum
     Lacrimal sac
     Nasolacrimal duct
Y   Lacrimal Duct, Left
     See X Lacrimal Duct, Right
	7 Via Natural or Artificial Opening
	8 Via Natural or Artificial Opening
	     Endoscopic
		D Intraluminal Device
		Z No Device
			Z No Qualifier

Non-OR Procedure   DRG Non-OR Procedure   Valid OR Procedure   HAC Associated Procedure   Combination Only   New/Revised April   New/Revised October

316   ICD-10-PCS 2023

Ø Medical and Surgical
8 Eye
W Revision   Definition: Correcting, to the extent possible, a portion of a malfunctioning device or the position of a displaced device

Explanation: Revision can include correcting a malfunctioning or displaced device by taking out or putting in components of the device such as a screw or pin

Body Part Character 4	Approach Character 5	Device Character 6	Qualifier Character 7
Ø Eye, Right Ciliary body Posterior chamber **1 Eye, Left** *See Ø Eye, Right*	**Ø Open** **3 Percutaneous** **7 Via Natural or Artificial Opening** **8 Via Natural or Artificial Opening** **Endoscopic**	**Ø Drainage Device** **3 Infusion Device** **7 Autologous Tissue Substitute** **C Extraluminal Device** **D Intraluminal Device** **J Synthetic Substitute** **K Nonautologous Tissue Substitute** **Y Other Device**	**Z No Qualifier**
Ø Eye, Right Ciliary body Posterior chamber **1 Eye, Left** *See Ø Eye, Right*	**X External**	**Ø Drainage Device** **3 Infusion Device** **7 Autologous Tissue Substitute** **C Extraluminal Device** **D Intraluminal Device** **J Synthetic Substitute** **K Nonautologous Tissue Substitute**	**Z No Qualifier**
J Lens, Right Zonule of Zinn **K Lens, Left** *See J Lens, Right*	**3 Percutaneous**	**J Synthetic Substitute** **Y Other Device**	**Z No Qualifier**
J Lens, Right Zonule of Zinn **K Lens, Left** *See J Lens, Right*	**X External**	**J Synthetic Substitute**	**Z No Qualifier**
L Extraocular Muscle, Right Inferior oblique muscle Inferior rectus muscle Lateral rectus muscle Medial rectus muscle Superior oblique muscle Superior rectus muscle **M Extraocular Muscle, Left** *See L Extraocular Muscle, Right*	**Ø Open** **3 Percutaneous**	**Ø Drainage Device** **7 Autologous Tissue Substitute** **J Synthetic Substitute** **K Nonautologous Tissue Substitute** **Y Other Device**	**Z No Qualifier**

Non-OR	Ø8W[Ø,1][3,7,8]YZ
Non-OR	Ø8W[Ø,1]X[Ø,3,7,C,D,J,K]Z
Non-OR	Ø8W[J,K]3YZ
Non-OR	Ø8W[J,K]XJZ
Non-OR	Ø8W[L,M]3YZ

Ø Medical and Surgical
8 Eye
X Transfer   Definition: Moving, without taking out, all or a portion of a body part to another location to take over the function of all or a portion of a body part

Explanation: The body part transferred remains connected to its vascular and nervous supply

Body Part Character 4	Approach Character 5	Device Character 6	Qualifier Character 7
L Extraocular Muscle, Right Inferior oblique muscle Inferior rectus muscle Lateral rectus muscle Medial rectus muscle Superior oblique muscle Superior rectus muscle **M Extraocular Muscle, Left** *See L Extraocular Muscle, Right*	**Ø Open** **3 Percutaneous**	**Z No Device**	**Z No Qualifier**

NC Noncovered Procedure   **LC** Limited Coverage   **QA** Questionable OB Admit   **NT** New Tech Add-on   ⊞ Combination Member   ♂ Male   ♀ Female

ICD-10-PCS 2023   317

Ø8W–Ø8X

Ear, Nose, Sinus Ø9Ø–Ø9W

Character Meanings*

This Character Meaning table is provided as a guide to assist the user in the identification of character members that may be found in this section of code tables. It **SHOULD NOT** be used to build a PCS code.

Operation–Character 3		Body Part–Character 4		Approach–Character 5		Device–Character 6		Qualifier–Character 7	
Ø	Alteration	Ø	External Ear, Right	Ø	Open	Ø	Drainage Device	Ø	Endolymphatic
1	Bypass	1	External Ear, Left	3	Percutaneous	1	Radioactive Element	X	Diagnostic
2	Change	2	External Ear, Bilateral	4	Percutaneous Endoscopic	4	Hearing Device, Bone Conduction	Z	No Qualifier
3	Control	3	External Auditory Canal, Right	7	Via Natural or Artificial Opening	5	Hearing Device, Single Channel Cochlear Prosthesis		
5	Destruction	4	External Auditory Canal, Left	8	Via Natural or Artificial Opening Endoscopic	6	Hearing Device, Multiple Channel Cochlear Prosthesis		
7	Dilation	5	Middle Ear, Right	X	External	7	Autologous Tissue Substitute		
8	Division	6	Middle Ear, Left			B	Intraluminal Device, Airway		
9	Drainage	7	Tympanic Membrane, Right			D	Intraluminal Device		
B	Excision	8	Tympanic Membrane, Left			J	Synthetic Substitute		
C	Extirpation	9	Auditory Ossicle, Right			K	Nonautologous Tissue Substitute		
D	Extraction	A	Auditory Ossicle, Left			S	Hearing Device		
H	Insertion	B	Mastoid Sinus, Right			Y	Other Device		
J	Inspection	C	Mastoid Sinus, Left			Z	No Device		
M	Reattachment	D	Inner Ear, Right						
N	Release	E	Inner Ear, Left						
P	Removal	F	Eustachian Tube, Right						
Q	Repair	G	Eustachian Tube, Left						
R	Replacement	H	Ear, Right						
S	Reposition	J	Ear, Left						
T	Resection	K	Nasal Mucosa and Soft Tissue						
U	Supplement	L	Nasal Turbinate						
W	Revision	M	Nasal Septum						
		N	Nasopharynx						
		P	Accessory Sinus						
		Q	Maxillary Sinus, Right						
		R	Maxillary Sinus, Left						
		S	Frontal Sinus, Right						
		T	Frontal Sinus, Left						
		U	Ethmoid Sinus, Right						
		V	Ethmoid Sinus, Left						
		W	Sphenoid Sinus, Right						
		X	Sphenoid Sinus, Left						
		Y	Sinus						

* Includes sinus ducts.

AHA Coding Clinic for table Ø93
2018, 4Q, 38   Control of epistaxis

AHA Coding Clinic for table Ø95
2018, 1Q, 19   Control of epistaxis via silver nitrate cauterization

AHA Coding Clinic for table Ø9H
2022, 2Q, 17   Congenital nasal pyriform aperture stenosis and repair
2020, 4Q, 43-44   Insertion of radioactive element

AHA Coding Clinic for table Ø9Q
2018, 1Q, 19   Control of epistaxis via silver nitrate cauterization
2017, 4Q, 106   Control of bleeding of external naris using suture
2014, 4Q, 20   Control of epistaxis
2014, 3Q, 22   Transsphenoidal removal of pituitary tumor and fat graft placement
2013, 4Q, 114   Balloon sinuplasty

AHA Coding Clinic for table Ø9U
2022, 1Q, 48   Repair of facial fractures of frontal sinus and orbital roof
2019, 4Q, 28-29   Sinus supplement

Ear Anatomy

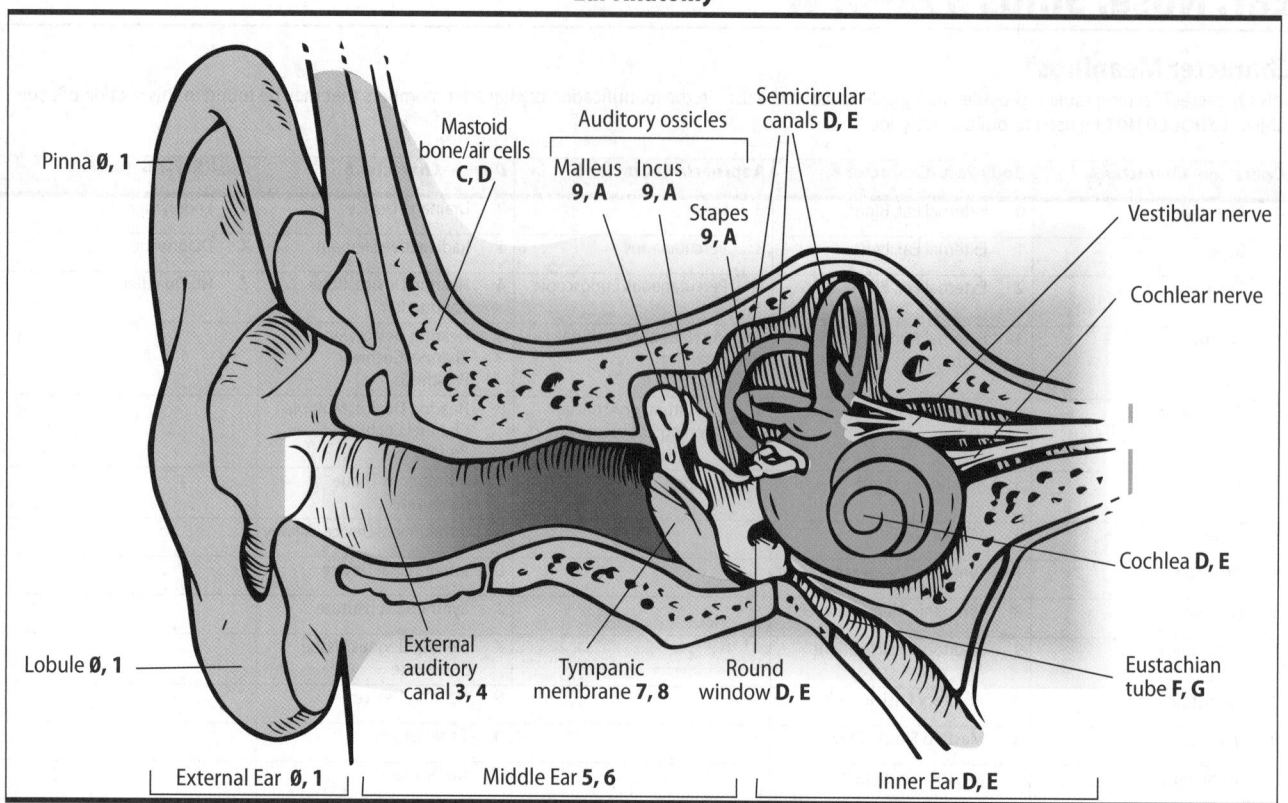

Pinna Ø, 1

Mastoid bone/air cells C, D

Auditory ossicles
Malleus 9, A
Incus 9, A
Stapes 9, A

Semicircular canals D, E

Vestibular nerve

Cochlear nerve

Lobule Ø, 1

External auditory canal 3, 4

Tympanic membrane 7, 8

Round window D, E

Cochlea D, E

Eustachian tube F, G

External Ear Ø, 1

Middle Ear 5, 6

Inner Ear D, E

Nasal Turbinates

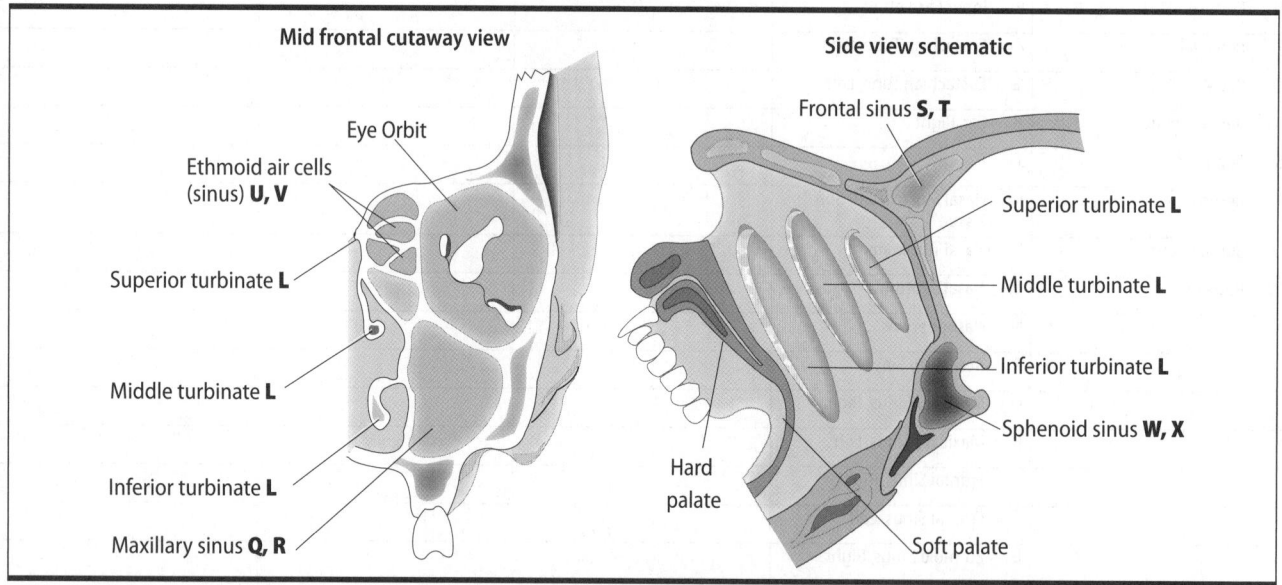

Mid frontal cutaway view

Side view schematic

Eye Orbit

Ethmoid air cells (sinus) U, V

Superior turbinate L

Middle turbinate L

Inferior turbinate L

Maxillary sinus Q, R

Frontal sinus S, T

Superior turbinate L

Middle turbinate L

Inferior turbinate L

Sphenoid sinus W, X

Hard palate

Soft palate

Paranasal Sinuses

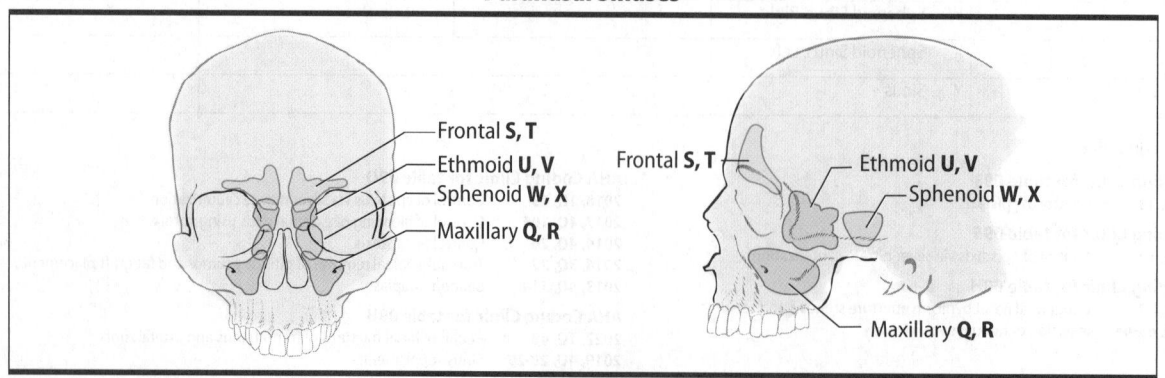

Frontal S, T
Ethmoid U, V
Sphenoid W, X
Maxillary Q, R

Frontal S, T

Ethmoid U, V
Sphenoid W, X

Maxillary Q, R

Ø **Medical and Surgical**
9 **Ear, Nose, Sinus**
Ø **Alteration**   Definition: Modifying the anatomic structure of a body part without affecting the function of the body part

Explanation: Principal purpose is to improve appearance

Body Part Character 4		Approach Character 5	Device Character 6	Qualifier Character 7
Ø **External Ear, Right** Antihelix Antitragus Auricle Earlobe Helix Pinna Tragus **1** **External Ear, Left** *See Ø External Ear, Right*	**2** **External Ear, Bilateral** *See Ø External Ear, Right* **K** **Nasal Mucosa and Soft Tissue** Columella External naris Greater alar cartilage Internal naris Lateral nasal cartilage Lesser alar cartilage Nasal cavity Nostril	**Ø** Open **3** Percutaneous **4** Percutaneous Endoscopic **X** External	**7** Autologous Tissue Substitute **J** Synthetic Substitute **K** Nonautologous Tissue Substitute **Z** No Device	**Z** No Qualifier

Ø **Medical and Surgical**
9 **Ear, Nose, Sinus**
1 **Bypass**   Definition: Altering the route of passage of the contents of a tubular body part

Explanation: Rerouting contents of a body part to a downstream area of the normal route, to a similar route and body part, or to an abnormal route and dissimilar body part. Includes one or more anastomoses, with or without the use of a device.

Body Part Character 4	Approach Character 5	Device Character 6	Qualifier Character 7
D **Inner Ear, Right** Bony labyrinth Bony vestibule Cochlea Round window Semicircular canal **E** **Inner Ear, Left** *See D Inner Ear, Right*	**Ø** Open	**7** Autologous Tissue Substitute **J** Synthetic Substitute **K** Nonautologous Tissue Substitute **Z** No Device	**Ø** Endolymphatic

Ø **Medical and Surgical**
9 **Ear, Nose, Sinus**
2 **Change**   Definition: Taking out or off a device from a body part and putting back an identical or similar device in or on the same body part without cutting or puncturing the skin or a mucous membrane

Explanation: All CHANGE procedures are coded using the approach EXTERNAL

Body Part Character 4	Approach Character 5	Device Character 6	Qualifier Character 7
H **Ear, Right** **J** **Ear, Left** **K** **Nasal Mucosa and Soft Tissue** Columella External naris Greater alar cartilage Internal naris Lateral nasal cartilage Lesser alar cartilage Nasal cavity Nostril **Y** **Sinus**	**X** External	**Ø** Drainage Device **Y** Other Device	**Z** No Qualifier

Non-OR   All body part, approach, device, and qualifier values

Ø **Medical and Surgical**
9 **Ear, Nose, Sinus**
3 **Control**   Definition: Stopping, or attempting to stop, postprocedural or other acute bleeding

Explanation: None

Body Part Character 4	Approach Character 5	Device Character 6	Qualifier Character 7
K **Nasal Mucosa and Soft Tissue** Columella External naris Greater alar cartilage Internal naris Lateral nasal cartilage Lesser alar cartilage Nasal cavity Nostril	**7** Via Natural or Artificial Opening **8** Via Natural or Artificial Opening Endoscopic	**Z** No Device	**Z** No Qualifier

Non-OR   Ø93K[7,8]ZZ

NC Noncovered Procedure   **LC** Limited Coverage   **QA** Questionable OB Admit   **NT** New Tech Add-on   ⊞ Combination Member   ♂ Male   ♀ Female

Ø **Medical and Surgical**
9 **Ear, Nose, Sinus**
5 **Destruction**   Definition: Physical eradication of all or a portion of a body part by the direct use of energy, force, or a destructive agent
Explanation: None of the body part is physically taken out

Body Part Character 4		Approach Character 5	Device Character 6	Qualifier Character 7
Ø **External Ear, Right** Antihelix Antitragus Auricle Earlobe Helix Pinna Tragus	**1** **External Ear, Left** *See Ø External Ear, Right*	**Ø** Open **3** Percutaneous **4** Percutaneous Endoscopic **X** External	**Z** No Device	**Z** No Qualifier
3 **External Auditory Canal, Right** External auditory meatus	**4** **External Auditory Canal, Left** *See 3 External Auditory Canal, Right*	**Ø** Open **3** Percutaneous **4** Percutaneous Endoscopic **7** Via Natural or Artificial Opening **8** Via Natural or Artificial Opening Endoscopic **X** External	**Z** No Device	**Z** No Qualifier
5 **Middle Ear, Right** Oval window Tympanic cavity **6** **Middle Ear, Left** *See 5 Middle Ear, Right* **9** **Auditory Ossicle, Right** Incus Malleus Stapes **A** **Auditory Ossicle, Left** *See 9 Auditory Ossicle, Right*	**D** **Inner Ear, Right** Bony labyrinth Bony vestibule Cochlea Round window Semicircular canal **E** **Inner Ear, Left** *See D Inner Ear, Right*	**Ø** Open **8** Via Natural or Artificial Opening Endoscopic	**Z** No Device	**Z** No Qualifier
7 **Tympanic Membrane, Right** Pars flaccida **8** **Tympanic Membrane, Left** *See 7 Tympanic Membrane, Right* **F** **Eustachian Tube, Right** Auditory tube Pharyngotympanic tube **G** **Eustachian Tube, Left** *See F Eustachian Tube, Right*	**L** **Nasal Turbinate** Inferior turbinate Middle turbinate Nasal concha Superior turbinate **N** **Nasopharynx** Choana Fossa of Rosenmuller Pharyngeal recess Rhinopharynx	**Ø** Open **3** Percutaneous **4** Percutaneous Endoscopic **7** Via Natural or Artificial Opening **8** Via Natural or Artificial Opening Endoscopic	**Z** No Device	**Z** No Qualifier
B **Mastoid Sinus, Right** Mastoid air cells **C** **Mastoid Sinus, Left** *See B Mastoid Sinus, Right* **M** **Nasal Septum** Quadrangular cartilage Septal cartilage Vomer bone **P** **Accessory Sinus** **Q** **Maxillary Sinus, Right** Antrum of Highmore	**R** **Maxillary Sinus, Left** *See Q Maxillary Sinus, Right* **S** **Frontal Sinus, Right** **T** **Frontal Sinus, Left** **U** **Ethmoid Sinus, Right** Ethmoidal air cell **V** **Ethmoid Sinus, Left** *See U Ethmoid Sinus, Right* **W** **Sphenoid Sinus, Right** **X** **Sphenoid Sinus, Left**	**Ø** Open **3** Percutaneous **4** Percutaneous Endoscopic **8** Via Natural or Artificial Opening Endoscopic	**Z** No Device	**Z** No Qualifier
K **Nasal Mucosa and Soft Tissue** Columella External naris Greater alar cartilage Internal naris Lateral nasal cartilage Lesser alar cartilage Nasal cavity Nostril		**Ø** Open **3** Percutaneous **4** Percutaneous Endoscopic **8** Via Natural or Artificial Opening Endoscopic **X** External	**Z** No Device	**Z** No Qualifier

Non-OR	Ø95[Ø,1][Ø,3,4,X]ZZ
Non-OR	Ø95[3,4][Ø,3,4,7,8,X]ZZ
Non-OR	Ø95[F,G][Ø,3,4,7,8]ZZ
Non-OR	Ø95M[Ø,3,4,8]ZZ
Non-OR	Ø95K[Ø,3,4,8,X]ZZ

Ø   **Medical and Surgical**
9   **Ear, Nose, Sinus**
7   **Dilation**   Definition: Expanding an orifice or the lumen of a tubular body part

Explanation: The orifice can be a natural orifice or an artificially created orifice. Accomplished by stretching a tubular body part using intraluminal pressure or by cutting part of the orifice or wall of the tubular body part.

Body Part Character 4	Approach Character 5	Device Character 6	Qualifier Character 7

F Eustachian Tube, Right
   Auditory tube
   Pharyngotympanic tube
G Eustachian Tube, Left
   See F Eustachian Tube, Right
	Ø Open
	7 Via Natural or Artificial Opening
	8 Via Natural or Artificial Opening
	    Endoscopic
		D Intraluminal Device
		Z No Device
			Z No Qualifier

F Eustachian Tube, Right
   Auditory tube
   Pharyngotympanic tube
G Eustachian Tube, Left
   See F Eustachian Tube, Right
	3 Percutaneous
	4 Percutaneous Endoscopic
		Z No Device	**Z** No Qualifier

Non-OR   All body part, approach, device, and qualifier values

Ø   **Medical and Surgical**
9   **Ear, Nose, Sinus**
8   **Division**   Definition: Cutting into a body part, without draining fluids and/or gases from the body part, in order to separate or transect a body part

Explanation: All or a portion of the body part is separated into two or more portions

Body Part Character 4	Approach Character 5	Device Character 6	Qualifier Character 7

L Nasal Turbinate
   Inferior turbinate
   Middle turbinate
   Nasal concha
   Superior turbinate
	Ø Open
	3 Percutaneous
	4 Percutaneous Endoscopic
	7 Via Natural or Artificial Opening
	8 Via Natural or Artificial Opening
	    Endoscopic
		Z No Device	**Z** No Qualifier

Ø   Medical and Surgical
9   Ear, Nose, Sinus
9   Drainage   Definition: Taking or letting out fluids and/or gases from a body part

Explanation: The qualifier DIAGNOSTIC is used to identify drainage procedures that are biopsies

Body Part Character 4		Approach Character 5	Device Character 6	Qualifier Character 7
Ø External Ear, Right Antihelix Antitragus Auricle Earlobe Helix Pinna Tragus	1 External Ear, Left See Ø External Ear, Right	Ø Open 3 Percutaneous 4 Percutaneous Endoscopic X External	Ø Drainage Device	Z No Qualifier
Ø External Ear, Right Antihelix Antitragus Auricle Earlobe Helix Pinna Tragus	1 External Ear, Left See Ø External Ear, Right	Ø Open 3 Percutaneous 4 Percutaneous Endoscopic X External	Z No Device	X Diagnostic Z No Qualifier
3 External Auditory Canal, Right External auditory meatus 4 External Auditory Canal, Left See 3 External Auditory Canal, Right	K Nasal Mucosa and Soft Tissue Columella External naris Greater alar cartilage Internal naris Lateral nasal cartilage Lesser alar cartilage Nasal cavity Nostril	Ø Open 3 Percutaneous 4 Percutaneous Endoscopic 7 Via Natural or Artificial Opening 8 Via Natural or Artificial Opening Endoscopic X External	Ø Drainage Device	Z No Qualifier
3 External Auditory Canal, Right External auditory meatus 4 External Auditory Canal, Left See 3 External Auditory Canal, Right	K Nasal Mucosa and Soft Tissue Columella External naris Greater alar cartilage Internal naris Lateral nasal cartilage Lesser alar cartilage Nasal cavity Nostril	Ø Open 3 Percutaneous 4 Percutaneous Endoscopic 7 Via Natural or Artificial Opening 8 Via Natural or Artificial Opening Endoscopic X External	Z No Device	X Diagnostic Z No Qualifier
5 Middle Ear, Right Oval window Tympanic cavity 6 Middle Ear, Left See 5 Middle Ear, Right 9 Auditory Ossicle, Right Incus Malleus Stapes	A Auditory Ossicle, Left See 9 Auditory Ossicle, Right D Inner Ear, Right Bony labyrinth Bony vestibule Cochlea Round window Semicircular canal E Inner Ear, Left See D Inner Ear, Right	Ø Open 7 Via Natural or Artificial Opening 8 Via Natural or Artificial Opening Endoscopic	Ø Drainage Device	Z No Qualifier
5 Middle Ear, Right Oval window Tympanic cavity 6 Middle Ear, Left See 5 Middle Ear, Right 9 Auditory Ossicle, Right Incus Malleus Stapes	A Auditory Ossicle, Left See 9 Auditory Ossicle, Right D Inner Ear, Right Bony labyrinth Bony vestibule Cochlea Round window Semicircular canal E Inner Ear, Left See D Inner Ear, Right	Ø Open 7 Via Natural or Artificial Opening 8 Via Natural or Artificial Opening Endoscopic	Z No Device	X Diagnostic Z No Qualifier

Non-OR	Ø99[Ø,1][Ø,3,4,X]ØZ
Non-OR	Ø99[Ø,1][Ø,3,4,X]Z[X,Z]
Non-OR	Ø99[3,4,K][Ø,3,4,7,8,X]ØZ
Non-OR	Ø99[3,4,K][Ø,3,4,7,8,X]Z[X,Z]
Non-OR	Ø99[5,6]8ØZ
Non-OR	Ø99[9,A,D,E][7,8]ØZ
Non-OR	Ø99[5,6]ØZZ
Non-OR	Ø99[5,6,9,A,D,E][7,8]Z[X,Z]

Ø99 Continued on next page

Non-OR Procedure   DRG Non-OR Procedure   Valid OR Procedure   HAC Associated Procedure   Combination Only   New/Revised April   New/Revised October

324   ICD-10-PCS 2023

Ø   **Medical and Surgical**   *099 Continued*
9   **Ear, Nose, Sinus**
9   **Drainage**   Definition: Taking or letting out fluids and/or gases from a body part
                        Explanation: The qualifier DIAGNOSTIC is used to identify drainage procedures that are biopsies

Body Part Character 4		Approach Character 5	Device Character 6	Qualifier Character 7
7 Tympanic Membrane, Right Pars flaccida **8 Tympanic Membrane, Left** *See 7 Tympanic Membrane, Right* **B Mastoid Sinus, Right** Mastoid air cells **C Mastoid Sinus, Left** *See B Mastoid Sinus, Right* **F Eustachian Tube, Right** Auditory tube Pharyngotympanic tube **G Eustachian Tube, Left** *See F Eustachian Tube, Right* **L Nasal Turbinate** Inferior turbinate Middle turbinate Nasal concha Superior turbinate **M Nasal Septum** Quadrangular cartilage Septal cartilage Vomer bone	**N Nasopharynx** Choana Fossa of Rosenmuller Pharyngeal recess Rhinopharynx **P Accessory Sinus** **Q Maxillary Sinus, Right** Antrum of Highmore **R Maxillary Sinus, Left** *See Q Maxillary Sinus, Right* **S Frontal Sinus, Right** **T Frontal Sinus, Left** **U Ethmoid Sinus, Right** Ethmoidal air cell **V Ethmoid Sinus, Left** *See U Ethmoid Sinus, Right* **W Sphenoid Sinus, Right** **X Sphenoid Sinus, Left**	**Ø Open** **3 Percutaneous** **4 Percutaneous Endoscopic** **7 Via Natural or Artificial Opening** **8 Via Natural or Artificial Opening Endoscopic**	**Ø Drainage Device**	**Z No Qualifier**
7 Tympanic Membrane, Right Pars flaccida **8 Tympanic Membrane, Left** *See 7 Tympanic Membrane, Right* **B Mastoid Sinus, Right** Mastoid air cells **C Mastoid Sinus, Left** *See B Mastoid Sinus, Right* **F Eustachian Tube, Right** Auditory tube Pharyngotympanic tube **G Eustachian Tube, Left** *See F Eustachian Tube, Right* **L Nasal Turbinate** Inferior turbinate Middle turbinate Nasal concha Superior turbinate **M Nasal Septum** Quadrangular cartilage Septal cartilage Vomer bone	**N Nasopharynx** Choana Fossa of Rosenmuller Pharyngeal recess Rhinopharynx **P Accessory Sinus** **Q Maxillary Sinus, Right** Antrum of Highmore **R Maxillary Sinus, Left** *See Q Maxillary Sinus, Right* **S Frontal Sinus, Right** **T Frontal Sinus, Left** **U Ethmoid Sinus, Right** Ethmoidal air cell **V Ethmoid Sinus, Left** *See U Ethmoid Sinus, Right* **W Sphenoid Sinus, Right** **X Sphenoid Sinus, Left**	**Ø Open** **3 Percutaneous** **4 Percutaneous Endoscopic** **7 Via Natural or Artificial Opening** **8 Via Natural or Artificial Opening Endoscopic**	**Z No Device**	**X Diagnostic** **Z No Qualifier**

Non-OR	099[B,C][3,7,8]ØZ
Non-OR	099[F,G,L,M][Ø,3,4,7,8]ØZ
Non-OR	099N3ØZ
Non-OR	099[P,Q,R,S,T,U,V,W,X][3,4,7,8]ØZ
Non-OR	099[7,8][Ø,3,4,7,8]ZZ
Non-OR	099[7,8][7,8]ZX
Non-OR	099[B,C]3ZZ
Non-OR	099[B,C][7,8]Z[X,Z]
Non-OR	099[F,G][Ø,3,4,7,8]ZZ
Non-OR	099[F,G][7,8]ZX
Non-OR	099[L,M][Ø,3,4,7,8]Z[X,Z]
Non-OR	099N[Ø,3,4,7,8]ZX
Non-OR	099N3ZZ
Non-OR	099[P,Q,R,S,T,U,V,W,X][3,4,7,8]Z[X,Z]

NC Noncovered Procedure   LC Limited Coverage   QA Questionable OB Admit   NT New Tech Add-on   ⊞ Combination Member   ♂ Male   ♀ Female

Ø   Medical and Surgical
9   Ear, Nose, Sinus
B   Excision   Definition: Cutting out or off, without replacement, a portion of a body part

                 Explanation: The qualifier DIAGNOSTIC is used to identify excision procedures that are biopsies

Body Part Character 4		Approach Character 5	Device Character 6	Qualifier Character 7
Ø External Ear, Right Antihelix Antitragus Auricle Earlobe Helix Pinna Tragus	**1 External Ear, Left** *See Ø External Ear, Right*	**Ø** Open **3** Percutaneous **4** Percutaneous Endoscopic **X** External	**Z** No Device	**X** Diagnostic **Z** No Qualifier
3 External Auditory Canal, Right External auditory meatus	**4 External Auditory Canal, Left** *See 3 External Auditory Canal, Right*	**Ø** Open **3** Percutaneous **4** Percutaneous Endoscopic **7** Via Natural or Artificial Opening **8** Via Natural or Artificial Opening Endoscopic **X** External	**Z** No Device	**X** Diagnostic **Z** No Qualifier
5 Middle Ear, Right Oval window Tympanic cavity **6 Middle Ear, Left** *See 5 Middle Ear, Right* **9 Auditory Ossicle, Right** Incus Malleus Stapes	**A Auditory Ossicle, Left** *See 9 Auditory Ossicle, Right* **D Inner Ear, Right** Bony labyrinth Bony vestibule Cochlea Round window Semicircular canal **E Inner Ear, Left** *See D Inner Ear, Right*	**Ø** Open **8** Via Natural or Artificial Opening Endoscopic	**Z** No Device	**X** Diagnostic **Z** No Qualifier
7 Tympanic Membrane, Right Pars flaccida **8 Tympanic Membrane, Left** *See 7 Tympanic Membrane, Right* **F Eustachian Tube, Right** Auditory tube Pharyngotympanic tube **G Eustachian Tube, Left** *See F Eustachian Tube, Right*	**L Nasal Turbinate** Inferior turbinate Middle turbinate Nasal concha Superior turbinate **N Nasopharynx** Choana Fossa of Rosenmuller Pharyngeal recess Rhinopharynx	**Ø** Open **3** Percutaneous **4** Percutaneous Endoscopic **7** Via Natural or Artificial Opening **8** Via Natural or Artificial Opening Endoscopic	**Z** No Device	**X** Diagnostic **Z** No Qualifier
B Mastoid Sinus, Right Mastoid air cells **C Mastoid Sinus, Left** *See B Mastoid Sinus, Right* **M Nasal Septum** Quadrangular cartilage Septal cartilage Vomer bone **P Accessory Sinus** **Q Maxillary Sinus, Right** Antrum of Highmore	**R Maxillary Sinus, Left** *See Q Maxillary Sinus, Right* **S Frontal Sinus, Right** **T Frontal Sinus, Left** **U Ethmoid Sinus, Right** Ethmoidal air cell **V Ethmoid Sinus, Left** *See U Ethmoid Sinus, Right* **W Sphenoid Sinus, Right** **X Sphenoid Sinus, Left**	**Ø** Open **3** Percutaneous **4** Percutaneous Endoscopic **8** Via Natural or Artificial Opening Endoscopic	**Z** No Device	**X** Diagnostic **Z** No Qualifier
K Nasal Mucosa and Soft Tissue Columella External naris Greater alar cartilage Internal naris Lateral nasal cartilage Lesser alar cartilage Nasal cavity Nostril		**Ø** Open **3** Percutaneous **4** Percutaneous Endoscopic **8** Via Natural or Artificial Opening Endoscopic **X** External	**Z** No Device	**X** Diagnostic **Z** No Qualifier

Non-OR	09B[Ø,1][Ø,3,4,X]Z[X,Z]
Non-OR	09B[3,4][Ø,3,4,7,8,X]Z[X,Z]
Non-OR	09B[F,G,L,N][Ø,3,4,7,8]Z[X,Z]
Non-OR	09BM[Ø,3,4,8]ZX
Non-OR	09B[P,Q,R,S,T,U,V,W,X][3,4,8]ZX
Non-OR	09BK8Z[X,Z]

Non-OR Procedure   DRG Non-OR Procedure   Valid OR Procedure   HAC Associated Procedure   Combination Only   New/Revised April   New/Revised October

326   ICD-10-PCS 2023

Ø   **Medical and Surgical**
9   **Ear, Nose, Sinus**
C   **Extirpation**   Definition: Taking or cutting out solid matter from a body part

Explanation: The solid matter may be an abnormal byproduct of a biological function or a foreign body; it may be imbedded in a body part or in the lumen of a tubular body part. The solid matter may or may not have been previously broken into pieces.

Body Part Character 4		Approach Character 5	Device Character 6	Qualifier Character 7
Ø External Ear, Right Antihelix Antitragus Auricle Earlobe Helix Pinna Tragus	**1 External Ear, Left** *See Ø External Ear, Right*	**Ø** Open **3** Percutaneous **4** Percutaneous Endoscopic **X** External	**Z** No Device	**Z** No Qualifier
3 External Auditory Canal, Right External auditory meatus	**4 External Auditory Canal, Left** *See 3 External Auditory Canal, Right*	**Ø** Open **3** Percutaneous **4** Percutaneous Endoscopic **7** Via Natural or Artificial Opening **8** Via Natural or Artificial Opening Endoscopic **X** External	**Z** No Device	**Z** No Qualifier
5 Middle Ear, Right Oval window Tympanic cavity **6 Middle Ear, Left** *See 5 Middle Ear, Right* **9 Auditory Ossicle, Right** Incus Malleus Stapes	**A Auditory Ossicle, Left** *See 9 Auditory Ossicle, Right* **D Inner Ear, Right** Bony labyrinth Bony vestibule Cochlea Round window Semicircular canal **E Inner Ear, Left** *See D Inner Ear, Right*	**Ø** Open **8** Via Natural or Artificial Opening Endoscopic	**Z** No Device	**Z** No Qualifier
7 Tympanic Membrane, Right Pars flaccida **8 Tympanic Membrane, Left** *See 7 Tympanic Membrane, Right* **F Eustachian Tube, Right** Auditory tube Pharyngotympanic tube **G Eustachian Tube, Left** *See F Eustachian Tube, Right*	**L Nasal Turbinate** Inferior turbinate Middle turbinate Nasal concha Superior turbinate **N Nasopharynx** Choana Fossa of Rosenmuller Pharyngeal recess Rhinopharynx	**Ø** Open **3** Percutaneous **4** Percutaneous Endoscopic **7** Via Natural or Artificial Opening **8** Via Natural or Artificial Opening Endoscopic	**Z** No Device	**Z** No Qualifier
B Mastoid Sinus, Right Mastoid air cells **C Mastoid Sinus, Left** *See B Mastoid Sinus, Right* **M Nasal Septum** Quadrangular cartilage Septal cartilage Vomer bone **P Accessory Sinus** **Q Maxillary Sinus, Right** Antrum of Highmore	**R Maxillary Sinus, Left** *See Q Maxillary Sinus, Right* **S Frontal Sinus, Right** **T Frontal Sinus, Left** **U Ethmoid Sinus, Right** Ethmoidal air cell **V Ethmoid Sinus, Left** *See U Ethmoid Sinus, Right* **W Sphenoid Sinus, Right** **X Sphenoid Sinus, Left**	**Ø** Open **3** Percutaneous **4** Percutaneous Endoscopic **8** Via Natural or Artificial Opening Endoscopic	**Z** No Device	**Z** No Qualifier
K Nasal Mucosa and Soft Tissue Columella External naris Greater alar cartilage Internal naris Lateral nasal cartilage Lesser alar cartilage Nasal cavity Nostril		**Ø** Open **3** Percutaneous **4** Percutaneous Endoscopic **8** Via Natural or Artificial Opening Endoscopic **X** External	**Z** No Device	**Z** No Qualifier

Non-OR	09C[Ø,1][Ø,3,4,X]ZZ
Non-OR	09C[3,4][Ø,3,4,7,8,X]ZZ
Non-OR	09C[7,8,F,G,L][Ø,3,4,7,8]ZZ
Non-OR	09CM[Ø,3,4,8]ZZ
Non-OR	09CK8ZZ

NC Noncovered Procedure   **LC** Limited Coverage   **QA** Questionable OB Admit   **NT** New Tech Add-on   ⊞ Combination Member   ♂ Male   ♀ Female

ICD-10-PCS 2023   327

Ø   **Medical and Surgical**
9   **Ear, Nose, Sinus**
D   **Extraction**   Definition: Pulling or stripping out or off all or a portion of a body part by the use of force
                  Explanation: The qualifier DIAGNOSTIC is used to identify extraction procedures that are biopsies

Body Part Character 4	Approach Character 5	Device Character 6	Qualifier Character 7

7 Tympanic Membrane, Right
  Pars flaccida
8 Tympanic Membrane, Left
  See 7 Tympanic Membrane, Right
L Nasal Turbinate
  Inferior turbinate
  Middle turbinate
  Nasal concha
  Superior turbinate
	Ø Open
	3 Percutaneous
	4 Percutaneous Endoscopic
	7 Via Natural or Artificial Opening
	8 Via Natural or Artificial Opening
	   Endoscopic
		Z No Device	**Z** No Qualifier

9 Auditory Ossicle, Right
  Incus
  Malleus
  Stapes
A Auditory Ossicle, Left
  See 9 Auditory Ossicle, Right
	Ø Open	**Z** No Device	**Z** No Qualifier

B Mastoid Sinus, Right
  Mastoid air cells
C Mastoid Sinus, Left
  See B Mastoid Sinus, Right
M Nasal Septum
  Quadrangular cartilage
  Septal cartilage
  Vomer bone
P Accessory Sinus
Q Maxillary Sinus, Right
  Antrum of Highmore
R Maxillary Sinus, Left
  See Q Maxillary Sinus, Right
S Frontal Sinus, Right
T Frontal Sinus, Left
U Ethmoid Sinus, Right
  Ethmoidal air cell
V Ethmoid Sinus, Left
  See U Ethmoid Sinus, Right
W Sphenoid Sinus, Right
X Sphenoid Sinus, Left
	Ø Open
	3 Percutaneous
	4 Percutaneous Endoscopic
		Z No Device	**Z** No Qualifier

Ø   **Medical and Surgical**
9   **Ear, Nose, Sinus**
H   **Insertion**   Definition: Putting in a nonbiological appliance that monitors, assists, performs, or prevents a physiological function but does not physically
                 take the place of a body part
                 Explanation: None

Body Part Character 4	Approach Character 5	Device Character 6	Qualifier Character 7

D Inner Ear, Right
  Bony labyrinth
  Bony vestibule
  Cochlea
  Round window
  Semicircular canal
E Inner Ear, Left
  See D Inner Ear, Right
	Ø Open
	3 Percutaneous
	4 Percutaneous Endoscopic
		1 Radioactive Element
		4 Hearing Device, Bone Conduction
		5 Hearing Device, Single Channel
		   Cochlear Prosthesis
		6 Hearing Device, Multiple Channel
		   Cochlear Prosthesis
		S Hearing Device
			Z No Qualifier

H Ear, Right
J Ear, Left
K Nasal Mucosa and Soft Tissue
  Columella
  External naris
  Greater alar cartilage
  Internal naris
  Lateral nasal cartilage
  Lesser alar cartilage
  Nasal cavity
  Nostril
Y Sinus
	Ø Open
	3 Percutaneous
	4 Percutaneous Endoscopic
	7 Via Natural or Artificial Opening
	8 Via Natural or Artificial Opening
	   Endoscopic
		1 Radioactive Element
		Y Other Device
			Z No Qualifier

N Nasopharynx
  Choana
  Fossa of Rosenmuller
  Pharyngeal recess
  Rhinopharynx
	7 Via Natural or Artificial Opening
	8 Via Natural or Artificial Opening
	   Endoscopic
		1 Radioactive Element
		B Intraluminal Device, Airway
			Z No Qualifier

Non-OR Ø9H[H,J,K]Ø1Z		**Non-OR** Ø9H[H,J,K,Y][3,4,7,8][1,Y]Z
Non-OR Ø9HKØYZ		**Non-OR** Ø9HN[7,8][1,B]Z

Ø   Medical and Surgical
9   Ear, Nose, Sinus
J   Inspection   Definition: Visually and/or manually exploring a body part

Explanation: Visual exploration may be performed with or without optical instrumentation. Manual exploration may be performed directly or through intervening body layers.

Body Part Character 4	Approach Character 5	Device Character 6	Qualifier Character 7

7   Tympanic Membrane, Right
   Pars flaccida
8   Tympanic Membrane, Left
   See 7 Tympanic Membrane, Right
H   Ear, Right
J   Ear, Left
	Ø Open
	3 Percutaneous
	4 Percutaneous Endoscopic
	7 Via Natural or Artificial Opening
	8 Via Natural or Artificial Opening
	   Endoscopic
	X External
		Z No Device	**Z** No Qualifier

D   Inner Ear, Right
   Bony labyrinth
   Bony vestibule
   Cochlea
   Round window
   Semicircular canal
E   Inner Ear, Left
   See D Inner Ear, Right
K   Nasal Mucosa and Soft Tissue
   Columella
   External naris
   Greater alar cartilage
   Internal naris
   Lateral nasal cartilage
   Lesser alar cartilage
   Nasal cavity
   Nostril
Y   Sinus
	Ø Open
	3 Percutaneous
	4 Percutaneous Endoscopic
	8 Via Natural or Artificial Opening
	   Endoscopic
	X External
		Z No Device	**Z** No Qualifier

Non-OR	09J[7,8][3,7,8,X]ZZ
Non-OR	09J[H,J][0,3,4,7,8,X]ZZ
Non-OR	09J[D,E][3,8,X]ZZ
Non-OR	09J[K,Y][0,3,4,8,X]ZZ

Ø   Medical and Surgical
9   Ear, Nose, Sinus
M   Reattachment   Definition: Putting back in or on all or a portion of a separated body part to its normal location or other suitable location

Explanation: Vascular circulation and nervous pathways may or may not be reestablished

Body Part Character 4	Approach Character 5	Device Character 6	Qualifier Character 7

Ø   External Ear, Right
   Antihelix
   Antitragus
   Auricle
   Earlobe
   Helix
   Pinna
   Tragus
1   External Ear, Left
   See Ø External Ear, Right
K   Nasal Mucosa and Soft Tissue
   Columella
   External naris
   Greater alar cartilage
   Internal naris
   Lateral nasal cartilage
   Lesser alar cartilage
   Nasal cavity
   Nostril
	X External	**Z** No Device	**Z** No Qualifier

NC Noncovered Procedure   **LC** Limited Coverage   **QA** Questionable OB Admit   **NT** New Tech Add-on   ⊞ Combination Member   ♂ Male   ♀ Female

ICD-10-PCS 2023   329

09J–09M

Ø Medical and Surgical
9 Ear, Nose, Sinus
N Release   Definition: Freeing a body part from an abnormal physical constraint by cutting or by the use of force

Explanation: Some of the restraining tissue may be taken out but none of the body part is taken out

Body Part Character 4		Approach Character 5	Device Character 6	Qualifier Character 7
Ø External Ear, Right Antihelix Antitragus Auricle Earlobe Helix Pinna Tragus	**1 External Ear, Left** *See Ø External Ear, Right*	**Ø** Open **3** Percutaneous **4** Percutaneous Endoscopic **X** External	**Z** No Device	**Z** No Qualifier
3 External Auditory Canal, Right External auditory meatus	**4 External Auditory Canal, Left** *See 3 External Auditory Canal, Right*	**Ø** Open **3** Percutaneous **4** Percutaneous Endoscopic **7** Via Natural or Artificial Opening **8** Via Natural or Artificial Opening Endoscopic **X** External	**Z** No Device	**Z** No Qualifier
5 Middle Ear, Right Oval window Tympanic cavity **6 Middle Ear, Left** *See 5 Middle Ear, Right* **9 Auditory Ossicle, Right** Incus Malleus Stapes	**A Auditory Ossicle, Left** *See 9 Auditory Ossicle, Right* **D Inner Ear, Right** Bony labyrinth Bony vestibule Cochlea Round window Semicircular canal **E Inner Ear, Left** *See D Inner Ear, Right*	**Ø** Open **8** Via Natural or Artificial Opening Endoscopic	**Z** No Device	**Z** No Qualifier
7 Tympanic Membrane, Right Pars flaccida **8 Tympanic Membrane, Left** *See 7 Tympanic Membrane, Right* **F Eustachian Tube, Right** Auditory tube Pharyngotympanic tube **G Eustachian Tube, Left** *See F Eustachian Tube, Right*	**L Nasal Turbinate** Inferior turbinate Middle turbinate Nasal concha Superior turbinate **N Nasopharynx** Choana Fossa of Rosenmuller Pharyngeal recess Rhinopharynx	**Ø** Open **3** Percutaneous **4** Percutaneous Endoscopic **7** Via Natural or Artificial Opening **8** Via Natural or Artificial Opening Endoscopic	**Z** No Device	**Z** No Qualifier
B Mastoid Sinus, Right Mastoid air cells **C Mastoid Sinus, Left** *See B Mastoid Sinus, Right* **M Nasal Septum** Quadrangular cartilage Septal cartilage Vomer bone **P Accessory Sinus** **Q Maxillary Sinus, Right** Antrum of Highmore	**R Maxillary Sinus, Left** *See Q Maxillary Sinus, Right* **S Frontal Sinus, Right** **T Frontal Sinus, Left** **U Ethmoid Sinus, Right** Ethmoidal air cell **V Ethmoid Sinus, Left** *See U Ethmoid Sinus, Right* **W Sphenoid Sinus, Right** **X Sphenoid Sinus, Left**	**Ø** Open **3** Percutaneous **4** Percutaneous Endoscopic **8** Via Natural or Artificial Opening Endoscopic	**Z** No Device	**Z** No Qualifier
K Nasal Mucosa and Soft Tissue Columella External naris Greater alar cartilage Internal naris Lateral nasal cartilage Lesser alar cartilage Nasal cavity Nostril		**Ø** Open **3** Percutaneous **4** Percutaneous Endoscopic **8** Via Natural or Artificial Opening Endoscopic **X** External	**Z** No Device	**Z** No Qualifier

Non-OR	Ø9N[Ø,1]XZZ
Non-OR	Ø9N[3,4]XZZ
Non-OR	Ø9N[F,G,L][Ø,3,4,7,8]ZZ
Non-OR	Ø9NM[Ø,3,4,8]ZZ
Non-OR	Ø9NK[Ø,3,4,8,X]ZZ

Non-OR Procedure   DRG Non-OR Procedure   Valid OR Procedure   HAC Associated Procedure   Combination Only   New/Revised April   New/Revised October

330   ICD-10-PCS 2023

Ø   **Medical and Surgical**
9   **Ear, Nose, Sinus**
P   **Removal**   Definition: Taking out or off a device from a body part

Explanation: If a device is taken out and a similar device put in without cutting or puncturing the skin or mucous membrane, the procedure is coded to the root operation CHANGE. Otherwise, the procedure for taking out a device is coded to the root operation REMOVAL.

Body Part Character 4	Approach Character 5	Device Character 6	Qualifier Character 7

7   **Tympanic Membrane, Right**
    Pars flaccida
8   **Tympanic Membrane, Left**
    See 7 Tympanic Membrane, Right
	Ø Open
	7 Via Natural or Artificial Opening
	8 Via Natural or Artificial Opening
	    Endoscopic
	X External
		Ø Drainage Device	**Z** No Qualifier

D   **Inner Ear, Right**
    Bony labyrinth
    Bony vestibule
    Cochlea
    Round window
    Semicircular canal
E   **Inner Ear, Left**
    See D Inner Ear, Right
	Ø Open
	7 Via Natural or Artificial Opening
	8 Via Natural or Artificial Opening
	    Endoscopic
		S Hearing Device	**Z** No Qualifier

H   **Ear, Right**
J   **Ear, Left**
K   **Nasal Mucosa and Soft Tissue**
    Columella
    External naris
    Greater alar cartilage
    Internal naris
    Lateral nasal cartilage
    Lesser alar cartilage
    Nasal cavity
    Nostril
	Ø Open
	3 Percutaneous
	4 Percutaneous Endoscopic
	7 Via Natural or Artificial Opening
	8 Via Natural or Artificial Opening
	    Endoscopic
		Ø Drainage Device
		7 Autologous Tissue Substitute
		D Intraluminal Device
		J Synthetic Substitute
		K Nonautologous Tissue Substitute
		Y Other Device
			Z No Qualifier

H   **Ear, Right**
J   **Ear, Left**
K   **Nasal Mucosa and Soft Tissue**
    Columella
    External naris
    Greater alar cartilage
    Internal naris
    Lateral nasal cartilage
    Lesser alar cartilage
    Nasal cavity
    Nostril
	X External	**Ø** Drainage Device
		7 Autologous Tissue Substitute
		D Intraluminal Device
		J Synthetic Substitute
		K Nonautologous Tissue Substitute
			Z No Qualifier

Y **Sinus**	**Ø** Open **3** Percutaneous **4** Percutaneous Endoscopic	**Ø** Drainage Device **Y** Other Device	**Z** No Qualifier
Y **Sinus**	**7** Via Natural or Artificial Opening **8** Via Natural or Artificial Opening Endoscopic	**Y** Other Device	**Z** No Qualifier
Y **Sinus**	**X** External	**Ø** Drainage Device	**Z** No Qualifier

Non-OR   09P[7,8][0,7,8,X]0Z
Non-OR   09P[H,J][3,4][0,J,K,Y]Z
Non-OR   09P[H,J][7,8][0,D,Y]Z
Non-OR   09PK[0,3,4,7,8][0,7,D,J,K,Y]Z
Non-OR   09P[H,J]X[0,7,D,J,K]Z
Non-OR   09PKX[0,7,D,J,K]Z
Non-OR   09PY[3,4]YZ
Non-OR   09PY[7,8]YZ
Non-OR   09PYX0Z

NC Noncovered Procedure   **LC** Limited Coverage   **QA** Questionable OB Admit   **NT** New Tech Add-on   ✚ Combination Member   ♂ Male   ♀ Female

ICD-10-PCS 2023   331

Ear, Nose, Sinus

Ø   Medical and Surgical
9   Ear, Nose, Sinus
Q   Repair   Definition: Restoring, to the extent possible, a body part to its normal anatomic structure and function

                           Explanation: Used only when the method to accomplish the repair is not one of the other root operations

Body Part Character 4		Approach Character 5	Device Character 6	Qualifier Character 7
Ø External Ear, Right Antihelix Antitragus Auricle Earlobe Helix Pinna Tragus	**1 External Ear, Left** *See Ø External Ear, Right* **2 External Ear, Bilateral** *See Ø External Ear, Right*	**Ø** Open **3** Percutaneous **4** Percutaneous Endoscopic **X** External	**Z** No Device	**Z** No Qualifier
3 External Auditory Canal, Right External auditory meatus **4 External Auditory Canal, Left** *See 3 External Auditory Canal, Right*	**F Eustachian Tube, Right** Auditory tube Pharyngotympanic tube **G Eustachian Tube, Left** *See F Eustachian Tube, Right*	**Ø** Open **3** Percutaneous **4** Percutaneous Endoscopic **7** Via Natural or Artificial Opening **8** Via Natural or Artificial Opening Endoscopic **X** External	**Z** No Device	**Z** No Qualifier
5 Middle Ear, Right Oval window Tympanic cavity **6 Middle Ear, Left** *See 5 Middle Ear, Right* **9 Auditory Ossicle, Right** Incus Malleus Stapes	**A Auditory Ossicle, Left** *See 9 Auditory Ossicle, Right* **D Inner Ear, Right** Bony labyrinth Bony vestibule Cochlea Round window Semicircular canal **E Inner Ear, Left** *See D Inner Ear, Right*	**Ø** Open **8** Via Natural or Artificial Opening Endoscopic	**Z** No Device	**Z** No Qualifier
7 Tympanic Membrane, Right Pars flaccida **8 Tympanic Membrane, Left** *See 7 Tympanic Membrane, Right* **L Nasal Turbinate** Inferior turbinate Middle turbinate Nasal concha Superior turbinate	**N Nasopharynx** Choana Fossa of Rosenmuller Pharyngeal recess Rhinopharynx	**Ø** Open **3** Percutaneous **4** Percutaneous Endoscopic **7** Via Natural or Artificial Opening **8** Via Natural or Artificial Opening Endoscopic	**Z** No Device	**Z** No Qualifier
B Mastoid Sinus, Right Mastoid air cells **C Mastoid Sinus, Left** *See B Mastoid Sinus, Right* **M Nasal Septum** Quadrangular cartilage Septal cartilage Vomer bone **P Accessory Sinus** **Q Maxillary Sinus, Right** Antrum of Highmore	**R Maxillary Sinus, Left** *See Q Maxillary Sinus, Right* **S Frontal Sinus, Right** **T Frontal Sinus, Left** **U Ethmoid Sinus, Right** Ethmoidal air cell **V Ethmoid Sinus, Left** *See U Ethmoid Sinus, Right* **W Sphenoid Sinus, Right** **X Sphenoid Sinus, Left**	**Ø** Open **3** Percutaneous **4** Percutaneous Endoscopic **8** Via Natural or Artificial Opening Endoscopic	**Z** No Device	**Z** No Qualifier
K Nasal Mucosa and Soft Tissue Columella External naris Greater alar cartilage Internal naris Lateral nasal cartilage Lesser alar cartilage Nasal cavity Nostril		**Ø** Open **3** Percutaneous **4** Percutaneous Endoscopic **8** Via Natural or Artificial Opening Endoscopic **X** External	**Z** No Device	**Z** No Qualifier

Non-OR   Ø9Q[Ø,1,2]XZZ
Non-OR   Ø9Q[3,4]XZZ
Non-OR   Ø9Q[F,G][Ø,3,4,7,8,X]ZZ
Non-OR   Ø9QKXZZ

Non-OR Procedure   DRG Non-OR Procedure   Valid OR Procedure   HAC Associated Procedure   Combination Only   New/Revised April   New/Revised October

332   ICD-10-PCS 2023

0   **Medical and Surgical**
9   **Ear, Nose, Sinus**
R   **Replacement**   Definition: Putting in or on biological or synthetic material that physically takes the place and/or function of all or a portion of a body part

Explanation: The body part may have been taken out or replaced, or may be taken out, physically eradicated, or rendered nonfunctional during the REPLACEMENT procedure. A REMOVAL procedure is coded for taking out the device used in a previous replacement procedure.

Body Part Character 4	Approach Character 5	Device Character 6	Qualifier Character 7

0   **External Ear, Right**
   Antihelix
   Antitragus
   Auricle
   Earlobe
   Helix
   Pinna
   Tragus
1   **External Ear, Left**
   See 0 External Ear, Right
2   **External Ear, Bilateral**
   See 0 External Ear, Right
K   **Nasal Mucosa and Soft Tissue**
   Columella
   External naris
   Greater alar cartilage
   Internal naris
   Lateral nasal cartilage
   Lesser alar cartilage
   Nasal cavity
   Nostril
	0 Open
	X External
		7 Autologous Tissue Substitute
		J Synthetic Substitute
		K Nonautologous Tissue Substitute
			Z No Qualifier

5   **Middle Ear, Right**
   Oval window
   Tympanic cavity
6   **Middle Ear, Left**
   See 5 Middle Ear, Right
9   **Auditory Ossicle, Right**
   Incus
   Malleus
   Stapes
A   **Auditory Ossicle, Left**
   See 9 Auditory Ossicle, Right
D   **Inner Ear, Right**
   Bony labyrinth
   Bony vestibule
   Cochlea
   Round window
   Semicircular canal
E   **Inner Ear, Left**
   See D Inner Ear, Right
	0 Open	**7** Autologous Tissue Substitute
		J Synthetic Substitute
		K Nonautologous Tissue Substitute
			Z No Qualifier

7   **Tympanic Membrane, Right**
   Pars flaccida
8   **Tympanic Membrane, Left**
   See 7 Tympanic Membrane, Right
N   **Nasopharynx**
   Choana
   Fossa of Rosenmuller
   Pharyngeal recess
   Rhinopharynx
	0 Open
	7 Via Natural or Artificial Opening
	8 Via Natural or Artificial Opening Endoscopic
		7 Autologous Tissue Substitute
		J Synthetic Substitute
		K Nonautologous Tissue Substitute
			Z No Qualifier

L   **Nasal Turbinate**
   Inferior turbinate
   Middle turbinate
   Nasal concha
   Superior turbinate
	0 Open
	3 Percutaneous
	4 Percutaneous Endoscopic
	7 Via Natural or Artificial Opening
	8 Via Natural or Artificial Opening Endoscopic
		7 Autologous Tissue Substitute
		J Synthetic Substitute
		K Nonautologous Tissue Substitute
			Z No Qualifier

M   **Nasal Septum**
   Quadrangular cartilage
   Septal cartilage
   Vomer bone
	0 Open
	3 Percutaneous
	4 Percutaneous Endoscopic
		7 Autologous Tissue Substitute
		J Synthetic Substitute
		K Nonautologous Tissue Substitute
			Z No Qualifier

NC Noncovered Procedure   **LC** Limited Coverage   **QA** Questionable OB Admit   **NT** New Tech Add-on   ⊞ Combination Member   ♂ Male   ♀ Female

ICD-10-PCS 2023   333

Ø **Medical and Surgical**
9 **Ear, Nose, Sinus**
S **Reposition**   Definition: Moving to its normal location, or other suitable location, all or a portion of a body part

Explanation: The body part is moved to a new location from an abnormal location, or from a normal location where it is not functioning correctly. The body part may or may not be cut out or off to be moved to the new location.

Body Part Character 4	Approach Character 5	Device Character 6	Qualifier Character 7
Ø **External Ear, Right** Antihelix Antitragus Auricle Earlobe Helix Pinna Tragus 1 **External Ear, Left** *See Ø External Ear, Right* 2 **External Ear, Bilateral** *See Ø External Ear, Right* K **Nasal Mucosa and Soft Tissue** Columella External naris Greater alar cartilage Internal naris Lateral nasal cartilage Lesser alar cartilage Nasal cavity Nostril	Ø Open 4 Percutaneous Endoscopic X External	Z No Device	Z No Qualifier
7 **Tympanic Membrane, Right** Pars flaccida 8 **Tympanic Membrane, Left** *See 7 Tympanic Membrane, Right* F **Eustachian Tube, Right** Auditory tube Pharyngotympanic tube G **Eustachian Tube, Left** *See F Eustachian Tube, Right* L **Nasal Turbinate** Inferior turbinate Middle turbinate Nasal concha Superior turbinate	Ø Open 4 Percutaneous Endoscopic 7 Via Natural or Artificial Opening 8 Via Natural or Artificial Opening Endoscopic	Z No Device	Z No Qualifier
9 **Auditory Ossicle, Right** Incus Malleus Stapes A **Auditory Ossicle, Left** *See 9 Auditory Ossicle, Right* M **Nasal Septum** Quadrangular cartilage Septal cartilage Vomer bone	Ø Open 4 Percutaneous Endoscopic	Z No Device	Z No Qualifier

Non-OR   09S[F,G][Ø,4,7,8]ZZ

Non-OR Procedure   DRG Non-OR Procedure   Valid OR Procedure   HAC Associated Procedure   Combination Only   New/Revised April   New/Revised October

334

ICD-10-PCS 2023

Ø	**Medical and Surgical**
9	**Ear, Nose, Sinus**
T	**Resection**	Definition: Cutting out or off, without replacement, all of a body part
		Explanation: None

Body Part Character 4		Approach Character 5	Device Character 6	Qualifier Character 7
Ø External Ear, Right Antihelix Antitragus Auricle Earlobe Helix Pinna Tragus	**1 External Ear, Left** *See Ø External Ear, Right*	**Ø Open** **4 Percutaneous Endoscopic** **X External**	**Z No Device**	**Z No Qualifier**
5 Middle Ear, Right Oval window Tympanic cavity **6 Middle Ear, Left** *See 5 Middle Ear, Right* **9 Auditory Ossicle, Right** Incus Malleus Stapes	**A Auditory Ossicle, Left** *See 9 Auditory Ossicle, Right* **D Inner Ear, Right** Bony labyrinth Bony vestibule Cochlea Round window Semicircular canal **E Inner Ear, Left** *See D Inner Ear, Right*	**Ø Open** **8 Via Natural or Artificial Opening Endoscopic**	**Z No Device**	**Z No Qualifier**
7 Tympanic Membrane, Right Pars flaccida **8 Tympanic Membrane, Left** *See 7 Tympanic Membrane, Right* **F Eustachian Tube, Right** Auditory tube Pharyngotympanic tube **G Eustachian Tube, Left** *See F Eustachian Tube, Right*	**L Nasal Turbinate** Inferior turbinate Middle turbinate Nasal concha Superior turbinate **N Nasopharynx** Choana Fossa of Rosenmuller Pharyngeal recess Rhinopharynx	**Ø Open** **4 Percutaneous Endoscopic** **7 Via Natural or Artificial Opening** **8 Via Natural or Artificial Opening Endoscopic**	**Z No Device**	**Z No Qualifier**
B Mastoid Sinus, Right Mastoid air cells **C Mastoid Sinus, Left** *See B Mastoid Sinus, Right* **M Nasal Septum** Quadrangular cartilage Septal cartilage Vomer bone **P Accessory Sinus** **Q Maxillary Sinus, Right** Antrum of Highmore	**R Maxillary Sinus, Left** *See Q Maxillary Sinus, Right* **S Frontal Sinus, Right** **T Frontal Sinus, Left** **U Ethmoid Sinus, Right** Ethmoidal air cell **V Ethmoid Sinus, Left** *See U Ethmoid Sinus, Right* **W Sphenoid Sinus, Right** **X Sphenoid Sinus, Left**	**Ø Open** **4 Percutaneous Endoscopic** **8 Via Natural or Artificial Opening Endoscopic**	**Z No Device**	**Z No Qualifier**
K Nasal Mucosa and Soft Tissue Columella External naris Greater alar cartilage Internal naris Lateral nasal cartilage Lesser alar cartilage Nasal cavity Nostril		**Ø Open** **4 Percutaneous Endoscopic** **8 Via Natural or Artificial Opening Endoscopic** **X External**	**Z No Device**	**Z No Qualifier**

Non-OR   Ø9T[F,G][Ø,4,7,8]ZZ

Ear, Nose, Sinus

Ø   **Medical and Surgical**
9   **Ear, Nose, Sinus**
U   **Supplement**   Definition: Putting in or on biological or synthetic material that physically reinforces and/or augments the function of a portion of a body part
Explanation: The biological material is non-living, or is living and from the same individual. The body part may have been previously replaced, and the SUPPLEMENT procedure is performed to physically reinforce and/or augment the function of the replaced body part.

Body Part Character 4		Approach Character 5	Device Character 6	Qualifier Character 7
Ø **External Ear, Right** Antihelix Antitragus Auricle Earlobe Helix Pinna Tragus	1 **External Ear, Left** *See Ø External Ear, Right* 2 **External Ear, Bilateral** *See Ø External Ear, Right*	Ø Open X External	7 Autologous Tissue Substitute J Synthetic Substitute K Nonautologous Tissue Substitute	Z No Qualifier
5 **Middle Ear, Right** Oval window Tympanic cavity 6 **Middle Ear, Left** *See 5 Middle Ear, Right* 9 **Auditory Ossicle, Right** Incus Malleus Stapes A **Auditory Ossicle, Left** *See 9 Auditory Ossicle, Right*	D **Inner Ear, Right** Bony labyrinth Bony vestibule Cochlea Round window Semicircular canal E **Inner Ear, Left** *See D Inner Ear, Right*	Ø Open 8 Via Natural or Artificial Opening Endoscopic	7 Autologous Tissue Substitute J Synthetic Substitute K Nonautologous Tissue Substitute	Z No Qualifier
7 **Tympanic Membrane, Right** Pars flaccida 8 **Tympanic Membrane, Left** *See 7 Tympanic Membrane, Right*	N **Nasopharynx** Choana Fossa of Rosenmuller Pharyngeal recess Rhinopharynx	Ø Open 7 Via Natural or Artificial Opening 8 Via Natural or Artificial Opening Endoscopic	7 Autologous Tissue Substitute J Synthetic Substitute K Nonautologous Tissue Substitute	Z No Qualifier
B **Mastoid Sinus, Right** Mastoid air cells C **Mastoid Sinus, Left** *See B Mastoid Sinus, Right* L **Nasal Turbinate** Inferior turbinate Middle turbinate Nasal concha Superior turbinate P **Accessory Sinus** Q **Maxillary Sinus, Right** Antrum of Highmore	R **Maxillary Sinus, Left** *See Q Maxillary Sinus, Right* S **Frontal Sinus, Right** T **Frontal Sinus, Left** U **Ethmoid Sinus, Right** Ethmoidal air cell V **Ethmoid Sinus, Left** *See U Ethmoid Sinus, Right* W **Sphenoid Sinus, Right** X **Sphenoid Sinus, Left**	Ø Open 3 Percutaneous 4 Percutaneous Endoscopic 7 Via Natural or Artificial Opening 8 Via Natural or Artificial Opening Endoscopic	7 Autologous Tissue Substitute J Synthetic Substitute K Nonautologous Tissue Substitute	Z No Qualifier
K **Nasal Mucosa and Soft Tissue** Columella External naris Greater alar cartilage Internal naris Lateral nasal cartilage Lesser alar cartilage Nasal cavity Nostril		Ø Open 8 Via Natural or Artificial Opening Endoscopic X External	7 Autologous Tissue Substitute J Synthetic Substitute K Nonautologous Tissue Substitute	Z No Qualifier
M **Nasal Septum** Quadrangular cartilage Septal cartilage Vomer bone		Ø Open 3 Percutaneous 4 Percutaneous Endoscopic 8 Via Natural or Artificial Opening Endoscopic	7 Autologous Tissue Substitute J Synthetic Substitute K Nonautologous Tissue Substitute	Z No Qualifier

Non-OR Procedure   DRG Non-OR Procedure   Valid OR Procedure   HAC Associated Procedure   Combination Only   New/Revised April   New/Revised October

336   ICD-10-PCS 2023

Ø Medical and Surgical
9 Ear, Nose, Sinus
W Revision   Definition: Correcting, to the extent possible, a portion of a malfunctioning device or the position of a displaced device

Explanation: Revision can include correcting a malfunctioning or displaced device by taking out or putting in components of the device such as a screw or pin

Body Part Character 4	Approach Character 5	Device Character 6	Qualifier Character 7
7 Tympanic Membrane, Right Pars flaccida **8 Tympanic Membrane, Left** *See 7 Tympanic Membrane, Right* **9 Auditory Ossicle, Right** Incus Malleus Stapes **A Auditory Ossicle, Left** *See 9 Auditory Ossicle, Right*	**Ø** Open **7** Via Natural or Artificial Opening **8** Via Natural or Artificial Opening Endoscopic	**7** Autologous Tissue Substitute **J** Synthetic Substitute **K** Nonautologous Tissue Substitute	**Z** No Qualifier
D Inner Ear, Right Bony labyrinth Bony vestibule Cochlea Round window Semicircular canal **E Inner Ear, Left** *See D Inner Ear, Right*	**Ø** Open **7** Via Natural or Artificial Opening **8** Via Natural or Artificial Opening Endoscopic	**S** Hearing Device	**Z** No Qualifier
H Ear, Right **J Ear, Left** **K Nasal Mucosa and Soft Tissue** Columella External naris Greater alar cartilage Internal naris Lateral nasal cartilage Lesser alar cartilage Nasal cavity Nostril	**Ø** Open **3** Percutaneous **4** Percutaneous Endoscopic **7** Via Natural or Artificial Opening **8** Via Natural or Artificial Opening Endoscopic	**Ø** Drainage Device **7** Autologous Tissue Substitute **D** Intraluminal Device **J** Synthetic Substitute **K** Nonautologous Tissue Substitute **Y** Other Device	**Z** No Qualifier
H Ear, Right **J Ear, Left** **K Nasal Mucosa and Soft Tissue** Columella External naris Greater alar cartilage Internal naris Lateral nasal cartilage Lesser alar cartilage Nasal cavity Nostril	**X** External	**Ø** Drainage Device **7** Autologous Tissue Substitute **D** Intraluminal Device **J** Synthetic Substitute **K** Nonautologous Tissue Substitute	**Z** No Qualifier
Y Sinus	**Ø** Open **3** Percutaneous **4** Percutaneous Endoscopic	**Ø** Drainage Device **Y** Other Device	**Z** No Qualifier
Y Sinus	**7** Via Natural or Artificial Opening **8** Via Natural or Artificial Opening Endoscopic	**Y** Other Device	**Z** No Qualifier
Y Sinus	**X** External	**Ø** Drainage Device	**Z** No Qualifier

Non-OR Ø9W[H,J][3,4][J,K,Y]Z
Non-OR Ø9W[H,J][7,8][D,Y]Z
Non-OR Ø9WK[Ø,3,4,7,8][Ø,7,D,J,K,Y]Z
Non-OR Ø9W[H,J,K]X[Ø,7,D,J,K]Z
Non-OR Ø9WY[3,4]YZ
Non-OR Ø9WY[7,8]YZ
Non-OR Ø9WYXØZ

NC Noncovered Procedure   LC Limited Coverage   QA Questionable OB Admit   NT New Tech Add-on   ⊞ Combination Member   ♂ Male   ♀ Female

ICD-10-PCS 2023   337

Respiratory System ØB1–ØBY

Respiratory System

Character Meanings

This Character Meaning table is provided as a guide to assist the user in the identification of character members that may be found in this section of code tables. It **SHOULD NOT** be used to build a PCS code.

Operation–Character 3		Body Part–Character 4		Approach–Character 5		Device–Character 6		Qualifier–Character 7	
1	Bypass	Ø	Tracheobronchial Tree	Ø	Open	Ø	Drainage Device	Ø	Allogeneic
2	Change	1	Trachea	3	Percutaneous	1	Radioactive Element	1	Syngeneic
5	Destruction	2	Carina	4	Percutaneous Endoscopic	2	Monitoring Device	2	Zooplastic
7	Dilation	3	Main Bronchus, Right	7	Via Natural or Artificial Opening	3	Infusion Device	3	Laser Interstitial Thermal Therapy
9	Drainage	4	Upper Lobe Bronchus, Right	8	Via Natural or Artificial Opening Endoscopic	7	Autologous Tissue Substitute	4	Cutaneous
B	Excision	5	Middle Lobe Bronchus, Right	X	External	C	Extraluminal Device	6	Esophagus
C	Extirpation	6	Lower Lobe Bronchus, Right			D	Intraluminal Device	X	Diagnostic
D	Extraction	7	Main Bronchus, Left			E	Intraluminal Device, Endotracheal Airway	Z	No Qualifier
F	Fragmentation	8	Upper Lobe Bronchus, Left			F	Tracheostomy Device		
H	Insertion	9	Lingula Bronchus			G	Intraluminal Device, Endobronchial Valve		
J	Inspection	B	Lower Lobe Bronchus, Left			J	Synthetic Substitute		
L	Occlusion	C	Upper Lung Lobe, Right			K	Nonautologous Tissue Substitute		
M	Reattachment	D	Middle Lung Lobe, Right			M	Diaphragmatic Pacemaker Lead		
N	Release	F	Lower Lung Lobe, Right			Y	Other Device		
P	Removal	G	Upper Lung Lobe, Left			Z	No Device		
Q	Repair	H	Lung Lingula						
R	Replacement	J	Lower Lung Lobe, Left						
S	Reposition	K	Lung, Right						
T	Resection	L	Lung, Left						
U	Supplement	M	Lungs, Bilateral						
V	Restriction	N	Pleura, Right						
W	Revision	P	Pleura, Left						
Y	Transplantation	Q	Pleura						
		T	Diaphragm						

AHA Coding Clinic for table ØB5
| 2016, 2Q, 17 | Photodynamic therapy for treatment of malignant mesothelioma |
| 2015, 2Q, 31 | Thoracoscopic talc pleurodesis |

AHA Coding Clinic for table ØB7
| 2020, 3Q, 43 | Tracheobronchomalacia with placement of tracheobronchial stent |

AHA Coding Clinic for table ØB9
2017, 3Q, 15	Bronchoscopy with suctioning for removal of retained secretions
2017, 1Q, 51	Bronchoalveolar lavage
2016, 1Q, 26	Bronchoalveolar lavage, endobronchial biopsy and transbronchial biopsy
2016, 1Q, 27	Fiberoptic bronchoscopy with brushings and bronchoalveolar lavage

AHA Coding Clinic for table ØBB
2022, 2Q, 19	Transbronchial lung biopsy using alligator forceps
2016, 1Q, 26	Bronchoalveolar lavage, endobronchial biopsy and transbronchial biopsy
2016, 1Q, 27	Fiberoptic bronchoscopy with brushings and bronchoalveolar lavage
2014, 1Q, 20	Fiducial marker placement

AHA Coding Clinic for table ØBC
| 2017, 3Q, 14 | Bronchoscopy with suctioning and washings for removal of mucus plug |

AHA Coding Clinic for table ØBD
| 2020, 3Q, 40 | Transbronchial cryobiopsy of upper, middle and lower lobes of lung |
| 2018, 3Q, 28 | Lung decortication for empyema |

AHA Coding Clinic for table ØBH
| 2019, 3Q, 33 | Insertion of endobronchial valve |
| 2014, 4Q, 3-10 | Mechanical ventilation |

AHA Coding Clinic for table ØBJ
| 2015, 2Q, 31 | Thoracoscopic talc pleurodesis |
| 2014, 1Q, 20 | Fiducial marker placement |

AHA Coding Clinic for table ØBL
| 2019, 3Q, 33 | Insertion of endobronchial valve |

AHA Coding Clinic for table ØBN
2019, 2Q, 20	Pericardiectomy for constrictive pericarditis
2018, 3Q, 28	Lung decortication
2018, 3Q, 28	Lung decortication for empyema
2015, 3Q, 15	Vascular ring surgery with release of esophagus and trachea

AHA Coding Clinic for table ØBQ
2020, 3Q, 41	Plication of diaphragm
2016, 2Q, 22	Esophageal lengthening Collis gastroplasty with Nissen fundoplication and hiatal hernia
2014, 3Q, 28	Laparoscopic Nissen fundoplication and diaphragmatic hernia repair

AHA Coding Clinic for table ØBU
| 2020, 3Q, 43 | Tracheobronchomalacia with placement of tracheobronchial stent |
| 2015, 1Q, 28 | Repair of bronchopleural fistula using omental pedicle graft |

AHA Coding Clinic for table ØBV
| 2020, 3Q, 41 | Plication of diaphragm |

Respiratory System

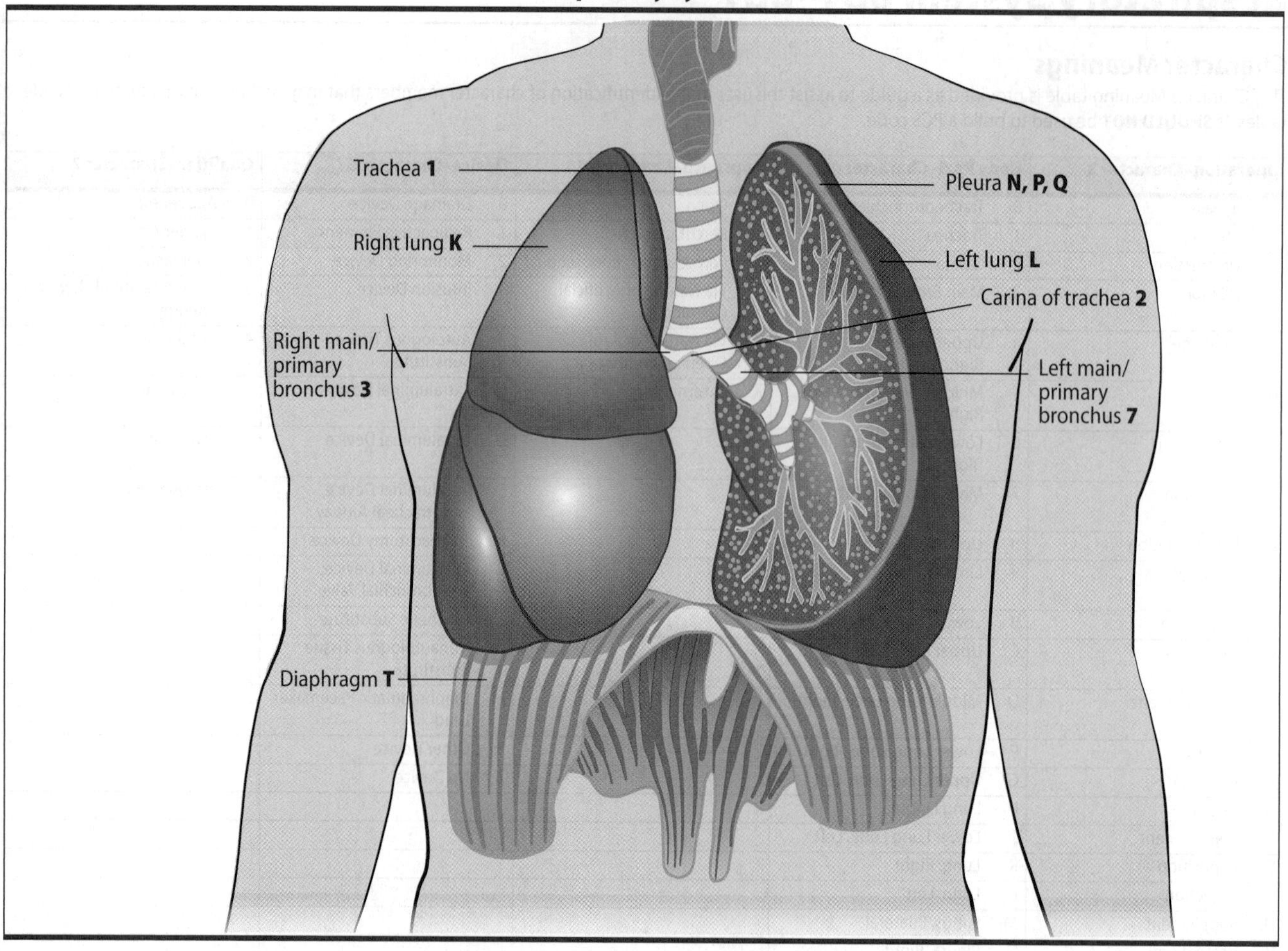

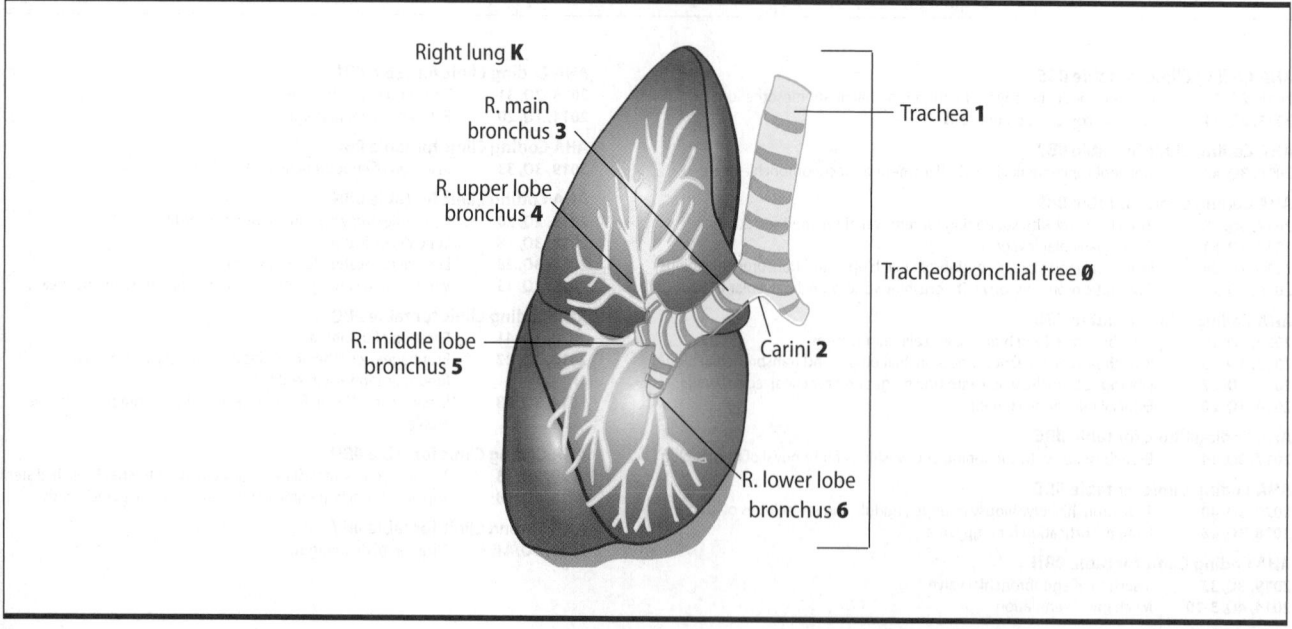

Right Lung Bronchi

Ø   **Medical and Surgical**
B   **Respiratory System**
1   **Bypass**   Definition: Altering the route of passage of the contents of a tubular body part

Explanation: Rerouting contents of a body part to a downstream area of the normal route, to a similar route and body part, or to an abnormal route and dissimilar body part. Includes one or more anastomoses, with or without the use of a device.

Body Part Character 4	Approach Character 5	Device Character 6	Qualifier Character 7
1 Trachea Cricoid cartilage	Ø Open	D Intraluminal Device	6 Esophagus
1 Trachea Cricoid cartilage	Ø Open	F Tracheostomy Device Z No Device	4 Cutaneous
1 Trachea Cricoid cartilage	3 Percutaneous 4 Percutaneous Endoscopic	F Tracheostomy Device Z No Device	4 Cutaneous

DRG Non-OR	ØB113[F,Z]4
Non-OR	ØB11ØD6

Ø   **Medical and Surgical**
B   **Respiratory System**
2   **Change**   Definition: Taking out or off a device from a body part and putting back an identical or similar device in or on the same body part without cutting or puncturing the skin or a mucous membrane

Explanation: All CHANGE procedures are coded using the approach EXTERNAL

Body Part Character 4	Approach Character 5	Device Character 6	Qualifier Character 7
Ø Tracheobronchial Tree K Lung, Right L Lung, Left Q Pleura T Diaphragm	X External	Ø Drainage Device Y Other Device	Z No Qualifier
1 Trachea Cricoid cartilage	X External	Ø Drainage Device E Intraluminal Device, Endotracheal Airway F Tracheostomy Device Y Other Device	Z No Qualifier

Non-OR	All body part, approach, device, and qualifier values

NC Noncovered Procedure   **LC** Limited Coverage   **QA** Questionable OB Admit   **NT** New Tech Add-on   ⊞ Combination Member   ♂ Male   ♀ Female

ICD-10-PCS 2023   **341**

ØB1–ØB2

Respiratory System *(side tab)*

Ø   **Medical and Surgical**
B   **Respiratory System**
5   **Destruction**   Definition: Physical eradication of all or a portion of a body part by the direct use of energy, force, or a destructive agent
                         Explanation: None of the body part is physically taken out

Body Part Character 4	Approach Character 5	Device Character 6	Qualifier Character 7

1 Trachea
   Cricoid cartilage
2 Carina
3 Main Bronchus, Right
   Bronchus intermedius
   Intermediate bronchus
4 Upper Lobe Bronchus, Right
5 Middle Lobe Bronchus, Right
6 Lower Lobe Bronchus, Right
7 Main Bronchus, Left
8 Upper Lobe Bronchus, Left
9 Lingula Bronchus
B Lower Lobe Bronchus, Left
	Ø Open
	3 Percutaneous
	4 Percutaneous Endoscopic
	7 Via Natural or Artificial Opening
	8 Via Natural or Artificial Opening
	   Endoscopic
		Z No Device	Z No Qualifier

C Upper Lung Lobe, Right D Middle Lung Lobe, Right F Lower Lung Lobe, Right G Upper Lung Lobe, Left H Lung Lingula J Lower Lung Lobe, Left K Lung, Right L Lung, Left M Lungs, Bilateral	Ø Open 3 Percutaneous 4 Percutaneous Endoscopic	Z No Device	3 Laser Interstitial Thermal Therapy Z No Qualifier
C Upper Lung Lobe, Right D Middle Lung Lobe, Right F Lower Lung Lobe, Right G Upper Lung Lobe, Left H Lung Lingula J Lower Lung Lobe, Left K Lung, Right L Lung, Left M Lungs, Bilateral	7 Via Natural or Artificial Opening 8 Via Natural or Artificial Opening Endoscopic	Z No Device	Z No Qualifier
N Pleura, Right P Pleura, Left T Diaphragm	Ø Open 3 Percutaneous 4 Percutaneous Endoscopic	Z No Device	Z No Qualifier

Non-OR   ØB5[3,4,5,6,7,8,9,B]4ZZ
Non-OR   ØB5[C,D,F,G,H,J,K,L,M]8ZZ

Ø   **Medical and Surgical**
B   **Respiratory System**
7   **Dilation**   Definition: Expanding an orifice or the lumen of a tubular body part
                      Explanation: The orifice can be a natural orifice or an artificially created orifice. Accomplished by stretching a tubular body part using
                      intraluminal pressure or by cutting part of the orifice or wall of the tubular body part.

Body Part Character 4	Approach Character 5	Device Character 6	Qualifier Character 7

1 Trachea
   Cricoid cartilage
2 Carina
3 Main Bronchus, Right
   Bronchus intermedius
   Intermediate bronchus
4 Upper Lobe Bronchus, Right
5 Middle Lobe Bronchus, Right
6 Lower Lobe Bronchus, Right
7 Main Bronchus, Left
8 Upper Lobe Bronchus, Left
9 Lingula Bronchus
B Lower Lobe Bronchus, Left
	Ø Open
	3 Percutaneous
	4 Percutaneous Endoscopic
	7 Via Natural or Artificial
	   Opening
	8 Via Natural or Artificial
	   Opening Endoscopic
		D Intraluminal Device
		Z No Device
			Z No Qualifier

Non-OR   ØB7[3,4,5,6,7,8,9,B][Ø,3,4,7,8][D,Z]Z

Non-OR Procedure   DRG Non-OR Procedure   Valid OR Procedure   HAC Associated Procedure   Combination Only   New/Revised April   New/Revised October

342   ICD-10-PCS 2023

ØB5–ØB7 *(side tab)*

0   **Medical and Surgical**
B   **Respiratory System**
9   **Drainage**   Definition: Taking or letting out fluids and/or gases from a body part

                       Explanation: The qualifier DIAGNOSTIC is used to identify drainage procedures that are biopsies

Body Part Character 4		Approach Character 5	Device Character 6	Qualifier Character 7

1 Trachea
  Cricoid cartilage
2 Carina
3 Main Bronchus, Right
  Bronchus intermedius
  Intermediate bronchus
4 Upper Lobe Bronchus, Right
5 Middle Lobe Bronchus, Right
6 Lower Lobe Bronchus, Right
7 Main Bronchus, Left
	8 Upper Lobe Bronchus, Left
	9 Lingula Bronchus
	B Lower Lobe Bronchus, Left
	C Upper Lung Lobe, Right
	D Middle Lung Lobe, Right
	F Lower Lung Lobe, Right
	G Upper Lung Lobe, Left
	H Lung Lingula
	J Lower Lung Lobe, Left
	K Lung, Right
	L Lung, Left
	M Lungs, Bilateral
		0 Open
		3 Percutaneous
		4 Percutaneous Endoscopic
		7 Via Natural or Artificial Opening
		8 Via Natural or Artificial Opening Endoscopic
			0 Drainage Device	Z No Qualifier

1 Trachea
  Cricoid cartilage
2 Carina
3 Main Bronchus, Right
  Bronchus intermedius
  Intermediate bronchus
4 Upper Lobe Bronchus, Right
5 Middle Lobe Bronchus, Right
6 Lower Lobe Bronchus, Right
7 Main Bronchus, Left
	8 Upper Lobe Bronchus, Left
	9 Lingula Bronchus
	B Lower Lobe Bronchus, Left
	C Upper Lung Lobe, Right
	D Middle Lung Lobe, Right
	F Lower Lung Lobe, Right
	G Upper Lung Lobe, Left
	H Lung Lingula
	J Lower Lung Lobe, Left
	K Lung, Right
	L Lung, Left
	M Lungs, Bilateral
		0 Open
		3 Percutaneous
		4 Percutaneous Endoscopic
		7 Via Natural or Artificial Opening
		8 Via Natural or Artificial Opening Endoscopic
			Z No Device	X Diagnostic
				Z No Qualifier

N Pleura, Right P Pleura, Left		0 Open 3 Percutaneous 4 Percutaneous Endoscopic 8 Via Natural or Artificial Opening Endoscopic	0 Drainage Device	Z No Qualifier
N Pleura, Right P Pleura, Left		0 Open 3 Percutaneous 4 Percutaneous Endoscopic 8 Via Natural or Artificial Opening Endoscopic	Z No Device	X Diagnostic Z No Qualifier
T Diaphragm		0 Open 3 Percutaneous 4 Percutaneous Endoscopic	0 Drainage Device	Z No Qualifier
T Diaphragm		0 Open 3 Percutaneous 4 Percutaneous Endoscopic	Z No Device	X Diagnostic Z No Qualifier

Non-OR	0B9[1,2,3,4,5,6,7,8,9,B][7,8]0Z		Non-OR	0B9[N,P][0,3,8]0Z
Non-OR	0B9[1,2,3,4,5,6,7,8,9,B][3,4]ZX		Non-OR	0B9[N,P][0,3,8]Z[X,Z]
Non-OR	0B9[1,2,3,4,5,6,7,8,9,B][7,8]Z[X,Z]		Non-OR	0B9[N,P]4ZX
Non-OR	0B9[C,D,F,G,H,J,K,L,M][3,4,7]ZX		Non-OR	0B9T[3,4]0Z
Non-OR	0B9[C,D,F,G,H,J,K,L,M]8Z[X,Z]		Non-OR	0B9T[3,4]Z[X,Z]

NC Noncovered Procedure   LC Limited Coverage   QA Questionable OB Admit   NT New Tech Add-on   ⊞ Combination Member   ♂ Male   ♀ Female

ICD-10-PCS 2023   343

0B9–0B9

Ø Medical and Surgical
B Respiratory System
B Excision   Definition: Cutting out or off, without replacement, a portion of a body part

Explanation: The qualifier DIAGNOSTIC is used to identify excision procedures that are biopsies

Body Part Character 4	Approach Character 5	Device Character 6	Qualifier Character 7

1 Trachea
  Cricoid cartilage
2 Carina
3 Main Bronchus, Right
  Bronchus intermedius
  Intermediate bronchus
4 Upper Lobe Bronchus, Right
5 Middle Lobe Bronchus, Right
6 Lower Lobe Bronchus, Right
7 Main Bronchus, Left
8 Upper Lobe Bronchus, Left
9 Lingula Bronchus
B Lower Lobe Bronchus, Left
C Upper Lung Lobe, Right
D Middle Lung Lobe, Right
F Lower Lung Lobe, Right
G Upper Lung Lobe, Left
H Lung Lingula
J Lower Lung Lobe, Left
K Lung, Right
L Lung, Left
M Lungs, Bilateral
	Ø Open
	3 Percutaneous
	4 Percutaneous Endoscopic
	7 Via Natural or Artificial Opening
	8 Via Natural or Artificial Opening Endoscopic
		Z No Device	X Diagnostic
			Z No Qualifier

N Pleura, Right P Pleura, Left	Ø Open 3 Percutaneous 4 Percutaneous Endoscopic 8 Via Natural or Artificial Opening Endoscopic	Z No Device	X Diagnostic Z No Qualifier
T Diaphragm	Ø Open 3 Percutaneous 4 Percutaneous Endoscopic	Z No Device	X Diagnostic Z No Qualifier

Non-OR   ØBB[1,2,3,4,5,6,7,8,9,B][3,4,7,8]ZX
Non-OR   ØBB[3,4,5,6,7,8,9,B,M][4,8]ZZ
Non-OR   ØBB[C,D,F,G,H,J,K,L,M]3ZX

Non-OR   ØBB[C,D,F,G,H,J,K,L]8ZZ
Non-OR   ØBB[N,P]3ZX

Ø Medical and Surgical
B Respiratory System
C Extirpation   Definition: Taking or cutting out solid matter from a body part

Explanation: The solid matter may be an abnormal byproduct of a biological function or a foreign body; it may be imbedded in a body part or in the lumen of a tubular body part. The solid matter may or may not have been previously broken into pieces.

Body Part Character 4	Approach Character 5	Device Character 6	Qualifier Character 7

1 Trachea
  Cricoid cartilage
2 Carina
3 Main Bronchus, Right
  Bronchus intermedius
  Intermediate bronchus
4 Upper Lobe Bronchus, Right
5 Middle Lobe Bronchus, Right
6 Lower Lobe Bronchus, Right
7 Main Bronchus, Left
8 Upper Lobe Bronchus, Left
9 Lingula Bronchus
B Lower Lobe Bronchus, Left
C Upper Lung Lobe, Right
D Middle Lung Lobe, Right
F Lower Lung Lobe, Right
G Upper Lung Lobe, Left
H Lung Lingula
J Lower Lung Lobe, Left
K Lung, Right
L Lung, Left
M Lungs, Bilateral
	Ø Open
	3 Percutaneous
	4 Percutaneous Endoscopic
	7 Via Natural or Artificial Opening
	8 Via Natural or Artificial Opening Endoscopic
		Z No Device	Z No Qualifier

N Pleura, Right P Pleura, Left T Diaphragm	Ø Open 3 Percutaneous 4 Percutaneous Endoscopic	Z No Device	Z No Qualifier

Non-OR   ØBC[1,2,3,4,5,6,7,8,9,B][7,8]ZZ
Non-OR   ØBC[N,P]3ZZ

Non-OR Procedure   DRG Non-OR Procedure   Valid OR Procedure   HAC Associated Procedure   Combination Only   New/Revised April   New/Revised October

Ø	Medical and Surgical
B	Respiratory System
D	Extraction Definition: Pulling or stripping out or off all or a portion of a body part by the use of force
	Explanation: The qualifier DIAGNOSTIC is used to identify extraction procedures that are biopsies

Body Part Character 4	Approach Character 5	Device Character 6	Qualifier Character 7

1 Trachea
   Cricoid cartilage
2 Carina
3 Main Bronchus, Right
   Bronchus intermedius
   Intermediate bronchus
4 Upper Lobe Bronchus, Right
5 Middle Lobe Bronchus, Right
6 Lower Lobe Bronchus, Right
7 Main Bronchus, Left
8 Upper Lobe Bronchus, Left
9 Lingula Bronchus
B Lower Lobe Bronchus, Left
C Upper Lung Lobe, Right
D Middle Lung Lobe, Right
F Lower Lung Lobe, Right
G Upper Lung Lobe, Left
H Lung Lingula
J Lower Lung Lobe, Left
K Lung, Right
L Lung, Left
M Lungs, Bilateral
	4 Percutaneous Endoscopic
	8 Via Natural or Artificial Opening
	   Endoscopic
		Z No Device	X Diagnostic

N Pleura, Right P Pleura, Left	Ø Open 3 Percutaneous 4 Percutaneous Endoscopic	Z No Device	X Diagnostic Z No Qualifier

Non-OR ØBD[1,2,3,4,5,6,7,8,9,B,C,D,F,G,H,J,K,L,M][4,8]ZX

Ø	Medical and Surgical
B	Respiratory System
F	Fragmentation Definition: Breaking solid matter in a body part into pieces
	Explanation: Physical force (e.g., manual, ultrasonic) applied directly or indirectly is used to break the solid matter into pieces. The solid matter may be an abnormal byproduct of a biological function or a foreign body. The pieces of solid matter are not taken out.

Body Part Character 4	Approach Character 5	Device Character 6	Qualifier Character 7

1 Trachea   `NC`
   Cricoid cartilage
2 Carina   `NC`
3 Main Bronchus, Right   `NC`
   Bronchus intermedius
   Intermediate bronchus
4 Upper Lobe Bronchus, Right   `NC`
5 Middle Lobe Bronchus, Right   `NC`
6 Lower Lobe Bronchus, Right   `NC`
7 Main Bronchus, Left   `NC`
8 Upper Lobe Bronchus, Left   `NC`
9 Lingula Bronchus   `NC`
B Lower Lobe Bronchus, Left   `NC`
	Ø Open
	3 Percutaneous
	4 Percutaneous Endoscopic
	7 Via Natural or Artificial Opening
	8 Via Natural or Artificial Opening
	   Endoscopic
	X External
		Z No Device	Z No Qualifier

Non-OR ØBF[1,2,3,4,5,6,7,8,9,B]XZZ
Non-OR ØBF[3,4,5,6,7,8,9,B][7,8]ZZ
`NC`   ØBF[1,2,3,4,5,6,7,8,9,B]XZZ

Respiratory System (side)

Ø Medical and Surgical
B Respiratory System
H Insertion   Definition: Putting in a nonbiological appliance that monitors, assists, performs, or prevents a physiological function but does not physically take the place of a body part
Explanation: None

Body Part Character 4	Approach Character 5	Device Character 6	Qualifier Character 7
Ø Tracheobronchial Tree	Ø Open 3 Percutaneous 4 Percutaneous Endoscopic 7 Via Natural or Artificial Opening 8 Via Natural or Artificial Opening Endoscopic	1 Radioactive Element 2 Monitoring Device 3 Infusion Device D Intraluminal Device Y Other Device	Z No Qualifier
1 Trachea Cricoid cartilage	Ø Open	2 Monitoring Device D Intraluminal Device Y Other Device	Z No Qualifier
1 Trachea Cricoid cartilage	3 Percutaneous	D Intraluminal Device E Intraluminal Device, Endotracheal Airway Y Other Device	Z No Qualifier
1 Trachea Cricoid cartilage	4 Percutaneous Endoscopic	D Intraluminal Device Y Other Device	Z No Qualifier
1 Trachea Cricoid cartilage	7 Via Natural or Artificial Opening 8 Via Natural or Artificial Opening Endoscopic	2 Monitoring Device D Intraluminal Device E Intraluminal Device, Endotracheal Airway Y Other Device	Z No Qualifier
3 Main Bronchus, Right Bronchus intermedius Intermediate bronchus 4 Upper Lobe Bronchus, Right 5 Middle Lobe Bronchus, Right 6 Lower Lobe Bronchus, Right 7 Main Bronchus, Left 8 Upper Lobe Bronchus, Left 9 Lingula Bronchus B Lower Lobe Bronchus, Left	Ø Open 3 Percutaneous 4 Percutaneous Endoscopic 7 Via Natural or Artificial Opening 8 Via Natural or Artificial Opening Endoscopic	G Intraluminal Device, Endobronchial Valve	Z No Qualifier
K Lung, Right L Lung, Left	Ø Open 3 Percutaneous 4 Percutaneous Endoscopic 7 Via Natural or Artificial Opening 8 Via Natural or Artificial Opening Endoscopic	1 Radioactive Element 2 Monitoring Device 3 Infusion Device Y Other Device	Z No Qualifier
Q Pleura	Ø Open 3 Percutaneous 4 Percutaneous Endoscopic 7 Via Natural or Artificial Opening 8 Via Natural or Artificial Opening Endoscopic	Y Other Device	Z No Qualifier
T Diaphragm	Ø Open 3 Percutaneous 4 Percutaneous Endoscopic	2 Monitoring Device M Diaphragmatic Pacemaker Lead Y Other Device	Z No Qualifier
T Diaphragm	7 Via Natural or Artificial Opening 8 Via Natural or Artificial Opening Endoscopic	Y Other Device	Z No Qualifier

DRG Non-OR   ØBH[3,4,5,6,7,8,9,B]8GZ
Non-OR   ØBHØ3YZ
Non-OR   ØBHØ[7,8][2,3,D,Y]Z
Non-OR   ØBH13[E,Y]Z
Non-OR   ØBH1[7,8][2,D,E,Y]Z
Non-OR   ØBH[K,L]3YZ
Non-OR   ØBH[K,L]7[2,3,Y]Z
Non-OR   ØBH[K,L]8[2,3]Z
Non-OR   ØBHQ[3,7]YZ
Non-OR   ØBHT3YZ
Non-OR   ØBHT[7,8]YZ

Non-OR Procedure   DRG Non-OR Procedure   Valid OR Procedure   HAC Associated Procedure   Combination Only   New/Revised April   New/Revised October

Ø   **Medical and Surgical**
B   **Respiratory System**
J   **Inspection**   Definition: Visually and/or manually exploring a body part

Explanation: Visual exploration may be performed with or without optical instrumentation. Manual exploration may be performed directly or through intervening body layers.

Body Part Character 4	Approach Character 5	Device Character 6	Qualifier Character 7

Ø Tracheobronchial Tree
1 Trachea
   Cricoid cartilage
K Lung, Right
L Lung, Left
Q Pleura
T Diaphragm
	Ø Open
	3 Percutaneous
	4 Percutaneous Endoscopic
	7 Via Natural or Artificial Opening
	8 Via Natural or Artificial Opening
	   Endoscopic
	X External
		Z No Device	**Z** No Qualifier

Non-OR   ØBJ[Ø,K,L,Q,T][3,7,8,X]ZZ
Non-OR   ØBJ1[3,4,7,8,X]ZZ

Ø   **Medical and Surgical**
B   **Respiratory System**
L   **Occlusion**   Definition: Completely closing an orifice or the lumen of a tubular body part

Explanation: The orifice can be a natural orifice or an artificially created orifice

Body Part Character 4	Approach Character 5	Device Character 6	Qualifier Character 7

1 Trachea
   Cricoid cartilage
2 Carina
3 Main Bronchus, Right
   Bronchus intermedius
   Intermediate bronchus
4 Upper Lobe Bronchus, Right
5 Middle Lobe Bronchus, Right
6 Lower Lobe Bronchus, Right
7 Main Bronchus, Left
8 Upper Lobe Bronchus, Left
9 Lingula Bronchus
B Lower Lobe Bronchus, Left
	Ø Open
	3 Percutaneous
	4 Percutaneous Endoscopic
		C Extraluminal Device
		D Intraluminal Device
		Z No Device
			Z No Qualifier

1 Trachea
   Cricoid cartilage
2 Carina
3 Main Bronchus, Right
   Bronchus intermedius
   Intermediate bronchus
4 Upper Lobe Bronchus, Right
5 Middle Lobe Bronchus, Right
6 Lower Lobe Bronchus, Right
7 Main Bronchus, Left
8 Upper Lobe Bronchus, Left
9 Lingula Bronchus
B Lower Lobe Bronchus, Left
	7 Via Natural or Artificial Opening
	8 Via Natural or Artificial Opening
	   Endoscopic
		D Intraluminal Device
		Z No Device
			Z No Qualifier

Ø   Medical and Surgical
B   Respiratory System
M   Reattachment   Definition: Putting back in or on all or a portion of a separated body part to its normal location or other suitable location

                          Explanation: Vascular circulation and nervous pathways may or may not be reestablished

Body Part Character 4	Approach Character 5	Device Character 6	Qualifier Character 7

1 Trachea
   Cricoid cartilage
2 Carina
3 Main Bronchus, Right
   Bronchus intermedius
   Intermediate bronchus
4 Upper Lobe Bronchus, Right
5 Middle Lobe Bronchus, Right
6 Lower Lobe Bronchus, Right
7 Main Bronchus, Left
8 Upper Lobe Bronchus, Left
9 Lingula Bronchus
B Lower Lobe Bronchus, Left
C Upper Lung Lobe, Right
D Middle Lung Lobe, Right
F Lower Lung Lobe, Right
G Upper Lung Lobe, Left
H Lung Lingula
J Lower Lung Lobe, Left
K Lung, Right
L Lung, Left
T Diaphragm
	Ø Open	Z No Device	Z No Qualifier

Ø   Medical and Surgical
B   Respiratory System
N   Release   Definition: Freeing a body part from an abnormal physical constraint by cutting or by the use of force

                          Explanation: Some of the restraining tissue may be taken out but none of the body part is taken out

Body Part Character 4	Approach Character 5	Device Character 6	Qualifier Character 7

1 Trachea
   Cricoid cartilage
2 Carina
3 Main Bronchus, Right
   Bronchus intermedius
   Intermediate bronchus
4 Upper Lobe Bronchus, Right
5 Middle Lobe Bronchus, Right
6 Lower Lobe Bronchus, Right
7 Main Bronchus, Left
8 Upper Lobe Bronchus, Left
9 Lingula Bronchus
B Lower Lobe Bronchus, Left
C Upper Lung Lobe, Right
D Middle Lung Lobe, Right
F Lower Lung Lobe, Right
G Upper Lung Lobe, Left
H Lung Lingula
J Lower Lung Lobe, Left
K Lung, Right
L Lung, Left
M Lungs, Bilateral
	Ø Open
	3 Percutaneous
	4 Percutaneous Endoscopic
	7 Via Natural or Artificial Opening
	8 Via Natural or Artificial Opening
	   Endoscopic
		Z No Device	Z No Qualifier

N Pleura, Right P Pleura, Left T Diaphragm	Ø Open 3 Percutaneous 4 Percutaneous Endoscopic	Z No Device	Z No Qualifier

Non-OR Procedure   DRG Non-OR Procedure   Valid OR Procedure   HAC Associated Procedure   Combination Only   New/Revised April   New/Revised October

348   ICD-10-PCS 2023

Ø   **Medical and Surgical**
B   **Respiratory System**
P   **Removal**   Definition: Taking out or off a device from a body part

Explanation: If a device is taken out and a similar device put in without cutting or puncturing the skin or mucous membrane, the procedure is coded to the root operation CHANGE. Otherwise, the procedure for taking out a device is coded to the root operation REMOVAL.

Body Part Character 4	Approach Character 5	Device Character 6	Qualifier Character 7
Ø Tracheobronchial Tree	Ø Open 3 Percutaneous 4 Percutaneous Endoscopic 7 Via Natural or Artificial Opening 8 Via Natural or Artificial Opening Endoscopic	Ø Drainage Device 1 Radioactive Element 2 Monitoring Device 3 Infusion Device 7 Autologous Tissue Substitute C Extraluminal Device D Intraluminal Device J Synthetic Substitute K Nonautologous Tissue Substitute Y Other Device	Z No Qualifier
Ø Tracheobronchial Tree	X External	Ø Drainage Device 1 Radioactive Element 2 Monitoring Device 3 Infusion Device D Intraluminal Device	Z No Qualifier
1 Trachea Cricoid cartilage	Ø Open 3 Percutaneous 4 Percutaneous Endoscopic 7 Via Natural or Artificial Opening 8 Via Natural or Artificial Opening Endoscopic	Ø Drainage Device 2 Monitoring Device 7 Autologous Tissue Substitute C Extraluminal Device D Intraluminal Device F Tracheostomy Device J Synthetic Substitute K Nonautologous Tissue Substitute	Z No Qualifier
1 Trachea Cricoid cartilage	X External	Ø Drainage Device 2 Monitoring Device D Intraluminal Device F Tracheostomy Device	Z No Qualifier
K Lung, Right L Lung, Left	Ø Open 3 Percutaneous 4 Percutaneous Endoscopic 7 Via Natural or Artificial Opening 8 Via Natural or Artificial Opening Endoscopic	Ø Drainage Device 1 Radioactive Element 2 Monitoring Device 3 Infusion Device Y Other Device	Z No Qualifier
K Lung, Right L Lung, Left	X External	Ø Drainage Device 1 Radioactive Element 2 Monitoring Device 3 Infusion Device	Z No Qualifier
Q Pleura	Ø Open 3 Percutaneous 4 Percutaneous Endoscopic 7 Via Natural or Artificial Opening 8 Via Natural or Artificial Opening Endoscopic	Ø Drainage Device 1 Radioactive Element 2 Monitoring Device Y Other Device	Z No Qualifier
Q Pleura	X External	Ø Drainage Device 1 Radioactive Element 2 Monitoring Device	Z No Qualifier
T Diaphragm	Ø Open 3 Percutaneous 4 Percutaneous Endoscopic 7 Via Natural or Artificial Opening 8 Via Natural or Artificial Opening Endoscopic	Ø Drainage Device 2 Monitoring Device 7 Autologous Tissue Substitute J Synthetic Substitute K Nonautologous Tissue Substitute M Diaphragmatic Pacemaker Lead Y Other Device	Z No Qualifier
T Diaphragm	X External	Ø Drainage Device 2 Monitoring Device M Diaphragmatic Pacemaker Lead	Z No Qualifier

Non-OR ØBPØ[3,4]YZ	Non-OR ØBPL7[Ø,2,3,Y]Z
Non-OR ØBPØ[7,8][Ø,2,3,D,Y]Z	Non-OR ØBPL8[Ø,2,3]Z
Non-OR ØBPØX[Ø,1,2,3,D]Z	Non-OR ØBP[K,L]X[Ø,1,2,3]Z
Non-OR ØBP1[Ø,3,4]FZ	Non-OR ØBPQ[Ø,3,4,7,8][Ø,1,2,]Z
Non-OR ØBP1[7,8][Ø,2,D,F]Z	Non-OR ØBPQ[3,7]YZ
Non-OR ØBP1X[Ø,2,D,F]Z	Non-OR ØBPQX[Ø,1,2]Z
Non-OR ØBP[K,L]3YZ	Non-OR ØBPT3YZ
Non-OR ØBPK7[Ø,1,2,3,Y]Z	Non-OR ØBPT[7,8][Ø,2,Y]Z
Non-OR ØBPK8[Ø,1,2,3]Z	Non-OR ØBPTX[Ø,2,M]Z

NC Noncovered Procedure   LC Limited Coverage   QA Questionable OB Admit   NT New Tech Add-on   ✚ Combination Member   ♂ Male   ♀ Female

ICD-10-PCS 2023   349

ØBP–ØBP

Ø **Medical and Surgical**
B **Respiratory System**
Q **Repair**   Definition: Restoring, to the extent possible, a body part to its normal anatomic structure and function
                 Explanation: Used only when the method to accomplish the repair is not one of the other root operations

Body Part Character 4	Approach Character 5	Device Character 6	Qualifier Character 7
1 Trachea 　Cricoid cartilage **2** Carina **3** Main Bronchus, Right 　Bronchus intermedius 　Intermediate bronchus **4** Upper Lobe Bronchus, Right **5** Middle Lobe Bronchus, Right **6** Lower Lobe Bronchus, Right **7** Main Bronchus, Left **8** Upper Lobe Bronchus, Left **9** Lingula Bronchus **B** Lower Lobe Bronchus, Left **C** Upper Lung Lobe, Right **D** Middle Lung Lobe, Right **F** Lower Lung Lobe, Right **G** Upper Lung Lobe, Left **H** Lung Lingula **J** Lower Lung Lobe, Left **K** Lung, Right **L** Lung, Left **M** Lungs, Bilateral	**Ø** Open **3** Percutaneous **4** Percutaneous Endoscopic **7** Via Natural or Artificial Opening **8** Via Natural or Artificial Opening 　Endoscopic	**Z** No Device	**Z** No Qualifier
N Pleura, Right **P** Pleura, Left **T** Diaphragm	**Ø** Open **3** Percutaneous **4** Percutaneous Endoscopic	**Z** No Device	**Z** No Qualifier

Ø **Medical and Surgical**
B **Respiratory System**
R **Replacement**   Definition: Putting in or on biological or synthetic material that physically takes the place and/or function of all or a portion of a body part
                    Explanation: The body part may have been taken out or replaced, or may be taken out, physically eradicated, or rendered nonfunctional during the REPLACEMENT procedure. A REMOVAL procedure is coded for taking out the device used in a previous replacement procedure.

Body Part Character 4	Approach Character 5	Device Character 6	Qualifier Character 7
1 Trachea 　Cricoid cartilage **2** Carina **3** Main Bronchus, Right 　Bronchus intermedius 　Intermediate bronchus **4** Upper Lobe Bronchus, Right **5** Middle Lobe Bronchus, Right **6** Lower Lobe Bronchus, Right **7** Main Bronchus, Left **8** Upper Lobe Bronchus, Left **9** Lingula Bronchus **B** Lower Lobe Bronchus, Left **T** Diaphragm	**Ø** Open **4** Percutaneous Endoscopic	**7** Autologous Tissue Substitute **J** Synthetic Substitute **K** Nonautologous Tissue Substitute	**Z** No Qualifier

Non-OR Procedure　　DRG Non-OR Procedure　　Valid OR Procedure　　HAC Associated Procedure　　Combination Only　　New/Revised April　　New/Revised October

350   ICD-10-PCS 2023

Ø Medical and Surgical
B Respiratory System
S Reposition   Definition: Moving to its normal location, or other suitable location, all or a portion of a body part

Explanation: The body part is moved to a new location from an abnormal location, or from a normal location where it is not functioning correctly. The body part may or may not be cut out or off to be moved to the new location.

Body Part Character 4	Approach Character 5	Device Character 6	Qualifier Character 7

1 Trachea
   Cricoid cartilage
2 Carina
3 Main Bronchus, Right
   Bronchus intermedius
   Intermediate bronchus
4 Upper Lobe Bronchus, Right
5 Middle Lobe Bronchus, Right
6 Lower Lobe Bronchus, Right
7 Main Bronchus, Left
8 Upper Lobe Bronchus, Left
9 Lingula Bronchus
B Lower Lobe Bronchus, Left
C Upper Lung Lobe, Right
D Middle Lung Lobe, Right
F Lower Lung Lobe, Right
G Upper Lung Lobe, Left
H Lung Lingula
J Lower Lung Lobe, Left
K Lung, Right
L Lung, Left
T Diaphragm
	Ø Open	Z No Device	Z No Qualifier

Ø Medical and Surgical
B Respiratory System
T Resection   Definition: Cutting out or off, without replacement, all of a body part

Explanation: None

Body Part Character 4	Approach Character 5	Device Character 6	Qualifier Character 7

1 Trachea
   Cricoid cartilage
2 Carina
3 Main Bronchus, Right
   Bronchus intermedius
   Intermediate bronchus
4 Upper Lobe Bronchus, Right
5 Middle Lobe Bronchus, Right
6 Lower Lobe Bronchus, Right
7 Main Bronchus, Left
8 Upper Lobe Bronchus, Left
9 Lingula Bronchus
B Lower Lobe Bronchus, Left
C Upper Lung Lobe, Right
D Middle Lung Lobe, Right
F Lower Lung Lobe, Right
G Upper Lung Lobe, Left
H Lung Lingula
J Lower Lung Lobe, Left
K Lung, Right
L Lung, Left
M Lungs, Bilateral
T Diaphragm
	Ø Open
	4 Percutaneous Endoscopic
		Z No Device	Z No Qualifier

Ø   Medical and Surgical
B   Respiratory System
U   Supplement   Definition: Putting in or on biological or synthetic material that physically reinforces and/or augments the function of a portion of a body part

Explanation: The biological material is non-living, or is living and from the same individual. The body part may have been previously replaced, and the SUPPLEMENT procedure is performed to physically reinforce and/or augment the function of the replaced body part.

Body Part Character 4	Approach Character 5	Device Character 6	Qualifier Character 7

1   Trachea
     Cricoid cartilage
2   Carina
3   Main Bronchus, Right
     Bronchus intermedius
     Intermediate bronchus
4   Upper Lobe Bronchus, Right
5   Middle Lobe Bronchus, Right
6   Lower Lobe Bronchus, Right
7   Main Bronchus, Left
8   Upper Lobe Bronchus, Left
9   Lingula Bronchus
B   Lower Lobe Bronchus, Left
	Ø Open
	4 Percutaneous Endoscopic
	8 Via Natural or Artificial Opening
	     Endoscopic
		7 Autologous Tissue Substitute
		J Synthetic Substitute
		K Nonautologous Tissue Substitute
			Z No Qualifier

T Diaphragm	Ø Open 4 Percutaneous Endoscopic	7 Autologous Tissue Substitute J Synthetic Substitute K Nonautologous Tissue Substitute	Z No Qualifier

Ø   Medical and Surgical
B   Respiratory System
V   Restriction   Definition: Partially closing an orifice or the lumen of a tubular body part

Explanation: The orifice can be a natural orifice or an artificially created orifice

Body Part Character 4	Approach Character 5	Device Character 6	Qualifier Character 7

1   Trachea
     Cricoid cartilage
2   Carina
3   Main Bronchus, Right
     Bronchus intermedius
     Intermediate bronchus
4   Upper Lobe Bronchus, Right
5   Middle Lobe Bronchus, Right
6   Lower Lobe Bronchus, Right
7   Main Bronchus, Left
8   Upper Lobe Bronchus, Left
9   Lingula Bronchus
B   Lower Lobe Bronchus, Left
	Ø Open
	3 Percutaneous
	4 Percutaneous Endoscopic
		C Extraluminal Device
		D Intraluminal Device
		Z No Device
			Z No Qualifier

1   Trachea
     Cricoid cartilage
2   Carina
3   Main Bronchus, Right
     Bronchus intermedius
     Intermediate bronchus
4   Upper Lobe Bronchus, Right
5   Middle Lobe Bronchus, Right
6   Lower Lobe Bronchus, Right
7   Main Bronchus, Left
8   Upper Lobe Bronchus, Left
9   Lingula Bronchus
B   Lower Lobe Bronchus, Left
	7 Via Natural or Artificial Opening
	8 Via Natural or Artificial Opening
	     Endoscopic
		D Intraluminal Device
		Z No Device
			Z No Qualifier

Non-OR Procedure   DRG Non-OR Procedure   Valid OR Procedure   HAC Associated Procedure   Combination Only   New/Revised April   New/Revised October

352   ICD-10-PCS 2023

Ø   **Medical and Surgical**
B   **Respiratory System**
W   **Revision**   Definition: Correcting, to the extent possible, a portion of a malfunctioning device or the position of a displaced device

                  Explanation: Revision can include correcting a malfunctioning or displaced device by taking out or putting in components of the device such as a screw or pin

Body Part Character 4	Approach Character 5	Device Character 6	Qualifier Character 7
Ø Tracheobronchial Tree	Ø Open 3 Percutaneous 4 Percutaneous Endoscopic 7 Via Natural or Artificial Opening 8 Via Natural or Artificial Opening Endoscopic	Ø Drainage Device 2 Monitoring Device 3 Infusion Device 7 Autologous Tissue Substitute C Extraluminal Device D Intraluminal Device J Synthetic Substitute K Nonautologous Tissue Substitute Y Other Device	Z No Qualifier
Ø Tracheobronchial Tree	X External	Ø Drainage Device 2 Monitoring Device 3 Infusion Device 7 Autologous Tissue Substitute C Extraluminal Device D Intraluminal Device J Synthetic Substitute K Nonautologous Tissue Substitute	Z No Qualifier

1   Trachea
    Cricoid cartilage
	Ø Open
	3 Percutaneous
	4 Percutaneous Endoscopic
	7 Via Natural or Artificial Opening
	8 Via Natural or Artificial Opening
	    Endoscopic
	X External
		Ø Drainage Device
		2 Monitoring Device
		7 Autologous Tissue Substitute
		C Extraluminal Device
		D Intraluminal Device
		F Tracheostomy Device
		J Synthetic Substitute
		K Nonautologous Tissue Substitute
			Z No Qualifier

K Lung, Right L Lung, Left	Ø Open 3 Percutaneous 4 Percutaneous Endoscopic 7 Via Natural or Artificial Opening 8 Via Natural or Artificial Opening Endoscopic	Ø Drainage Device 2 Monitoring Device 3 Infusion Device Y Other Device	Z No Qualifier
K Lung, Right L Lung, Left	X External	Ø Drainage Device 2 Monitoring Device 3 Infusion Device	Z No Qualifier
Q Pleura	Ø Open 3 Percutaneous 4 Percutaneous Endoscopic 7 Via Natural or Artificial Opening 8 Via Natural or Artificial Opening Endoscopic	Ø Drainage Device 2 Monitoring Device Y Other Device	Z No Qualifier
Q Pleura	X External	Ø Drainage Device 2 Monitoring Device	Z No Qualifier
T Diaphragm	Ø Open 3 Percutaneous 4 Percutaneous Endoscopic 7 Via Natural or Artificial Opening 8 Via Natural or Artificial Opening Endoscopic	Ø Drainage Device 2 Monitoring Device 7 Autologous Tissue Substitute J Synthetic Substitute K Nonautologous Tissue Substitute M Diaphragmatic Pacemaker Lead Y Other Device	Z No Qualifier
T Diaphragm	X External	Ø Drainage Device 2 Monitoring Device 7 Autologous Tissue Substitute J Synthetic Substitute K Nonautologous Tissue Substitute M Diaphragmatic Pacemaker Lead	Z No Qualifier

Non-OR   ØBWØ[3,4]YZ
Non-OR   ØBWØ[7,8][2,3,D,Y]Z
Non-OR   ØBWØX[Ø,2,3,7,C,D,J,K]Z
Non-OR   ØBW1X[Ø,2,7,C,D,F,J,K]Z
Non-OR   ØBW[K,L]3YZ
Non-OR   ØBW[K,L]7[Ø,2,3,Y]Z
Non-OR   ØBW[K,L]8[Ø,2,3]Z
Non-OR   ØBW[K,L]X[Ø,2,3]Z
Non-OR   ØBWQ[Ø,3,4,7,8][Ø,2]Z
Non-OR   ØBWQ[Ø,3,7]YZ
Non-OR   ØBWQX[Ø,2]Z
Non-OR   ØBWT[3,7,8]YZ
Non-OR   ØBWTX[Ø,2,7,J,K,M]Z

NC Noncovered Procedure   LC Limited Coverage   QA Questionable OB Admit   NT New Tech Add-on   ⊞ Combination Member   ♂ Male   ♀ Female

Ø   Medical and Surgical
B   Respiratory System
Y   Transplantation   Definition: Putting in or on all or a portion of a living body part taken from another individual or animal to physically take the place and/or
                         function of all or a portion of a similar body part

                     Explanation: The native body part may or may not be taken out, and the transplanted body part may take over all or a portion of its function

Body Part Character 4		Approach Character 5	Device Character 6	Qualifier Character 7
C Upper Lung Lobe, Right	LC	Ø Open	Z No Device	Ø Allogeneic
D Middle Lung Lobe, Right	LC			1 Syngeneic
F Lower Lung Lobe, Right	LC			2 Zooplastic
G Upper Lung Lobe, Left	LC			
H Lung Lingula	LC			
J Lower Lung Lobe, Left	LC			
K Lung, Right	LC			
L Lung, Left	LC			
M Lungs, Bilateral	LC			

LC   ØBY[C,D,F,G,H,J,K,L,M]ØZ[Ø,1,2]

Non-OR Procedure   DRG Non-OR Procedure   Valid OR Procedure   HAC Associated Procedure   Combination Only   New/Revised April   New/Revised October

354   ICD-10-PCS 2023

Mouth and Throat 0C0–0CX

Character Meanings

This Character Meaning table is provided as a guide to assist the user in the identification of character members that may be found in this section of code tables. It **SHOULD NOT** be used to build a PCS code.

Operation–Character 3		Body Part–Character 4		Approach–Character 5		Device–Character 6		Qualifier–Character 7	
0	Alteration	0	Upper Lip	0	Open	0	Drainage Device	0	Single
2	Change	1	Lower Lip	3	Percutaneous	1	Radioactive Element	1	Multiple
5	Destruction	2	Hard Palate	4	Percutaneous Endoscopic	5	External Fixation Device	2	All
7	Dilation	3	Soft Palate	7	Via Natural or Artificial Opening	7	Autologous Tissue Substitute	X	Diagnostic
9	Drainage	4	Buccal Mucosa	8	Via Natural or Artificial Opening Endoscopic	B	Intraluminal Device, Airway	Z	No Qualifier
B	Excision	5	Upper Gingiva	X	External	C	Extraluminal Device		
C	Extirpation	6	Lower Gingiva			D	Intraluminal Device		
D	Extraction	7	Tongue			J	Synthetic Substitute		
F	Fragmentation	8	Parotid Gland, Right			K	Nonautologous Tissue Substitute		
H	Insertion	9	Parotid Gland, Left			Y	Other Device		
J	Inspection	A	Salivary Gland			Z	No Device		
L	Occlusion	B	Parotid Duct, Right						
M	Reattachment	C	Parotid Duct, Left						
N	Release	D	Sublingual Gland, Right						
P	Removal	F	Sublingual Gland, Left						
Q	Repair	G	Submaxillary Gland, Right						
R	Replacement	H	Submaxillary Gland, Left						
S	Reposition	J	Minor Salivary Gland						
T	Resection	M	Pharynx						
U	Supplement	N	Uvula						
V	Restriction	P	Tonsils						
W	Revision	Q	Adenoids						
X	Transfer	R	Epiglottis						
		S	Larynx						
		T	Vocal Cord, Right						
		V	Vocal Cord, Left						
		W	Upper Tooth						
		X	Lower Tooth						
		Y	Mouth and Throat						

AHA Coding Clinic for table 0C9
2017, 2Q, 16   Incision and drainage of floor of mouth

AHA Coding Clinic for table 0CB
2017, 2Q, 16   Excision of floor of mouth
2016, 3Q, 28   Lingual tonsillectomy, tongue base excision and epiglottopexy
2016, 2Q, 19   Biopsy of the base of tongue
2014, 3Q, 21   Superficial parotidectomy

AHA Coding Clinic for table 0CC
2016, 2Q, 20   Sialendoscopy with stone removal

AHA Coding Clinic for table 0CH
2020, 4Q, 43-44   Insertion of radioactive element

AHA Coding Clinic for table 0CQ
2017, 1Q, 20   Preparatory nasal adhesion repair before definitive cleft palate repair

AHA Coding Clinic for table 0CR
2014, 3Q, 25   Excision of soft palate with placement of surgical obturator
2014, 2Q, 5   Oasis acellular matrix graft
2014, 2Q, 6   Composite grafting (synthetic versus nonautologous tissue substitute)

AHA Coding Clinic for table 0CS
2022, 2Q, 24   Palatoplasty with intravelar veloplasty
2016, 3Q, 28   Lingual tonsillectomy, tongue base excision and epiglottopexy

AHA Coding Clinic for table 0CT
2016, 2Q, 12   Resection of malignant neoplasm of infratemporal fossa
2014, 3Q, 21   Superficial parotidectomy
2014, 3Q, 23   Le Fort I osteotomy

Salivary Glands

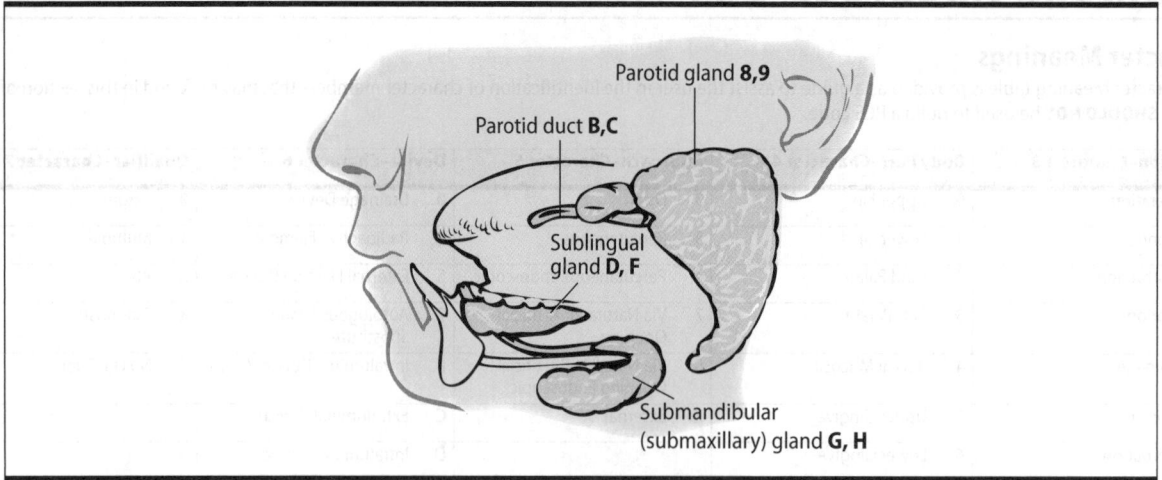

Parotid gland **8,9**

Parotid duct **B,C**

Sublingual gland **D, F**

Submandibular (submaxillary) gland **G, H**

Oral Anatomy

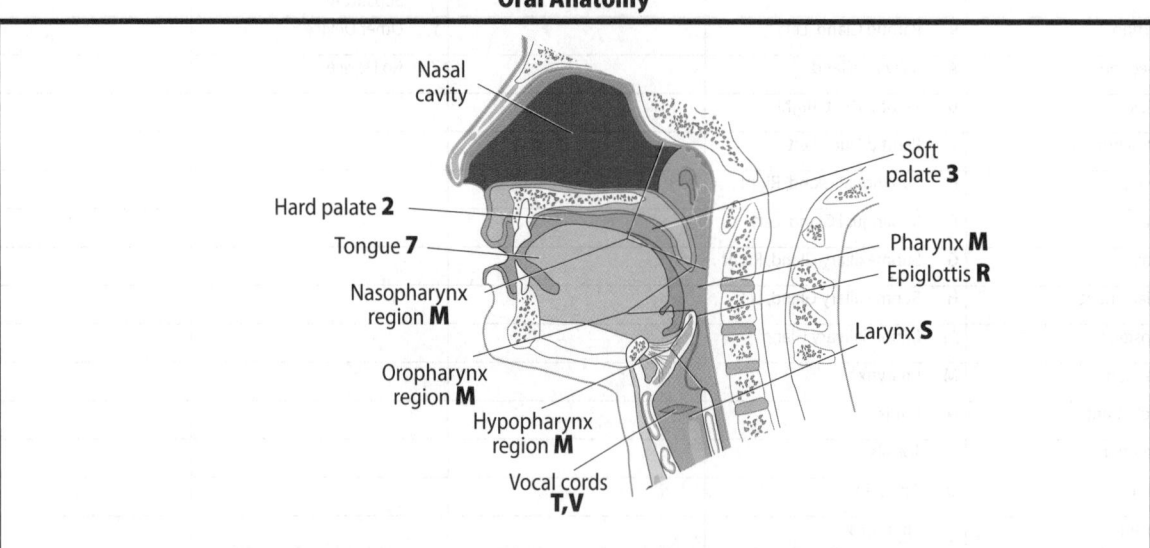

Nasal cavity

Hard palate **2**

Tongue **7**

Nasopharynx region **M**

Oropharynx region **M**

Hypopharynx region **M**

Vocal cords **T,V**

Soft palate **3**

Pharynx **M**

Epiglottis **R**

Larynx **S**

Mouth Frontal View (Upper)

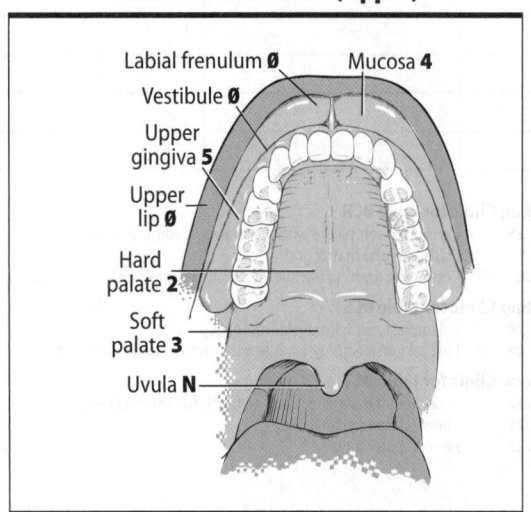

Labial frenulum **Ø**

Vestibule **Ø**

Upper gingiva **5**

Upper lip **Ø**

Hard palate **2**

Soft palate **3**

Uvula **N**

Mucosa **4**

Mouth Frontal View (Lower)

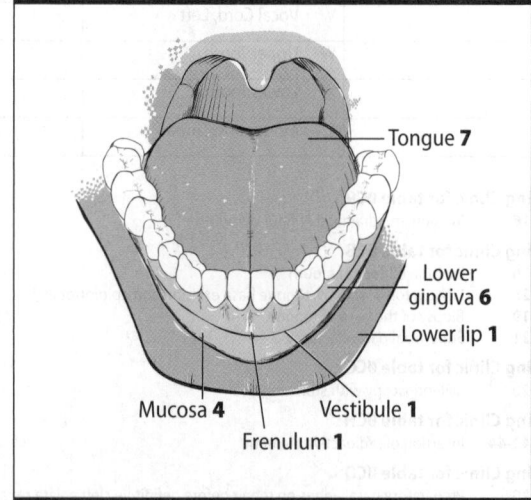

Tongue **7**

Lower gingiva **6**

Lower lip **1**

Vestibule **1**

Frenulum **1**

Mucosa **4**

Ø **Medical and Surgical**
C **Mouth and Throat**
Ø **Alteration**   Definition: Modifying the anatomic structure of a body part without affecting the function of the body part
          Explanation: Principal purpose is to improve appearance

Body Part Character 4	Approach Character 5	Device Character 6	Qualifier Character 7

Ø Upper Lip
   Frenulum labii superioris
   Labial gland
   Vermilion border
1 Lower Lip
   Frenulum labii inferioris
   Labial gland
   Vermilion border
	X External	**7 Autologous Tissue Substitute**
		J Synthetic Substitute
		K Nonautologous Tissue Substitute
		Z No Device
			Z No Qualifier

Ø **Medical and Surgical**
C **Mouth and Throat**
2 **Change**   Definition: Taking out or off a device from a body part and putting back an identical or similar device in or on the same body part without cutting or puncturing the skin or a mucous membrane
          Explanation: All CHANGE procedures are coded using the approach EXTERNAL

Body Part Character 4	Approach Character 5	Device Character 6	Qualifier Character 7

A Salivary Gland
S Larynx
   Aryepiglottic fold
   Arytenoid cartilage
   Corniculate cartilage
   Cuneiform cartilage
   False vocal cord
   Glottis
   Rima glottidis
   Thyroid cartilage
   Ventricular fold
Y Mouth and Throat
	X External	**Ø Drainage Device**
		Y Other Device
			Z No Qualifier

Non-OR All body part, approach, device, and qualifier values

Mouth and Throat

Ø Medical and Surgical
C Mouth and Throat
5 Destruction   Definition: Physical eradication of all or a portion of a body part by the direct use of energy, force, or a destructive agent
                     Explanation: None of the body part is physically taken out

Body Part Character 4		Approach Character 5	Device Character 6	Qualifier Character 7

Ø Upper Lip
   Frenulum labii superioris
   Labial gland
   Vermilion border
1 Lower Lip
   Frenulum labii inferioris
   Labial gland
   Vermilion border
2 Hard Palate
3 Soft Palate
4 Buccal Mucosa
   Buccal gland
   Molar gland
   Palatine gland
	5 Upper Gingiva
	6 Lower Gingiva
	7 Tongue
	   Frenulum linguae
	N Uvula
	   Palatine uvula
	P Tonsils
	   Palatine tonsil
	Q Adenoids
	   Pharyngeal tonsil
		Ø Open
		3 Percutaneous
		X External
			Z No Device	Z No Qualifier

8 Parotid Gland, Right
9 Parotid Gland, Left
B Parotid Duct, Right
   Stensen's duct
C Parotid Duct, Left
   See B Parotid Duct, Right
D Sublingual Gland, Right
	F Sublingual Gland, Left
	G Submaxillary Gland, Right
	   Submandibular gland
	H Submaxillary Gland, Left
	   See G Submaxillary Gland, Right
	J Minor Salivary Gland
	   Anterior lingual gland
		Ø Open
		3 Percutaneous
			Z No Device	Z No Qualifier

M Pharynx
   Base of tongue
   Hypopharynx
   Laryngopharynx
   Lingual tonsil
   Oropharynx
   Piriform recess (sinus)
   Tongue, base of
R Epiglottis
   Glossoepiglottic fold
	S Larynx
	   Aryepiglottic fold
	   Arytenoid cartilage
	   Corniculate cartilage
	   Cuneiform cartilage
	   False vocal cord
	   Glottis
	   Rima glottidis
	   Thyroid cartilage
	   Ventricular fold
	T Vocal Cord, Right
	   Vocal fold
	V Vocal Cord, Left
	   See T Vocal Cord, Right
		Ø Open
		3 Percutaneous
		4 Percutaneous Endoscopic
		7 Via Natural or Artificial Opening
		8 Via Natural or Artificial Opening Endoscopic
			Z No Device	Z No Qualifier

W Upper Tooth X Lower Tooth		Ø Open X External	Z No Device	Ø Single 1 Multiple 2 All

Non-OR   ØC5[5,6][Ø,3,X]ZZ
Non-OR   ØC5[W,X][Ø,X]Z[Ø,1,2]

Ø Medical and Surgical
C Mouth and Throat
7 Dilation   Definition: Expanding an orifice or the lumen of a tubular body part
               Explanation: The orifice can be a natural orifice or an artificially created orifice. Accomplished by stretching a tubular body part using intraluminal pressure or by cutting part of the orifice or wall of the tubular body part.

Body Part Character 4	Approach Character 5	Device Character 6	Qualifier Character 7

B Parotid Duct, Right
   Stensen's duct
C Parotid Duct, Left
   See B Parotid Duct, Right
	Ø Open
	3 Percutaneous
	7 Via Natural or Artificial Opening
		D Intraluminal Device
		Z No Device
			Z No Qualifier

M Pharynx
   Base of tongue
   Hypopharynx
   Laryngopharynx
   Lingual tonsil
   Oropharynx
   Piriform recess (sinus)
   Tongue, base of
	7 Via Natural or Artificial Opening
	8 Via Natural or Artificial Opening Endoscopic
		D Intraluminal Device
		Z No Device
			Z No Qualifier

S Larynx
   Aryepiglottic fold
   Arytenoid cartilage
   Corniculate cartilage
   Cuneiform cartilage
   False vocal cord
   Glottis
   Rima glottidis
   Thyroid cartilage
   Ventricular fold
	Ø Open
	3 Percutaneous
	4 Percutaneous Endoscopic
	7 Via Natural or Artificial Opening
	8 Via Natural or Artificial Opening Endoscopic
		D Intraluminal Device
		Z No Device
			Z No Qualifier

Non-OR   ØC7[B,C][Ø,3,7][D,Z]Z
Non-OR   ØC7M[7,8][D,Z]Z

Non-OR Procedure   DRG Non-OR Procedure   Valid OR Procedure   HAC Associated Procedure   Combination Only   New/Revised April   New/Revised October

Ø Medical and Surgical
C Mouth and Throat
9 Drainage   Definition: Taking or letting out fluids and/or gases from a body part

Explanation: The qualifier DIAGNOSTIC is used to identify drainage procedures that are biopsies

Body Part Character 4		Approach Character 5	Device Character 6	Qualifier Character 7

Ø Upper Lip
  Frenulum labii superioris
  Labial gland
  Vermilion border
1 Lower Lip
  Frenulum labii inferioris
  Labial gland
  Vermilion border
2 Hard Palate
3 Soft Palate
4 Buccal Mucosa
  Buccal gland
  Molar gland
  Palatine gland
	5 Upper Gingiva
	6 Lower Gingiva
	7 Tongue
	  Frenulum linguae
	N Uvula
	  Palatine uvula
	P Tonsils
	  Palatine tonsil
	Q Adenoids
	  Pharyngeal tonsil
		Ø Open
		3 Percutaneous
		X External
			Ø Drainage Device	Z No Qualifier

Ø Upper Lip
  Frenulum labii superioris
  Labial gland
  Vermilion border
1 Lower Lip
  Frenulum labii inferioris
  Labial gland
  Vermilion border
2 Hard Palate
3 Soft Palate
4 Buccal Mucosa
  Buccal gland
  Molar gland
  Palatine gland
	5 Upper Gingiva
	6 Lower Gingiva
	7 Tongue
	  Frenulum linguae
	N Uvula
	  Palatine uvula
	P Tonsils
	  Palatine tonsil
	Q Adenoids
	  Pharyngeal tonsil
		Ø Open
		3 Percutaneous
		X External
			Z No Device	X Diagnostic
				Z No Qualifier

8 Parotid Gland, Right
9 Parotid Gland, Left
B Parotid Duct, Right
  Stensen's duct
C Parotid Duct, Left
  See B Parotid Duct, Right
D Sublingual Gland, Right
	F Sublingual Gland, Left
	G Submaxillary Gland, Right
	  Submandibular gland
	H Submaxillary Gland, Left
	  See G Submaxillary Gland, Right
	J Minor Salivary Gland
	  Anterior lingual gland
		Ø Open
		3 Percutaneous
			Ø Drainage Device	Z No Qualifier

8 Parotid Gland, Right
9 Parotid Gland, Left
B Parotid Duct, Right
  Stensen's duct
C Parotid Duct, Left
  See B Parotid Duct, Right
	D Sublingual Gland, Right
	F Sublingual Gland, Left
	G Submaxillary Gland, Right
	  Submandibular gland
	H Submaxillary Gland, Left
	  See G Submaxillary Gland, Right
	J Minor Salivary Gland
	  Anterior lingual gland
		Ø Open
		3 Percutaneous
			Z No Device	X Diagnostic
				Z No Qualifier

M Pharynx
  Base of tongue
  Hypopharynx
  Laryngopharynx
  Lingual tonsil
  Oropharynx
  Piriform recess (sinus)
  Tongue, base of
R Epiglottis
  Glossoepiglottic fold
	S Larynx
	  Aryepiglottic fold
	  Arytenoid cartilage
	  Corniculate cartilage
	  Cuneiform cartilage
	  False vocal cord
	  Glottis
	  Rima glottidis
	  Thyroid cartilage
	  Ventricular fold
	T Vocal Cord, Right
	  Vocal fold
	V Vocal Cord, Left
	  See T Vocal Cord, Right
		Ø Open
		3 Percutaneous
		4 Percutaneous Endoscopic
		7 Via Natural or Artificial Opening
		8 Via Natural or Artificial Opening Endoscopic
			Ø Drainage Device	Z No Qualifier

Non-OR	ØC9[Ø,1,2,3,4,7,N,P,Q]3ØZ
Non-OR	ØC9[5,6][Ø,3,X]ØZ
Non-OR	ØC9[Ø,1,4][Ø,3,X]ZX
Non-OR	ØC9[Ø,1,2,3,4,7,N,P,Q]3ZZ
Non-OR	ØC9[5,6][Ø,3,X]Z[X,Z]
Non-OR	ØC97[3,X]ZX
Non-OR	ØC9[8,9,B,C,D,F,G,H,J][Ø,3]ØZ
Non-OR	ØC9[8,9,B,C,D,F,G,H,J]3ZX
Non-OR	ØC9[8,9,G,H]3ZZ
Non-OR	ØC9[B,C,D, F,J][Ø,3]ZZ
Non-OR	ØC9[M,R,S,T,V]3ØZ

ØC9 Continued on next page

Mouth and Throat

0C9 Continued

0   **Medical and Surgical**
C   **Mouth and Throat**
9   **Drainage**   Definition: Taking or letting out fluids and/or gases from a body part

            Explanation: The qualifier DIAGNOSTIC is used to identify drainage procedures that are biopsies

Body Part Character 4		Approach Character 5	Device Character 6	Qualifier Character 7

M Pharynx
   Base of tongue
   Hypopharynx
   Laryngopharynx
   Lingual tonsil
   Oropharynx
   Piriform recess (sinus)
   Tongue, base of
R Epiglottis
   Glossoepiglottic fold
	S Larynx
	   Aryepiglottic fold
	   Arytenoid cartilage
	   Corniculate cartilage
	   Cuneiform cartilage
	   False vocal cord
	   Glottis
	   Rima glottidis
	   Thyroid cartilage
	   Ventricular fold
	T Vocal Cord, Right
	   Vocal fold
	V Vocal Cord, Left
	   See T Vocal Cord, Right
		0 Open
		3 Percutaneous
		4 Percutaneous Endoscopic
		7 Via Natural or Artificial Opening
		8 Via Natural or Artificial Opening Endoscopic
			Z No Device	**X** Diagnostic
				Z No Qualifier

W Upper Tooth **X** Lower Tooth		**0** Open **X** External	**0** Drainage Device **Z** No Device	**0** Single **1** Multiple **2** All

Non-OR	0C9M[0,3,4,7,8]ZX
Non-OR	0C9[M,R,S,T,V]3ZZ
Non-OR	0C9[R,S,T,V][3,4,7,8]ZX
Non-OR	0C9[W,X][0,X][0,Z][0,1,2]

0   **Medical and Surgical**
C   **Mouth and Throat**
B   **Excision**   Definition: Cutting out or off, without replacement, a portion of a body part

            Explanation: The qualifier DIAGNOSTIC is used to identify excision procedures that are biopsies

Body Part Character 4		Approach Character 5	Device Character 6	Qualifier Character 7

0 Upper Lip
   Frenulum labii superioris
   Labial gland
   Vermilion border
1 Lower Lip
   Frenulum labii inferioris
   Labial gland
   Vermilion border
2 Hard Palate
3 Soft Palate
4 Buccal Mucosa
   Buccal gland
   Molar gland
   Palatine gland
	5 Upper Gingiva
	6 Lower Gingiva
	7 Tongue
	   Frenulum linguae
	N Uvula
	   Palatine uvula
	P Tonsils
	   Palatine tonsil
	Q Adenoids
	   Pharyngeal tonsil
		0 Open
		3 Percutaneous
		X External
			Z No Device	**X** Diagnostic
				Z No Qualifier

8 Parotid Gland, Right
9 Parotid Gland, Left
B Parotid Duct, Right
   Stensen's duct
C Parotid Duct, Left
   See B Parotid Duct, Right
D Sublingual Gland, Right
	F Sublingual Gland, Left
	G Submaxillary Gland, Right
	   Submandibular gland
	H Submaxillary Gland, Left
	   See G Submaxillary Gland, Right
	J Minor Salivary Gland
	   Anterior lingual gland
		0 Open
		3 Percutaneous
			Z No Device	**X** Diagnostic
				Z No Qualifier

M Pharynx
   Base of tongue
   Hypopharynx
   Laryngopharynx
   Lingual tonsil
   Oropharynx
   Piriform recess (sinus)
   Tongue, base of
R Epiglottis
   Glossoepiglottic fold
	S Larynx
	   Aryepiglottic fold
	   Arytenoid cartilage
	   Corniculate cartilage
	   Cuneiform cartilage
	   False vocal cord
	   Glottis
	   Rima glottidis
	   Thyroid cartilage
	   Ventricular fold
	T Vocal Cord, Right
	   Vocal fold
	V Vocal Cord, Left
	   See T Vocal Cord, Right
		0 Open
		3 Percutaneous
		4 Percutaneous Endoscopic
		7 Via Natural or Artificial Opening
		8 Via Natural or Artificial Opening Endoscopic
			Z No Device	**X** Diagnostic
				Z No Qualifier

W Upper Tooth **X** Lower Tooth		**0** Open **X** External	**Z** No Device	**0** Single **1** Multiple **2** All

Non-OR	0CB[0,1,4][0,3,X]ZX
Non-OR	0CB[5,6][0,3,X]Z[X,Z]
Non-OR	0CB7[3,X]ZX
Non-OR	0CB[8,9,B,C,D,F,G,H,J]3ZX

Non-OR	0CBM[0,3,4,7,8]ZX
Non-OR	0CB[R,S,T,V][3,4,7,8]ZX
Non-OR	0CB[W,X][0,X]Z[0,1,2]

Non-OR Procedure   DRG Non-OR Procedure   Valid OR Procedure   HAC Associated Procedure   Combination Only   New/Revised April   New/Revised October

360   ICD-10-PCS 2023

Ø   **Medical and Surgical**
C   **Mouth and Throat**
C   **Extirpation**   Definition: Taking or cutting out solid matter from a body part

                              Explanation: The solid matter may be an abnormal byproduct of a biological function or a foreign body; it may be imbedded in a body part or in the lumen of a tubular body part. The solid matter may or may not have been previously broken into pieces.

Body Part Character 4		Approach Character 5	Device Character 6	Qualifier Character 7

Ø Upper Lip
   Frenulum labii superioris
   Labial gland
   Vermilion border
1 Lower Lip
   Frenulum labii inferioris
   Labial gland
   Vermilion border
2 Hard Palate
3 Soft Palate
4 Buccal Mucosa
   Buccal gland
   Molar gland
   Palatine gland
	5 Upper Gingiva
	6 Lower Gingiva
	7 Tongue
	   Frenulum linguae
	N Uvula
	   Palatine uvula
	P Tonsils
	   Palatine tonsil
	Q Adenoids
	   Pharyngeal tonsil
		Ø Open
		3 Percutaneous
		X External
			Z No Device	**Z** No Qualifier

8 Parotid Gland, Right
9 Parotid Gland, Left
B Parotid Duct, Right
   Stensen's duct
C Parotid Duct, Left
   See B Parotid Duct, Right
D Sublingual Gland, Right
	F Sublingual Gland, Left
	G Submaxillary Gland, Right
	   Submandibular gland
	H Submaxillary Gland, Left
	   See G Submaxillary Gland, Right
	J Minor Salivary Gland
	   Anterior lingual gland
		Ø Open
		3 Percutaneous
			Z No Device	**Z** No Qualifier

M Pharynx
   Base of tongue
   Hypopharynx
   Laryngopharynx
   Lingual tonsil
   Oropharynx
   Piriform recess (sinus)
   Tongue, base of
R Epiglottis
   Glossoepiglottic fold
	S Larynx
	   Aryepiglottic fold
	   Arytenoid cartilage
	   Corniculate cartilage
	   Cuneiform cartilage
	   False vocal cord
	   Glottis
	   Rima glottidis
	   Thyroid cartilage
	   Ventricular fold
	T Vocal Cord, Right
	   Vocal fold
	V Vocal Cord, Left
	   See T Vocal Cord, Right
		Ø Open
		3 Percutaneous
		4 Percutaneous Endoscopic
		7 Via Natural or Artificial Opening
		8 Via Natural or Artificial Opening Endoscopic
			Z No Device	**Z** No Qualifier

W Upper Tooth **X** Lower Tooth		**Ø** Open **X** External	**Z** No Device	**Ø** Single **1** Multiple **2** All

Non-OR	ØCC[Ø,1,2,3,4,7,N,P,Q]XZZ
Non-OR	ØCC[5,6][Ø,3,X]ZZ
Non-OR	ØCC[8,9,G,H]3ZZ
Non-OR	ØCC[B,C,D,F,J][Ø,3]ZZ
Non-OR	ØCC[M,S][7,8]ZZ
Non-OR	ØCC[W,X][Ø,X]Z[Ø,1,2]

Ø   **Medical and Surgical**
C   **Mouth and Throat**
D   **Extraction**   Definition: Pulling or stripping out or off all or a portion of a body part by the use of force

                              Explanation: The qualifier DIAGNOSTIC is used to identify extraction procedures that are biopsies

Body Part Character 4	Approach Character 5	Device Character 6	Qualifier Character 7

T Vocal Cord, Right
   Vocal fold
V Vocal Cord, Left
   See T Vocal Cord, Right
	Ø Open
	3 Percutaneous
	4 Percutaneous Endoscopic
	7 Via Natural or Artificial Opening
	8 Via Natural or Artificial Opening Endoscopic
		Z No Device	**Z** No Qualifier

W Upper Tooth **X** Lower Tooth	**X** External	**Z** No Device	**Ø** Single **1** Multiple **2** All

Non-OR	ØCD[W,X]XZ[Ø,1,2]

NC Noncovered Procedure   **LC** Limited Coverage   **QA** Questionable OB Admit   **NT** New Tech Add-on   ⊞ Combination Member   ♂ Male   ♀ Female

ICD-10-PCS 2023   361

Mouth and Throat

Ø   **Medical and Surgical**
C   **Mouth and Throat**
F   **Fragmentation**   Definition: Breaking solid matter in a body part into pieces

Explanation: Physical force (e.g., manual, ultrasonic) applied directly or indirectly is used to break the solid matter into pieces. The solid matter may be an abnormal byproduct of a biological function or a foreign body. The pieces of solid matter are not taken out.

Body Part Character 4	Approach Character 5	Device Character 6	Qualifier Character 7

B   Parotid Duct, Right   **NC**
    Stensen's duct
C   Parotid Duct, Left   **NC**
    See B Parotid Duct, Right
	Ø Open
	3 Percutaneous
	7 Via Natural or Artificial Opening
	X External
		Z No Device	**Z** No Qualifier

Non-OR **NC**	All body part, approach, device, and qualifier values ØCF[B,C]XZZ

Ø   **Medical and Surgical**
C   **Mouth and Throat**
H   **Insertion**   Definition: Putting in a nonbiological appliance that monitors, assists, performs, or prevents a physiological function but does not physically take the place of a body part

Explanation: None

Body Part Character 4	Approach Character 5	Device Character 6	Qualifier Character 7
7 Tongue Frenulum linguae	**Ø** Open **3** Percutaneous **X** External	**1** Radioactive Element	**Z** No Qualifier

A   Salivary Gland
S   Larynx
    Aryepiglottic fold
    Arytenoid cartilage
    Corniculate cartilage
    Cuneiform cartilage
    False vocal cord
    Glottis
    Rima glottidis
    Thyroid cartilage
    Ventricular fold
	Ø Open
	3 Percutaneous
	7 Via Natural or Artificial Opening
	8 Via Natural or Artificial Opening Endoscopic
		1 Radioactive Element
		Y Other Device
			Z No Qualifier

Y Mouth and Throat	**Ø** Open **3** Percutaneous	**1** Radioactive Element **Y** Other Device	**Z** No Qualifier
Y Mouth and Throat	**7** Via Natural or Artificial Opening **8** Via Natural or Artificial Opening Endoscopic	**1** Radioactive Element **B** Intraluminal Device, Airway **Y** Other Device	**Z** No Qualifier

Non-OR	ØCH[A,S]Ø1Z
Non-OR	ØCHSØYZ
Non-OR	ØCH[A,S][3,7,8][1,Y]Z
Non-OR	ØCHY[Ø,3][1,Y]Z
Non-OR	ØCHY[7,8][1,B,Y]Z

Ø   **Medical and Surgical**
C   **Mouth and Throat**
J   **Inspection**   Definition: Visually and/or manually exploring a body part

Explanation: Visual exploration may be performed with or without optical instrumentation. Manual exploration may be performed directly or through intervening body layers.

Body Part Character 4	Approach Character 5	Device Character 6	Qualifier Character 7
A Salivary Gland	**Ø** Open **3** Percutaneous **X** External	**Z** No Device	**Z** No Qualifier

S   Larynx
    Aryepiglottic fold
    Arytenoid cartilage
    Corniculate cartilage
    Cuneiform cartilage
    False vocal cord
    Glottis
    Rima glottidis
    Thyroid cartilage
    Ventricular fold
Y   Mouth and Throat
	Ø Open
	3 Percutaneous
	4 Percutaneous Endoscopic
	7 Via Natural or Artificial Opening
	8 Via Natural or Artificial Opening Endoscopic
	X External
		Z No Device	**Z** No Qualifier

Non-OR	All body part, approach, device, and qualifier values

Non-OR Procedure   DRG Non-OR Procedure   Valid OR Procedure   HAC Associated Procedure   Combination Only   New/Revised April   New/Revised October

362   ICD-10-PCS 2023

Ø   Medical and Surgical
C   Mouth and Throat
L   Occlusion   Definition: Completely closing an orifice or the lumen of a tubular body part

Explanation: The orifice can be a natural orifice or an artificially created orifice

Body Part Character 4	Approach Character 5	Device Character 6	Qualifier Character 7

B Parotid Duct, Right
   Stensen's duct
C Parotid Duct, Left
   See B Parotid Duct, Right
	Ø Open
	3 Percutaneous
	4 Percutaneous Endoscopic
		C Extraluminal Device
		D Intraluminal Device
		Z No Device
			Z No Qualifier

B Parotid Duct, Right
   Stensen's duct
C Parotid Duct, Left
   See B Parotid Duct, Right
	7 Via Natural or Artificial Opening
	8 Via Natural or Artificial Opening Endoscopic
		D Intraluminal Device
		Z No Device
			Z No Qualifier

Ø   Medical and Surgical
C   Mouth and Throat
M   Reattachment   Definition: Putting back in or on all or a portion of a separated body part to its normal location or other suitable location

Explanation: Vascular circulation and nervous pathways may or may not be reestablished

Body Part Character 4	Approach Character 5	Device Character 6	Qualifier Character 7

Ø Upper Lip
   Frenulum labii superioris
   Labial gland
   Vermilion border
1 Lower Lip
   Frenulum labii inferioris
   Labial gland
   Vermilion border
3 Soft Palate
7 Tongue
   Frenulum linguae
N Uvula
   Palatine uvula
	Ø Open	**Z** No Device	**Z** No Qualifier

W Upper Tooth **X** Lower Tooth	**Ø** Open **X** External	**Z** No Device	**Ø** Single **1** Multiple **2** All

Non-OR   ØCM[W,X][Ø,X]Z[Ø,1,2]

NC Noncovered Procedure   LC Limited Coverage   QA Questionable OB Admit   NT New Tech Add-on   ⊞ Combination Member   ♂ Male   ♀ Female

ICD-10-PCS 2023   363

Mouth and Throat

Ø   Medical and Surgical
C   Mouth and Throat
N   Release   Definition: Freeing a body part from an abnormal physical constraint by cutting or by the use of force
           Explanation: Some of the restraining tissue may be taken out but none of the body part is taken out

Body Part Character 4	Approach Character 5	Device Character 6	Qualifier Character 7
Ø Upper Lip Frenulum labii superioris Labial gland Vermilion border **1 Lower Lip** Frenulum labii inferioris Labial gland Vermilion border **2 Hard Palate** **3 Soft Palate** **4 Buccal Mucosa** Buccal gland Molar gland Palatine gland **5 Upper Gingiva** **6 Lower Gingiva** **7 Tongue** Frenulum linguae **N Uvula** Palatine uvula **P Tonsils** Palatine tonsil **Q Adenoids** Pharyngeal tonsil	**Ø Open** **3 Percutaneous** **X External**	**Z No Device**	**Z No Qualifier**
8 Parotid Gland, Right **9 Parotid Gland, Left** **B Parotid Duct, Right** Stensen's duct **C Parotid Duct, Left** *See B Parotid Duct, Right* **D Sublingual Gland, Right** **F Sublingual Gland, Left** **G Submaxillary Gland, Right** Submandibular gland **H Submaxillary Gland, Left** *See G Submaxillary Gland, Right* **J Minor Salivary Gland** Anterior lingual gland	**Ø Open** **3 Percutaneous**	**Z No Device**	**Z No Qualifier**
M Pharynx Base of tongue Hypopharynx Laryngopharynx Lingual tonsil Oropharynx Piriform recess (sinus) Tongue, base of **R Epiglottis** Glossoepiglottic fold **S Larynx** Aryepiglottic fold Arytenoid cartilage Corniculate cartilage Cuneiform cartilage False vocal cord Glottis Rima glottidis Thyroid cartilage Ventricular fold **T Vocal Cord, Right** Vocal fold **V Vocal Cord, Left** *See T Vocal Cord, Right*	**Ø Open** **3 Percutaneous** **4 Percutaneous Endoscopic** **7 Via Natural or Artificial Opening** **8 Via Natural or Artificial Opening Endoscopic**	**Z No Device**	**Z No Qualifier**
W Upper Tooth **X Lower Tooth**	**Ø Open** **X External**	**Z No Device**	**Ø Single** **1 Multiple** **2 All**

Non-OR   ØCN[Ø,1,5,6,7][Ø,3,X]ZZ
Non-OR   ØCN[W,X][Ø,X]Z[Ø,1,2]

0   **Medical and Surgical**
C   **Mouth and Throat**
P   **Removal**   Definition: Taking out or off a device from a body part

Explanation: If a device is taken out and a similar device put in without cutting or puncturing the skin or mucous membrane, the procedure is coded to the root operation CHANGE. Otherwise, the procedure for taking out a device is coded to the root operation REMOVAL.

Body Part Character 4	Approach Character 5	Device Character 6	Qualifier Character 7
A Salivary Gland	**0** Open **3** Percutaneous	**0** Drainage Device **C** Extraluminal Device **Y** Other Device	**Z** No Qualifier
A Salivary Gland	**7** Via Natural or Artificial Opening **8** Via Natural or Artificial Opening Endoscopic	**Y** Other Device	**Z** No Qualifier

S Larynx
  Aryepiglottic fold
  Arytenoid cartilage
  Corniculate cartilage
  Cuneiform cartilage
  False vocal cord
  Glottis
  Rima glottidis
  Thyroid cartilage
  Ventricular fold
	0 Open
	3 Percutaneous
	7 Via Natural or Artificial Opening
	8 Via Natural or Artificial Opening Endoscopic
		0 Drainage Device
		7 Autologous Tissue Substitute
		D Intraluminal Device
		J Synthetic Substitute
		K Nonautologous Tissue Substitute
		Y Other Device
			Z No Qualifier

S Larynx
  Aryepiglottic fold
  Arytenoid cartilage
  Corniculate cartilage
  Cuneiform cartilage
  False vocal cord
  Glottis
  Rima glottidis
  Thyroid cartilage
  Ventricular fold
	X External	**0** Drainage Device
		7 Autologous Tissue Substitute
		D Intraluminal Device
		J Synthetic Substitute
		K Nonautologous Tissue Substitute
			Z No Qualifier

Y Mouth and Throat	**0** Open **3** Percutaneous **7** Via Natural or Artificial Opening **8** Via Natural or Artificial Opening Endoscopic	**0** Drainage Device **1** Radioactive Element **7** Autologous Tissue Substitute **D** Intraluminal Device **J** Synthetic Substitute **K** Nonautologous Tissue Substitute **Y** Other Device	**Z** No Qualifier
Y Mouth and Throat	**X** External	**0** Drainage Device **1** Radioactive Element **7** Autologous Tissue Substitute **D** Intraluminal Device **J** Synthetic Substitute **K** Nonautologous Tissue Substitute	**Z** No Qualifier

Non-OR	0CPA[0,3][0,C,Y]Z
Non-OR	0CPA[7,8]YZ
Non-OR	0CPS3YZ
Non-OR	0CPS[7,8][0,D,Y]Z
Non-OR	0CPSX[0,7,D,J,K]Z
Non-OR	0CPY3YZ
Non-OR	0CPY[7,8][0,D,Y]Z
Non-OR	0CPYX[0,1,7,D,J,K]Z

NC Noncovered Procedure   **LC** Limited Coverage   **QA** Questionable OB Admit   **NT** New Tech Add-on   ⊞ Combination Member   ♂ Male   ♀ Female

ICD-10-PCS 2023

365

0CP–0CP

Mouth and Throat

Ø   **Medical and Surgical**
C   **Mouth and Throat**
Q   **Repair**   Definition: Restoring, to the extent possible, a body part to its normal anatomic structure and function
                        Explanation: Used only when the method to accomplish the repair is not one of the other root operations

Body Part Character 4	Approach Character 5	Device Character 6	Qualifier Character 7

Ø **Upper Lip**
     Frenulum labii superioris
     Labial gland
     Vermilion border
1 **Lower Lip**
     Frenulum labii inferioris
     Labial gland
     Vermilion border
2 **Hard Palate**
3 **Soft Palate**
4 **Buccal Mucosa**
     Buccal gland
     Molar gland
     Palatine gland
5 **Upper Gingiva**
6 **Lower Gingiva**
7 **Tongue**
     Frenulum linguae
N **Uvula**
     Palatine uvula
P **Tonsils**
     Palatine tonsil
Q **Adenoids**
     Pharyngeal tonsil
	Ø **Open**
	3 **Percutaneous**
	X **External**
		Z **No Device**	Z **No Qualifier**

8 **Parotid Gland, Right**
9 **Parotid Gland, Left**
B **Parotid Duct, Right**
     Stensen's duct
C **Parotid Duct, Left**
     See B Parotid Duct, Right
D **Sublingual Gland, Right**
F **Sublingual Gland, Left**
G **Submaxillary Gland, Right**
     Submandibular gland
H **Submaxillary Gland, Left**
     See G Submaxillary Gland, Right
J **Minor Salivary Gland**
     Anterior lingual gland
	Ø **Open**
	3 **Percutaneous**
		Z **No Device**	Z **No Qualifier**

M **Pharynx**
     Base of tongue
     Hypopharynx
     Laryngopharynx
     Lingual tonsil
     Oropharynx
     Piriform recess (sinus)
     Tongue, base of
R **Epiglottis**
     Glossoepiglottic fold
S **Larynx**
     Aryepiglottic fold
     Arytenoid cartilage
     Corniculate cartilage
     Cuneiform cartilage
     False vocal cord
     Glottis
     Rima glottidis
     Thyroid cartilage
     Ventricular fold
T **Vocal Cord, Right**
     Vocal fold
V **Vocal Cord, Left**
     See T Vocal Cord, Right
	Ø **Open**
	3 **Percutaneous**
	4 **Percutaneous Endoscopic**
	7 **Via Natural or Artificial Opening**
	8 **Via Natural or Artificial Opening
	    Endoscopic**
		Z **No Device**	Z **No Qualifier**

W **Upper Tooth** X **Lower Tooth**	Ø **Open** X **External**	Z **No Device**	Ø **Single** 1 **Multiple** 2 **All**

Non-OR	ØCQ[Ø,1,4,7]XZZ
Non-OR	ØCQ[5,6][Ø,3,X]ZZ
Non-OR	ØCQ[W,X][Ø,X]Z[Ø,1,2]

Non-OR Procedure   DRG Non-OR Procedure   Valid OR Procedure   HAC Associated Procedure   Combination Only   New/Revised April   New/Revised October

366   ICD-10-PCS 2023

Ø   **Medical and Surgical**
C   **Mouth and Throat**
R   **Replacement**   Definition: Putting in or on biological or synthetic material that physically takes the place and/or function of all or a portion of a body part
                          Explanation: The body part may have been taken out or replaced, or may be taken out, physically eradicated, or rendered nonfunctional during
                          the REPLACEMENT procedure. A REMOVAL procedure is coded for taking out the device used in a previous replacement procedure.

Body Part Character 4	Approach Character 5	Device Character 6	Qualifier Character 7

Ø **Upper Lip**
   Frenulum labii superioris
   Labial gland
   Vermilion border
1 **Lower Lip**
   Frenulum labii inferioris
   Labial gland
   Vermilion border
2 **Hard Palate**
3 **Soft Palate**
4 **Buccal Mucosa**
   Buccal gland
   Molar gland
   Palatine gland
5 **Upper Gingiva**
6 **Lower Gingiva**
7 **Tongue**
   Frenulum linguae
N **Uvula**
   Palatine uvula
	Ø Open
	3 Percutaneous
	X External
		7 Autologous Tissue Substitute
		J Synthetic Substitute
		K Nonautologous Tissue Substitute
			Z No Qualifier

B **Parotid Duct, Right**
   Stensen's duct
C **Parotid Duct, Left**
   See B Parotid Duct, Right
	Ø Open
	3 Percutaneous
		7 Autologous Tissue Substitute
		J Synthetic Substitute
		K Nonautologous Tissue Substitute
			Z No Qualifier

M **Pharynx**
   Base of tongue
   Hypopharynx
   Laryngopharynx
   Lingual tonsil
   Oropharynx
   Piriform recess (sinus)
   Tongue, base of
R **Epiglottis**
   Glossoepiglottic fold
S **Larynx**
   Aryepiglottic fold
   Arytenoid cartilage
   Corniculate cartilage
   Cuneiform cartilage
   False vocal cord
   Glottis
   Rima glottidis
   Thyroid cartilage
   Ventricular fold
T **Vocal Cord, Right**
   Vocal fold
V **Vocal Cord, Left**
   See T Vocal Cord, Right
	Ø Open
	7 Via Natural or Artificial Opening
	8 Via Natural or Artificial Opening Endoscopic
		7 Autologous Tissue Substitute
		J Synthetic Substitute
		K Nonautologous Tissue Substitute
			Z No Qualifier

W **Upper Tooth** **X** **Lower Tooth**	**Ø** Open **X** External	**7** Autologous Tissue Substitute **J** Synthetic Substitute **K** Nonautologous Tissue Substitute	**Ø** Single **1** Multiple **2** All

Non-OR   ØCR[W,X][Ø,X][7,J,K][Ø,1,2]

NC Noncovered Procedure   **LC** Limited Coverage   **QA** Questionable OB Admit   **NT** New Tech Add-on   ⊞ Combination Member   ♂ Male   ♀ Female

ICD-10-PCS 2023   367

Ø Medical and Surgical
C Mouth and Throat
S Reposition   Definition: Moving to its normal location, or other suitable location, all or a portion of a body part

Explanation: The body part is moved to a new location from an abnormal location, or from a normal location where it is not functioning correctly. The body part may or may not be cut out or off to be moved to the new location.

Body Part Character 4	Approach Character 5	Device Character 6	Qualifier Character 7
Ø Upper Lip Frenulum labii superioris Labial gland Vermilion border **1 Lower Lip** Frenulum labii inferioris Labial gland Vermilion border **2 Hard Palate** **3 Soft Palate** **7 Tongue** Frenulum linguae **N Uvula** Palatine uvula	**Ø Open** **X External**	**Z No Device**	**Z No Qualifier**
B Parotid Duct, Right Stensen's duct **C Parotid Duct, Left** *See B Parotid Duct, Right*	**Ø Open** **3 Percutaneous**	**Z No Device**	**Z No Qualifier**
R Epiglottis Glossoepiglottic fold **T Vocal Cord, Right** Vocal fold **V Vocal Cord, Left** *See T Vocal Cord, Right*	**Ø Open** **7 Via Natural or Artificial Opening** **8 Via Natural or Artificial Opening Endoscopic**	**Z No Device**	**Z No Qualifier**
W Upper Tooth **X Lower Tooth**	**Ø Open** **X External**	**5 External Fixation Device** **Z No Device**	**Ø Single** **1 Multiple** **2 All**

Non-OR   ØCS[W,X][Ø,X][5,Z][Ø,1,2]

Ø **Medical and Surgical**
C **Mouth and Throat**
T **Resection**   Definition: Cutting out or off, without replacement, all of a body part
            Explanation: None

Body Part Character 4	Approach Character 5	Device Character 6	Qualifier Character 7
Ø **Upper Lip** Frenulum labii superioris Labial gland Vermilion border **1** **Lower Lip** Frenulum labii inferioris Labial gland Vermilion border **2** **Hard Palate** **3** **Soft Palate** **7** **Tongue** Frenulum linguae **N** **Uvula** Palatine uvula **P** **Tonsils** Palatine tonsil **Q** **Adenoids** Pharyngeal tonsil	**Ø** Open **X** External	**Z** No Device	**Z** No Qualifier
8 **Parotid Gland, Right** **9** **Parotid Gland, Left** **B** **Parotid Duct, Right** Stensen's duct **C** **Parotid Duct, Left** See B Parotid Duct, Right **D** **Sublingual Gland, Right** **F** **Sublingual Gland, Left** **G** **Submaxillary Gland, Right** Submandibular gland **H** **Submaxillary Gland, Left** See G Submaxillary Gland, Right **J** **Minor Salivary Gland** Anterior lingual gland	**Ø** Open	**Z** No Device	**Z** No Qualifier
M **Pharynx** Base of tongue Hypopharynx Laryngopharynx Lingual tonsil Oropharynx Piriform recess (sinus) Tongue, base of **R** **Epiglottis** Glossoepiglottic fold **S** **Larynx** Aryepiglottic fold Arytenoid cartilage Corniculate cartilage Cuneiform cartilage False vocal cord Glottis Rima glottidis Thyroid cartilage Ventricular fold **T** **Vocal Cord, Right** Vocal fold **V** **Vocal Cord, Left** See T Vocal Cord, Right	**Ø** Open **4** Percutaneous Endoscopic **7** Via Natural or Artificial Opening **8** Via Natural or Artificial Opening Endoscopic	**Z** No Device	**Z** No Qualifier
W **Upper Tooth** **X** **Lower Tooth**	**Ø** Open	**Z** No Device	**Ø** Single **1** Multiple **2** All

Non-OR   ØCT[W,X]ØZ[Ø,1,2]

NC Noncovered Procedure   LC Limited Coverage   QA Questionable OB Admit   NT New Tech Add-on   ⊞ Combination Member   ♂ Male   ♀ Female

ICD-10-PCS 2023   **369**

Mouth and Throat

Ø   **Medical and Surgical**
C   **Mouth and Throat**
U   **Supplement**   Definition: Putting in or on biological or synthetic material that physically reinforces and/or augments the function of a portion of a body part
                         Explanation: The biological material is non-living, or is living and from the same individual. The body part may have been previously replaced, and the SUPPLEMENT procedure is performed to physically reinforce and/or augment the function of the replaced body part.

Body Part Character 4	Approach Character 5	Device Character 6	Qualifier Character 7

Ø Upper Lip
   Frenulum labii superioris
   Labial gland
   Vermilion border
1 Lower Lip
   Frenulum labii inferioris
   Labial gland
   Vermilion border
2 Hard Palate
3 Soft Palate
4 Buccal Mucosa
   Buccal gland
   Molar gland
   Palatine gland
5 Upper Gingiva
6 Lower Gingiva
7 Tongue
   Frenulum linguae
N Uvula
   Palatine uvula
	Ø Open
	3 Percutaneous
	X External
		7 Autologous Tissue Substitute
		J Synthetic Substitute
		K Nonautologous Tissue Substitute
			Z No Qualifier

M Pharynx
   Base of tongue
   Hypopharynx
   Laryngopharynx
   Lingual tonsil
   Oropharynx
   Piriform recess (sinus)
   Tongue, base of
R Epiglottis
   Glossoepiglottic fold
S Larynx
   Aryepiglottic fold
   Arytenoid cartilage
   Corniculate cartilage
   Cuneiform cartilage
   False vocal cord
   Glottis
   Rima glottidis
   Thyroid cartilage
   Ventricular fold
T Vocal Cord, Right
   Vocal fold
V Vocal Cord, Left
   See T Vocal Cord, Right
	Ø Open
	7 Via Natural or Artificial Opening
	8 Via Natural or Artificial Opening
	   Endoscopic
		7 Autologous Tissue Substitute
		J Synthetic Substitute
		K Nonautologous Tissue Substitute
			Z No Qualifier

Non-OR   ØCU2[Ø,3]JZ

Ø   **Medical and Surgical**
C   **Mouth and Throat**
V   **Restriction**   Definition: Partially closing an orifice or the lumen of a tubular body part
               Explanation: The orifice can be a natural orifice or an artificially created orifice

Body Part Character 4	Approach Character 5	Device Character 6	Qualifier Character 7

B Parotid Duct, Right
   Stensen's duct
C Parotid Duct, Left
   See B Parotid Duct, Right
	Ø Open
	3 Percutaneous
		C Extraluminal Device
		D Intraluminal Device
		Z No Device
			Z No Qualifier

B Parotid Duct, Right
   Stensen's duct
C Parotid Duct, Left
   See B Parotid Duct, Right
	7 Via Natural or Artificial Opening
	8 Via Natural or Artificial Opening
	   Endoscopic
		D Intraluminal Device
		Z No Device
			Z No Qualifier

Non-OR Procedure   DRG Non-OR Procedure   Valid OR Procedure   HAC Associated Procedure   Combination Only   New/Revised April   New/Revised October

370   ICD-10-PCS 2023

0   **Medical and Surgical**
C   **Mouth and Throat**
W   **Revision**   Definition: Correcting, to the extent possible, a portion of a malfunctioning device or the position of a displaced device

                      Explanation: Revision can include correcting a malfunctioning or displaced device by taking out or putting in components of the device such as a screw or pin

Body Part Character 4	Approach Character 5	Device Character 6	Qualifier Character 7
A Salivary Gland	**0** Open **3** Percutaneous	**0** Drainage Device **C** Extraluminal Device **Y** Other Device	**Z** No Qualifier
A Salivary Gland	**7** Via Natural or Artificial Opening **8** Via Natural or Artificial Opening Endoscopic	**Y** Other Device	**Z** No Qualifier
A Salivary Gland	**X** External	**0** Drainage Device **C** Extraluminal Device	**Z** No Qualifier

S   Larynx
    Aryepiglottic fold
    Arytenoid cartilage
    Corniculate cartilage
    Cuneiform cartilage
    False vocal cord
    Glottis
    Rima glottidis
    Thyroid cartilage
    Ventricular fold
	0 Open
	3 Percutaneous
	7 Via Natural or Artificial Opening
	8 Via Natural or Artificial Opening Endoscopic
		0 Drainage Device
		7 Autologous Tissue Substitute
		D Intraluminal Device
		J Synthetic Substitute
		K Nonautologous Tissue Substitute
		Y Other Device
			Z No Qualifier

S   Larynx
    Aryepiglottic fold
    Arytenoid cartilage
    Corniculate cartilage
    Cuneiform cartilage
    False vocal cord
    Glottis
    Rima glottidis
    Thyroid cartilage
    Ventricular fold
	X External	**0** Drainage Device
		7 Autologous Tissue Substitute
		D Intraluminal Device
		J Synthetic Substitute
		K Nonautologous Tissue Substitute
			Z No Qualifier

Y Mouth and Throat	**0** Open **3** Percutaneous **7** Via Natural or Artificial Opening **8** Via Natural or Artificial Opening Endoscopic	**0** Drainage Device **1** Radioactive Element **7** Autologous Tissue Substitute **D** Intraluminal Device **J** Synthetic Substitute **K** Nonautologous Tissue Substitute **Y** Other Device	**Z** No Qualifier
Y Mouth and Throat	**X** External	**0** Drainage Device **1** Radioactive Element **7** Autologous Tissue Substitute **D** Intraluminal Device **J** Synthetic Substitute **K** Nonautologous Tissue Substitute	**Z** No Qualifier

Non-OR	0CWA[0,3][0,C,Y]Z
Non-OR	0CWA[7,8]YZ
Non-OR	0CWAX[0,C]Z
Non-OR	0CWS[3,7,8]YZ
Non-OR	0CWSX[0,7,D,J,K]Z
Non-OR	0CWY07Z
Non-OR	0CWY[3,7,8]YZ
Non-OR	0CWYX[0,1,7,D,J,K]Z

NC Noncovered Procedure   **LC** Limited Coverage   **QA** Questionable OB Admit   **NT** New Tech Add-on   ⊞ Combination Member   ♂ Male   ♀ Female

ICD-10-PCS 2023   371

Ø   **Medical and Surgical**
C   **Mouth and Throat**
X   **Transfer**   Definition: Moving, without taking out, all or a portion of a body part to another location to take over the function of all or a portion of a body part
                 Explanation: The body part transferred remains connected to its vascular and nervous supply

Body Part Character 4	Approach Character 5	Device Character 6	Qualifier Character 7

Ø   **Upper Lip**
    Frenulum labii superioris
    Labial gland
    Vermilion border
1   **Lower Lip**
    Frenulum labii inferioris
    Labial gland
    Vermilion border
3   **Soft Palate**
4   **Buccal Mucosa**
    Buccal gland
    Molar gland
    Palatine gland
5   **Upper Gingiva**
6   **Lower Gingiva**
7   **Tongue**
    Frenulum linguae
	Ø **Open**
	X **External**
		Z **No Device**	Z **No Qualifier**

Gastrointestinal System ØD1–ØDY

Character Meanings

This Character Meaning table is provided as a guide to assist the user in the identification of character members that may be found in this section of code tables. It **SHOULD NOT** be used to build a PCS code.

Operation–Character 3	Body Part–Character 4	Approach–Character 5	Device–Character 6	Qualifier–Character 7
1 Bypass	Ø Upper Intestinal Tract	Ø Open	Ø Drainage Device	Ø Allogeneic
2 Change	1 Esophagus, Upper	3 Percutaneous	1 Radioactive Element	1 Syngeneic
5 Destruction	2 Esophagus, Middle	4 Percutaneous Endoscopic	2 Monitoring Device	2 Zooplastic
7 Dilation	3 Esophagus, Lower	7 Via Natural or Artificial Opening	3 Infusion Device	3 Vertical OR Laser Interstitial Thermal Therapy
8 Division	4 Esophagogastric Junction	8 Via Natural or Artificial Opening Endoscopic	7 Autologous Tissue Substitute	4 Cutaneous
9 Drainage	5 Esophagus	F Via Natural or Artificial Opening with Percutaneous Endoscopic Assistance	B Intraluminal Device, Airway	5 Esophagus
B Excision	6 Stomach	X External	C Extraluminal Device	6 Stomach
C Extirpation	7 Stomach, Pylorus		D Intraluminal Device	7 Vagina
D Extraction	8 Small Intestine		J Synthetic Substitute	8 Small Intestine
F Fragmentation	9 Duodenum		K Nonautologous Tissue Substitute	9 Duodenum
H Insertion	A Jejunum		L Artificial Sphincter	A Jejunum
J Inspection	B Ileum		M Stimulator Lead	B Ileum OR Bladder
L Occlusion	C Ileocecal Valve		U Feeding Device	C Ureter, Right
M Reattachment	D Lower Intestinal Tract		Y Other Device	D Ureter, Left
N Release	E Large Intestine		Z No Device	E Large Intestine
P Removal	F Large Intestine, Right			F Ureters, Bilateral
Q Repair	G Large Intestine, Left			H Cecum
R Replacement	H Cecum			K Ascending Colon
S Reposition	J Appendix			L Transverse Colon
T Resection	K Ascending Colon			M Descending Colon
U Supplement	L Transverse Colon			N Sigmoid Colon
V Restriction	M Descending Colon			P Rectum
W Revision	N Sigmoid Colon			Q Anus
X Transfer	P Rectum			X Diagnostic
Y Transplantation	Q Anus			Z No Qualifier
	R Anal Sphincter			
	U Omentum			
	V Mesentery			
	W Peritoneum			

AHA Coding Clinic for Gastrointestinal System

2022, 1Q, 11	Procedures performed on a continuous vessel, ICD-10-PCS Guideline B4.1c

AHA Coding Clinic for table ØD1

2021, 1Q, 19	Kock pouch revision surgery
2019, 4Q, 29	Intestinal bypass
2017, 2Q, 17	Billroth II (distal gastrectomy and gastrojejunostomy)
2016, 2Q, 31	Laparoscopic biliopancreatic diversion with duodenal switch
2014, 4Q, 41	Abdominoperineal resection (APR) with flap closure of perineum and colostomy

AHA Coding Clinic for table ØD2

2022, 1Q, 45	Insertion, removal and replacement of endoluminal vacuum application
2019, 1Q, 26	Exchange of clogged gastrojejunostomy tube

AHA Coding Clinic for table ØD5

2017, 1Q, 34	Debulking of tumor and peritoneum ablation

AHA Coding Clinic for table ØD7

2020, 3Q, 45	Dilation versus drainage of perirectal cyst
2017, 3Q, 23	Laparoscopic pyloromyotomy
2014, 4Q, 40	Dilation of gastrojejunostomy anastomosis stricture

AHA Coding Clinic for table ØD8

2019, 2Q, 15	Reversal of Roux-en-Y bypass
2017, 3Q, 22	Laparoscopic esophagomyotomy (Heller type) and Toupet fundoplication
2017, 3Q, 23	Laparoscopic pyloromyotomy

AHA Coding Clinic for table ØD9

2020, 3Q, 45	Dilation versus drainage of perirectal cyst
2015, 2Q, 29	Insertion of nasogastric tube for drainage and feeding

AHA Coding Clinic for table ØDB

2021, 3Q, 28	Retrieval of capsule via small bowel excision
2021, 2Q, 11	Serosal injury with excision of small intestine
2021, 1Q, 20	Rectal suction biopsy
2021, 1Q, 22	Total proctocolectomy with creation of J-pouch
2019, 2Q, 15	Reversal of Roux-en-Y bypass
2019, 1Q, 3-8	Whipple procedure
2019, 1Q, 27	Excision of pelvic sidewall mass
2017, 2Q, 17	Billroth II (distal gastrectomy and gastrojejunostomy)
2017, 1Q, 16	Hepatic flexure versus transverse colon
2016, 3Q, 3-7	Stoma creation & takedown procedures
2016, 2Q, 31	Laparoscopic biliopancreatic diversion with duodenal switch
2016, 1Q, 22	Perineal proctectomy
2016, 1Q, 24	Endoscopic brush biopsy of esophagus
2014, 4Q, 40	Abdominoperineal resection (APR) with flap closure of perineum and colostomy
2014, 3Q, 28	Ileostomy takedown and parastomal hernia repair
2014, 3Q, 32	Pyloric-sparing Whipple procedure

AHA Coding Clinic for table ØDD

2021, 1Q, 20	Rectal suction biopsy
2017, 4Q, 41-42	Extraction procedures

AHA Coding Clinic for table ØDH

2022, 1Q, 44	Insertion, removal and replacement of endoluminal vacuum application
2020, 4Q, 43-44	Insertion of radioactive element
2020, 3Q, 43	Staged laparoscopic gastric conduit and placement of feeding tube
2019, 2Q, 18	Endoscopic wound VAC placement
2016, 3Q, 26	Insertion of gastrostomy tube
2013, 4Q, 117	Percutaneous endoscopic placement of gastrostomy tube

AHA Coding Clinic for table ØDJ

2019, 1Q, 25	Laparoscopic appendectomy converted to open procedure
2019, 1Q, 25	Milking of inspissated material from ileum to colon
2017, 2Q, 15	Low anterior resection with sigmoidoscopy
2016, 2Q, 20	Capsule endoscopy of small intestine
2015, 3Q, 24	Esophagogastroduodenoscopy with epinephrine injection for control of bleeding

AHA Coding Clinic for table ØDL

2013, 4Q, 112	Endoscopic banding of esophageal varices

AHA Coding Clinic for table ØDN

2017, 4Q, 49-50	New and revised body part values - Repositioning of the intestine
2017, 1Q, 35	Lysis of omental and peritoneal adhesions
2015, 3Q, 15	Vascular ring surgery with release of esophagus and trachea
2015, 3Q, 16	Vascular ring surgery and double aortic arch

AHA Coding Clinic for table ØDP

2019, 2Q, 18	Removal of wound VAC

AHA Coding Clinic for table ØDQ

2019, 2Q, 15	Reversal of Roux-en-Y bypass
2018, 2Q, 25	Third and fourth degree obstetric lacerations
2018, 1Q, 11	Repair of internal hernia at Petersen space
2017, 3Q, 17	Posterior sagittal anorectoplasty
2016, 3Q, 3-7	Stoma creation & takedown procedures
2016, 3Q, 26	Insertion of gastrostomy tube
2016, 1Q, 7	Obstetrical perineal laceration repair
2016, 1Q, 8	Obstetrical perineal laceration repair
2014, 4Q, 20	Control of bleeding duodenal ulcer

AHA Coding Clinic for table ØDS

2019, 1Q, 30	Laparoscopic-assisted rectopexy with manual reduction of prolapse
2017, 4Q, 49-50	New and revised body part values - Repositioning of the intestine
2017, 3Q, 9	Ileocolic intussusception reduction via air enema
2017, 3Q, 17	Posterior sagittal anorectoplasty
2016, 3Q, 3-5	Stoma creation & takedown procedures

AHA Coding Clinic for table ØDT

2022, 1Q, 49	Robotic-assisted low anterior resection of colon
2021, 1Q, 22	Total proctocolectomy with creation of J-pouch
2020, 4Q, 100	Robotic-assisted sigmoid colectomy with extension of incision for specimen removal
2019, 1Q, 3-8	Whipple procedure
2019, 1Q, 14	Esophagectomy with colon interposition
2017, 4Q, 49-50	New and revised body part values - Repositioning of the intestine
2014, 4Q, 40	Abdominoperineal resection (APR) with flap closure of perineum and colostomy
2014, 4Q, 42	Right colectomy with side-to-side functional end-to-end anastomosis
2014, 3Q, 6	Ileocecectomy including cecum, terminal ileum and appendix
2014, 3Q, 6	Right colectomy

AHA Coding Clinic for table ØDU

2021, 2Q, 20	Malone antegrade continence enema procedure
2021, 1Q, 22	Total proctocolectomy with creation of J-pouch
2019, 1Q, 30	Laparoscopic-assisted rectopexy with manual reduction of prolapse

AHA Coding Clinic for table ØDV

2017, 3Q, 22	Laparoscopic esophagomyotomy (Heller type) and Toupet fundoplication
2016, 2Q, 22	Esophageal lengthening Collis gastroplasty with Nissen fundoplication and hiatal hernia
2014, 3Q, 28	Laparoscopic Nissen fundoplication and diaphragmatic hernia repair

AHA Coding Clinic for table ØDW

2021, 1Q, 19	Kock pouch revision surgery
2018, 1Q, 20	Adjustment of gastric band

AHA Coding Clinic for table ØDX

2019, 4Q, 29-30	Transfer large intestine to vagina
2019, 1Q, 14	Esophagectomy with colon interposition
2017, 2Q, 18	Esophagectomy and esophagogastrectomy with cervical esophagogastrostomy
2016, 2Q, 22	Esophageal lengthening Collis gastroplasty with Nissen fundoplication and hiatal hernia
2015, 1Q, 28	Repair of bronchopleural fistula using omental pedicle graft

Upper Intestinal Tract (Ø) and Lower Intestinal Tract (D)

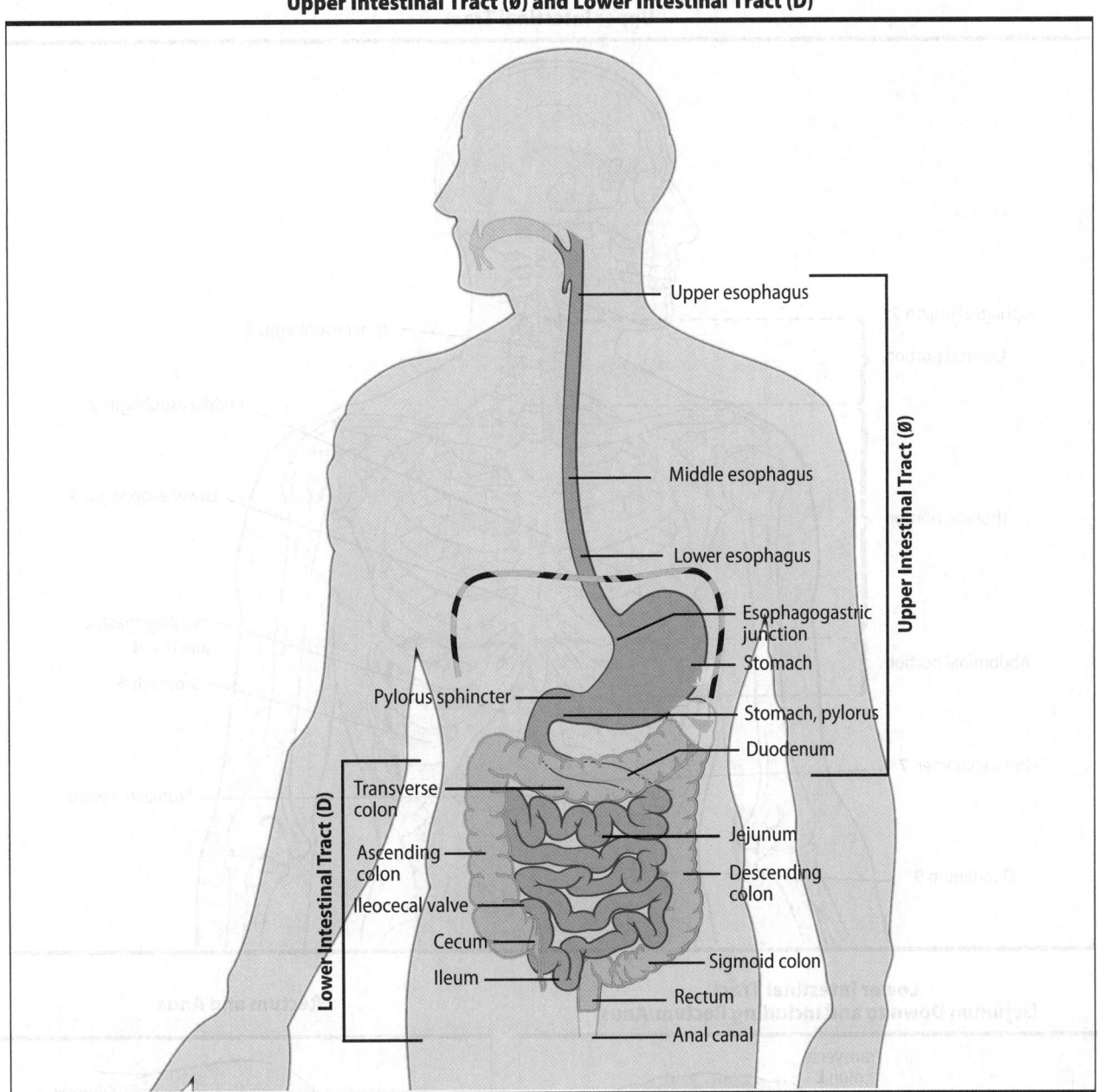

Gastrointestinal System

Upper Intestinal Tract

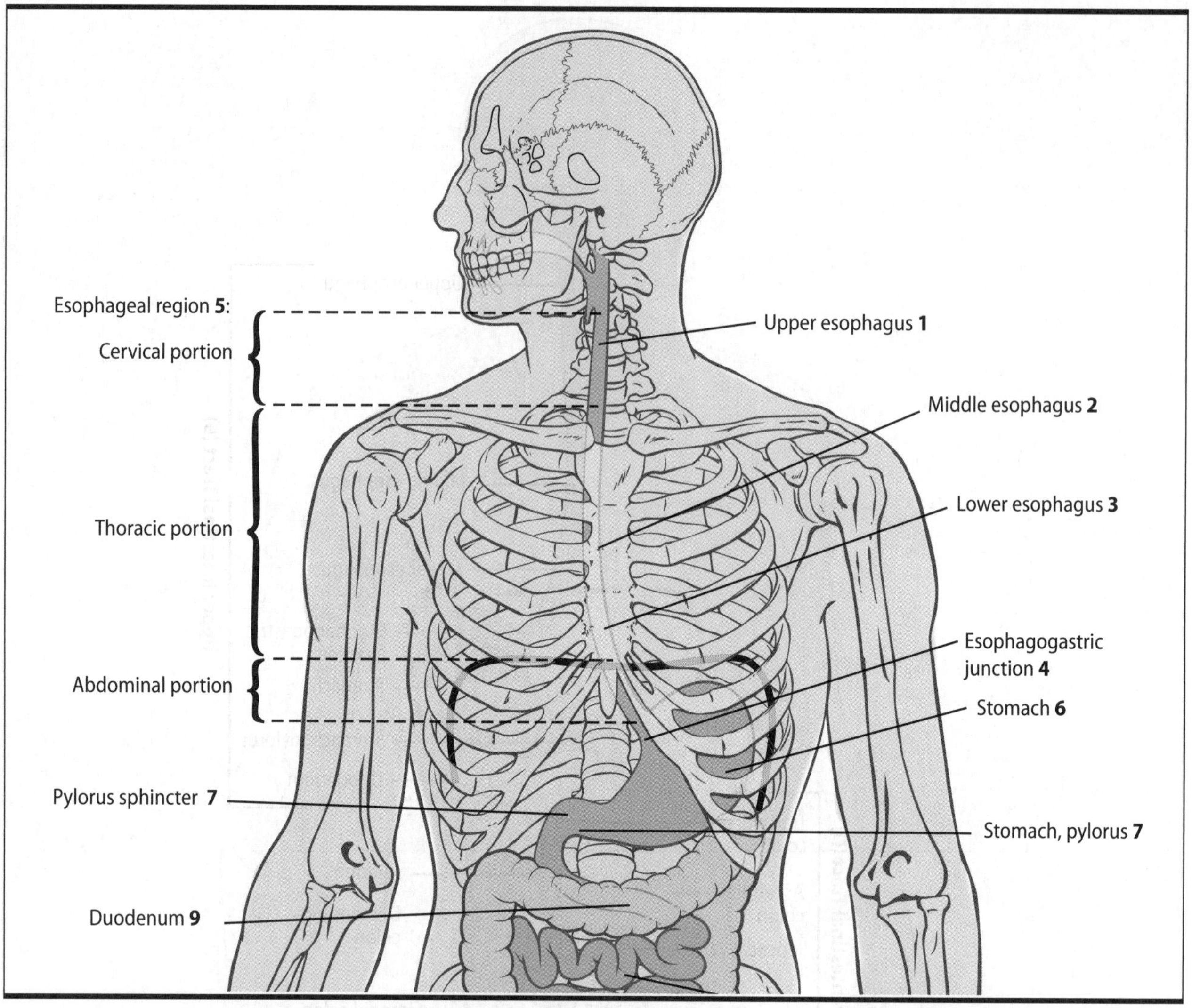

Esophageal region **5**:

Cervical portion

Thoracic portion

Abdominal portion

Pylorus sphincter **7**

Duodenum **9**

Upper esophagus **1**

Middle esophagus **2**

Lower esophagus **3**

Esophagogastric junction **4**

Stomach **6**

Stomach, pylorus **7**

Lower Intestinal Tract
(Jejunum Down to and Including Rectum/Anus)

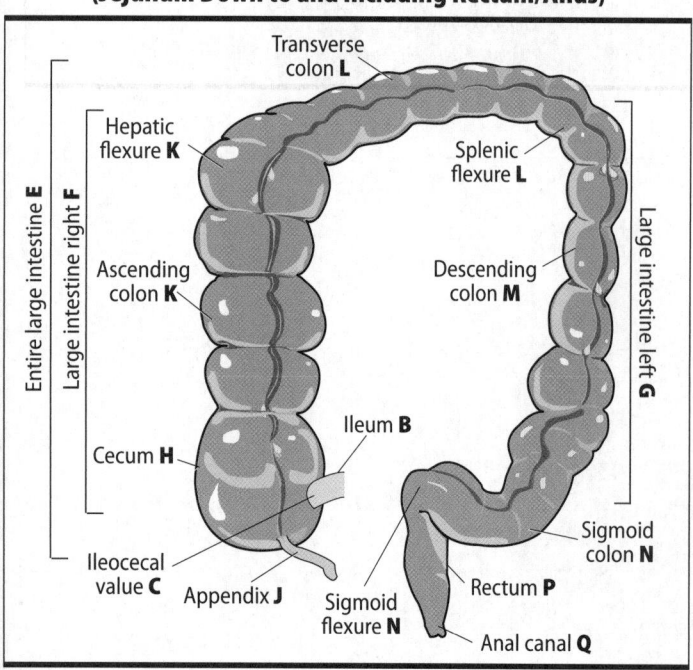

Transverse colon **L**

Hepatic flexure **K**

Splenic flexure **L**

Ascending colon **K**

Descending colon **M**

Entire large intestine **E**

Large intestine right **F**

Large intestine left **G**

Cecum **H**

Ileum **B**

Ileocecal value **C**

Appendix **J**

Sigmoid flexure **N**

Rectum **P**

Sigmoid colon **N**

Anal canal **Q**

Rectum and Anus

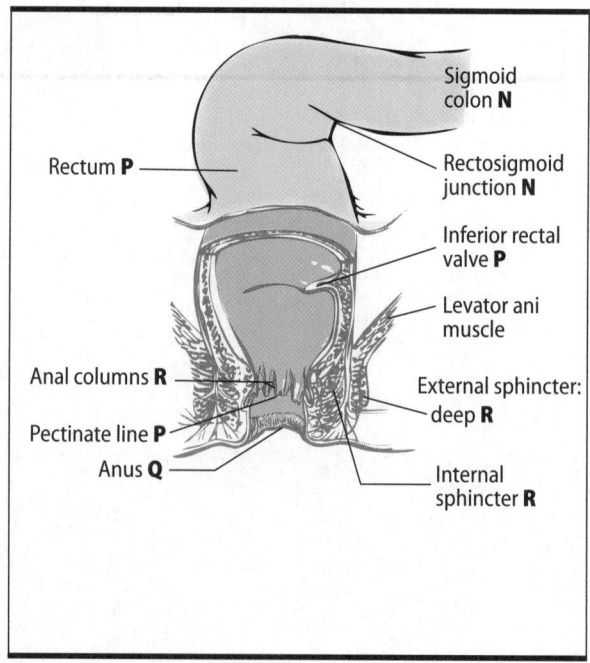

Rectum **P**

Sigmoid colon **N**

Rectosigmoid junction **N**

Inferior rectal valve **P**

Levator ani muscle

Anal columns **R**

Pectinate line **P**

Anus **Q**

External sphincter: deep **R**

Internal sphincter **R**

Ø   **Medical and Surgical**
D   **Gastrointestinal System**
1   **Bypass**   Definition: Altering the route of passage of the contents of a tubular body part
                Explanation: Rerouting contents of a body part to a downstream area of the normal route, to a similar route and body part, or to an abnormal route and dissimilar body part. Includes one or more anastomoses, with or without the use of a device.

Body Part Character 4	Approach Character 5	Device Character 6	Qualifier Character 7

1 Esophagus, Upper
   Cervical esophagus
2 Esophagus, Middle
   Thoracic esophagus
3 Esophagus, Lower
   Abdominal esophagus
5 Esophagus
	Ø Open
	4 Percutaneous Endoscopic
	8 Via Natural or Artificial Opening
	   Endoscopic
		7 Autologous Tissue Substitute
		J Synthetic Substitute
		K Nonautologous Tissue Substitute
		Z No Device
			4 Cutaneous
			6 Stomach
			9 Duodenum
			A Jejunum
			B Ileum

1 Esophagus, Upper
   Cervical esophagus
2 Esophagus, Middle
   Thoracic esophagus
3 Esophagus, Lower
   Abdominal esophagus
5 Esophagus
	3 Percutaneous	J Synthetic Substitute	4 Cutaneous

6 Stomach 9 Duodenum	Ø Open 4 Percutaneous Endoscopic 8 Via Natural or Artificial Opening Endoscopic	7 Autologous Tissue Substitute J Synthetic Substitute K Nonautologous Tissue Substitute Z No Device	4 Cutaneous 9 Duodenum A Jejunum B Ileum L Transverse Colon
6 Stomach 9 Duodenum	3 Percutaneous	J Synthetic Substitute	4 Cutaneous
8 Small Intestine	Ø Open 4 Percutaneous Endoscopic 8 Via Natural or Artificial Opening Endoscopic	7 Autologous Tissue Substitute J Synthetic Substitute K Nonautologous Tissue Substitute Z No Device	4 Cutaneous 8 Small Intestine H Cecum K Ascending Colon L Transverse Colon M Descending Colon N Sigmoid Colon P Rectum Q Anus

A Jejunum
   Duodenojejunal flexure
	Ø Open
	4 Percutaneous Endoscopic
	8 Via Natural or Artificial Opening
	   Endoscopic
		7 Autologous Tissue Substitute
		J Synthetic Substitute
		K Nonautologous Tissue Substitute
		Z No Device
			4 Cutaneous
			A Jejunum
			B Ileum
			H Cecum
			K Ascending Colon
			L Transverse Colon
			M Descending Colon
			N Sigmoid Colon
			P Rectum
			Q Anus

A Jejunum Duodenojejunal flexure	3 Percutaneous	J Synthetic Substitute	4 Cutaneous
B Ileum	Ø Open 4 Percutaneous Endoscopic 8 Via Natural or Artificial Opening Endoscopic	7 Autologous Tissue Substitute J Synthetic Substitute K Nonautologous Tissue Substitute Z No Device	4 Cutaneous B Ileum H Cecum K Ascending Colon L Transverse Colon M Descending Colon N Sigmoid Colon P Rectum Q Anus
B Ileum	3 Percutaneous	J Synthetic Substitute	4 Cutaneous
E Large Intestine	Ø Open 4 Percutaneous Endoscopic 8 Via Natural or Artificial Opening Endoscopic	7 Autologous Tissue Substitute J Synthetic Substitute K Nonautologous Tissue Substitute Z No Device	4 Cutaneous E Large Intestine P Rectum
H Cecum	Ø Open 4 Percutaneous Endoscopic 8 Via Natural or Artificial Opening Endoscopic	7 Autologous Tissue Substitute J Synthetic Substitute K Nonautologous Tissue Substitute Z No Device	4 Cutaneous H Cecum K Ascending Colon L Transverse Colon M Descending Colon N Sigmoid Colon P Rectum
H Cecum	3 Percutaneous	J Synthetic Substitute	4 Cutaneous

Non-OR   ØD16[Ø,4,8][7,J,K,Z]4
Non-OR   ØD163J4
HAC   ØD16[Ø,4,8][7,J,K,Z][9,A,B,L] when reported with PDx E66.Ø1 and SDx K68.11, K95.Ø1, K95.81 or T81.4Ø–T81.49 with 7th character A

ØD1 Continued on next page

NC Noncovered Procedure   **LC** Limited Coverage   **QA** Questionable OB Admit   **NT** New Tech Add-on   ✚ Combination Member   ♂ Male   ♀ Female

ICD-10-PCS 2023   **377**

ØD1–ØD1

ØD1 Continued

Ø **Medical and Surgical**
D **Gastrointestinal System**
1 **Bypass**   Definition: Altering the route of passage of the contents of a tubular body part

Explanation: Rerouting contents of a body part to a downstream area of the normal route, to a similar route and body part, or to an abnormal route and dissimilar body part. Includes one or more anastomoses, with or without the use of a device.

Body Part Character 4	Approach Character 5	Device Character 6	Qualifier Character 7
K Ascending Colon	Ø Open 4 Percutaneous Endoscopic 8 Via Natural or Artificial Opening Endoscopic	7 Autologous Tissue Substitute J Synthetic Substitute K Nonautologous Tissue Substitute Z No Device	4 Cutaneous K Ascending Colon L Transverse Colon M Descending Colon N Sigmoid Colon P Rectum
K Ascending Colon	3 Percutaneous	J Synthetic Substitute	4 Cutaneous
L Transverse Colon Hepatic flexure Splenic flexure	Ø Open 4 Percutaneous Endoscopic 8 Via Natural or Artificial Opening Endoscopic	7 Autologous Tissue Substitute J Synthetic Substitute K Nonautologous Tissue Substitute Z No Device	4 Cutaneous L Transverse Colon M Descending Colon N Sigmoid Colon P Rectum
L Transverse Colon Hepatic flexure Splenic flexure	3 Percutaneous	J Synthetic Substitute	4 Cutaneous
M Descending Colon	Ø Open 4 Percutaneous Endoscopic 8 Via Natural or Artificial Opening Endoscopic	7 Autologous Tissue Substitute J Synthetic Substitute K Nonautologous Tissue Substitute Z No Device	4 Cutaneous M Descending Colon N Sigmoid Colon P Rectum
M Descending Colon	3 Percutaneous	J Synthetic Substitute	4 Cutaneous
N Sigmoid Colon Rectosigmoid junction Sigmoid flexure	Ø Open 4 Percutaneous Endoscopic 8 Via Natural or Artificial Opening Endoscopic	7 Autologous Tissue Substitute J Synthetic Substitute K Nonautologous Tissue Substitute Z No Device	4 Cutaneous N Sigmoid Colon P Rectum
N Sigmoid Colon Rectosigmoid junction Sigmoid flexure	3 Percutaneous	J Synthetic Substitute	4 Cutaneous

Ø **Medical and Surgical**
D **Gastrointestinal System**
2 **Change**   Definition: Taking out or off a device from a body part and putting back an identical or similar device in or on the same body part without cutting or puncturing the skin or a mucous membrane

Explanation: All CHANGE procedures are coded using the approach EXTERNAL

Body Part Character 4	Approach Character 5	Device Character 6	Qualifier Character 7
Ø Upper Intestinal Tract D Lower Intestinal Tract	X External	Ø Drainage Device U Feeding Device Y Other Device	Z No Qualifier

U Omentum
  Gastrocolic ligament
  Gastrocolic omentum
  Gastrohepatic omentum
  Gastrophrenic ligament
  Gastrosplenic ligament
  Greater Omentum
  Hepatogastric ligament
  Lesser Omentum
V Mesentery
  Mesoappendix
  Mesocolon
W Peritoneum
  Epiploic foramen
	X External	Ø Drainage Device
		Y Other Device
			Z No Qualifier

Non-OR   All body part, approach, device, and qualifier values

Non-OR Procedure   DRG Non-OR Procedure   Valid OR Procedure   HAC Associated Procedure   Combination Only   New/Revised April   New/Revised October

378   ICD-10-PCS 2023

ØD1–ØD2

Ø   Medical and Surgical
D   Gastrointestinal System
5   Destruction   Definition: Physical eradication of all or a portion of a body part by the direct use of energy, force, or a destructive agent
                  Explanation: None of the body part is physically taken out

Body Part Character 4	Approach Character 5	Device Character 6	Qualifier Character 7

1 Esophagus, Upper
  Cervical esophagus
2 Esophagus, Middle
  Thoracic esophagus
3 Esophagus, Lower
  Abdominal esophagus
4 Esophagogastric Junction
  Cardia
  Cardioesophageal junction
  Gastroesophageal (GE)
    junction
5 Esophagus
6 Stomach
7 Stomach, Pylorus
  Pyloric antrum
  Pyloric canal
  Pyloric sphincter
8 Small Intestine
9 Duodenum
	A Jejunum
	  Duodenojejunal flexure
	B Ileum
	C Ileocecal Valve
	E Large Intestine
	F Large Intestine, Right
	G Large Intestine, Left
	H Cecum
	J Appendix
	  Vermiform appendix
	K Ascending Colon
	L Transverse Colon
	  Hepatic flexure
	  Splenic flexure
	M Descending Colon
	N Sigmoid Colon
	  Rectosigmoid junction
	  Sigmoid flexure
	P Rectum
	  Anorectal junction
		Ø Open
		3 Percutaneous
		4 Percutaneous Endoscopic
			Z No Device	**3 Laser Interstitial Thermal**
				  Therapy
				Z No Qualifier

1 Esophagus, Upper
  Cervical esophagus
2 Esophagus, Middle
  Thoracic esophagus
3 Esophagus, Lower
  Abdominal esophagus
4 Esophagogastric Junction
  Cardia
  Cardioesophageal junction
  Gastroesophageal (GE)
    junction
5 Esophagus
6 Stomach
7 Stomach, Pylorus
  Pyloric antrum
  Pyloric canal
  Pyloric sphincter
8 Small Intestine
9 Duodenum
	A Jejunum
	  Duodenojejunal flexure
	B Ileum
	C Ileocecal Valve
	E Large Intestine
	F Large Intestine, Right
	G Large Intestine, Left
	H Cecum
	J Appendix
	  Vermiform appendix
	K Ascending Colon
	L Transverse Colon
	  Hepatic flexure
	  Splenic flexure
	M Descending Colon
	N Sigmoid Colon
	  Rectosigmoid junction
	  Sigmoid flexure
	P Rectum
	  Anorectal junction
		7 Via Natural or Artificial
		  Opening
		8 Via Natural or Artificial
		  Opening Endoscopic
			Z No Device	**Z No Qualifier**

Q Anus
  Anal orifice
	Ø Open
	3 Percutaneous
	4 Percutaneous Endoscopic
		Z No Device	**3 Laser Interstitial Thermal**
			  Therapy
			Z No Qualifier

Q Anus
  Anal orifice
	7 Via Natural or Artificial
	  Opening
	8 Via Natural or Artificial
	  Opening Endoscopic
	X External
		Z No Device	**Z No Qualifier**

R Anal Sphincter
  External anal sphincter
  Internal anal sphincter
U Omentum
  Gastrocolic ligament
  Gastrocolic omentum
  Gastrohepatic omentum
  Gastrophrenic ligament
  Gastrosplenic ligament
  Greater Omentum
  Hepatogastric ligament
  Lesser Omentum
V Mesentery
  Mesoappendix
  Mesocolon
W Peritoneum
  Epiploic foramen
	Ø Open
	3 Percutaneous
	4 Percutaneous Endoscopic
		Z No Device	**Z No Qualifier**

Non-OR	ØD5[1,2,3,4,5,6,7,9,E,F,G,H,K,L,M,N]4ZZ
Non-OR	ØD5P[Ø,3,4]ZZ
Non-OR	ØD5[1,2,3,4,5,6,7,8,9,A,B,C,E,F,G,H,K,L,M,N]8ZZ
Non-OR	ØD5P[7,8]ZZ
Non-OR	ØD5Q4ZZ
Non-OR	ØD5Q8ZZ
Non-OR	ØD5R4ZZ

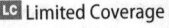 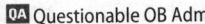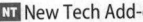

0   Medical and Surgical
D   Gastrointestinal System
7   Dilation   Definition: Expanding an orifice or the lumen of a tubular body part

Explanation: The orifice can be a natural orifice or an artificially created orifice. Accomplished by stretching a tubular body part using intraluminal pressure or by cutting part of the orifice or wall of the tubular body part.

Body Part Character 4	Approach Character 5	Device Character 6	Qualifier Character 7

1 Esophagus, Upper
   Cervical esophagus
2 Esophagus, Middle
   Thoracic esophagus
3 Esophagus, Lower
   Abdominal esophagus
4 Esophagogastric Junction
   Cardia
   Cardioesophageal junction
   Gastroesophageal (GE) junction
5 Esophagus
6 Stomach
7 Stomach, Pylorus
   Pyloric antrum
   Pyloric canal
   Pyloric sphincter
8 Small Intestine
9 Duodenum
A Jejunum
   Duodenojejunal flexure
B Ileum
C Ileocecal Valve
E Large Intestine
F Large Intestine, Right
G Large Intestine, Left
H Cecum
K Ascending Colon
L Transverse Colon
   Hepatic flexure
   Splenic flexure
M Descending Colon
N Sigmoid Colon
   Rectosigmoid junction
   Sigmoid flexure
P Rectum
   Anorectal junction
Q Anus
   Anal orifice
	Ø Open
	3 Percutaneous
	4 Percutaneous Endoscopic
	7 Via Natural or Artificial Opening
	8 Via Natural or Artificial Opening
	   Endoscopic
		D Intraluminal Device
		Z No Device
			Z No Qualifier

Non-OR	ØD7[1,2,3,4,5,6,8,9,A,B,C,E,F,G,H,K,L,M,N,P,Q][7,8][D,Z]Z
Non-OR	ØD77[4,8]DZ
Non-OR	ØD777[D,Z]Z
Non-OR	ØD7[8,9,A,B,C,E,F,G,H,K,L,M,N][Ø,3,4]DZ

0   Medical and Surgical
D   Gastrointestinal System
8   Division   Definition: Cutting into a body part, without draining fluids and/or gases from the body part, in order to separate or transect a body part

Explanation: All or a portion of the body part is separated into two or more portions

Body Part Character 4	Approach Character 5	Device Character 6	Qualifier Character 7

4 Esophagogastric Junction
   Cardia
   Cardioesophageal junction
   Gastroesophageal (GE) junction
7 Stomach, Pylorus
   Pyloric antrum
   Pyloric canal
   Pyloric sphincter
	Ø Open
	3 Percutaneous
	4 Percutaneous Endoscopic
	7 Via Natural or Artificial Opening
	8 Via Natural or Artificial Opening
	   Endoscopic
		Z No Device	Z No Qualifier

R Anal Sphincter
   External anal sphincter
   Internal anal sphincter
	Ø Open
	3 Percutaneous
		Z No Device	Z No Qualifier

Non-OR Procedure   DRG Non-OR Procedure   Valid OR Procedure   HAC Associated Procedure   Combination Only   New/Revised April   New/Revised October

380

ICD-10-PCS 2023

Ø **Medical and Surgical**
D **Gastrointestinal System**
9 **Drainage** Definition: Taking or letting out fluids and/or gases from a body part
  Explanation: The qualifier DIAGNOSTIC is used to identify drainage procedures that are biopsies

Body Part Character 4		Approach Character 5	Device Character 6	Qualifier Character 7
1 Esophagus, Upper Cervical esophagus 2 Esophagus, Middle Thoracic esophagus 3 Esophagus, Lower Abdominal esophagus 4 Esophagogastric Junction Cardia Cardioesophageal junction Gastroesophageal (GE) junction 5 Esophagus 6 Stomach 7 Stomach, Pylorus Pyloric antrum Pyloric canal Pyloric sphincter 8 Small Intestine 9 Duodenum	A Jejunum Duodenojejunal flexure B Ileum C Ileocecal Valve E Large Intestine F Large Intestine, Right G Large Intestine, Left H Cecum J Appendix Vermiform appendix K Ascending Colon L Transverse Colon Hepatic flexure Splenic flexure M Descending Colon N Sigmoid Colon Rectosigmoid junction Sigmoid flexure P Rectum Anorectal junction	Ø Open 3 Percutaneous 4 Percutaneous Endoscopic 7 Via Natural or Artificial Opening 8 Via Natural or Artificial Opening Endoscopic	Ø Drainage Device	Z No Qualifier
1 Esophagus, Upper Cervical esophagus 2 Esophagus, Middle Thoracic esophagus 3 Esophagus, Lower Abdominal esophagus 4 Esophagogastric Junction Cardia Cardioesophageal junction Gastroesophageal (GE) junction 5 Esophagus 6 Stomach 7 Stomach, Pylorus Pyloric antrum Pyloric canal Pyloric sphincter 8 Small Intestine 9 Duodenum	A Jejunum Duodenojejunal flexure B Ileum C Ileocecal Valve E Large Intestine F Large Intestine, Right G Large Intestine, Left H Cecum J Appendix Vermiform appendix K Ascending Colon L Transverse Colon Hepatic flexure Splenic flexure M Descending Colon N Sigmoid Colon Rectosigmoid junction Sigmoid flexure P Rectum Anorectal junction	Ø Open 3 Percutaneous 4 Percutaneous Endoscopic 7 Via Natural or Artificial Opening 8 Via Natural or Artificial Opening Endoscopic	Z No Device	X Diagnostic Z No Qualifier
Q Anus Anal orifice		Ø Open 3 Percutaneous 4 Percutaneous Endoscopic 7 Via Natural or Artificial Opening 8 Via Natural or Artificial Opening Endoscopic X External	Ø Drainage Device	Z No Qualifier
Q Anus Anal orifice		Ø Open 3 Percutaneous 4 Percutaneous Endoscopic 7 Via Natural or Artificial Opening 8 Via Natural or Artificial Opening Endoscopic X External	Z No Device	X Diagnostic Z No Qualifier

Non-OR ØD9[1,2,3,4,5,C,J]3ØZ
Non-OR ØD9[6,7,8,9,A,B,E,F,G,H,K,L,M,N,P][3,7,8]ØZ
Non-OR ØD9[1,2,3,4,5,6,7,8,9,A,B,C,E,F,G,H,K,L,M,N,P][3,4,7,8]ZX
Non-OR ØD9[1,2,3,4,5,6,7,8,9,A,B,C,E,F,G,H,J,K,L,M,N,P]3ZZ
Non-OR ØD9Q3ØZ
Non-OR ØD9Q[Ø,3,4,7,8,X]ZX
Non-OR ØD9Q3ZZ

ØD9 Continued on next page

NC Noncovered Procedure LC Limited Coverage OA Questionable OB Admit NT New Tech Add-on ⊞ Combination Member ♂ Male ♀ Female

Ø   **Medical and Surgical**
D   **Gastrointestinal System**
9   **Drainage**   Definition: Taking or letting out fluids and/or gases from a body part
                       Explanation: The qualifier DIAGNOSTIC is used to identify drainage procedures that are biopsies

Body Part Character 4	Approach Character 5	Device Character 6	Qualifier Character 7

R Anal Sphincter
   External anal sphincter
   Internal anal sphincter
U Omentum
   Gastrocolic ligament
   Gastrocolic omentum
   Gastrohepatic omentum
   Gastrophrenic ligament
   Gastrosplenic ligament
   Greater Omentum
   Hepatogastric ligament
   Lesser Omentum
V Mesentery
   Mesoappendix
   Mesocolon
W Peritoneum
   Epiploic foramen
	Ø Open
	3 Percutaneous
	4 Percutaneous Endoscopic
		Ø Drainage Device	**Z** No Qualifier

R Anal Sphincter
   External anal sphincter
   Internal anal sphincter
U Omentum
   Gastrocolic ligament
   Gastrocolic omentum
   Gastrohepatic omentum
   Gastrophrenic ligament
   Gastrosplenic ligament
   Greater Omentum
   Hepatogastric ligament
   Lesser Omentum
V Mesentery
   Mesoappendix
   Mesocolon
W Peritoneum
   Epiploic foramen
	Ø Open
	3 Percutaneous
	4 Percutaneous Endoscopic
		Z No Device	**X** Diagnostic
			Z No Qualifier

Non-OR	ØD9[R,W]3ØZ
Non-OR	ØD9[U,V][3,4]ØZ
Non-OR	ØD9[R,U,V,W]3Z[X,Z]
Non-OR	ØD9R[Ø,4]ZX
Non-OR	ØD9[U,V]4ZZ

Non-OR Procedure   DRG Non-OR Procedure   Valid OR Procedure   HAC Associated Procedure   Combination Only   New/Revised April   New/Revised October

382

ICD-10-PCS 2023

Ø   **Medical and Surgical**
D   **Gastrointestinal System**
B   **Excision**   Definition: Cutting out or off, without replacement, a portion of a body part
          Explanation: The qualifier DIAGNOSTIC is used to identify excision procedures that are biopsies

Body Part Character 4	Approach Character 5	Device Character 6	Qualifier Character 7

1 Esophagus, Upper
  Cervical esophagus
2 Esophagus, Middle
  Thoracic esophagus
3 Esophagus, Lower
  Abdominal esophagus
4 Esophagogastric Junction
  Cardia
  Cardioesophageal junction
  Gastroesophageal (GE) junction
5 Esophagus
7 Stomach, Pylorus
  Pyloric antrum
  Pyloric canal
  Pyloric sphincter
 	
8 Small Intestine
9 Duodenum
A Jejunum
  Duodenojejunal flexure
B Ileum
C Ileocecal Valve
E Large Intestine
F Large Intestine, Right
H Cecum
J Appendix
  Vermiform appendix
K Ascending Colon
P Rectum
  Anorectal junction
	Ø Open
	3 Percutaneous
	4 Percutaneous Endoscopic
	7 Via Natural or Artificial Opening
	8 Via Natural or Artificial Opening Endoscopic
		Z No Device	X Diagnostic
			Z No Qualifier

6 Stomach	Ø Open 3 Percutaneous 4 Percutaneous Endoscopic 7 Via Natural or Artificial Opening 8 Via Natural or Artificial Opening Endoscopic	Z No Device	3 Vertical X Diagnostic Z No Qualifier

G Large Intestine, Left
L Transverse Colon
  Hepatic flexure
  Splenic flexure
M Descending Colon
N Sigmoid Colon
  Rectosigmoid junction
  Sigmoid flexure
	Ø Open
	3 Percutaneous
	4 Percutaneous Endoscopic
	7 Via Natural or Artificial Opening
	8 Via Natural or Artificial Opening Endoscopic
		Z No Device	X Diagnostic
			Z No Qualifier

G Large Intestine, Left
L Transverse Colon
  Hepatic flexure
  Splenic flexure
M Descending Colon
N Sigmoid Colon
  Rectosigmoid junction
  Sigmoid flexure
	F Via Natural or Artificial Opening with Percutaneous Endoscopic Assistance	Z No Device	Z No Qualifier

Q Anus Anal orifice	Ø Open 3 Percutaneous 4 Percutaneous Endoscopic 7 Via Natural or Artificial Opening 8 Via Natural or Artificial Opening Endoscopic X External	Z No Device	X Diagnostic Z No Qualifier

R Anal Sphincter
  External anal sphincter
  Internal anal sphincter
U Omentum
  Gastrocolic ligament
  Gastrocolic omentum
  Gastrohepatic omentum
  Gastrophrenic ligament
  Gastrosplenic ligament
  Greater Omentum
  Hepatogastric ligament
  Lesser Omentum
V Mesentery
  Mesoappendix
  Mesocolon
W Peritoneum
  Epiploic foramen
	Ø Open
	3 Percutaneous
	4 Percutaneous Endoscopic
		Z No Device	X Diagnostic
			Z No Qualifier

Non-OR   ØDB[1,2,3,4,5,7,8,9,A,B,C,E,F,H,K,P][3,4,7,8]ZX
Non-OR   ØDB[1,2,3,5,7,9][4,8]ZZ
Non-OR   ØDB[4,E,F,H,K,P]8ZZ
Non-OR   ØDB6[3,7]ZX
Non-OR   ØDB68Z[X,Z]
Non-OR   ØDB[G,L,M,N][3,4,7,8]ZX

Non-OR   ØDB[G,L,M,N]8ZZ
Non-OR   ØDBQ[Ø,3,4,7,8,X]ZX
Non-OR   ØDBQ8ZZ
Non-OR   ØDBR[Ø,3,4]ZX
Non-OR   ØDB[U,V,W][3,4]ZX

NC Noncovered Procedure   **LC** Limited Coverage   **QA** Questionable OB Admit   **NT** New Tech Add-on   ⊞ Combination Member   ♂ Male   ♀ Female

ICD-10-PCS 2023   383   ØDB–ØDB

Ø **Medical and Surgical**
D **Gastrointestinal System**
C **Extirpation**   Definition: Taking or cutting out solid matter from a body part

Explanation: The solid matter may be an abnormal byproduct of a biological function or a foreign body; it may be imbedded in a body part or in the lumen of a tubular body part. The solid matter may or may not have been previously broken into pieces.

Body Part Character 4	Approach Character 5	Device Character 6	Qualifier Character 7
1 Esophagus, Upper Cervical esophagus **2** Esophagus, Middle Thoracic esophagus **3** Esophagus, Lower Abdominal esophagus **4** Esophagogastric Junction Cardia Cardioesophageal junction Gastroesophageal (GE) junction **5** Esophagus **6** Stomach **7** Stomach, Pylorus Pyloric antrum Pyloric canal Pyloric sphincter **8** Small Intestine **9** Duodenum **A** Jejunum Duodenojejunal flexure **B** Ileum **C** Ileocecal Valve **E** Large Intestine **F** Large Intestine, Right **G** Large Intestine, Left **H** Cecum **J** Appendix Vermiform appendix **K** Ascending Colon **L** Transverse Colon Hepatic flexure Splenic flexure **M** Descending Colon **N** Sigmoid Colon Rectosigmoid junction Sigmoid flexure **P** Rectum Anorectal junction	**Ø** Open **3** Percutaneous **4** Percutaneous Endoscopic **7** Via Natural or Artificial Opening **8** Via Natural or Artificial Opening Endoscopic	**Z** No Device	**Z** No Qualifier
Q Anus Anal orifice	**Ø** Open **3** Percutaneous **4** Percutaneous Endoscopic **7** Via Natural or Artificial Opening **8** Via Natural or Artificial Opening Endoscopic **X** External	**Z** No Device	**Z** No Qualifier
R Anal Sphincter External anal sphincter Internal anal sphincter **U** Omentum Gastrocolic ligament Gastrocolic omentum Gastrohepatic omentum Gastrophrenic ligament Gastrosplenic ligament Greater Omentum Hepatogastric ligament Lesser Omentum **V** Mesentery Mesoappendix Mesocolon **W** Peritoneum Epiploic foramen	**Ø** Open **3** Percutaneous **4** Percutaneous Endoscopic	**Z** No Device	**Z** No Qualifier

Non-OR ØDC[1,2,3,4,5,6,7,8,9,A,B,C,E,F,G,H,K,L,M,N,P][7,8]ZZ
Non-OR ØDCQ[7,8,X]ZZ

Ø   **Medical and Surgical**
D   **Gastrointestinal System**
D   **Extraction**   Definition: Pulling or stripping out or off all or a portion of a body part by the use of force
                  Explanation: The qualifier DIAGNOSTIC is used to identify extraction procedures that are biopsies

Body Part Character 4	Approach Character 5	Device Character 6	Qualifier Character 7

1 Esophagus, Upper
   Cervical esophagus
2 Esophagus, Middle
   Thoracic esophagus
3 Esophagus, Lower
   Abdominal esophagus
4 Esophagogastric Junction
   Cardia
   Cardioesophageal junction
   Gastroesophageal (GE) junction
5 Esophagus
6 Stomach
7 Stomach, Pylorus
   Pyloric antrum
   Pyloric canal
   Pyloric sphincter
8 Small Intestine
9 Duodenum
A Jejunum
   Duodenojejunal flexure
B Ileum
C Ileocecal Valve
E Large Intestine
F Large Intestine, Right
G Large Intestine, Left
H Cecum
J Appendix
   Vermiform appendix
K Ascending Colon
L Transverse Colon
   Hepatic flexure
   Splenic flexure
M Descending Colon
N Sigmoid Colon
   Rectosigmoid junction
   Sigmoid flexure
P Rectum
   Anorectal junction
	3 Percutaneous
	4 Percutaneous Endoscopic
	8 Via Natural or Artificial Opening
	   Endoscopic
		Z No Device	X Diagnostic

Q Anus
   Anal orifice
	3 Percutaneous
	4 Percutaneous Endoscopic
	8 Via Natural or Artificial Opening
	   Endoscopic
	X External
		Z No Device	X Diagnostic

Non-OR   ØDD[1,2,3,4,5,6,7,8,9,A,B,C,E,F,G,H,K,L,M,N,P][3,4,8]ZX
Non-OR   ØDDQ[3,4,8,X]ZX

NC Noncovered Procedure   LC Limited Coverage   QA Questionable OB Admit   NT New Tech Add-on   ⊞ Combination Member   ♂ Male   ♀ Female

ICD-10-PCS 2023   **385**

ØDD–ØDD

Ø Medical and Surgical
D Gastrointestinal System
F Fragmentation Definition: Breaking solid matter in a body part into pieces
Explanation: Physical force (e.g., manual, ultrasonic) applied directly or indirectly is used to break the solid matter into pieces. The solid matter may be an abnormal byproduct of a biological function or a foreign body. The pieces of solid matter are not taken out.

Body Part Character 4		Approach Character 5	Device Character 6	Qualifier Character 7
5 Esophagus	NC	Ø Open	Z No Device	Z No Qualifier
6 Stomach	NC	3 Percutaneous		
8 Small Intestine	NC	4 Percutaneous Endoscopic		
9 Duodenum	NC	7 Via Natural or Artificial Opening		
A Jejunum	NC	8 Via Natural or Artificial Opening Endoscopic		
Duodenojejunal flexure		X External		
B Ileum	NC			
E Large Intestine	NC			
F Large Intestine, Right	NC			
G Large Intestine, Left	NC			
H Cecum	NC			
J Appendix	NC			
Vermiform appendix				
K Ascending Colon	NC			
L Transverse Colon	NC			
Hepatic flexure				
Splenic flexure				
M Descending Colon	NC			
N Sigmoid Colon	NC			
Rectosigmoid junction				
Sigmoid flexure				
P Rectum	NC			
Anorectal junction				
Q Anus	NC			
Anal orifice				

Non-OR ØDF[5,6,8,9,A,B,E,F,G,H,J,K,L,M,N,P,Q]XZZ
NC ØDF[5,6,8,9,A,B,E,F,G,H,J,K,L,M,N,P,Q]XZZ

Non-OR Procedure   DRG Non-OR Procedure   Valid OR Procedure   HAC Associated Procedure   Combination Only   New/Revised April   New/Revised October
386

ICD-10-PCS 2023

Ø   **Medical and Surgical**
D   **Gastrointestinal System**
H   **Insertion**   Definition: Putting in a nonbiological appliance that monitors, assists, performs, or prevents a physiological function but does not physically take the place of a body part
                  Explanation: None

Body Part Character 4	Approach Character 5	Device Character 6	Qualifier Character 7
Ø Upper Intestinal Tract **D** Lower Intestinal Tract	**Ø** Open **3** Percutaneous **4** Percutaneous Endoscopic **7** Via Natural or Artificial Opening **8** Via Natural or Artificial Opening Endoscopic	**Y** Other Device	**Z** No Qualifier
5 Esophagus	**Ø** Open **3** Percutaneous **4** Percutaneous Endoscopic	**1** Radioactive Element **2** Monitoring Device **3** Infusion Device **D** Intraluminal Device **U** Feeding Device **Y** Other Device	**Z** No Qualifier
5 Esophagus	**7** Via Natural or Artificial Opening **8** Via Natural or Artificial Opening Endoscopic	**1** Radioactive Element **2** Monitoring Device **3** Infusion Device **B** Intraluminal Device, Airway **D** Intraluminal Device **U** Feeding Device **Y** Other Device	**Z** No Qualifier
6 Stomach ⊞	**Ø** Open **3** Percutaneous **4** Percutaneous Endoscopic	**1** Radioactive Element **2** Monitoring Device **3** Infusion Device **D** Intraluminal Device **M** Stimulator Lead **U** Feeding Device **Y** Other Device	**Z** No Qualifier
6 Stomach	**7** Via Natural or Artificial Opening **8** Via Natural or Artificial Opening Endoscopic	**1** Radioactive Element **2** Monitoring Device **3** Infusion Device **D** Intraluminal Device **U** Feeding Device **Y** Other Device	**Z** No Qualifier
8 Small Intestine **9** Duodenum **A** Jejunum Duodenojejunal flexure **B** Ileum	**Ø** Open **3** Percutaneous **4** Percutaneous Endoscopic **7** Via Natural or Artificial Opening **8** Via Natural or Artificial Opening Endoscopic	**1** Radioactive Element **2** Monitoring Device **3** Infusion Device **D** Intraluminal Device **U** Feeding Device	**Z** No Qualifier
E Large Intestine **P** Rectum Anorectal junction	**Ø** Open **3** Percutaneous **4** Percutaneous Endoscopic **7** Via Natural or Artificial Opening **8** Via Natural or Artificial Opening Endoscopic	**1** Radioactive Element **D** Intraluminal Device	**Z** No Qualifier
Q Anus Anal orifice	**Ø** Open **3** Percutaneous **4** Percutaneous Endoscopic	**D** Intraluminal Device **L** Artificial Sphincter	**Z** No Qualifier
Q Anus Anal orifice	**7** Via Natural or Artificial Opening **8** Via Natural or Artificial Opening Endoscopic	**D** Intraluminal Device	**Z** No Qualifier

R Anal Sphincter
    External anal sphincter
    Internal anal sphincter
	Ø Open
	3 Percutaneous
	4 Percutaneous Endoscopic
		M Stimulator Lead	**Z** No Qualifier

Non-OR ØDH[Ø,D][Ø,3,4,7,8]YZ	**See Appendix L for Procedure Combinations**
Non-OR ØDH5[Ø,3,4][D,U]Z	⊞ ØDH6[Ø,3,4]MZ
Non-OR ØDH5[3,4]YZ	
Non-OR ØDH5[7,8][2,3,B,D,U,Y]Z	
Non-OR ØDH631Z	
Non-OR ØDH6[Ø,3,4]UZ	
Non-OR ØDH6[3,4]YZ	
Non-OR ØDH6[7,8][1,2,3,D,U,Y]Z	
Non-OR ØDH[8,9,A,B][Ø,3,4,7,8][1,D,U]Z	
Non-OR ØDH[8,9,A,B][7,8][2,3]Z	
Non-OR ØDHE[Ø,3,4,7,8][1,D]Z	
Non-OR ØDHP[Ø,3,4,7,8]DZ	

NC Noncovered Procedure   **LC** Limited Coverage   **QA** Questionable OB Admit   **NT** New Tech Add-on   ⊞ Combination Member   ♂ Male   ♀ Female

ICD-10-PCS 2023   387

ØDH–ØDH

Gastrointestinal System

Ø   Medical and Surgical
D   Gastrointestinal System
J   Inspection   Definition: Visually and/or manually exploring a body part

Explanation: Visual exploration may be performed with or without optical instrumentation. Manual exploration may be performed directly or through intervening body layers.

Body Part Character 4	Approach Character 5	Device Character 6	Qualifier Character 7
Ø Upper Intestinal Tract **6** Stomach **D** Lower Intestinal Tract	**Ø** Open **3** Percutaneous **4** Percutaneous Endoscopic **7** Via Natural or Artificial Opening **8** Via Natural or Artificial Opening Endoscopic **X** External	**Z** No Device	**Z** No Qualifier

U Omentum
    Gastrocolic ligament
    Gastrocolic omentum
    Gastrohepatic omentum
    Gastrophrenic ligament
    Gastrosplenic ligament
    Greater Omentum
    Hepatogastric ligament
    Lesser Omentum
V Mesentery
    Mesoappendix
    Mesocolon
W Peritoneum
    Epiploic foramen
	Ø Open
	3 Percutaneous
	4 Percutaneous Endoscopic
	X External
		Z No Device	**Z** No Qualifier

Non-OR	ØDJ[Ø,6,D][3,7,8,X]ZZ
Non-OR	ØDJ[U,V,W][3,X]ZZ

Non-OR Procedure   DRG Non-OR Procedure   Valid OR Procedure   HAC Associated Procedure   Combination Only   New/Revised April   New/Revised October

388   ICD-10-PCS 2023

Ø Medical and Surgical
D Gastrointestinal System
L Occlusion   Definition: Completely closing an orifice or the lumen of a tubular body part
        Explanation: The orifice can be a natural orifice or an artificially created orifice

Body Part Character 4		Approach Character 5	Device Character 6	Qualifier Character 7

1 Esophagus, Upper
  Cervical esophagus
2 Esophagus, Middle
  Thoracic esophagus
3 Esophagus, Lower
  Abdominal esophagus
4 Esophagogastric
  Junction
  Cardia
  Cardioesophageal
    junction
  Gastroesophageal (GE)
    junction
5 Esophagus
6 Stomach
7 Stomach, Pylorus
  Pyloric antrum
  Pyloric canal
  Pyloric sphincter
8 Small Intestine
	9 Duodenum
	A Jejunum
	  Duodenojejunal flexure
	B Ileum
	C Ileocecal Valve
	E Large Intestine
	F Large Intestine, Right
	G Large Intestine, Left
	H Cecum
	K Ascending Colon
	L Transverse Colon
	  Hepatic flexure
	  Splenic flexure
	M Descending Colon
	N Sigmoid Colon
	  Rectosigmoid junction
	  Sigmoid flexure
	P Rectum
	  Anorectal junction
		Ø Open
		3 Percutaneous
		4 Percutaneous Endoscopic
			C Extraluminal Device
			D Intraluminal Device
			Z No Device
				Z No Qualifier

1 Esophagus, Upper
  Cervical esophagus
2 Esophagus, Middle
  Thoracic esophagus
3 Esophagus, Lower
  Abdominal esophagus
4 Esophagogastric
  Junction
  Cardia
  Cardioesophageal
    junction
  Gastroesophageal (GE)
    junction
5 Esophagus
6 Stomach
7 Stomach, Pylorus
  Pyloric antrum
  Pyloric canal
  Pyloric sphincter
8 Small Intestine
	9 Duodenum
	A Jejunum
	  Duodenojejunal flexure
	B Ileum
	C Ileocecal Valve
	E Large Intestine
	F Large Intestine, Right
	G Large Intestine, Left
	H Cecum
	K Ascending Colon
	L Transverse Colon
	  Hepatic flexure
	  Splenic flexure
	M Descending Colon
	N Sigmoid Colon
	  Rectosigmoid junction
	  Sigmoid flexure
	P Rectum
	  Anorectal junction
		7 Via Natural or Artificial
		  Opening
		8 Via Natural or Artificial
		  Opening Endoscopic
			D Intraluminal Device
			Z No Device
				Z No Qualifier

Q Anus Anal orifice		Ø Open 3 Percutaneous 4 Percutaneous Endoscopic X External	C Extraluminal Device D Intraluminal Device Z No Device	Z No Qualifier

Q Anus
  Anal orifice
		7 Via Natural or Artificial
		  Opening
		8 Via Natural or Artificial
		  Opening Endoscopic
			D Intraluminal Device
			Z No Device
				Z No Qualifier

Non-OR ØDL[1,2,3,4,5][Ø,3,4][C,D,Z]Z
Non-OR ØDL[1,2,3,4,5][7,8][D,Z]Z

Ø **Medical and Surgical**
D **Gastrointestinal System**
M **Reattachment**   Definition: Putting back in or on all or a portion of a separated body part to its normal location or other suitable location
Explanation: Vascular circulation and nervous pathways may or may not be reestablished

Body Part Character 4	Approach Character 5	Device Character 6	Qualifier Character 7

5 Esophagus
6 Stomach
8 Small Intestine
9 Duodenum
A Jejunum
   Duodenojejunal flexure
B Ileum
E Large Intestine
F Large Intestine, Right
G Large Intestine, Left
H Cecum
K Ascending Colon
L Transverse Colon
   Hepatic flexure
   Splenic flexure
M Descending Colon
N Sigmoid Colon
   Rectosigmoid junction
   Sigmoid flexure
P Rectum
   Anorectal junction
	Ø Open
	4 Percutaneous Endoscopic
		Z No Device	**Z** No Qualifier

Ø **Medical and Surgical**
D **Gastrointestinal System**
N **Release**   Definition: Freeing a body part from an abnormal physical constraint by cutting or by the use of force
Explanation: Some of the restraining tissue may be taken out but none of the body part is taken out

Body Part Character 4	Approach Character 5	Device Character 6	Qualifier Character 7

1 Esophagus, Upper
   Cervical esophagus
2 Esophagus, Middle
   Thoracic esophagus
3 Esophagus, Lower
   Abdominal esophagus
4 Esophagogastric
   Junction
   Cardia
   Cardioesophageal
     junction
   Gastroesophageal (GE)
     junction
5 Esophagus
6 Stomach
7 Stomach, Pylorus
   Pyloric antrum
   Pyloric canal
   Pyloric sphincter
8 Small Intestine
9 Duodenum
 	
A Jejunum
   Duodenojejunal flexure
B Ileum
C Ileocecal Valve
E Large Intestine
F Large Intestine, Right
G Large Intestine, Left
H Cecum
J Appendix
   Vermiform appendix
K Ascending Colon
L Transverse Colon
   Hepatic flexure
   Splenic flexure
M Descending Colon
N Sigmoid Colon
   Rectosigmoid junction
   Sigmoid flexure
P Rectum
   Anorectal junction
	Ø Open
	3 Percutaneous
	4 Percutaneous Endoscopic
	7 Via Natural or Artificial
	   Opening
	8 Via Natural or Artificial
	   Opening Endoscopic
		Z No Device	**Z** No Qualifier

Q Anus
   Anal orifice
	Ø Open
	3 Percutaneous
	4 Percutaneous Endoscopic
	7 Via Natural or Artificial
	   Opening
	8 Via Natural or Artificial
	   Opening Endoscopic
	X External
		Z No Device	**Z** No Qualifier

R Anal Sphincter
   External anal sphincter
   Internal anal sphincter
U Omentum
   Gastrocolic ligament
   Gastrocolic omentum
   Gastrohepatic omentum
   Gastrophrenic ligament
   Gastrosplenic ligament
   Greater Omentum
   Hepatogastric ligament
   Lesser Omentum
V Mesentery
   Mesoappendix
   Mesocolon
W Peritoneum
   Epiploic foramen
	Ø Open
	3 Percutaneous
	4 Percutaneous Endoscopic
		Z No Device	**Z** No Qualifier

Non-OR   ØDN[8,9,A,B,E,F,G,H,K,L,M,N][7,8]ZZ

Ø **Medical and Surgical**
D **Gastrointestinal System**
P **Removal**　　　Definition: Taking out or off a device from a body part

Explanation: If a device is taken out and a similar device put in without cutting or puncturing the skin or mucous membrane, the procedure is coded to the root operation CHANGE. Otherwise, the procedure for taking out a device is coded to the root operation REMOVAL.

Body Part Character 4	Approach Character 5	Device Character 6	Qualifier Character 7
Ø Upper Intestinal Tract D Lower Intestinal Tract	Ø Open 3 Percutaneous 4 Percutaneous Endoscopic 7 Via Natural or Artificial Opening 8 Via Natural or Artificial Opening Endoscopic	Ø Drainage Device 2 Monitoring Device 3 Infusion Device 7 Autologous Tissue Substitute C Extraluminal Device D Intraluminal Device J Synthetic Substitute K Nonautologous Tissue Substitute U Feeding Device Y Other Device	Z No Qualifier
Ø Upper Intestinal Tract D Lower Intestinal Tract	X External	Ø Drainage Device 2 Monitoring Device 3 Infusion Device D Intraluminal Device U Feeding Device	Z No Qualifier
5 Esophagus	Ø Open 3 Percutaneous 4 Percutaneous Endoscopic	1 Radioactive Element 2 Monitoring Device 3 Infusion Device U Feeding Device Y Other Device	Z No Qualifier
5 Esophagus	7 Via Natural or Artificial Opening 8 Via Natural or Artificial Opening Endoscopic	1 Radioactive Element D Intraluminal Device Y Other Device	Z No Qualifier
5 Esophagus	X External	1 Radioactive Element 2 Monitoring Device 3 Infusion Device D Intraluminal Device U Feeding Device	Z No Qualifier
6 Stomach	Ø Open 3 Percutaneous 4 Percutaneous Endoscopic	Ø Drainage Device 2 Monitoring Device 3 Infusion Device 7 Autologous Tissue Substitute C Extraluminal Device D Intraluminal Device J Synthetic Substitute K Nonautologous Tissue Substitute M Stimulator Lead U Feeding Device Y Other Device	Z No Qualifier
6 Stomach	7 Via Natural or Artificial Opening 8 Via Natural or Artificial Opening Endoscopic	Ø Drainage Device 2 Monitoring Device 3 Infusion Device 7 Autologous Tissue Substitute C Extraluminal Device D Intraluminal Device J Synthetic Substitute K Nonautologous Tissue Substitute U Feeding Device Y Other Device	Z No Qualifier
6 Stomach	X External	Ø Drainage Device 2 Monitoring Device 3 Infusion Device D Intraluminal Device U Feeding Device	Z No Qualifier

Non-OR	ØDP[Ø,D][3,4]YZ
Non-OR	ØDP[Ø,D][7,8][Ø,2,3,D,U,Y]Z
Non-OR	ØDP[Ø,D]X[Ø,2,3,D,U]Z
Non-OR	ØDP5[3,4]YZ
Non-OR	ØDP5[7,8][1,D,Y]Z
Non-OR	ØDP5X[1,2,3,D,U]Z
Non-OR	ØDP6[3,4]YZ
Non-OR	ØDP6[7,8][Ø,2,3,D,U,Y]Z
Non-OR	ØDP6X[Ø,2,3,D,U]Z

ØDP Continued on next page

Gastrointestinal System

Ø   **Medical and Surgical**
D   **Gastrointestinal System**
P   **Removal**   Definition: Taking out or off a device from a body part

ØDP Continued

Explanation: If a device is taken out and a similar device put in without cutting or puncturing the skin or mucous membrane, the procedure is coded to the root operation CHANGE. Otherwise, the procedure for taking out a device is coded to the root operation REMOVAL.

Body Part Character 4	Approach Character 5	Device Character 6	Qualifier Character 7

P   **Rectum**
     Anorectal junction
	Ø Open
	3 Percutaneous
	4 Percutaneous Endoscopic
	7 Via Natural or Artificial Opening
	8 Via Natural or Artificial Opening
	     Endoscopic
	X External
		1 Radioactive Element	**Z** No Qualifier

Q   **Anus**
     Anal orifice
	Ø Open
	3 Percutaneous
	4 Percutaneous Endoscopic
	7 Via Natural or Artificial Opening
	8 Via Natural or Artificial Opening
	     Endoscopic
		L Artificial Sphincter	**Z** No Qualifier

R   **Anal Sphincter**
     External anal sphincter
     Internal anal sphincter
	Ø Open
	3 Percutaneous
	4 Percutaneous Endoscopic
		M Stimulator Lead	**Z** No Qualifier

U   **Omentum**
     Gastrocolic ligament
     Gastrocolic omentum
     Gastrohepatic omentum
     Gastrophrenic ligament
     Gastrosplenic ligament
     Greater Omentum
     Hepatogastric ligament
     Lesser Omentum
V   **Mesentery**
     Mesoappendix
     Mesocolon
W   **Peritoneum**
     Epiploic foramen
	Ø Open
	3 Percutaneous
	4 Percutaneous Endoscopic
		Ø Drainage Device
		1 Radioactive Element
		7 Autologous Tissue Substitute
		J Synthetic Substitute
		K Nonautologous Tissue Substitute
			Z No Qualifier

Non-OR   ØDPP[7,8,X]1Z

Non-OR Procedure   DRG Non-OR Procedure   Valid OR Procedure   HAC Associated Procedure   Combination Only   New/Revised April   New/Revised October

392   ICD-10-PCS 2023

Gastrointestinal System (side tab)

Ø   **Medical and Surgical**
D   **Gastrointestinal System**
Q   **Repair**   Definition: Restoring, to the extent possible, a body part to its normal anatomic structure and function
                    Explanation: Used only when the method to accomplish the repair is not one of the other root operations

Body Part Character 4	Approach Character 5	Device Character 6	Qualifier Character 7

1 **Esophagus, Upper**
   Cervical esophagus
2 **Esophagus, Middle**
   Thoracic esophagus
3 **Esophagus, Lower**
   Abdominal esophagus
4 **Esophagogastric Junction**
   Cardia
   Cardioesophageal junction
   Gastroesophageal (GE) junction
5 **Esophagus**
6 **Stomach**
7 **Stomach, Pylorus**
   Pyloric antrum
   Pyloric canal
   Pyloric sphincter
8 **Small Intestine** ⊞
9 **Duodenum** ⊞
A **Jejunum** ⊞
   Duodenojejunal flexure
B **Ileum** ⊞
C **Ileocecal Valve**
E **Large Intestine** ⊞
F **Large Intestine, Right** ⊞
G **Large Intestine, Left** ⊞
H **Cecum** ⊞
J **Appendix**
   Vermiform appendix
K **Ascending Colon** ⊞
L **Transverse Colon** ⊞
   Hepatic flexure
   Splenic flexure
M **Descending Colon** ⊞
N **Sigmoid Colon** ⊞
   Rectosigmoid junction
   Sigmoid flexure
P **Rectum**
   Anorectal junction
	Ø **Open**
	3 **Percutaneous**
	4 **Percutaneous Endoscopic**
	7 **Via Natural or Artificial Opening**
	8 **Via Natural or Artificial Opening**
	   Endoscopic
		Z **No Device**	Z **No Qualifier**

Q **Anus**
   Anal orifice
	Ø **Open**
	3 **Percutaneous**
	4 **Percutaneous Endoscopic**
	7 **Via Natural or Artificial Opening**
	8 **Via Natural or Artificial Opening**
	   Endoscopic
	X **External**
		Z **No Device**	Z **No Qualifier**

R **Anal Sphincter**
   External anal sphincter
   Internal anal sphincter
U **Omentum**
   Gastrocolic ligament
   Gastrocolic omentum
   Gastrohepatic omentum
   Gastrophrenic ligament
   Gastrosplenic ligament
   Greater Omentum
   Hepatogastric ligament
   Lesser Omentum
V **Mesentery**
   Mesoappendix
   Mesocolon
W **Peritoneum**
   Epiploic foramen
	Ø **Open**
	3 **Percutaneous**
	4 **Percutaneous Endoscopic**
		Z **No Device**	Z **No Qualifier**

Non-OR   ØDQU[Ø,3,4]ZZ

⊞   **See Appendix L for Procedure Combinations**
     ØDQ[8,9,A,B,E,F,G,H,K,L,M,N]ØZZ

NC Noncovered Procedure   **LC** Limited Coverage   **QA** Questionable OB Admit   **NT** New Tech Add-on   ⊞ Combination Member   ♂ Male   ♀ Female

ICD-10-PCS 2023   393

Gastrointestinal System

Ø   **Medical and Surgical**
D   **Gastrointestinal System**
R   **Replacement**   Definition: Putting in or on biological or synthetic material that physically takes the place and/or function of all or a portion of a body part

                   Explanation: The body part may have been taken out or replaced, or may be taken out, physically eradicated, or rendered nonfunctional during the REPLACEMENT procedure. A REMOVAL procedure is coded for taking out the device used in a previous replacement procedure.

Body Part Character 4	Approach Character 5	Device Character 6	Qualifier Character 7
5 Esophagus	Ø Open 4 Percutaneous Endoscopic 7 Via Natural or Artificial Opening 8 Via Natural or Artificial Opening Endoscopic	7 Autologous Tissue Substitute J Synthetic Substitute K Nonautologous Tissue Substitute	Z No Qualifier

R Anal Sphincter
   External anal sphincter
   Internal anal sphincter
U Omentum
   Gastrocolic ligament
   Gastrocolic omentum
   Gastrohepatic omentum
   Gastrophrenic ligament
   Gastrosplenic ligament
   Greater Omentum
   Hepatogastric ligament
   Lesser Omentum
V Mesentery
   Mesoappendix
   Mesocolon
W Peritoneum
   Epiploic foramen
	Ø Open
	4 Percutaneous Endoscopic
		7 Autologous Tissue Substitute
		J Synthetic Substitute
		K Nonautologous Tissue Substitute
			Z No Qualifier

Ø   **Medical and Surgical**
D   **Gastrointestinal System**
S   **Reposition**   Definition: Moving to its normal location, or other suitable location, all or a portion of a body part

                   Explanation: The body part is moved to a new location from an abnormal location, or from a normal location where it is not functioning correctly. The body part may or may not be cut out or off to be moved to the new location.

Body Part Character 4	Approach Character 5	Device Character 6	Qualifier Character 7

5 Esophagus
6 Stomach
9 Duodenum
A Jejunum
   Duodenojejunal flexure
B Ileum
H Cecum
K Ascending Colon
L Transverse Colon
   Hepatic flexure
   Splenic flexure
M Descending Colon
N Sigmoid Colon
   Rectosigmoid junction
   Sigmoid flexure
P Rectum
   Anorectal junction
Q Anus
   Anal orifice
	Ø Open
	4 Percutaneous Endoscopic
	7 Via Natural or Artificial Opening
	8 Via Natural or Artificial Opening Endoscopic
	X External
		Z No Device	Z No Qualifier

8 Small Intestine E Large Intestine	Ø Open 4 Percutaneous Endoscopic 7 Via Natural or Artificial Opening 8 Via Natural or Artificial Opening Endoscopic	Z No Device	Z No Qualifier

    Non-OR   ØDS[5,6,9,A,B,H,K,L,M,N,P,Q]XZZ

Non-OR Procedure   DRG Non-OR Procedure   Valid OR Procedure   HAC Associated Procedure   Combination Only   New/Revised April   New/Revised October

394   ICD-10-PCS 2023

Ø   **Medical and Surgical**
D   **Gastrointestinal System**
T   **Resection**   Definition: Cutting out or off, without replacement, all of a body part
                   Explanation: None

Body Part Character 4	Approach Character 5	Device Character 6	Qualifier Character 7

1 Esophagus, Upper
   Cervical esophagus
2 Esophagus, Middle
   Thoracic esophagus
3 Esophagus, Lower
   Abdominal esophagus
4 Esophagogastric Junction
   Cardia
   Cardioesophageal junction
   Gastroesophageal (GE) junction
5 Esophagus
6 Stomach
7 Stomach, Pylorus
   Pyloric antrum
   Pyloric canal
   Pyloric sphincter
8 Small Intestine
9 Duodenum ⊞
A Jejunum
   Duodenojejunal flexure
B Ileum
C Ileocecal Valve
E Large Intestine
F Large Intestine, Right
H Cecum
J Appendix
   Vermiform appendix
K Ascending Colon
P Rectum
   Anorectal junction
Q Anus
   Anal orifice
	Ø Open
	4 Percutaneous Endoscopic
	7 Via Natural or Artificial Opening
	8 Via Natural or Artificial Opening
	   Endoscopic
		Z No Device	**Z** No Qualifier

G Large Intestine, Left
L Transverse Colon
   Hepatic flexure
   Splenic flexure
M Descending Colon
N Sigmoid Colon
   Rectosigmoid junction
   Sigmoid flexure
	Ø Open
	4 Percutaneous Endoscopic
	7 Via Natural or Artificial Opening
	8 Via Natural or Artificial Opening
	   Endoscopic
	F Via Natural or Artificial Opening
	   with Percutaneous Endoscopic
	   Assistance
		Z No Device	**Z** No Qualifier

R Anal Sphincter
   External anal sphincter
   Internal anal sphincter
U Omentum
   Gastrocolic ligament
   Gastrocolic omentum
   Gastrohepatic omentum
   Gastrophrenic ligament
   Gastrosplenic ligament
   Greater Omentum
   Hepatogastric ligament
   Lesser Omentum
	Ø Open
	4 Percutaneous Endoscopic
		Z No Device	**Z** No Qualifier

See Appendix L for Procedure Combinations
⊞   ØDT9ØZZ

NC Noncovered Procedure   LC Limited Coverage   QA Questionable OB Admit   NT New Tech Add-on   ⊞ Combination Member   ♂ Male   ♀ Female

ICD-10-PCS 2023   **395**

Ø   Medical and Surgical
D   Gastrointestinal System
U   Supplement   Definition: Putting in or on biological or synthetic material that physically reinforces and/or augments the function of a portion of a body part
Explanation: The biological material is non-living, or is living and from the same individual. The body part may have been previously replaced, and the SUPPLEMENT procedure is performed to physically reinforce and/or augment the function of the replaced body part.

Body Part Character 4	Approach Character 5	Device Character 6	Qualifier Character 7

1 Esophagus, Upper
   Cervical esophagus
2 Esophagus, Middle
   Thoracic esophagus
3 Esophagus, Lower
   Abdominal esophagus
4 Esophagogastric Junction
   Cardia
   Cardioesophageal junction
   Gastroesophageal (GE) junction
5 Esophagus
6 Stomach
7 Stomach, Pylorus
   Pyloric antrum
   Pyloric canal
   Pyloric sphincter
8 Small Intestine
9 Duodenum
A Jejunum
   Duodenojejunal flexure
B Ileum
C Ileocecal Valve
E Large Intestine
F Large Intestine, Right
G Large Intestine, Left
H Cecum
K Ascending Colon
L Transverse Colon
   Hepatic flexure
   Splenic flexure
M Descending Colon
N Sigmoid Colon
   Rectosigmoid junction
   Sigmoid flexure
P Rectum
   Anorectal junction
	Ø Open
	4 Percutaneous Endoscopic
	7 Via Natural or Artificial Opening
	8 Via Natural or Artificial Opening Endoscopic
		7 Autologous Tissue Substitute
		J Synthetic Substitute
		K Nonautologous Tissue Substitute
			Z No Qualifier

Q Anus Anal orifice	Ø Open 4 Percutaneous Endoscopic 7 Via Natural or Artificial Opening 8 Via Natural or Artificial Opening Endoscopic X External	7 Autologous Tissue Substitute J Synthetic Substitute K Nonautologous Tissue Substitute	Z No Qualifier

R Anal Sphincter
   External anal sphincter
   Internal anal sphincter
U Omentum
   Gastrocolic ligament
   Gastrocolic omentum
   Gastrohepatic omentum
   Gastrophrenic ligament
   Gastrosplenic ligament
   Greater Omentum
   Hepatogastric ligament
   Lesser Omentum
V Mesentery
   Mesoappendix
   Mesocolon
W Peritoneum
   Epiploic foramen
	Ø Open
	4 Percutaneous Endoscopic
		7 Autologous Tissue Substitute
		J Synthetic Substitute
		K Nonautologous Tissue Substitute
			Z No Qualifier

Ø   **Medical and Surgical**
D   **Gastrointestinal System**
V   **Restriction**   Definition: Partially closing an orifice or the lumen of a tubular body part
                       Explanation: The orifice can be a natural orifice or an artificially created orifice

Body Part Character 4		Approach Character 5	Device Character 6	Qualifier Character 7
1 Esophagus, Upper Cervical esophagus 2 Esophagus, Middle Thoracic esophagus 3 Esophagus, Lower Abdominal esophagus 4 Esophagogastric Junction Cardia Cardioesophageal junction Gastroesophageal (GE) junction 5 Esophagus 6 Stomach 7 Stomach, Pylorus Pyloric antrum Pyloric canal Pyloric sphincter 8 Small Intestine	9 Duodenum A Jejunum Duodenojejunal flexure B Ileum C Ileocecal Valve E Large Intestine F Large Intestine, Right G Large Intestine, Left H Cecum K Ascending Colon L Transverse Colon Hepatic flexure Splenic flexure M Descending Colon N Sigmoid Colon Rectosigmoid junction Sigmoid flexure P Rectum Anorectal junction	Ø Open 3 Percutaneous 4 Percutaneous Endoscopic	C Extraluminal Device D Intraluminal Device Z No Device	Z No Qualifier
1 Esophagus, Upper Cervical esophagus 2 Esophagus, Middle Thoracic esophagus 3 Esophagus, Lower Abdominal esophagus 4 Esophagogastric Junction Cardia Cardioesophageal junction Gastroesophageal (GE) junction 5 Esophagus 6 Stomach **NC** 7 Stomach, Pylorus Pyloric antrum Pyloric canal Pyloric sphincter 8 Small Intestine	9 Duodenum A Jejunum Duodenojejunal flexure B Ileum C Ileocecal Valve E Large Intestine F Large Intestine, Right G Large Intestine, Left H Cecum K Ascending Colon L Transverse Colon Hepatic flexure Splenic flexure M Descending Colon N Sigmoid Colon Rectosigmoid junction Sigmoid flexure P Rectum Anorectal junction	7 Via Natural or Artificial Opening 8 Via Natural or Artificial Opening Endoscopic	D Intraluminal Device Z No Device	Z No Qualifier
Q Anus Anal orifice		Ø Open 3 Percutaneous 4 Percutaneous Endoscopic X External	C Extraluminal Device D Intraluminal Device Z No Device	Z No Qualifier
Q Anus Anal orifice		7 Via Natural or Artificial Opening 8 Via Natural or Artificial Opening Endoscopic	D Intraluminal Device Z No Device	Z No Qualifier

Non-OR   ØDV6[7,8]DZ
HAC   ØDV64CZ when reported with PDx E66.Ø1 and SDx K68.11, K95.Ø1, K95.81, or T81.4Ø–T81.49 with 7th character A
NC   ØDV6[7,8]DZ

NC Noncovered Procedure   **LC** Limited Coverage   **QA** Questionable OB Admit   **NT** New Tech Add-on   ✛ Combination Member   ♂ Male   ♀ Female

ICD-10-PCS 2023   397

ØDV–ØDV

Gastrointestinal System

Ø   **Medical and Surgical**
D   **Gastrointestinal System**
W   **Revision**   Definition: Correcting, to the extent possible, a portion of a malfunctioning device or the position of a displaced device
                 Explanation: Revision can include correcting a malfunctioning or displaced device by taking out or putting in components of the device such as a screw or pin

Body Part Character 4	Approach Character 5	Device Character 6	Qualifier Character 7
Ø Upper Intestinal Tract D Lower Intestinal Tract	Ø Open 3 Percutaneous 4 Percutaneous Endoscopic 7 Via Natural or Artificial Opening 8 Via Natural or Artificial Opening Endoscopic	Ø Drainage Device 2 Monitoring Device 3 Infusion Device 7 Autologous Tissue Substitute C Extraluminal Device D Intraluminal Device J Synthetic Substitute K Nonautologous Tissue Substitute U Feeding Device Y Other Device	Z No Qualifier
Ø Upper Intestinal Tract D Lower Intestinal Tract	X External	Ø Drainage Device 2 Monitoring Device 3 Infusion Device 7 Autologous Tissue Substitute C Extraluminal Device D Intraluminal Device J Synthetic Substitute K Nonautologous Tissue Substitute U Feeding Device	Z No Qualifier
5 Esophagus	Ø Open 3 Percutaneous 4 Percutaneous Endoscopic	Y Other Device	Z No Qualifier
5 Esophagus	7 Via Natural or Artificial Opening 8 Via Natural or Artificial Opening Endoscopic	D Intraluminal Device Y Other Device	Z No Qualifier
5 Esophagus	X External	D Intraluminal Device	Z No Qualifier
6 Stomach	Ø Open 3 Percutaneous 4 Percutaneous Endoscopic	Ø Drainage Device 2 Monitoring Device 3 Infusion Device 7 Autologous Tissue Substitute C Extraluminal Device D Intraluminal Device J Synthetic Substitute K Nonautologous Tissue Substitute M Stimulator Lead U Feeding Device Y Other Device	Z No Qualifier
6 Stomach	7 Via Natural or Artificial Opening 8 Via Natural or Artificial Opening Endoscopic	Ø Drainage Device 2 Monitoring Device 3 Infusion Device 7 Autologous Tissue Substitute C Extraluminal Device D Intraluminal Device J Synthetic Substitute K Nonautologous Tissue Substitute U Feeding Device Y Other Device	Z No Qualifier
6 Stomach	X External	Ø Drainage Device 2 Monitoring Device 3 Infusion Device 7 Autologous Tissue Substitute C Extraluminal Device D Intraluminal Device J Synthetic Substitute K Nonautologous Tissue Substitute U Feeding Device	Z No Qualifier

Non-OR   ØDW[Ø,D][3,4,7,8]YZ
Non-OR   ØDW[Ø,D]8UZ
Non-OR   ØDW[Ø,D]X[Ø,2,3,7,C,D,J,K,U]Z
Non-OR   ØDW5[Ø,3,4]YZ
Non-OR   ØDW5[7,8]YZ
Non-OR   ØDW5XDZ
Non-OR   ØDW6[3,4]YZ
Non-OR   ØDW68UZ
Non-OR   ØDW6[7,8]YZ
Non-OR   ØDW6X[Ø,2,3,7,C,D,J,K,U]Z

ØDW Continued on next page

Non-OR Procedure   DRG Non-OR Procedure   Valid OR Procedure   HAC Associated Procedure   Combination Only   New/Revised April   New/Revised October

Ø   Medical and Surgical   *ØDW Continued*
D   Gastrointestinal System
W   Revision   Definition: Correcting, to the extent possible, a portion of a malfunctioning device or the position of a displaced device

                     Explanation: Revision can include correcting a malfunctioning or displaced device by taking out or putting in components of the device such as a screw or pin

Body Part Character 4	Approach Character 5	Device Character 6	Qualifier Character 7
8 Small Intestine E Large Intestine	Ø Open 4 Percutaneous Endoscopic 7 Via Natural or Artificial Opening 8 Via Natural or Artificial Opening Endoscopic	7 Autologous Tissue Substitute J Synthetic Substitute K Nonautologous Tissue Substitute	Z No Qualifier
Q Anus Anal orifice	Ø Open 3 Percutaneous 4 Percutaneous Endoscopic 7 Via Natural or Artificial Opening 8 Via Natural or Artificial Opening Endoscopic	L Artificial Sphincter	Z No Qualifier

R   Anal Sphincter
      External anal sphincter
      Internal anal sphincter
	Ø Open
	3 Percutaneous
	4 Percutaneous Endoscopic
		M Stimulator Lead	Z No Qualifier

U   Omentum
      Gastrocolic ligament
      Gastrocolic omentum
      Gastrohepatic omentum
      Gastrophrenic ligament
      Gastrosplenic ligament
      Greater Omentum
      Hepatogastric ligament
      Lesser Omentum
V   Mesentery
      Mesoappendix
      Mesocolon
W   Peritoneum
      Epiploic foramen
	Ø Open
	3 Percutaneous
	4 Percutaneous Endoscopic
		Ø Drainage Device
		7 Autologous Tissue Substitute
		J Synthetic Substitute
		K Nonautologous Tissue Substitute
			Z No Qualifier

Non-OR   ØDW[U,V,W][Ø,3,4]ØZ

Ø   Medical and Surgical
D   Gastrointestinal System
X   Transfer   Definition: Moving, without taking out, all or a portion of a body part to another location to take over the function of all or a portion of a body part

                     Explanation: The body part transferred remains connected to its vascular and nervous supply

Body Part Character 4	Approach Character 5	Device Character 6	Qualifier Character 7
6 Stomach	Ø Open 4 Percutaneous Endoscopic	Z No Device	5 Esophagus
8 Small Intestine	Ø Open 4 Percutaneous Endoscopic	Z No Device	5 Esophagus B Bladder C Ureter, Right D Ureter, Left F Ureters, Bilateral
E Large Intestine	Ø Open 4 Percutaneous Endoscopic	Z No Device	5 Esophagus 7 Vagina ♀ B Bladder

♀   ØDXE[Ø,4]Z7

Ø   Medical and Surgical
D   Gastrointestinal System
Y   Transplantation   Definition: Putting in or on all or a portion of a living body part taken from another individual or animal to physically take the place and/or function of all or a portion of a similar body part

                     Explanation: The native body part may or may not be taken out, and the transplanted body part may take over all or a portion of its function

Body Part Character 4	Approach Character 5	Device Character 6	Qualifier Character 7
5 Esophagus 6 Stomach 8 Small Intestine LC E Large Intestine LC	Ø Open	Z No Device	Ø Allogeneic 1 Syngeneic 2 Zooplastic

Non-OR   ØDY5ØZ[Ø,1,2]
LC   ØDY[8,E]ØZ[Ø,1,2]

NC Noncovered Procedure   **LC** Limited Coverage   **QA** Questionable OB Admit   **NT** New Tech Add-on   ⊞ Combination Member   ♂ Male   ♀ Female

ICD-10-PCS 2023   **399**

Hepatobiliary System and Pancreas ØF1–ØFY

Character Meanings

This Character Meaning table is provided as a guide to assist the user in the identification of character members that may be found in this section of code tables. It **SHOULD NOT** be used to build a PCS code.

Operation–Character 3		Body Part–Character 4		Approach–Character 5		Device–Character 6		Qualifier–Character 7	
1	Bypass	Ø	Liver	Ø	Open	Ø	Drainage Device	Ø	Allogeneic
2	Change	1	Liver, Right Lobe	3	Percutaneous	1	Radioactive Element	1	Syngeneic
5	Destruction	2	Liver, Left Lobe	4	Percutaneous Endoscopic	2	Monitoring Device	2	Zooplastic
7	Dilation	4	Gallbladder	7	Via Natural or Artificial Opening	3	Infusion Device	3	Duodenum OR Laser Interstitial Thermal Therapy
8	Division	5	Hepatic Duct, Right	8	Via Natural or Artificial Opening Endoscopic	7	Autologous Tissue Substitute	4	Stomach
9	Drainage	6	Hepatic Duct, Left	X	External	C	Extraluminal Device	5	Hepatic Duct, Right
B	Excision	7	Hepatic Duct, Common			D	Intraluminal Device	6	Hepatic Duct, Left
C	Extirpation	8	Cystic Duct			J	Synthetic Substitute	7	Hepatic Duct, Caudate
D	Extraction	9	Common Bile Duct			K	Nonautologous Tissue Substitute	8	Cystic Duct
F	Fragmentation	B	Hepatobiliary Duct			Y	Other Device	9	Common Bile Duct
H	Insertion	C	Ampulla of Vater			Z	No Device	B	Small Intestine
J	Inspection	D	Pancreatic Duct					C	Large Intestine
L	Occlusion	F	Pancreatic Duct, Accessory					F	Irreversible Electroporation
M	Reattachment	G	Pancreas					X	Diagnostic
N	Release							Z	No Qualifier
P	Removal								
Q	Repair								
R	Replacement								
S	Reposition								
T	Resection								
U	Supplement								
V	Restriction								
W	Revision								
Y	Transplantation								

AHA Coding Clinic for table ØF1
2020, 4Q, 53   Bypass pancreatic duct to stomach

AHA Coding Clinic for table ØF5
2018, 4Q, 39   Irreversible electroporation

AHA Coding Clinic for table ØF7
2016, 3Q, 27   Endoscopic retrograde cholangiopancreatography with sphincterotomy and insertion of pancreatic stent
2016, 1Q, 25   Endoscopic retrograde cholangiopancreatography with brush biopsy of pancreatic and common bile ducts
2015, 1Q, 32   Percutaneous transhepatic biliary drainage catheter placement
2014, 3Q, 15   Drainage of pancreatic pseudocyst

AHA Coding Clinic for table ØF8
2021, 4Q, 48-49   Division of liver for staged hepatectomy

AHA Coding Clinic for table ØF9
2020, 3Q, 34   Cystogastrostomy with stent insertion
2015, 1Q, 32   Percutaneous transhepatic biliary drainage catheter placement
2014, 3Q, 15   Drainage of pancreatic pseudocyst

AHA Coding Clinic for table ØFB
2019, 1Q, 3-8   Whipple procedure
2016, 3Q, 41   Open cholecystectomy with needle biopsy of liver
2016, 1Q, 23   Endoscopic ultrasound with aspiration biopsy of common hepatic duct
2016, 1Q, 25   Endoscopic retrograde cholangiopancreatography with brush biopsy of pancreatic and common bile ducts
2014, 3Q, 32   Pyloric-sparing Whipple procedure

AHA Coding Clinic for table ØFC
2016, 3Q, 27   Endoscopic retrograde cholangiopancreatography with sphincterotomy and insertion of pancreatic stent

AHA Coding Clinic for table ØFH
2022, 2Q, 26   Radioembolization of right hepatic lobe
2020, 4Q, 43-44   Insertion of radioactive element

AHA Coding Clinic for table ØFQ
2016, 3Q, 27   Revision of common bile duct anastomosis
2013, 4Q, 109   Separating conjoined twins

AHA Coding Clinic for table ØFT
2021, 4Q, 49   Division of liver for staged hepatectomy
2019, 1Q, 3-8   Whipple procedure
2012, 4Q, 99   Domino liver transplant

AHA Coding Clinic for table ØFY
2014, 3Q, 13   Orthotopic liver transplant with end to side cavoplasty
2012, 4Q, 99   Domino liver transplant

Liver

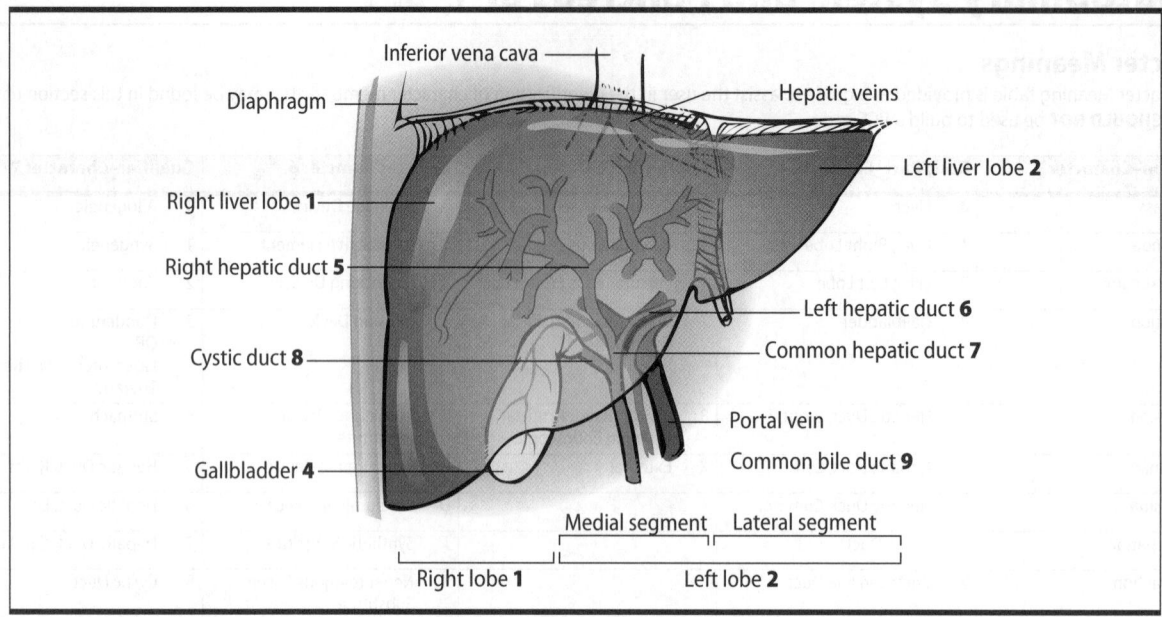

Inferior vena cava

Hepatic veins

Diaphragm

Left liver lobe **2**

Right liver lobe **1**

Right hepatic duct **5**

Left hepatic duct **6**

Common hepatic duct **7**

Cystic duct **8**

Portal vein

Common bile duct **9**

Gallbladder **4**

Medial segment   Lateral segment

Right lobe **1**   Left lobe **2**

Pancreas

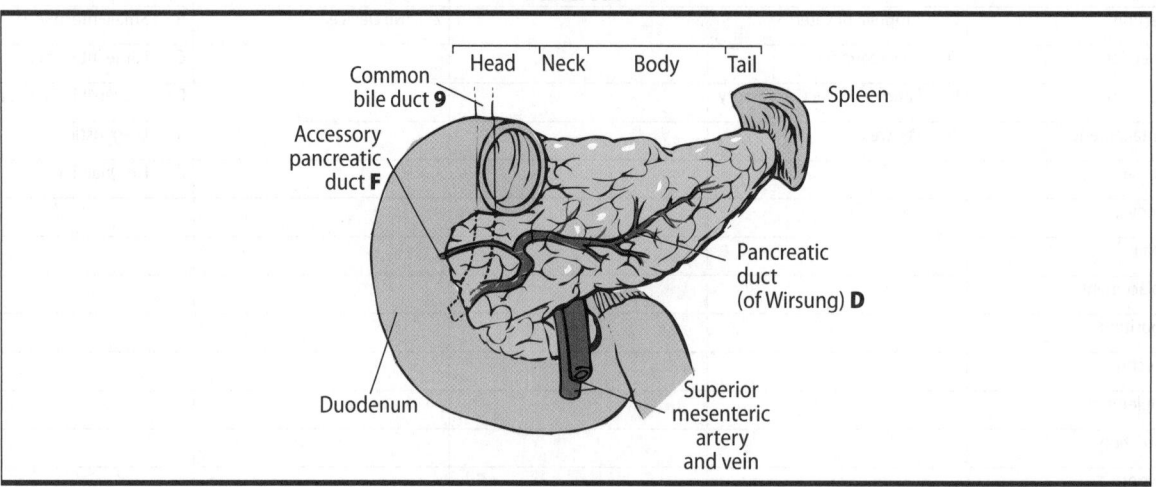

Head   Neck   Body   Tail

Common bile duct **9**

Spleen

Accessory pancreatic duct **F**

Pancreatic duct (of Wirsung) **D**

Duodenum

Superior mesenteric artery and vein

Gallbladder and Ducts

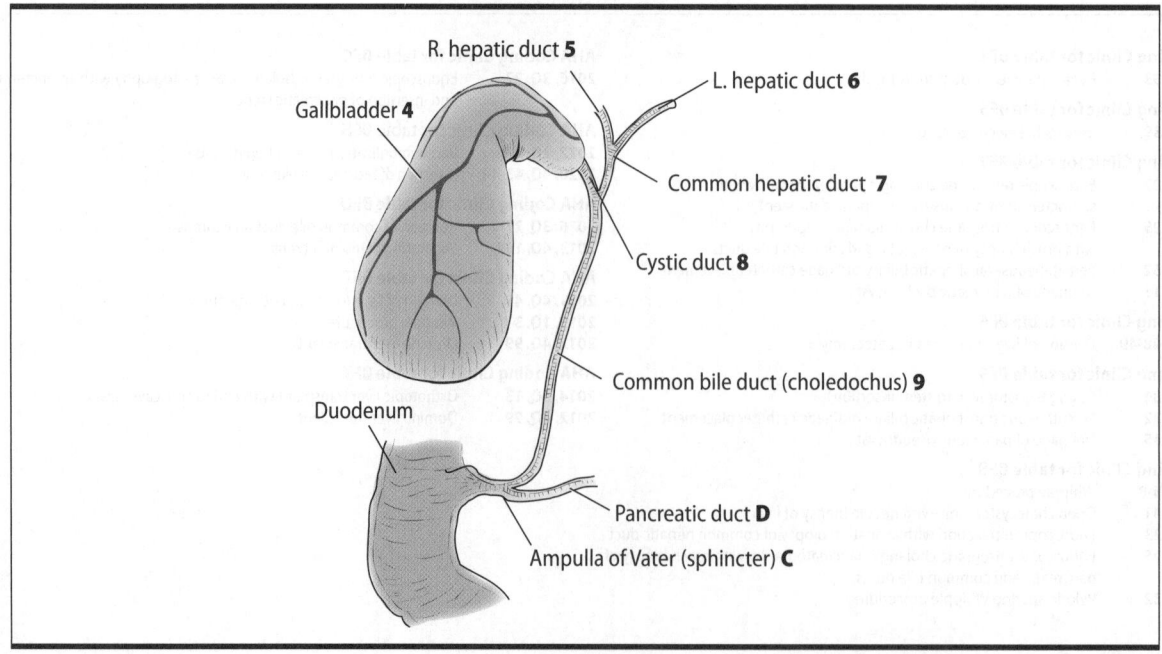

R. hepatic duct **5**

L. hepatic duct **6**

Gallbladder **4**

Common hepatic duct **7**

Cystic duct **8**

Common bile duct (choledochus) **9**

Duodenum

Pancreatic duct **D**

Ampulla of Vater (sphincter) **C**

Ø   **Medical and Surgical**
F   **Hepatobiliary System and Pancreas**
1   **Bypass**   Definition: Altering the route of passage of the contents of a tubular body part

             Explanation: Rerouting contents of a body part to a downstream area of the normal route, to a similar route and body part, or to an abnormal route and dissimilar body part. Includes one or more anastomoses, with or without the use of a device.

Body Part Character 4	Approach Character 5	Device Character 6	Qualifier Character 7
4 Gallbladder 5 Hepatic Duct, Right 6 Hepatic Duct, Left 7 Hepatic Duct, Common 8 Cystic Duct 9 Common Bile Duct	Ø Open 4 Percutaneous Endoscopic	D Intraluminal Device Z No Device	3 Duodenum 4 Stomach 5 Hepatic Duct, Right 6 Hepatic Duct, Left 7 Hepatic Duct, Caudate 8 Cystic Duct 9 Common Bile Duct B Small Intestine
D Pancreatic Duct Duct of Wirsung	Ø Open 4 Percutaneous Endoscopic	D Intraluminal Device Z No Device	3 Duodenum 4 Stomach B Small Intestine C Large Intestine
F Pancreatic Duct, Accessory Duct of Santorini G Pancreas	Ø Open 4 Percutaneous Endoscopic	D Intraluminal Device Z No Device	3 Duodenum B Small Intestine C Large Intestine

Ø   **Medical and Surgical**
F   **Hepatobiliary System and Pancreas**
2   **Change**   Definition: Taking out or off a device from a body part and putting back an identical or similar device in or on the same body part without cutting or puncturing the skin or a mucous membrane

             Explanation: All CHANGE procedures are coded using the approach EXTERNAL

Body Part Character 4	Approach Character 5	Device Character 6	Qualifier Character 7

Ø Liver
   Quadrate lobe
4 Gallbladder
B Hepatobiliary Duct
D Pancreatic Duct
   Duct of Wirsung
G Pancreas
	X External	Ø Drainage Device
		Y Other Device
			Z No Qualifier

Non-OR   All body part, approach, device, and qualifier values

NC Noncovered Procedure   **LC** Limited Coverage   **QA** Questionable OB Admit   **NT** New Tech Add-on   ⊞ Combination Member   ♂ Male   ♀ Female

ICD-10-PCS 2023   **403**

Ø   Medical and Surgical
F   Hepatobiliary System and Pancreas
5   Destruction   Definition: Physical eradication of all or a portion of a body part by the direct use of energy, force, or a destructive agent
                         Explanation: None of the body part is physically taken out

Body Part Character 4	Approach Character 5	Device Character 6	Qualifier Character 7
Ø Liver Quadrate lobe 1 Liver, Right Lobe 2 Liver, Left Lobe	Ø Open 3 Percutaneous 4 Percutaneous Endoscopic	Z No Device	3 Laser Interstitial Thermal Therapy F Irreversible Electroporation Z No Qualifier
4 Gallbladder	Ø Open 3 Percutaneous 4 Percutaneous Endoscopic	Z No Device	3 Laser Interstitial Thermal Therapy Z No Qualifier
4 Gallbladder	8 Via Natural or Artificial Opening Endoscopic	Z No Device	Z No Qualifier

5   Hepatic Duct, Right
6   Hepatic Duct, Left
7   Hepatic Duct, Common
8   Cystic Duct
9   Common Bile Duct
C   Ampulla of Vater
     Duodenal ampulla
     Hepatopancreatic ampulla
D   Pancreatic Duct
     Duct of Wirsung
F   Pancreatic Duct, Accessory
     Duct of Santorini
	Ø Open
	3 Percutaneous
	4 Percutaneous Endoscopic
		Z No Device	3 Laser Interstitial Thermal Therapy
			Z No Qualifier

5   Hepatic Duct, Right
6   Hepatic Duct, Left
7   Hepatic Duct, Common
8   Cystic Duct
9   Common Bile Duct
C   Ampulla of Vater
     Duodenal ampulla
     Hepatopancreatic ampulla
D   Pancreatic Duct
     Duct of Wirsung
F   Pancreatic Duct, Accessory
     Duct of Santorini
	7 Via Natural or Artificial Opening
	8 Via Natural or Artificial Opening
	     Endoscopic
		Z No Device	Z No Qualifier

G Pancreas	Ø Open 3 Percutaneous 4 Percutaneous Endoscopic	Z No Device	3 Laser Interstitial Thermal Therapy F Irreversible Electroporation Z No Qualifier
G Pancreas	8 Via Natural or Artificial Opening Endoscopic	Z No Device	Z No Qualifier

Non-OR   ØF5[5,6,7,8,9,C,D,F]4ZZ
Non-OR   ØF5[5,6,7,8,9,C,D,F]8ZZ
Non-OR   ØF5G4Z[F,Z]
Non-OR   ØF5G8ZZ

Ø   Medical and Surgical
F   Hepatobiliary System and Pancreas
7   Dilation   Definition: Expanding an orifice or the lumen of a tubular body part
                       Explanation: The orifice can be a natural orifice or an artificially created orifice. Accomplished by stretching a tubular body part using intraluminal pressure or by cutting part of the orifice or wall of the tubular body part.

Body Part Character 4	Approach Character 5	Device Character 6	Qualifier Character 7

5   Hepatic Duct, Right
6   Hepatic Duct, Left
7   Hepatic Duct, Common
8   Cystic Duct
9   Common Bile Duct
C   Ampulla of Vater
     Duodenal ampulla
     Hepatopancreatic ampulla
D   Pancreatic Duct
     Duct of Wirsung
F   Pancreatic Duct, Accessory
     Duct of Santorini
	Ø Open
	3 Percutaneous
	4 Percutaneous Endoscopic
	7 Via Natural or Artificial Opening
	8 Via Natural or Artificial Opening
	     Endoscopic
		D Intraluminal Device
		Z No Device
			Z No Qualifier

Non-OR   ØF7[5,6,7,8,9][3,4,8][D,Z]Z
Non-OR   ØF7[5,6,7,8,9,D]]7DZ
Non-OR   ØF7C8[D,Z]Z
Non-OR   ØF7[D,F][4,8][D,Z]Z

Non-OR Procedure   DRG Non-OR Procedure   Valid OR Procedure   HAC Associated Procedure   Combination Only   New/Revised April   New/Revised October

0   **Medical and Surgical**
F   **Hepatobiliary System and Pancreas**
8   **Division**   Definition: Cutting into a body part, without draining fluids and/or gases from the body part, in order to separate or transect a body part
                       Explanation: All or a portion of the body part is separated into two or more portions

Body Part Character 4	Approach Character 5	Device Character 6	Qualifier Character 7
0 Liver **1** Liver, Right Lobe **2** Liver, Left Lobe **G** Pancreas	**0** Open **3** Percutaneous **4** Percutaneous Endoscopic	**Z** No Device	**Z** No Qualifier

Non-OR   0F8[0,1,2]3ZZ

0   **Medical and Surgical**
F   **Hepatobiliary System and Pancreas**
9   **Drainage**   Definition: Taking or letting out fluids and/or gases from a body part
                        Explanation: The qualifier DIAGNOSTIC is used to identify drainage procedures that are biopsies

Body Part Character 4	Approach Character 5	Device Character 6	Qualifier Character 7
0 Liver Quadrate lobe **1** Liver, Right Lobe **2** Liver, Left Lobe	**0** Open **3** Percutaneous **4** Percutaneous Endoscopic	**0** Drainage Device	**Z** No Qualifier
0 Liver Quadrate lobe **1** Liver, Right Lobe **2** Liver, Left Lobe	**0** Open **3** Percutaneous **4** Percutaneous Endoscopic	**Z** No Device	**X** Diagnostic **Z** No Qualifier
4 Gallbladder **G** Pancreas	**0** Open **3** Percutaneous **4** Percutaneous Endoscopic **8** Via Natural or Artificial Opening Endoscopic	**0** Drainage Device	**Z** No Qualifier
4 Gallbladder **G** Pancreas	**0** Open **3** Percutaneous **4** Percutaneous Endoscopic **8** Via Natural or Artificial Opening Endoscopic	**Z** No Device	**X** Diagnostic **Z** No Qualifier

5   Hepatic Duct, Right
6   Hepatic Duct, Left
7   Hepatic Duct, Common
8   Cystic Duct
9   Common Bile Duct
C   Ampulla of Vater
     Duodenal ampulla
     Hepatopancreatic ampulla
D   Pancreatic Duct
     Duct of Wirsung
F   Pancreatic Duct, Accessory
     Duct of Santorini
	0 Open
	3 Percutaneous
	4 Percutaneous Endoscopic
	7 Via Natural or Artificial Opening
	8 Via Natural or Artificial Opening
	     Endoscopic
		0 Drainage Device	**Z** No Qualifier

5   Hepatic Duct, Right
6   Hepatic Duct, Left
7   Hepatic Duct, Common
8   Cystic Duct
9   Common Bile Duct
C   Ampulla of Vater
     Duodenal ampulla
     Hepatopancreatic ampulla
D   Pancreatic Duct
     Duct of Wirsung
F   Pancreatic Duct, Accessory
     Duct of Santorini
	0 Open
	3 Percutaneous
	4 Percutaneous Endoscopic
	7 Via Natural or Artificial Opening
	8 Via Natural or Artificial Opening
	     Endoscopic
		Z No Device	**X** Diagnostic
			Z No Qualifier

Non-OR 0F9[0,1,2][3,4]0Z	**Non-OR** 0F99[3,8]0Z
Non-OR 0F9[0,1,2][3,4]Z[X,Z]	**Non-OR** 0F9C[3,4,8]0Z
Non-OR 0F9[4,G]80Z	**Non-OR** 0F9[D,F][3,8]0Z
Non-OR 0F9G30Z	**Non-OR** 0F9[5,6,8,9,C,D,F]3Z[X,Z]
Non-OR 0F9[4,G]8Z[X,Z]	**Non-OR** 0F9[5,6,8,9,C,D,F][4,7,8]ZX
Non-OR 0F9G3Z[XZ]	**Non-OR** 0F9[5,6,8,D,F]8ZZ
Non-OR 0F9G4ZX	**Non-OR** 0F97[3,4,7,8]Z[X,Z]
Non-OR 0F9[5,6,8][3,8]0Z	**Non-OR** 0F99[4,7,8]ZZ
Non-OR 0F97[3,4,7,8]0Z	**Non-OR** 0F9C[4,8]ZZ

NC Noncovered Procedure   **LC** Limited Coverage   **QA** Questionable OB Admit   **NT** New Tech Add-on   ⊞ Combination Member   ♂ Male   ♀ Female

ICD-10-PCS 2023   405

Ø   Medical and Surgical
F   Hepatobiliary System and Pancreas
B   Excision   Definition: Cutting out or off, without replacement, a portion of a body part

                 Explanation: The qualifier DIAGNOSTIC is used to identify excision procedures that are biopsies

Body Part Character 4	Approach Character 5	Device Character 6	Qualifier Character 7
Ø Liver Quadrate lobe 1 Liver, Right Lobe 2 Liver, Left Lobe	Ø Open 3 Percutaneous 4 Percutaneous Endoscopic	Z No Device	X Diagnostic Z No Qualifier
4 Gallbladder G Pancreas	Ø Open 3 Percutaneous 4 Percutaneous Endoscopic 8 Via Natural or Artificial Opening Endoscopic	Z No Device	X Diagnostic Z No Qualifier

5   Hepatic Duct, Right
6   Hepatic Duct, Left
7   Hepatic Duct, Common
8   Cystic Duct
9   Common Bile Duct
C   Ampulla of Vater
     Duodenal ampulla
     Hepatopancreatic ampulla
D   Pancreatic Duct
     Duct of Wirsung
F   Pancreatic Duct, Accessory
     Duct of Santorini
	Ø Open
	3 Percutaneous
	4 Percutaneous Endoscopic
	7 Via Natural or Artificial Opening
	8 Via Natural or Artificial Opening
	     Endoscopic
		Z No Device	X Diagnostic
			Z No Qualifier

Non-OR   ØFB[Ø,1,2]3ZX
Non-OR   ØFB[4,G][3,4,8]ZX
Non-OR   ØFB[5,6,7,8,9,C,D,F][3,4,7,8]ZX
Non-OR   ØFB[5,6,7,8,9,C,D,F][4,8]ZZ

Ø   Medical and Surgical
F   Hepatobiliary System and Pancreas
C   Extirpation   Definition: Taking or cutting out solid matter from a body part

                 Explanation: The solid matter may be an abnormal byproduct of a biological function or a foreign body; it may be imbedded in a body part or in the lumen of a tubular body part. The solid matter may or may not have been previously broken into pieces.

Body Part Character 4	Approach Character 5	Device Character 6	Qualifier Character 7
Ø Liver Quadrate lobe 1 Liver, Right Lobe 2 Liver, Left Lobe	Ø Open 3 Percutaneous 4 Percutaneous Endoscopic	Z No Device	Z No Qualifier
4 Gallbladder G Pancreas	Ø Open 3 Percutaneous 4 Percutaneous Endoscopic 8 Via Natural or Artificial Opening Endoscopic	Z No Device	Z No Qualifier

5   Hepatic Duct, Right
6   Hepatic Duct, Left
7   Hepatic Duct, Common
8   Cystic Duct
9   Common Bile Duct
C   Ampulla of Vater
     Duodenal ampulla
     Hepatopancreatic ampulla
D   Pancreatic Duct
     Duct of Wirsung
F   Pancreatic Duct, Accessory
     Duct of Santorini
	Ø Open
	3 Percutaneous
	4 Percutaneous Endoscopic
	7 Via Natural or Artificial Opening
	8 Via Natural or Artificial Opening
	     Endoscopic
		Z No Device	Z No Qualifier

Non-OR   ØFC[5,6,7,8][3,4,7,8]ZZ
Non-OR   ØFC9[3,7,8]ZZ
Non-OR   ØFCC[4,8]ZZ
Non-OR   ØFC[D,F][3,4,8]ZZ

Non-OR Procedure   DRG Non-OR Procedure   Valid OR Procedure   HAC Associated Procedure   Combination Only   New/Revised April   New/Revised October

406   ICD-10-PCS 2023

Ø   Medical and Surgical
F   Hepatobiliary System and Pancreas
D   Extraction   Definition: Pulling or stripping out or off all or a portion of a body part by the use of force

            Explanation: The qualifier DIAGNOSTIC is used to identify extraction procedures that are biopsies

Body Part Character 4	Approach Character 5	Device Character 6	Qualifier Character 7
Ø Liver Quadrate lobe 1 Liver, Right Lobe 2 Liver, Left Lobe	3 Percutaneous 4 Percutaneous Endoscopic	Z No Device	X Diagnostic

4   Gallbladder
5   Hepatic Duct, Right
6   Hepatic Duct, Left
7   Hepatic Duct, Common
8   Cystic Duct
9   Common Bile Duct
C   Ampulla of Vater
     Duodenal ampulla
     Hepatopancreatic ampulla
D   Pancreatic Duct
     Duct of Wirsung
F   Pancreatic Duct, Accessory
     Duct of Santorini
G   Pancreas
	3 Percutaneous
	4 Percutaneous Endoscopic
	8 Via Natural or Artificial Opening
	     Endoscopic
		Z No Device	X Diagnostic

Non-OR   ØFD[Ø,1,2]3ZX
Non-OR   ØFD[4,5,6,7,8,9,C,D,F,G][3,4,8]ZX

Ø   Medical and Surgical
F   Hepatobiliary System and Pancreas
F   Fragmentation   Definition: Breaking solid matter in a body part into pieces

            Explanation: Physical force (e.g., manual, ultrasonic) applied directly or indirectly is used to break the solid matter into pieces. The solid matter may be an abnormal byproduct of a biological function or a foreign body. The pieces of solid matter are not taken out.

Body Part Character 4	Approach Character 5	Device Character 6	Qualifier Character 7

4   Gallbladder   NC
5   Hepatic Duct, Right   NC
6   Hepatic Duct, Left   NC
7   Hepatic Duct, Common
8   Cystic Duct   NC
9   Common Bile Duct   NC
C   Ampulla of Vater   NC
     Duodenal ampulla
     Hepatopancreatic ampulla
D   Pancreatic Duct   NC
     Duct of Wirsung
F   Pancreatic Duct, Accessory   NC
     Duct of Santorini
	Ø Open
	3 Percutaneous
	4 Percutaneous Endoscopic
	7 Via Natural or Artificial Opening
	8 Via Natural or Artificial Opening
	     Endoscopic
	X External
		Z No Device	Z No Qualifier

Non-OR   ØFF[4,5,6,7,8,9,C,D,F][8,X]ZZ
NC   ØFF[4,5,6,8,9,C,D,F]XZZ

Ø   Medical and Surgical
F   Hepatobiliary System and Pancreas
H   Insertion   Definition: Putting in a nonbiological appliance that monitors, assists, performs, or prevents a physiological function but does not physically take the place of a body part

            Explanation: None

Body Part Character 4	Approach Character 5	Device Character 6	Qualifier Character 7
Ø Liver Quadrate lobe 4 Gallbladder G Pancreas	Ø Open 3 Percutaneous 4 Percutaneous Endoscopic	1 Radioactive Element 2 Monitoring Device 3 Infusion Device Y Other Device	Z No Qualifier
1 Liver, Right Lobe 2 Liver, Left Lobe	Ø Open 3 Percutaneous 4 Percutaneous Endoscopic	2 Monitoring Device 3 Infusion Device	Z No Qualifier

B   Hepatobiliary Duct   ⊞
D   Pancreatic Duct
     Duct of Wirsung
	Ø Open
	3 Percutaneous
	4 Percutaneous Endoscopic
	7 Via Natural or Artificial Opening
	8 Via Natural or Artificial Opening
	     Endoscopic
		1 Radioactive Element
		2 Monitoring Device
		3 Infusion Device
		D Intraluminal Device
		Y Other Device
			Z No Qualifier

Non-OR ØFH[Ø,4,G]31Z **Non-OR** ØFH[Ø,4,G][Ø,3,4]3Z **Non-OR** ØFH[Ø,4,G][3,4]YZ **Non-OR** ØFH[1,2][Ø,3,4]3Z	**Non-OR** ØFH[B,D][Ø,3,4]3Z **Non-OR** ØFH[B,D][4,8]DZ **Non-OR** ØFH[B,D][7,8][2,3]Z **Non-OR** ØFH[B,D][3,4,7,8]YZ	**See Appendix L for Procedure Combinations** ⊞ ØFHB7DZ

NC Noncovered Procedure   **LC** Limited Coverage   **QA** Questionable OB Admit   **NT** New Tech Add-on   ⊞ Combination Member   ♂ Male   ♀ Female

Ø   **Medical and Surgical**
F   **Hepatobiliary System and Pancreas**
J   **Inspection**   Definition: Visually and/or manually exploring a body part

         Explanation: Visual exploration may be performed with or without optical instrumentation. Manual exploration may be performed directly or through intervening body layers.

Body Part Character 4	Approach Character 5	Device Character 6	Qualifier Character 7
Ø Liver Quadrate lobe	**Ø** Open **3** Percutaneous **4** Percutaneous Endoscopic **X** External	**Z** No Device	**Z** No Qualifier
4 Gallbladder **G** Pancreas	**Ø** Open **3** Percutaneous **4** Percutaneous Endoscopic **8** Via Natural or Artificial Opening Endoscopic **X** External	**Z** No Device	**Z** No Qualifier

B Hepatobiliary Duct
D Pancreatic Duct
    Duct of Wirsung
	Ø Open
	3 Percutaneous
	4 Percutaneous Endoscopic
	7 Via Natural or Artificial Opening
	8 Via Natural or Artificial Opening
	    Endoscopic
		Z No Device	**Z** No Qualifier

Non-OR   ØFJØ[3,X]ZZ
Non-OR   ØFJ[4,G][3,8,X]ZZ
Non-OR   ØFJ[B,D][3,7,8]ZZ

Ø   **Medical and Surgical**
F   **Hepatobiliary System and Pancreas**
L   **Occlusion**   Definition: Completely closing an orifice or the lumen of a tubular body part

         Explanation: The orifice can be a natural orifice or an artificially created orifice

Body Part Character 4	Approach Character 5	Device Character 6	Qualifier Character 7

5 Hepatic Duct, Right
6 Hepatic Duct, Left
7 Hepatic Duct, Common
8 Cystic Duct
9 Common Bile Duct
C Ampulla of Vater
    Duodenal ampulla
    Hepatopancreatic ampulla
D Pancreatic Duct
    Duct of Wirsung
F Pancreatic Duct, Accessory
    Duct of Santorini
	Ø Open
	3 Percutaneous
	4 Percutaneous Endoscopic
		C Extraluminal Device
		D Intraluminal Device
		Z No Device
			Z No Qualifier

5 Hepatic Duct, Right
6 Hepatic Duct, Left
7 Hepatic Duct, Common
8 Cystic Duct
9 Common Bile Duct
C Ampulla of Vater
    Duodenal ampulla
    Hepatopancreatic ampulla
D Pancreatic Duct
    Duct of Wirsung
F Pancreatic Duct, Accessory
    Duct of Santorini
	7 Via Natural or Artificial Opening
	8 Via Natural or Artificial Opening
	    Endoscopic
		D Intraluminal Device
		Z No Device
			Z No Qualifier

Non-OR   ØFL[5,6,7,8,9][3,4][C,D,Z]Z
Non-OR   ØFL[5,6,7,8,9][7,8][D,Z]Z

Non-OR Procedure   DRG Non-OR Procedure   Valid OR Procedure   HAC Associated Procedure   Combination Only   New/Revised April   New/Revised October

Ø   **Medical and Surgical**
F   **Hepatobiliary System and Pancreas**
M   **Reattachment**   Definition: Putting back in or on all or a portion of a separated body part to its normal location or other suitable location
             Explanation: Vascular circulation and nervous pathways may or may not be reestablished

Body Part Character 4	Approach Character 5	Device Character 6	Qualifier Character 7

Ø   Liver
     Quadrate lobe
1   Liver, Right Lobe
2   Liver, Left Lobe
4   Gallbladder
5   Hepatic Duct, Right
6   Hepatic Duct, Left
7   Hepatic Duct, Common
8   Cystic Duct
9   Common Bile Duct
C   Ampulla of Vater
     Duodenal ampulla
     Hepatopancreatic ampulla
D   Pancreatic Duct
     Duct of Wirsung
F   Pancreatic Duct, Accessory
     Duct of Santorini
G   Pancreas
	Ø Open
	4 Percutaneous Endoscopic
		Z No Device	Z No Qualifier

Non-OR   ØFM[4,5,6,7,8,9]4ZZ

Ø   **Medical and Surgical**
F   **Hepatobiliary System and Pancreas**
N   **Release**   Definition: Freeing a body part from an abnormal physical constraint by cutting or by the use of force
             Explanation: Some of the restraining tissue may be taken out but none of the body part is taken out

Body Part Character 4	Approach Character 5	Device Character 6	Qualifier Character 7
Ø Liver Quadrate lobe 1 Liver, Right Lobe 2 Liver, Left Lobe	Ø Open 3 Percutaneous 4 Percutaneous Endoscopic	Z No Device	Z No Qualifier
4 Gallbladder G Pancreas	Ø Open 3 Percutaneous 4 Percutaneous Endoscopic 8 Via Natural or Artificial Opening Endoscopic	Z No Device	Z No Qualifier

5   Hepatic Duct, Right
6   Hepatic Duct, Left
7   Hepatic Duct, Common
8   Cystic Duct
9   Common Bile Duct
C   Ampulla of Vater
     Duodenal ampulla
     Hepatopancreatic ampulla
D   Pancreatic Duct
     Duct of Wirsung
F   Pancreatic Duct, Accessory
     Duct of Santorini
	Ø Open
	3 Percutaneous
	4 Percutaneous Endoscopic
	7 Via Natural or Artificial Opening
	8 Via Natural or Artificial Opening
	     Endoscopic
		Z No Device	Z No Qualifier

NC Noncovered Procedure   **LC** Limited Coverage   **QA** Questionable OB Admit   **NT** New Tech Add-on   ⊞ Combination Member   ♂ Male   ♀ Female

ICD-10-PCS 2023   **409**

Ø Medical and Surgical
F Hepatobiliary System and Pancreas
P Removal Definition: Taking out or off a device from a body part

Explanation: If a device is taken out and a similar device put in without cutting or puncturing the skin or mucous membrane, the procedure is coded to the root operation CHANGE. Otherwise, the procedure for taking out a device is coded to the root operation REMOVAL.

Body Part Character 4		Approach Character 5		Device Character 6		Qualifier Character 7	
Ø	Liver Quadrate lobe	Ø 3 4	Open Percutaneous Percutaneous Endoscopic	Ø 2 3 Y	Drainage Device Monitoring Device Infusion Device Other Device	Z	No Qualifier
Ø	Liver Quadrate lobe	X	External	Ø 2 3	Drainage Device Monitoring Device Infusion Device	Z	No Qualifier
4 G	Gallbladder Pancreas	Ø 3 4	Open Percutaneous Percutaneous Endoscopic	Ø 2 3 D Y	Drainage Device Monitoring Device Infusion Device Intraluminal Device Other Device	Z	No Qualifier
4 G	Gallbladder Pancreas	X	External	Ø 2 3 D	Drainage Device Monitoring Device Infusion Device Intraluminal Device	Z	No Qualifier
B D	Hepatobiliary Duct Pancreatic Duct Duct of Wirsung	Ø 3 4 7 8	Open Percutaneous Percutaneous Endoscopic Via Natural or Artificial Opening Via Natural or Artificial Opening Endoscopic	Ø 1 2 3 7 C D J K Y	Drainage Device Radioactive Element Monitoring Device Infusion Device Autologous Tissue Substitute Extraluminal Device Intraluminal Device Synthetic Substitute Nonautologous Tissue Substitute Other Device	Z	No Qualifier
B D	Hepatobiliary Duct Pancreatic Duct Duct of Wirsung	X	External	Ø 1 2 3 D	Drainage Device Radioactive Element Monitoring Device Infusion Device Intraluminal Device	Z	No Qualifier

Non-OR	ØFPØ[3,4]YZ	
Non-OR	ØFPØX[Ø,2,3]Z	
Non-OR	ØFPG3ØZ	
Non-OR	ØFP[4,G][3,4]YZ	
Non-OR	ØFP4X[Ø,2,3,D]Z	
Non-OR	ØFPGX[Ø,2,3]Z	
Non-OR	ØFP[B,D][3,4]YZ	
Non-OR	ØFP[B,D][7,8][Ø,2,3,D,Y]Z	
Non-OR	ØFP[B,D]X[Ø,1,2,3,D]Z	

See Appendix L for Procedure Combinations
Combo-only	ØFP[B,D][7,8]DZ
Combo-only	ØFP[B,D]XDZ

Ø   Medical and Surgical
F   Hepatobiliary System and Pancreas
Q   Repair   Definition: Restoring, to the extent possible, a body part to its normal anatomic structure and function
                Explanation: Used only when the method to accomplish the repair is not one of the other root operations

Body Part Character 4	Approach Character 5	Device Character 6	Qualifier Character 7
Ø Liver Quadrate lobe 1 Liver, Right Lobe 2 Liver, Left Lobe	Ø Open 3 Percutaneous 4 Percutaneous Endoscopic	Z No Device	Z No Qualifier
4 Gallbladder G Pancreas	Ø Open 3 Percutaneous 4 Percutaneous Endoscopic 8 Via Natural or Artificial Opening Endoscopic	Z No Device	Z No Qualifier

5 Hepatic Duct, Right
6 Hepatic Duct, Left
7 Hepatic Duct, Common
8 Cystic Duct
9 Common Bile Duct
C Ampulla of Vater
   Duodenal ampulla
   Hepatopancreatic ampulla
D Pancreatic Duct
   Duct of Wirsung
F Pancreatic Duct, Accessory
   Duct of Santorini
	Ø Open
	3 Percutaneous
	4 Percutaneous Endoscopic
	7 Via Natural or Artificial Opening
	8 Via Natural or Artificial Opening
	   Endoscopic
		Z No Device	Z No Qualifier

Ø   Medical and Surgical
F   Hepatobiliary System and Pancreas
R   Replacement   Definition: Putting in or on biological or synthetic material that physically takes the place and/or function of all or a portion of a body part
                Explanation: The body part may have been taken out or replaced, or may be taken out, physically eradicated, or rendered nonfunctional during the REPLACEMENT procedure. A REMOVAL procedure is coded for taking out the device used in a previous replacement procedure.

Body Part Character 4	Approach Character 5	Device Character 6	Qualifier Character 7

5 Hepatic Duct, Right
6 Hepatic Duct, Left
7 Hepatic Duct, Common
8 Cystic Duct
9 Common Bile Duct
C Ampulla of Vater
   Duodenal ampulla
   Hepatopancreatic ampulla
D Pancreatic Duct
   Duct of Wirsung
F Pancreatic Duct, Accessory
   Duct of Santorini
	Ø Open
	4 Percutaneous Endoscopic
	8 Via Natural or Artificial Opening
	   Endoscopic
		7 Autologous Tissue Substitute
		J Synthetic Substitute
		K Nonautologous Tissue Substitute
			Z No Qualifier

Ø   Medical and Surgical
F   Hepatobiliary System and Pancreas
S   Reposition   Definition: Moving to its normal location, or other suitable location, all or a portion of a body part
                Explanation: The body part is moved to a new location from an abnormal location, or from a normal location where it is not functioning correctly. The body part may or may not be cut out or off to be moved to the new location.

Body Part Character 4	Approach Character 5	Device Character 6	Qualifier Character 7

Ø Liver
   Quadrate lobe
4 Gallbladder
5 Hepatic Duct, Right
6 Hepatic Duct, Left
7 Hepatic Duct, Common
8 Cystic Duct
9 Common Bile Duct
C Ampulla of Vater
   Duodenal ampulla
   Hepatopancreatic ampulla
D Pancreatic Duct
   Duct of Wirsung
F Pancreatic Duct, Accessory
   Duct of Santorini
G Pancreas
	Ø Open
	4 Percutaneous Endoscopic
		Z No Device	Z No Qualifier

Ø   **Medical and Surgical**
F   **Hepatobiliary System and Pancreas**
T   **Resection**   Definition: Cutting out or off, without replacement, all of a body part
                         Explanation: None

Body Part Character 4	Approach Character 5	Device Character 6	Qualifier Character 7
Ø Liver Quadrate lobe 1 Liver, Right Lobe 2 Liver, Left Lobe 4 Gallbladder G Pancreas ⊞	Ø Open 4 Percutaneous Endoscopic	Z No Device	Z No Qualifier

5   Hepatic Duct, Right
6   Hepatic Duct, Left
7   Hepatic Duct, Common
8   Cystic Duct
9   Common Bile Duct
C   Ampulla of Vater
     Duodenal ampulla
     Hepatopancreatic ampulla
D   Pancreatic Duct
     Duct of Wirsung
F   Pancreatic Duct, Accessory
     Duct of Santorini
	Ø Open
	4 Percutaneous Endoscopic
	7 Via Natural or Artificial Opening
	8 Via Natural or Artificial Opening
	     Endoscopic
		Z No Device	Z No Qualifier

Non-OR   ØFT[D,F][4,8]ZZ

See Appendix L for Procedure Combinations
⊞   ØFTGØZZ

Ø   **Medical and Surgical**
F   **Hepatobiliary System and Pancreas**
U   **Supplement**   Definition: Putting in or on biological or synthetic material that physically reinforces and/or augments the function of a portion of a body part
                         Explanation: The biological material is non-living, or is living and from the same individual. The body part may have been previously replaced, and the SUPPLEMENT procedure is performed to physically reinforce and/or augment the function of the replaced body part.

Body Part Character 4	Approach Character 5	Device Character 6	Qualifier Character 7

5   Hepatic Duct, Right
6   Hepatic Duct, Left
7   Hepatic Duct, Common
8   Cystic Duct
9   Common Bile Duct
C   Ampulla of Vater
     Duodenal ampulla
     Hepatopancreatic ampulla
D   Pancreatic Duct
     Duct of Wirsung
F   Pancreatic Duct, Accessory
     Duct of Santorini
	Ø Open
	3 Percutaneous
	4 Percutaneous Endoscopic
	8 Via Natural or Artificial Opening
	     Endoscopic
		7 Autologous Tissue Substitute
		J Synthetic Substitute
		K Nonautologous Tissue Substitute
			Z No Qualifier

Ø   Medical and Surgical
F   Hepatobiliary System and Pancreas
V   Restriction   Definition: Partially closing an orifice or the lumen of a tubular body part

                      Explanation: The orifice can be a natural orifice or an artificially created orifice

Body Part Character 4	Approach Character 5	Device Character 6	Qualifier Character 7

5   Hepatic Duct, Right
6   Hepatic Duct, Left
7   Hepatic Duct, Common
8   Cystic Duct
9   Common Bile Duct
C   Ampulla of Vater
     Duodenal ampulla
     Hepatopancreatic ampulla
D   Pancreatic Duct
     Duct of Wirsung
F   Pancreatic Duct, Accessory
     Duct of Santorini
	Ø Open
	3 Percutaneous
	4 Percutaneous Endoscopic
		C Extraluminal Device
		D Intraluminal Device
		Z No Device
			Z No Qualifier

5   Hepatic Duct, Right
6   Hepatic Duct, Left
7   Hepatic Duct, Common
8   Cystic Duct
9   Common Bile Duct
C   Ampulla of Vater
     Duodenal ampulla
     Hepatopancreatic ampulla
D   Pancreatic Duct
     Duct of Wirsung
F   Pancreatic Duct, Accessory
     Duct of Santorini
	7 Via Natural or Artificial Opening
	8 Via Natural or Artificial Opening
	     Endoscopic
		D Intraluminal Device
		Z No Device
			Z No Qualifier

Non-OR   ØFV[5,6,7,8,9][3,4][C,D,Z]Z
Non-OR   ØFV[5,6,7,8,9][7,8][D,Z]Z

Hepatobiliary System and Pancreas *(side tab)*

Ø   **Medical and Surgical**
F   **Hepatobiliary System and Pancreas**
W   **Revision**   Definition: Correcting, to the extent possible, a portion of a malfunctioning device or the position of a displaced device

                       Explanation: Revision can include correcting a malfunctioning or displaced device by taking out or putting in components of the device such as a screw or pin

Body Part Character 4	Approach Character 5	Device Character 6	Qualifier Character 7
Ø Liver Quadrate lobe	**Ø** Open **3** Percutaneous **4** Percutaneous Endoscopic	**Ø** Drainage Device **2** Monitoring Device **3** Infusion Device **Y** Other Device	**Z** No Qualifier
Ø Liver Quadrate lobe	**X** External	**Ø** Drainage Device **2** Monitoring Device **3** Infusion Device	**Z** No Qualifier
4 Gallbladder **G** Pancreas	**Ø** Open **3** Percutaneous **4** Percutaneous Endoscopic	**Ø** Drainage Device **2** Monitoring Device **3** Infusion Device **D** Intraluminal Device **Y** Other Device	**Z** No Qualifier
4 Gallbladder **G** Pancreas	**X** External	**Ø** Drainage Device **2** Monitoring Device **3** Infusion Device **D** Intraluminal Device	**Z** No Qualifier
B Hepatobiliary Duct **D** Pancreatic Duct Duct of Wirsung	**Ø** Open **3** Percutaneous **4** Percutaneous Endoscopic **7** Via Natural or Artificial Opening **8** Via Natural or Artificial Opening Endoscopic	**Ø** Drainage Device **2** Monitoring Device **3** Infusion Device **7** Autologous Tissue Substitute **C** Extraluminal Device **D** Intraluminal Device **J** Synthetic Substitute **K** Nonautologous Tissue Substitute **Y** Other Device	**Z** No Qualifier
B Hepatobiliary Duct **D** Pancreatic Duct Duct of Wirsung	**X** External	**Ø** Drainage Device **2** Monitoring Device **3** Infusion Device **7** Autologous Tissue Substitute **C** Extraluminal Device **D** Intraluminal Device **J** Synthetic Substitute **K** Nonautologous Tissue Substitute	**Z** No Qualifier

Non-OR	ØFWØ[3,4]YZ
Non-OR	ØFWØX[Ø,2,3]Z
Non-OR	ØFW[4,G][3,4]YZ
Non-OR	ØFW[4,G]X[Ø,2,3,D]Z
Non-OR	ØFW[B,D][3,4,7,8]YZ
Non-OR	ØFW[B,D]X[Ø,2,3,7,C,D,J,K]Z

Ø   **Medical and Surgical**
F   **Hepatobiliary System and Pancreas**
Y   **Transplantation**   Definition: Putting in or on all or a portion of a living body part taken from another individual or animal to physically take the place and/or function of all or a portion of a similar body part

                              Explanation: The native body part may or may not be taken out, and the transplanted body part may take over all or a portion of its function

Body Part Character 4	Approach Character 5	Device Character 6	Qualifier Character 7
Ø Liver `LC` Quadrate lobe **G** Pancreas `LC` `NC` ⊞	**Ø** Open	**Z** No Device	**Ø** Allogeneic **1** Syngeneic **2** Zooplastic

`LC` ØFYØØZ[Ø,1,2]	**See Appendix L for Procedure Combinations**
`LC` ØFYGØZ[Ø,1]	⊞ ØFYGØZ[Ø,1,2]
`NC` ØFYGØZ2	

`NC`   ØFYGØZ[Ø,1] If reported alone without one of the following procedures
    ØTYØØZ[Ø,1,2], ØTY1ØZ[Ø,1,2] and without one of the following
    diagnoses E1Ø.1Ø-E1Ø.9, E89.1	

Non-OR Procedure   DRG Non-OR Procedure   Valid OR Procedure   HAC Associated Procedure   Combination Only   New/Revised April   New/Revised October

414   ICD-10-PCS 2023

ØFW–ØFY *(side tab)*

Endocrine System 0G2–0GW

Character Meanings

This Character Meaning table is provided as a guide to assist the user in the identification of character members that may be found in this section of code tables. It **SHOULD NOT** be used to build a PCS code.

Operation–Character 3	Body Part–Character 4	Approach–Character 5	Device–Character 6	Qualifier–Character 7
2 Change	0 Pituitary Gland	0 Open	0 Drainage Device	3 Laser Interstitial Thermal Therapy
5 Destruction	1 Pineal Body	3 Percutaneous	1 Radioactive Element	X Diagnostic
8 Division	2 Adrenal Gland, Left	4 Percutaneous Endoscopic	2 Monitoring Device	Z No Qualifier
9 Drainage	3 Adrenal Gland, Right	X External	3 Infusion Device	
B Excision	4 Adrenal Glands, Bilateral		Y Other Device	
C Extirpation	5 Adrenal Gland		Z No Device	
H Insertion	6 Carotid Body, Left			
J Inspection	7 Carotid Body, Right			
M Reattachment	8 Carotid Bodies, Bilateral			
N Release	9 Para-aortic Body			
P Removal	B Coccygeal Glomus			
Q Repair	C Glomus Jugulare			
S Reposition	D Aortic Body			
T Resection	F Paraganglion Extremity			
W Revision	G Thyroid Gland Lobe, Left			
	H Thyroid Gland Lobe, Right			
	J Thyroid Gland Isthmus			
	K Thyroid Gland			
	L Superior Parathyroid Gland, Right			
	M Superior Parathyroid Gland, Left			
	N Inferior Parathyroid Gland, Right			
	P Inferior Parathyroid Gland, Left			
	Q Parathyroid Glands, Multiple			
	R Parathyroid Gland			
	S Endocrine Gland			

AHA Coding Clinic for table 0GB

2021, 2Q, 7   Infrarenal para-aortic paraganglioma with excision
2017, 2Q, 20   Near total thyroidectomy
2014, 3Q, 22   Transsphenoidal removal of pituitary tumor and fat graft placement

AHA Coding Clinic for table 0GH

2020, 4Q, 43-44   Insertion of radioactive element

AHA Coding Clinic for table 0GT

2017, 2Q, 20   Near total thyroidectomy

Endocrine System

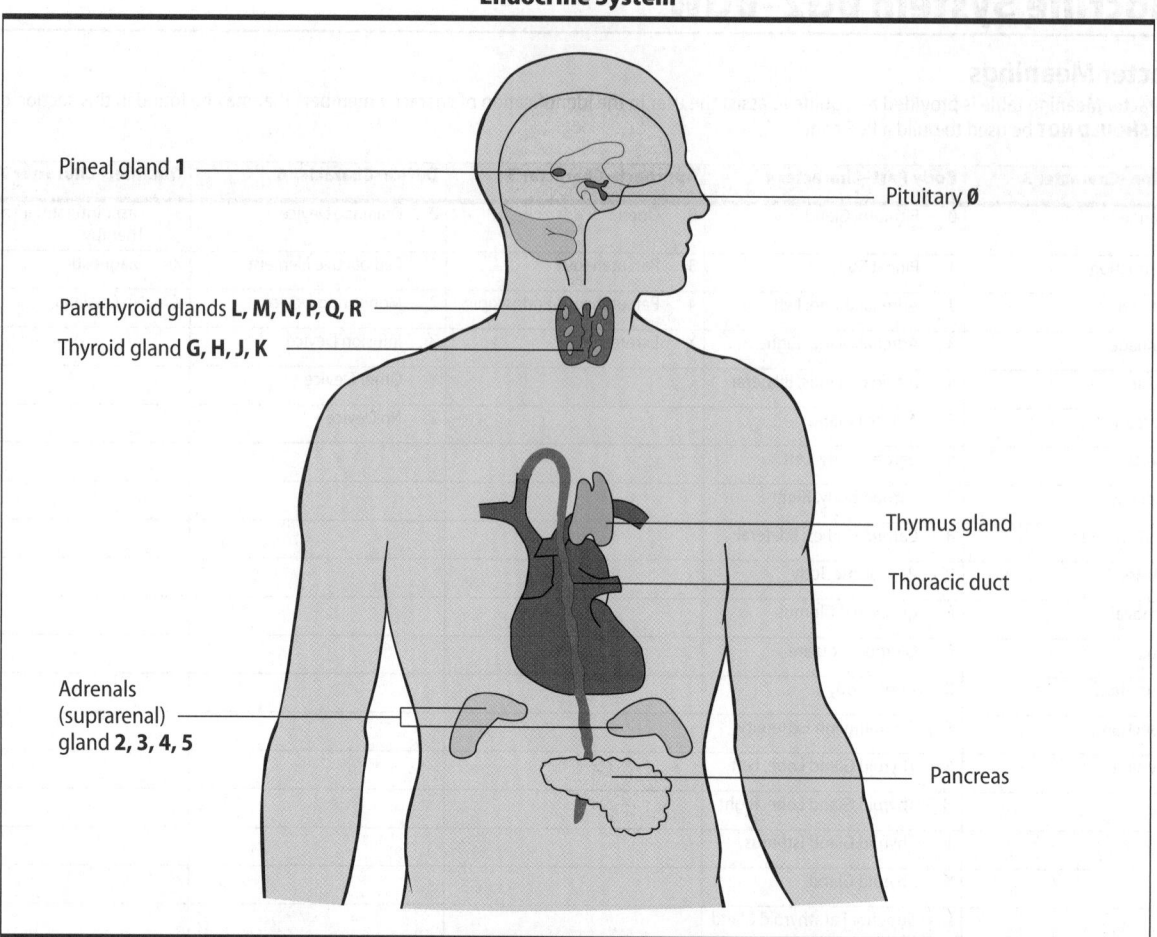

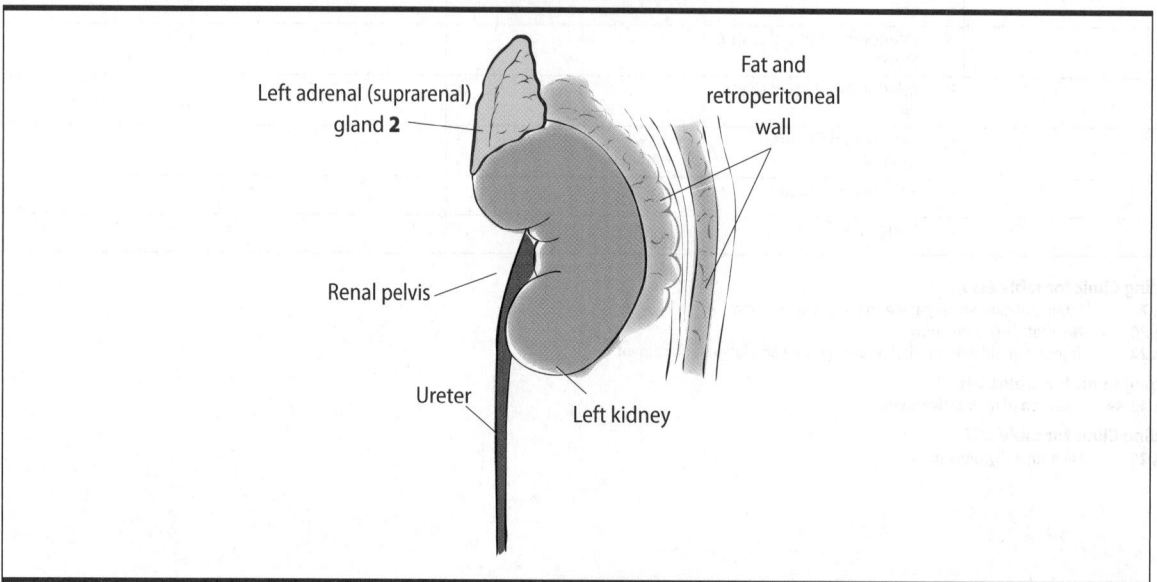

Thyroid

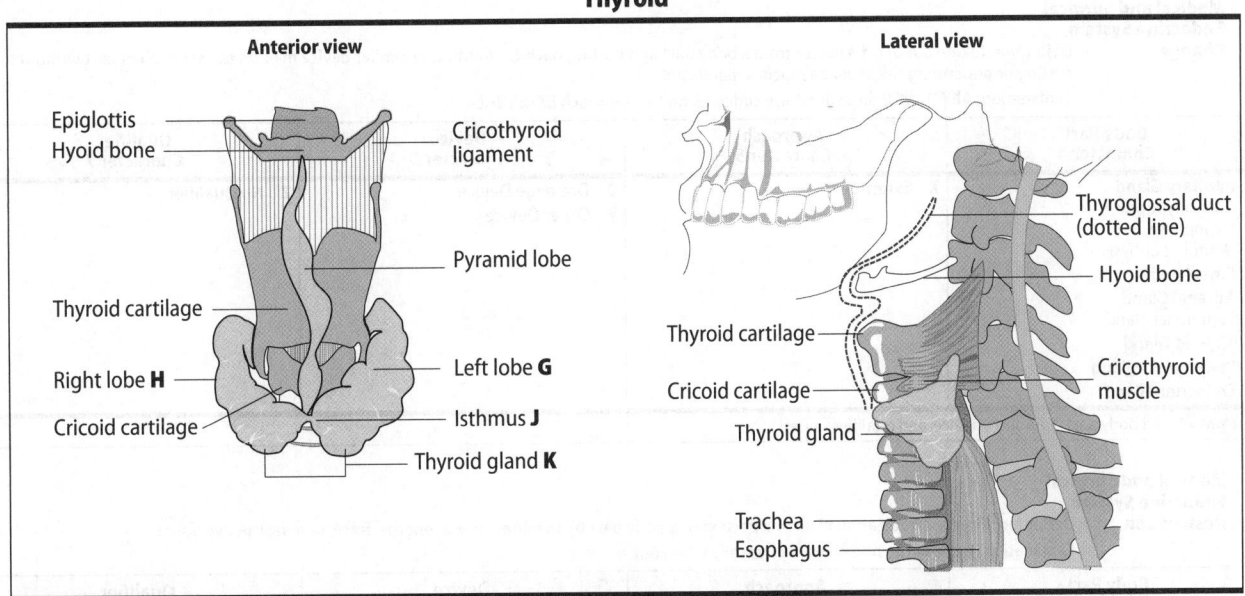

Anterior view

Epiglottis
Hyoid bone
Cricothyroid ligament
Pyramid lobe
Thyroid cartilage
Right lobe **H**
Left lobe **G**
Cricoid cartilage
Isthmus **J**
Thyroid gland **K**

Lateral view

Thyroglossal duct (dotted line)
Hyoid bone
Thyroid cartilage
Cricoid cartilage
Cricothyroid muscle
Thyroid gland
Trachea
Esophagus

Thyroid and Parathyroid Glands

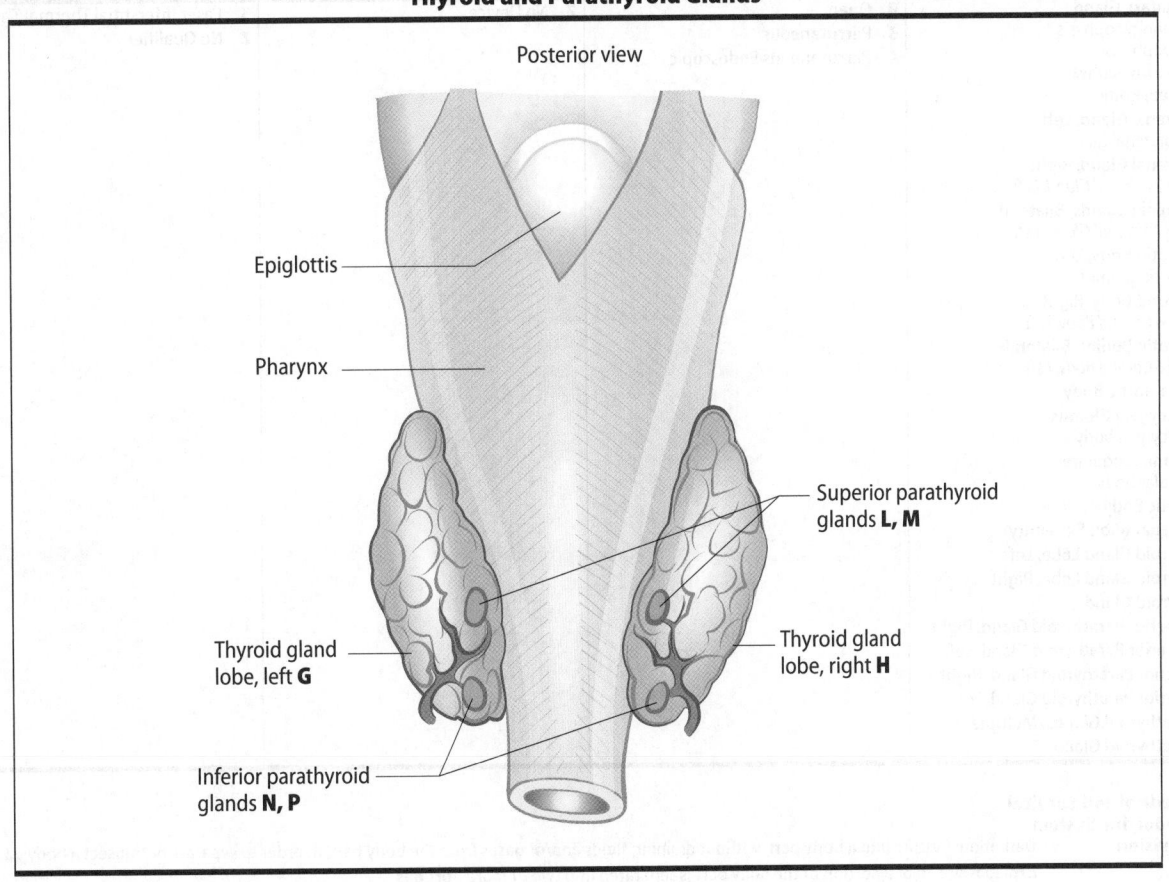

Posterior view

Epiglottis
Pharynx
Superior parathyroid glands **L, M**
Thyroid gland lobe, left **G**
Thyroid gland lobe, right **H**
Inferior parathyroid glands **N, P**

Endocrine System

0   **Medical and Surgical**
G   **Endocrine System**
2   **Change**   Definition: Taking out or off a device from a body part and putting back an identical or similar device in or on the same body part without cutting or puncturing the skin or a mucous membrane

Explanation: All CHANGE procedures are coded using the approach EXTERNAL

Body Part Character 4	Approach Character 5	Device Character 6	Qualifier Character 7

0 Pituitary Gland
    Adenohypophysis
    Hypophysis
    Neurohypophysis
1 Pineal Body
5 Adrenal Gland
    Suprarenal gland
K Thyroid Gland
R Parathyroid Gland
S Endocrine Gland
	X External	**0** Drainage Device
		Y Other Device
			Z No Qualifier

> **Non-OR**   All body part, approach, device, and qualifier values

0   **Medical and Surgical**
G   **Endocrine System**
5   **Destruction**   Definition: Physical eradication of all or a portion of a body part by the direct use of energy, force, or a destructive agent

Explanation: None of the body part is physically taken out

Body Part Character 4	Approach Character 5	Device Character 6	Qualifier Character 7

0 Pituitary Gland
    Adenohypophysis
    Hypophysis
    Neurohypophysis
1 Pineal Body
2 Adrenal Gland, Left
    Suprarenal gland
3 Adrenal Gland, Right
    See 2 Adrenal Gland, Left
4 Adrenal Glands, Bilateral
    See 2 Adrenal Gland, Left
6 Carotid Body, Left
    Carotid glomus
7 Carotid Body, Right
    See 6 Carotid Body, Left
8 Carotid Bodies, Bilateral
    See 6 Carotid Body, Left
9 Para-aortic Body
B Coccygeal Glomus
    Coccygeal body
C Glomus Jugulare
    Jugular body
D Aortic Body
F Paraganglion Extremity
G Thyroid Gland Lobe, Left
H Thyroid Gland Lobe, Right
K Thyroid Gland
L Superior Parathyroid Gland, Right
M Superior Parathyroid Gland, Left
N Inferior Parathyroid Gland, Right
P Inferior Parathyroid Gland, Left
Q Parathyroid Glands, Multiple
R Parathyroid Gland
	0 Open
	3 Percutaneous
	4 Percutaneous Endoscopic
		Z No Device	**3** Laser Interstitial Thermal Therapy
			Z No Qualifier

0   **Medical and Surgical**
G   **Endocrine System**
8   **Division**   Definition: Cutting into a body part, without draining fluids and/or gases from the body part, in order to separate or transect a body part

Explanation: All or a portion of the body part is separated into two or more portions

Body Part Character 4	Approach Character 5	Device Character 6	Qualifier Character 7

0 Pituitary Gland
    Adenohypophysis
    Hypophysis
    Neurohypophysis
J Thyroid Gland Isthmus
	0 Open
	3 Percutaneous
	4 Percutaneous Endoscopic
		Z No Device	**Z** No Qualifier

Non-OR Procedure   DRG Non-OR Procedure   Valid OR Procedure   HAC Associated Procedure   Combination Only   New/Revised April   New/Revised October

418   ICD-10-PCS 2023

0   **Medical and Surgical**
G   **Endocrine System**
9   **Drainage**   Definition: Taking or letting out fluids and/or gases from a body part
                      Explanation: The qualifier DIAGNOSTIC is used to identify drainage procedures that are biopsies

Body Part Character 4	Approach Character 5	Device Character 6	Qualifier Character 7
0 Pituitary Gland Adenohypophysis Hypophysis Neurohypophysis **1** Pineal Body **2** Adrenal Gland, Left Suprarenal gland **3** Adrenal Gland, Right *See 2 Adrenal Gland, Left* **4** Adrenal Glands, Bilateral *See 2 Adrenal Gland, Left* **6** Carotid Body, Left Carotid glomus **7** Carotid Body, Right *See 6 Carotid Body, Left* **8** Carotid Bodies, Bilateral *See 6 Carotid Body, Left* **9** Para-aortic Body **B** Coccygeal Glomus Coccygeal body **C** Glomus Jugulare Jugular body **D** Aortic Body **F** Paraganglion Extremity **G** Thyroid Gland Lobe, Left **H** Thyroid Gland Lobe, Right **K** Thyroid Gland **L** Superior Parathyroid Gland, Right **M** Superior Parathyroid Gland, Left **N** Inferior Parathyroid Gland, Right **P** Inferior Parathyroid Gland, Left **Q** Parathyroid Glands, Multiple **R** Parathyroid Gland	**0** Open **3** Percutaneous **4** Percutaneous Endoscopic	**0** Drainage Device	**Z** No Qualifier
0 Pituitary Gland Adenohypophysis Hypophysis Neurohypophysis **1** Pineal Body **2** Adrenal Gland, Left Suprarenal gland **3** Adrenal Gland, Right *See 2 Adrenal Gland, Left* **4** Adrenal Glands, Bilateral *See 2 Adrenal Gland, Left* **6** Carotid Body, Left Carotid glomus **7** Carotid Body, Right *See 6 Carotid Body, Left* **8** Carotid Bodies, Bilateral *See 6 Carotid Body, Left* **9** Para-aortic Body **B** Coccygeal Glomus Coccygeal body **C** Glomus Jugulare Jugular body **D** Aortic Body **F** Paraganglion Extremity **G** Thyroid Gland Lobe, Left **H** Thyroid Gland Lobe, Right **K** Thyroid Gland **L** Superior Parathyroid Gland, Right **M** Superior Parathyroid Gland, Left **N** Inferior Parathyroid Gland, Right **P** Inferior Parathyroid Gland, Left **Q** Parathyroid Glands, Multiple **R** Parathyroid Gland	**0** Open **3** Percutaneous **4** Percutaneous Endoscopic	**Z** No Device	**X** Diagnostic **Z** No Qualifier

Non-OR	0G9[0,1,2,3,4,6,7,8,9,B,C,D,F,G,H,K,L,M,N,P,Q,R]30Z
Non-OR	0G9[G,H,K,L,M,N,P,Q,R]40Z
Non-OR	0G9[2,3,4,G,H,K][3,4]ZX
Non-OR	0G9[0,1,2,3,4,6,7,8,9,B,C,D,F,G,H,K,L,M,N,P,Q,R]3ZZ
Non-OR	0G9[G,H,K,L,M,N,P,Q,R]4ZZ

NC Noncovered Procedure   **LC** Limited Coverage   **QA** Questionable OB Admit   **NT** New Tech Add-on   ⊞ Combination Member   ♂ Male   ♀ Female

ICD-10-PCS 2023   419   0G9–0G9

Ø   **Medical and Surgical**
G   **Endocrine System**
B   **Excision**   Definition: Cutting out or off, without replacement, a portion of a body part

Explanation: The qualifier DIAGNOSTIC is used to identify excision procedures that are biopsies

Body Part Character 4	Approach Character 5	Device Character 6	Qualifier Character 7

Ø Pituitary Gland
  Adenohypophysis
  Hypophysis
  Neurohypophysis
1 Pineal Body
2 Adrenal Gland, Left
  Suprarenal gland
3 Adrenal Gland, Right
  See 2 Adrenal Gland, Left
4 Adrenal Glands, Bilateral
  See 2 Adrenal Gland, Left
6 Carotid Body, Left
  Carotid glomus
7 Carotid Body, Right
  See 6 Carotid Body, Left
8 Carotid Bodies, Bilateral
  See 6 Carotid Body, Left
9 Para-aortic Body
B Coccygeal Glomus
  Coccygeal body
C Glomus Jugulare
  Jugular body
D Aortic Body
F Paraganglion Extremity
G Thyroid Gland Lobe, Left
H Thyroid Gland Lobe, Right
J Thyroid Gland Isthmus
L Superior Parathyroid Gland, Right
M Superior Parathyroid Gland, Left
N Inferior Parathyroid Gland, Right
P Inferior Parathyroid Gland, Left
Q Parathyroid Glands, Multiple
R Parathyroid Gland
	Ø Open
	3 Percutaneous
	4 Percutaneous Endoscopic
		Z No Device	**X** Diagnostic
			Z No Qualifier

Non-OR   ØGB[2,3,4,G,H,J][3,4]ZX

Ø   **Medical and Surgical**
G   **Endocrine System**
C   **Extirpation**   Definition: Taking or cutting out solid matter from a body part

Explanation: The solid matter may be an abnormal byproduct of a biological function or a foreign body; it may be imbedded in a body part or in the lumen of a tubular body part. The solid matter may or may not have been previously broken into pieces.

Body Part Character 4	Approach Character 5	Device Character 6	Qualifier Character 7

Ø Pituitary Gland
  Adenohypophysis
  Hypophysis
  Neurohypophysis
1 Pineal Body
2 Adrenal Gland, Left
  Suprarenal gland
3 Adrenal Gland, Right
  See 2 Adrenal Gland, Left
4 Adrenal Glands, Bilateral
  See 2 Adrenal Gland, Left
6 Carotid Body, Left
  Carotid glomus
7 Carotid Body, Right
  See 6 Carotid Body, Left
8 Carotid Bodies, Bilateral
  See 6 Carotid Body, Left
9 Para-aortic Body
B Coccygeal Glomus
  Coccygeal body
C Glomus Jugulare
  Jugular body
D Aortic Body
F Paraganglion Extremity
G Thyroid Gland Lobe, Left
H Thyroid Gland Lobe, Right
K Thyroid Gland
L Superior Parathyroid Gland, Right
M Superior Parathyroid Gland, Left
N Inferior Parathyroid Gland, Right
P Inferior Parathyroid Gland, Left
Q Parathyroid Glands, Multiple
R Parathyroid Gland
	Ø Open
	3 Percutaneous
	4 Percutaneous Endoscopic
		Z No Device	**Z** No Qualifier

Non-OR Procedure   DRG Non-OR Procedure   Valid OR Procedure   HAC Associated Procedure   Combination Only   New/Revised April   New/Revised October

Ø   Medical and Surgical
G   Endocrine System
H   Insertion   Definition: Putting in a nonbiological appliance that monitors, assists, performs, or prevents a physiological function but does not physically take the place of a body part

               Explanation: None

Body Part Character 4	Approach Character 5	Device Character 6	Qualifier Character 7
S Endocrine Gland	Ø Open 3 Percutaneous 4 Percutaneous Endoscopic	1 Radioactive Element 2 Monitoring Device 3 Infusion Device Y Other Device	Z No Qualifier

Non-OR   ØGHS31Z
Non-OR   ØGHS[3,4]YZ

Ø   Medical and Surgical
G   Endocrine System
J   Inspection   Definition: Visually and/or manually exploring a body part

               Explanation: Visual exploration may be performed with or without optical instrumentation. Manual exploration may be performed directly or through intervening body layers.

Body Part Character 4	Approach Character 5	Device Character 6	Qualifier Character 7

Ø   Pituitary Gland
    Adenohypophysis
    Hypophysis
    Neurohypophysis
1   Pineal Body
5   Adrenal Gland
    Suprarenal gland
K   Thyroid Gland
R   Parathyroid Gland
S   Endocrine Gland
	Ø Open
	3 Percutaneous
	4 Percutaneous Endoscopic
		Z No Device	Z No Qualifier

Non-OR   ØGJ[Ø,1,5,K,R,S]3ZZ

Ø   Medical and Surgical
G   Endocrine System
M   Reattachment   Definition: Putting back in or on all or a portion of a separated body part to its normal location or other suitable location

               Explanation: Vascular circulation and nervous pathways may or may not be reestablished

Body Part Character 4	Approach Character 5	Device Character 6	Qualifier Character 7

2   Adrenal Gland, Left
    Suprarenal gland
3   Adrenal Gland, Right
    See 2 Adrenal Gland, Left
G   Thyroid Gland Lobe, Left
H   Thyroid Gland Lobe, Right
L   Superior Parathyroid Gland, Right
M   Superior Parathyroid Gland, Left
N   Inferior Parathyroid Gland, Right
P   Inferior Parathyroid Gland, Left
Q   Parathyroid Glands, Multiple
R   Parathyroid Gland
	Ø Open
	4 Percutaneous Endoscopic
		Z No Device	Z No Qualifier

NC Noncovered Procedure   LC Limited Coverage   OA Questionable OB Admit   NT New Tech Add-on   ⊞ Combination Member   ♂ Male   ♀ Female

ICD-10-PCS 2023   421

ØGH–ØGM

Endocrine System

Ø **Medical and Surgical**
G **Endocrine System**
N **Release**   Definition: Freeing a body part from an abnormal physical constraint by cutting or by the use of force
                 Explanation: Some of the restraining tissue may be taken out but none of the body part is taken out

Body Part Character 4	Approach Character 5	Device Character 6	Qualifier Character 7

Ø **Pituitary Gland**
     Adenohypophysis
     Hypophysis
     Neurohypophysis
 1 **Pineal Body**
 2 **Adrenal Gland, Left**
     Suprarenal gland
 3 **Adrenal Gland, Right**
     See 2 Adrenal Gland, Left
 4 **Adrenal Glands, Bilateral**
     See 2 Adrenal Gland, Left
 6 **Carotid Body, Left**
     Carotid glomus
 7 **Carotid Body, Right**
     See 6 Carotid Body, Left
 8 **Carotid Bodies, Bilateral**
     See 6 Carotid Body, Left
 9 **Para-aortic Body**
 B **Coccygeal Glomus**
     Coccygeal body
 C **Glomus Jugulare**
     Jugular body
 D **Aortic Body**
 F **Paraganglion Extremity**
 G **Thyroid Gland Lobe, Left**
 H **Thyroid Gland Lobe, Right**
 K **Thyroid Gland**
 L **Superior Parathyroid Gland, Right**
 M **Superior Parathyroid Gland, Left**
 N **Inferior Parathyroid Gland, Right**
 P **Inferior Parathyroid Gland, Left**
 Q **Parathyroid Glands, Multiple**
 R **Parathyroid Gland**
	Ø Open
	 3 Percutaneous
	 4 Percutaneous Endoscopic
		Z No Device	Z No Qualifier

Non-OR   ØGN[6,7,8,9,B,C,D,F][Ø,3,4]ZZ

Ø **Medical and Surgical**
G **Endocrine System**
P **Removal**   Definition: Taking out or off a device from a body part
                 Explanation: If a device is taken out and a similar device put in without cutting or puncturing the skin or mucous membrane, the procedure is coded to the root operation CHANGE. Otherwise, the procedure for taking out a device is coded to the root operation REMOVAL.

Body Part Character 4	Approach Character 5	Device Character 6	Qualifier Character 7

Ø **Pituitary Gland**
     Adenohypophysis
     Hypophysis
     Neurohypophysis
 1 **Pineal Body**
 5 **Adrenal Gland**
     Suprarenal gland
 K **Thyroid Gland**
 R **Parathyroid Gland**
	Ø Open
	 3 Percutaneous
	 4 Percutaneous Endoscopic
	 X External
		Ø Drainage Device	Z No Qualifier

S **Endocrine Gland**	Ø Open 3 Percutaneous 4 Percutaneous Endoscopic	Ø Drainage Device 2 Monitoring Device 3 Infusion Device Y Other Device	Z No Qualifier
S **Endocrine Gland**	X External	Ø Drainage Device 2 Monitoring Device 3 Infusion Device	Z No Qualifier

Non-OR   ØGP[Ø,1,5,K,R]XØZ
Non-OR   ØGPS[3,4]YZ
Non-OR   ØGPSX[Ø,2,3]Z

Non-OR Procedure   DRG Non-OR Procedure   Valid OR Procedure   HAC Associated Procedure   Combination Only   New/Revised April   New/Revised October

422   ICD-10-PCS 2023

Ø   **Medical and Surgical**
G   **Endocrine System**
Q   **Repair**   Definition: Restoring, to the extent possible, a body part to its normal anatomic structure and function

                         Explanation: Used only when the method to accomplish the repair is not one of the other root operations

Body Part Character 4	Approach Character 5	Device Character 6	Qualifier Character 7

Ø **Pituitary Gland**
    Adenohypophysis
    Hypophysis
    Neurohypophysis
1 **Pineal Body**
2 **Adrenal Gland, Left**
    Suprarenal gland
3 **Adrenal Gland, Right**
    See 2 Adrenal Gland, Left
4 **Adrenal Glands, Bilateral**
    See 2 Adrenal Gland, Left
6 **Carotid Body, Left**
    Carotid glomus
7 **Carotid Body, Right**
    See 6 Carotid Body, Left
8 **Carotid Bodies, Bilateral**
    See 6 Carotid Body, Left
9 **Para-aortic Body**
B **Coccygeal Glomus**
    Coccygeal body
C **Glomus Jugulare**
    Jugular body
D **Aortic Body**
F **Paraganglion Extremity**
G **Thyroid Gland Lobe, Left**
H **Thyroid Gland Lobe, Right**
J **Thyroid Gland Isthmus**
K **Thyroid Gland**
L **Superior Parathyroid Gland, Right**
M **Superior Parathyroid Gland, Left**
N **Inferior Parathyroid Gland, Right**
P **Inferior Parathyroid Gland, Left**
Q **Parathyroid Glands, Multiple**
R **Parathyroid Gland**
	Ø Open
	3 Percutaneous
	4 Percutaneous Endoscopic
		Z No Device	**Z** No Qualifier

Ø   **Medical and Surgical**
G   **Endocrine System**
S   **Reposition**   Definition: Moving to its normal location, or other suitable location, all or a portion of a body part

                         Explanation: The body part is moved to a new location from an abnormal location, or from a normal location where it is not functioning correctly. The body part may or may not be cut out or off to be moved to the new location.

Body Part Character 4	Approach Character 5	Device Character 6	Qualifier Character 7

2 **Adrenal Gland, Left**
    Suprarenal gland
3 **Adrenal Gland, Right**
    See 2 Adrenal Gland, Left
G **Thyroid Gland Lobe, Left**
H **Thyroid Gland Lobe, Right**
L **Superior Parathyroid Gland, Right**
M **Superior Parathyroid Gland, Left**
N **Inferior Parathyroid Gland, Right**
P **Inferior Parathyroid Gland, Left**
Q **Parathyroid Glands, Multiple**
R **Parathyroid Gland**
	Ø Open
	4 Percutaneous Endoscopic
		Z No Device	**Z** No Qualifier

NC Noncovered Procedure   **LC** Limited Coverage   **QA** Questionable OB Admit   **NT** New Tech Add-on   ⊞ Combination Member   ♂ Male   ♀ Female

ICD-10-PCS 2023   423

ØGQ–ØGS

Ø Medical and Surgical
G Endocrine System
T Resection   Definition: Cutting out or off, without replacement, all of a body part
                 Explanation: None

Body Part Character 4	Approach Character 5	Device Character 6	Qualifier Character 7

Ø   Pituitary Gland
    Adenohypophysis
    Hypophysis
    Neurohypophysis
1   Pineal Body
2   Adrenal Gland, Left
    Suprarenal gland
3   Adrenal Gland, Right
    See 2 Adrenal Gland, Left
4   Adrenal Glands, Bilateral
    See 2 Adrenal Gland, Left
6   Carotid Body, Left
    Carotid glomus
7   Carotid Body, Right
    See 6 Carotid Body, Left
8   Carotid Bodies, Bilateral
    See 6 Carotid Body, Left
9   Para-aortic Body
B   Coccygeal Glomus
    Coccygeal body
C   Glomus Jugulare
    Jugular body
D   Aortic Body
F   Paraganglion Extremity
G   Thyroid Gland Lobe, Left
H   Thyroid Gland Lobe, Right
J   Thyroid Gland Isthmus
K   Thyroid Gland
L   Superior Parathyroid Gland, Right
M   Superior Parathyroid Gland, Left
N   Inferior Parathyroid Gland, Right
P   Inferior Parathyroid Gland, Left
Q   Parathyroid Glands, Multiple
R   Parathyroid Gland
	Ø Open
	4 Percutaneous Endoscopic
		Z No Device	Z No Qualifier

Non-OR   ØGT[6,7,8,9,B,C,D,F][Ø,4]ZZ

Ø Medical and Surgical
G Endocrine System
W Revision   Definition: Correcting, to the extent possible, a portion of a malfunctioning device or the position of a displaced device
                 Explanation: Revision can include correcting a malfunctioning or displaced device by taking out or putting in components of the device such as a screw or pin

Body Part Character 4	Approach Character 5	Device Character 6	Qualifier Character 7

Ø   Pituitary Gland
    Adenohypophysis
    Hypophysis
    Neurohypophysis
1   Pineal Body
5   Adrenal Gland
    Suprarenal gland
K   Thyroid Gland
R   Parathyroid Gland
	Ø Open
	3 Percutaneous
	4 Percutaneous Endoscopic
	X External
		Ø Drainage Device	Z No Qualifier

S Endocrine Gland	Ø Open 3 Percutaneous 4 Percutaneous Endoscopic	Ø Drainage Device 2 Monitoring Device 3 Infusion Device Y Other Device	Z No Qualifier
S Endocrine Gland	X External	Ø Drainage Device 2 Monitoring Device 3 Infusion Device	Z No Qualifier

Non-OR   ØGW[Ø,1,5,K,R]XØZ
Non-OR   ØGWS[3,4]YZ
Non-OR   ØGWSX[Ø,2,3]Z

Skin and Breast ØHØ–ØHX

Character Meanings*

This Character Meaning table is provided as a guide to assist the user in the identification of character members that may be found in this section of code tables. It **SHOULD NOT** be used to build a PCS code.

Operation–Character 3		Body Part–Character 4		Approach–Character 5		Device–Character 6		Qualifier–Character 7	
Ø	Alteration	Ø	Skin, Scalp	Ø	Open	Ø	Drainage Device	2	Cell Suspension Technique
2	Change	1	Skin, Face	3	Percutaneous	1	Radioactive Element	3	Full Thickness OR Laser Interstitial Thermal Therapy
5	Destruction	2	Skin, Right Ear	7	Via Natural or Artificial Opening	7	Autologous Tissue Substitute	4	Partial Thickness
8	Division	3	Skin, Left Ear	8	Via Natural or Artificial Opening Endoscopic	J	Synthetic Substitute	5	Latissimus Dorsi Myocutaneous Flap
9	Drainage	4	Skin, Neck	X	External	K	Nonautologous Tissue Substitute	6	Transverse Rectus Abdominis Myocutaneous Flap
B	Excision	5	Skin, Chest			N	Tissue Expander	7	Deep Inferior Epigastric Artery Perforator Flap
C	Extirpation	6	Skin, Back			Y	Other Device	8	Superficial Inferior Epigastric Artery Flap
D	Extraction	7	Skin, Abdomen			Z	No Device	9	Gluteal Artery Perforator Flap
H	Insertion	8	Skin, Buttock					D	Multiple
J	Inspection	9	Skin, Perineum					X	Diagnostic
M	Reattachment	A	Skin, Inguinal					Z	No Qualifier
N	Release	B	Skin, Right Upper Arm						
P	Removal	C	Skin, Left Upper Arm						
Q	Repair	D	Skin, Right Lower Arm						
R	Replacement	E	Skin, Left Lower Arm						
S	Reposition	F	Skin, Right Hand						
T	Resection	G	Skin, Left Hand						
U	Supplement	H	Skin, Right Upper Leg						
W	Revision	J	Skin, Left Upper Leg						
X	Transfer	K	Skin, Right Lower Leg						
		L	Skin, Left Lower Leg						
		M	Skin, Right Foot						
		N	Skin, Left Foot						
		P	Skin						
		Q	Finger Nail						
		R	Toe Nail						
		S	Hair						
		T	Breast, Right						
		U	Breast, Left						
		V	Breast, Bilateral						
		W	Nipple, Right						
		X	Nipple, Left						
		Y	Supernumerary Breast						

* Includes skin and breast glands and ducts.

AHA Coding Clinic for table ØHØ

2022, 1Q, 14	Reduction mammoplasty for breast symmetry
2022, 1Q, 15	Nipple reconstruction and breast reduction
2019, 4Q, 30-31	Breast procedures

AHA Coding Clinic for table ØH5

2019, 4Q, 30-31	Breast procedures

AHA Coding Clinic for table ØH9

2019, 4Q, 30-31	Breast procedures

AHA Coding Clinic for table ØHB

2022, 1Q, 14	Reduction mammoplasty for breast symmetry
2020, 1Q, 31	Repair of buried penis
2019, 4Q, 30-31	Breast procedures
2018, 1Q, 14	Excisional debridement of breast tissue and skin
2016, 3Q, 29	Closure of bilateral alveolar clefts
2015, 3Q, 3-8	Excisional and nonexcisional debridement

AHA Coding Clinic for table ØHC

2019, 4Q, 30-31	Breast procedures

AHA Coding Clinic for table ØHD

2019, 4Q, 30-31	Breast procedures
2016, 1Q, 40	Nonexcisional debridement of skin and subcutaneous tissue
2015, 3Q, 3-8	Excisional and nonexcisional debridement

AHA Coding Clinic for table ØHH

2019, 4Q, 30-31	Breast procedures
2017, 4Q, 67	New qualifier values - Pedicle flap procedures
2014, 2Q, 12	Pedicle latissimus myocutaneous flap with placement of breast tissue expanders
2013, 4Q, 107	Breast tissue expander placement using acellular dermal matrix

AHA Coding Clinic for table ØHJ

2019, 4Q, 30-31	Breast procedures

AHA Coding Clinic for table ØHN

2019, 4Q, 30-31	Breast procedures

AHA Coding Clinic for table ØHP

2019, 4Q, 30-31	Breast procedures
2018, 3Q, 13	Deep inferior epigastric artery perforator flap breast reconstruction
2016, 2Q, 27	Removal of nonviable transverse rectus abdominis myocutaneous (TRAM) flaps

AHA Coding Clinic for table ØHQ

2019, 4Q, 30-31	Breast procedures
2018, 2Q, 25	Third and fourth degree obstetric lacerations
2016, 1Q, 7	Obstetrical perineal laceration repair
2014, 4Q, 31	Delayed wound closure following fracture treatment

AHA Coding Clinic for table ØHR

2022, 1Q, 15	Nipple reconstruction and breast reduction
2020, 1Q, 27	Delayed reconstruction following mastectomy using gracilis musculocutaneous free flap
2020, 1Q, 28	Free flap microvascular breast reconstruction
2020, 1Q, 30	Polarity Skin TE™ application
2019, 4Q, 30-31	Breast procedures
2019, 4Q, 32	Cell suspension epithelial autograft
2019, 3Q, 32	Breast reconstruction with neurotization
2018, 3Q, 13	Deep inferior epigastric artery perforator flap breast reconstruction
2017, 1Q, 35	Epifix® allograft
2014, 3Q, 14	Application of TheraSkin® and excisional debridement

AHA Coding Clinic for table ØHT

2021, 2Q, 16	Goldilocks breast reconstruction
2018, 3Q, 13	Deep inferior epigastric artery perforator flap breast reconstruction
2014, 4Q, 34	Skin-sparing mastectomy

AHA Coding Clinic for table ØHU

2019, 4Q, 30-31	Breast procedures

AHA Coding Clinic for table ØHW

2019, 4Q, 30-31	Breast procedures

Integumentary Anatomy

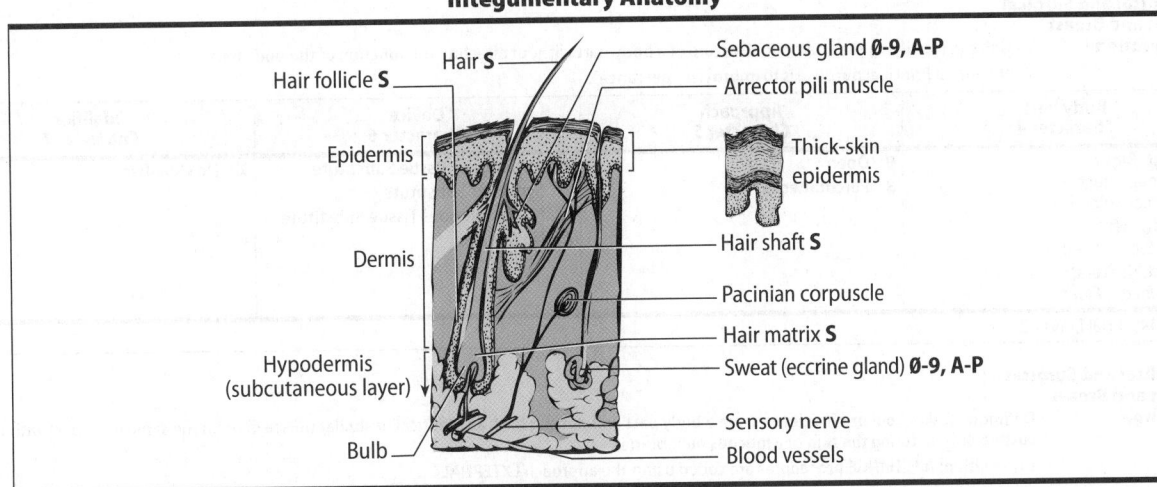

Nail Anatomy

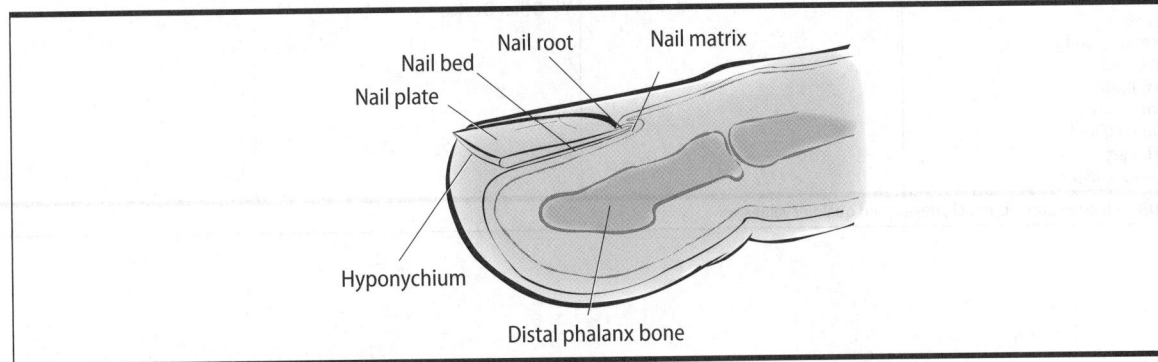

Breast

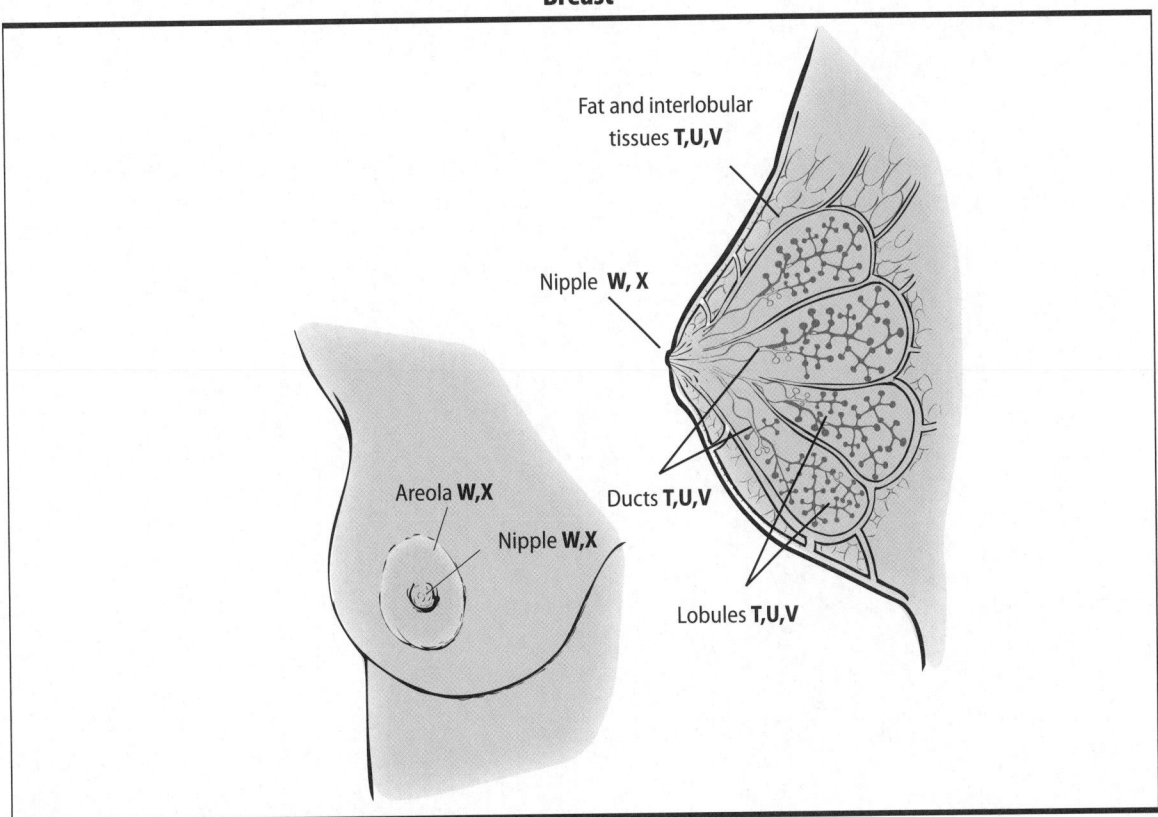

Ø Medical and Surgical
H Skin and Breast
Ø Alteration

Definition: Modifying the anatomic structure of a body part without affecting the function of the body part
Explanation: Principal purpose is to improve appearance

Body Part Character 4	Approach Character 5	Device Character 6	Qualifier Character 7
T Breast, Right Mammary duct Mammary gland **U** Breast, Left *See T Breast, Right* **V** Breast, Bilateral *See T Breast, Right*	**Ø** Open **3** Percutaneous	**7** Autologous Tissue Substitute **J** Synthetic Substitute **K** Nonautologous Tissue Substitute **Z** No Device	**Z** No Qualifier

Non-OR   ØHØ[T,U,V]3JZ

Ø Medical and Surgical
H Skin and Breast
2 Change

Definition: Taking out or off a device from a body part and putting back an identical or similar device in or on the same body part without cutting or puncturing the skin or a mucous membrane
Explanation: All CHANGE procedures are coded using the approach EXTERNAL

Body Part Character 4	Approach Character 5	Device Character 6	Qualifier Character 7
P Skin Dermis Epidermis Sebaceous gland Sweat gland **T** Breast, Right Mammary duct Mammary gland **U** Breast, Left *See T Breast, Right*	**X** External	**Ø** Drainage Device **Y** Other Device	**Z** No Qualifier

Non-OR   All body part, approach, device, and qualifier values

Non-OR Procedure   DRG Non-OR Procedure   Valid OR Procedure   HAC Associated Procedure   Combination Only   New/Revised April   New/Revised October

428

ICD-10-PCS 2023

Ø　**Medical and Surgical**
H　**Skin and Breast**
5　**Destruction**　　Definition: Physical eradication of all or a portion of a body part by the direct use of energy, force, or a destructive agent
　　　　　　　　　　Explanation: None of the body part is physically taken out

Body Part Character 4	Approach Character 5	Device Character 6	Qualifier Character 7
Ø　Skin, Scalp 1　Skin, Face 2　Skin, Right Ear 3　Skin, Left Ear 4　Skin, Neck 5　Skin, Chest 　　Breast procedures, skin only 6　Skin, Back 7　Skin, Abdomen 8　Skin, Buttock 9　Skin, Perineum 　　Perianal skin A　Skin, Inguinal B　Skin, Right Upper Arm C　Skin, Left Upper Arm D　Skin, Right Lower Arm E　Skin, Left Lower Arm F　Skin, Right Hand G　Skin, Left Hand H　Skin, Right Upper Leg J　Skin, Left Upper Leg K　Skin, Right Lower Leg L　Skin, Left Lower Leg M　Skin, Right Foot N　Skin, Left Foot	X　External	Z　No Device	D　Multiple Z　No Qualifier
Q　Finger Nail 　　Nail bed 　　Nail plate R　Toe Nail 　　*See Q Finger Nail*	X　External	Z　No Device	Z　No Qualifier
T　Breast, Right 　　Mammary duct 　　Mammary gland U　Breast, Left 　　*See T Breast, Right* V　Breast, Bilateral 　　*See T Breast, Right*	Ø　Open 3　Percutaneous	Z　No Device	3　Laser Interstitial Thermal Therapy Z　No Qualifier
T　Breast, Right 　　Mammary duct 　　Mammary gland U　Breast, Left 　　*See T Breast, Right* V　Breast, Bilateral 　　*See T Breast, Right*	7　Via Natural or Artificial Opening 8　Via Natural or Artificial Opening 　　Endoscopic	Z　No Device	Z　No Qualifier
W　Nipple, Right 　　Areola X　Nipple, Left 　　*See W Nipple, Right*	Ø　Open 3　Percutaneous 7　Via Natural or Artificial Opening 8　Via Natural or Artificial Opening 　　Endoscopic X　External	Z　No Device	Z　No Qualifier

DRG Non-OR	ØH5[Ø,1,4,5,6,7,8,9,A,B,C,D,E,F,G,H,J,K,L,M,N]XZ[D,Z]
DRG Non-OR	ØH5[Q,R]XZZ
Non-OR	ØH5[2,3]XZ[D,Z]

NC Noncovered Procedure　　LC Limited Coverage　　QA Questionable OB Admit　　NT New Tech Add-on　　⊞ Combination Member　　♂Male　　♀Female

ICD-10-PCS 2023　　429

ØH5–ØH5

Ø **Medical and Surgical**
H **Skin and Breast**
8 **Division**   Definition: Cutting into a body part, without draining fluids and/or gases from the body part, in order to separate or transect a body part
                      Explanation: All or a portion of the body part is separated into two or more portions

Body Part Character 4	Approach Character 5	Device Character 6	Qualifier Character 7
Ø Skin, Scalp	**X** External	**Z** No Device	**Z** No Qualifier
1 Skin, Face			
2 Skin, Right Ear			
3 Skin, Left Ear			
4 Skin, Neck			
5 Skin, Chest Breast procedures, skin only			
6 Skin, Back			
7 Skin, Abdomen			
8 Skin, Buttock			
9 Skin, Perineum Perianal skin			
A Skin, Inguinal			
B Skin, Right Upper Arm			
C Skin, Left Upper Arm			
D Skin, Right Lower Arm			
E Skin, Left Lower Arm			
F Skin, Right Hand			
G Skin, Left Hand			
H Skin, Right Upper Leg			
J Skin, Left Upper Leg			
K Skin, Right Lower Leg			
L Skin, Left Lower Leg			
M Skin, Right Foot			
N Skin, Left Foot			

Non-OR   All body part, approach, device, and qualifier values

Non-OR Procedure   DRG Non-OR Procedure   Valid OR Procedure   HAC Associated Procedure   Combination Only   New/Revised April   New/Revised October

430   ICD-10-PCS 2023

Ø   Medical and Surgical
H   Skin and Breast
9   Drainage   Definition: Taking or letting out fluids and/or gases from a body part

Explanation: The qualifier DIAGNOSTIC is used to identify drainage procedures that are biopsies

Body Part Character 4	Approach Character 5	Device Character 6	Qualifier Character 7

Ø Skin, Scalp   **E** Skin, Left Lower Arm
1 Skin, Face   **F** Skin, Right Hand
2 Skin, Right Ear   **G** Skin, Left Hand
3 Skin, Left Ear   **H** Skin, Right Upper Leg
4 Skin, Neck   **J** Skin, Left Upper Leg
5 Skin, Chest   **K** Skin, Right Lower Leg
    Breast procedures, skin   **L** Skin, Left Lower Leg
      only   **M** Skin, Right Foot
6 Skin, Back   **N** Skin, Left Foot
7 Skin, Abdomen   **Q** Finger Nail
8 Skin, Buttock   Nail bed
9 Skin, Perineum   Nail plate
    Perianal skin   **R** Toe Nail
A Skin, Inguinal   *See Q Finger Nail*
B Skin, Right Upper Arm
C Skin, Left Upper Arm
D Skin, Right Lower Arm
	X External	**Ø** Drainage Device	**Z** No Qualifier

Ø Skin, Scalp   **E** Skin, Left Lower Arm
1 Skin, Face   **F** Skin, Right Hand
2 Skin, Right Ear   **G** Skin, Left Hand
3 Skin, Left Ear   **H** Skin, Right Upper Leg
4 Skin, Neck   **J** Skin, Left Upper Leg
5 Skin, Chest   **K** Skin, Right Lower Leg
    Breast procedures, skin   **L** Skin, Left Lower Leg
      only   **M** Skin, Right Foot
6 Skin, Back   **N** Skin, Left Foot
7 Skin, Abdomen   **Q** Finger Nail
8 Skin, Buttock   Nail bed
9 Skin, Perineum   Nail plate
    Perianal skin   **R** Toe Nail
A Skin, Inguinal   *See Q Finger Nail*
B Skin, Right Upper Arm
C Skin, Left Upper Arm
D Skin, Right Lower Arm
	X External	**Z** No Device	**X** Diagnostic
			Z No Qualifier

T Breast, Right
    Mammary duct
    Mammary gland
U Breast, Left
    See T Breast, Right
V Breast, Bilateral
    See T Breast, Right
	Ø Open
	3 Percutaneous
	7 Via Natural or Artificial Opening
	8 Via Natural or Artificial Opening Endoscopic
		Ø Drainage Device	**Z** No Qualifier

T Breast, Right
    Mammary duct
    Mammary gland
U Breast, Left
    See T Breast, Right
V Breast, Bilateral
    See T Breast, Right
	Ø Open
	3 Percutaneous
	7 Via Natural or Artificial Opening
	8 Via Natural or Artificial Opening Endoscopic
		Z No Device	**X** Diagnostic
			Z No Qualifier

W Nipple, Right
    Areola
X Nipple, Left
    See W Nipple, Right
	Ø Open
	3 Percutaneous
	7 Via Natural or Artificial Opening
	8 Via Natural or Artificial Opening Endoscopic
	X External
		Ø Drainage Device	**Z** No Qualifier

W Nipple, Right
    Areola
X Nipple, Left
    See W Nipple, Right
	Ø Open
	3 Percutaneous
	7 Via Natural or Artificial Opening
	8 Via Natural or Artificial Opening Endoscopic
	X External
		Z No Device	**X** Diagnostic
			Z No Qualifier

Non-OR   ØH9[Ø,1,2,3,4,5,6,7,8,A,B,C,D,E,F,G,H,J,K,L,M,N,Q,R]XØZ
Non-OR   ØH9[Ø,1,2,3,4,5,6,7,8,A,B,C,D,E,F,G,H,J,K,L,M,N,Q,R]XZ[X,Z]
Non-OR   ØH99XZX
Non-OR   ØH9[T,U,V][Ø,3,7,8]ØZ
Non-OR   ØH9[T,U,V][3,7,8]Z[X,Z]
Non-OR   ØH9[W,X][Ø,3,7,8,X]ØZ
Non-OR   ØH9[W,X][3,7,8,X]Z[X,Z]

NC Noncovered Procedure   **LC** Limited Coverage   **QA** Questionable OB Admit   **NT** New Tech Add-on   ⊞ Combination Member   ♂ Male   ♀ Female

ICD-10-PCS 2023   431

ØH9–ØH9

Ø   Medical and Surgical
H   Skin and Breast
B   Excision   Definition: Cutting out or off, without replacement, a portion of a body part
                          Explanation: The qualifier DIAGNOSTIC is used to identify excision procedures that are biopsies

Body Part Character 4	Approach Character 5	Device Character 6	Qualifier Character 7

Ø Skin, Scalp
1 Skin, Face
2 Skin, Right Ear
3 Skin, Left Ear
4 Skin, Neck
5 Skin, Chest
    Breast procedures, skin only
6 Skin, Back
7 Skin, Abdomen
8 Skin, Buttock
9 Skin, Perineum
    Perianal skin
A Skin, Inguinal
B Skin, Right Upper Arm
C Skin, Left Upper Arm
D Skin, Right Lower Arm
E Skin, Left Lower Arm
F Skin, Right Hand
G Skin, Left Hand
H Skin, Right Upper Leg
J Skin, Left Upper Leg
K Skin, Right Lower Leg
L Skin, Left Lower Leg
M Skin, Right Foot
N Skin, Left Foot
Q Finger Nail
    Nail bed
    Nail plate
R Toe Nail
    See Q Finger Nail
	X External	**Z** No Device	**X** Diagnostic
			Z No Qualifier

T Breast, Right
    Mammary duct
    Mammary gland
U Breast, Left
    See T Breast, Right
V Breast, Bilateral
    See T Breast, Right
Y Supernumerary Breast
	Ø Open
	3 Percutaneous
	7 Via Natural or Artificial Opening
	8 Via Natural or Artificial Opening
	    Endoscopic
		Z No Device	**X** Diagnostic
			Z No Qualifier

W Nipple, Right
    Areola
X Nipple, Left
    See W Nipple, Right
	Ø Open
	3 Percutaneous
	7 Via Natural or Artificial Opening
	8 Via Natural or Artificial Opening
	    Endoscopic
	X External
		Z No Device	**X** Diagnostic
			Z No Qualifier

DRG Non-OR	ØHB9XZZ
Non-OR	ØHB[Ø,1,2,3,4,5,6,7,8,A,B,C,D,E,F,G,H,J,K,L,M,N,Q,R]XZ[X,Z]
Non-OR	ØHB9XZX
Non-OR	ØHB[T,U,V,Y][3,7,8]ZX
Non-OR	ØHB[W,X][3,7,8,X]ZX

Non-OR Procedure   DRG Non-OR Procedure   Valid OR Procedure   HAC Associated Procedure   Combination Only   New/Revised April   New/Revised October

Ø   Medical and Surgical
H   Skin and Breast
C   Extirpation   Definition: Taking or cutting out solid matter from a body part

Explanation: The solid matter may be an abnormal byproduct of a biological function or a foreign body; it may be imbedded in a body part or in the lumen of a tubular body part. The solid matter may or may not have been previously broken into pieces.

Body Part Character 4	Approach Character 5	Device Character 6	Qualifier Character 7

Ø   Skin, Scalp
1   Skin, Face
2   Skin, Right Ear
3   Skin, Left Ear
4   Skin, Neck
5   Skin, Chest
     Breast procedures, skin only
6   Skin, Back
7   Skin, Abdomen
8   Skin, Buttock
9   Skin, Perineum
     Perianal skin
A   Skin, Inguinal
B   Skin, Right Upper Arm
C   Skin, Left Upper Arm
D   Skin, Right Lower Arm
E   Skin, Left Lower Arm
F   Skin, Right Hand
G   Skin, Left Hand
H   Skin, Right Upper Leg
J   Skin, Left Upper Leg
K   Skin, Right Lower Leg
L   Skin, Left Lower Leg
M   Skin, Right Foot
N   Skin, Left Foot
Q   Finger Nail
     Nail bed
     Nail plate
R   Toe Nail
     See Q Finger Nail
	X External	**Z** No Device	**Z** No Qualifier

T   Breast, Right
     Mammary duct
     Mammary gland
U   Breast, Left
     See T Breast, Right
V   Breast, Bilateral
     See T Breast, Right
	Ø Open
	3 Percutaneous
	7 Via Natural or Artificial Opening
	8 Via Natural or Artificial Opening Endoscopic
		Z No Device	**Z** No Qualifier

W   Nipple, Right
     Areola
X   Nipple, Left
     See W Nipple, Right
	Ø Open
	3 Percutaneous
	7 Via Natural or Artificial Opening
	8 Via Natural or Artificial Opening Endoscopic
	X External
		Z No Device	**Z** No Qualifier

Non-OR   ØHC[Ø,1,2,3,4,5,6,7,8,9,A,B,C,D,E,F,G,H,J,K,L,M,N,Q,R]XZZ
Non-OR   ØHC[T,U,V][3,7,8]ZZ
Non-OR   ØHC[W,X][3,7,8,X]ZZ

NC Noncovered Procedure   LC Limited Coverage   QA Questionable OB Admit   NT New Tech Add-on   ⊞ Combination Member   ♂Male   ♀Female

ICD-10-PCS 2023   433

Skin and Breast

Ø   **Medical and Surgical**
H   **Skin and Breast**
D   **Extraction**   Definition: Pulling or stripping out or off all or a portion of a body part by the use of force
                       Explanation: The qualifier DIAGNOSTIC is used to identify extraction procedures that are biopsies

Body Part Character 4	Approach Character 5	Device Character 6	Qualifier Character 7

Ø   Skin, Scalp
1   Skin, Face
2   Skin, Right Ear
3   Skin, Left Ear
4   Skin, Neck
5   Skin, Chest
     Breast procedures, skin only
6   Skin, Back
7   Skin, Abdomen
8   Skin, Buttock
9   Skin, Perineum
     Perianal skin
A   Skin, Inguinal
B   Skin, Right Upper Arm
C   Skin, Left Upper Arm
D   Skin, Right Lower Arm
E   Skin, Left Lower Arm
F   Skin, Right Hand
G   Skin, Left Hand
H   Skin, Right Upper Leg
J   Skin, Left Upper Leg
K   Skin, Right Lower Leg
L   Skin, Left Lower Leg
M   Skin, Right Foot
N   Skin, Left Foot
Q   Finger Nail
     Nail bed
     Nail plate
R   Toe Nail
     See Q Finger Nail
S   Hair
	X External	Z No Device	Z No Qualifier

T   Breast, Right
     Mammary duct
     Mammary gland
U   Breast, Left
     See T Breast, Right
V   Breast, Bilateral
     See T Breast, Right
Y   Supernumerary Breast
	Ø Open	Z No Device	Z No Qualifier

Non-OR   All body part, approach, device, and qualifier values

Non-OR Procedure   DRG Non-OR Procedure   Valid OR Procedure   HAC Associated Procedure   Combination Only   New/Revised April   New/Revised October

434   ICD-10-PCS 2023

Ø   **Medical and Surgical**
H   **Skin and Breast**
H   **Insertion**   Definition: Putting in a nonbiological appliance that monitors, assists, performs, or prevents a physiological function but does not physically take the place of a body part
                        Explanation: None

Body Part Character 4	Approach Character 5	Device Character 6	Qualifier Character 7
P Skin	**X** External	**Y** Other Device	**Z** No Qualifier
T Breast, Right Mammary duct Mammary gland **U** Breast, Left *See T Breast, Right*	**Ø** Open **3** Percutaneous **7** Via Natural or Artificial Opening **8** Via Natural or Artificial Opening Endoscopic	**1** Radioactive Element **N** Tissue Expander **Y** Other Device	**Z** No Qualifier
V Breast, Bilateral Mammary duct Mammary gland	**Ø** Open **3** Percutaneous **7** Via Natural or Artificial Opening **8** Via Natural or Artificial Opening Endoscopic	**1** Radioactive Element **N** Tissue Expander	**Z** No Qualifier
W Nipple, Right Areola **X** Nipple, Left *See W Nipple, Right*	**Ø** Open **3** Percutaneous **7** Via Natural or Artificial Opening **8** Via Natural or Artificial Opening Endoscopic	**1** Radioactive Element **N** Tissue Expander	**Z** No Qualifier
W Nipple, Right Areola **X** Nipple, Left *See W Nipple, Right*	**X** External	**1** Radioactive Element	**Z** No Qualifier

Non-OR   ØHHPXYZ
Non-OR   ØHH[T,U][3,7,8]YZ

Ø   **Medical and Surgical**
H   **Skin and Breast**
J   **Inspection**   Definition: Visually and/or manually exploring a body part
                        Explanation: Visual exploration may be performed with or without optical instrumentation. Manual exploration may be performed directly or through intervening body layers.

Body Part Character 4	Approach Character 5	Device Character 6	Qualifier Character 7
P Skin Dermis Epidermis Sebaceous gland Sweat gland **Q** Finger Nail Nail bed Nail plate **R** Toe Nail *See Q Finger Nail*	**X** External	**Z** No Device	**Z** No Qualifier
T Breast, Right Mammary duct Mammary gland **U** Breast, Left *See T Breast, Right*	**Ø** Open **3** Percutaneous **7** Via Natural or Artificial Opening **8** Via Natural or Artificial Opening Endoscopic	**Z** No Device	**Z** No Qualifier

Non-OR   All body part, approach, device and qualifier values

Skin and Breast

Ø **Medical and Surgical**
H **Skin and Breast**
M **Reattachment**   Definition: Putting back in or on all or a portion of a separated body part to its normal location or other suitable location
Explanation: Vascular circulation and nervous pathways may or may not be reestablished

Body Part Character 4	Approach Character 5	Device Character 6	Qualifier Character 7
Ø Skin, Scalp	X External	Z No Device	Z No Qualifier
1 Skin, Face			
2 Skin, Right Ear			
3 Skin, Left Ear			
4 Skin, Neck			
5 Skin, Chest 　 Breast procedures, skin only			
6 Skin, Back			
7 Skin, Abdomen			
8 Skin, Buttock			
9 Skin, Perineum 　 Perianal skin			
A Skin, Inguinal			
B Skin, Right Upper Arm			
C Skin, Left Upper Arm			
D Skin, Right Lower Arm			
E Skin, Left Lower Arm			
F Skin, Right Hand			
G Skin, Left Hand			
H Skin, Right Upper Leg			
J Skin, Left Upper Leg			
K Skin, Right Lower Leg			
L Skin, Left Lower Leg			
M Skin, Right Foot			
N Skin, Left Foot			
T Breast, Right 　 Mammary duct 　 Mammary gland			
U Breast, Left 　 See T Breast, Right			
V Breast, Bilateral 　 See T Breast, Right			
W Nipple, Right 　 Areola			
X Nipple, Left 　 See W Nipple, Right			

Non-OR   ØHMØXZZ

Non-OR Procedure   DRG Non-OR Procedure   Valid OR Procedure   HAC Associated Procedure   Combination Only   New/Revised April   New/Revised October

436

ICD-10-PCS 2023

Ø **Medical and Surgical**
H **Skin and Breast**
N **Release**   Definition: Freeing a body part from an abnormal physical constraint by cutting or by the use of force
               Explanation: Some of the restraining tissue may be taken out but none of the body part is taken out

Body Part Character 4	Approach Character 5	Device Character 6	Qualifier Character 7

Ø Skin, Scalp
1 Skin, Face
2 Skin, Right Ear
3 Skin, Left Ear
4 Skin, Neck
5 Skin, Chest
   Breast procedures, skin only
6 Skin, Back
7 Skin, Abdomen
8 Skin, Buttock
9 Skin, Perineum
   Perianal skin
A Skin, Inguinal
B Skin, Right Upper Arm
C Skin, Left Upper Arm
D Skin, Right Lower Arm
E Skin, Left Lower Arm
F Skin, Right Hand
G Skin, Left Hand
H Skin, Right Upper Leg
J Skin, Left Upper Leg
K Skin, Right Lower Leg
L Skin, Left Lower Leg
M Skin, Right Foot
N Skin, Left Foot
Q Finger Nail
   Nail bed
   Nail plate
R Toe Nail
   See Q Finger Nail
	X External	Z No Device	Z No Qualifier

T Breast, Right
   Mammary duct
   Mammary gland
U Breast, Left
   See T Breast, Right
V Breast, Bilateral
   See T Breast, Right
	Ø Open
	3 Percutaneous
	7 Via Natural or Artificial Opening
	8 Via Natural or Artificial Opening
	   Endoscopic
		Z No Device	Z No Qualifier

W Nipple, Right
   Areola
X Nipple, Left
   See W Nipple, Right
	Ø Open
	3 Percutaneous
	7 Via Natural or Artificial Opening
	8 Via Natural or Artificial Opening
	   Endoscopic
	X External
		Z No Device	Z No Qualifier

Ø Medical and Surgical
H Skin and Breast
P Removal   Definition: Taking out or off a device from a body part

Explanation: If a device is taken out and a similar device put in without cutting or puncturing the skin or mucous membrane, the procedure is coded to the root operation CHANGE. Otherwise, the procedure for taking out a device is coded to the root operation REMOVAL.

Body Part Character 4	Approach Character 5	Device Character 6	Qualifier Character 7
P Skin Dermis Epidermis Sebaceous gland Sweat gland	**X External**	**Ø Drainage Device** **7 Autologous Tissue Substitute** **J Synthetic Substitute** **K Nonautologous Tissue Substitute** **Y Other Device**	**Z No Qualifier**
Q Finger Nail Nail bed Nail plate **R Toe Nail** *See Q Finger Nail*	**X External**	**Ø Drainage Device** **7 Autologous Tissue Substitute** **J Synthetic Substitute** **K Nonautologous Tissue Substitute**	**Z No Qualifier**
S Hair	**X External**	**7 Autologous Tissue Substitute** **J Synthetic Substitute** **K Nonautologous Tissue Substitute**	**Z No Qualifier**
T Breast, Right Mammary duct Mammary gland **U Breast, Left** *See T Breast, Right*	**Ø Open** **3 Percutaneous** **7 Via Natural or Artificial Opening** **8 Via Natural or Artificial Opening Endoscopic**	**Ø Drainage Device** **1 Radioactive Element** **7 Autologous Tissue Substitute** **J Synthetic Substitute** **K Nonautologous Tissue Substitute** **N Tissue Expander** **Y Other Device**	**Z No Qualifier**

Non-OR	ØHPPX[Ø,7,J,K,Y]Z
Non-OR	ØHP[Q,R]X[Ø,7,J,K]Z
Non-OR	ØHPSX[7,J,K]Z
Non-OR	ØHP[T,U]Ø[Ø,1,7,K]Z
Non-OR	ØHP[T,U]3[Ø,1,7,K,Y]Z
Non-OR	ØHP[T,U][7,8][Ø,1,7,J,K,N,Y]Z

Non-OR Procedure   DRG Non-OR Procedure   Valid OR Procedure   HAC Associated Procedure   Combination Only   New/Revised April   New/Revised October

438   ICD-10-PCS 2023

Ø   **Medical and Surgical**
H   **Skin and Breast**
Q   **Repair**   Definition: Restoring, to the extent possible, a body part to its normal anatomic structure and function
                Explanation: Used only when the method to accomplish the repair is not one of the other root operations

Body Part Character 4	Approach Character 5	Device Character 6	Qualifier Character 7

Ø Skin, Scalp
1 Skin, Face
2 Skin, Right Ear
3 Skin, Left Ear
4 Skin, Neck
5 Skin, Chest
    Breast procedures, skin only
6 Skin, Back
7 Skin, Abdomen
8 Skin, Buttock
9 Skin, Perineum
    Perianal skin
A Skin, Inguinal
B Skin, Right Upper Arm
C Skin, Left Upper Arm
D Skin, Right Lower Arm
E Skin, Left Lower Arm
F Skin, Right Hand
G Skin, Left Hand
H Skin, Right Upper Leg
J Skin, Left Upper Leg
K Skin, Right Lower Leg
L Skin, Left Lower Leg
M Skin, Right Foot
N Skin, Left Foot
Q Finger Nail
    Nail bed
    Nail plate
R Toe Nail
    See Q Finger Nail
	X External	**Z** No Device	**Z** No Qualifier

T Breast, Right
    Mammary duct
    Mammary gland
U Breast, Left
    See T Breast, Right
V Breast, Bilateral
    See T Breast, Right
Y Supernumerary Breast
	Ø Open
	3 Percutaneous
	7 Via Natural or Artificial Opening
	8 Via Natural or Artificial Opening
	    Endoscopic
		Z No Device	**Z** No Qualifier

W Nipple, Right
    Areola
X Nipple, Left
    See W Nipple, Right
	Ø Open
	3 Percutaneous
	7 Via Natural or Artificial Opening
	8 Via Natural or Artificial Opening
	    Endoscopic
	X External
		Z No Device	**Z** No Qualifier

DRG Non-OR   ØHQ9XZZ
Non-OR   ØHQ[Ø,1,2,3,4,5,6,7,8,A,B,C,D,E,F,G,H,J,K,L,M,N]XZZ

NC Noncovered Procedure   **LC** Limited Coverage   **QA** Questionable OB Admit   **NT** New Tech Add-on   ⊞ Combination Member   ♂ Male   ♀ Female

ICD-10-PCS 2023   **439**

ØHQ–ØHQ

Ø Medical and Surgical
H Skin and Breast
R Replacement   Definition: Putting in or on biological or synthetic material that physically takes the place and/or function of all or a portion of a body part

Explanation: The body part may have been taken out or replaced, or may be taken out, physically eradicated, or rendered nonfunctional during the REPLACEMENT procedure. A REMOVAL procedure is coded for taking out the device used in a previous replacement procedure.

Body Part Character 4		Approach Character 5	Device Character 6	Qualifier Character 7

Ø Skin, Scalp
 1 Skin, Face
 2 Skin, Right Ear
 3 Skin, Left Ear
 4 Skin, Neck
 5 Skin, Chest
    Breast procedures, skin only
 6 Skin, Back
 7 Skin, Abdomen
 8 Skin, Buttock
 9 Skin, Perineum
    Perianal skin
 A Skin, Inguinal
	B Skin, Right Upper Arm
	 C Skin, Left Upper Arm
	 D Skin, Right Lower Arm
	 E Skin, Left Lower Arm
	 F Skin, Right Hand
	 G Skin, Left Hand
	 H Skin, Right Upper Leg
	 J Skin, Left Upper Leg
	 K Skin, Right Lower Leg
	 L Skin, Left Lower Leg
	 M Skin, Right Foot
	 N Skin, Left Foot
		X External	7 Autologous Tissue Substitute	2 Cell Suspension Technique
				 3 Full Thickness
				 4 Partial Thickness

Ø Skin, Scalp
 1 Skin, Face
 2 Skin, Right Ear
 3 Skin, Left Ear
 4 Skin, Neck
 5 Skin, Chest
    Breast procedures, skin only
 6 Skin, Back
 7 Skin, Abdomen
 8 Skin, Buttock
 9 Skin, Perineum
    Perianal skin
 A Skin, Inguinal
	B Skin, Right Upper Arm
	 C Skin, Left Upper Arm
	 D Skin, Right Lower Arm
	 E Skin, Left Lower Arm
	 F Skin, Right Hand
	 G Skin, Left Hand
	 H Skin, Right Upper Leg
	 J Skin, Left Upper Leg
	 K Skin, Right Lower Leg
	 L Skin, Left Lower Leg
	 M Skin, Right Foot
	 N Skin, Left Foot
		X External	J Synthetic Substitute	3 Full Thickness
				 4 Partial Thickness
				 Z No Qualifier

Ø Skin, Scalp
 1 Skin, Face
 2 Skin, Right Ear
 3 Skin, Left Ear
 4 Skin, Neck
 5 Skin, Chest
    Breast procedures, skin only
 6 Skin, Back
 7 Skin, Abdomen
 8 Skin Buttock
 9 Skin, Perineum
    Perianal skin
 A Skin, Inguinal
	B Skin, Right Upper Arm
	 C Skin, Left Upper Arm
	 D Skin, Right Lower Arm
	 E Skin, Left Lower Arm
	 F Skin, Right Hand
	 G Skin, Left Hand
	 H Skin, Right Upper Leg
	 J Skin, Left Upper Leg
	 K Skin, Right Lower Leg
	 L Skin, Left Lower Leg
	 M Skin, Right Foot
	 N Skin, Left Foot
		X External	K Nonautologous Tissue Substitute	3 Full Thickness
				 4 Partial Thickness

Q Finger Nail
    Nail bed
    Nail plate
	R Toe Nail
	    See Q Finger Nail
	 S Hair
		X External	7 Autologous Tissue Substitute
			 J Synthetic Substitute
			 K Nonautologous Tissue Substitute
				Z No Qualifier

T Breast, Right
    Mammary duct
    Mammary gland
	U Breast, Left
	    See T Breast, Right
	 V Breast, Bilateral
	    See T Breast, Right
		Ø Open	7 Autologous Tissue Substitute	5 Latissimus Dorsi Myocutaneous Flap
				 6 Transverse Rectus Abdominis Myocutaneous Flap
				 7 Deep Inferior Epigastric Artery Perforator Flap
				 8 Superficial Inferior Epigastric Artery Flap
				 9 Gluteal Artery Perforator Flap
				 Z No Qualifier

T Breast, Right
    Mammary duct
    Mammary gland
	U Breast, Left
	    See T Breast, Right
	 V Breast, Bilateral
	    See T Breast, Right
		Ø Open	J Synthetic Substitute
			 K Nonautologous Tissue Substitute
				Z No Qualifier

T Breast, Right ⊞
    Mammary duct
    Mammary gland
 U Breast, Left ⊞
    See T Breast, Right
	V Breast, Bilateral ⊞
	    See T Breast, Right
		3 Percutaneous	7 Autologous Tissue Substitute
			 J Synthetic Substitute
			 K Nonautologous Tissue Substitute
				Z No Qualifier

W Nipple, Right
    Areola
	X Nipple, Left
	    See W Nipple, Right
		Ø Open
		 3 Percutaneous
		 X External
			7 Autologous Tissue Substitute
			 J Synthetic Substitute
			 K Nonautologous Tissue Substitute
				Z No Qualifier

Non-OR   ØHRSX7Z

See Appendix L for Procedure Combinations
   ⊞   ØHR[T,U,V]37Z

Non-OR Procedure   DRG Non-OR Procedure   Valid OR Procedure   HAC Associated Procedure   Combination Only   New/Revised April   New/Revised October

Ø Medical and Surgical
H Skin and Breast
S Reposition — Definition: Moving to its normal location, or other suitable location, all or a portion of a body part

Explanation: The body part is moved to a new location from an abnormal location, or from a normal location where it is not functioning correctly. The body part may or may not be cut out or off to be moved to the new location.

Body Part Character 4	Approach Character 5	Device Character 6	Qualifier Character 7

S Hair
W Nipple, Right
  Areola
X Nipple, Left
  See W Nipple, Right
	X External	**Z** No Device	**Z** No Qualifier

T Breast, Right
  Mammary duct
  Mammary gland
U Breast, Left
  See T Breast, Right
V Breast, Bilateral
  See T Breast, Right
	Ø Open	**Z** No Device	**Z** No Qualifier

Non-OR ØHSSXZZ

Ø Medical and Surgical
H Skin and Breast
T Resection — Definition: Cutting out or off, without replacement, all of a body part

Explanation: None

Body Part Character 4	Approach Character 5	Device Character 6	Qualifier Character 7

Q Finger Nail
  Nail bed
  Nail plate
R Toe Nail
  See Q Finger Nail
W Nipple, Right
  Areola
X Nipple, Left
  See W Nipple, Right
	X External	**Z** No Device	**Z** No Qualifier

T Breast, Right ⊞
  Mammary duct
  Mammary gland
U Breast, Left ⊞
  See T Breast, Right
V Breast, Bilateral ⊞
  See T Breast, Right
Y Supernumerary Breast
	Ø Open	**Z** No Device	**Z** No Qualifier

Non-OR ØHT[Q,R]XZZ

See Appendix L for Procedure Combinations
⊞ ØHT[T,U,V]ØZZ

Ø Medical and Surgical
H Skin and Breast
U Supplement — Definition: Putting in or on biological or synthetic material that physically reinforces and/or augments the function of a portion of a body part

Explanation: The biological material is non-living, or is living and from the same individual. The body part may have been previously replaced, and the SUPPLEMENT procedure is performed to physically reinforce and/or augment the function of the replaced body part.

Body Part Character 4	Approach Character 5	Device Character 6	Qualifier Character 7

T Breast, Right
  Mammary duct
  Mammary gland
U Breast, Left
  See T Breast, Right
V Breast, Bilateral
  See T Breast, Right
	Ø Open
	3 Percutaneous
	7 Via Natural or Artificial Opening
	8 Via Natural or Artificial Opening Endoscopic
		7 Autologous Tissue Substitute
		J Synthetic Substitute
		K Nonautologous Tissue Substitute
			Z No Qualifier

W Nipple, Right
  Areola
X Nipple, Left
  See W Nipple, Right
	Ø Open
	3 Percutaneous
	7 Via Natural or Artificial Opening
	8 Via Natural or Artificial Opening Endoscopic
	X External
		7 Autologous Tissue Substitute
		J Synthetic Substitute
		K Nonautologous Tissue Substitute
			Z No Qualifier

Non-OR ØHU[T,U,V]3JZ

NC Noncovered Procedure **LC** Limited Coverage **QA** Questionable OB Admit **NT** New Tech Add-on ⊞ Combination Member ♂ Male ♀ Female

ICD-10-PCS 2023 **441**

Ø   Medical and Surgical
H   Skin and Breast
W   Revision   Definition: Correcting, to the extent possible, a portion of a malfunctioning device or the position of a displaced device

Explanation: Revision can include correcting a malfunctioning or displaced device by taking out or putting in components of the device such as a screw or pin

Body Part Character 4	Approach Character 5	Device Character 6	Qualifier Character 7

P Skin
   Dermis
   Epidermis
   Sebaceous gland
   Sweat gland
	X External	**Ø Drainage Device**
		7 Autologous Tissue Substitute
		J Synthetic Substitute
		K Nonautologous Tissue Substitute
		Y Other Device
			Z No Qualifier

Q Finger Nail
   Nail bed
   Nail plate
R Toe Nail
   See Q Finger Nail
	X External	**Ø Drainage Device**
		7 Autologous Tissue Substitute
		J Synthetic Substitute
		K Nonautologous Tissue Substitute
			Z No Qualifier

S Hair	**X External**	**7 Autologous Tissue Substitute** **J Synthetic Substitute** **K Nonautologous Tissue Substitute**	**Z No Qualifier**

T Breast, Right
   Mammary duct
   Mammary gland
U Breast, Left
   See T Breast, Right
	Ø Open
	3 Percutaneous
	7 Via Natural or Artificial Opening
	8 Via Natural or Artificial Opening
	   Endoscopic
		Ø Drainage Device
		7 Autologous Tissue Substitute
		J Synthetic Substitute
		K Nonautologous Tissue Substitute
		N Tissue Expander
		Y Other Device
			Z No Qualifier

Non-OR	ØHWPX[Ø,7,J,K,Y]Z
Non-OR	ØHW[Q,R]X[Ø,7,J,K]Z
Non-OR	ØHWSX[7,J,K]Z
Non-OR	ØHW[T,U]Ø[Ø,7,K,N]Z
Non-OR	ØHW[T,U]3[Ø,7,K,N,Y]Z
Non-OR	ØHW[T,U][7,8][Ø,7,J,K,N,Y]Z

Ø   Medical and Surgical
H   Skin and Breast
X   Transfer   Definition: Moving, without taking out, all or a portion of a body part to another location to take over the function of all or a portion of a body part

Explanation: The body part transferred remains connected to its vascular and nervous supply

Body Part Character 4	Approach Character 5	Device Character 6	Qualifier Character 7

Ø Skin, Scalp
1 Skin, Face
2 Skin, Right Ear
3 Skin, Left Ear
4 Skin, Neck
5 Skin, Chest
   Breast procedures, skin only
6 Skin, Back
7 Skin, Abdomen
8 Skin, Buttock
9 Skin, Perineum
   Perianal skin
A Skin, Inguinal
B Skin, Right Upper Arm
C Skin, Left Upper Arm
D Skin, Right Lower Arm
E Skin, Left Lower Arm
F Skin, Right Hand
G Skin, Left Hand
H Skin, Right Upper Leg
J Skin, Left Upper Leg
K Skin, Right Lower Leg
L Skin, Left Lower Leg
M Skin, Right Foot
N Skin, Left Foot
	X External	**Z No Device**	**Z No Qualifier**

Non-OR Procedure   DRG Non-OR Procedure   Valid OR Procedure   HAC Associated Procedure   Combination Only   New/Revised April   New/Revised October

442   ICD-10-PCS 2023

Subcutaneous Tissue and Fascia ØJØ–ØJX

Character Meanings

This Character Meaning table is provided as a guide to assist the user in the identification of character members that may be found in this section of code tables. It **SHOULD NOT** be used to build a PCS code.

Operation–Character 3	Body Part–Character 4	Approach–Character 5	Device–Character 6	Qualifier–Character 7
Ø Alteration	Ø Subcutaneous Tissue and Fascia, Scalp	Ø Open	Ø Drainage Device OR Monitoring Device, Hemodynamic	B Skin and Subcutaneous Tissue
2 Change	1 Subcutaneous Tissue and Fascia, Face	3 Percutaneous	1 Radioactive Element	C Skin, Subcutaneous Tissue and Fascia
5 Destruction	4 Subcutaneous Tissue and Fascia, Right Neck	X External	2 Monitoring Device	X Diagnostic
8 Division	5 Subcutaneous Tissue and Fascia, Left Neck		3 Infusion Device	Z No Qualifier
9 Drainage	6 Subcutaneous Tissue and Fascia, Chest		4 Pacemaker, Single Chamber	
B Excision	7 Subcutaneous Tissue and Fascia, Back		5 Pacemaker, Single Chamber Rate Responsive	
C Extirpation	8 Subcutaneous Tissue and Fascia, Abdomen		6 Pacemaker, Dual Chamber	
D Extraction	9 Subcutaneous Tissue and Fascia, Buttock		7 Autologous Tissue Substitute OR Cardiac Resynchronization Pacemaker Pulse Generator	
H Insertion	B Subcutaneous Tissue and Fascia, Perineum		8 Defibrillator Generator	
J Inspection	C Subcutaneous Tissue and Fascia, Pelvic Region		9 Cardiac Resynchronization Defibrillator Pulse Generator	
N Release	D Subcutaneous Tissue and Fascia, Right Upper Arm		A Contractility Modulation Device	
P Removal	F Subcutaneous Tissue and Fascia, Left Upper Arm		B Stimulator Generator, Single Array	
Q Repair	G Subcutaneous Tissue and Fascia, Right Lower Arm		C Stimulator Generator, Single Array Rechargeable	
R Replacement	H Subcutaneous Tissue and Fascia, Left Lower Arm		D Stimulator Generator, Multiple Array	
U Supplement	J Subcutaneous Tissue and Fascia, Right Hand		E Stimulator Generator, Multiple Array Rechargeable	
W Revision	K Subcutaneous Tissue and Fascia, Left Hand		F Subcutaneous Defibrillator Lead	
X Transfer	L Subcutaneous Tissue and Fascia, Right Upper Leg		H Contraceptive Device	
	M Subcutaneous Tissue and Fascia, Left Upper Leg		J Synthetic Substitute	
	N Subcutaneous Tissue and Fascia, Right Lower Leg		K Nonautologous Tissue Substitute	
	P Subcutaneous Tissue and Fascia, Left Lower Leg		M Stimulator Generator	
	Q Subcutaneous Tissue and Fascia, Right Foot		N Tissue Expander	
	R Subcutaneous Tissue and Fascia, Left Foot		P Cardiac Rhythm Related Device	
	S Subcutaneous Tissue and Fascia, Head and Neck		V Infusion Device, Pump	
	T Subcutaneous Tissue and Fascia, Trunk		W Vascular Access Device, Totally Implantable	
	V Subcutaneous Tissue and Fascia, Upper Extremity		X Vascular Access Device, Tunneled	
	W Subcutaneous Tissue and Fascia, Lower Extremity		Y Other Device	
			Z No Device	

AHA Coding Clinic for table ØJ2

2018, 3Q, 10	Disruption of perma-catheter fibrin sheath via angioplasty of superior vena cava
2017, 2Q, 26	Exchange of tunneled catheter

AHA Coding Clinic for table ØJ5

2019, 3Q, 25	Endoscopic removal of pilonidal sinus and cyst

AHA Coding Clinic for table ØJ8

2017, 3Q, 11	Bilateral escharotomy of leg, thigh and foot

AHA Coding Clinic for table ØJ9

2018, 3Q, 16	Incision and drainage of submandibular space
2018, 3Q, 16	Incision and drainage of neck abscess
2015, 3Q, 23	Incision and drainage of multiple abscess cavities using vessel loop

AHA Coding Clinic for table ØJB

2020, 1Q, 31	Repair of buried penis
2019, 3Q, 25	Endoscopic removal of pilonidal sinus and cyst
2018, 3Q, 17	Excisional debridement of periosteum
2018, 1Q, 7	Placement of fat graft following lumbar decompression surgery
2015, 3Q, 3-8	Excisional and nonexcisional debridement
2015, 2Q, 13	Transfer of free flap to reconstruct orbital defect
2015, 1Q, 29	Fistulectomy with placement of seton
2014, 4Q, 38	Abdominoplasty and abdominal wall plication for hernia repair
2014, 3Q, 22	Transsphenoidal removal of pituitary tumor and fat graft placement

AHA Coding Clinic for table ØJC

2017, 3Q, 22	Replacement of native skull bone flap

AHA Coding Clinic for table ØJD

2016, 3Q, 20	VersaJet™ nonexcisional debridement of leg muscle
2016, 3Q, 21	Nonexcisional debridement of infected lumbar wound
2016, 3Q, 21	Nonexcisional pulsed lavage debridement
2016, 3Q, 22	Debridement of bone and tendon using Tenex ultrasound device
2016, 1Q, 40	Nonexcisional debridement of skin and subcutaneous tissue
2015, 3Q, 3-8	Excisional and nonexcisional debridement
2015, 1Q, 23	Non-Excisional debridement with lavage of wound

AHA Coding Clinic for table ØJH

2020, 4Q, 54	Insertion of other device into subcutaneous tissue and fascia
2020, 4Q, 55	Insertion of subcutaneous pump system for ascites drainage
2020, 2Q, 15	Ommaya reservoir with ventricular catheter placement
2020, 2Q, 16	Ommaya reservoir placement for cerebrospinal fluid infusion therapy
2019, 4Q, 33	Subcutaneous implantable cardioverter defibrillator lead
2017, 4Q, 63-64	Added and revised device values - Vascular access reservoir
2017, 2Q, 24	Tunneled catheter versus totally implantable catheter
2017, 2Q, 26	Exchange of tunneled catheter
2016, 4Q, 97-98	Phrenic neurostimulator
2016, 2Q, 14	Insertion of peritoneal totally implantable venous access device
2016, 2Q, 15	Removal and replacement of tunneled internal jugular catheter
2015, 4Q, 14	New Section X codes—New Technology procedures
2015, 4Q, 30-31	Vascular access devices
2015, 2Q, 33	Totally implantable central venous access device (Port-a-Cath)
2014, 3Q, 19	End of life replacement of Baclofen pump
2013, 4Q, 116	Device character for Port-A-Cath placement
2012, 4Q, 104	Placement of subcutaneous implantable cardioverter defibrillator

AHA Coding Clinic for table ØJN

2017, 3Q, 11	Bilateral escharotomy of leg, thigh and foot

AHA Coding Clinic for table ØJP

2019, 4Q, 33	Subcutaneous implantable cardioverter defibrillator lead
2018, 4Q, 86	Placement of lumboatrial shunt
2018, 3Q, 29	Decommissioning of left ventricular assist device with exploration of mediastinum
2016, 2Q, 15	Removal and replacement of tunneled internal jugular catheter
2015, 4Q, 31	Vascular access devices
2014, 3Q, 19	End of life replacement of Baclofen pump
2013, 4Q, 109	Separating conjoined twins
2012, 4Q, 104	Placement of subcutaneous implantable cardioverter defibrillator

AHA Coding Clinic for table ØJQ

2017, 3Q, 19	Anterior repair of cystocele
2014, 4Q, 44	Posterior colporrhaphy/rectocele repair

AHA Coding Clinic for table ØJR

2015, 2Q, 13	Transfer of free flap to reconstruct orbital defect

AHA Coding Clinic for table ØJU

2018, 2Q, 20	Prelaminated free flap graft using Alloderm™
2018, 1Q, 7	Placement of fat graft following lumbar decompression surgery

AHA Coding Clinic for table ØJW

2019, 4Q, 33	Subcutaneous implantable cardioverter defibrillator lead
2018, 1Q, 8	Ventricular peritoneal shunt ligation
2015, 4Q, 33	Externalization of peritoneal dialysis catheter
2015, 2Q, 9	Revision of ventriculoperitoneal (VP) shunt
2012, 4Q, 104	Placement of subcutaneous implantable cardioverter defibrillator

AHA Coding Clinic for table ØJX

2022, 1Q, 48	Repair of facial fractures of frontal sinus and orbital roof
2021, 3Q, 19	Elbow amputation and targeted muscle reinnervation
2021, 2Q, 16	Goldilocks breast reconstruction
2018, 1Q, 10	Complex wound closure using pericranial flap
2014, 3Q, 18	Placement of reverse sural fasciocutaneous pedicle flap
2013, 4Q, 109	Separating conjoined twins

Ø   Medical and Surgical
J   Subcutaneous Tissue and Fascia
Ø   Alteration   Definition: Modifying the anatomic structure of a body part without affecting the function of the body part
                 Explanation: Principal purpose is to improve appearance

Body Part Character 4		Approach Character 5	Device Character 6	Qualifier Character 7

**1   Subcutaneous Tissue and
    Fascia, Face**
    Masseteric fascia
    Orbital fascia
    Submandibular space
**4   Subcutaneous Tissue and
    Fascia, Right Neck**
    Deep cervical fascia
    Pretracheal fascia
    Prevertebral fascia
**5   Subcutaneous Tissue and
    Fascia, Left Neck**
    *See 4 Subcutaneous Tissue and
      Fascia, Right Neck*
**6   Subcutaneous Tissue and
    Fascia, Chest**
    Pectoral fascia
**7   Subcutaneous Tissue and
    Fascia, Back**
**8   Subcutaneous Tissue and
    Fascia, Abdomen**
**9   Subcutaneous Tissue and
    Fascia, Buttock**
**D   Subcutaneous Tissue and
    Fascia, Right Upper Arm**
    Axillary fascia
    Deltoid fascia
    Infraspinatus fascia
    Subscapular aponeurosis
    Supraspinatus fascia
	**F Subcutaneous Tissue and
	    Fascia, Left Upper Arm**
	    *See D Subcutaneous Tissue and
	      Fascia, Right Upper Arm*
	**G Subcutaneous Tissue and
	    Fascia, Right Lower Arm**
	    Antebrachial fascia
	    Bicipital aponeurosis
	**H Subcutaneous Tissue and
	    Fascia, Left Lower Arm**
	    *See G Subcutaneous Tissue and
	      Fascia, Right Lower Arm*
	**L Subcutaneous Tissue and
	    Fascia, Right Upper Leg**
	    Crural fascia
	    Fascia lata
	    Iliac fascia
	    Iliotibial tract (band)
	**M Subcutaneous Tissue and
	    Fascia, Left Upper Leg**
	    *See L Subcutaneous Tissue and
	      Fascia, Right Upper Leg*
	**N Subcutaneous Tissue and
	    Fascia, Right Lower Leg**
	**P Subcutaneous Tissue and
	    Fascia, Left Lower Leg**
		Ø Open
		3 Percutaneous
			Z No Device	**Z** No Qualifier

Ø   Medical and Surgical
J   Subcutaneous Tissue and Fascia
2   Change   Definition: Taking out or off a device from a body part and putting back an identical or similar device in or on the same body part without
                 cutting or puncturing the skin or a mucous membrane
                 Explanation: All CHANGE procedures are coded using the approach EXTERNAL

Body Part Character 4	Approach Character 5	Device Character 6	Qualifier Character 7

S   Subcutaneous Tissue and Fascia, Head and Neck
T   Subcutaneous Tissue and Fascia, Trunk
    External oblique aponeurosis
    Transversalis fascia
V   Subcutaneous Tissue and Fascia, Upper Extremity
W   Subcutaneous Tissue and Fascia, Lower Extremity
	X External	**Ø** Drainage Device
		Y Other Device
			Z No Qualifier

Non-OR   All body part, approach, device, and qualifier values

NC Noncovered Procedure   **LC** Limited Coverage   **QA** Questionable OB Admit   **NT** New Tech Add-on   ⊞ Combination Member   ♂ Male   ♀ Female

ICD-10-PCS 2023   **445**

Ø   Medical and Surgical
J   Subcutaneous Tissue and Fascia
5   Destruction   Definition: Physical eradication of all or a portion of a body part by the direct use of energy, force, or a destructive agent
                      Explanation: None of the body part is physically taken out

Body Part Character 4		Approach Character 5	Device Character 6	Qualifier Character 7
Ø Subcutaneous Tissue and Fascia, Scalp Galea aponeurotica	**G Subcutaneous Tissue and Fascia, Right Lower Arm** Antebrachial fascia Bicipital aponeurosis	**Ø Open** **3 Percutaneous**	**Z No Device**	**Z No Qualifier**
1 Subcutaneous Tissue and Fascia, Face Masseteric fascia Orbital fascia Submandibular space	**H Subcutaneous Tissue and Fascia, Left Lower Arm** *See G Subcutaneous Tissue and Fascia, Right Lower Arm*			
4 Subcutaneous Tissue and Fascia, Right Neck Deep cervical fascia Pretracheal fascia Prevertebral fascia	**J Subcutaneous Tissue and Fascia, Right Hand** Palmar fascia (aponeurosis)			
5 Subcutaneous Tissue and Fascia, Left Neck *See 4 Subcutaneous Tissue and Fascia, Right Neck*	**K Subcutaneous Tissue and Fascia, Left Hand** *See J Subcutaneous Tissue and Fascia, Right Hand*			
6 Subcutaneous Tissue and Fascia, Chest Pectoral fascia	**L Subcutaneous Tissue and Fascia, Right Upper Leg** Crural fascia Fascia lata Iliac fascia Iliotibial tract (band)			
7 Subcutaneous Tissue and Fascia, Back	**M Subcutaneous Tissue and Fascia, Left Upper Leg** *See L Subcutaneous Tissue and Fascia, Right Upper Leg*			
8 Subcutaneous Tissue and Fascia, Abdomen	**N Subcutaneous Tissue and Fascia, Right Lower Leg**			
9 Subcutaneous Tissue and Fascia, Buttock	**P Subcutaneous Tissue and Fascia, Left Lower Leg**			
B Subcutaneous Tissue and Fascia, Perineum	**Q Subcutaneous Tissue and Fascia, Right Foot** Plantar fascia (aponeurosis)			
C Subcutaneous Tissue and Fascia, Pelvic Region	**R Subcutaneous Tissue and Fascia, Left Foot** *See Q Subcutaneous Tissue and Fascia, Right Foot*			
D Subcutaneous Tissue and Fascia, Right Upper Arm Axillary fascia Deltoid fascia Infraspinatus fascia Subscapular aponeurosis Supraspinatus fascia				
F Subcutaneous Tissue and Fascia, Left Upper Arm *See D Subcutaneous Tissue and Fascia, Right Upper Arm*				

DRG Non-OR   All body part, approach, device, and qualifier values

Ø   **Medical and Surgical**
J   **Subcutaneous Tissue and Fascia**
8   **Division**   Definition: Cutting into a body part, without draining fluids and/or gases from the body part, in order to separate or transect a body part
                           Explanation: All or a portion of the body part is separated into two or more portions

Body Part Character 4		Approach Character 5	Device Character 6	Qualifier Character 7
Ø Subcutaneous Tissue and Fascia, Scalp Galea aponeurotica **1** Subcutaneous Tissue and Fascia, Face Masseteric fascia Orbital fascia Submandibular space **4** Subcutaneous Tissue and Fascia, Right Neck Deep cervical fascia Pretracheal fascia Prevertebral fascia **5** Subcutaneous Tissue and Fascia, Left Neck *See 4 Subcutaneous Tissue and Fascia, Right Neck* **6** Subcutaneous Tissue and Fascia, Chest Pectoral fascia **7** Subcutaneous Tissue and Fascia, Back **8** Subcutaneous Tissue and Fascia, Abdomen **9** Subcutaneous Tissue and Fascia, Buttock **B** Subcutaneous Tissue and Fascia, Perineum **C** Subcutaneous Tissue and Fascia, Pelvic Region **D** Subcutaneous Tissue and Fascia, Right Upper Arm Axillary fascia Deltoid fascia Infraspinatus fascia Subscapular aponeurosis Supraspinatus fascia **F** Subcutaneous Tissue and Fascia, Left Upper Arm *See D Subcutaneous Tissue and Fascia, Right Upper Arm* **G** Subcutaneous Tissue and Fascia, Right Lower Arm Antebrachial fascia Bicipital aponeurosis	**H** Subcutaneous Tissue and Fascia, Left Lower Arm *See G Subcutaneous Tissue and Fascia, Right Lower Arm* **J** Subcutaneous Tissue and Fascia, Right Hand Palmar fascia (aponeurosis) **K** Subcutaneous Tissue and Fascia, Left Hand *See J Subcutaneous Tissue and Fascia, Right Hand* **L** Subcutaneous Tissue and Fascia, Right Upper Leg Crural fascia Fascia lata Iliac fascia Iliotibial tract (band) **M** Subcutaneous Tissue and Fascia, Left Upper Leg *See L Subcutaneous Tissue and Fascia, Right Upper Leg* **N** Subcutaneous Tissue and Fascia, Right Lower Leg **P** Subcutaneous Tissue and Fascia, Left Lower Leg **Q** Subcutaneous Tissue and Fascia, Right Foot Plantar fascia (aponeurosis) **R** Subcutaneous Tissue and Fascia, Left Foot *See Q Subcutaneous Tissue and Fascia, Right Foot* **S** Subcutaneous Tissue and Fascia, Head and Neck **T** Subcutaneous Tissue and Fascia, Trunk External oblique aponeurosis Transversalis fascia **V** Subcutaneous Tissue and Fascia, Upper Extremity **W** Subcutaneous Tissue and Fascia, Lower Extremity	**Ø** Open **3** Percutaneous	**Z** No Device	**Z** No Qualifier

Ø   Medical and Surgical
J   Subcutaneous Tissue and Fascia
9   Drainage   Definition: Taking or letting out fluids and/or gases from a body part

Explanation: The qualifier DIAGNOSTIC is used to identify drainage procedures that are biopsies

Body Part Character 4		Approach Character 5	Device Character 6	Qualifier Character 7
Ø **Subcutaneous Tissue and Fascia, Scalp** Galea aponeurotica	**G** **Subcutaneous Tissue and Fascia, Right Lower Arm** Antebrachial fascia Bicipital aponeurosis	**Ø** Open **3** Percutaneous	**Ø** Drainage Device	**Z** No Qualifier
1 **Subcutaneous Tissue and Fascia, Face** Masseteric fascia Orbital fascia Submandibular space	**H** **Subcutaneous Tissue and Fascia, Left Lower Arm** *See G Subcutaneous Tissue and Fascia, Right Lower Arm*			
4 **Subcutaneous Tissue and Fascia, Right Neck** Deep cervical fascia Pretracheal fascia Prevertebral fascia	**J** **Subcutaneous Tissue and Fascia, Right Hand** Palmar fascia (aponeurosis)			
5 **Subcutaneous Tissue and Fascia, Left Neck** *See 4 Subcutaneous Tissue and Fascia, Right Neck*	**K** **Subcutaneous Tissue and Fascia, Left Hand** *See J Subcutaneous Tissue and Fascia, Right Hand*			
6 **Subcutaneous Tissue and Fascia, Chest** Pectoral fascia	**L** **Subcutaneous Tissue and Fascia, Right Upper Leg** Crural fascia Fascia lata Iliac fascia Iliotibial tract (band)			
7 **Subcutaneous Tissue and Fascia, Back**	**M** **Subcutaneous Tissue and Fascia, Left Upper Leg** *See L Subcutaneous Tissue and Fascia, Right Upper Leg*			
8 **Subcutaneous Tissue and Fascia, Abdomen**	**N** **Subcutaneous Tissue and Fascia, Right Lower Leg**			
9 **Subcutaneous Tissue and Fascia, Buttock**	**P** **Subcutaneous Tissue and Fascia, Left Lower Leg**			
B **Subcutaneous Tissue and Fascia, Perineum**	**Q** **Subcutaneous Tissue and Fascia, Right Foot** Plantar fascia (aponeurosis)			
C **Subcutaneous Tissue and Fascia, Pelvic Region**	**R** **Subcutaneous Tissue and Fascia, Left Foot** *See Q Subcutaneous Tissue and Fascia, Right Foot*			
D **Subcutaneous Tissue and Fascia, Right Upper Arm** Axillary fascia Deltoid fascia Infraspinatus fascia Subscapular aponeurosis Supraspinatus fascia				
F **Subcutaneous Tissue and Fascia, Left Upper Arm** *See D Subcutaneous Tissue and Fascia, Right Upper Arm*				

Non-OR	All body part, approach, device, and qualifier values

ØJ9 Continued on next page

Non-OR Procedure   DRG Non-OR Procedure   Valid OR Procedure   HAC Associated Procedure   Combination Only   New/Revised April   New/Revised October

448   ICD-10-PCS 2023

Ø   **Medical and Surgical**   *ØJ9 Continued*

J   **Subcutaneous Tissue and Fascia**

9   **Drainage**   Definition: Taking or letting out fluids and/or gases from a body part

                          Explanation: The qualifier DIAGNOSTIC is used to identify drainage procedures that are biopsies

Body Part Character 4		Approach Character 5	Device Character 6	Qualifier Character 7
Ø **Subcutaneous Tissue and Fascia, Scalp** Galea aponeurotica **1** **Subcutaneous Tissue and Fascia, Face** Masseteric fascia Orbital fascia Submandibular space **4** **Subcutaneous Tissue and Fascia, Right Neck** Deep cervical fascia Pretracheal fascia Prevertebral fascia **5** **Subcutaneous Tissue and Fascia, Left Neck** *See 4 Subcutaneous Tissue and Fascia, Right Neck* **6** **Subcutaneous Tissue and Fascia, Chest** Pectoral fascia **7** **Subcutaneous Tissue and Fascia, Back** **8** **Subcutaneous Tissue and Fascia, Abdomen** **9** **Subcutaneous Tissue and Fascia, Buttock** **B** **Subcutaneous Tissue and Fascia, Perineum** **C** **Subcutaneous Tissue and Fascia, Pelvic Region** **D** **Subcutaneous Tissue and Fascia, Right Upper Arm** Axillary fascia Deltoid fascia Infraspinatus fascia Subscapular aponeurosis Supraspinatus fascia **F** **Subcutaneous Tissue and Fascia, Left Upper Arm** *See D Subcutaneous Tissue and Fascia, Right Upper Arm*	**G** **Subcutaneous Tissue and Fascia, Right Lower Arm** Antebrachial fascia Bicipital aponeurosis **H** **Subcutaneous Tissue and Fascia, Left Lower Arm** *See G Subcutaneous Tissue and Fascia, Right Lower Arm* **J** **Subcutaneous Tissue and Fascia, Right Hand** Palmar fascia (aponeurosis) **K** **Subcutaneous Tissue and Fascia, Left Hand** *See J Subcutaneous Tissue and Fascia, Right Hand* **L** **Subcutaneous Tissue and Fascia, Right Upper Leg** Crural fascia Fascia lata Iliac fascia Iliotibial tract (band) **M** **Subcutaneous Tissue and Fascia, Left Upper Leg** *See L Subcutaneous Tissue and Fascia, Right Upper Leg* **N** **Subcutaneous Tissue and Fascia, Right Lower Leg** **P** **Subcutaneous Tissue and Fascia, Left Lower Leg** **Q** **Subcutaneous Tissue and Fascia, Right Foot** Plantar fascia (aponeurosis) **R** **Subcutaneous Tissue and Fascia, Left Foot** *See Q Subcutaneous Tissue and Fascia, Right Foot*	**Ø** Open **3** Percutaneous	**Z** No Device	**X** Diagnostic **Z** No Qualifier

Non-OR	All body part, approach, device, and qualifier values

NC Noncovered Procedure   **LC** Limited Coverage   **QA** Questionable OB Admit   **NT** New Tech Add-on   ⊞ Combination Member   ♂ Male   ♀ Female

ICD-10-PCS 2023   **449**

Subcutaneous Tissue and Fascia *(left margin)*

Ø   **Medical and Surgical**
J   **Subcutaneous Tissue and Fascia**
B   **Excision**   Definition: Cutting out or off, without replacement, a portion of a body part
                      Explanation: The qualifier DIAGNOSTIC is used to identify excision procedures that are biopsies

Body Part Character 4		Approach Character 5	Device Character 6	Qualifier Character 7

Ø   Subcutaneous Tissue and Fascia, Scalp
    Galea aponeurotica
1   Subcutaneous Tissue and Fascia, Face
    Masseteric fascia
    Orbital fascia
    Submandibular space
4   Subcutaneous Tissue and Fascia, Right Neck
    Deep cervical fascia
    Pretracheal fascia
    Prevertebral fascia
5   Subcutaneous Tissue and Fascia, Left Neck
    See 4 Subcutaneous Tissue and Fascia, Right Neck
6   Subcutaneous Tissue and Fascia, Chest
    Pectoral fascia
7   Subcutaneous Tissue and Fascia, Back
8   Subcutaneous Tissue and Fascia, Abdomen
9   Subcutaneous Tissue and Fascia, Buttock
B   Subcutaneous Tissue and Fascia, Perineum
C   Subcutaneous Tissue and Fascia, Pelvic Region
D   Subcutaneous Tissue and Fascia, Right Upper Arm
    Axillary fascia
    Deltoid fascia
    Infraspinatus fascia
    Subscapular aponeurosis
    Supraspinatus fascia
F   Subcutaneous Tissue and Fascia, Left Upper Arm
    See D Subcutaneous Tissue and Fascia, Right Upper Arm
	G Subcutaneous Tissue and Fascia, Right Lower Arm
	    Antebrachial fascia
	    Bicipital aponeurosis
	H Subcutaneous Tissue and Fascia, Left Lower Arm
	    See G Subcutaneous Tissue and Fascia, Right Lower Arm
	J Subcutaneous Tissue and Fascia, Right Hand
	    Palmar fascia (aponeurosis)
	K Subcutaneous Tissue and Fascia, Left Hand
	    See J Subcutaneous Tissue and Fascia, Right Hand
	L Subcutaneous Tissue and Fascia, Right Upper Leg
	    Crural fascia
	    Fascia lata
	    Iliac fascia
	    Iliotibial tract (band)
	M Subcutaneous Tissue and Fascia, Left Upper Leg
	    See L Subcutaneous Tissue and Fascia, Right Upper Leg
	N Subcutaneous Tissue and Fascia, Right Lower Leg
	P Subcutaneous Tissue and Fascia, Left Lower Leg
	Q Subcutaneous Tissue and Fascia, Right Foot
	    Plantar fascia (aponeurosis)
	R Subcutaneous Tissue and Fascia, Left Foot
	    See Q Subcutaneous Tissue and Fascia, Right Foot
		Ø Open
		3 Percutaneous
			Z No Device	X Diagnostic
				Z No Qualifier

DRG Non-OR   ØJB[Ø,4,5,6,7,8,9,B,C,D,F,G,H,L,M,N,P,Q,R]3ZZ
Non-OR   ØJB[Ø,1,4,5,6,7,8,9,B,C,D,F,G,H,J,K,L,M,N,P,Q,R][Ø,3]ZX

Non-OR Procedure   DRG Non-OR Procedure   Valid OR Procedure   HAC Associated Procedure   Combination Only   New/Revised April   New/Revised October

450   ICD-10-PCS 2023

ØJB–ØJB *(left margin bottom)*

Ø   Medical and Surgical
J   Subcutaneous Tissue and Fascia
C   Extirpation   Definition: Taking or cutting out solid matter from a body part

Explanation: The solid matter may be an abnormal byproduct of a biological function or a foreign body; it may be imbedded in a body part or in the lumen of a tubular body part. The solid matter may or may not have been previously broken into pieces.

Body Part Character 4		Approach Character 5	Device Character 6	Qualifier Character 7
Ø Subcutaneous Tissue and Fascia, Scalp Galea aponeurotica **1 Subcutaneous Tissue and Fascia, Face** Masseteric fascia Orbital fascia Submandibular space **4 Subcutaneous Tissue and Fascia, Right Neck** Deep cervical fascia Pretracheal fascia Prevertebral fascia **5 Subcutaneous Tissue and Fascia, Left Neck** *See 4 Subcutaneous Tissue and Fascia, Right Neck* **6 Subcutaneous Tissue and Fascia, Chest** Pectoral fascia **7 Subcutaneous Tissue and Fascia, Back** **8 Subcutaneous Tissue and Fascia, Abdomen** **9 Subcutaneous Tissue and Fascia, Buttock** **B Subcutaneous Tissue and Fascia, Perineum** **C Subcutaneous Tissue and Fascia, Pelvic Region** **D Subcutaneous Tissue and Fascia, Right Upper Arm** Axillary fascia Deltoid fascia Infraspinatus fascia Subscapular aponeurosis Supraspinatus fascia **F Subcutaneous Tissue and Fascia, Left Upper Arm** *See D Subcutaneous Tissue and Fascia, Right Upper Arm*	**G Subcutaneous Tissue and Fascia, Right Lower Arm** Antebrachial fascia Bicipital aponeurosis **H Subcutaneous Tissue and Fascia, Left Lower Arm** *See G Subcutaneous Tissue and Fascia, Right Lower Arm* **J Subcutaneous Tissue and Fascia, Right Hand** Palmar fascia (aponeurosis) **K Subcutaneous Tissue and Fascia, Left Hand** *See J Subcutaneous Tissue and Fascia, Right Hand* **L Subcutaneous Tissue and Fascia, Right Upper Leg** Crural fascia Fascia lata Iliac fascia Iliotibial tract (band) **M Subcutaneous Tissue and Fascia, Left Upper Leg** *See L Subcutaneous Tissue and Fascia, Right Upper Leg* **N Subcutaneous Tissue and Fascia, Right Lower Leg** **P Subcutaneous Tissue and Fascia, Left Lower Leg** **Q Subcutaneous Tissue and Fascia, Right Foot** Plantar fascia (aponeurosis) **R Subcutaneous Tissue and Fascia, Left Foot** *See Q Subcutaneous Tissue and Fascia, Right Foot*	**Ø Open** **3 Percutaneous**	**Z No Device**	**Z No Qualifier**

Non-OR   ØJC[Ø,1,4,5,6,7,8,9,B,C,D,F,G,H,J,K,L,M,N,P,Q,R]3ZZ

Subcutaneous Tissue and Fascia

Ø	Medical and Surgical
J	Subcutaneous Tissue and Fascia
D	Extraction

Definition: Pulling or stripping out or off all or a portion of a body part by the use of force

Explanation: The qualifier DIAGNOSTIC is used to identify extraction procedures that are biopsies

Body Part Character 4		Approach Character 5	Device Character 6	Qualifier Character 7

Ø Subcutaneous Tissue and Fascia, Scalp
   Galea aponeurotica
	G Subcutaneous Tissue and Fascia, Right Lower Arm
	   Antebrachial fascia
	   Bicipital aponeurosis
		Ø Open
		3 Percutaneous
			Z No Device	**Z** No Qualifier

1 Subcutaneous Tissue and Fascia, Face
   Masseteric fascia
   Orbital fascia
   Submandibular space
	H Subcutaneous Tissue and Fascia, Left Lower Arm
	   See G Subcutaneous Tissue and Fascia, Right Lower Arm			

4 Subcutaneous Tissue and Fascia, Right Neck
   Deep cervical fascia
   Pretracheal fascia
   Prevertebral fascia
	J Subcutaneous Tissue and Fascia, Right Hand
	   Palmar fascia (aponeurosis)
	K Subcutaneous Tissue and Fascia, Left Hand			

5 Subcutaneous Tissue and Fascia, Left Neck
   See 4 Subcutaneous Tissue and Fascia, Right Neck
	See J Subcutaneous Tissue and Fascia, Right Hand
	L Subcutaneous Tissue and Fascia, Right Upper Leg
	   Crural fascia			

6 Subcutaneous Tissue and Fascia, Chest
   Pectoral fascia
	Fascia lata
	   Iliac fascia
	   Iliotibial tract (band)			

7 Subcutaneous Tissue and Fascia, Back	**M** Subcutaneous Tissue and Fascia, Left Upper Leg *See L Subcutaneous Tissue and Fascia, Right Upper Leg*			
8 Subcutaneous Tissue and Fascia, Abdomen	**N** Subcutaneous Tissue and Fascia, Right Lower Leg			
9 Subcutaneous Tissue and Fascia, Buttock	**P** Subcutaneous Tissue and Fascia, Left Lower Leg			
B Subcutaneous Tissue and Fascia, Perineum	**Q** Subcutaneous Tissue and Fascia, Right Foot Plantar fascia (aponeurosis)			
C Subcutaneous Tissue and Fascia, Pelvic Region	**R** Subcutaneous Tissue and Fascia, Left Foot *See Q Subcutaneous Tissue and Fascia, Right Foot*			

D Subcutaneous Tissue and Fascia, Right Upper Arm
   Axillary fascia
   Deltoid fascia
   Infraspinatus fascia
   Subscapular aponeurosis
   Supraspinatus fascia				

F Subcutaneous Tissue and Fascia, Left Upper Arm *See D Subcutaneous Tissue and Fascia, Right Upper Arm*				

Non-OR   ØJD[Ø,1,4,5,B,C,D,F,G,H,J,K,N,P,Q,R]3ZZ

See Appendix L for Procedure Combinations
Combo-only   ØJD[6,7,8,9,L,M]3ZZ

Non-OR Procedure   DRG Non-OR Procedure   Valid OR Procedure   HAC Associated Procedure   Combination Only   New/Revised April   New/Revised October

452   ICD-10-PCS 2023

Ø   **Medical and Surgical**
J   **Subcutaneous Tissue and Fascia**
H   **Insertion**   Definition: Putting in a nonbiological appliance that monitors, assists, performs, or prevents a physiological function but does not physically take the place of a body part
                           Explanation: None

Body Part Character 4		Approach Character 5	Device Character 6	Qualifier Character 7
Ø Subcutaneous Tissue and Fascia, Scalp Galea aponeurotica **1** Subcutaneous Tissue and Fascia, Face Masseteric fascia Orbital fascia Submandibular space **4** Subcutaneous Tissue and Fascia, Right Neck Deep cervical fascia Pretracheal fascia Prevertebral fascia **5** Subcutaneous Tissue and Fascia, Left Neck *See 4 Subcutaneous Tissue and Fascia, Right Neck* **9** Subcutaneous Tissue and Fascia, Buttock **B** Subcutaneous Tissue and Fascia, Perineum	**C** Subcutaneous Tissue and Fascia, Pelvic Region **J** Subcutaneous Tissue and Fascia, Right Hand Palmar fascia (aponeurosis) **K** Subcutaneous Tissue and Fascia, Left Hand *See J Subcutaneous Tissue and Fascia, Right Hand* **Q** Subcutaneous Tissue and Fascia, Right Foot Plantar fascia (aponeurosis) **R** Subcutaneous Tissue and Fascia, Left Foot *See Q Subcutaneous Tissue and Fascia, Right Foot*	**Ø** Open **3** Percutaneous	**N** Tissue Expander	**Z** No Qualifier
6 Subcutaneous Tissue and Fascia, Chest ⊞ Pectoral fascia		**Ø** Open **3** Percutaneous	**Ø** Monitoring Device, Hemodynamic **2** Monitoring Device **4** Pacemaker, Single Chamber **5** Pacemaker, Single Chamber Rate Responsive **6** Pacemaker, Dual Chamber **7** Cardiac Resynchronization Pacemaker Pulse Generator **8** Defibrillator Generator **9** Cardiac Resynchronization Defibrillator Pulse Generator **A** Contractility Modulation Device **B** Stimulator Generator, Single Array **C** Stimulator Generator, Single Array Rechargeable **D** Stimulator Generator, Multiple Array **E** Stimulator Generator, Multiple Array Rechargeable **F** Subcutaneous Defibrillator Lead **H** Contraceptive Device **M** Stimulator Generator **N** Tissue Expander **P** Cardiac Rhythm Related Device **V** Infusion Device, Pump **W** Vascular Access Device, Totally Implantable **X** Vascular Access Device, Tunneled **Y** Other Device	**Z** No Qualifier
7 Subcutaneous Tissue and Fascia, Back ᴺᶜ ⊞		**Ø** Open **3** Percutaneous	**B** Stimulator Generator, Single Array **C** Stimulator Generator, Single Array Rechargeable **D** Stimulator Generator, Multiple Array **E** Stimulator Generator, Multiple Array Rechargeable **M** Stimulator Generator **N** Tissue Expander **V** Infusion Device, Pump **Y** Other Device	**Z** No Qualifier

DRG Non-OR ØJH6[Ø,3][4,5,6,7,H,P,X]Z	
DRG Non-OR ØJH63WX	
Non-OR ØJH63YZ	ᴺᶜ ØJH7[Ø,3]MZ
Non-OR ØJH73YZ	**See Appendix L for Procedure Combinations**
HAC ØJH6[Ø,3][4,5,6,7,8,9,P]Z when reported with SDx K68.11 or T81.4Ø-T81.49, T82.7 with 7th character A	⊞ ØJH6[Ø,3][4,5,6,7,8,9,A,B,C,D,E,F,M,P]Z
HAC ØJH63XZ when reported with SDx J95.811	⊞ ØJH7[Ø,3][B,C,D,E,M]Z

ØJH Continued on next page

ᴺᶜ Noncovered Procedure   ᴸᶜ Limited Coverage   � Questionable OB Admit   ᴺᵀ New Tech Add-on   ⊞ Combination Member   ♂Male   ♀Female

ICD-10-PCS 2023   453

Subcutaneous Tissue and Fascia

Ø   **Medical and Surgical**   *ØJH Continued*
J   **Subcutaneous Tissue and Fascia**
H   **Insertion**   Definition: Putting in a nonbiological appliance that monitors, assists, performs, or prevents a physiological function but does not physically
                       take the place of a body part
                       Explanation: None

Body Part Character 4		Approach Character 5	Device Character 6	Qualifier Character 7
8 Subcutaneous Tissue and Fascia, Abdomen NC ⊞		Ø Open 3 Percutaneous	Ø Monitoring Device, Hemodynamic 2 Monitoring Device 4 Pacemaker, Single Chamber 5 Pacemaker, Single Chamber Rate Responsive 6 Pacemaker, Dual Chamber 7 Cardiac Resynchronization Pacemaker Pulse Generator 8 Defibrillator Generator 9 Cardiac Resynchronization Defibrillator Pulse Generator A Contractility Modulation Device B Stimulator Generator, Single Array C Stimulator Generator, Single Array Rechargeable D Stimulator Generator, Multiple Array E Stimulator Generator, Multiple Array Rechargeable H Contraceptive Device M Stimulator Generator N Tissue Expander P Cardiac Rhythm Related Device V Infusion Device, Pump W Vascular Access Device, Totally Implantable X Vascular Access Device, Tunneled Y Other Device	Z No Qualifier
D Subcutaneous Tissue and Fascia, Right Upper Arm Axillary fascia Deltoid fascia Infraspinatus fascia Subscapular aponeurosis Supraspinatus fascia F Subcutaneous Tissue and Fascia, Left Upper Arm *See D Subcutaneous Tissue and Fascia, Right Upper Arm* G Subcutaneous Tissue and Fascia, Right Lower Arm Antebrachial fascia Bicipital aponeurosis H Subcutaneous Tissue and Fascia, Left Lower Arm *See G Subcutaneous Tissue and Fascia, Right Lower Arm*	L Subcutaneous Tissue and Fascia, Right Upper Leg Crural fascia Fascia lata Iliac fascia Iliotibial tract (band) M Subcutaneous Tissue and Fascia, Left Upper Leg *See L Subcutaneous Tissue and Fascia, Right Upper Leg* N Subcutaneous Tissue and Fascia, Right Lower Leg P Subcutaneous Tissue and Fascia, Left Lower Leg	Ø Open 3 Percutaneous	H Contraceptive Device N Tissue Expander V Infusion Device, Pump W Vascular Access Device, Totally Implantable X Vascular Access Device, Tunneled	Z No Qualifier
S Subcutaneous Tissue and Fascia, Head and Neck V Subcutaneous Tissue and Fascia, Upper Extremity W Subcutaneous Tissue and Fascia, Lower Extremity		Ø Open 3 Percutaneous	1 Radioactive Element 3 Infusion Device Y Other Device	Z No Qualifier
T Subcutaneous Tissue and Fascia, Trunk External oblique aponeurosis Transversalis fascia		Ø Open 3 Percutaneous	1 Radioactive Element 3 Infusion Device V Infusion Device, Pump Y Other Device	Z No Qualifier

DRG Non-OR	ØJH8[Ø,3][2,4,5,6,7,H,P,X]Z	**Non-OR** ØJH83YZ	**HAC** ØJH8[Ø,3][4,5,6,7,8,9,P]Z when reported with SDx K68.11 or
DRG Non-OR	ØJH83WX	**Non-OR** ØJH[D,F,G,H,L,M][Ø,3]HZ	T81.4Ø-T81.49, T82.7 with 7th character A
DRG Non-OR	ØJH[D,F,G,H,L,M,N,P]ØXZ	**Non-OR** ØJHNØHZ	**NC** ØJH8[Ø,3]MZ
DRG Non-OR	ØJH[D,F,G,H,L,M,N,P]3[W,X]Z	**Non-OR** ØJH[S,V,W]Ø3Z	**See Appendix L for Procedure Combinations**
DRG Non-OR	ØJHN3HZ	**Non-OR** ØJH[S,V,W]3[3,Y]Z	⊞ ØJH8[Ø,3][4,5,6,7,8,9,A,B,C,D,E,M,P]Z
DRG Non-OR	ØJHP[Ø,3]HZ	**Non-OR** ØJHTØ3Z	
		Non-OR ØJHT3[3,Y]Z	

Ø　**Medical and Surgical**
J　**Subcutaneous Tissue and Fascia**
J　**Inspection**　　　Definition: Visually and/or manually exploring a body part

　　　　　Explanation: Visual exploration may be performed with or without optical instrumentation. Manual exploration may be performed directly or through intervening body layers.

Body Part Character 4	Approach Character 5	Device Character 6	Qualifier Character 7
S Subcutaneous Tissue and Fascia, Head and Neck **T** Subcutaneous Tissue and Fascia, Trunk 　　External oblique aponeurosis 　　Transversalis fascia **V** Subcutaneous Tissue and Fascia, Upper Extremity **W** Subcutaneous Tissue and Fascia, Lower Extremity	**Ø** Open **3** Percutaneous **X** External	**Z** No Device	**Z** No Qualifier

Non-OR　All body part, approach, device, and qualifier values

Ø　**Medical and Surgical**
J　**Subcutaneous Tissue and Fascia**
N　**Release**　　　Definition: Freeing a body part from an abnormal physical constraint by cutting or by the use of force

　　　　　Explanation: Some of the restraining tissue may be taken out but none of the body part is taken out

Body Part Character 4	Approach Character 5	Device Character 6	Qualifier Character 7
Ø Subcutaneous Tissue and Fascia, Scalp 　　Galea aponeurotica **1** Subcutaneous Tissue and Fascia, Face 　　Masseteric fascia 　　Orbital fascia 　　Submandibular space **4** Subcutaneous Tissue and Fascia, Right Neck 　　Deep cervical fascia 　　Pretracheal fascia 　　Prevertebral fascia **5** Subcutaneous Tissue and Fascia, Left Neck 　　*See 4 Subcutaneous Tissue and Fascia, Right Neck* **6** Subcutaneous Tissue and Fascia, Chest 　　Pectoral fascia **7** Subcutaneous Tissue and Fascia, Back **8** Subcutaneous Tissue and Fascia, Abdomen **9** Subcutaneous Tissue and Fascia, Buttock **B** Subcutaneous Tissue and Fascia, Perineum **C** Subcutaneous Tissue and Fascia, Pelvic Region **D** Subcutaneous Tissue and Fascia, Right Upper Arm 　　Axillary fascia 　　Deltoid fascia 　　Infraspinatus fascia 　　Subscapular aponeurosis 　　Supraspinatus fascia **F** Subcutaneous Tissue and Fascia, Left Upper Arm 　　*See D Subcutaneous Tissue and Fascia, Right Upper Arm* **G** Subcutaneous Tissue and Fascia, Right Lower Arm 　　Antebrachial fascia 　　Bicipital aponeurosis **H** Subcutaneous Tissue and Fascia, Left Lower Arm 　　*See G Subcutaneous Tissue and Fascia, Right Lower Arm* **J** Subcutaneous Tissue and Fascia, Right Hand 　　Palmar fascia (aponeurosis) **K** Subcutaneous Tissue and Fascia, Left Hand 　　*See J Subcutaneous Tissue and Fascia, Right Hand* **L** Subcutaneous Tissue and Fascia, Right Upper Leg 　　Crural fascia 　　Fascia lata 　　Iliac fascia 　　Iliotibial tract (band) **M** Subcutaneous Tissue and Fascia, Left Upper Leg 　　*See L Subcutaneous Tissue and Fascia, Right Upper Leg* **N** Subcutaneous Tissue and Fascia, Right Lower Leg **P** Subcutaneous Tissue and Fascia, Left Lower Leg **Q** Subcutaneous Tissue and Fascia, Right Foot 　　Plantar fascia (aponeurosis) **R** Subcutaneous Tissue and Fascia, Left Foot 　　*See Q Subcutaneous Tissue and Fascia, Right Foot*	**Ø** Open **3** Percutaneous **X** External	**Z** No Device	**Z** No Qualifier

Non-OR　ØJN[Ø,1,4,5,6,7,8,9,B,C,D,F,G,H,J,K,L,M,N,P,Q,R]XZZ

NC Noncovered Procedure　　**LC** Limited Coverage　　**QA** Questionable OB Admit　　**NT** New Tech Add-on　　⊞ Combination Member　　♂ Male　　♀ Female

ICD-10-PCS 2023　　　　　　　　　　　　　　　　　　　　　　　　　　　　　　　455

Subcutaneous Tissue and Fascia (side tab)

Ø Medical and Surgical
J Subcutaneous Tissue and Fascia
P Removal   Definition: Taking out or off a device from a body part

Explanation: If a device is taken out and a similar device put in without cutting or puncturing the skin or mucous membrane, the procedure is coded to the root operation CHANGE. Otherwise, the procedure for taking out a device is coded to the root operation REMOVAL.

Body Part Character 4	Approach Character 5	Device Character 6	Qualifier Character 7
S Subcutaneous Tissue and Fascia, Head and Neck	**Ø** Open **3** Percutaneous	**Ø** Drainage Device **1** Radioactive Element **3** Infusion Device **7** Autologous Tissue Substitute **J** Synthetic Substitute **K** Nonautologous Tissue Substitute **N** Tissue Expander **Y** Other Device	**Z** No Qualifier
S Subcutaneous Tissue and Fascia, Head and Neck	**X** External	**Ø** Drainage Device **1** Radioactive Element **3** Infusion Device	**Z** No Qualifier
T Subcutaneous Tissue and Fascia, Trunk External oblique aponeurosis Transversalis fascia	**Ø** Open **3** Percutaneous	**Ø** Drainage Device **1** Radioactive Element **2** Monitoring Device **3** Infusion Device **7** Autologous Tissue Substitute **F** Subcutaneous Defibrillator Lead **H** Contraceptive Device **J** Synthetic Substitute **K** Nonautologous Tissue Substitute **M** Stimulator Generator **N** Tissue Expander **P** Cardiac Rhythm Related Device **V** Infusion Device, Pump **W** Vascular Access Device, Totally Implantable **X** Vascular Access Device, Tunneled **Y** Other Device	**Z** No Qualifier
T Subcutaneous Tissue and Fascia, Trunk External oblique aponeurosis Transversalis fascia	**X** External	**Ø** Drainage Device **1** Radioactive Element **2** Monitoring Device **3** Infusion Device **H** Contraceptive Device **V** Infusion Device, Pump **X** Vascular Access Device, Tunneled	**Z** No Qualifier
V Subcutaneous Tissue and Fascia, Upper Extremity **W** Subcutaneous Tissue and Fascia, Lower Extremity	**Ø** Open **3** Percutaneous	**Ø** Drainage Device **1** Radioactive Element **3** Infusion Device **7** Autologous Tissue Substitute **H** Contraceptive Device **J** Synthetic Substitute **K** Nonautologous Tissue Substitute **N** Tissue Expander **V** Infusion Device, Pump **W** Vascular Access Device, Totally Implantable **X** Vascular Access Device, Tunneled **Y** Other Device	**Z** No Qualifier
V Subcutaneous Tissue and Fascia, Upper Extremity **W** Subcutaneous Tissue and Fascia, Lower Extremity	**X** External	**Ø** Drainage Device **1** Radioactive Element **3** Infusion Device **H** Contraceptive Device **V** Infusion Device, Pump **X** Vascular Access Device, Tunneled	**Z** No Qualifier

Non-OR	ØJPS[Ø,3][Ø,1,3,7,J,K,N,Y]Z
Non-OR	ØJPSX[Ø,1,3]Z
Non-OR	ØJPT[Ø,3][Ø,1,2,3,7,H,J,K,M,N,V,W,X,Y]Z
Non-OR	ØJPTX[Ø,1,2,3,H,V,X]Z
Non-OR	ØJP[V,W][Ø,3][Ø,1,3,7,H,J,K,N,V,W,X,Y]Z
Non-OR	ØJP[V,W]X[Ø,1,3,H,V,X]Z
HAC	ØJPT[Ø,3][F,P]Z when reported with SDx K68.11 or T81.4Ø-T81.49, T82.7 with 7th character A

Non-OR Procedure   DRG Non-OR Procedure   Valid OR Procedure   HAC Associated Procedure   Combination Only   New/Revised April   New/Revised October

Ø Medical and Surgical
J Subcutaneous Tissue and Fascia
Q Repair   Definition: Restoring, to the extent possible, a body part to its normal anatomic structure and function
                  Explanation: Used only when the method to accomplish the repair is not one of the other root operations

Body Part Character 4		Approach Character 5	Device Character 6	Qualifier Character 7
Ø Subcutaneous Tissue and Fascia, Scalp Galea aponeurotica **1 Subcutaneous Tissue and Fascia, Face** Masseteric fascia Orbital fascia Submandibular space **4 Subcutaneous Tissue and Fascia, Right Neck** Deep cervical fascia Pretracheal fascia Prevertebral fascia **5 Subcutaneous Tissue and Fascia, Left Neck** *See 4 Subcutaneous Tissue and Fascia, Right Neck* **6 Subcutaneous Tissue and Fascia, Chest** Pectoral fascia **7 Subcutaneous Tissue and Fascia, Back** **8 Subcutaneous Tissue and Fascia, Abdomen** **9 Subcutaneous Tissue and Fascia, Buttock** **B Subcutaneous Tissue and Fascia, Perineum** **C Subcutaneous Tissue and Fascia, Pelvic Region** **D Subcutaneous Tissue and Fascia, Right Upper Arm** Axillary fascia Deltoid fascia Infraspinatus fascia Subscapular aponeurosis Supraspinatus fascia **F Subcutaneous Tissue and Fascia, Left Upper Arm** *See D Subcutaneous Tissue and Fascia, Right Upper Arm*	**G Subcutaneous Tissue and Fascia, Right Lower Arm** Antebrachial fascia Bicipital aponeurosis **H Subcutaneous Tissue and Fascia, Left Lower Arm** *See G Subcutaneous Tissue and Fascia, Right Lower Arm* **J Subcutaneous Tissue and Fascia, Right Hand** Palmar fascia (aponeurosis) **K Subcutaneous Tissue and Fascia, Left Hand** *See J Subcutaneous Tissue and Fascia, Right Hand* **L Subcutaneous Tissue and Fascia, Right Upper Leg** Crural fascia Fascia lata Iliac fascia Iliotibial tract (band) **M Subcutaneous Tissue and Fascia, Left Upper Leg** *See L Subcutaneous Tissue and Fascia, Right Upper Leg* **N Subcutaneous Tissue and Fascia, Right Lower Leg** **P Subcutaneous Tissue and Fascia, Left Lower Leg** **Q Subcutaneous Tissue and Fascia, Right Foot** Plantar fascia (aponeurosis) **R Subcutaneous Tissue and Fascia, Left Foot** *See Q Subcutaneous Tissue and Fascia, Right Foot*	**Ø Open** **3 Percutaneous**	**Z No Device**	**Z No Qualifier**

Non-OR   ØJQ[Ø,1,4,5,6,7,8,9,B,C,D,F,G,H,J,K,L,M,N,P,Q,R]3ZZ

NC Noncovered Procedure   **LC** Limited Coverage   **QA** Questionable OB Admit   **NT** New Tech Add-on   ⊞ Combination Member   ♂ Male   ♀ Female

ICD-10-PCS 2023   457

Subcutaneous Tissue and Fascia *(left margin)*

Ø Medical and Surgical
J Subcutaneous Tissue and Fascia
R Replacement   Definition: Putting in or on biological or synthetic material that physically takes the place and/or function of all or a portion of a body part

         Explanation: The body part may have been taken out or replaced, or may be taken out, physically eradicated, or rendered nonfunctional during the REPLACEMENT procedure. A REMOVAL procedure is coded for taking out the device used in a previous replacement procedure.

Body Part Character 4		Approach Character 5	Device Character 6	Qualifier Character 7
Ø Subcutaneous Tissue and Fascia, Scalp Galea aponeurotica **1 Subcutaneous Tissue and Fascia, Face** Masseteric fascia Orbital fascia Submandibular space **4 Subcutaneous Tissue and Fascia, Right Neck** Deep cervical fascia Pretracheal fascia Prevertebral fascia **5 Subcutaneous Tissue and Fascia, Left Neck** *See 4 Subcutaneous Tissue and Fascia, Right Neck* **6 Subcutaneous Tissue and Fascia, Chest** Pectoral fascia **7 Subcutaneous Tissue and Fascia, Back** **8 Subcutaneous Tissue and Fascia, Abdomen** **9 Subcutaneous Tissue and Fascia, Buttock** **B Subcutaneous Tissue and Fascia, Perineum** **C Subcutaneous Tissue and Fascia, Pelvic Region** **D Subcutaneous Tissue and Fascia, Right Upper Arm** Axillary fascia Deltoid fascia Infraspinatus fascia Subscapular aponeurosis Supraspinatus fascia **F Subcutaneous Tissue and Fascia, Left Upper Arm** *See D Subcutaneous Tissue and Fascia, Right Upper Arm*	**G Subcutaneous Tissue and Fascia, Right Lower Arm** Antebrachial fascia Bicipital aponeurosis **H Subcutaneous Tissue and Fascia, Left Lower Arm** *See G Subcutaneous Tissue and Fascia, Right Lower Arm* **J Subcutaneous Tissue and Fascia, Right Hand** Palmar fascia (aponeurosis) **K Subcutaneous Tissue and Fascia, Left Hand** *See J Subcutaneous Tissue and Fascia, Right Hand* **L Subcutaneous Tissue and Fascia, Right Upper Leg** Crural fascia Fascia lata Iliac fascia Iliotibial tract (band) **M Subcutaneous Tissue and Fascia, Left Upper Leg** *See L Subcutaneous Tissue and Fascia, Right Upper Leg* **N Subcutaneous Tissue and Fascia, Right Lower Leg** **P Subcutaneous Tissue and Fascia, Left Lower Leg** **Q Subcutaneous Tissue and Fascia, Right Foot** Plantar fascia (aponeurosis) **R Subcutaneous Tissue and Fascia, Left Foot** *See Q Subcutaneous Tissue and Fascia, Right Foot*	**Ø Open** **3 Percutaneous**	**7 Autologous Tissue Substitute** **J Synthetic Substitute** **K Nonautologous Tissue Substitute**	**Z No Qualifier**

Ø   **Medical and Surgical**
J   **Subcutaneous Tissue and Fascia**
U   **Supplement:**   Definition: Putting in or on biological or synthetic material that physically reinforces and/or augments the function of a portion of a body part

             Explanation: The biological material is non-living, or is living and from the same individual. The body part may have been previously replaced, and the SUPPLEMENT procedure is performed to physically reinforce and/or augment the function of the replaced body part.

Body Part Character 4		Approach Character 5	Device Character 6	Qualifier Character 7

Ø   **Subcutaneous Tissue and Fascia, Scalp**
    Galea aponeurotica
1   **Subcutaneous Tissue and Fascia, Face**
    Masseteric fascia
    Orbital fascia
    Submandibular space
4   **Subcutaneous Tissue and Fascia, Right Neck**
    Deep cervical fascia
    Pretracheal fascia
    Prevertebral fascia
5   **Subcutaneous Tissue and Fascia, Left Neck**
    See 4 Subcutaneous Tissue and Fascia, Right Neck
6   **Subcutaneous Tissue and Fascia, Chest**
    Pectoral fascia
7   **Subcutaneous Tissue and Fascia, Back**
8   **Subcutaneous Tissue and Fascia, Abdomen**
9   **Subcutaneous Tissue and Fascia, Buttock**
B   **Subcutaneous Tissue and Fascia, Perineum**
C   **Subcutaneous Tissue and Fascia, Pelvic Region**
D   **Subcutaneous Tissue and Fascia, Right Upper Arm**
    Axillary fascia
    Deltoid fascia
    Infraspinatus fascia
    Subscapular aponeurosis
    Supraspinatus fascia
F   **Subcutaneous Tissue and Fascia, Left Upper Arm**
    See D Subcutaneous Tissue and Fascia, Right Upper Arm
	G **Subcutaneous Tissue and Fascia, Right Lower Arm**
	    Antebrachial fascia
	    Bicipital aponeurosis
	H **Subcutaneous Tissue and Fascia, Left Lower Arm**
	    See G Subcutaneous Tissue and Fascia, Right Lower Arm
	J **Subcutaneous Tissue and Fascia, Right Hand**
	    Palmar fascia (aponeurosis)
	K **Subcutaneous Tissue and Fascia, Left Hand**
	    See J Subcutaneous Tissue and Fascia, Right Hand
	L **Subcutaneous Tissue and Fascia, Right Upper Leg**
	    Crural fascia
	    Fascia lata
	    Iliac fascia
	    Iliotibial tract (band)
	M **Subcutaneous Tissue and Fascia, Left Upper Leg**
	    See L Subcutaneous Tissue and Fascia, Right Upper Leg
	N **Subcutaneous Tissue and Fascia, Right Lower Leg**
	P **Subcutaneous Tissue and Fascia, Left Lower Leg**
	Q **Subcutaneous Tissue and Fascia, Right Foot**
	    Plantar fascia (aponeurosis)
	R **Subcutaneous Tissue and Fascia, Left Foot**
	    See Q Subcutaneous Tissue and Fascia, Right Foot
		Ø Open
		3 Percutaneous
			7 Autologous Tissue Substitute
			J Synthetic Substitute
			K Nonautologous Tissue Substitute
				Z No Qualifier

NC Noncovered Procedure   **LC** Limited Coverage   **QA** Questionable OB Admit   **NT** New Tech Add-on   ⊞ Combination Member   ♂ Male   ♀ Female

ICD-10-PCS 2023   **459**

Subcutaneous Tissue and Fascia *(left margin)*

Ø Medical and Surgical
J Subcutaneous Tissue and Fascia
W Revision   Definition: Correcting, to the extent possible, a portion of a malfunctioning device or the position of a displaced device

Explanation: Revision can include correcting a malfunctioning or displaced device by taking out or putting in components of the device such as a screw or pin

Body Part Character 4	Approach Character 5	Device Character 6	Qualifier Character 7
S Subcutaneous Tissue and Fascia, Head and Neck	**Ø** Open **3** Percutaneous	**Ø** Drainage Device **3** Infusion Device **7** Autologous Tissue Substitute **J** Synthetic Substitute **K** Nonautologous Tissue Substitute **N** Tissue Expander **Y** Other Device	**Z** No Qualifier
S Subcutaneous Tissue and Fascia, Head and Neck	**X** External	**Ø** Drainage Device **3** Infusion Device **7** Autologous Tissue Substitute **J** Synthetic Substitute **K** Nonautologous Tissue Substitute **N** Tissue Expander	**Z** No Qualifier
T Subcutaneous Tissue and Fascia, Trunk External oblique aponeurosis Transversalis fascia	**Ø** Open **3** Percutaneous	**Ø** Drainage Device **2** Monitoring Device **3** Infusion Device **7** Autologous Tissue Substitute **F** Subcutaneous Defibrillator Lead **H** Contraceptive Device **J** Synthetic Substitute **K** Nonautologous Tissue Substitute **M** Stimulator Generator **N** Tissue Expander **P** Cardiac Rhythm Related Device **V** Infusion Device, Pump **W** Vascular Access Device, Totally Implantable **X** Vascular Access Device, Tunneled **Y** Other Device	**Z** No Qualifier
T Subcutaneous Tissue and Fascia, Trunk External oblique aponeurosis Transversalis fascia	**X** External	**Ø** Drainage Device **2** Monitoring Device **3** Infusion Device **7** Autologous Tissue Substitute **F** Subcutaneous Defibrillator Lead **H** Contraceptive Device **J** Synthetic Substitute **K** Nonautologous Tissue Substitute **M** Stimulator Generator **N** Tissue Expander **P** Cardiac Rhythm Related Device **V** Infusion Device, Pump **W** Vascular Access Device, Totally Implantable **X** Vascular Access Device, Tunneled	**Z** No Qualifier
V Subcutaneous Tissue and Fascia, Upper Extremity **W** Subcutaneous Tissue and Fascia, Lower Extremity	**Ø** Open **3** Percutaneous	**Ø** Drainage Device **3** Infusion Device **7** Autologous Tissue Substitute **H** Contraceptive Device **J** Synthetic Substitute **K** Nonautologous Tissue Substitute **N** Tissue Expander **V** Infusion Device, Pump **W** Vascular Access Device, Totally Implantable **X** Vascular Access Device, Tunneled **Y** Other Device	**Z** No Qualifier
V Subcutaneous Tissue and Fascia, Upper Extremity **W** Subcutaneous Tissue and Fascia, Lower Extremity	**X** External	**Ø** Drainage Device **3** Infusion Device **7** Autologous Tissue Substitute **H** Contraceptive Device **J** Synthetic Substitute **K** Nonautologous Tissue Substitute **N** Tissue Expander **V** Infusion Device, Pump **W** Vascular Access Device, Totally Implantable **X** Vascular Access Device, Tunneled	**Z** No Qualifier

DRG Non-OR	ØJWS[Ø,3][Ø,3,7,J,K,N,Y]Z	
DRG Non-OR	ØJWT[Ø,3][Ø,3,7,H,J,K,M,N,V,W,X]Z	
DRG Non-OR	ØJWTXMZ	
DRG Non-OR	ØJW[V,W][Ø,3][Ø,3,7,H,J,K,N,V,W,X,Y]Z	
Non-OR	ØJWSX[Ø,3,7,J,K,N]Z	
Non-OR	ØJWT3YZ	
Non-OR	ØJWTX[Ø,2,3,7,F,H,J,K,N,P,V,W,X]Z	
Non-OR	ØJW[V,W]X[Ø,3,7,H,J,K,N,V,W,X]Z	

HAC   ØJWT[Ø,3][F,P]Z when reported with SDx K68.11 or T81.4Ø-T81.49, T82.7 with 7th character A

Non-OR Procedure   DRG Non-OR Procedure   Valid OR Procedure   HAC Associated Procedure   Combination Only   New/Revised April   New/Revised October

460   ICD-10-PCS 2023

Ø   Medical and Surgical
J   Subcutaneous Tissue and Fascia
X   Transfer   Definition: Moving, without taking out, all or a portion of a body part to another location to take over the function of all or a portion of a body part
        Explanation: The body part transferred remains connected to its vascular and nervous supply

Body Part Character 4		Approach Character 5	Device Character 6	Qualifier Character 7
Ø **Subcutaneous Tissue and Fascia, Scalp** Galea aponeurotica **1** **Subcutaneous Tissue and Fascia, Face** Masseteric fascia Orbital fascia Submandibular space **4** **Subcutaneous Tissue and Fascia, Right Neck** Deep cervical fascia Pretracheal fascia Prevertebral fascia **5** **Subcutaneous Tissue and Fascia, Left Neck** *See 4 Subcutaneous Tissue and Fascia, Right Neck* **6** **Subcutaneous Tissue and Fascia, Chest** Pectoral fascia **7** **Subcutaneous Tissue and Fascia, Back** **8** **Subcutaneous Tissue and Fascia, Abdomen** **9** **Subcutaneous Tissue and Fascia, Buttock** **B** **Subcutaneous Tissue and Fascia, Perineum** **C** **Subcutaneous Tissue and Fascia, Pelvic Region** **D** **Subcutaneous Tissue and Fascia, Right Upper Arm** Axillary fascia Deltoid fascia Infraspinatus fascia Subscapular aponeurosis Supraspinatus fascia **F** **Subcutaneous Tissue and Fascia, Left Upper Arm** *See D Subcutaneous Tissue and Fascia, Right Upper Arm*	**G** **Subcutaneous Tissue and Fascia, Right Lower Arm** Antebrachial fascia Bicipital aponeurosis **H** **Subcutaneous Tissue and Fascia, Left Lower Arm** *See G Subcutaneous Tissue and Fascia, Right Lower Arm* **J** **Subcutaneous Tissue and Fascia, Right Hand** Palmar fascia (aponeurosis) **K** **Subcutaneous Tissue and Fascia, Left Hand** *See J Subcutaneous Tissue and Fascia, Right Hand* **L** **Subcutaneous Tissue and Fascia, Right Upper Leg** Crural fascia Fascia lata Iliac fascia Iliotibial tract (band) **M** **Subcutaneous Tissue and Fascia, Left Upper Leg** *See L Subcutaneous Tissue and Fascia, Right Upper Leg* **N** **Subcutaneous Tissue and Fascia, Right Lower Leg** **P** **Subcutaneous Tissue and Fascia, Left Lower Leg** **Q** **Subcutaneous Tissue and Fascia, Right Foot** Plantar fascia (aponeurosis) **R** **Subcutaneous Tissue and Fascia, Left Foot** *See Q Subcutaneous Tissue and Fascia, Right Foot*	**Ø** Open **3** Percutaneous	**Z** No Device	**B** Skin and Subcutaneous Tissue **C** Skin, Subcutaneous Tissue and Fascia **Z** No Qualifier

Muscles 0K2–0KX

Character Meanings

This Character Meaning table is provided as a guide to assist the user in the identification of character members that may be found in this section of code tables. It **SHOULD NOT** be used to build a PCS code.

Operation–Character 3	Body Part–Character 4	Approach–Character 5	Device–Character 6	Qualifier–Character 7
2 Change	0 Head Muscle	0 Open	0 Drainage Device	0 Skin
5 Destruction	1 Facial Muscle	3 Percutaneous	7 Autologous Tissue Substitute	1 Subcutaneous Tissue
8 Division	2 Neck Muscle, Right	4 Percutaneous Endoscopic	J Synthetic Substitute	2 Skin and Subcutaneous Tissue
9 Drainage	3 Neck Muscle, Left	7 Via Natural or Artificial Opening	K Nonautologous Tissue Substitute	5 Latissimus Dorsi Myocutaneous Flap
B Excision	4 Tongue, Palate, Pharynx Muscle	8 Via Natural or Artificial Opening Endoscopic	M Stimulator Lead	6 Transverse Rectus Abdominis Myocutaneous Flap
C Extirpation	5 Shoulder Muscle, Right	X External	Y Other Device	7 Deep Inferior Epigastric Artery Perforator Flap
D Extraction	6 Shoulder Muscle, Left		Z No Device	8 Superficial Inferior Epigastric Artery Flap
H Insertion	7 Upper Arm Muscle, Right			9 Gluteal Artery Perforator Flap
J Inspection	8 Upper Arm Muscle, Left			X Diagnostic
M Reattachment	9 Lower Arm and Wrist Muscle, Right			Z No Qualifier
N Release	B Lower Arm and Wrist Muscle, Left			
P Removal	C Hand Muscle, Right			
Q Repair	D Hand Muscle, Left			
R Replacement	F Trunk Muscle, Right			
S Reposition	G Trunk Muscle, Left			
T Resection	H Thorax Muscle, Right			
U Supplement	J Thorax Muscle, Left			
W Revision	K Abdomen Muscle, Right			
X Transfer	L Abdomen Muscle, Left			
	M Perineum Muscle			
	N Hip Muscle, Right			
	P Hip Muscle, Left			
	Q Upper Leg Muscle, Right			
	R Upper Leg Muscle, Left			
	S Lower Leg Muscle, Right			
	T Lower Leg Muscle, Left			
	V Foot Muscle, Right			
	W Foot Muscle, Left			
	X Upper Muscle			
	Y Lower Muscle			

AHA Coding Clinic for table 0K8
2021, 4Q, 50   Endoscopic division of tongue, palate and pharynx muscle
2020, 2Q, 25   Endoscopic stapling of Zenker's diverticulum

AHA Coding Clinic for table 0KB
2020, 1Q, 27   Delayed reconstruction following mastectomy using gracilis musculocutaneous free flap
2016, 3Q, 20   Excisional debridement of sacrum
2015, 3Q, 3-8   Excisional and nonexcisional debridement

AHA Coding Clinic for table 0KD
2017, 4Q, 41-42   Extraction procedures

AHA Coding Clinic for table 0KH
2020, 4Q, 63   Intercompartmental pressure measurement

AHA Coding Clinic for table 0KN
2017, 2Q, 12   Compartment syndrome and fasciotomy of foot
2017, 2Q, 13   Compartment syndrome and fasciotomy of leg
2015, 2Q, 22   Arthroscopic subacromial decompression
2014, 4Q, 39   Abdominal component release with placement of mesh for hernia repair

AHA Coding Clinic for table 0KQ
2018, 2Q, 25   Third and fourth degree obstetric lacerations
2016, 2Q, 34   Assisted vaginal delivery
2016, 1Q, 7   Obstetrical perineal laceration repair
2014, 4Q, 43   Second degree obstetric perineal laceration
2013, 4Q, 120   Repair of second degree perineum obstetric laceration

AHA Coding Clinic for table 0KS
2017, 1Q, 41   Manual reduction of hernia

AHA Coding Clinic for table 0KT
2016, 2Q, 12   Resection of malignant neoplasm of infratemporal fossa
2015, 1Q, 38   Abdominoperineal resection with flap closure of the perineum and colostomy

AHA Coding Clinic for table 0KX
2018, 2Q, 18   Transverse rectus abdominis myocutaneous (TRAM) delay
2017, 4Q, 67   New qualifier values - Pedicle flap procedures
2016, 3Q, 30   Resection of femur with interposition arthroplasty
2015, 3Q, 33   Cleft lip repair using Millard rotation advancement
2015, 2Q, 26   Pharyngeal flap to soft palate
2014, 4Q, 41   Abdominoperineal resection (APR) with flap closure of perineum and colostomy
2014, 2Q, 10   Transverse abdominomyocutaneous (TRAM) breast reconstruction
2014, 2Q, 12   Pedicle latissimus myocutaneous flap with placement of breast tissue expanders

Muscles

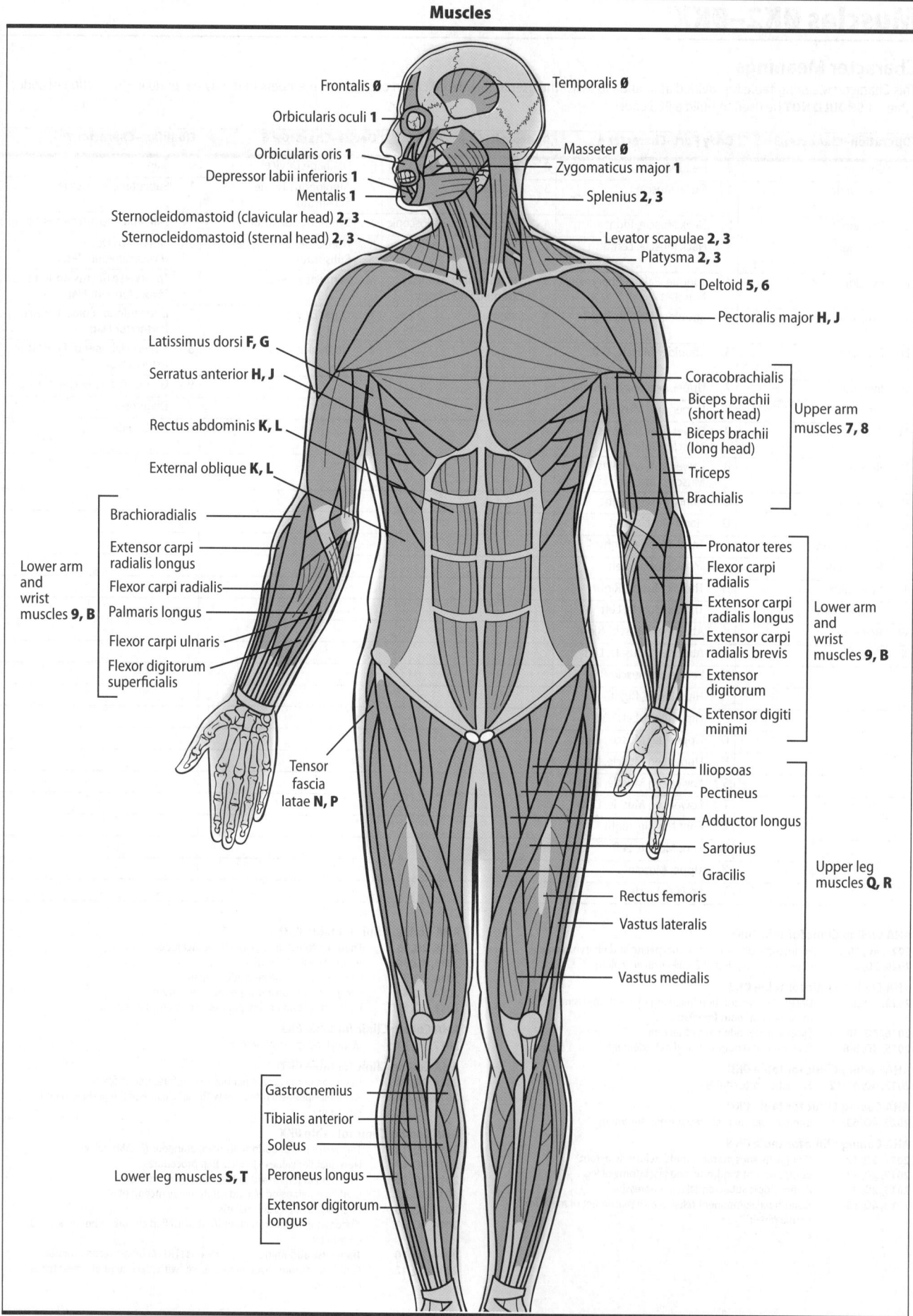

Frontalis **Ø**
Temporalis **Ø**
Orbicularis oculi **1**
Orbicularis oris **1**
Masseter **Ø**
Depressor labii inferioris **1**
Zygomaticus major **1**
Mentalis **1**
Splenius **2, 3**
Sternocleidomastoid (clavicular head) **2, 3**
Sternocleidomastoid (sternal head) **2, 3**
Levator scapulae **2, 3**
Platysma **2, 3**
Deltoid **5, 6**
Pectoralis major **H, J**
Latissimus dorsi **F, G**
Serratus anterior **H, J**
Coracobrachialis
Biceps brachii (short head)
Biceps brachii (long head)
Rectus abdominis **K, L**
Upper arm muscles **7, 8**
External oblique **K, L**
Triceps
Brachialis
Brachioradialis
Pronator teres
Extensor carpi radialis longus
Flexor carpi radialis
Flexor carpi radialis
Extensor carpi radialis longus
Palmaris longus
Extensor carpi radialis brevis
Lower arm and wrist muscles **9, B**
Flexor carpi ulnaris
Extensor digitorum
Flexor digitorum superficialis
Extensor digiti minimi
Lower arm and wrist muscles **9, B**
Iliopsoas
Pectineus
Adductor longus
Tensor fascia latae **N, P**
Sartorius
Gracilis
Rectus femoris
Upper leg muscles **Q, R**
Vastus lateralis
Vastus medialis
Gastrocnemius
Tibialis anterior
Soleus
Lower leg muscles **S, T**
Peroneus longus
Extensor digitorum longus

Ø   **Medical and Surgical**
K   **Muscles**
2   **Change**   Definition: Taking out or off a device from a body part and putting back an identical or similar device in or on the same body part without cutting or puncturing the skin or a mucous membrane

Explanation: All CHANGE procedures are coded using the approach EXTERNAL

Body Part Character 4	Approach Character 5	Device Character 6	Qualifier Character 7
X Upper Muscle **Y** Lower Muscle	**X** External	**Ø** Drainage Device **Y** Other Device	**Z** No Qualifier

Non-OR	All body part, approach, device, and qualifier values

Ø   **Medical and Surgical**
K   **Muscles**
5   **Destruction**   Definition: Physical eradication of all or a portion of a body part by the direct use of energy, force, or a destructive agent

Explanation: None of the body part is physically taken out

Body Part Character 4			Approach Character 5	Device Character 6	Qualifier Character 7

Ø **Head Muscle**
   Auricularis muscle
   Masseter muscle
   Pterygoid muscle
   Splenius capitis muscle
   Temporalis muscle
   Temporoparietalis muscle
1 **Facial Muscle**
   Buccinator muscle
   Corrugator supercilii muscle
   Depressor anguli oris muscle
   Depressor labii inferioris muscle
   Depressor septi nasi muscle
   Depressor supercilii muscle
   Levator anguli oris muscle
   Levator labii superioris alaeque
     nasi muscle
   Levator labii superioris muscle
   Mentalis muscle
   Nasalis muscle
   Occipitofrontalis muscle
   Orbicularis oris muscle
   Procerus muscle
   Risorius muscle
   Zygomaticus muscle
2 **Neck Muscle, Right**
   Anterior vertebral muscle
   Arytenoid muscle
   Cricothyroid muscle
   Infrahyoid muscle
   Levator scapulae muscle
   Platysma muscle
   Scalene muscle
   Splenius cervicis muscle
   Sternocleidomastoid muscle
   Suprahyoid muscle
   Thyroarytenoid muscle
3 **Neck Muscle, Left**
   See 2 Neck Muscle, Right
4 **Tongue, Palate, Pharynx**
   Muscle
   Chondroglossus muscle
   Genioglossus muscle
   Hyoglossus muscle
   Inferior longitudinal muscle
   Levator veli palatini muscle
   Palatoglossal muscle
   Palatopharyngeal muscle
   Pharyngeal constrictor muscle
   Salpingopharyngeus muscle
   Styloglossus muscle
   Stylopharyngeus muscle
   Superior longitudinal muscle
   Tensor veli palatini muscle
5 **Shoulder Muscle, Right**
   Deltoid muscle
   Infraspinatus muscle
   Subscapularis muscle
   Supraspinatus muscle
   Teres major muscle
   Teres minor muscle
6 **Shoulder Muscle, Left**
   See 5 Shoulder Muscle, Right
	7 **Upper Arm Muscle, Right**
	   Biceps brachii muscle
	   Brachialis muscle
	   Coracobrachialis muscle
	   Triceps brachii muscle
	8 **Upper Arm Muscle, Left**
	   See 7 Upper Arm Muscle, Right
	9 **Lower Arm and Wrist Muscle,**
	   Right
	   Anatomical snuffbox
	   Brachioradialis muscle
	   Extensor carpi radialis muscle
	   Extensor carpi ulnaris muscle
	   Flexor carpi radialis muscle
	   Flexor carpi ulnaris muscle
	   Flexor pollicis longus muscle
	   Palmaris longus muscle
	   Pronator quadratus muscle
	   Pronator teres muscle
	B **Lower Arm and Wrist Muscle,**
	   Left
	   See 9 Lower Arm and Wrist
	     Muscle, Right
	C **Hand Muscle, Right**
	   Hypothenar muscle
	   Palmar interosseous muscle
	   Thenar muscle
	D **Hand Muscle, Left**
	   See C Hand Muscle, Right
	F **Trunk Muscle, Right**
	   Coccygeus muscle
	   Erector spinae muscle
	   Interspinalis muscle
	   Intertransversarius muscle
	   Latissimus dorsi muscle
	   Quadratus lumborum muscle
	   Rhomboid major muscle
	   Rhomboid minor muscle
	   Serratus posterior muscle
	   Transversospinalis muscle
	   Trapezius muscle
	G **Trunk Muscle, Left**
	   See F Trunk Muscle, Right
	H **Thorax Muscle, Right**
	   Intercostal muscle
	   Levatores costarum muscle
	   Pectoralis major muscle
	   Pectoralis minor muscle
	   Serratus anterior muscle
	   Subclavius muscle
	   Subcostal muscle
	   Transverse thoracis muscle
	J **Thorax Muscle, Left**
	   See H Thorax Muscle, Right
	K **Abdomen Muscle, Right**
	   External oblique muscle
	   Internal oblique muscle
	   Pyramidalis muscle
	   Rectus abdominis muscle
	   Transversus abdominis muscle
	L **Abdomen Muscle, Left**
	   See K Abdomen Muscle, Right
		M **Perineum Muscle**
		   Bulbospongiosus muscle
		   Cremaster muscle
		   Deep transverse perineal muscle
		   Ischiocavernosus muscle
		   Levator ani muscle
		   Superficial transverse perineal
		     muscle
		N **Hip Muscle, Right**
		   Gemellus muscle
		   Gluteus maximus muscle
		   Gluteus medius muscle
		   Gluteus minimus muscle
		   Iliacus muscle
		   Obturator muscle
		   Piriformis muscle
		   Psoas muscle
		   Quadratus femoris muscle
		   Tensor fasciae latae muscle
		P **Hip Muscle, Left**
		   See N Hip Muscle, Right
		Q **Upper Leg Muscle, Right**
		   Adductor brevis muscle
		   Adductor longus muscle
		   Adductor magnus muscle
		   Biceps femoris muscle
		   Gracilis muscle
		   Pectineus muscle
		   Quadriceps (femoris)
		   Rectus femoris muscle
		   Sartorius muscle
		   Semimembranosus muscle
		   Semitendinosus muscle
		   Vastus intermedius muscle
		   Vastus lateralis muscle
		   Vastus medialis muscle
		R **Upper Leg Muscle, Left**
		   See Q Upper Leg Muscle, Right
		S **Lower Leg Muscle, Right**
		   Extensor digitorum longus muscle
		   Extensor hallucis longus muscle
		   Fibularis brevis muscle
		   Fibularis longus muscle
		   Flexor digitorum longus muscle
		   Flexor hallucis longus muscle
		   Gastrocnemius muscle
		   Peroneus brevis muscle
		   Peroneus longus muscle
		   Popliteus muscle
		   Soleus muscle
		   Tibialis anterior muscle
		   Tibialis posterior muscle
		T **Lower Leg Muscle, Left**
		   See S Lower Leg Muscle, Right
		V **Foot Muscle, Right**
		   Abductor hallucis muscle
		   Adductor hallucis muscle
		   Extensor digitorum brevis muscle
		   Extensor hallucis brevis muscle
		   Flexor digitorum brevis muscle
		   Flexor hallucis brevis muscle
		   Quadratus plantae muscle
		W **Foot Muscle, Left**
		   See V Foot Muscle, Right
			Ø Open
			3 Percutaneous
			4 Percutaneous
			   Endoscopic
				Z No Device	**Z** No Qualifier

NC Noncovered Procedure   LC Limited Coverage   QA Questionable OB Admit   NT New Tech Add-on   ⊞ Combination Member   ♂ Male   ♀ Female

ICD-10-PCS 2023   465

ØK2–ØK5

Ø   **Medical and Surgical**
K   **Muscles**
8   **Division**   Definition: Cutting into a body part, without draining fluids and/or gases from the body part, in order to separate or transect a body part
                   Explanation: All or a portion of the body part is separated into two or more portions

Body Part — Character 4			Approach — Character 5	Device — Character 6	Qualifier — Character 7
Ø Head Muscle Auricularis muscle Masseter muscle Pterygoid muscle Splenius capitis muscle Temporalis muscle Temporoparietalis muscle **1 Facial Muscle** Buccinator muscle Corrugator supercilii muscle Depressor anguli oris muscle Depressor labii inferioris muscle Depressor septi nasi muscle Depressor supercilii muscle Levator anguli oris muscle Levator labii superioris alaeque nasi muscle Levator labii superioris muscle Mentalis muscle Nasalis muscle Occipitofrontalis muscle Orbicularis oris muscle Procerus muscle Risorius muscle Zygomaticus muscle **2 Neck Muscle, Right** Anterior vertebral muscle Arytenoid muscle Cricothyroid muscle Infrahyoid muscle Levator scapulae muscle Platysma muscle Scalene muscle Splenius cervicis muscle Sternocleidomastoid muscle Suprahyoid muscle Thyroarytenoid muscle **3 Neck Muscle, Left** *See 2 Neck Muscle, Right* Tensor veli palatini muscle **5 Shoulder Muscle, Right** Deltoid muscle Infraspinatus muscle Subscapularis muscle Supraspinatus muscle Teres major muscle Teres minor muscle **6 Shoulder Muscle, Left** *See 5 Shoulder Muscle, Right* **7 Upper Arm Muscle, Right** Biceps brachii muscle Brachialis muscle Coracobrachialis muscle Triceps brachii muscle **8 Upper Arm Muscle, Left** *See 7 Upper Arm Muscle, Right*	**9 Lower Arm and Wrist Muscle, Right** Anatomical snuffbox Brachioradialis muscle Extensor carpi radialis muscle Extensor carpi ulnaris muscle Flexor carpi radialis muscle Flexor carpi ulnaris muscle Flexor pollicis longus muscle Palmaris longus muscle Pronator quadratus muscle Pronator teres muscle **B Lower Arm and Wrist Muscle, Left** *See 9 Lower Arm and Wrist Muscle, Right* **C Hand Muscle, Right** Hypothenar muscle Palmar interosseous muscle Thenar muscle **D Hand Muscle, Left** *See C Hand Muscle, Right* **F Trunk Muscle, Right** Coccygeus muscle Erector spinae muscle Interspinalis muscle Intertransversarius muscle Latissimus dorsi muscle Quadratus lumborum muscle Rhomboid major muscle Rhomboid minor muscle Serratus posterior muscle Transversospinalis muscle Trapezius muscle **G Trunk Muscle, Left** *See F Trunk Muscle, Right* **H Thorax Muscle, Right** Intercostal muscle Levatores costarum muscle Pectoralis major muscle Pectoralis minor muscle Serratus anterior muscle Subclavius muscle Subcostal muscle Transverse thoracis muscle **J Thorax Muscle, Left** *See H Thorax Muscle, Right* **K Abdomen Muscle, Right** External oblique muscle Internal oblique muscle Pyramidalis muscle Rectus abdominis muscle Transversus abdominis muscle **L Abdomen Muscle, Left** *See K Abdomen Muscle, Right* **M Perineum Muscle** Bulbospongiosus muscle Cremaster muscle Deep transverse perineal muscle Ischiocavernosus muscle Levator ani muscle Superficial transverse perineal muscle	**N Hip Muscle, Right** Gemellus muscle Gluteus maximus muscle Gluteus medius muscle Gluteus minimus muscle Iliacus muscle Obturator muscle Piriformis muscle Psoas muscle Quadratus femoris muscle Tensor fasciae latae muscle **P Hip Muscle, Left** *See N Hip Muscle, Right* **Q Upper Leg Muscle, Right** Adductor brevis muscle Adductor longus muscle Adductor magnus muscle Biceps femoris muscle Gracilis muscle Pectineus muscle Quadriceps (femoris) Rectus femoris muscle Sartorius muscle Semimembranosus muscle Semitendinosus muscle Vastus intermedius muscle Vastus lateralis muscle Vastus medialis muscle **R Upper Leg Muscle, Left** *See Q Upper Leg Muscle, Right* **S Lower Leg Muscle, Right** Extensor digitorum longus muscle Extensor hallucis longus muscle Fibularis brevis muscle Fibularis longus muscle Flexor digitorum longus muscle Flexor hallucis longus muscle Gastrocnemius muscle Peroneus brevis muscle Peroneus longus muscle Popliteus muscle Soleus muscle Tibialis anterior muscle Tibialis posterior muscle **T Lower Leg Muscle, Left** *See S Lower Leg Muscle, Right* **V Foot Muscle, Right** Abductor hallucis muscle Adductor hallucis muscle Extensor digitorum brevis muscle Extensor hallucis brevis muscle Flexor digitorum brevis muscle Flexor hallucis brevis muscle Quadratus plantae muscle **W Foot Muscle, Left** *See V Foot Muscle, Right*	**Ø** Open **3** Percutaneous **4** Percutaneous Endoscopic	**Z** No Device	**Z** No Qualifier
4 Tongue, Palate, Pharynx Muscle Chondroglossus muscle Genioglossus muscle Hyoglossus muscle Inferior longitudinal muscle Levator veli palatini muscle Palatoglossal muscle Palatopharyngeal muscle Pharyngeal constrictor muscle Salpingopharyngeus muscle Styloglossus muscle Stylopharyngeus muscle Superior longitudinal muscle Tensor veli palatini muscle			**Ø** Open **3** Percutaneous **4** Percutaneous Endoscopic **7** Via Natural or Artificial Opening **8** Via Natural or Artificial Opening Endoscopic	**Z** No Device	**Z** No Qualifier

Non-OR Procedure   DRG Non-OR Procedure   Valid OR Procedure   HAC Associated Procedure   Combination Only   New/Revised April   New/Revised October

466   ICD-10-PCS 2023

ØK8–ØK8

Ø   **Medical and Surgical**
K   **Muscles**
9   **Drainage**   Definition: Taking or letting out fluids and/or gases from a body part
                   Explanation: The qualifier DIAGNOSTIC is used to identify drainage procedures that are biopsies

Body Part Character 4			Approach Character 5	Device Character 6	Qualifier Character 7
Ø Head Muscle Auricularis muscle Masseter muscle Pterygoid muscle Splenius capitis muscle Temporalis muscle Temporoparietalis muscle **1 Facial Muscle** Buccinator muscle Corrugator supercilii muscle Depressor anguli oris muscle Depressor labii inferioris muscle Depressor septi nasi muscle Depressor supercilii muscle Levator anguli oris muscle Levator labii superioris alaeque nasi muscle Levator labii superioris muscle Mentalis muscle Nasalis muscle Occipitofrontalis muscle Orbicularis oris muscle Procerus muscle Risorius muscle Zygomaticus muscle **2 Neck Muscle, Right** Anterior vertebral muscle Arytenoid muscle Cricothyroid muscle Infrahyoid muscle Levator scapulae muscle Platysma muscle Scalene muscle Splenius cervicis muscle Sternocleidomastoid muscle Suprahyoid muscle Thyroarytenoid muscle **3 Neck Muscle, Left** *See 2 Neck Muscle, Right* **4 Tongue, Palate, Pharynx Muscle** Chondroglossus muscle Genioglossus muscle Hyoglossus muscle Inferior longitudinal muscle Levator veli palatini muscle Palatoglossal muscle Palatopharyngeal muscle Pharyngeal constrictor muscle Salpingopharyngeus muscle Styloglossus muscle Stylopharyngeus muscle Superior longitudinal muscle Tensor veli palatini muscle **5 Shoulder Muscle, Right** Deltoid muscle Infraspinatus muscle Subscapularis muscle Supraspinatus muscle Teres major muscle Teres minor muscle **6 Shoulder Muscle, Left** *See 5 Shoulder Muscle, Right*	**7 Upper Arm Muscle, Right** Biceps brachii muscle Brachialis muscle Coracobrachialis muscle Triceps brachii muscle **8 Upper Arm Muscle, Left** *See 7 Upper Arm Muscle, Right* **9 Lower Arm and Wrist Muscle, Right** Anatomical snuffbox Brachioradialis muscle Extensor carpi radialis muscle Extensor carpi ulnaris muscle Flexor carpi radialis muscle Flexor carpi ulnaris muscle Flexor pollicis longus muscle Palmaris longus muscle Pronator quadratus muscle Pronator teres muscle **B Lower Arm and Wrist Muscle, Left** *See 9 Lower Arm and Wrist Muscle, Right* **C Hand Muscle, Right** Hypothenar muscle Palmar interosseous muscle Thenar muscle **D Hand Muscle, Left** *See C Hand Muscle, Right* **F Trunk Muscle, Right** Coccygeus muscle Erector spinae muscle Interspinalis muscle Intertransversarius muscle Latissimus dorsi muscle Quadratus lumborum muscle Rhomboid major muscle Rhomboid minor muscle Serratus posterior muscle Transversospinalis muscle Trapezius muscle **G Trunk Muscle, Left** *See F Trunk Muscle, Right* **H Thorax Muscle, Right** Intercostal muscle Levatores costarum muscle Pectoralis major muscle Pectoralis minor muscle Serratus anterior muscle Subclavius muscle Subcostal muscle Transverse thoracis muscle **J Thorax Muscle, Left** *See H Thorax Muscle, Right* **K Abdomen Muscle, Right** External oblique muscle Internal oblique muscle Pyramidalis muscle Rectus abdominis muscle Transversus abdominis muscle **L Abdomen Muscle, Left** *See K Abdomen Muscle, Right*	**M Perineum Muscle** Bulbospongiosus muscle Cremaster muscle Deep transverse perineal muscle Ischiocavernosus muscle Levator ani muscle Superficial transverse perineal muscle **N Hip Muscle, Right** Gemellus muscle Gluteus maximus muscle Gluteus medius muscle Gluteus minimus muscle Iliacus muscle Obturator muscle Piriformis muscle Psoas muscle Quadratus femoris muscle Tensor fasciae latae muscle **P Hip Muscle, Left** *See N Hip Muscle, Right* **Q Upper Leg Muscle, Right** Adductor brevis muscle Adductor longus muscle Adductor magnus muscle Biceps femoris muscle Gracilis muscle Pectineus muscle Quadriceps (femoris) Rectus femoris muscle Sartorius muscle Semimembranosus muscle Semitendinosus muscle Vastus intermedius muscle Vastus lateralis muscle Vastus medialis muscle **R Upper Leg Muscle, Left** *See Q Upper Leg Muscle, Right* **S Lower Leg Muscle, Right** Extensor digitorum longus muscle Extensor hallucis longus muscle Fibularis brevis muscle Fibularis longus muscle Flexor digitorum longus muscle Flexor hallucis longus muscle Gastrocnemius muscle Peroneus brevis muscle Peroneus longus muscle Popliteus muscle Soleus muscle Tibialis anterior muscle Tibialis posterior muscle **T Lower Leg Muscle, Left** *See S Lower Leg Muscle, Right* **V Foot Muscle, Right** Abductor hallucis muscle Adductor hallucis muscle Extensor digitorum brevis muscle Extensor hallucis brevis muscle Flexor digitorum brevis muscle Flexor hallucis brevis muscle Quadratus plantae muscle **W Foot Muscle, Left** *See V Foot Muscle, Right*	**Ø Open** **3 Percutaneous** **4 Percutaneous Endoscopic**	**Ø Drainage Device**	**Z No Qualifier**

Non-OR   ØK9[Ø,1,2,3,4,5,6,7,8,9,B,C,D,F,G,H,J,K,L,M,N,P,Q,R,S,T,V,W]3ØZ

ØK9 Continued on next page

NC Noncovered Procedure   **LC** Limited Coverage   **QA** Questionable OB Admit   **NT** New Tech Add-on   ✛ Combination Member   ♂ Male   ♀ Female

Ø	**Medical and Surgical**
K	**Muscles**
9	**Drainage**

ØK9 Continued

Definition: Taking or letting out fluids and/or gases from a body part
Explanation: The qualifier DIAGNOSTIC is used to identify drainage procedures that are biopsies

Body Part Character 4			Approach Character 5	Device Character 6	Qualifier Character 7
Ø Head Muscle Auricularis muscle Masseter muscle Pterygoid muscle Splenius capitis muscle Temporalis muscle Temporoparietalis muscle **1 Facial Muscle** Buccinator muscle Corrugator supercilii muscle Depressor anguli oris muscle Depressor labii inferioris muscle Depressor septi nasi muscle Depressor supercilii muscle Levator anguli oris muscle Levator labii superioris alaeque nasi muscle Levator labii superioris muscle Mentalis muscle Nasalis muscle Occipitofrontalis muscle Orbicularis oris muscle Procerus muscle Risorius muscle Zygomaticus muscle **2 Neck Muscle, Right** Anterior vertebral muscle Arytenoid muscle Cricothyroid muscle Infrahyoid muscle Levator scapulae muscle Platysma muscle Scalene muscle Splenius cervicis muscle Sternocleidomastoid muscle Suprahyoid muscle Thyroarytenoid muscle **3 Neck Muscle, Left** *See 2 Neck Muscle, Right* **4 Tongue, Palate, Pharynx Muscle** Chondroglossus muscle Genioglossus muscle Hyoglossus muscle Inferior longitudinal muscle Levator veli palatini muscle Palatoglossal muscle Palatopharyngeal muscle Pharyngeal constrictor muscle Salpingopharyngeus muscle Styloglossus muscle Stylopharyngeus muscle Superior longitudinal muscle Tensor veli palatini muscle **5 Shoulder Muscle, Right** Deltoid muscle Infraspinatus muscle Subscapularis muscle Supraspinatus muscle Teres major muscle Teres minor muscle **6 Shoulder Muscle, Left** *See 5 Shoulder Muscle, Right*	**7 Upper Arm Muscle, Right** Biceps brachii muscle Brachialis muscle Coracobrachialis muscle Triceps brachii muscle **8 Upper Arm Muscle, Left** *See 7 Upper Arm Muscle, Right* **9 Lower Arm and Wrist Muscle, Right** Anatomical snuffbox Brachioradialis muscle Extensor carpi radialis muscle Extensor carpi ulnaris muscle Flexor carpi radialis muscle Flexor carpi ulnaris muscle Flexor pollicis longus muscle Palmaris longus muscle Pronator quadratus muscle Pronator teres muscle **B Lower Arm and Wrist Muscle, Left** *See 9 Lower Arm and Wrist Muscle, Right* **C Hand Muscle, Right** Hypothenar muscle Palmar interosseous muscle Thenar muscle **D Hand Muscle, Left** *See C Hand Muscle, Right* **F Trunk Muscle, Right** Coccygeus muscle Erector spinae muscle Interspinalis muscle Intertransversarius muscle Latissimus dorsi muscle Quadratus lumborum muscle Rhomboid major muscle Rhomboid minor muscle Serratus posterior muscle Transversospinalis muscle Trapezius muscle **G Trunk Muscle, Left** *See F Trunk Muscle, Right* **H Thorax Muscle, Right** Intercostal muscle Levatores costarum muscle Pectoralis major muscle Pectoralis minor muscle Serratus anterior muscle Subclavius muscle Subcostal muscle Transverse thoracis muscle **J Thorax Muscle, Left** *See H Thorax Muscle, Right* **K Abdomen Muscle, Right** External oblique muscle Internal oblique muscle Pyramidalis muscle Rectus abdominis muscle Transversus abdominis muscle **L Abdomen Muscle, Left** *See K Abdomen Muscle, Right*	**M Perineum Muscle** Bulbospongiosus muscle Cremaster muscle Deep transverse perineal muscle Ischiocavernosus muscle Levator ani muscle Superficial transverse perineal muscle **N Hip Muscle, Right** Gemellus muscle Gluteus maximus muscle Gluteus medius muscle Gluteus minimus muscle Iliacus muscle Obturator muscle Piriformis muscle Psoas muscle Quadratus femoris muscle Tensor fasciae latae muscle **P Hip Muscle, Left** *See N Hip Muscle, Right* **Q Upper Leg Muscle, Right** Adductor brevis muscle Adductor longus muscle Adductor magnus muscle Biceps femoris muscle Gracilis muscle Pectineus muscle Quadriceps (femoris) Rectus femoris muscle Sartorius muscle Semimembranosus muscle Semitendinosus muscle Vastus intermedius muscle Vastus lateralis muscle Vastus medialis muscle **R Upper Leg Muscle, Left** *See Q Upper Leg Muscle, Right* **S Lower Leg Muscle, Right** Extensor digitorum longus muscle Extensor hallucis longus muscle Fibularis brevis muscle Fibularis longus muscle Flexor digitorum longus muscle Flexor hallucis longus muscle Gastrocnemius muscle Peroneus brevis muscle Peroneus longus muscle Popliteus muscle Soleus muscle Tibialis anterior muscle Tibialis posterior muscle **T Lower Leg Muscle, Left** *See S Lower Leg Muscle, Right* **V Foot Muscle, Right** Abductor hallucis muscle Adductor hallucis muscle Extensor digitorum brevis muscle Extensor hallucis brevis muscle Flexor digitorum brevis muscle Flexor hallucis brevis muscle Quadratus plantae muscle **W Foot Muscle, Left** *See V Foot Muscle, Right*	**Ø** Open **3** Percutaneous **4** Percutaneous Endoscopic	**Z** No Device	**X** Diagnostic **Z** No Qualifier

Non-OR   ØK9[Ø,1,2,3,4,5,6,7,8,9,B,F,G,H,J,K,L,M,N,P,Q,R,S,T,V,W]3ZZ
Non-OR   ØK9[C,D][3,4]ZZ

Non-OR Procedure   DRG Non-OR Procedure   Valid OR Procedure   HAC Associated Procedure   Combination Only   New/Revised April   New/Revised October

468   ICD-10-PCS 2023

Ø	Medical and Surgical
K	Muscles
B	Excision

Definition: Cutting out or off, without replacement, a portion of a body part

Explanation: The qualifier DIAGNOSTIC is used to identify excision procedures that are biopsies

Body Part Character 4			Approach Character 5	Device Character 6	Qualifier Character 7
Ø Head Muscle Auricularis muscle Masseter muscle Pterygoid muscle Splenius capitis muscle Temporalis muscle Temporoparietalis muscle **1 Facial Muscle** Buccinator muscle Corrugator supercilii muscle Depressor anguli oris muscle Depressor labii inferioris muscle Depressor septi nasi muscle Depressor supercilii muscle Levator anguli oris muscle Levator labii superioris alaeque nasi muscle Levator labii superioris muscle Mentalis muscle Nasalis muscle Occipitofrontalis muscle Orbicularis oris muscle Procerus muscle Risorius muscle Zygomaticus muscle **2 Neck Muscle, Right** Anterior vertebral muscle Arytenoid muscle Cricothyroid muscle Infrahyoid muscle Levator scapulae muscle Platysma muscle Scalene muscle Splenius cervicis muscle Sternocleidomastoid muscle Suprahyoid muscle Thyroarytenoid muscle **3 Neck Muscle, Left** *See 2 Neck Muscle, Right* **4 Tongue, Palate, Pharynx Muscle** Chondroglossus muscle Genioglossus muscle Hyoglossus muscle Inferior longitudinal muscle Levator veli palatini muscle Palatoglossal muscle Palatopharyngeal muscle Pharyngeal constrictor muscle Salpingopharyngeus muscle Styloglossus muscle Stylopharyngeus muscle Superior longitudinal muscle Tensor veli palatini muscle **5 Shoulder Muscle, Right** Deltoid muscle Infraspinatus muscle Subscapularis muscle Supraspinatus muscle Teres major muscle Teres minor muscle **6 Shoulder Muscle, Left** *See 5 Shoulder Muscle, Right*	**7 Upper Arm Muscle, Right** Biceps brachii muscle Brachialis muscle Coracobrachialis muscle Triceps brachii muscle **8 Upper Arm Muscle, Left** *See 7 Upper Arm Muscle, Right* **9 Lower Arm and Wrist Muscle, Right** Anatomical snuffbox Brachioradialis muscle Extensor carpi radialis muscle Extensor carpi ulnaris muscle Flexor carpi radialis muscle Flexor carpi ulnaris muscle Flexor pollicis longus muscle Palmaris longus muscle Pronator quadratus muscle Pronator teres muscle **B Lower Arm and Wrist Muscle, Left** *See 9 Lower Arm and Wrist Muscle, Right* **C Hand Muscle, Right** Hypothenar muscle Palmar interosseous muscle Thenar muscle **D Hand Muscle, Left** *See C Hand Muscle, Right* **F Trunk Muscle, Right** Coccygeus muscle Erector spinae muscle Interspinalis muscle Intertransversarius muscle Latissimus dorsi muscle Quadratus lumborum muscle Rhomboid major muscle Rhomboid minor muscle Serratus posterior muscle Transversospinalis muscle Trapezius muscle **G Trunk Muscle, Left** *See F Trunk Muscle, Right* **H Thorax Muscle, Right** Intercostal muscle Levatores costarum muscle Pectoralis major muscle Pectoralis minor muscle Serratus anterior muscle Subclavius muscle Subcostal muscle Transverse thoracis muscle **J Thorax Muscle, Left** *See H Thorax Muscle, Right* **K Abdomen Muscle, Right** External oblique muscle Internal oblique muscle Pyramidalis muscle Rectus abdominis muscle Transversus abdominis muscle **L Abdomen Muscle, Left** *See K Abdomen Muscle, Right*	**M Perineum Muscle** Bulbospongiosus muscle Cremaster muscle Deep transverse perineal muscle Ischiocavernosus muscle Levator ani muscle Superficial transverse perineal muscle **N Hip Muscle, Right** Gemellus muscle Gluteus maximus muscle Gluteus medius muscle Gluteus minimus muscle Iliacus muscle Obturator muscle Piriformis muscle Psoas muscle Quadratus femoris muscle Tensor fasciae latae muscle **P Hip Muscle, Left** *See N Hip Muscle, Right* **Q Upper Leg Muscle, Right** Adductor brevis muscle Adductor longus muscle Adductor magnus muscle Biceps femoris muscle Gracilis muscle Pectineus muscle Quadriceps (femoris) Rectus femoris muscle Sartorius muscle Semimembranosus muscle Semitendinosus muscle Vastus intermedius muscle Vastus lateralis muscle Vastus medialis muscle **R Upper Leg Muscle, Left** *See Q Upper Leg Muscle, Right* **S Lower Leg Muscle, Right** Extensor digitorum longus muscle Extensor hallucis longus muscle Fibularis brevis muscle Fibularis longus muscle Flexor digitorum longus muscle Flexor hallucis longus muscle Gastrocnemius muscle Peroneus brevis muscle Peroneus longus muscle Popliteus muscle Soleus muscle Tibialis anterior muscle Tibialis posterior muscle **T Lower Leg Muscle, Left** *See S Lower Leg Muscle, Right* **V Foot Muscle, Right** Abductor hallucis muscle Adductor hallucis muscle Extensor digitorum brevis muscle Extensor hallucis brevis muscle Flexor digitorum brevis muscle Flexor hallucis brevis muscle Quadratus plantae muscle **W Foot Muscle, Left** *See V Foot Muscle, Right*	**Ø** Open **3** Percutaneous **4** Percutaneous Endoscopic	**Z** No Device	**X** Diagnostic **Z** No Qualifier

Non-OR   ØKB[N,P]3Z[X,Z]

NC Noncovered Procedure   **LC** Limited Coverage   **QA** Questionable OB Admit   **NT** New Tech Add-on   ⊞ Combination Member   ♂ Male   ♀ Female

ICD-10-PCS 2023   469

ØKB–ØKB

Ø	**Medical and Surgical**
K	**Muscles**
C	**Extirpation**

Definition: Taking or cutting out solid matter from a body part

Explanation: The solid matter may be an abnormal byproduct of a biological function or a foreign body; it may be imbedded in a body part or in the lumen of a tubular body part. The solid matter may or may not have been previously broken into pieces.

Body Part Character 4			Approach Character 5	Device Character 6	Qualifier Character 7
Ø Head Muscle Auricularis muscle Masseter muscle Pterygoid muscle Splenius capitis muscle Temporalis muscle Temporoparietalis muscle **1 Facial Muscle** Buccinator muscle Corrugator supercilii muscle Depressor anguli oris muscle Depressor labii inferioris muscle Depressor septi nasi muscle Depressor supercilii muscle Levator anguli oris muscle Levator labii superioris alaeque nasi muscle Levator labii superioris muscle Mentalis muscle Nasalis muscle Occipitofrontalis muscle Orbicularis oris muscle Procerus muscle Risorius muscle Zygomaticus muscle **2 Neck Muscle, Right** Anterior vertebral muscle Arytenoid muscle Cricothyroid muscle Infrahyoid muscle Levator scapulae muscle Platysma muscle Scalene muscle Splenius cervicis muscle Sternocleidomastoid muscle Suprahyoid muscle Thyroarytenoid muscle **3 Neck Muscle, Left** *See 2 Neck Muscle, Right* **4 Tongue, Palate, Pharynx Muscle** Chondroglossus muscle Genioglossus muscle Hyoglossus muscle Inferior longitudinal muscle Levator veli palatini muscle Palatoglossal muscle Palatopharyngeal muscle Pharyngeal constrictor muscle Salpingopharyngeus muscle Styloglossus muscle Stylopharyngeus muscle Superior longitudinal muscle Tensor veli palatini muscle **5 Shoulder Muscle, Right** Deltoid muscle Infraspinatus muscle Subscapularis muscle Supraspinatus muscle Teres major muscle Teres minor muscle **6 Shoulder Muscle, Left** *See 5 Shoulder Muscle, Right*	**7 Upper Arm Muscle, Right** Biceps brachii muscle Brachialis muscle Coracobrachialis muscle Triceps brachii muscle **8 Upper Arm Muscle, Left** *See 7 Upper Arm Muscle, Right* **9 Lower Arm and Wrist Muscle, Right** Anatomical snuffbox Brachioradialis muscle Extensor carpi radialis muscle Extensor carpi ulnaris muscle Flexor carpi radialis muscle Flexor carpi ulnaris muscle Flexor pollicis longus muscle Palmaris longus muscle Pronator quadratus muscle Pronator teres muscle **B Lower Arm and Wrist Muscle, Left** *See 9 Lower Arm and Wrist Muscle, Right* **C Hand Muscle, Right** Hypothenar muscle Palmar interosseous muscle Thenar muscle **D Hand Muscle, Left** *See C Hand Muscle, Right* **F Trunk Muscle, Right** Coccygeus muscle Erector spinae muscle Interspinalis muscle Intertransversarius muscle Latissimus dorsi muscle Quadratus lumborum muscle Rhomboid major muscle Rhomboid minor muscle Serratus posterior muscle Transversospinalis muscle Trapezius muscle **G Trunk Muscle, Left** *See F Trunk Muscle, Right* **H Thorax Muscle, Right** Intercostal muscle Levatores costarum muscle Pectoralis major muscle Pectoralis minor muscle Serratus anterior muscle Subclavius muscle Subcostal muscle Transverse thoracis muscle **J Thorax Muscle, Left** *See H Thorax Muscle, Right* **K Abdomen Muscle, Right** External oblique muscle Internal oblique muscle Pyramidalis muscle Rectus abdominis muscle Transversus abdominis muscle **L Abdomen Muscle, Left** *See K Abdomen Muscle, Right*	**M Perineum Muscle** Bulbospongiosus muscle Cremaster muscle Deep transverse perineal muscle Ischiocavernosus muscle Levator ani muscle Superficial transverse perineal muscle **N Hip Muscle, Right** Gemellus muscle Gluteus maximus muscle Gluteus medius muscle Gluteus minimus muscle Iliacus muscle Obturator muscle Piriformis muscle Psoas muscle Quadratus femoris muscle Tensor fasciae latae muscle **P Hip Muscle, Left** *See N Hip Muscle, Right* **Q Upper Leg Muscle, Right** Adductor brevis muscle Adductor longus muscle Adductor magnus muscle Biceps femoris muscle Gracilis muscle Pectineus muscle Quadriceps (femoris) Rectus femoris muscle Sartorius muscle Semimembranosus muscle Semitendinosus muscle Vastus intermedius muscle Vastus lateralis muscle Vastus medialis muscle **R Upper Leg Muscle, Left** *See Q Upper Leg Muscle, Right* **S Lower Leg Muscle, Right** Extensor digitorum longus muscle Extensor hallucis longus muscle Fibularis brevis muscle Fibularis longus muscle Flexor digitorum longus muscle Flexor hallucis longus muscle Gastrocnemius muscle Peroneus brevis muscle Peroneus longus muscle Popliteus muscle Soleus muscle Tibialis anterior muscle Tibialis posterior muscle **T Lower Leg Muscle, Left** *See S Lower Leg Muscle, Right* **V Foot Muscle, Right** Abductor hallucis muscle Adductor hallucis muscle Extensor digitorum brevis muscle Extensor hallucis brevis muscle Flexor digitorum brevis muscle Flexor hallucis brevis muscle Quadratus plantae muscle **W Foot Muscle, Left** *See V Foot Muscle, Right*	**Ø Open** **3 Percutaneous** **4 Percutaneous Endoscopic**	**Z No Device**	**Z No Qualifier**

Non-OR Procedure   DRG Non-OR Procedure   Valid OR Procedure   HAC Associated Procedure   Combination Only   New/Revised April   New/Revised October

470

ØKC–ØKC

ICD-10-PCS 2023

Ø Medical and Surgical
K Muscles
D Extraction

Definition: Pulling or stripping out or off all or a portion of a body part by the use of force
Explanation: The qualifier DIAGNOSTIC is used to identify extraction procedures that are biopsies

Body Part Character 4			Approach Character 5	Device Character 6	Qualifier Character 7
0 Head Muscle Auricularis muscle Masseter muscle Pterygoid muscle Splenius capitis muscle Temporalis muscle Temporoparietalis muscle **1 Facial Muscle** Buccinator muscle Corrugator supercilii muscle Depressor anguli oris muscle Depressor labii inferioris muscle Depressor septi nasi muscle Depressor supercilii muscle Levator anguli oris muscle Levator labii superioris alaeque nasi muscle Levator labii superioris muscle Mentalis muscle Nasalis muscle Occipitofrontalis muscle Orbicularis oris muscle Procerus muscle Risorius muscle Zygomaticus muscle **2 Neck Muscle, Right** Anterior vertebral muscle Arytenoid muscle Cricothyroid muscle Infrahyoid muscle Levator scapulae muscle Platysma muscle Scalene muscle Splenius cervicis muscle Sternocleidomastoid muscle Suprahyoid muscle Thyroarytenoid muscle **3 Neck Muscle, Left** *See 2 Neck Muscle, Right* **4 Tongue, Palate, Pharynx Muscle** Chondroglossus muscle Genioglossus muscle Hyoglossus muscle Inferior longitudinal muscle Levator veli palatini muscle Palatoglossal muscle Palatopharyngeal muscle Pharyngeal constrictor muscle Salpingopharyngeus muscle Styloglossus muscle Stylopharyngeus muscle Superior longitudinal muscle Tensor veli palatini muscle **5 Shoulder Muscle, Right** Deltoid muscle Infraspinatus muscle Subscapularis muscle Supraspinatus muscle Teres major muscle Teres minor muscle **6 Shoulder Muscle, Left** *See 5 Shoulder Muscle, Right*	**7 Upper Arm Muscle, Right** Biceps brachii muscle Brachialis muscle Coracobrachialis muscle Triceps brachii muscle **8 Upper Arm Muscle, Left** *See 7 Upper Arm Muscle, Right* **9 Lower Arm and Wrist Muscle, Right** Anatomical snuffbox Brachioradialis muscle Extensor carpi radialis muscle Extensor carpi ulnaris muscle Flexor carpi radialis muscle Flexor carpi ulnaris muscle Flexor pollicis longus muscle Palmaris longus muscle Pronator quadratus muscle Pronator teres muscle **B Lower Arm and Wrist Muscle, Left** *See 9 Lower Arm and Wrist Muscle, Right* **C Hand Muscle, Right** Hypothenar muscle Palmar interosseous muscle Thenar muscle **D Hand Muscle, Left** *See C Hand Muscle, Right* **F Trunk Muscle, Right** Coccygeus muscle Erector spinae muscle Interspinalis muscle Intertransversarius muscle Latissimus dorsi muscle Quadratus lumborum muscle Rhomboid major muscle Rhomboid minor muscle Serratus posterior muscle Transversospinalis muscle Trapezius muscle **G Trunk Muscle, Left** *See F Trunk Muscle, Right* **H Thorax Muscle, Right** Intercostal muscle Levatores costarum muscle Pectoralis major muscle Pectoralis minor muscle Serratus anterior muscle Subclavius muscle Subcostal muscle Transverse thoracis muscle **J Thorax Muscle, Left** *See H Thorax Muscle, Right* **K Abdomen Muscle, Right** External oblique muscle Internal oblique muscle Pyramidalis muscle Rectus abdominis muscle Transversus abdominis muscle **L Abdomen Muscle, Left** *See K Abdomen Muscle, Right*	**M Perineum Muscle** Bulbospongiosus muscle Cremaster muscle Deep transverse perineal muscle Ischiocavernosus muscle Levator ani muscle Superficial transverse perineal muscle **N Hip Muscle, Right** Gemellus muscle Gluteus maximus muscle Gluteus medius muscle Gluteus minimus muscle Iliacus muscle Obturator muscle Piriformis muscle Psoas muscle Quadratus femoris muscle Tensor fasciae latae muscle **P Hip Muscle, Left** *See N Hip Muscle, Right* **Q Upper Leg Muscle, Right** Adductor brevis muscle Adductor longus muscle Adductor magnus muscle Biceps femoris muscle Gracilis muscle Pectineus muscle Quadriceps (femoris) Rectus femoris muscle Sartorius muscle Semimembranosus muscle Semitendinosus muscle Vastus intermedius muscle Vastus lateralis muscle Vastus medialis muscle **R Upper Leg Muscle, Left** *See Q Upper Leg Muscle, Right* **S Lower Leg Muscle, Right** Extensor digitorum longus muscle Extensor hallucis longus muscle Fibularis brevis muscle Fibularis longus muscle Flexor digitorum longus muscle Flexor hallucis longus muscle Gastrocnemius muscle Peroneus brevis muscle Peroneus longus muscle Popliteus muscle Soleus muscle Tibialis anterior muscle Tibialis posterior muscle **T Lower Leg Muscle, Left** *See S Lower Leg Muscle, Right* **V Foot Muscle, Right** Abductor hallucis muscle Adductor hallucis muscle Extensor digitorum brevis muscle Extensor hallucis brevis muscle Flexor digitorum brevis muscle Flexor hallucis brevis muscle Quadratus plantae muscle **W Foot Muscle, Left** *See V Foot Muscle, Right*	**0 Open**	**Z No Device**	**Z No Qualifier**

NC Noncovered Procedure   LC Limited Coverage   QA Questionable OB Admit   NT New Tech Add-on   ⊞ Combination Member   ♂ Male   ♀ Female

ICD-10-PCS 2023   471

ØKD–ØKD

Ø **Medical and Surgical**
K **Muscles**
H **Insertion**   Definition: Putting in a nonbiological appliance that monitors, assists, performs, or prevents a physiological function but does not physically take the place of a body part
Explanation: None

Body Part Character 4	Approach Character 5	Device Character 6	Qualifier Character 7
X Upper Muscle **Y** Lower Muscle	**Ø** Open **3** Percutaneous **4** Percutaneous Endoscopic	**M** Stimulator Lead **Y** Other Device	**Z** No Qualifier

Non-OR   ØKH[X,Y][3,4]YZ

Ø **Medical and Surgical**
K **Muscles**
J **Inspection**   Definition: Visually and/or manually exploring a body part
Explanation: Visual exploration may be performed with or without optical instrumentation. Manual exploration may be performed directly or through intervening body layers.

Body Part Character 4	Approach Character 5	Device Character 6	Qualifier Character 7
X Upper Muscle **Y** Lower Muscle	**Ø** Open **3** Percutaneous **4** Percutaneous Endoscopic **X** External	**Z** No Device	**Z** No Qualifier

Non-OR   ØKJ[X,Y][3,X]ZZ

Non-OR Procedure   DRG Non-OR Procedure   Valid OR Procedure   HAC Associated Procedure   Combination Only   New/Revised April   New/Revised October

472

ICD-10-PCS 2023

Ø   **Medical and Surgical**
K   **Muscles**
M   **Reattachment**   Definition: Putting back in or on all or a portion of a separated body part to its normal location or other suitable location

Explanation: Vascular circulation and nervous pathways may or may not be reestablished

Body Part Character 4			Approach Character 5	Device Character 6	Qualifier Character 7
Ø Head Muscle Auricularis muscle Masseter muscle Pterygoid muscle Splenius capitis muscle Temporalis muscle Temporoparietalis muscle **1 Facial Muscle** Buccinator muscle Corrugator supercilii muscle Depressor anguli oris muscle Depressor labii inferioris muscle Depressor septi nasi muscle Depressor supercilii muscle Levator anguli oris muscle Levator labii superioris alaeque nasi muscle Levator labii superioris muscle Mentalis muscle Nasalis muscle Occipitofrontalis muscle Orbicularis oris muscle Procerus muscle Risorius muscle Zygomaticus muscle **2 Neck Muscle, Right** Anterior vertebral muscle Arytenoid muscle Cricothyroid muscle Infrahyoid muscle Levator scapulae muscle Platysma muscle Scalene muscle Splenius cervicis muscle Sternocleidomastoid muscle Suprahyoid muscle Thyroarytenoid muscle **3 Neck Muscle, Left** *See 2 Neck Muscle, Right* **4 Tongue, Palate, Pharynx Muscle** Chondroglossus muscle Genioglossus muscle Hyoglossus muscle Inferior longitudinal muscle Levator veli palatini muscle Palatoglossal muscle Palatopharyngeal muscle Pharyngeal constrictor muscle Salpingopharyngeus muscle Styloglossus muscle Stylopharyngeus muscle Superior longitudinal muscle Tensor veli palatini muscle **5 Shoulder Muscle, Right** Deltoid muscle Infraspinatus muscle Subscapularis muscle Supraspinatus muscle Teres major muscle Teres minor muscle **6 Shoulder Muscle, Left** *See 5 Shoulder Muscle, Right*	**7 Upper Arm Muscle, Right** Biceps brachii muscle Brachialis muscle Coracobrachialis muscle Triceps brachii muscle **8 Upper Arm Muscle, Left** *See 7 Upper Arm Muscle, Right* **9 Lower Arm and Wrist Muscle, Right** Anatomical snuffbox Brachioradialis muscle Extensor carpi radialis muscle Extensor carpi ulnaris muscle Flexor carpi radialis muscle Flexor carpi ulnaris muscle Flexor pollicis longus muscle Palmaris longus muscle Pronator quadratus muscle Pronator teres muscle **B Lower Arm and Wrist Muscle, Left** *See 9 Lower Arm and Wrist Muscle, Right* **C Hand Muscle, Right** Hypothenar muscle Palmar interosseous muscle Thenar muscle **D Hand Muscle, Left** *See C Hand Muscle, Right* **F Trunk Muscle, Right** Coccygeus muscle Erector spinae muscle Interspinalis muscle Intertransversarius muscle Latissimus dorsi muscle Quadratus lumborum muscle Rhomboid major muscle Rhomboid minor muscle Serratus posterior muscle Transversospinalis muscle Trapezius muscle **G Trunk Muscle, Left** *See F Trunk Muscle, Right* **H Thorax Muscle, Right** Intercostal muscle Levatores costarum muscle Pectoralis major muscle Pectoralis minor muscle Serratus anterior muscle Subclavius muscle Subcostal muscle Transverse thoracis muscle **J Thorax Muscle, Left** *See H Thorax Muscle, Right* **K Abdomen Muscle, Right** External oblique muscle Internal oblique muscle Pyramidalis muscle Rectus abdominis muscle Transversus abdominis muscle **L Abdomen Muscle, Left** *See K Abdomen Muscle, Right*	**M Perineum Muscle** Bulbospongiosus muscle Cremaster muscle Deep transverse perineal muscle Ischiocavernosus muscle Levator ani muscle Superficial transverse perineal muscle **N Hip Muscle, Right** Gemellus muscle Gluteus maximus muscle Gluteus medius muscle Gluteus minimus muscle Iliacus muscle Obturator muscle Piriformis muscle Psoas muscle Quadratus femoris muscle Tensor fasciae latae muscle **P Hip Muscle, Left** *See N Hip Muscle, Right* **Q Upper Leg Muscle, Right** Adductor brevis muscle Adductor longus muscle Adductor magnus muscle Biceps femoris muscle Gracilis muscle Pectineus muscle Quadriceps (femoris) Rectus femoris muscle Sartorius muscle Semimembranosus muscle Semitendinosus muscle Vastus intermedius muscle Vastus lateralis muscle Vastus medialis muscle **R Upper Leg Muscle, Left** *See Q Upper Leg Muscle, Right* **S Lower Leg Muscle, Right** Extensor digitorum longus muscle Extensor hallucis longus muscle Fibularis brevis muscle Fibularis longus muscle Flexor digitorum longus muscle Flexor hallucis longus muscle Gastrocnemius muscle Peroneus brevis muscle Peroneus longus muscle Popliteus muscle Soleus muscle Tibialis anterior muscle Tibialis posterior muscle **T Lower Leg Muscle, Left** *See S Lower Leg Muscle, Right* **V Foot Muscle, Right** Abductor hallucis muscle Adductor hallucis muscle Extensor digitorum brevis muscle Extensor hallucis brevis muscle Flexor digitorum brevis muscle Flexor hallucis brevis muscle Quadratus plantae muscle **W Foot Muscle, Left** *See V Foot Muscle, Right*	**Ø Open** **4 Percutaneous Endoscopic**	**Z No Device**	**Z No Qualifier**

NC Noncovered Procedure   **LC** Limited Coverage   **QA** Questionable OB Admit   **NT** New Tech Add-on   ⊞ Combination Member   ♂ Male   ♀ Female

Ø Medical and Surgical
K Muscles
N Release

Definition: Freeing a body part from an abnormal physical constraint by cutting or by the use of force
Explanation: Some of the restraining tissue may be taken out but none of the body part is taken out

Body Part Character 4		Approach Character 5	Device Character 6	Qualifier Character 7

Body Part — Character 4

Ø Head Muscle
Auricularis muscle
Masseter muscle
Pterygoid muscle
Splenius capitis muscle
Temporalis muscle
Temporoparietalis muscle

1 Facial Muscle
Buccinator muscle
Corrugator supercilii muscle
Depressor anguli oris muscle
Depressor labii inferioris muscle
Depressor septi nasi muscle
Depressor supercilii muscle
Levator anguli oris muscle
Levator labii superioris alaeque nasi muscle
Levator labii superioris muscle
Mentalis muscle
Nasalis muscle
Occipitofrontalis muscle
Orbicularis oris muscle
Procerus muscle
Risorius muscle
Zygomaticus muscle

2 Neck Muscle, Right
Anterior vertebral muscle
Arytenoid muscle
Cricothyroid muscle
Infrahyoid muscle
Levator scapulae muscle
Platysma muscle
Scalene muscle
Splenius cervicis muscle
Sternocleidomastoid muscle
Suprahyoid muscle
Thyroarytenoid muscle

3 Neck Muscle, Left
See 2 Neck Muscle, Right

4 Tongue, Palate, Pharynx Muscle
Chondroglossus muscle
Genioglossus muscle
Hyoglossus muscle
Inferior longitudinal muscle
Levator veli palatini muscle
Palatoglossal muscle
Palatopharyngeal muscle
Pharyngeal constrictor muscle
Salpingopharyngeus muscle
Styloglossus muscle
Stylopharyngeus muscle
Superior longitudinal muscle
Tensor veli palatini muscle

5 Shoulder Muscle, Right
Deltoid muscle
Infraspinatus muscle
Subscapularis muscle
Supraspinatus muscle
Teres major muscle
Teres minor muscle

6 Shoulder Muscle, Left
See 5 Shoulder Muscle, Right

7 Upper Arm Muscle, Right
Biceps brachii muscle
Brachialis muscle
Coracobrachialis muscle
Triceps brachii muscle

8 Upper Arm Muscle, Left
See 7 Upper Arm Muscle, Right

9 Lower Arm and Wrist Muscle, Right
Anatomical snuffbox
Brachioradialis muscle
Extensor carpi radialis muscle
Extensor carpi ulnaris muscle
Flexor carpi radialis muscle
Flexor carpi ulnaris muscle
Flexor pollicis longus muscle
Palmaris longus muscle
Pronator quadratus muscle
Pronator teres muscle

B Lower Arm and Wrist Muscle, Left
See 9 Lower Arm and Wrist Muscle, Right

C Hand Muscle, Right
Hypothenar muscle
Palmar interosseous muscle
Thenar muscle

D Hand Muscle, Left
See C Hand Muscle, Right

F Trunk Muscle, Right
Coccygeus muscle
Erector spinae muscle
Interspinalis muscle
Intertransversarius muscle
Latissimus dorsi muscle
Quadratus lumborum muscle
Rhomboid major muscle
Rhomboid minor muscle
Serratus posterior muscle
Transversospinalis muscle
Trapezius muscle

G Trunk Muscle, Left
See F Trunk Muscle, Right

H Thorax Muscle, Right
Intercostal muscle
Levatores costarum muscle
Pectoralis major muscle
Pectoralis minor muscle
Serratus anterior muscle
Subclavius muscle
Subcostal muscle
Transverse thoracis muscle

J Thorax Muscle, Left
See H Thorax Muscle, Right

K Abdomen Muscle, Right
External oblique muscle
Internal oblique muscle
Pyramidalis muscle
Rectus abdominis muscle
Transversus abdominis muscle

L Abdomen Muscle, Left
See K Abdomen Muscle, Right

M Perineum Muscle
Bulbospongiosus muscle
Cremaster muscle
Deep transverse perineal muscle
Ischiocavernosus muscle
Levator ani muscle
Superficial transverse perineal muscle

N Hip Muscle, Right
Gemellus muscle
Gluteus maximus muscle
Gluteus medius muscle
Gluteus minimus muscle
Iliacus muscle
Obturator muscle
Piriformis muscle
Psoas muscle
Quadratus femoris muscle
Tensor fasciae latae muscle

P Hip Muscle, Left
See N Hip Muscle, Right

Q Upper Leg Muscle, Right
Adductor brevis muscle
Adductor longus muscle
Adductor magnus muscle
Biceps femoris muscle
Gracilis muscle
Pectineus muscle
Quadriceps (femoris)
Rectus femoris muscle
Sartorius muscle
Semimembranosus muscle
Semitendinosus muscle
Vastus intermedius muscle
Vastus lateralis muscle
Vastus medialis muscle

R Upper Leg Muscle, Left
See Q Upper Leg Muscle, Right

S Lower Leg Muscle, Right
Extensor digitorum longus muscle
Extensor hallucis longus muscle
Fibularis brevis muscle
Fibularis longus muscle
Flexor digitorum longus muscle
Flexor hallucis longus muscle
Gastrocnemius muscle
Peroneus brevis muscle
Peroneus longus muscle
Popliteus muscle
Soleus muscle
Tibialis anterior muscle
Tibialis posterior muscle

T Lower Leg Muscle, Left
See S Lower Leg Muscle, Right

V Foot Muscle, Right
Abductor hallucis muscle
Adductor hallucis muscle
Extensor digitorum brevis muscle
Extensor hallucis brevis muscle
Flexor digitorum brevis muscle
Flexor hallucis brevis muscle
Quadratus plantae muscle

W Foot Muscle, Left
See V Foot Muscle, Right

Approach — Character 5
Ø Open
3 Percutaneous
4 Percutaneous Endoscopic
X External

Device — Character 6
Z No Device

Qualifier — Character 7
Z No Qualifier

Non-OR ØKN[Ø,1,2,3,4,5,6,7,8,9,B,C,D,F,G,H,J,K,L,M,N,P,Q,R,S,T,V,W]XZZ

Non-OR Procedure   DRG Non-OR Procedure   Valid OR Procedure   HAC Associated Procedure   Combination Only   New/Revised April   New/Revised October

Ø   **Medical and Surgical**
K   **Muscles**
P   **Removal**   Definition: Taking out or off a device from a body part

Explanation: If a device is taken out and a similar device put in without cutting or puncturing the skin or mucous membrane, the procedure is coded to the root operation CHANGE. Otherwise, the procedure for taking out a device is coded to the root operation REMOVAL.

Body Part Character 4	Approach Character 5	Device Character 6	Qualifier Character 7
X Upper Muscle Y Lower Muscle	Ø Open 3 Percutaneous 4 Percutaneous Endoscopic	Ø Drainage Device 7 Autologous Tissue Substitute J Synthetic Substitute K Nonautologous Tissue Substitute M Stimulator Lead Y Other Device	Z No Qualifier
X Upper Muscle Y Lower Muscle	X External	Ø Drainage Device M Stimulator Lead	Z No Qualifier

Non-OR   ØKP[X,Y][3,4]YZ
Non-OR   ØKP[X,Y]X[Ø,M]Z

NC Noncovered Procedure   LC Limited Coverage   QA Questionable OB Admit   NT New Tech Add-on   ⊞ Combination Member   ♂ Male   ♀ Female

ICD-10-PCS 2023   475

ØKP–ØKP

Ø   Medical and Surgical
K   Muscles
Q   Repair

Definition: Restoring, to the extent possible, a body part to its normal anatomic structure and function

Explanation: Used only when the method to accomplish the repair is not one of the other root operations

Body Part Character 4			Approach Character 5	Device Character 6	Qualifier Character 7
Ø Head Muscle Auricularis muscle Masseter muscle Pterygoid muscle Splenius capitis muscle Temporalis muscle Temporoparietalis muscle **1 Facial Muscle** Buccinator muscle Corrugator supercilii muscle Depressor anguli oris muscle Depressor labii inferioris muscle Depressor septi nasi muscle Depressor supercilii muscle Levator anguli oris muscle Levator labii superioris alaeque nasi muscle Levator labii superioris muscle Mentalis muscle Nasalis muscle Occipitofrontalis muscle Orbicularis oris muscle Procerus muscle Risorius muscle Zygomaticus muscle **2 Neck Muscle, Right** Anterior vertebral muscle Arytenoid muscle Cricothyroid muscle Infrahyoid muscle Levator scapulae muscle Platysma muscle Scalene muscle Splenius cervicis muscle Sternocleidomastoid muscle Suprahyoid muscle Thyroarytenoid muscle **3 Neck Muscle, Left** *See 2 Neck Muscle, Right* **4 Tongue, Palate, Pharynx Muscle** Chondroglossus muscle Genioglossus muscle Hyoglossus muscle Inferior longitudinal muscle Levator veli palatini muscle Palatoglossal muscle Palatopharyngeal muscle Pharyngeal constrictor muscle Salpingopharyngeus muscle Styloglossus muscle Stylopharyngeus muscle Superior longitudinal muscle Tensor veli palatini muscle **5 Shoulder Muscle, Right** Deltoid muscle Infraspinatus muscle Subscapularis muscle Supraspinatus muscle Teres major muscle Teres minor muscle **6 Shoulder Muscle, Left** *See 5 Shoulder Muscle, Right*	**7 Upper Arm Muscle, Right** Biceps brachii muscle Brachialis muscle Coracobrachialis muscle Triceps brachii muscle **8 Upper Arm Muscle, Left** *See 7 Upper Arm Muscle, Right* **9 Lower Arm and Wrist Muscle, Right** Anatomical snuffbox Brachioradialis muscle Extensor carpi radialis muscle Extensor carpi ulnaris muscle Flexor carpi radialis muscle Flexor carpi ulnaris muscle Flexor pollicis longus muscle Palmaris longus muscle Pronator quadratus muscle Pronator teres muscle **B Lower Arm and Wrist Muscle, Left** *See 9 Lower Arm and Wrist Muscle, Right* **C Hand Muscle, Right** Hypothenar muscle Palmar interosseous muscle Thenar muscle **D Hand Muscle, Left** *See C Hand Muscle, Right* **F Trunk Muscle, Right** Coccygeus muscle Erector spinae muscle Interspinalis muscle Intertransversarius muscle Latissimus dorsi muscle Quadratus lumborum muscle Rhomboid major muscle Rhomboid minor muscle Serratus posterior muscle Transversospinalis muscle Trapezius muscle **G Trunk Muscle, Left** *See F Trunk Muscle, Right* **H Thorax Muscle, Right** Intercostal muscle Levatores costarum muscle Pectoralis major muscle Pectoralis minor muscle Serratus anterior muscle Subclavius muscle Subcostal muscle Transverse thoracis muscle **J Thorax Muscle, Left** *See H Thorax Muscle, Right* **K Abdomen Muscle, Right** External oblique muscle Internal oblique muscle Pyramidalis muscle Rectus abdominis muscle Transversus abdominis muscle **L Abdomen Muscle, Left** *See K Abdomen Muscle, Right*	**M Perineum Muscle** Bulbospongiosus muscle Cremaster muscle Deep transverse perineal muscle Ischiocavernosus muscle Levator ani muscle Superficial transverse perineal muscle **N Hip Muscle, Right** Gemellus muscle Gluteus maximus muscle Gluteus medius muscle Gluteus minimus muscle Iliacus muscle Obturator muscle Piriformis muscle Psoas muscle Quadratus femoris muscle Tensor fasciae latae muscle **P Hip Muscle, Left** *See N Hip Muscle, Right* **Q Upper Leg Muscle, Right** Adductor brevis muscle Adductor longus muscle Adductor magnus muscle Biceps femoris muscle Gracilis muscle Pectineus muscle Quadriceps (femoris) Rectus femoris muscle Sartorius muscle Semimembranosus muscle Semitendinosus muscle Vastus intermedius muscle Vastus lateralis muscle Vastus medialis muscle **R Upper Leg Muscle, Left** *See Q Upper Leg Muscle, Right* **S Lower Leg Muscle, Right** Extensor digitorum longus muscle Extensor hallucis longus muscle Fibularis brevis muscle Fibularis longus muscle Flexor digitorum longus muscle Flexor hallucis longus muscle Gastrocnemius muscle Peroneus brevis muscle Peroneus longus muscle Popliteus muscle Soleus muscle Tibialis anterior muscle Tibialis posterior muscle **T Lower Leg Muscle, Left** *See S Lower Leg Muscle, Right* **V Foot Muscle, Right** Abductor hallucis muscle Adductor hallucis muscle Extensor digitorum brevis muscle Extensor hallucis brevis muscle Flexor digitorum brevis muscle Flexor hallucis brevis muscle Quadratus plantae muscle **W Foot Muscle, Left** *See V Foot Muscle, Right*	**Ø Open** **3 Percutaneous** **4 Percutaneous Endoscopic**	**Z No Device**	**Z No Qualifier**

Non-OR Procedure   DRG Non-OR Procedure   Valid OR Procedure   HAC Associated Procedure   Combination Only   New/Revised April   New/Revised October

476   ICD-10-PCS 2023

Ø Medical and Surgical
K Muscles
R Replacement   Definition: Putting in or on biological or synthetic material that physically takes the place and/or function of all or a portion of a body part

Explanation: The body part may have been taken out or replaced, or may be taken out, physically eradicated, or rendered nonfunctional during the REPLACEMENT procedure. A REMOVAL procedure is coded for taking out the device used in a previous replacement procedure.

Body Part Character 4			Approach Character 5	Device Character 6	Qualifier Character 7
Ø Head Muscle Auricularis muscle Masseter muscle Pterygoid muscle Splenius capitis muscle Temporalis muscle Temporoparietalis muscle **1 Facial Muscle** Buccinator muscle Corrugator supercilii muscle Depressor anguli oris muscle Depressor labii inferioris muscle Depressor septi nasi muscle Depressor supercilii muscle Levator anguli oris muscle Levator labii superioris alaeque nasi muscle Levator labii superioris muscle Mentalis muscle Nasalis muscle Occipitofrontalis muscle Orbicularis oris muscle Procerus muscle Risorius muscle Zygomaticus muscle **2 Neck Muscle, Right** Anterior vertebral muscle Arytenoid muscle Cricothyroid muscle Infrahyoid muscle Levator scapulae muscle Platysma muscle Scalene muscle Splenius cervicis muscle Sternocleidomastoid muscle Suprahyoid muscle Thyroarytenoid muscle **3 Neck Muscle, Left** *See 2 Neck Muscle, Right* **4 Tongue, Palate, Pharynx Muscle** Chondroglossus muscle Genioglossus muscle Hyoglossus muscle Inferior longitudinal muscle Levator veli palatini muscle Palatoglossal muscle Palatopharyngeal muscle Pharyngeal constrictor muscle Salpingopharyngeus muscle Styloglossus muscle Stylopharyngeus muscle Superior longitudinal muscle Tensor veli palatini muscle **5 Shoulder Muscle, Right** Deltoid muscle Infraspinatus muscle Subscapularis muscle Supraspinatus muscle Teres major muscle Teres minor muscle **6 Shoulder Muscle, Left** *See 5 Shoulder Muscle, Right*	**7 Upper Arm Muscle, Right** Biceps brachii muscle Brachialis muscle Coracobrachialis muscle Triceps brachii muscle **8 Upper Arm Muscle, Left** *See 7 Upper Arm Muscle, Right* **9 Lower Arm and Wrist Muscle, Right** Anatomical snuffbox Brachioradialis muscle Extensor carpi radialis muscle Extensor carpi ulnaris muscle Flexor carpi radialis muscle Flexor carpi ulnaris muscle Flexor pollicis longus muscle Palmaris longus muscle Pronator quadratus muscle Pronator teres muscle **B Lower Arm and Wrist Muscle, Left** *See 9 Lower Arm and Wrist Muscle, Right* **C Hand Muscle, Right** Hypothenar muscle Palmar interosseous muscle Thenar muscle **D Hand Muscle, Left** *See C Hand Muscle, Right* **F Trunk Muscle, Right** Coccygeus muscle Erector spinae muscle Interspinalis muscle Intertransversarius muscle Latissimus dorsi muscle Quadratus lumborum muscle Rhomboid major muscle Rhomboid minor muscle Serratus posterior muscle Transversospinalis muscle Trapezius muscle **G Trunk Muscle, Left** *See F Trunk Muscle, Right* **H Thorax Muscle, Right** Intercostal muscle Levatores costarum muscle Pectoralis major muscle Pectoralis minor muscle Serratus anterior muscle Subclavius muscle Subcostal muscle Transverse thoracis muscle **J Thorax Muscle, Left** *See H Thorax Muscle, Right* **K Abdomen Muscle, Right** External oblique muscle Internal oblique muscle Pyramidalis muscle Rectus abdominis muscle Transversus abdominis muscle **L Abdomen Muscle, Left** *See K Abdomen Muscle, Right*	**M Perineum Muscle** Bulbospongiosus muscle Cremaster muscle Deep transverse perineal muscle Ischiocavernosus muscle Levator ani muscle Superficial transverse perineal muscle **N Hip Muscle, Right** Gemellus muscle Gluteus maximus muscle Gluteus medius muscle Gluteus minimus muscle Iliacus muscle Obturator muscle Piriformis muscle Psoas muscle Quadratus femoris muscle Tensor fasciae latae muscle **P Hip Muscle, Left** *See N Hip Muscle, Right* **Q Upper Leg Muscle, Right** Adductor brevis muscle Adductor longus muscle Adductor magnus muscle Biceps femoris muscle Gracilis muscle Pectineus muscle Quadriceps (femoris) Rectus femoris muscle Sartorius muscle Semimembranosus muscle Semitendinosus muscle Vastus intermedius muscle Vastus lateralis muscle Vastus medialis muscle **R Upper Leg Muscle, Left** *See Q Upper Leg Muscle, Right* **S Lower Leg Muscle, Right** Extensor digitorum longus muscle Extensor hallucis longus muscle Fibularis brevis muscle Fibularis longus muscle Flexor digitorum longus muscle Flexor hallucis longus muscle Gastrocnemius muscle Peroneus brevis muscle Peroneus longus muscle Popliteus muscle Soleus muscle Tibialis anterior muscle Tibialis posterior muscle **T Lower Leg Muscle, Left** *See S Lower Leg Muscle, Right* **V Foot Muscle, Right** Abductor hallucis muscle Adductor hallucis muscle Extensor digitorum brevis muscle Extensor hallucis brevis muscle Flexor digitorum brevis muscle Flexor hallucis brevis muscle Quadratus plantae muscle **W Foot Muscle, Left** *See V Foot Muscle, Right*	**Ø Open** **4 Percutaneous Endoscopic**	**7 Autologous Tissue Substitute** **J Synthetic Substitute** **K Nonautologous Tissue Substitute**	**Z No Qualifier**

NC Noncovered Procedure   **LC** Limited Coverage   **QA** Questionable OB Admit   **NT** New Tech Add-on   ⊞ Combination Member   ♂ Male   ♀ Female

ICD-10-PCS 2023   477

ØKR–ØKR

Ø   Medical and Surgical
K   Muscles
S   Reposition   Definition: Moving to its normal location, or other suitable location, all or a portion of a body part

Explanation: The body part is moved to a new location from an abnormal location, or from a normal location where it is not functioning correctly. The body part may or may not be cut out or off to be moved to the new location.

Body Part Character 4			Approach Character 5	Device Character 6	Qualifier Character 7

Ø Head Muscle
Auricularis muscle
Masseter muscle
Pterygoid muscle
Splenius capitis muscle
Temporalis muscle
Temporoparietalis muscle
1 Facial Muscle
Buccinator muscle
Corrugator supercilii
  muscle
Depressor anguli oris
  muscle
Depressor labii inferioris
  muscle
Depressor septi nasi
  muscle
Depressor supercilii
  muscle
Levator anguli oris muscle
Levator labii superioris
  alaeque nasi muscle
Levator labii superioris
  muscle
Mentalis muscle
Nasalis muscle
Occipitofrontalis muscle
Orbicularis oris muscle
Procerus muscle
Risorius muscle
Zygomaticus muscle
2 Neck Muscle, Right
Anterior vertebral muscle
Arytenoid muscle
Cricothyroid muscle
Infrahyoid muscle
Levator scapulae muscle
Platysma muscle
Scalene muscle
Splenius cervicis muscle
Sternocleidomastoid
  muscle
Suprahyoid muscle
Thyroarytenoid muscle
3 Neck Muscle, Left
See 2 Neck Muscle, Right
4 Tongue, Palate, Pharynx
  Muscle
Chondroglossus muscle
Genioglossus muscle
Hyoglossus muscle
Inferior longitudinal
  muscle
Levator veli palatini
  muscle
Palatoglossal muscle
Palatopharyngeal muscle
Pharyngeal constrictor
  muscle
Salpingopharyngeus
  muscle
Styloglossus muscle
Stylopharyngeus muscle
Superior longitudinal
  muscle
Tensor veli palatini muscle
5 Shoulder Muscle, Right
Deltoid muscle
Infraspinatus muscle
Subscapularis muscle
Supraspinatus muscle
Teres major muscle
Teres minor muscle
6 Shoulder Muscle, Left
*See 5 Shoulder Muscle,
  Right*
	7 Upper Arm Muscle, Right
	Biceps brachii muscle
	Brachialis muscle
	Coracobrachialis muscle
	Triceps brachii muscle
	8 Upper Arm Muscle, Left
	*See 7 Upper Arm Muscle,
	  Right*
	9 Lower Arm and Wrist
	  Muscle, Right
	Anatomical snuffbox
	Brachioradialis muscle
	Extensor carpi radialis
	  muscle
	Extensor carpi ulnaris
	  muscle
	Flexor carpi radialis
	  muscle
	Flexor carpi ulnaris muscle
	Flexor pollicis longus
	  muscle
	Palmaris longus muscle
	Pronator quadratus
	  muscle
	Pronator teres muscle
	B Lower Arm and Wrist
	  Muscle, Left
	*See 9 Lower Arm and Wrist
	  Muscle, Right*
	C Hand Muscle, Right
	Hypothenar muscle
	Palmar interosseous
	  muscle
	Thenar muscle
	D Hand Muscle, Left
	See C Hand Muscle, Right
	F Trunk Muscle, Right
	Coccygeus muscle
	Erector spinae muscle
	Interspinalis muscle
	Intertransversarius muscle
	Latissimus dorsi muscle
	Quadratus lumborum
	  muscle
	Rhomboid major muscle
	Rhomboid minor muscle
	Serratus posterior muscle
	Transversospinalis muscle
	Trapezius muscle
	G Trunk Muscle, Left
	See F Trunk Muscle, Right
	H Thorax Muscle, Right
	Intercostal muscle
	Levatores costarum
	  muscle
	Pectoralis major muscle
	Pectoralis minor muscle
	Serratus anterior muscle
	Subclavius muscle
	Subcostal muscle
	Transverse thoracis
	  muscle
	J Thorax Muscle, Left
	See H Thorax Muscle, Right
	K Abdomen Muscle, Right
	External oblique muscle
	Internal oblique muscle
	Pyramidalis muscle
	Rectus abdominis muscle
	Transversus abdominis
	  muscle
	L Abdomen Muscle, Left
	*See K Abdomen Muscle,
	  Right*
		M Perineum Muscle
		Bulbospongiosus muscle
		Cremaster muscle
		Deep transverse perineal
		  muscle
		Ischiocavernosus muscle
		Levator ani muscle
		Superficial transverse
		  perineal muscle
		N Hip Muscle, Right
		Gemellus muscle
		Gluteus maximus muscle
		Gluteus medius muscle
		Gluteus minimus muscle
		Iliacus muscle
		Obturator muscle
		Piriformis muscle
		Psoas muscle
		Quadratus femoris muscle
		Tensor fasciae latae
		  muscle
		P Hip Muscle, Left
		See N Hip Muscle, Right
		Q Upper Leg Muscle, Right
		Adductor brevis muscle
		Adductor longus muscle
		Adductor magnus muscle
		Biceps femoris muscle
		Gracilis muscle
		Pectineus muscle
		Quadriceps (femoris)
		Rectus femoris muscle
		Sartorius muscle
		Semimembranosus
		  muscle
		Semitendinosus muscle
		Vastus intermedius muscle
		Vastus lateralis muscle
		Vastus medialis muscle
		R Upper Leg Muscle, Left
		*See Q Upper Leg Muscle,
		  Right*
		S Lower Leg Muscle, Right
		Extensor digitorum longus
		  muscle
		Extensor hallucis longus
		  muscle
		Fibularis brevis muscle
		Fibularis longus muscle
		Flexor digitorum longus
		  muscle
		Flexor hallucis longus
		  muscle
		Gastrocnemius muscle
		Peroneus brevis muscle
		Peroneus longus muscle
		Popliteus muscle
		Soleus muscle
		Tibialis anterior muscle
		Tibialis posterior muscle
		T Lower Leg Muscle, Left
		*See S Lower Leg Muscle,
		  Right*
		V Foot Muscle, Right
		Abductor hallucis muscle
		Adductor hallucis muscle
		Extensor digitorum brevis
		  muscle
		Extensor hallucis brevis
		  muscle
		Flexor digitorum brevis
		  muscle
		Flexor hallucis brevis
		  muscle
		Quadratus plantae muscle
		W Foot Muscle, Left
		See V Foot Muscle, Right
			Ø Open
			**4 Percutaneous
			  Endoscopic**
				Z No Device	**Z No Qualifier**

Non-OR Procedure   DRG Non-OR Procedure   Valid OR Procedure   HAC Associated Procedure   Combination Only   New/Revised April   New/Revised October

478

ICD-10-PCS 2023

Ø   **Medical and Surgical**
K   **Muscles**
T   **Resection**   Definition: Cutting out or off, without replacement, all of a body part

Explanation: None

Body Part Character 4			Approach Character 5	Device Character 6	Qualifier Character 7
Ø Head Muscle	**7 Upper Arm Muscle, Right**	**M Perineum Muscle**	**Ø Open**	**Z No Device**	**Z No Qualifier**
Auricularis muscle	Biceps brachii muscle	Bulbospongiosus muscle	**4 Percutaneous Endoscopic**		
Masseter muscle	Brachialis muscle	Cremaster muscle			
Pterygoid muscle	Coracobrachialis muscle	Deep transverse perineal muscle			
Splenius capitis muscle	Triceps brachii muscle	Ischiocavernosus muscle			
Temporalis muscle	**8 Upper Arm Muscle, Left**	Levator ani muscle			
Temporoparietalis muscle	*See 7 Upper Arm Muscle, Right*	Superficial transverse perineal muscle			
1 Facial Muscle	**9 Lower Arm and Wrist Muscle, Right**	**N Hip Muscle, Right**			
Buccinator muscle	Anatomical snuffbox	Gemellus muscle			
Corrugator supercilii muscle	Brachioradialis muscle	Gluteus maximus muscle			
Depressor anguli oris muscle	Extensor carpi radialis muscle	Gluteus medius muscle			
Depressor labii inferioris muscle	Extensor carpi ulnaris muscle	Gluteus minimus muscle			
Depressor septi nasi muscle	Flexor carpi radialis muscle	Iliacus muscle			
Depressor supercilii muscle	Flexor carpi ulnaris muscle	Obturator muscle			
Levator anguli oris muscle	Flexor pollicis longus muscle	Piriformis muscle			
Levator labii superioris alaeque nasi muscle	Palmaris longus muscle	Psoas muscle			
Levator labii superioris muscle	Pronator quadratus muscle	Quadratus femoris muscle			
Mentalis muscle	Pronator teres muscle	Tensor fasciae latae muscle			
Nasalis muscle	**B Lower Arm and Wrist Muscle, Left**	**P Hip Muscle, Left**			
Occipitofrontalis muscle	*See 9 Lower Arm and Wrist Muscle, Right*	*See N Hip Muscle, Right*			
Orbicularis oris muscle	**C Hand Muscle, Right**	**Q Upper Leg Muscle, Right**			
Procerus muscle	Hypothenar muscle	Adductor brevis muscle			
Risorius muscle	Palmar interosseous muscle	Adductor longus muscle			
Zygomaticus muscle	Thenar muscle	Adductor magnus muscle			
2 Neck Muscle, Right	**D Hand Muscle, Left**	Biceps femoris muscle			
Anterior vertebral muscle	*See C Hand Muscle, Right*	Gracilis muscle			
Arytenoid muscle	**F Trunk Muscle, Right**	Pectineus muscle			
Cricothyroid muscle	Coccygeus muscle	Quadriceps (femoris)			
Infrahyoid muscle	Erector spinae muscle	Rectus femoris muscle			
Levator scapulae muscle	Interspinalis muscle	Sartorius muscle			
Platysma muscle	Intertransversarius muscle	Semimembranosus muscle			
Scalene muscle	Latissimus dorsi muscle	Semitendinosus muscle			
Splenius cervicis muscle	Quadratus lumborum muscle	Vastus intermedius muscle			
Sternocleidomastoid muscle	Rhomboid major muscle	Vastus lateralis muscle			
Suprahyoid muscle	Rhomboid minor muscle	Vastus medialis muscle			
Thyroarytenoid muscle	Serratus posterior muscle	**R Upper Leg Muscle, Left**			
3 Neck Muscle, Left	Transversospinalis muscle	*See Q Upper Leg Muscle, Right*			
See 2 Neck Muscle, Right	Trapezius muscle	**S Lower Leg Muscle, Right**			
4 Tongue, Palate, Pharynx Muscle	**G Trunk Muscle, Left**	Extensor digitorum longus muscle			
Chondroglossus muscle	*See F Trunk Muscle, Right*	Extensor hallucis longus muscle			
Genioglossus muscle	**H Thorax Muscle, Right** ⊞	Fibularis brevis muscle			
Hyoglossus muscle	Intercostal muscle	Fibularis longus muscle			
Inferior longitudinal muscle	Levatores costarum muscle	Flexor digitorum longus muscle			
Levator veli palatini muscle	Pectoralis major muscle	Flexor hallucis longus muscle			
Palatoglossal muscle	Pectoralis minor muscle	Gastrocnemius muscle			
Palatopharyngeal muscle	Serratus anterior muscle	Peroneus brevis muscle			
Pharyngeal constrictor muscle	Subclavius muscle	Peroneus longus muscle			
Salpingopharyngeus muscle	Subcostal muscle	Popliteus muscle			
Styloglossus muscle	Transverse thoracis muscle	Soleus muscle			
Stylopharyngeus muscle	**J Thorax Muscle, Left** ⊞	Tibialis anterior muscle			
Superior longitudinal muscle	*See H Thorax Muscle, Right*	Tibialis posterior muscle			
Tensor veli palatini muscle	**K Abdomen Muscle, Right**	**T Lower Leg Muscle, Left**			
5 Shoulder Muscle, Right	External oblique muscle	*See S Lower Leg Muscle, Right*			
Deltoid muscle	Internal oblique muscle	**V Foot Muscle, Right**			
Infraspinatus muscle	Pyramidalis muscle	Abductor hallucis muscle			
Subscapularis muscle	Rectus abdominis muscle	Adductor hallucis muscle			
Supraspinatus muscle	Transversus abdominis muscle	Extensor digitorum brevis muscle			
Teres major muscle	**L Abdomen Muscle, Left**	Extensor hallucis brevis muscle			
Teres minor muscle	*See K Abdomen Muscle, Right*	Flexor digitorum brevis muscle			
6 Shoulder Muscle, Left		Flexor hallucis brevis muscle			
See 5 Shoulder Muscle, Right		Quadratus plantae muscle			
		W Foot Muscle, Left			
		See V Foot Muscle, Right			

See Appendix L for Procedure Combinations
⊞   ØKT[H,J]ØZZ

NC Noncovered Procedure   LC Limited Coverage   QA Questionable OB Admit   NT New Tech Add-on   ⊞ Combination Member   ♂ Male   ♀ Female

ICD-10-PCS 2023   ØKT–ØKT   479

Ø   **Medical and Surgical**
K   **Muscles**
U   **Supplement**   Definition: Putting in or on biological or synthetic material that physically reinforces and/or augments the function of a portion of a body part

Explanation: The biological material is non-living, or is living and from the same individual. The body part may have been previously replaced, and the SUPPLEMENT procedure is performed to physically reinforce and/or augment the function of the replaced body part.

Body Part Character 4			Approach Character 5	Device Character 6	Qualifier Character 7

Ø **Head Muscle**
Auricularis muscle
Masseter muscle
Pterygoid muscle
Splenius capitis muscle
Temporalis muscle
Temporoparietalis muscle
1 **Facial Muscle**
Buccinator muscle
Corrugator supercilii
  muscle
Depressor anguli oris
  muscle
Depressor labii inferioris
  muscle
Depressor septi nasi
  muscle
Depressor supercilii
  muscle
Levator anguli oris muscle
Levator labii superioris
  alaeque nasi muscle
Levator labii superioris
  muscle
Mentalis muscle
Nasalis muscle
Occipitofrontalis muscle
Orbicularis oris muscle
Procerus muscle
Risorius muscle
Zygomaticus muscle
2 **Neck Muscle, Right**
Anterior vertebral muscle
Arytenoid muscle
Cricothyroid muscle
Infrahyoid muscle
Levator scapulae muscle
Platysma muscle
Scalene muscle
Splenius cervicis muscle
Sternocleidomastoid
  muscle
Suprahyoid muscle
Thyroarytenoid muscle
3 **Neck Muscle, Left**
See 2 Neck Muscle, Right
4 **Tongue, Palate, Pharynx**
  Muscle
Chondroglossus muscle
Genioglossus muscle
Hyoglossus muscle
Inferior longitudinal
  muscle
Levator veli palatini
  muscle
Palatoglossal muscle
Palatopharyngeal muscle
Pharyngeal constrictor
  muscle
Salpingopharyngeus
  muscle
Styloglossus muscle
Stylopharyngeus muscle
Superior longitudinal
  muscle
Tensor veli palatini muscle
5 **Shoulder Muscle, Right**
Deltoid muscle
Infraspinatus muscle
Subscapularis muscle
Supraspinatus muscle
Teres major muscle
Teres minor muscle
6 **Shoulder Muscle, Left**
See 5 Shoulder Muscle,
  Right
	7 **Upper Arm Muscle, Right**
	Biceps brachii muscle
	Brachialis muscle
	Coracobrachialis muscle
	Triceps brachii muscle
	8 **Upper Arm Muscle, Left**
	See 7 Upper Arm Muscle,
	  Right
	9 **Lower Arm and Wrist**
	  Muscle, Right
	Anatomical snuffbox
	Brachioradialis muscle
	Extensor carpi radialis
	  muscle
	Extensor carpi ulnaris
	  muscle
	Flexor carpi radialis
	  muscle
	Flexor carpi ulnaris muscle
	Flexor pollicis longus
	  muscle
	Palmaris longus muscle
	Pronator quadratus
	  muscle
	Pronator teres muscle
	B **Lower Arm and Wrist**
	  Muscle, Left
	See 9 Lower Arm and Wrist
	  Muscle, Right
	C **Hand Muscle, Right**
	Hypothenar muscle
	Palmar interosseous
	  muscle
	Thenar muscle
	D **Hand Muscle, Left**
	See C Hand Muscle, Right
	F **Trunk Muscle, Right**
	Coccygeus muscle
	Erector spinae muscle
	Interspinalis muscle
	Intertransversarius muscle
	Latissimus dorsi muscle
	Quadratus lumborum
	  muscle
	Rhomboid major muscle
	Rhomboid minor muscle
	Serratus posterior muscle
	Transversospinalis muscle
	Trapezius muscle
	G **Trunk Muscle, Left**
	See F Trunk Muscle, Right
	H **Thorax Muscle, Right**
	Intercostal muscle
	Levatores costarum
	  muscle
	Pectoralis major muscle
	Pectoralis minor muscle
	Serratus anterior muscle
	Subclavius muscle
	Subcostal muscle
	Transverse thoracis
	  muscle
	J **Thorax Muscle, Left**
	See H Thorax Muscle, Right
	K **Abdomen Muscle, Right**
	External oblique muscle
	Internal oblique muscle
	Pyramidalis muscle
	Rectus abdominis muscle
	Transversus abdominis
	  muscle
	L **Abdomen Muscle, Left**
	See K Abdomen Muscle,
	  Right
		M **Perineum Muscle**
		Bulbospongiosus muscle
		Cremaster muscle
		Deep transverse perineal
		  muscle
		Ischiocavernosus muscle
		Levator ani muscle
		Superficial transverse
		  perineal muscle
		N **Hip Muscle, Right**
		Gemellus muscle
		Gluteus maximus muscle
		Gluteus medius muscle
		Gluteus minimus muscle
		Iliacus muscle
		Obturator muscle
		Piriformis muscle
		Psoas muscle
		Quadratus femoris muscle
		Tensor fasciae latae
		  muscle
		P **Hip Muscle, Left**
		See N Hip Muscle, Right
		Q **Upper Leg Muscle, Right**
		Adductor brevis muscle
		Adductor longus muscle
		Adductor magnus muscle
		Biceps femoris muscle
		Gracilis muscle
		Pectineus muscle
		Quadriceps (femoris)
		Rectus femoris muscle
		Sartorius muscle
		Semimembranosus
		  muscle
		Semitendinosus muscle
		Vastus intermedius muscle
		Vastus lateralis muscle
		Vastus medialis muscle
		R **Upper Leg Muscle, Left**
		See Q Upper Leg Muscle,
		  Right
		S **Lower Leg Muscle, Right**
		Extensor digitorum longus
		  muscle
		Extensor hallucis longus
		  muscle
		Fibularis brevis muscle
		Fibularis longus muscle
		Flexor digitorum longus
		  muscle
		Flexor hallucis longus
		  muscle
		Gastrocnemius muscle
		Peroneus brevis muscle
		Peroneus longus muscle
		Popliteus muscle
		Soleus muscle
		Tibialis anterior muscle
		Tibialis posterior muscle
		T **Lower Leg Muscle, Left**
		See S Lower Leg Muscle,
		  Right
		V **Foot Muscle, Right**
		Abductor hallucis muscle
		Adductor hallucis muscle
		Extensor digitorum brevis
		  muscle
		Extensor hallucis brevis
		  muscle
		Flexor digitorum brevis
		  muscle
		Flexor hallucis brevis
		  muscle
		Quadratus plantae muscle
		W **Foot Muscle, Left**
		See V Foot Muscle, Right
			Ø **Open**
			4 **Percutaneous**
			  Endoscopic
				7 **Autologous Tissue**
				  Substitute
				J **Synthetic**
				  Substitute
				K **Nonautologous**
				  Tissue Substitute
					Z **No Qualifier**

Non-OR Procedure   DRG Non-OR Procedure   Valid OR Procedure   HAC Associated Procedure   Combination Only   New/Revised April   New/Revised October

480

ICD-10-PCS 2023

ØKU–ØKU

Ø   Medical and Surgical
K   Muscles
W   Revision   Definition: Correcting, to the extent possible, a portion of a malfunctioning device or the position of a displaced device

                 Explanation: Revision can include correcting a malfunctioning or displaced device by taking out or putting in components of the device such as a screw or pin

Body Part Character 4	Approach Character 5	Device Character 6	Qualifier Character 7
X Upper Muscle Y Lower Muscle	Ø Open 3 Percutaneous 4 Percutaneous Endoscopic	Ø Drainage Device 7 Autologous Tissue Substitute J Synthetic Substitute K Nonautologous Tissue Substitute M Stimulator Lead Y Other Device	Z No Qualifier
X Upper Muscle Y Lower Muscle	X External	Ø Drainage Device 7 Autologous Tissue Substitute J Synthetic Substitute K Nonautologous Tissue Substitute M Stimulator Lead	Z No Qualifier

Non-OR   ØKW[X,Y][3,4]YZ
Non-OR   ØKW[X,Y]X[Ø,7,J,K,M]Z

NC Noncovered Procedure   LC Limited Coverage   QA Questionable OB Admit   NT New Tech Add-on   ⊞ Combination Member   ♂ Male   ♀ Female

ICD-10-PCS 2023   481

Ø Medical and Surgical
K Muscles
X Transfer

Definition: Moving, without taking out, all or a portion of a body part to another location to take over the function of all or a portion of a body part
Explanation: The body part transferred remains connected to its vascular and nervous supply

Body Part Character 4			Approach Character 5	Device Character 6	Qualifier Character 7
Ø Head Muscle Auricularis muscle Masseter muscle Pterygoid muscle Splenius capitis muscle Temporalis muscle Temporoparietalis muscle **1 Facial Muscle** Buccinator muscle Corrugator supercilii muscle Depressor anguli oris muscle Depressor labii inferioris muscle Depressor septi nasi muscle Depressor supercilii muscle Levator anguli oris muscle Levator labii superioris alaeque nasi muscle Levator labii superioris muscle Mentalis muscle Nasalis muscle Occipitofrontalis muscle Orbicularis oris muscle Procerus muscle Risorius muscle Zygomaticus muscle **2 Neck Muscle, Right** Anterior vertebral muscle Arytenoid muscle Cricothyroid muscle Infrahyoid muscle Levator scapulae muscle Platysma muscle Scalene muscle Splenius cervicis muscle Sternocleidomastoid muscle Suprahyoid muscle Thyroarytenoid muscle **3 Neck Muscle, Left** *See 2 Neck Muscle, Right* **4 Tongue, Palate, Pharynx Muscle** Chondroglossus muscle Genioglossus muscle Hyoglossus muscle Inferior longitudinal muscle Levator veli palatini muscle Palatoglossal muscle Palatopharyngeal muscle Pharyngeal constrictor muscle Salpingopharyngeus muscle Styloglossus muscle Stylopharyngeus muscle Superior longitudinal muscle Tensor veli palatini muscle **5 Shoulder Muscle, Right** Deltoid muscle Infraspinatus muscle Subscapularis muscle Supraspinatus muscle Teres major muscle Teres minor muscle	**6 Shoulder Muscle, Left** *See 5 Shoulder Muscle, Right* **7 Upper Arm Muscle, Right** Biceps brachii muscle Brachialis muscle Coracobrachialis muscle Triceps brachii muscle **8 Upper Arm Muscle, Left** *See 7 Upper Arm Muscle, Right* **9 Lower Arm and Wrist Muscle, Right** Anatomical snuffbox Brachioradialis muscle Extensor carpi radialis muscle Extensor carpi ulnaris muscle Flexor carpi radialis muscle Flexor carpi ulnaris muscle Flexor pollicis longus muscle Palmaris longus muscle Pronator quadratus muscle Pronator teres muscle **B Lower Arm and Wrist Muscle, Left** *See 9 Lower Arm and Wrist Muscle, Right* **C Hand Muscle, Right** Hypothenar muscle Palmar interosseous muscle Thenar muscle **D Hand Muscle, Left** *See C Hand Muscle, Right* **H Thorax Muscle, Right** Intercostal muscle Levatores costarum muscle Pectoralis major muscle Pectoralis minor muscle Serratus anterior muscle Subclavius muscle Subcostal muscle Transverse thoracis muscle **J Thorax Muscle, Left** *See H Thorax Muscle, Right* **M Perineum Muscle** Bulbospongiosus muscle Cremaster muscle Deep transverse perineal muscle Ischiocavernosus muscle Levator ani muscle Superficial transverse perineal muscle **N Hip Muscle, Right** Gemellus muscle Gluteus maximus muscle Gluteus medius muscle Gluteus minimus muscle Iliacus muscle Obturator muscle Piriformis muscle Psoas muscle Quadratus femoris muscle Tensor fasciae latae muscle	**P Hip Muscle, Left** *See N Hip Muscle, Right* **Q Upper Leg Muscle, Right** Adductor brevis muscle Adductor longus muscle Adductor magnus muscle Biceps femoris muscle Gracilis muscle Pectineus muscle Quadriceps (femoris) Rectus femoris muscle Sartorius muscle Semimembranosus muscle Semitendinosus muscle Vastus intermedius muscle Vastus lateralis muscle Vastus medialis muscle **R Upper Leg Muscle, Left** *See Q Upper Leg Muscle, Right* **S Lower Leg Muscle, Right** Extensor digitorum longus muscle Extensor hallucis longus muscle Fibularis brevis muscle Fibularis longus muscle Flexor digitorum longus muscle Flexor hallucis longus muscle Gastrocnemius muscle Peroneus brevis muscle Peroneus longus muscle Popliteus muscle Soleus muscle Tibialis anterior muscle Tibialis posterior muscle **T Lower Leg Muscle, Left** *See S Lower Leg Muscle, Right* **V Foot Muscle, Right** Abductor hallucis muscle Adductor hallucis muscle Extensor digitorum brevis muscle Extensor hallucis brevis muscle Flexor digitorum brevis muscle Flexor hallucis brevis muscle Quadratus plantae muscle **W Foot Muscle, Left** *See V Foot Muscle, Right*	**Ø Open** **4 Percutaneous Endoscopic**	**Z No Device**	**Ø Skin** **1 Subcutaneous Tissue** **2 Skin and Subcutaneous Tissue** **Z No Qualifier**

ØKX Continued on next page

Non-OR Procedure   DRG Non-OR Procedure   Valid OR Procedure   HAC Associated Procedure   Combination Only   New/Revised April   New/Revised October

482   ICD-10-PCS 2023

Ø   **Medical and Surgical**   *ØKX Continued*
K   **Muscles**
X   **Transfer**   Definition: Moving, without taking out, all or a portion of a body part to another location to take over the function of all or a portion of a body part

Explanation: The body part transferred remains connected to its vascular and nervous supply

Body Part Character 4	Approach Character 5	Device Character 6	Qualifier Character 7

F **Trunk Muscle, Right**
    Coccygeus muscle
    Erector spinae muscle
    Interspinalis muscle
    Intertransversarius muscle
    Latissimus dorsi muscle
    Quadratus lumborum muscle
    Rhomboid major muscle
    Rhomboid minor muscle
    Serratus posterior muscle
    Transversospinalis muscle
    Trapezius muscle
G **Trunk Muscle, Left**
    See F Trunk Muscle, Right
	Ø Open
	4 Percutaneous Endoscopic
		Z No Device	**Ø** Skin
			1 Subcutaneous Tissue
			2 Skin and Subcutaneous Tissue
			5 Latissimus Dorsi Myocutaneous
			    Flap
			7 Deep Inferior Epigastric Artery
			    Perforator Flap
			8 Superficial Inferior Epigastric
			    Artery Flap
			9 Gluteal Artery Perforator Flap
			Z No Qualifier

K **Abdomen Muscle, Right**
    External oblique muscle
    Internal oblique muscle
    Pyramidalis muscle
    Rectus abdominis muscle
    Transversus abdominis muscle
L **Abdomen Muscle, Left**
    See K Abdomen Muscle, Right
	Ø Open
	4 Percutaneous Endoscopic
		Z No Device	**Ø** Skin
			1 Subcutaneous Tissue
			2 Skin and Subcutaneous Tissue
			6 Transverse Rectus Abdominis
			    Myocutaneous Flap
			Z No Qualifier

Tendons ØL2–ØLX

Character Meanings*

This Character Meaning table is provided as a guide to assist the user in the identification of character members that may be found in this section of code tables. It **SHOULD NOT** be used to build a PCS code.

Operation–Character 3	Body Part–Character 4	Approach–Character 5	Device–Character 6	Qualifier–Character 7
2 Change	Ø Head and Neck Tendon	Ø Open	Ø Drainage Device	X Diagnostic
5 Destruction	1 Shoulder Tendon, Right	3 Percutaneous	7 Autologous Tissue Substitute	Z No Qualifier
8 Division	2 Shoulder Tendon, Left	4 Percutaneous Endoscopic	J Synthetic Substitute	
9 Drainage	3 Upper Arm Tendon, Right	X External	K Nonautologous Tissue Substitute	
B Excision	4 Upper Arm Tendon, Left		Y Other Device	
C Extirpation	5 Lower Arm and Wrist Tendon, Right		Z No Device	
D Extraction	6 Lower Arm and Wrist Tendon, Left			
H Insertion	7 Hand Tendon, Right			
J Inspection	8 Hand Tendon, Left			
M Reattachment	9 Trunk Tendon, Right			
N Release	B Trunk Tendon, Left			
P Removal	C Thorax Tendon, Right			
Q Repair	D Thorax Tendon, Left			
R Replacement	F Abdomen Tendon, Right			
S Reposition	G Abdomen Tendon, Left			
T Resection	H Perineum Tendon			
U Supplement	J Hip Tendon, Right			
W Revision	K Hip Tendon, Left			
X Transfer	L Upper Leg Tendon, Right			
	M Upper Leg Tendon, Left			
	N Lower Leg Tendon, Right			
	P Lower Leg Tendon, Left			
	Q Knee Tendon, Right			
	R Knee Tendon, Left			
	S Ankle Tendon, Right			
	T Ankle Tendon, Left			
	V Foot Tendon, Right			
	W Foot Tendon, Left			
	X Upper Tendon			
	Y Lower Tendon			

* Includes synovial membrane.

AHA Coding Clinic for table ØL8
2016, 3Q, 30   Resection of femur with interposition arthroplasty

AHA Coding Clinic for table ØLB
2017, 2Q, 21   Arthroscopic anterior cruciate ligament revision using autograft with anterolateral ligament reconstruction
2015, 3Q, 26   Thumb arthroplasty with resection of trapezium
2014, 3Q, 14   Application of TheraSkin® and excisional debridement
2014, 3Q, 18   Placement of reverse sural fasciocutaneous pedicle flap

AHA Coding Clinic for table ØLD
2017, 4Q, 41   Extraction procedures

AHA Coding Clinic for table ØLQ
2016, 3Q, 32   Rotator cuff repair, tenodesis, decompression, acromioplasty and coracoplasty
2015, 2Q, 11   Repair of patellar and quadriceps tendons with allograft
2013, 3Q, 20   Superior labrum anterior posterior (SLAP) repair and subacromial decompression

AHA Coding Clinic for table ØLS
2016, 3Q, 32   Rotator cuff repair, tenodesis, decompression, acromioplasty and coracoplasty
2015, 3Q, 14   Endoprosthetic replacement of humerus and tendon reattachment

AHA Coding Clinic for table ØLU
2015, 2Q, 11   Repair of patellar and quadriceps tendons with allograft

Foot Tendons

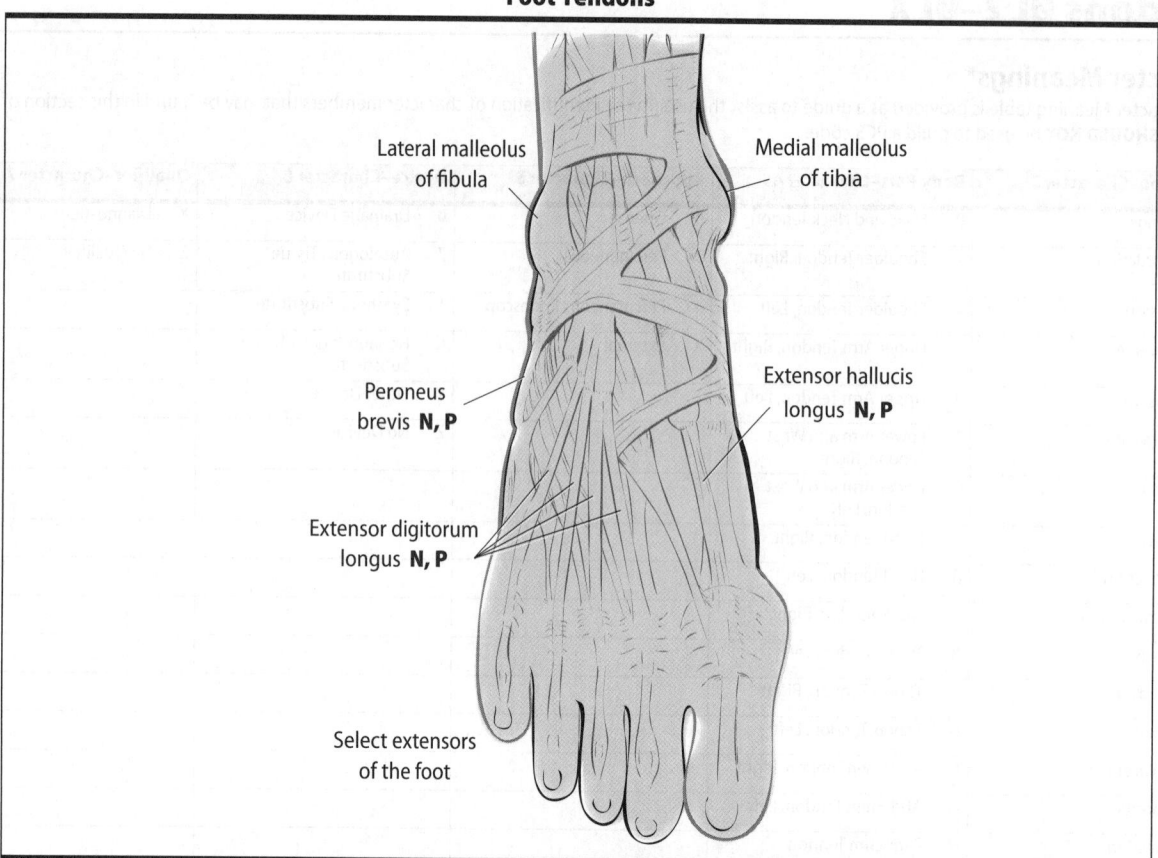

Lateral malleolus of fibula

Medial malleolus of tibia

Peroneus brevis **N, P**

Extensor hallucis longus **N, P**

Extensor digitorum longus **N, P**

Select extensors of the foot

Shoulder Tendons

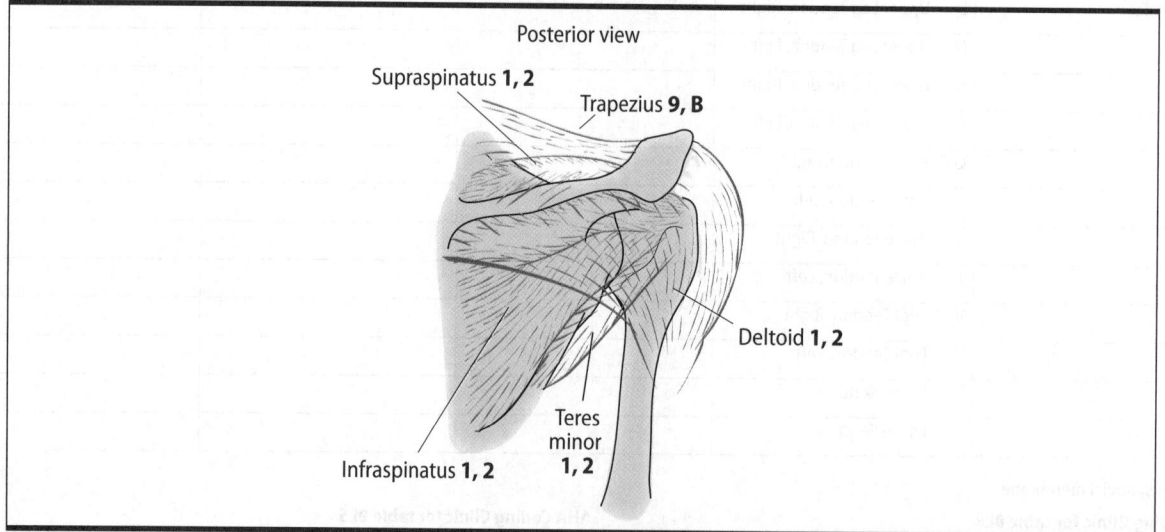

Posterior view

Supraspinatus **1, 2**

Trapezius **9, B**

Deltoid **1, 2**

Teres minor **1, 2**

Infraspinatus **1, 2**

Tendons of Wrist and Hand

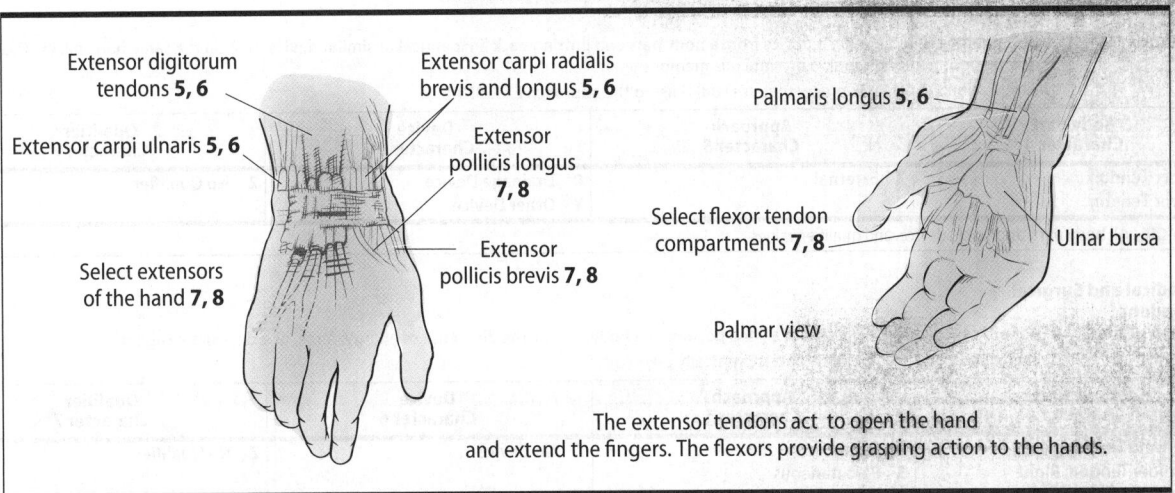

Extensor digitorum tendons **5, 6**

Extensor carpi ulnaris **5, 6**

Select extensors of the hand **7, 8**

Extensor carpi radialis brevis and longus **5, 6**

Extensor pollicis longus **7, 8**

Extensor pollicis brevis **7, 8**

Palmaris longus **5, 6**

Select flexor tendon compartments **7, 8**

Ulnar bursa

Palmar view

The extensor tendons act to open the hand and extend the fingers. The flexors provide grasping action to the hands.

Leg Muscles and Tendons

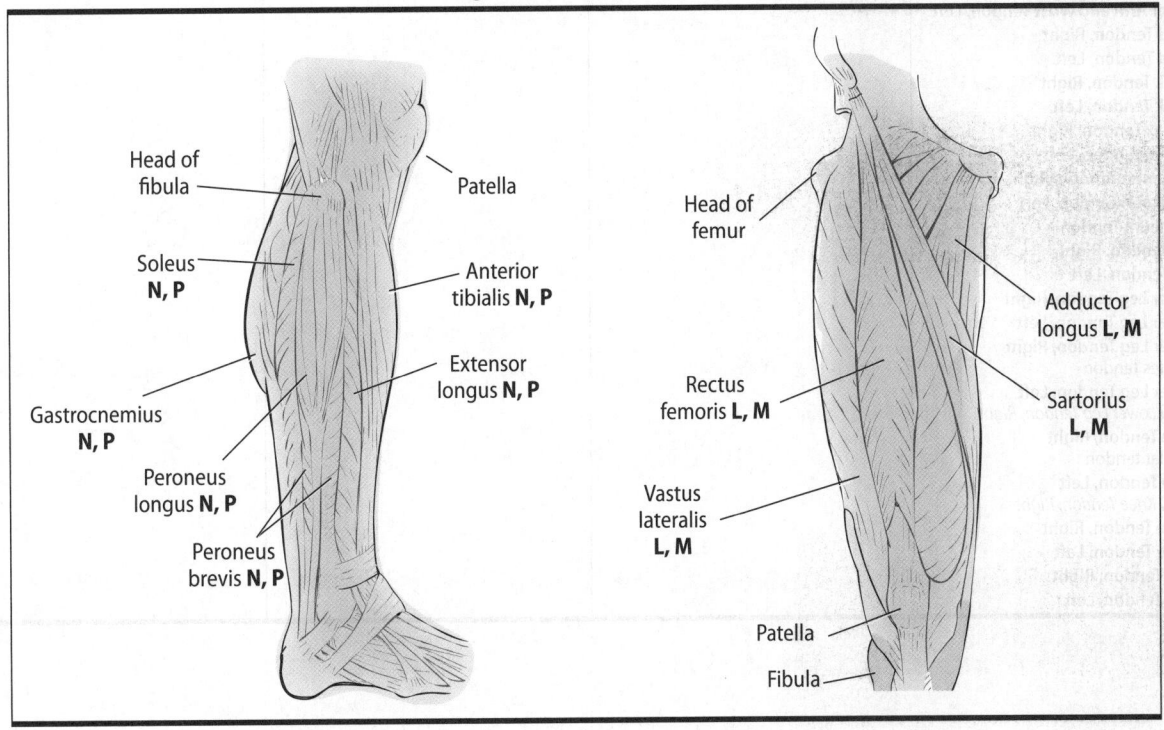

Head of fibula

Soleus **N, P**

Gastrocnemius **N, P**

Peroneus longus **N, P**

Peroneus brevis **N, P**

Patella

Anterior tibialis **N, P**

Extensor longus **N, P**

Head of femur

Rectus femoris **L, M**

Vastus lateralis **L, M**

Adductor longus **L, M**

Sartorius **L, M**

Patella

Fibula

Ø   Medical and Surgical
L   Tendons
2   Change   Definition: Taking out or off a device from a body part and putting back an identical or similar device in or on the same body part without cutting or puncturing the skin or a mucous membrane

Explanation: All CHANGE procedures are coded using the approach EXTERNAL

Body Part Character 4	Approach Character 5	Device Character 6	Qualifier Character 7
X Upper Tendon Y Lower Tendon	X External	Ø Drainage Device Y Other Device	Z No Qualifier

Non-OR	All body part, approach, device, and qualifier values

Ø   Medical and Surgical
L   Tendons
5   Destruction   Definition: Physical eradication of all or a portion of a body part by the direct use of energy, force, or a destructive agent

Explanation: None of the body part is physically taken out

Body Part Character 4	Approach Character 5	Device Character 6	Qualifier Character 7

Ø Head and Neck Tendon
1 Shoulder Tendon, Right
2 Shoulder Tendon, Left
3 Upper Arm Tendon, Right
4 Upper Arm Tendon, Left
5 Lower Arm and Wrist Tendon, Right
6 Lower Arm and Wrist Tendon, Left
7 Hand Tendon, Right
8 Hand Tendon, Left
9 Trunk Tendon, Right
B Trunk Tendon, Left
C Thorax Tendon, Right
D Thorax Tendon, Left
F Abdomen Tendon, Right
G Abdomen Tendon, Left
H Perineum Tendon
J Hip Tendon, Right
K Hip Tendon, Left
L Upper Leg Tendon, Right
M Upper Leg Tendon, Left
N Lower Leg Tendon, Right
   Achilles tendon
P Lower Leg Tendon, Left
   See N Lower Leg Tendon, Right
Q Knee Tendon, Right
   Patellar tendon
R Knee Tendon, Left
   See Q Knee Tendon, Right
S Ankle Tendon, Right
T Ankle Tendon, Left
V Foot Tendon, Right
W Foot Tendon, Left
	Ø Open
	3 Percutaneous
	4 Percutaneous Endoscopic
		Z No Device	Z No Qualifier

Non-OR Procedure   DRG Non-OR Procedure   Valid OR Procedure   HAC Associated Procedure   Combination Only   New/Revised April   New/Revised October

488   ICD-10-PCS 2023

0   Medical and Surgical
L   Tendons
8   Division   Definition: Cutting into a body part, without draining fluids and/or gases from the body part, in order to separate or transect a body part
      Explanation: All or a portion of the body part is separated into two or more portions

Body Part Character 4	Approach Character 5	Device Character 6	Qualifier Character 7
0 Head and Neck Tendon	0 Open	Z No Device	Z No Qualifier
1 Shoulder Tendon, Right	3 Percutaneous		
2 Shoulder Tendon, Left	4 Percutaneous Endoscopic		
3 Upper Arm Tendon, Right			
4 Upper Arm Tendon, Left			
5 Lower Arm and Wrist Tendon, Right			
6 Lower Arm and Wrist Tendon, Left			
7 Hand Tendon, Right			
8 Hand Tendon, Left			
9 Trunk Tendon, Right			
B Trunk Tendon, Left			
C Thorax Tendon, Right			
D Thorax Tendon, Left			
F Abdomen Tendon, Right			
G Abdomen Tendon, Left			
H Perineum Tendon			
J Hip Tendon, Right			
K Hip Tendon, Left			
L Upper Leg Tendon, Right			
M Upper Leg Tendon, Left			
N Lower Leg Tendon, Right Achilles tendon			
P Lower Leg Tendon, Left *See N Lower Leg Tendon, Right*			
Q Knee Tendon, Right Patellar tendon			
R Knee Tendon, Left *See Q Knee Tendon, Right*			
S Ankle Tendon, Right			
T Ankle Tendon, Left			
V Foot Tendon, Right			
W Foot Tendon, Left			

Ø   **Medical and Surgical**
L   **Tendons**
9   **Drainage**   Definition: Taking or letting out fluids and/or gases from a body part
          Explanation: The qualifier DIAGNOSTIC is used to identify drainage procedures that are biopsies

Body Part Character 4	Approach Character 5	Device Character 6	Qualifier Character 7

Ø   Head and Neck Tendon
1   Shoulder Tendon, Right
2   Shoulder Tendon, Left
3   Upper Arm Tendon, Right
4   Upper Arm Tendon, Left
5   Lower Arm and Wrist Tendon, Right
6   Lower Arm and Wrist Tendon, Left
7   Hand Tendon, Right
8   Hand Tendon, Left
9   Trunk Tendon, Right
B   Trunk Tendon, Left
C   Thorax Tendon, Right
D   Thorax Tendon, Left
F   Abdomen Tendon, Right
G   Abdomen Tendon, Left
H   Perineum Tendon
J   Hip Tendon, Right
K   Hip Tendon, Left
L   Upper Leg Tendon, Right
M   Upper Leg Tendon, Left
N   Lower Leg Tendon, Right
     Achilles tendon
P   Lower Leg Tendon, Left
     See N Lower Leg Tendon, Right
Q   Knee Tendon, Right
     Patellar tendon
R   Knee Tendon, Left
     See Q Knee Tendon, Right
S   Ankle Tendon, Right
T   Ankle Tendon, Left
V   Foot Tendon, Right
W   Foot Tendon, Left
	Ø Open
	3 Percutaneous
	4 Percutaneous Endoscopic
		Ø Drainage Device	Z No Qualifier

Ø   Head and Neck Tendon
1   Shoulder Tendon, Right
2   Shoulder Tendon, Left
3   Upper Arm Tendon, Right
4   Upper Arm Tendon, Left
5   Lower Arm and Wrist Tendon, Right
6   Lower Arm and Wrist Tendon, Left
7   Hand Tendon, Right
8   Hand Tendon, Left
9   Trunk Tendon, Right
B   Trunk Tendon, Left
C   Thorax Tendon, Right
D   Thorax Tendon, Left
F   Abdomen Tendon, Right
G   Abdomen Tendon, Left
H   Perineum Tendon
J   Hip Tendon, Right
K   Hip Tendon, Left
L   Upper Leg Tendon, Right
M   Upper Leg Tendon, Left
N   Lower Leg Tendon, Right
     Achilles tendon
P   Lower Leg Tendon, Left
     See N Lower Leg Tendon, Right
Q   Knee Tendon, Right
     Patellar tendon
R   Knee Tendon, Left
     See Q Knee Tendon, Right
S   Ankle Tendon, Right
T   Ankle Tendon, Left
V   Foot Tendon, Right
W   Foot Tendon, Left
	Ø Open
	3 Percutaneous
	4 Percutaneous Endoscopic
		Z No Device	X Diagnostic
			Z No Qualifier

Non-OR   ØL9[Ø,1,2,3,4,5,6,7,8,9,B,C,D,F,G,H,J,K,L,M,N,P,Q,R,S,T,V,W]3ØZ
Non-OR   ØL9[Ø,1,2,3,4,5,6,7,8,9,B,C,D,F,G,H,J,K,L,M,N,P,Q,R,S,T,V,W]3ZZ

Non-OR   ØL9[7,8]4ZZ

Non-OR Procedure   DRG Non-OR Procedure   Valid OR Procedure   HAC Associated Procedure   Combination Only   New/Revised April   New/Revised October

490   ICD-10-PCS 2023

ØL9–ØL9

Ø   **Medical and Surgical**
L   **Tendons**
B   **Excision**   Definition: Cutting out or off, without replacement, a portion of a body part

                                       Explanation: The qualifier DIAGNOSTIC is used to identify excision procedures that are biopsies

Body Part Character 4	Approach Character 5	Device Character 6	Qualifier Character 7

Ø Head and Neck Tendon
1 Shoulder Tendon, Right
2 Shoulder Tendon, Left
3 Upper Arm Tendon, Right
4 Upper Arm Tendon, Left
5 Lower Arm and Wrist Tendon, Right
6 Lower Arm and Wrist Tendon, Left
7 Hand Tendon, Right
8 Hand Tendon, Left
9 Trunk Tendon, Right
B Trunk Tendon, Left
C Thorax Tendon, Right
D Thorax Tendon, Left
F Abdomen Tendon, Right
G Abdomen Tendon, Left
H Perineum Tendon
J Hip Tendon, Right
K Hip Tendon, Left
L Upper Leg Tendon, Right
M Upper Leg Tendon, Left
N Lower Leg Tendon, Right
     Achilles tendon
P Lower Leg Tendon, Left
     See N Lower Leg Tendon, Right
Q Knee Tendon, Right
     Patellar tendon
R Knee Tendon, Left
     See Q Knee Tendon, Right
S Ankle Tendon, Right
T Ankle Tendon, Left
V Foot Tendon, Right
W Foot Tendon, Left
	Ø Open
	3 Percutaneous
	4 Percutaneous Endoscopic
		Z No Device	**X** Diagnostic
			Z No Qualifier

Tendons

Ø   **Medical and Surgical**
L   **Tendons**
C   **Extirpation**   Definition: Taking or cutting out solid matter from a body part

Explanation: The solid matter may be an abnormal byproduct of a biological function or a foreign body; it may be imbedded in a body part or in the lumen of a tubular body part. The solid matter may or may not have been previously broken into pieces.

Body Part Character 4	Approach Character 5	Device Character 6	Qualifier Character 7
Ø Head and Neck Tendon	**Ø** Open	**Z** No Device	**Z** No Qualifier
1 Shoulder Tendon, Right	**3** Percutaneous		
2 Shoulder Tendon, Left	**4** Percutaneous Endoscopic		
3 Upper Arm Tendon, Right			
4 Upper Arm Tendon, Left			
5 Lower Arm and Wrist Tendon, Right			
6 Lower Arm and Wrist Tendon, Left			
7 Hand Tendon, Right			
8 Hand Tendon, Left			
9 Trunk Tendon, Right			
B Trunk Tendon, Left			
C Thorax Tendon, Right			
D Thorax Tendon, Left			
F Abdomen Tendon, Right			
G Abdomen Tendon, Left			
H Perineum Tendon			
J Hip Tendon, Right			
K Hip Tendon, Left			
L Upper Leg Tendon, Right			
M Upper Leg Tendon, Left			
N Lower Leg Tendon, Right Achilles tendon			
P Lower Leg Tendon, Left *See N Lower Leg Tendon, Right*			
Q Knee Tendon, Right Patellar tendon			
R Knee Tendon, Left *See Q Knee Tendon, Right*			
S Ankle Tendon, Right			
T Ankle Tendon, Left			
V Foot Tendon, Right			
W Foot Tendon, Left			

Non-OR Procedure   DRG Non-OR Procedure   Valid OR Procedure   HAC Associated Procedure   Combination Only   New/Revised April   New/Revised October

492   ICD-10-PCS 2023

Ø Medical and Surgical
L Tendons
D Extraction   Definition: Pulling or stripping out or off all or a portion of a body part by the use of force
      Explanation: The qualifier DIAGNOSTIC is used to identify extraction procedures that are biopsies

Body Part Character 4	Approach Character 5	Device Character 6	Qualifier Character 7
Ø Head and Neck Tendon	Ø Open	Z No Device	Z No Qualifier
1 Shoulder Tendon, Right			
2 Shoulder Tendon, Left			
3 Upper Arm Tendon, Right			
4 Upper Arm Tendon, Left			
5 Lower Arm and Wrist Tendon, Right			
6 Lower Arm and Wrist Tendon, Left			
7 Hand Tendon, Right			
8 Hand Tendon, Left			
9 Trunk Tendon, Right			
B Trunk Tendon, Left			
C Thorax Tendon, Right			
D Thorax Tendon, Left			
F Abdomen Tendon, Right			
G Abdomen Tendon, Left			
H Perineum Tendon			
J Hip Tendon, Right			
K Hip Tendon, Left			
L Upper Leg Tendon, Right			
M Upper Leg Tendon, Left			
N Lower Leg Tendon, Right Achilles tendon			
P Lower Leg Tendon, Left See N Lower Leg Tendon, Right			
Q Knee Tendon, Right Patellar tendon			
R Knee Tendon, Left See Q Knee Tendon, Right			
S Ankle Tendon, Right			
T Ankle Tendon, Left			
V Foot Tendon, Right			
W Foot Tendon, Left			

Ø Medical and Surgical
L Tendons
H Insertion   Definition: Putting in a nonbiological appliance that monitors, assists, performs, or prevents a physiological function but does not physically take the place of a body part
      Explanation: None

Body Part Character 4	Approach Character 5	Device Character 6	Qualifier Character 7
X Upper Tendon	Ø Open	Y Other Device	Z No Qualifier
Y Lower Tendon	3 Percutaneous		
	4 Percutaneous Endoscopic		

Non-OR   ØLH[X,Y][3,4]YZ

Ø Medical and Surgical
L Tendons
J Inspection   Definition: Visually and/or manually exploring a body part
      Explanation: Visual exploration may be performed with or without optical instrumentation. Manual exploration may be performed directly or through intervening body layers.

Body Part Character 4	Approach Character 5	Device Character 6	Qualifier Character 7
X Upper Tendon	Ø Open	Z No Device	Z No Qualifier
Y Lower Tendon	3 Percutaneous		
	4 Percutaneous Endoscopic		
	X External		

Non-OR   ØLJ[X,Y][3,X]ZZ

Ø Medical and Surgical
L Tendons
M Reattachment Definition: Putting back in or on all or a portion of a separated body part to its normal location or other suitable location

Explanation: Vascular circulation and nervous pathways may or may not be reestablished

Body Part Character 4	Approach Character 5	Device Character 6	Qualifier Character 7

Ø Head and Neck Tendon
1 Shoulder Tendon, Right
2 Shoulder Tendon, Left
3 Upper Arm Tendon, Right
4 Upper Arm Tendon, Left
5 Lower Arm and Wrist Tendon, Right
6 Lower Arm and Wrist Tendon, Left
7 Hand Tendon, Right
8 Hand Tendon, Left
9 Trunk Tendon, Right
B Trunk Tendon, Left
C Thorax Tendon, Right
D Thorax Tendon, Left
F Abdomen Tendon, Right
G Abdomen Tendon, Left
H Perineum Tendon
J Hip Tendon, Right
K Hip Tendon, Left
L Upper Leg Tendon, Right
M Upper Leg Tendon, Left
N Lower Leg Tendon, Right
   Achilles tendon
P Lower Leg Tendon, Left
   See N Lower Leg Tendon, Right
Q Knee Tendon, Right
   Patellar tendon
R Knee Tendon, Left
   See Q Knee Tendon, Right
S Ankle Tendon, Right
T Ankle Tendon, Left
V Foot Tendon, Right
W Foot Tendon, Left
	Ø Open
	4 Percutaneous Endoscopic
		Z No Device	Z No Qualifier

Ø Medical and Surgical
L Tendons
N Release Definition: Freeing a body part from an abnormal physical constraint by cutting or by the use of force

Explanation: Some of the restraining tissue may be taken out but none of the body part is taken out

Body Part Character 4	Approach Character 5	Device Character 6	Qualifier Character 7

Ø Head and Neck Tendon
1 Shoulder Tendon, Right
2 Shoulder Tendon, Left
3 Upper Arm Tendon, Right
4 Upper Arm Tendon, Left
5 Lower Arm and Wrist Tendon, Right
6 Lower Arm and Wrist Tendon, Left
7 Hand Tendon, Right
8 Hand Tendon, Left
9 Trunk Tendon, Right
B Trunk Tendon, Left
C Thorax Tendon, Right
D Thorax Tendon, Left
F Abdomen Tendon, Right
G Abdomen Tendon, Left
H Perineum Tendon
J Hip Tendon, Right
K Hip Tendon, Left
L Upper Leg Tendon, Right
M Upper Leg Tendon, Left
N Lower Leg Tendon, Right
   Achilles tendon
P Lower Leg Tendon, Left
   See N Lower Leg Tendon, Right
Q Knee Tendon, Right
   Patellar tendon
R Knee Tendon, Left
   See Q Knee Tendon, Right
S Ankle Tendon, Right
T Ankle Tendon, Left
V Foot Tendon, Right
W Foot Tendon, Left
	Ø Open
	3 Percutaneous
	4 Percutaneous Endoscopic
	X External
		Z No Device	Z No Qualifier

Non-OR ØLN[Ø,1,2,3,4,5,6,7,8,9,B,C,D,F,G,H,J,K,L,M,N,P,Q,R,S,T,V,W]XZZ

Non-OR Procedure DRG Non-OR Procedure Valid OR Procedure HAC Associated Procedure Combination Only New/Revised April New/Revised October

Ø   **Medical and Surgical**
L   **Tendons**
P   **Removal**   Definition: Taking out or off a device from a body part

Explanation: If a device is taken out and a similar device put in without cutting or puncturing the skin or mucous membrane, the procedure is coded to the root operation CHANGE. Otherwise, the procedure for taking out a device is coded to the root operation REMOVAL.

Body Part Character 4	Approach Character 5	Device Character 6	Qualifier Character 7
X Upper Tendon Y Lower Tendon	Ø Open 3 Percutaneous 4 Percutaneous Endoscopic	Ø Drainage Device 7 Autologous Tissue Substitute J Synthetic Substitute K Nonautologous Tissue Substitute Y Other Device	Z No Qualifier
X Upper Tendon Y Lower Tendon	X External	Ø Drainage Device	Z No Qualifier

Non-OR	ØLP[X,Y]3ØZ
Non-OR	ØLP[X,Y][3,4]YZ
Non-OR	ØLP[X,Y]XØZ

Ø   **Medical and Surgical**
L   **Tendons**
Q   **Repair**   Definition: Restoring, to the extent possible, a body part to its normal anatomic structure and function

Explanation: Used only when the method to accomplish the repair is not one of the other root operations

Body Part Character 4	Approach Character 5	Device Character 6	Qualifier Character 7

Ø Head and Neck Tendon
1 Shoulder Tendon, Right
2 Shoulder Tendon, Left
3 Upper Arm Tendon, Right
4 Upper Arm Tendon, Left
5 Lower Arm and Wrist Tendon, Right
6 Lower Arm and Wrist Tendon, Left
7 Hand Tendon, Right
8 Hand Tendon, Left
9 Trunk Tendon, Right
B Trunk Tendon, Left
C Thorax Tendon, Right
D Thorax Tendon, Left
F Abdomen Tendon, Right
G Abdomen Tendon, Left
H Perineum Tendon
J Hip Tendon, Right
K Hip Tendon, Left
L Upper Leg Tendon, Right
M Upper Leg Tendon, Left
N Lower Leg Tendon, Right
   Achilles tendon
P Lower Leg Tendon, Left
   See N Lower Leg Tendon, Right
Q Knee Tendon, Right
   Patellar tendon
R Knee Tendon, Left
   See Q Knee Tendon, Right
S Ankle Tendon, Right
T Ankle Tendon, Left
V Foot Tendon, Right
W Foot Tendon, Left
	Ø Open
	3 Percutaneous
	4 Percutaneous Endoscopic
		Z No Device	Z No Qualifier

Ø **Medical and Surgical**
L **Tendons**
R **Replacement**   Definition: Putting in or on biological or synthetic material that physically takes the place and/or function of all or a portion of a body part
                           Explanation: The body part may have been taken out or replaced, or may be taken out, physically eradicated, or rendered nonfunctional during
                           the REPLACEMENT procedure. A REMOVAL procedure is coded for taking out the device used in a previous replacement procedure.

Body Part Character 4	Approach Character 5	Device Character 6	Qualifier Character 7

Ø Head and Neck Tendon
1 Shoulder Tendon, Right
2 Shoulder Tendon, Left
3 Upper Arm Tendon, Right
4 Upper Arm Tendon, Left
5 Lower Arm and Wrist Tendon, Right
6 Lower Arm and Wrist Tendon, Left
7 Hand Tendon, Right
8 Hand Tendon, Left
9 Trunk Tendon, Right
B Trunk Tendon, Left
C Thorax Tendon, Right
D Thorax Tendon, Left
F Abdomen Tendon, Right
G Abdomen Tendon, Left
H Perineum Tendon
J Hip Tendon, Right
K Hip Tendon, Left
L Upper Leg Tendon, Right
M Upper Leg Tendon, Left
N Lower Leg Tendon, Right
   Achilles tendon
P Lower Leg Tendon, Left
   See N Lower Leg Tendon, Right
Q Knee Tendon, Right
   Patellar tendon
R Knee Tendon, Left
   See Q Knee Tendon, Right
S Ankle Tendon, Right
T Ankle Tendon, Left
V Foot Tendon, Right
W Foot Tendon, Left
	Ø Open
	4 Percutaneous Endoscopic
		7 Autologous Tissue Substitute
		J Synthetic Substitute
		K Nonautologous Tissue Substitute
			Z No Qualifier

Ø **Medical and Surgical**
L **Tendons**
S **Reposition**   Definition: Moving to its normal location, or other suitable location, all or a portion of a body part
                         Explanation: The body part is moved to a new location from an abnormal location, or from a normal location where it is not functioning
                         correctly. The body part may or may not be cut out or off to be moved to the new location.

Body Part Character 4	Approach Character 5	Device Character 6	Qualifier Character 7

Ø Head and Neck Tendon
1 Shoulder Tendon, Right
2 Shoulder Tendon, Left
3 Upper Arm Tendon, Right
4 Upper Arm Tendon, Left
5 Lower Arm and Wrist Tendon, Right
6 Lower Arm and Wrist Tendon, Left
7 Hand Tendon, Right
8 Hand Tendon, Left
9 Trunk Tendon, Right
B Trunk Tendon, Left
C Thorax Tendon, Right
D Thorax Tendon, Left
F Abdomen Tendon, Right
G Abdomen Tendon, Left
H Perineum Tendon
J Hip Tendon, Right
K Hip Tendon, Left
L Upper Leg Tendon, Right
M Upper Leg Tendon, Left
N Lower Leg Tendon, Right
   Achilles tendon
P Lower Leg Tendon, Left
   See N Lower Leg Tendon, Right
Q Knee Tendon, Right
   Patellar tendon
R Knee Tendon, Left
   See Q Knee Tendon, Right
S Ankle Tendon, Right
T Ankle Tendon, Left
V Foot Tendon, Right
W Foot Tendon, Left
	Ø Open
	4 Percutaneous Endoscopic
		Z No Device	Z No Qualifier

ØLR–ØLS

Non-OR Procedure   DRG Non-OR Procedure   Valid OR Procedure   HAC Associated Procedure   Combination Only   New/Revised April   New/Revised October
496
ICD-10-PCS 2023

0   **Medical and Surgical**
L   **Tendons**
T   **Resection**   Definition: Cutting out or off, without replacement, all of a body part
                      Explanation: None

Body Part Character 4	Approach Character 5	Device Character 6	Qualifier Character 7

0   Head and Neck Tendon
1   Shoulder Tendon, Right
2   Shoulder Tendon, Left
3   Upper Arm Tendon, Right
4   Upper Arm Tendon, Left
5   Lower Arm and Wrist Tendon, Right
6   Lower Arm and Wrist Tendon, Left
7   Hand Tendon, Right
8   Hand Tendon, Left
9   Trunk Tendon, Right
B   Trunk Tendon, Left
C   Thorax Tendon, Right
D   Thorax Tendon, Left
F   Abdomen Tendon, Right
G   Abdomen Tendon, Left
H   Perineum Tendon
J   Hip Tendon, Right
K   Hip Tendon, Left
L   Upper Leg Tendon, Right
M   Upper Leg Tendon, Left
N   Lower Leg Tendon, Right
     Achilles tendon
P   Lower Leg Tendon, Left
     See N Lower Leg Tendon, Right
Q   Knee Tendon, Right
     Patellar tendon
R   Knee Tendon, Left
     See Q Knee Tendon, Right
S   Ankle Tendon, Right
T   Ankle Tendon, Left
V   Foot Tendon, Right
W   Foot Tendon, Left
	0 Open
	4 Percutaneous Endoscopic
		Z No Device	Z No Qualifier

0   **Medical and Surgical**
L   **Tendons**
U   **Supplement**   Definition: Putting in or on biological or synthetic material that physically reinforces and/or augments the function of a portion of a body part
                      Explanation: The biological material is non-living, or is living and from the same individual. The body part may have been previously replaced, and the SUPPLEMENT procedure is performed to physically reinforce and/or augment the function of the replaced body part.

Body Part Character 4	Approach Character 5	Device Character 6	Qualifier Character 7

0   Head and Neck Tendon
1   Shoulder Tendon, Right
2   Shoulder Tendon, Left
3   Upper Arm Tendon, Right
4   Upper Arm Tendon, Left
5   Lower Arm and Wrist Tendon, Right
6   Lower Arm and Wrist Tendon, Left
7   Hand Tendon, Right
8   Hand Tendon, Left
9   Trunk Tendon, Right
B   Trunk Tendon, Left
C   Thorax Tendon, Right
D   Thorax Tendon, Left
F   Abdomen Tendon, Right
G   Abdomen Tendon, Left
H   Perineum Tendon
J   Hip Tendon, Right
K   Hip Tendon, Left
L   Upper Leg Tendon, Right
M   Upper Leg Tendon, Left
N   Lower Leg Tendon, Right
     Achilles tendon
P   Lower Leg Tendon, Left
     See N Lower Leg Tendon, Right
Q   Knee Tendon, Right
     Patellar tendon
R   Knee Tendon, Left
     See Q Knee Tendon, Right
S   Ankle Tendon, Right
T   Ankle Tendon, Left
V   Foot Tendon, Right
W   Foot Tendon, Left
	0 Open
	4 Percutaneous Endoscopic
		7 Autologous Tissue Substitute
		J Synthetic Substitute
		K Nonautologous Tissue Substitute
			Z No Qualifier

Ø   **Medical and Surgical**
L   **Tendons**
W   **Revision**   Definition: Correcting, to the extent possible, a portion of a malfunctioning device or the position of a displaced device
                      Explanation: Revision can include correcting a malfunctioning or displaced device by taking out or putting in components of the device such as a screw or pin

Body Part Character 4	Approach Character 5	Device Character 6	Qualifier Character 7
X Upper Tendon **Y** Lower Tendon	**Ø** Open **3** Percutaneous **4** Percutaneous Endoscopic	**Ø** Drainage Device **7** Autologous Tissue Substitute **J** Synthetic Substitute **K** Nonautologous Tissue Substitute **Y** Other Device	**Z** No Qualifier
X Upper Tendon **Y** Lower Tendon	**X** External	**Ø** Drainage Device **7** Autologous Tissue Substitute **J** Synthetic Substitute **K** Nonautologous Tissue Substitute	**Z** No Qualifier

Non-OR   ØLW[X,Y][3,4]YZ
Non-OR   ØLW[X,Y]X[Ø,7,J,K]Z

Ø   **Medical and Surgical**
L   **Tendons**
X   **Transfer**   Definition: Moving, without taking out, all or a portion of a body part to another location to take over the function of all or a portion of a body part
                     Explanation: The body part transferred remains connected to its vascular and nervous supply

Body Part Character 4	Approach Character 5	Device Character 6	Qualifier Character 7

Ø Head and Neck Tendon
1 Shoulder Tendon, Right
2 Shoulder Tendon, Left
3 Upper Arm Tendon, Right
4 Upper Arm Tendon, Left
5 Lower Arm and Wrist Tendon, Right
6 Lower Arm and Wrist Tendon, Left
7 Hand Tendon, Right
8 Hand Tendon, Left
9 Trunk Tendon, Right
B Trunk Tendon, Left
C Thorax Tendon, Right
D Thorax Tendon, Left
F Abdomen Tendon, Right
G Abdomen Tendon, Left
H Perineum Tendon
J Hip Tendon, Right
K Hip Tendon, Left
L Upper Leg Tendon, Right
M Upper Leg Tendon, Left
N Lower Leg Tendon, Right
    Achilles tendon
P Lower Leg Tendon, Left
    See N Lower Leg Tendon, Right
Q Knee Tendon, Right
    Patellar tendon
R Knee Tendon, Left
    See Q Knee Tendon, Right
S Ankle Tendon, Right
T Ankle Tendon, Left
V Foot Tendon, Right
W Foot Tendon, Left
	Ø Open
	4 Percutaneous Endoscopic
		Z No Device	**Z** No Qualifier

Non-OR Procedure   DRG Non-OR Procedure   Valid OR Procedure   HAC Associated Procedure   Combination Only   New/Revised April   New/Revised October

498   ØLW–ØLX   ICD-10-PCS 2023

Bursae and Ligaments ØM2–ØMX

Character Meanings*

This Character Meaning table is provided as a guide to assist the user in the identification of character members that may be found in this section of code tables. It **SHOULD NOT** be used to build a PCS code.

Operation–Character 3		Body Part–Character 4		Approach–Character 5		Device–Character 6		Qualifier–Character 7	
2	Change	Ø	Head and Neck Bursa and Ligament	Ø	Open	Ø	Drainage Device	X	Diagnostic
5	Destruction	1	Shoulder Bursa and Ligament, Right	3	Percutaneous	7	Autologous Tissue Substitute	Z	No Qualifier
8	Division	2	Shoulder Bursa and Ligament, Left	4	Percutaneous Endoscopic	J	Synthetic Substitute		
9	Drainage	3	Elbow Bursa and Ligament, Right	X	External	K	Nonautologous Tissue Substitute		
B	Excision	4	Elbow Bursa and Ligament, Left			Y	Other Device		
C	Extirpation	5	Wrist Bursa and Ligament, Right			Z	No Device		
D	Extraction	6	Wrist Bursa and Ligament, Left						
H	Insertion	7	Hand Bursa and Ligament, Right						
J	Inspection	8	Hand Bursa and Ligament, Left						
M	Reattachment	9	Upper Extremity Bursa and Ligament, Right						
N	Release	B	Upper Extremity Bursa and Ligament, Left						
P	Removal	C	Upper Spine Bursa and Ligament						
Q	Repair	D	Lower Spine Bursa and Ligament						
R	Replacement	F	Sternum Bursa and Ligament						
S	Reposition	G	Rib(s) Bursa and Ligament						
T	Resection	H	Abdomen Bursa and Ligament, Right						
U	Supplement	J	Abdomen Bursa and Ligament, Left						
W	Revision	K	Perineum Bursa and Ligament						
X	Transfer	L	Hip Bursa and Ligament, Right						
		M	Hip Bursa and Ligament, Left						
		N	Knee Bursa and Ligament, Right						
		P	Knee Bursa and Ligament, Left						
		Q	Ankle Bursa and Ligament, Right						
		R	Ankle Bursa and Ligament, Left						
		S	Foot Bursa and Ligament, Right						
		T	Foot Bursa and Ligament, Left						
		V	Lower Extremity Bursa and Ligament, Right						
		W	Lower Extremity Bursa and Ligament, Left						
		X	Upper Bursa and Ligament						
		Y	Lower Bursa and Ligament						

* Includes synovial membrane.

AHA Coding Clinic for table ØMB
2018, 3Q, 17   Excisional debridement of periosteum

AHA Coding Clinic for table ØMM
2013, 3Q, 20   Superior labrum anterior posterior (SLAP) repair and subacromial decompression

AHA Coding Clinic for table ØMQ
2014, 3Q, 9   Interspinous ligamentoplasty

AHA Coding Clinic for table ØMT
2017, 2Q, 21   Arthroscopic anterior cruciate ligament revision using autograft with anterolateral ligament reconstruction

AHA Coding Clinic for table ØMU
2017, 2Q, 21   Arthroscopic anterior cruciate ligament revision using autograft with anterolateral ligament reconstruction

Shoulder Ligaments

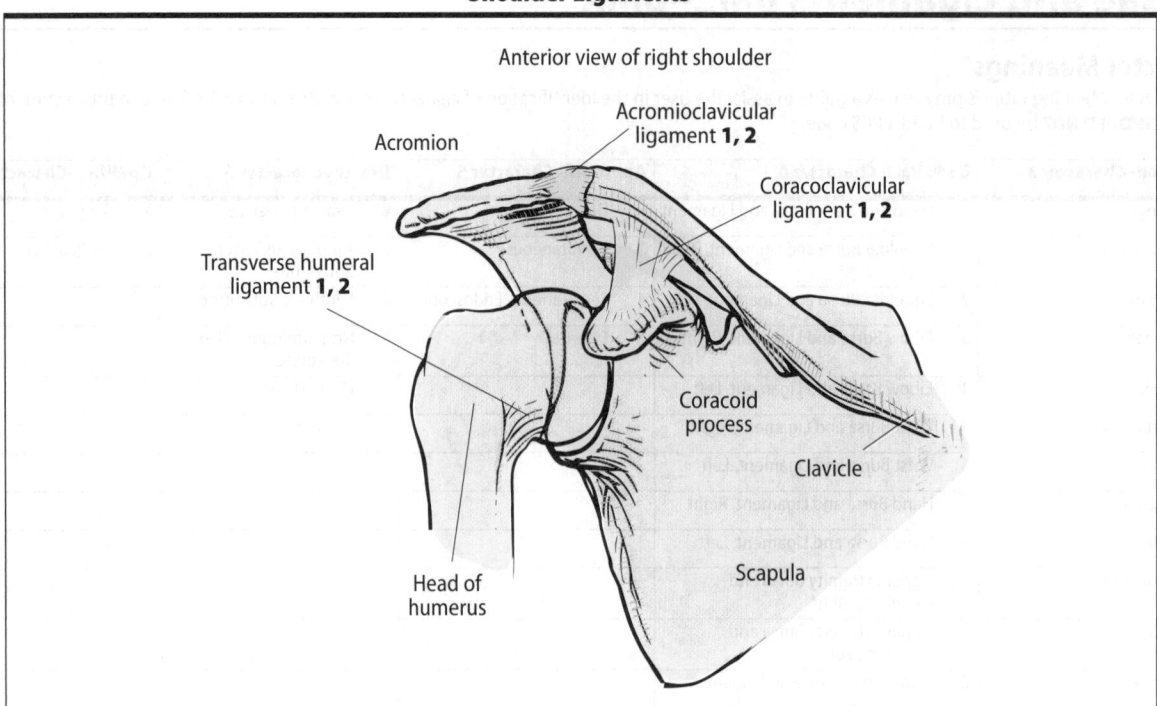

Anterior view of right shoulder

Acromion

Acromioclavicular ligament **1, 2**

Coracoclavicular ligament **1, 2**

Transverse humeral ligament **1, 2**

Coracoid process

Clavicle

Head of humerus

Scapula

Knee Bursae

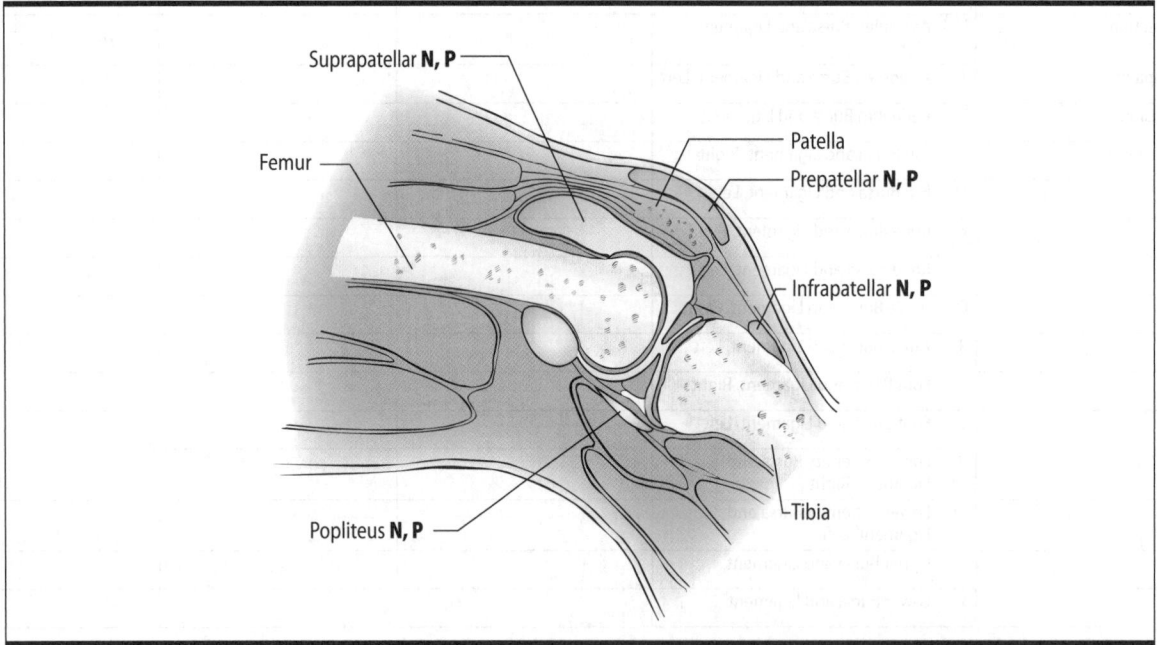

Suprapatellar **N, P**

Femur

Patella

Prepatellar **N, P**

Infrapatellar **N, P**

Popliteus **N, P**

Tibia

Knee Ligaments

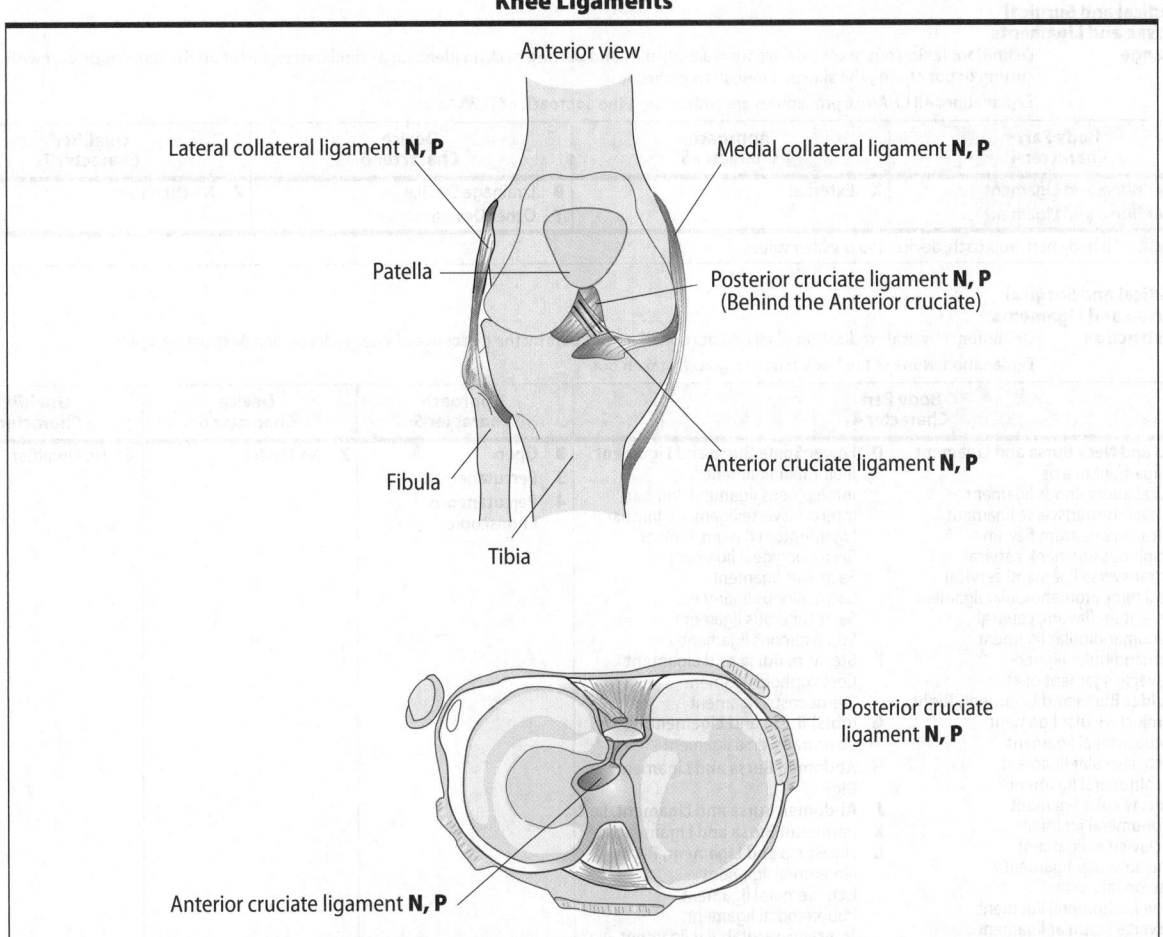

Anterior view

Lateral collateral ligament **N, P**

Medial collateral ligament **N, P**

Patella

Posterior cruciate ligament **N, P**
(Behind the Anterior cruciate)

Anterior cruciate ligament **N, P**

Fibula

Tibia

Posterior cruciate ligament **N, P**

Anterior cruciate ligament **N, P**

Wrist Ligaments

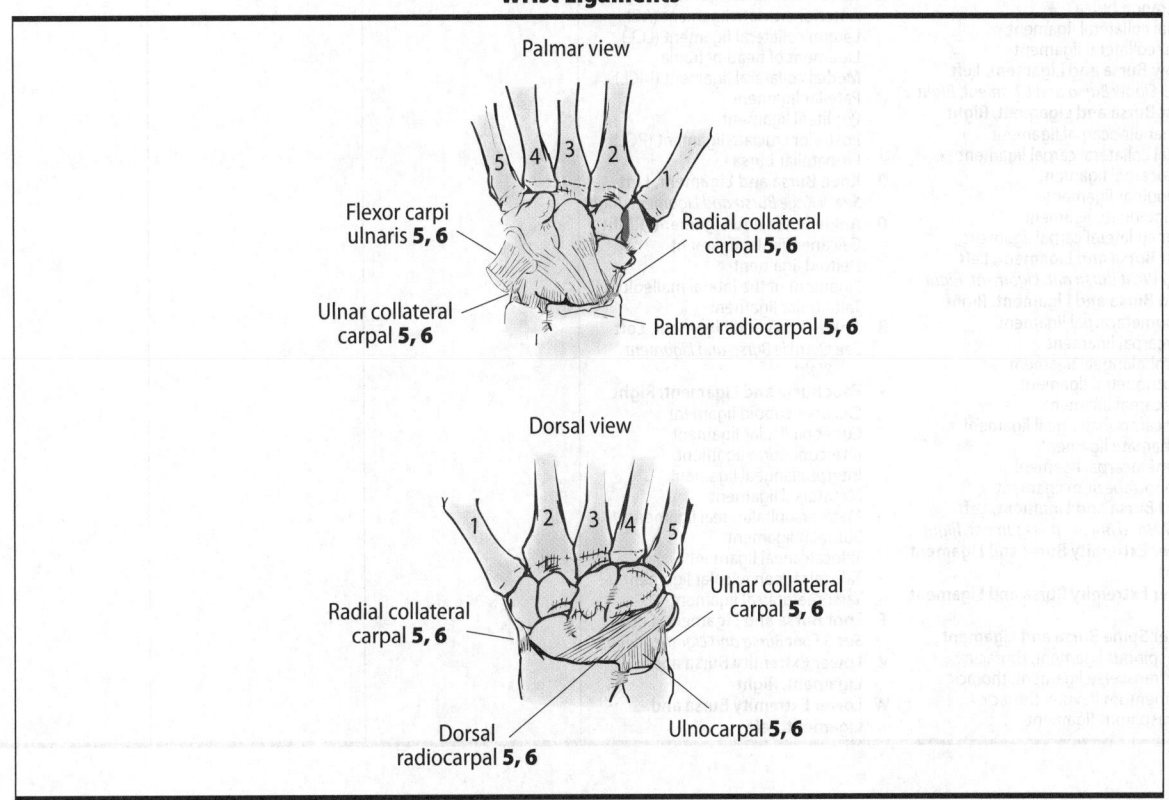

Palmar view

5 4 3 2 1

Flexor carpi ulnaris **5, 6**

Radial collateral carpal **5, 6**

Ulnar collateral carpal **5, 6**

Palmar radiocarpal **5, 6**

Dorsal view

1 2 3 4 5

Radial collateral carpal **5, 6**

Ulnar collateral carpal **5, 6**

Dorsal radiocarpal **5, 6**

Ulnocarpal **5, 6**

Bursae and Ligaments

Ø   **Medical and Surgical**
M   **Bursae and Ligaments**
2   **Change**   Definition: Taking out or off a device from a body part and putting back an identical or similar device in or on the same body part without cutting or puncturing the skin or a mucous membrane

                           Explanation: All CHANGE procedures are coded using the approach EXTERNAL

Body Part Character 4	Approach Character 5	Device Character 6	Qualifier Character 7
X Upper Bursa and Ligament Y Lower Bursa and Ligament	X External	Ø Drainage Device Y Other Device	Z No Qualifier

> **Non-OR**   All body part, approach, device, and qualifier values

Ø   **Medical and Surgical**
M   **Bursae and Ligaments**
5   **Destruction**   Definition: Physical eradication of all or a portion of a body part by the direct use of energy, force, or a destructive agent

                           Explanation: None of the body part is physically taken out

Body Part Character 4	Approach Character 5	Device Character 6	Qualifier Character 7

Ø   **Head and Neck Bursa and Ligament**
    Alar ligament of axis
    Cervical interspinous ligament
    Cervical intertransverse ligament
    Cervical ligamentum flavum
    Interspinous ligament, cervical
    Intertransverse ligament, cervical
    Lateral temporomandibular ligament
    Ligamentum flavum, cervical
    Sphenomandibular ligament
    Stylomandibular ligament
    Transverse ligament of atlas
1   **Shoulder Bursa and Ligament, Right**
    Acromioclavicular ligament
    Coracoacromial ligament
    Coracoclavicular ligament
    Coracohumeral ligament
    Costoclavicular ligament
    Glenohumeral ligament
    Interclavicular ligament
    Sternoclavicular ligament
    Subacromial bursa
    Transverse humeral ligament
    Transverse scapular ligament
2   **Shoulder Bursa and Ligament, Left**
    See 1 Shoulder Bursa and Ligament, Right
3   **Elbow Bursa and Ligament, Right**
    Annular ligament
    Olecranon bursa
    Radial collateral ligament
    Ulnar collateral ligament
4   **Elbow Bursa and Ligament, Left**
    See 3 Elbow Bursa and Ligament, Right
5   **Wrist Bursa and Ligament, Right**
    Palmar ulnocarpal ligament
    Radial collateral carpal ligament
    Radiocarpal ligament
    Radioulnar ligament
    Scapholunate ligament
    Ulnar collateral carpal ligament
6   **Wrist Bursa and Ligament, Left**
    See 5 Wrist Bursa and Ligament, Right
7   **Hand Bursa and Ligament, Right**
    Carpometacarpal ligament
    Intercarpal ligament
    Interphalangeal ligament
    Lunotriquetral ligament
    Metacarpal ligament
    Metacarpophalangeal ligament
    Pisohamate ligament
    Pisometacarpal ligament
    Scaphotrapezium ligament
8   **Hand Bursa and Ligament, Left**
    See 7 Hand Bursa and Ligament, Right
9   **Upper Extremity Bursa and Ligament, Right**
B   **Upper Extremity Bursa and Ligament, Left**
C   **Upper Spine Bursa and Ligament**
    Interspinous ligament, thoracic
    Intertransverse ligament, thoracic
    Ligamentum flavum, thoracic
    Supraspinous ligament
 	
D   **Lower Spine Bursa and Ligament**
    Iliolumbar ligament
    Interspinous ligament, lumbar
    Intertransverse ligament, lumbar
    Ligamentum flavum, lumbar
    Sacrococcygeal ligament
    Sacroiliac ligament
    Sacrospinous ligament
    Sacrotuberous ligament
    Supraspinous ligament
F   **Sternum Bursa and Ligament**
    Costoxiphoid ligament
    Sternocostal ligament
G   **Rib(s) Bursa and Ligament**
    Costotransverse ligament
H   **Abdomen Bursa and Ligament, Right**
J   **Abdomen Bursa and Ligament, Left**
K   **Perineum Bursa and Ligament**
L   **Hip Bursa and Ligament, Right**
    Iliofemoral ligament
    Ischiofemoral ligament
    Pubofemoral ligament
    Transverse acetabular ligament
    Trochanteric bursa
M   **Hip Bursa and Ligament, Left**
    See L Hip Bursa and Ligament, Right
N   **Knee Bursa and Ligament, Right**
    Anterior cruciate ligament (ACL)
    Lateral collateral ligament (LCL)
    Ligament of head of fibula
    Medial collateral ligament (MCL)
    Patellar ligament
    Popliteal ligament
    Posterior cruciate ligament (PCL)
    Prepatellar bursa
P   **Knee Bursa and Ligament, Left**
    See N Knee Bursa and Ligament, Right
Q   **Ankle Bursa and Ligament, Right**
    Calcaneofibular ligament
    Deltoid ligament
    Ligament of the lateral malleolus
    Talofibular ligament
R   **Ankle Bursa and Ligament, Left**
    See Q Ankle Bursa and Ligament, Right
S   **Foot Bursa and Ligament, Right**
    Calcaneocuboid ligament
    Cuneonavicular ligament
    Intercuneiform ligament
    Interphalangeal ligament
    Metatarsal ligament
    Metatarsophalangeal ligament
    Subtalar ligament
    Talocalcaneal ligament
    Talocalcaneonavicular ligament
    Tarsometatarsal ligament
T   **Foot Bursa and Ligament, Left**
    See S Foot Bursa and Ligament, Right
V   **Lower Extremity Bursa and Ligament, Right**
W   **Lower Extremity Bursa and Ligament, Left**
	Ø Open
	3 Percutaneous
	4 Percutaneous Endoscopic
		Z No Device	Z No Qualifier

Non-OR Procedure   DRG Non-OR Procedure   Valid OR Procedure   HAC Associated Procedure   Combination Only   New/Revised April   New/Revised October

502   ICD-10-PCS 2023

Bursae and Ligaments

Ø   **Medical and Surgical**
M   **Bursae and Ligaments**
8   **Division**   Definition: Cutting into a body part, without draining fluids and/or gases from the body part, in order to separate or transect a body part
                 Explanation: All or a portion of the body part is separated into two or more portions

Body Part Character 4		Approach Character 5	Device Character 6	Qualifier Character 7

Ø   **Head and Neck Bursa and Ligament**
    Alar ligament of axis
    Cervical interspinous ligament
    Cervical intertransverse ligament
    Cervical ligamentum flavum
    Interspinous ligament, cervical
    Intertransverse ligament, cervical
    Lateral temporomandibular ligament
    Ligamentum flavum, cervical
    Sphenomandibular ligament
    Stylomandibular ligament
    Transverse ligament of atlas
	D **Lower Spine Bursa and Ligament**
	    Iliolumbar ligament
	    Interspinous ligament, lumbar
	    Intertransverse ligament, lumbar
	    Ligamentum flavum, lumbar
	    Sacrococcygeal ligament
	    Sacroiliac ligament
	    Sacrospinous ligament
	    Sacrotuberous ligament
	    Supraspinous ligament
		Ø Open
		3 Percutaneous
		4 Percutaneous Endoscopic
			Z No Device	**Z** No Qualifier

1   **Shoulder Bursa and Ligament, Right**
    Acromioclavicular ligament
    Coracoacromial ligament
    Coracoclavicular ligament
    Coracohumeral ligament
    Costoclavicular ligament
    Glenohumeral ligament
    Interclavicular ligament
    Sternoclavicular ligament
    Subacromial bursa
    Transverse humeral ligament
    Transverse scapular ligament
	F **Sternum Bursa and Ligament**
	    Costoxiphoid ligament
	    Sternocostal ligament
	
	G **Rib(s) Bursa and Ligament**
	    Costotransverse ligament
	
	H **Abdomen Bursa and Ligament, Right**
	
	J **Abdomen Bursa and Ligament, Left**			

2   **Shoulder Bursa and Ligament, Left**
    See 1 Shoulder Bursa and Ligament, Right
	K **Perineum Bursa and Ligament**
	
	L **Hip Bursa and Ligament, Right**
	    Iliofemoral ligament
	    Ischiofemoral ligament
	    Pubofemoral ligament
	    Transverse acetabular ligament
	    Trochanteric bursa			

3   **Elbow Bursa and Ligament, Right**
    Annular ligament
    Olecranon bursa
    Radial collateral ligament
    Ulnar collateral ligament
	M **Hip Bursa and Ligament, Left**
	    See L Hip Bursa and Ligament, Right			

4   **Elbow Bursa and Ligament, Left**
    See 3 Elbow Bursa and Ligament, Right
	N **Knee Bursa and Ligament, Right**
	    Anterior cruciate ligament (ACL)
	    Lateral collateral ligament (LCL)
	    Ligament of head of fibula
	    Medial collateral ligament (MCL)
	    Patellar ligament
	    Popliteal ligament
	    Posterior cruciate ligament (PCL)
	    Prepatellar bursa			

5   **Wrist Bursa and Ligament, Right**
    Palmar ulnocarpal ligament
    Radial collateral carpal ligament
    Radiocarpal ligament
    Radioulnar ligament
    Scapholunate ligament
    Ulnar collateral carpal ligament
	P **Knee Bursa and Ligament, Left**
	    See N Knee Bursa and Ligament, Right			

6   **Wrist Bursa and Ligament, Left**
    See 5 Wrist Bursa and Ligament, Right
	Q **Ankle Bursa and Ligament, Right**
	    Calcaneofibular ligament
	    Deltoid ligament
	    Ligament of the lateral malleolus
	    Talofibular ligament			

7   **Hand Bursa and Ligament, Right**
    Carpometacarpal ligament
    Intercarpal ligament
    Interphalangeal ligament
    Lunotriquetral ligament
    Metacarpal ligament
    Metacarpophalangeal ligament
    Pisohamate ligament
    Pisometacarpal ligament
    Scaphotrapezium ligament
	R **Ankle Bursa and Ligament, Left**
	    See Q Ankle Bursa and Ligament, Right
	
	S **Foot Bursa and Ligament, Right**
	    Calcaneocuboid ligament
	    Cuneonavicular ligament
	    Intercuneiform ligament
	    Interphalangeal ligament
	    Metatarsal ligament
	    Metatarsophalangeal ligament
	    Subtalar ligament
	    Talocalcaneal ligament
	    Talocalcaneonavicular ligament
	    Tarsometatarsal ligament			

8   **Hand Bursa and Ligament, Left**
    See 7 Hand Bursa and Ligament, Right
	T **Foot Bursa and Ligament, Left**
	    See S Foot Bursa and Ligament, Right			

9 **Upper Extremity Bursa and Ligament, Right**	**V** **Lower Extremity Bursa and Ligament, Right**			
B **Upper Extremity Bursa and Ligament, Left**	**W** **Lower Extremity Bursa and Ligament, Left**			

C   **Upper Spine Bursa and Ligament**
    Interspinous ligament, thoracic
    Intertransverse ligament, thoracic
    Ligamentum flavum, thoracic
    Supraspinous ligament				

NC Noncovered Procedure   **LC** Limited Coverage   **OA** Questionable OB Admit   **NT** New Tech Add-on   **⊞** Combination Member   ♂ Male   ♀ Female

ICD-10-PCS 2023   **503**

Ø   Medical and Surgical
M   Bursae and Ligaments
9   Drainage   Definition: Taking or letting out fluids and/or gases from a body part
                          Explanation: The qualifier DIAGNOSTIC is used to identify drainage procedures that are biopsies

Body Part Character 4		Approach Character 5	Device Character 6	Qualifier Character 7
Ø Head and Neck Bursa and Ligament	**D Lower Spine Bursa and Ligament**	**Ø Open**	**Ø Drainage Device**	**Z No Qualifier**
Alar ligament of axis	Iliolumbar ligament	**3 Percutaneous**		
Cervical interspinous ligament	Interspinous ligament, lumbar	**4 Percutaneous Endoscopic**		
Cervical intertransverse ligament	Intertransverse ligament, lumbar			
Cervical ligamentum flavum	Ligamentum flavum, lumbar			
Interspinous ligament, cervical	Sacrococcygeal ligament			
Intertransverse ligament, cervical	Sacroiliac ligament			
Lateral temporomandibular ligament	Sacrospinous ligament			
Ligamentum flavum, cervical	Sacrotuberous ligament			
Sphenomandibular ligament	Supraspinous ligament			
Stylomandibular ligament	**F Sternum Bursa and Ligament**			
Transverse ligament of atlas	Costoxiphoid ligament			
1 Shoulder Bursa and Ligament, Right	Sternocostal ligament			
Acromioclavicular ligament	**G Rib(s) Bursa and Ligament**			
Coracoacromial ligament	Costotransverse ligament			
Coracoclavicular ligament	**H Abdomen Bursa and Ligament, Right**			
Coracohumeral ligament	**J Abdomen Bursa and Ligament, Left**			
Costoclavicular ligament	**K Perineum Bursa and Ligament**			
Glenohumeral ligament	**L Hip Bursa and Ligament, Right**			
Interclavicular ligament	Iliofemoral ligament			
Sternoclavicular ligament	Ischiofemoral ligament			
Subacromial bursa	Pubofemoral ligament			
Transverse humeral ligament	Transverse acetabular ligament			
Transverse scapular ligament	Trochanteric bursa			
2 Shoulder Bursa and Ligament, Left	**M Hip Bursa and Ligament, Left**			
See 1 Shoulder Bursa and Ligament, Right	*See L Hip Bursa and Ligament, Right*			
3 Elbow Bursa and Ligament, Right	**N Knee Bursa and Ligament, Right**			
Annular ligament	Anterior cruciate ligament (ACL)			
Olecranon bursa	Lateral collateral ligament (LCL)			
Radial collateral ligament	Ligament of head of fibula			
Ulnar collateral ligament	Medial collateral ligament (MCL)			
4 Elbow Bursa and Ligament, Left	Patellar ligament			
See 3 Elbow Bursa and Ligament, Right	Popliteal ligament			
5 Wrist Bursa and Ligament, Right	Posterior cruciate ligament (PCL)			
Palmar ulnocarpal ligament	Prepatellar bursa			
Radial collateral carpal ligament	**P Knee Bursa and Ligament, Left**			
Radiocarpal ligament	*See N Knee Bursa and Ligament, Right*			
Radioulnar ligament	**Q Ankle Bursa and Ligament, Right**			
Scapholunate ligament	Calcaneofibular ligament			
Ulnar collateral carpal ligament	Deltoid ligament			
6 Wrist Bursa and Ligament, Left	Ligament of the lateral malleolus			
See 5 Wrist Bursa and Ligament, Right	Talofibular ligament			
7 Hand Bursa and Ligament, Right	**R Ankle Bursa and Ligament, Left**			
Carpometacarpal ligament	*See Q Ankle Bursa and Ligament, Right*			
Intercarpal ligament	**S Foot Bursa and Ligament, Right**			
Interphalangeal ligament	Calcaneocuboid ligament			
Lunotriquetral ligament	Cuneonavicular ligament			
Metacarpal ligament	Intercuneiform ligament			
Metacarpophalangeal ligament	Interphalangeal ligament			
Pisohamate ligament	Metatarsal ligament			
Pisometacarpal ligament	Metatarsophalangeal ligament			
Scaphotrapezium ligament	Subtalar ligament			
8 Hand Bursa and Ligament, Left	Talocalcaneal ligament			
See 7 Hand Bursa and Ligament, Right	Talocalcaneonavicular ligament			
9 Upper Extremity Bursa and Ligament, Right	Tarsometatarsal ligament			
B Upper Extremity Bursa and Ligament, Left	**T Foot Bursa and Ligament, Left**			
C Upper Spine Bursa and Ligament	*See S Foot Bursa and Ligament, Right*			
Interspinous ligament, thoracic	**V Lower Extremity Bursa and Ligament, Right**			
Intertransverse ligament, thoracic	**W Lower Extremity Bursa and Ligament, Left**			
Ligamentum flavum, thoracic				
Supraspinous ligament				

Non-OR   ØM9[Ø,1,2,3,4,5,6,7,8,9,B,C,D,F,G,H,J,K,L,M,N,P,Q,R,S,T,V,W]3ØZ
Non-OR   ØM9[1,2,3,4,7,8,9,B,C,D,F,G,H,J,K,L,M,V,W]4ØZ

ØM9 Continued on next page

Ø Medical and Surgical
M Bursae and Ligaments
9 Drainage   Definition: Taking or letting out fluids and/or gases from a body part

Explanation: The qualifier DIAGNOSTIC is used to identify drainage procedures that are biopsies

Body Part Character 4		Approach Character 5	Device Character 6	Qualifier Character 7
Ø Head and Neck Bursa and Ligament Alar ligament of axis Cervical interspinous ligament Cervical intertransverse ligament Cervical ligamentum flavum Interspinous ligament, cervical Intertransverse ligament, cervical Lateral temporomandibular ligament Ligamentum flavum, cervical Sphenomandibular ligament Stylomandibular ligament Transverse ligament of atlas **1 Shoulder Bursa and Ligament, Right** Acromioclavicular ligament Coracoacromial ligament Coracoclavicular ligament Coracohumeral ligament Costoclavicular ligament Glenohumeral ligament Interclavicular ligament Sternoclavicular ligament Subacromial bursa Transverse humeral ligament Transverse scapular ligament **2 Shoulder Bursa and Ligament, Left** *See 1 Shoulder Bursa and Ligament, Right* **3 Elbow Bursa and Ligament, Right** Annular ligament Olecranon bursa Radial collateral ligament Ulnar collateral ligament **4 Elbow Bursa and Ligament, Left** *See 3 Elbow Bursa and Ligament, Right* **5 Wrist Bursa and Ligament, Right** Palmar ulnocarpal ligament Radial collateral carpal ligament Radiocarpal ligament Radioulnar ligament Scapholunate ligament Ulnar collateral carpal ligament **6 Wrist Bursa and Ligament, Left** *See 5 Wrist Bursa and Ligament, Right* **7 Hand Bursa and Ligament, Right** Carpometacarpal ligament Intercarpal ligament Interphalangeal ligament Lunotriquetral ligament Metacarpal ligament Metacarpophalangeal ligament Pisohamate ligament Pisometacarpal ligament Scaphotrapezium ligament **8 Hand Bursa and Ligament, Left** *See 7 Hand Bursa and Ligament, Right* **9 Upper Extremity Bursa and Ligament, Right** **B Upper Extremity Bursa and Ligament, Left** **C Upper Spine Bursa and Ligament** Interspinous ligament, thoracic Intertransverse ligament, thoracic Ligamentum flavum, thoracic Supraspinous ligament	**D Lower Spine Bursa and Ligament** Iliolumbar ligament Interspinous ligament, lumbar Intertransverse ligament, lumbar Ligamentum flavum, lumbar Sacrococcygeal ligament Sacroiliac ligament Sacrospinous ligament Sacrotuberous ligament Supraspinous ligament **F Sternum Bursa and Ligament** Costoxiphoid ligament Sternocostal ligament **G Rib(s) Bursa and Ligament** Costotransverse ligament **H Abdomen Bursa and Ligament, Right** **J Abdomen Bursa and Ligament, Left** **K Perineum Bursa and Ligament** **L Hip Bursa and Ligament, Right** Iliofemoral ligament Ischiofemoral ligament Pubofemoral ligament Transverse acetabular ligament Trochanteric bursa **M Hip Bursa and Ligament, Left** *See L Hip Bursa and Ligament, Left* **N Knee Bursa and Ligament, Right** Anterior cruciate ligament (ACL) Lateral collateral ligament (LCL) Ligament of head of fibula Medial collateral ligament (MCL) Patellar ligament Popliteal ligament Posterior cruciate ligament (PCL) Prepatellar bursa **P Knee Bursa and Ligament, Left** *See N Knee Bursa and Ligament, Right* **Q Ankle Bursa and Ligament, Right** Calcaneofibular ligament Deltoid ligament Ligament of the lateral malleolus Talofibular ligament **R Ankle Bursa and Ligament, Left** *See Q Ankle Bursa and Ligament, Right* **S Foot Bursa and Ligament, Right** Calcaneocuboid ligament Cuneonavicular ligament Intercuneiform ligament Interphalangeal ligament Metatarsal ligament Metatarsophalangeal ligament Subtalar ligament Talocalcaneal ligament Talocalcaneonavicular ligament Tarsometatarsal ligament **T Foot Bursa and Ligament, Left** *See S Foot Bursa and Ligament, Right* **V Lower Extremity Bursa and Ligament, Right** **W Lower Extremity Bursa and Ligament, Left**	**Ø Open** **3 Percutaneous** **4 Percutaneous Endoscopic**	**Z No Device**	**X Diagnostic** **Z No Qualifier**

Non-OR	ØM9[Ø,1,2,3,4,5,6,7,8,C,D,F,G,L,M,N,P,Q,R,S,T][Ø,3,4]ZX
Non-OR	ØM9[Ø,1,2,3,4,5,6,7,8,9,B,C,D,F,G,H,J,K,L,M,N,P,Q,R,S,T,V,W]3ZZ
Non-OR	ØM9[Ø,5,6,7,8,9,B,C,D,F,G,H,J,K,N,P,Q,R,S,T,V,W]4ZZ

NC Noncovered Procedure   LC Limited Coverage   QA Questionable OB Admit   NT New Tech Add-on   ⊞ Combination Member   ♂ Male   ♀ Female

ICD-10-PCS 2023   505

Bursae and Ligaments

Ø   Medical and Surgical
M   Bursae and Ligaments
B   Excision   Definition: Cutting out or off, without replacement, a portion of a body part
                Explanation: The qualifier DIAGNOSTIC is used to identify excision procedures that are biopsies

Body Part Character 4		Approach Character 5	Device Character 6	Qualifier Character 7

Ø Head and Neck Bursa and Ligament
  Alar ligament of axis
  Cervical interspinous ligament
  Cervical intertransverse ligament
  Cervical ligamentum flavum
  Interspinous ligament, cervical
  Intertransverse ligament, cervical
  Lateral temporomandibular
    ligament
  Ligamentum flavum, cervical
  Sphenomandibular ligament
  Stylomandibular ligament
  Transverse ligament of atlas
1 Shoulder Bursa and Ligament, Right
  Acromioclavicular ligament
  Coracoacromial ligament
  Coracoclavicular ligament
  Coracohumeral ligament
  Costoclavicular ligament
  Glenohumeral ligament
  Interclavicular ligament
  Sternoclavicular ligament
  Subacromial bursa
  Transverse humeral ligament
  Transverse scapular ligament
2 Shoulder Bursa and Ligament, Left
  See 1 Shoulder Bursa and Ligament, Right
3 Elbow Bursa and Ligament, Right
  Annular ligament
  Olecranon bursa
  Radial collateral ligament
  Ulnar collateral ligament
4 Elbow Bursa and Ligament, Left
  See 3 Elbow Bursa and Ligament, Right
5 Wrist Bursa and Ligament, Right
  Palmar ulnocarpal ligament
  Radial collateral carpal ligament
  Radiocarpal ligament
  Radioulnar ligament
  Scapholunate ligament
  Ulnar collateral carpal ligament
6 Wrist Bursa and Ligament, Left
  See 5 Wrist Bursa and Ligament, Right
7 Hand Bursa and Ligament, Right
  Carpometacarpal ligament
  Intercarpal ligament
  Interphalangeal ligament
  Lunotriquetral ligament
  Metacarpal ligament
  Metacarpophalangeal ligament
  Pisohamate ligament
  Pisometacarpal ligament
  Scaphotrapezium ligament
8 Hand Bursa and Ligament, Left
  See 7 Hand Bursa and Ligament, Right
9 Upper Extremity Bursa and Ligament, Right
B Upper Extremity Bursa and Ligament, Left
C Upper Spine Bursa and Ligament
  Interspinous ligament, thoracic
  Intertransverse ligament, thoracic
  Ligamentum flavum, thoracic
  Supraspinous ligament
	D Lower Spine Bursa and Ligament
	  Iliolumbar ligament
	  Interspinous ligament, lumbar
	  Intertransverse ligament, lumbar
	  Ligamentum flavum, lumbar
	  Sacrococcygeal ligament
	  Sacroiliac ligament
	  Sacrospinous ligament
	  Sacrotuberous ligament
	  Supraspinous ligament
	F Sternum Bursa and Ligament
	  Costoxiphoid ligament
	  Sternocostal ligament
	G Rib(s) Bursa and Ligament
	  Costotransverse ligament
	H Abdomen Bursa and Ligament, Right
	J Abdomen Bursa and Ligament, Left
	K Perineum Bursa and Ligament
	L Hip Bursa and Ligament, Right
	  Iliofemoral ligament
	  Ischiofemoral ligament
	  Pubofemoral ligament
	  Transverse acetabular ligament
	  Trochanteric bursa
	M Hip Bursa and Ligament, Left
	  See L Hip Bursa and Ligament, Right
	N Knee Bursa and Ligament, Right
	  Anterior cruciate ligament (ACL)
	  Lateral collateral ligament (LCL)
	  Ligament of head of fibula
	  Medial collateral ligament (MCL)
	  Patellar ligament
	  Popliteal ligament
	  Posterior cruciate ligament (PCL)
	  Prepatellar bursa
	P Knee Bursa and Ligament, Left
	  See N Knee Bursa and Ligament, Right
	Q Ankle Bursa and Ligament, Right
	  Calcaneofibular ligament
	  Deltoid ligament
	  Ligament of the lateral malleolus
	  Talofibular ligament
	R Ankle Bursa and Ligament, Left
	  See Q Ankle Bursa and Ligament, Right
	S Foot Bursa and Ligament, Right
	  Calcaneocuboid ligament
	  Cuneonavicular ligament
	  Intercuneiform ligament
	  Interphalangeal ligament
	  Metatarsal ligament
	  Metatarsophalangeal ligament
	  Subtalar ligament
	  Talocalcaneal ligament
	  Talocalcaneonavicular ligament
	  Tarsometatarsal ligament
	T Foot Bursa and Ligament, Left
	  See S Foot Bursa and Ligament, Right
	V Lower Extremity Bursa and Ligament, Right
	W Lower Extremity Bursa and Ligament, Left
		Ø Open
		3 Percutaneous
		4 Percutaneous Endoscopic
			Z No Device	**X Diagnostic**
				Z No Qualifier

Non-OR   ØMB[Ø,1,2,3,4,5,6,7,8,B,C,D,F,G,L,M,N,P,Q,R,S,T][Ø,3,4]ZX
Non-OR   ØMB94ZX

Ø   **Medical and Surgical**
M   **Bursae and Ligaments**
C   **Extirpation**   Definition: Taking or cutting out solid matter from a body part

Explanation: The solid matter may be an abnormal byproduct of a biological function or a foreign body; it may be imbedded in a body part or in the lumen of a tubular body part. The solid matter may or may not have been previously broken into pieces.

Body Part Character 4		Approach Character 5	Device Character 6	Qualifier Character 7
Ø Head and Neck Bursa and Ligament Alar ligament of axis Cervical interspinous ligament Cervical intertransverse ligament Cervical ligamentum flavum Interspinous ligament, cervical Intertransverse ligament, cervical Lateral temporomandibular ligament Ligamentum flavum, cervical Sphenomandibular ligament Stylomandibular ligament Transverse ligament of atlas	**D** Lower Spine Bursa and Ligament Iliolumbar ligament Interspinous ligament, lumbar Intertransverse ligament, lumbar Ligamentum flavum, lumbar Sacrococcygeal ligament Sacroiliac ligament Sacrospinous ligament Sacrotuberous ligament Supraspinous ligament	**Ø** Open **3** Percutaneous **4** Percutaneous Endoscopic	**Z** No Device	**Z** No Qualifier
1 Shoulder Bursa and Ligament, Right Acromioclavicular ligament Coracoacromial ligament Coracoclavicular ligament Coracohumeral ligament Costoclavicular ligament Glenohumeral ligament Interclavicular ligament Sternoclavicular ligament Subacromial bursa Transverse humeral ligament Transverse scapular ligament	**F** Sternum Bursa and Ligament Costoxiphoid ligament Sternocostal ligament **G** Rib(s) Bursa and Ligament Costotransverse ligament **H** Abdomen Bursa and Ligament, Right **J** Abdomen Bursa and Ligament, Left **K** Perineum Bursa and Ligament **L** Hip Bursa and Ligament, Right Iliofemoral ligament Ischiofemoral ligament Pubofemoral ligament Transverse acetabular ligament Trochanteric bursa			
2 Shoulder Bursa and Ligament, Left *See 1 Shoulder Bursa and Ligament, Right*	**M** Hip Bursa and Ligament, Left *See L Hip Bursa and Ligament, Right*			
3 Elbow Bursa and Ligament, Right Annular ligament Olecranon bursa Radial collateral ligament Ulnar collateral ligament	**N** Knee Bursa and Ligament, Right Anterior cruciate ligament (ACL) Lateral collateral ligament (LCL) Ligament of head of fibula Medial collateral ligament (MCL) Patellar ligament Popliteal ligament Posterior cruciate ligament (PCL) Prepatellar bursa			
4 Elbow Bursa and Ligament, Left *See 3 Elbow Bursa and Ligament, Right*	**P** Knee Bursa and Ligament, Left *See N Knee Bursa and Ligament, Right*			
5 Wrist Bursa and Ligament, Right Palmar ulnocarpal ligament Radial collateral carpal ligament Radiocarpal ligament Radioulnar ligament Scapholunate ligament Ulnar collateral carpal ligament	**Q** Ankle Bursa and Ligament, Right Calcaneofibular ligament Deltoid ligament Ligament of the lateral malleolus Talofibular ligament			
6 Wrist Bursa and Ligament, Left *See 5 Wrist Bursa and Ligament, Right*	**R** Ankle Bursa and Ligament, Left *See Q Ankle Bursa and Ligament, Right*			
7 Hand Bursa and Ligament, Right Carpometacarpal ligament Intercarpal ligament Interphalangeal ligament Lunotriquetral ligament Metacarpal ligament Metacarpophalangeal ligament Pisohamate ligament Pisometacarpal ligament Scaphotrapezium ligament	**S** Foot Bursa and Ligament, Right Calcaneocuboid ligament Cuneonavicular ligament Intercuneiform ligament Interphalangeal ligament Metatarsal ligament Metatarsophalangeal ligament Subtalar ligament Talocalcaneal ligament Talocalcaneonavicular ligament Tarsometatarsal ligament			
8 Hand Bursa and Ligament, Left *See 7 Hand Bursa and Ligament, Right*	**T** Foot Bursa and Ligament, Left *See S Foot Bursa and Ligament, Right*			
9 Upper Extremity Bursa and Ligament, Right	**V** Lower Extremity Bursa and Ligament, Right			
B Upper Extremity Bursa and Ligament, Left	**W** Lower Extremity Bursa and Ligament, Left			
C Upper Spine Bursa and Ligament Interspinous ligament, thoracic Intertransverse ligament, thoracic Ligamentum flavum, thoracic Supraspinous ligament				

Ø   Medical and Surgical
M   Bursae and Ligaments
D   Extraction   Definition: Pulling or stripping out or off all or a portion of a body part by the use of force
Explanation: The qualifier DIAGNOSTIC is used to identify extraction procedures that are biopsies

Body Part Character 4		Approach Character 5	Device Character 6	Qualifier Character 7
Ø Head and Neck Bursa and Ligament Alar ligament of axis Cervical interspinous ligament Cervical intertransverse ligament Cervical ligamentum flavum Interspinous ligament, cervical Intertransverse ligament, cervical Lateral temporomandibular ligament Ligamentum flavum, cervical Sphenomandibular ligament Stylomandibular ligament Transverse ligament of atlas	**D** Lower Spine Bursa and Ligament Iliolumbar ligament Interspinous ligament, lumbar Intertransverse ligament, lumbar Ligamentum flavum, lumbar Sacrococcygeal ligament Sacroiliac ligament Sacrospinous ligament Sacrotuberous ligament Supraspinous ligament	**Ø** Open **3** Percutaneous **4** Percutaneous Endoscopic	**Z** No Device	**Z** No Qualifier
1 Shoulder Bursa and Ligament, Right Acromioclavicular ligament Coracoacromial ligament Coracoclavicular ligament Coracohumeral ligament Costoclavicular ligament Glenohumeral ligament Interclavicular ligament Sternoclavicular ligament Subacromial bursa Transverse humeral ligament Transverse scapular ligament	**F** Sternum Bursa and Ligament Costoxiphoid ligament Sternocostal ligament **G** Rib(s) Bursa and Ligament Costotransverse ligament **H** Abdomen Bursa and Ligament, Right **J** Abdomen Bursa and Ligament, Left			
2 Shoulder Bursa and Ligament, Left *See 1 Shoulder Bursa and Ligament, Right*	**K** Perineum Bursa and Ligament **L** Hip Bursa and Ligament, Right Iliofemoral ligament Ischiofemoral ligament Pubofemoral ligament Transverse acetabular ligament Trochanteric bursa			
3 Elbow Bursa and Ligament, Right Annular ligament Olecranon bursa Radial collateral ligament Ulnar collateral ligament	**M** Hip Bursa and Ligament, Left *See L Hip Bursa and Ligament, Right*			
4 Elbow Bursa and Ligament, Left *See 3 Elbow Bursa and Ligament, Right*	**N** Knee Bursa and Ligament, Right Anterior cruciate ligament (ACL) Lateral collateral ligament (LCL) Ligament of head of fibula Medial collateral ligament (MCL) Patellar ligament Popliteal ligament Posterior cruciate ligament (PCL) Prepatellar bursa			
5 Wrist Bursa and Ligament, Right Palmar ulnocarpal ligament Radial collateral carpal ligament Radiocarpal ligament Radioulnar ligament Scapholunate ligament Ulnar collateral carpal ligament	**P** Knee Bursa and Ligament, Left *See N Knee Bursa and Ligament, Right*			
6 Wrist Bursa and Ligament, Left *See 5 Wrist Bursa and Ligament, Right*	**Q** Ankle Bursa and Ligament, Right Calcaneofibular ligament Deltoid ligament Ligament of the lateral malleolus Talofibular ligament			
7 Hand Bursa and Ligament, Right Carpometacarpal ligament Intercarpal ligament Interphalangeal ligament Lunotriquetral ligament Metacarpal ligament Metacarpophalangeal ligament Pisohamate ligament Pisometacarpal ligament Scaphotrapezium ligament	**R** Ankle Bursa and Ligament, Left *See Q Ankle Bursa and Ligament, Right* **S** Foot Bursa and Ligament, Right Calcaneocuboid ligament Cuneonavicular ligament Intercuneiform ligament Interphalangeal ligament Metatarsal ligament Metatarsophalangeal ligament Subtalar ligament Talocalcaneal ligament Talocalcaneonavicular ligament Tarsometatarsal ligament			
8 Hand Bursa and Ligament, Left *See 7 Hand Bursa and Ligament, Right*	**T** Foot Bursa and Ligament, Left *See S Foot Bursa and Ligament, Right*			
9 Upper Extremity Bursa and Ligament, Right **B** Upper Extremity Bursa and Ligament, Left **C** Upper Spine Bursa and Ligament Interspinous ligament, thoracic Intertransverse ligament, thoracic Ligamentum flavum, thoracic Supraspinous ligament	**V** Lower Extremity Bursa and Ligament, Right **W** Lower Extremity Bursa and Ligament, Left			

Ø   Medical and Surgical
M   Bursae and Ligaments
H   Insertion   Definition: Putting in a nonbiological appliance that monitors, assists, performs, or prevents a physiological function but does not physically take the place of a body part

                        Explanation: None

Body Part Character 4	Approach Character 5	Device Character 6	Qualifier Character 7
X Upper Bursa and Ligament Y Lower Bursa and Ligament	Ø Open 3 Percutaneous 4 Percutaneous Endoscopic	Y Other Device	Z No Qualifier

Non-OR   ØMH[X,Y][3,4]YZ

Ø   Medical and Surgical
M   Bursae and Ligaments
J   Inspection   Definition: Visually and/or manually exploring a body part

                        Explanation: Visual exploration may be performed with or without optical instrumentation. Manual exploration may be performed directly or through intervening body layers.

Body Part Character 4	Approach Character 5	Device Character 6	Qualifier Character 7
X Upper Bursa and Ligament Y Lower Bursa and Ligament	Ø Open 3 Percutaneous 4 Percutaneous Endoscopic X External	Z No Device	Z No Qualifier

Non-OR   ØMJ[X,Y][3,X]ZZ

NC Noncovered Procedure   **LC** Limited Coverage   **QA** Questionable OB Admit   **NT** New Tech Add-on   ⊞ Combination Member   ♂ Male   ♀ Female

ICD-10-PCS 2023   **509**

Ø   **Medical and Surgical**
M   **Bursae and Ligaments**
M   **Reattachment**   Definition: Putting back in or on all or a portion of a separated body part to its normal location or other suitable location
                       Explanation: Vascular circulation and nervous pathways may or may not be reestablished

Body Part — Character 4		Approach — Character 5	Device — Character 6	Qualifier — Character 7
Ø **Head and Neck Bursa and Ligament** Alar ligament of axis Cervical interspinous ligament Cervical intertransverse ligament Cervical ligamentum flavum Interspinous ligament, cervical Intertransverse ligament, cervical Lateral temporomandibular ligament Ligamentum flavum, cervical Sphenomandibular ligament Stylomandibular ligament Transverse ligament of atlas **1** **Shoulder Bursa and Ligament, Right** Acromioclavicular ligament Coracoacromial ligament Coracoclavicular ligament Coracohumeral ligament Costoclavicular ligament Glenohumeral ligament Interclavicular ligament Sternoclavicular ligament Subacromial bursa Transverse humeral ligament Transverse scapular ligament **2** **Shoulder Bursa and Ligament, Left** *See* 1 Shoulder Bursa and Ligament, Right **3** **Elbow Bursa and Ligament, Right** Annular ligament Olecranon bursa Radial collateral ligament Ulnar collateral ligament **4** **Elbow Bursa and Ligament, Left** *See* 3 Elbow Bursa and Ligament, Right **5** **Wrist Bursa and Ligament, Right** Palmar ulnocarpal ligament Radial collateral carpal ligament Radiocarpal ligament Radioulnar ligament Scapholunate ligament Ulnar collateral carpal ligament **6** **Wrist Bursa and Ligament, Left** *See* 5 Wrist Bursa and Ligament, Right **7** **Hand Bursa and Ligament, Right** Carpometacarpal ligament Intercarpal ligament Interphalangeal ligament Lunotriquetral ligament Metacarpal ligament Metacarpophalangeal ligament Pisohamate ligament Pisometacarpal ligament Scaphotrapezium ligament **8** **Hand Bursa and Ligament, Left** *See* 7 Hand Bursa and Ligament, Right **9** **Upper Extremity Bursa and Ligament, Right** **B** **Upper Extremity Bursa and Ligament, Left** **C** **Upper Spine Bursa and Ligament** Interspinous ligament, thoracic Intertransverse ligament, thoracic Ligamentum flavum, thoracic Supraspinous ligament	**D** **Lower Spine Bursa and Ligament** Iliolumbar ligament Interspinous ligament, lumbar Intertransverse ligament, lumbar Ligamentum flavum, lumbar Sacrococcygeal ligament Sacroiliac ligament Sacrospinous ligament Sacrotuberous ligament Supraspinous ligament **F** **Sternum Bursa and Ligament** Costoxiphoid ligament Sternocostal ligament **G** **Rib(s) Bursa and Ligament** Costotransverse ligament **H** **Abdomen Bursa and Ligament, Right** **J** **Abdomen Bursa and Ligament, Left** **K** **Perineum Bursa and Ligament** **L** **Hip Bursa and Ligament, Right** Iliofemoral ligament Ischiofemoral ligament Pubofemoral ligament Transverse acetabular ligament Trochanteric bursa **M** **Hip Bursa and Ligament, Left** *See* L Hip Bursa and Ligament, Right **N** **Knee Bursa and Ligament, Right** Anterior cruciate ligament (ACL) Lateral collateral ligament (LCL) Ligament of head of fibula Medial collateral ligament (MCL) Patellar ligament Popliteal ligament Posterior cruciate ligament (PCL) Prepatellar bursa **P** **Knee Bursa and Ligament, Left** *See* N Knee Bursa and Ligament, Right **Q** **Ankle Bursa and Ligament, Right** Calcaneofibular ligament Deltoid ligament Ligament of the lateral malleolus Talofibular ligament **R** **Ankle Bursa and Ligament, Left** *See* Q Ankle Bursa and Ligament, Right **S** **Foot Bursa and Ligament, Right** Calcaneocuboid ligament Cuneonavicular ligament Intercuneiform ligament Interphalangeal ligament Metatarsal ligament Metatarsophalangeal ligament Subtalar ligament Talocalcaneal ligament Talocalcaneonavicular ligament Tarsometatarsal ligament **T** **Foot Bursa and Ligament, Left** *See* S Foot Bursa and Ligament, Right **V** **Lower Extremity Bursa and Ligament, Right** **W** **Lower Extremity Bursa and Ligament, Left**	**Ø** Open **4** Percutaneous Endoscopic	**Z** No Device	**Z** No Qualifier

Non-OR Procedure   DRG Non-OR Procedure   Valid OR Procedure   HAC Associated Procedure   Combination Only   New/Revised April   New/Revised October

510   ICD-10-PCS 2023

Ø   Medical and Surgical
M   Bursae and Ligaments
N   Release   Definition: Freeing a body part from an abnormal physical constraint by cutting or by the use of force
                 Explanation: Some of the restraining tissue may be taken out but none of the body part is taken out

Body Part Character 4		Approach Character 5	Device Character 6	Qualifier Character 7
Ø Head and Neck Bursa and Ligament Alar ligament of axis Cervical interspinous ligament Cervical intertransverse ligament Cervical ligamentum flavum Interspinous ligament, cervical Intertransverse ligament, cervical Lateral temporomandibular ligament Ligamentum flavum, cervical Sphenomandibular ligament Stylomandibular ligament Transverse ligament of atlas	**D Lower Spine Bursa and Ligament** Iliolumbar ligament Interspinous ligament, lumbar Intertransverse ligament, lumbar Ligamentum flavum, lumbar Sacrococcygeal ligament Sacroiliac ligament Sacrospinous ligament Sacrotuberous ligament Supraspinous ligament	**Ø Open** **3 Percutaneous** **4 Percutaneous Endoscopic** **X External**	**Z No Device**	**Z No Qualifier**
1 Shoulder Bursa and Ligament, Right Acromioclavicular ligament Coracoacromial ligament Coracoclavicular ligament Coracohumeral ligament Costoclavicular ligament Glenohumeral ligament Interclavicular ligament Sternoclavicular ligament Subacromial bursa Transverse humeral ligament Transverse scapular ligament	**F Sternum Bursa and Ligament** Costoxiphoid ligament Sternocostal ligament **G Rib(s) Bursa and Ligament** Costotransverse ligament **H Abdomen Bursa and Ligament, Right** **J Abdomen Bursa and Ligament, Left** **K Perineum Bursa and Ligament** **L Hip Bursa and Ligament, Right** Iliofemoral ligament Ischiofemoral ligament Pubofemoral ligament Transverse acetabular ligament Trochanteric bursa			
2 Shoulder Bursa and Ligament, Left *See 1 Shoulder Bursa and Ligament, Right*	**M Hip Bursa and Ligament, Left** *See L Hip Bursa and Ligament, Right*			
3 Elbow Bursa and Ligament, Right Annular ligament Olecranon bursa Radial collateral ligament Ulnar collateral ligament	**N Knee Bursa and Ligament, Right** Anterior cruciate ligament (ACL) Lateral collateral ligament (LCL) Ligament of head of fibula Medial collateral ligament (MCL) Patellar ligament Popliteal ligament Posterior cruciate ligament (PCL) Prepatellar bursa			
4 Elbow Bursa and Ligament, Left *See 3 Elbow Bursa and Ligament, Right*	**P Knee Bursa and Ligament, Left** *See N Knee Bursa and Ligament, Right*			
5 Wrist Bursa and Ligament, Right Palmar ulnocarpal ligament Radial collateral carpal ligament Radiocarpal ligament Radioulnar ligament Scapholunate ligament Ulnar collateral carpal ligament	**Q Ankle Bursa and Ligament, Right** Calcaneofibular ligament Deltoid ligament Ligament of the lateral malleolus Talofibular ligament			
6 Wrist Bursa and Ligament, Left *See 5 Wrist Bursa and Ligament, Right*	**R Ankle Bursa and Ligament, Left** *See Q Ankle Bursa and Ligament, Right*			
7 Hand Bursa and Ligament, Right Carpometacarpal ligament Intercarpal ligament Interphalangeal ligament Lunotriquetral ligament Metacarpal ligament Metacarpophalangeal ligament Pisohamate ligament Pisometacarpal ligament Scaphotrapezium ligament	**S Foot Bursa and Ligament, Right** Calcaneocuboid ligament Cuneonavicular ligament Intercuneiform ligament Interphalangeal ligament Metatarsal ligament Metatarsophalangeal ligament Subtalar ligament Talocalcaneal ligament Talocalcaneonavicular ligament Tarsometatarsal ligament			
8 Hand Bursa and Ligament, Left *See 7 Hand Bursa and Ligament, Right*	**T Foot Bursa and Ligament, Left** *See S Foot Bursa and Ligament, Right*			
9 Upper Extremity Bursa and Ligament, Right **B Upper Extremity Bursa and Ligament, Left** **C Upper Spine Bursa and Ligament** Interspinous ligament, thoracic Intertransverse ligament, thoracic Ligamentum flavum, thoracic Supraspinous ligament	**V Lower Extremity Bursa and Ligament, Right** **W Lower Extremity Bursa and Ligament, Left**			

Non-OR   ØMN[Ø,1,2,3,4,5,6,7,8,9,B,C,D,F,G,H,J,K,L,M,N,P,Q,R,S,T,V,W]XZZ

NC Noncovered Procedure   **LC** Limited Coverage   **QA** Questionable OB Admit   **NT** New Tech Add-on   ⊞ Combination Member   ♂ Male   ♀ Female

ICD-10-PCS 2023   **511**

Bursae and Ligaments

Ø   **Medical and Surgical**
M   **Bursae and Ligaments**
P   **Removal**   Definition: Taking out or off a device from a body part

Explanation: If a device is taken out and a similar device put in without cutting or puncturing the skin or mucous membrane, the procedure is coded to the root operation CHANGE. Otherwise, the procedure for taking out a device is coded to the root operation REMOVAL.

Body Part Character 4	Approach Character 5	Device Character 6	Qualifier Character 7
X Upper Bursa and Ligament Y Lower Bursa and Ligament	Ø Open 3 Percutaneous 4 Percutaneous Endoscopic	Ø Drainage Device 7 Autologous Tissue Substitute J Synthetic Substitute K Nonautologous Tissue Substitute Y Other Device	Z No Qualifier
X Upper Bursa and Ligament Y Lower Bursa and Ligament	X External	Ø Drainage Device	Z No Qualifier

Non-OR   ØMP[X,Y]3ØZ
Non-OR   ØMP[X,Y][3,4]YZ
Non-OR   ØMP[X,Y]XØZ

Ø   **Medical and Surgical**
M   **Bursae and Ligaments**
Q   **Repair**   Definition: Restoring, to the extent possible, a body part to its normal anatomic structure and function
                     Explanation: Used only when the method to accomplish the repair is not one of the other root operations

Body Part — Character 4		Approach — Character 5	Device — Character 6	Qualifier — Character 7
Ø Head and Neck Bursa and Ligament Alar ligament of axis Cervical interspinous ligament Cervical intertransverse ligament Cervical ligamentum flavum Interspinous ligament, cervical Intertransverse ligament, cervical Lateral temporomandibular ligament Ligamentum flavum, cervical Sphenomandibular ligament Stylomandibular ligament Transverse ligament of atlas	**D** Lower Spine Bursa and Ligament Iliolumbar ligament Interspinous ligament, lumbar Intertransverse ligament, lumbar Ligamentum flavum, lumbar Sacrococcygeal ligament Sacroiliac ligament Sacrospinous ligament Sacrotuberous ligament Supraspinous ligament	**Ø** Open **3** Percutaneous **4** Percutaneous Endoscopic	**Z** No Device	**Z** No Qualifier
1 Shoulder Bursa and Ligament, Right Acromioclavicular ligament Coracoacromial ligament Coracoclavicular ligament Coracohumeral ligament Costoclavicular ligament Glenohumeral ligament Interclavicular ligament Sternoclavicular ligament Subacromial bursa Transverse humeral ligament Transverse scapular ligament	**F** Sternum Bursa and Ligament Costoxiphoid ligament Sternocostal ligament **G** Rib(s) Bursa and Ligament Costotransverse ligament **H** Abdomen Bursa and Ligament, Right **J** Abdomen Bursa and Ligament, Left **K** Perineum Bursa and Ligament			
2 Shoulder Bursa and Ligament, Left *See 1 Shoulder Bursa and Ligament, Right*	**L** Hip Bursa and Ligament, Right Iliofemoral ligament Ischiofemoral ligament Pubofemoral ligament Transverse acetabular ligament Trochanteric bursa			
3 Elbow Bursa and Ligament, Right Annular ligament Olecranon bursa Radial collateral ligament Ulnar collateral ligament	**M** Hip Bursa and Ligament, Left *See L Hip Bursa and Ligament, Right*			
4 Elbow Bursa and Ligament, Left *See 3 Elbow Bursa and Ligament, Right*	**N** Knee Bursa and Ligament, Right Anterior cruciate ligament (ACL) Lateral collateral ligament (LCL) Ligament of head of fibula Medial collateral ligament (MCL) Patellar ligament Popliteal ligament Posterior cruciate ligament (PCL) Prepatellar bursa			
5 Wrist Bursa and Ligament, Right Palmar ulnocarpal ligament Radial collateral carpal ligament Radiocarpal ligament Radioulnar ligament Scapholunate ligament Ulnar collateral carpal ligament	**P** Knee Bursa and Ligament, Left *See N Knee Bursa and Ligament, Right*			
6 Wrist Bursa and Ligament, Left *See 5 Wrist Bursa and Ligament, Right*	**Q** Ankle Bursa and Ligament, Right Calcaneofibular ligament Deltoid ligament Ligament of the lateral malleolus Talofibular ligament			
7 Hand Bursa and Ligament, Right Carpometacarpal ligament Intercarpal ligament Interphalangeal ligament Lunotriquetral ligament Metacarpal ligament Metacarpophalangeal ligament Pisohamate ligament Pisometacarpal ligament Scaphotrapezium ligament	**R** Ankle Bursa and Ligament, Left *See Q Ankle Bursa and Ligament, Right* **S** Foot Bursa and Ligament, Right Calcaneocuboid ligament Cuneonavicular ligament Intercuneiform ligament Interphalangeal ligament Metatarsal ligament Metatarsophalangeal ligament Subtalar ligament Talocalcaneal ligament Talocalcaneonavicular ligament Tarsometatarsal ligament			
8 Hand Bursa and Ligament, Left *See 7 Hand Bursa and Ligament, Right*				
9 Upper Extremity Bursa and Ligament, Right	**T** Foot Bursa and Ligament, Left *See S Foot Bursa and Ligament, Right*			
B Upper Extremity Bursa and Ligament, Left	**V** Lower Extremity Bursa and Ligament, Right			
C Upper Spine Bursa and Ligament Interspinous ligament, thoracic Intertransverse ligament, thoracic Ligamentum flavum, thoracic Supraspinous ligament	**W** Lower Extremity Bursa and Ligament, Left			

NC Noncovered Procedure   **LC** Limited Coverage   **QA** Questionable OB Admit   **NT** New Tech Add-on   ⊞ Combination Member   ♂ Male   ♀ Female

ICD-10-PCS 2023   513

Bursae and Ligaments *(side tab)*

Ø   **Medical and Surgical**
M   **Bursae and Ligaments**
R   **Replacement**   Definition: Putting in or on biological or synthetic material that physically takes the place and/or function of all or a portion of a body part

Explanation: The body part may have been taken out or replaced, or may be taken out, physically eradicated, or rendered nonfunctional during the REPLACEMENT procedure. A REMOVAL procedure is coded for taking out the device used in a previous replacement procedure.

Body Part Character 4		Approach Character 5	Device Character 6	Qualifier Character 7
Ø **Head and Neck Bursa and Ligament** Alar ligament of axis Cervical interspinous ligament Cervical intertransverse ligament Cervical ligamentum flavum Interspinous ligament, cervical Intertransverse ligament, cervical Lateral temporomandibular ligament Ligamentum flavum, cervical Sphenomandibular ligament Stylomandibular ligament Transverse ligament of atlas **1** **Shoulder Bursa and Ligament, Right** Acromioclavicular ligament Coracoacromial ligament Coracoclavicular ligament Coracohumeral ligament Costoclavicular ligament Glenohumeral ligament Interclavicular ligament Sternoclavicular ligament Subacromial bursa Transverse humeral ligament Transverse scapular ligament **2** **Shoulder Bursa and Ligament, Left** *See 1 Shoulder Bursa and Ligament, Right* **3** **Elbow Bursa and Ligament, Right** Annular ligament Olecranon bursa Radial collateral ligament Ulnar collateral ligament **4** **Elbow Bursa and Ligament, Left** *See 3 Elbow Bursa and Ligament, Right* **5** **Wrist Bursa and Ligament, Right** Palmar ulnocarpal ligament Radial collateral carpal ligament Radiocarpal ligament Radioulnar ligament Scapholunate ligament Ulnar collateral carpal ligament **6** **Wrist Bursa and Ligament, Left** *See 5 Wrist Bursa and Ligament, Right* **7** **Hand Bursa and Ligament, Right** Carpometacarpal ligament Intercarpal ligament Interphalangeal ligament Lunotriquetral ligament Metacarpal ligament Metacarpophalangeal ligament Pisohamate ligament Pisometacarpal ligament Scaphotrapezium ligament **8** **Hand Bursa and Ligament, Left** *See 7 Hand Bursa and Ligament, Right* **9** **Upper Extremity Bursa and Ligament, Right** **B** **Upper Extremity Bursa and Ligament, Left** **C** **Upper Spine Bursa and Ligament** Interspinous ligament, thoracic Intertransverse ligament, thoracic Ligamentum flavum, thoracic Supraspinous ligament	**D** **Lower Spine Bursa and Ligament** Iliolumbar ligament Interspinous ligament, lumbar Intertransverse ligament, lumbar Ligamentum flavum, lumbar Sacrococcygeal ligament Sacroiliac ligament Sacrospinous ligament Sacrotuberous ligament Supraspinous ligament **F** **Sternum Bursa and Ligament** Costoxiphoid ligament Sternocostal ligament **G** **Rib(s) Bursa and Ligament** Costotransverse ligament **H** **Abdomen Bursa and Ligament, Right** **J** **Abdomen Bursa and Ligament, Left** **K** **Perineum Bursa and Ligament** **L** **Hip Bursa and Ligament, Right** Iliofemoral ligament Ischiofemoral ligament Pubofemoral ligament Transverse acetabular ligament Trochanteric bursa **M** **Hip Bursa and Ligament, Left** *See L Hip Bursa and Ligament, Right* **N** **Knee Bursa and Ligament, Right** Anterior cruciate ligament (ACL) Lateral collateral ligament (LCL) Ligament of head of fibula Medial collateral ligament (MCL) Patellar ligament Popliteal ligament Posterior cruciate ligament (PCL) Prepatellar bursa **P** **Knee Bursa and Ligament, Left** *See N Knee Bursa and Ligament, Right* **Q** **Ankle Bursa and Ligament, Right** Calcaneofibular ligament Deltoid ligament Ligament of the lateral malleolus Talofibular ligament **R** **Ankle Bursa and Ligament, Left** *See Q Ankle Bursa and Ligament, Right* **S** **Foot Bursa and Ligament, Right** Calcaneocuboid ligament Cuneonavicular ligament Intercuneiform ligament Interphalangeal ligament Metatarsal ligament Metatarsophalangeal ligament Subtalar ligament Talocalcaneal ligament Talocalcaneonavicular ligament Tarsometatarsal ligament **T** **Foot Bursa and Ligament, Left** *See S Foot Bursa and Ligament, Right* **V** **Lower Extremity Bursa and Ligament, Right** **W** **Lower Extremity Bursa and Ligament, Left**	**Ø** Open **4** Percutaneous Endoscopic	**7** Autologous Tissue Substitute **J** Synthetic Substitute **K** Nonautologous Tissue Substitute	**Z** No Qualifier

Non-OR Procedure   DRG Non-OR Procedure   Valid OR Procedure   HAC Associated Procedure   Combination Only   New/Revised April   New/Revised October

514   ICD-10-PCS 2023

Ø   **Medical and Surgical**
M   **Bursae and Ligaments**
S   **Reposition**   Definition: Moving to its normal location, or other suitable location, all or a portion of a body part

Explanation: The body part is moved to a new location from an abnormal location, or from a normal location where it is not functioning correctly. The body part may or may not be cut out or off to be moved to the new location.

Body Part Character 4		Approach Character 5	Device Character 6	Qualifier Character 7
Ø Head and Neck Bursa and Ligament Alar ligament of axis Cervical interspinous ligament Cervical intertransverse ligament Cervical ligamentum flavum Interspinous ligament, cervical Intertransverse ligament, cervical Lateral temporomandibular ligament Ligamentum flavum, cervical Sphenomandibular ligament Stylomandibular ligament Transverse ligament of atlas **1** Shoulder Bursa and Ligament, Right Acromioclavicular ligament Coracoacromial ligament Coracoclavicular ligament Coracohumeral ligament Costoclavicular ligament Glenohumeral ligament Interclavicular ligament Sternoclavicular ligament Subacromial bursa Transverse humeral ligament Transverse scapular ligament **2** Shoulder Bursa and Ligament, Left *See 1 Shoulder Bursa and Ligament, Right* **3** Elbow Bursa and Ligament, Right Annular ligament Olecranon bursa Radial collateral ligament Ulnar collateral ligament **4** Elbow Bursa and Ligament, Left *See 3 Elbow Bursa and Ligament, Right* **5** Wrist Bursa and Ligament, Right Palmar ulnocarpal ligament Radial collateral carpal ligament Radiocarpal ligament Radioulnar ligament Scapholunate ligament Ulnar collateral carpal ligament **6** Wrist Bursa and Ligament, Left *See 5 Wrist Bursa and Ligament, Right* **7** Hand Bursa and Ligament, Right Carpometacarpal ligament Intercarpal ligament Interphalangeal ligament Lunotriquetral ligament Metacarpal ligament Metacarpophalangeal ligament Pisohamate ligament Pisometacarpal ligament Scaphotrapezium ligament **8** Hand Bursa and Ligament, Left *See 7 Hand Bursa and Ligament, Right* **9** Upper Extremity Bursa and Ligament, Right **B** Upper Extremity Bursa and Ligament, Left **C** Upper Spine Bursa and Ligament Interspinous ligament, thoracic Intertransverse ligament, thoracic Ligamentum flavum, thoracic Supraspinous ligament	**D** Lower Spine Bursa and Ligament Iliolumbar ligament Interspinous ligament, lumbar Intertransverse ligament, lumbar Ligamentum flavum, lumbar Sacrococcygeal ligament Sacroiliac ligament Sacrospinous ligament Sacrotuberous ligament Supraspinous ligament **F** Sternum Bursa and Ligament Costoxiphoid ligament Sternocostal ligament **G** Rib(s) Bursa and Ligament Costotransverse ligament **H** Abdomen Bursa and Ligament, Right **J** Abdomen Bursa and Ligament, Left **K** Perineum Bursa and Ligament **L** Hip Bursa and Ligament, Right Iliofemoral ligament Ischiofemoral ligament Pubofemoral ligament Transverse acetabular ligament Trochanteric bursa **M** Hip Bursa and Ligament, Left *See L Hip Bursa and Ligament, Right* **N** Knee Bursa and Ligament, Right Anterior cruciate ligament (ACL) Lateral collateral ligament (LCL) Ligament of head of fibula Medial collateral ligament (MCL) Patellar ligament Popliteal ligament Posterior cruciate ligament (PCL) Prepatellar bursa **P** Knee Bursa and Ligament, Left *See N Knee Bursa and Ligament, Right* **Q** Ankle Bursa and Ligament, Right Calcaneofibular ligament Deltoid ligament Ligament of the lateral malleolus Talofibular ligament **R** Ankle Bursa and Ligament, Left *See Q Ankle Bursa and Ligament, Right* **S** Foot Bursa and Ligament, Right Calcaneocuboid ligament Cuneonavicular ligament Intercuneiform ligament Interphalangeal ligament Metatarsal ligament Metatarsophalangeal ligament Subtalar ligament Talocalcaneal ligament Talocalcaneonavicular ligament Tarsometatarsal ligament **T** Foot Bursa and Ligament, Left *See S Foot Bursa and Ligament, Right* **V** Lower Extremity Bursa and Ligament, Right **W** Lower Extremity Bursa and Ligament, Left	**Ø** Open **4** Percutaneous Endoscopic	**Z** No Device	**Z** No Qualifier

Ø Medical and Surgical
M Bursae and Ligaments
T Resection   Definition: Cutting out or off, without replacement, all of a body part
          Explanation: None

Body Part Character 4		Approach Character 5	Device Character 6	Qualifier Character 7
Ø Head and Neck Bursa and Ligament Alar ligament of axis Cervical interspinous ligament Cervical intertransverse ligament Cervical ligamentum flavum Interspinous ligament, cervical Intertransverse ligament, cervical Lateral temporomandibular ligament Ligamentum flavum, cervical Sphenomandibular ligament Stylomandibular ligament Transverse ligament of atlas **1 Shoulder Bursa and Ligament, Right** Acromioclavicular ligament Coracoacromial ligament Coracoclavicular ligament Coracohumeral ligament Costoclavicular ligament Glenohumeral ligament Interclavicular ligament Sternoclavicular ligament Subacromial bursa Transverse humeral ligament Transverse scapular ligament **2 Shoulder Bursa and Ligament, Left** *See 1 Shoulder Bursa and Ligament, Right* **3 Elbow Bursa and Ligament, Right** Annular ligament Olecranon bursa Radial collateral ligament Ulnar collateral ligament **4 Elbow Bursa and Ligament, Left** *See 3 Elbow Bursa and Ligament, Right* **5 Wrist Bursa and Ligament, Right** Palmar ulnocarpal ligament Radial collateral carpal ligament Radiocarpal ligament Radioulnar ligament Scapholunate ligament Ulnar collateral carpal ligament **6 Wrist Bursa and Ligament, Left** *See 5 Wrist Bursa and Ligament, Right* **7 Hand Bursa and Ligament, Right** Carpometacarpal ligament Intercarpal ligament Interphalangeal ligament Lunotriquetral ligament Metacarpal ligament Metacarpophalangeal ligament Pisohamate ligament Pisometacarpal ligament Scaphotrapezium ligament **8 Hand Bursa and Ligament, Left** *See 7 Hand Bursa and Ligament, Right* **9 Upper Extremity Bursa and Ligament, Right** **B Upper Extremity Bursa and Ligament, Left** **C Upper Spine Bursa and Ligament** Interspinous ligament, thoracic Intertransverse ligament, thoracic Ligamentum flavum, thoracic Supraspinous ligament	**D Lower Spine Bursa and Ligament** Iliolumbar ligament Interspinous ligament, lumbar Intertransverse ligament, lumbar Ligamentum flavum, lumbar Sacrococcygeal ligament Sacroiliac ligament Sacrospinous ligament Sacrotuberous ligament Supraspinous ligament **F Sternum Bursa and Ligament** Costoxiphoid ligament Sternocostal ligament **G Rib(s) Bursa and Ligament** Costotransverse ligament **H Abdomen Bursa and Ligament, Right** **J Abdomen Bursa and Ligament, Left** **K Perineum Bursa and Ligament** **L Hip Bursa and Ligament, Right** Iliofemoral ligament Ischiofemoral ligament Pubofemoral ligament Transverse acetabular ligament Trochanteric bursa **M Hip Bursa and Ligament, Left** *See L Hip Bursa and Ligament, Right* **N Knee Bursa and Ligament, Right** Anterior cruciate ligament (ACL) Lateral collateral ligament (LCL) Ligament of head of fibula Medial collateral ligament (MCL) Patellar ligament Popliteal ligament Posterior cruciate ligament (PCL) Prepatellar bursa **P Knee Bursa and Ligament, Left** *See N Knee Bursa and Ligament, Right* **Q Ankle Bursa and Ligament, Right** Calcaneofibular ligament Deltoid ligament Ligament of the lateral malleolus Talofibular ligament **R Ankle Bursa and Ligament, Left** *See Q Ankle Bursa and Ligament, Right* **S Foot Bursa and Ligament, Right** Calcaneocuboid ligament Cuneonavicular ligament Intercuneiform ligament Interphalangeal ligament Metatarsal ligament Metatarsophalangeal ligament Subtalar ligament Talocalcaneal ligament Talocalcaneonavicular ligament Tarsometatarsal ligament **T Foot Bursa and Ligament, Left** *See S Foot Bursa and Ligament, Right* **V Lower Extremity Bursa and Ligament, Right** **W Lower Extremity Bursa and Ligament, Left**	**Ø Open** **4 Percutaneous Endoscopic**	**Z No Device**	**Z No Qualifier**

Ø Medical and Surgical
M Bursae and Ligaments
U Supplement　Definition: Putting in or on biological or synthetic material that physically reinforces and/or augments the function of a portion of a body part
Explanation: The biological material is non-living, or is living and from the same individual. The body part may have been previously replaced, and the SUPPLEMENT procedure is performed to physically reinforce and/or augment the function of the replaced body part.

Body Part Character 4		Approach Character 5	Device Character 6	Qualifier Character 7
Ø Head and Neck Bursa and Ligament Alar ligament of axis Cervical interspinous ligament Cervical intertransverse ligament Cervical ligamentum flavum Interspinous ligament, cervical Intertransverse ligament, cervical Lateral temporomandibular ligament Ligamentum flavum, cervical Sphenomandibular ligament Stylomandibular ligament Transverse ligament of atlas	**D Lower Spine Bursa and Ligament** Iliolumbar ligament Interspinous ligament, lumbar Intertransverse ligament, lumbar Ligamentum flavum, lumbar Sacrococcygeal ligament Sacroiliac ligament Sacrospinous ligament Sacrotuberous ligament Supraspinous ligament	**Ø Open** **4 Percutaneous Endoscopic**	**7 Autologous Tissue Substitute** **J Synthetic Substitute** **K Nonautologous Tissue Substitute**	**Z No Qualifier**
1 Shoulder Bursa and Ligament, Right Acromioclavicular ligament Coracoacromial ligament Coracoclavicular ligament Coracohumeral ligament Costoclavicular ligament Glenohumeral ligament Interclavicular ligament Sternoclavicular ligament Subacromial bursa Transverse humeral ligament Transverse scapular ligament	**F Sternum Bursa and Ligament** Costoxiphoid ligament Sternocostal ligament **G Rib(s) Bursa and Ligament** Costotransverse ligament **H Abdomen Bursa and Ligament, Right** **J Abdomen Bursa and Ligament, Left** **K Perineum Bursa and Ligament**			
2 Shoulder Bursa and Ligament, Left *See 1 Shoulder Bursa and Ligament, Right*	**L Hip Bursa and Ligament, Right** Iliofemoral ligament Ischiofemoral ligament Pubofemoral ligament Transverse acetabular ligament Trochanteric bursa			
3 Elbow Bursa and Ligament, Right Annular ligament Olecranon bursa Radial collateral ligament Ulnar collateral ligament	**M Hip Bursa and Ligament, Left** *See L Hip Bursa and Ligament, Right*			
4 Elbow Bursa and Ligament, Left *See 3 Elbow Bursa and Ligament, Right*	**N Knee Bursa and Ligament, Right** Anterior cruciate ligament (ACL) Lateral collateral ligament (LCL) Ligament of head of fibula Medial collateral ligament (MCL) Patellar ligament Popliteal ligament Posterior cruciate ligament (PCL) Prepatellar bursa			
5 Wrist Bursa and Ligament, Right Palmar ulnocarpal ligament Radial collateral carpal ligament Radiocarpal ligament Radioulnar ligament Scapholunate ligament Ulnar collateral carpal ligament	**P Knee Bursa and Ligament, Left** *See N Knee Bursa and Ligament, Right*			
6 Wrist Bursa and Ligament, Left *See 5 Wrist Bursa and Ligament, Right*	**Q Ankle Bursa and Ligament, Right** Calcaneofibular ligament Deltoid ligament Ligament of the lateral malleolus Talofibular ligament			
7 Hand Bursa and Ligament, Right Carpometacarpal ligament Intercarpal ligament Interphalangeal ligament Lunotriquetral ligament Metacarpal ligament Metacarpophalangeal ligament Pisohamate ligament Pisometacarpal ligament Scaphotrapezium ligament	**R Ankle Bursa and Ligament, Left** *See Q Ankle Bursa and Ligament, Right*			
8 Hand Bursa and Ligament, Left *See 7 Hand Bursa and Ligament, Right*	**S Foot Bursa and Ligament, Right** Calcaneocuboid ligament Cuneonavicular ligament Intercuneiform ligament Interphalangeal ligament Metatarsal ligament Metatarsophalangeal ligament Subtalar ligament Talocalcaneal ligament Talocalcaneonavicular ligament Tarsometatarsal ligament			
9 Upper Extremity Bursa and Ligament, Right **B Upper Extremity Bursa and Ligament, Left**	**T Foot Bursa and Ligament, Left** *See S Foot Bursa and Ligament, Right*			
C Upper Spine Bursa and Ligament Interspinous ligament, thoracic Intertransverse ligament, thoracic Ligamentum flavum, thoracic Supraspinous ligament	**V Lower Extremity Bursa and Ligament, Right** **W Lower Extremity Bursa and Ligament, Left**			

NC Noncovered Procedure　LC Limited Coverage　OA Questionable OB Admit　NT New Tech Add-on　⊞ Combination Member　♂ Male　♀ Female

ICD-10-PCS 2023　　517

Bursae and Ligaments

Ø   **Medical and Surgical**
M   **Bursae and Ligaments**
W   **Revision**   Definition: Correcting, to the extent possible, a portion of a malfunctioning device or the position of a displaced device

                          Explanation: Revision can include correcting a malfunctioning or displaced device by taking out or putting in components of the device such as a screw or pin

Body Part Character 4	Approach Character 5	Device Character 6	Qualifier Character 7
X Upper Bursa and Ligament Y Lower Bursa and Ligament	Ø Open 3 Percutaneous 4 Percutaneous Endoscopic	Ø Drainage Device 7 Autologous Tissue Substitute J Synthetic Substitute K Nonautologous Tissue Substitute Y Other Device	Z No Qualifier
X Upper Bursa and Ligament Y Lower Bursa and Ligament	X External	Ø Drainage Device 7 Autologous Tissue Substitute J Synthetic Substitute K Nonautologous Tissue Substitute	Z No Qualifier

Non-OR   ØMW[X,Y][3,4]YZ
Non-OR   ØMW[X,Y]X[Ø,7,J,K]Z

Ø **Medical and Surgical**
M **Bursae and Ligaments**
X **Transfer**   Definition: Moving, without taking out, all or a portion of a body part to another location to take over the function of all or a portion of a body part
               Explanation: The body part transferred remains connected to its vascular and nervous supply

Body Part Character 4		Approach Character 5	Device Character 6	Qualifier Character 7
Ø **Head and Neck Bursa and Ligament** Alar ligament of axis Cervical interspinous ligament Cervical intertransverse ligament Cervical ligamentum flavum Interspinous ligament, cervical Intertransverse ligament, cervical Lateral temporomandibular ligament Ligamentum flavum, cervical Sphenomandibular ligament Stylomandibular ligament Transverse ligament of atlas 1 **Shoulder Bursa and Ligament, Right** Acromioclavicular ligament Coracoacromial ligament Coracoclavicular ligament Coracohumeral ligament Costoclavicular ligament Glenohumeral ligament Interclavicular ligament Sternoclavicular ligament Subacromial bursa Transverse humeral ligament Transverse scapular ligament 2 **Shoulder Bursa and Ligament, Left** *See 1 Shoulder Bursa and Ligament, Right* 3 **Elbow Bursa and Ligament, Right** Annular ligament Olecranon bursa Radial collateral ligament Ulnar collateral ligament 4 **Elbow Bursa and Ligament, Left** *See 3 Elbow Bursa and Ligament, Right* 5 **Wrist Bursa and Ligament, Right** Palmar ulnocarpal ligament Radial collateral carpal ligament Radiocarpal ligament Radioulnar ligament Scapholunate ligament Ulnar collateral carpal ligament 6 **Wrist Bursa and Ligament, Left** *See 5 Wrist Bursa and Ligament, Right* 7 **Hand Bursa and Ligament, Right** Carpometacarpal ligament Intercarpal ligament Interphalangeal ligament Lunotriquetral ligament Metacarpal ligament Metacarpophalangeal ligament Pisohamate ligament Pisometacarpal ligament Scaphotrapezium ligament 8 **Hand Bursa and Ligament, Left** *See 7 Hand Bursa and Ligament, Right* 9 **Upper Extremity Bursa and Ligament, Right** B **Upper Extremity Bursa and Ligament, Left** C **Upper Spine Bursa and Ligament** Interspinous ligament, thoracic Intertransverse ligament, thoracic Ligamentum flavum, thoracic Supraspinous ligament	D **Lower Spine Bursa and Ligament** Iliolumbar ligament Interspinous ligament, lumbar Intertransverse ligament, lumbar Ligamentum flavum, lumbar Sacrococcygeal ligament Sacroiliac ligament Sacrospinous ligament Sacrotuberous ligament Supraspinous ligament F **Sternum Bursa and Ligament** Costoxiphoid ligament Sternocostal ligament G **Rib(s) Bursa and Ligament** Costotransverse ligament H **Abdomen Bursa and Ligament, Right** J **Abdomen Bursa and Ligament, Left** K **Perineum Bursa and Ligament** L **Hip Bursa and Ligament, Right** Iliofemoral ligament Ischiofemoral ligament Pubofemoral ligament Transverse acetabular ligament Trochanteric bursa M **Hip Bursa and Ligament, Left** *See L Hip Bursa and Ligament, Right* N **Knee Bursa and Ligament, Right** Anterior cruciate ligament (ACL) Lateral collateral ligament (LCL) Ligament of head of fibula Medial collateral ligament (MCL) Patellar ligament Popliteal ligament Posterior cruciate ligament (PCL) Prepatellar bursa P **Knee Bursa and Ligament, Left** *See N Knee Bursa and Ligament, Right* Q **Ankle Bursa and Ligament, Right** Calcaneofibular ligament Deltoid ligament Ligament of the lateral malleolus Talofibular ligament R **Ankle Bursa and Ligament, Left** *See Q Ankle Bursa and Ligament, Right* S **Foot Bursa and Ligament, Right** Calcaneocuboid ligament Cuneonavicular ligament Intercuneiform ligament Interphalangeal ligament Metatarsal ligament Metatarsophalangeal ligament Subtalar ligament Talocalcaneal ligament Talocalcaneonavicular ligament Tarsometatarsal ligament T **Foot Bursa and Ligament, Left** *See S Foot Bursa and Ligament, Right* V **Lower Extremity Bursa and Ligament, Right** W **Lower Extremity Bursa and Ligament, Left**	Ø Open 4 Percutaneous Endoscopic	Z No Device	Z No Qualifier

NC Noncovered Procedure   LC Limited Coverage   QA Questionable OB Admit   NT New Tech Add-on   ⊞ Combination Member   ♂ Male   ♀ Female

ICD-10-PCS 2023   519

ØMX–ØMX

Head and Facial Bones ØN2–ØNW

Character Meanings

This Character Meaning table is provided as a guide to assist the user in the identification of character members that may be found in this section of code tables. It **SHOULD NOT** be used to build a PCS code.

Operation–Character 3	Body Part–Character 4	Approach–Character 5	Device–Character 6	Qualifier–Character 7
2 Change	Ø Skull	Ø Open	Ø Drainage Device	X Diagnostic
5 Destruction	1 Frontal Bone	3 Percutaneous	3 Infusion Device	Z No Qualifier
8 Division	3 Parietal Bone, Right	4 Percutaneous Endoscopic	4 Internal Fixation Device	
9 Drainage	4 Parietal Bone, Left	X External	5 External Fixation Device	
B Excision	5 Temporal Bone, Right		7 Autologous Tissue Substitute	
C Extirpation	6 Temporal Bone, Left		J Synthetic Substitute	
D Extraction	7 Occipital Bone		K Nonautologous Tissue Substitute	
H Insertion	B Nasal Bone		M Bone Growth Stimulator	
J Inspection	C Sphenoid Bone		N Neurostimulator Generator	
N Release	F Ethmoid Bone, Right		S Hearing Device	
P Removal	G Ethmoid Bone, Left		Y Other Device	
Q Repair	H Lacrimal Bone, Right		Z No Device	
R Replacement	J Lacrimal Bone, Left			
S Reposition	K Palatine Bone, Right			
T Resection	L Palatine Bone, Left			
U Supplement	M Zygomatic Bone, Right			
W Revision	N Zygomatic Bone, Left			
	P Orbit, Right			
	Q Orbit, Left			
	R Maxilla			
	T Mandible, Right			
	V Mandible, Left			
	W Facial Bone			
	X Hyoid Bone			

AHA Coding Clinic for table ØNB

2022, 2Q, 17	Congenital nasal pyriform aperture stenosis and repair
2021, 3Q, 21	Excision of thyroglossal duct cyst
2021, 1Q, 21	Maxillectomy with reconstruction of maxilla
2017, 1Q, 20	Preparatory nasal adhesion repair before definitive cleft palate repair
2015, 3Q, 3-8	Excisional and nonexcisional debridement
2015, 2Q, 12	Orbital exenteration

AHA Coding Clinic for table ØND

2017, 4Q, 41	Extraction procedures

AHA Coding Clinic for table ØNH

2021, 4Q, 51	Insertion of infusion device in skull
2015, 3Q, 13	Nonexcisional debridement of cranial wound with removal and replacement of hardware

AHA Coding Clinic for table ØNP

2015, 3Q, 13	Nonexcisional debridement of cranial wound with removal and replacement of hardware

AHA Coding Clinic for table ØNQ

2016, 3Q, 29	Closure of bilateral alveolar clefts

AHA Coding Clinic for table ØNR

2021, 3Q, 29	Repair of superior semicircular canal dehiscence
2021, 1Q, 21	Maxillectomy with reconstruction of maxilla
2017, 3Q, 17	Resection of schwannoma and placement of DuraGen and Lorenz cranial plating system
2017, 3Q, 22	Replacement of native skull bone flap
2017, 1Q, 23	Reconstruction of mandible using titanium and bone
2014, 3Q, 7	Hemi-cranioplasty for repair of cranial defect

AHA Coding Clinic for table ØNS

2022, 1Q, 48	Repair of facial fractures of frontal sinus and orbital roof
2017, 3Q, 22	Replacement of native skull bone flap
2017, 1Q, 20	Preparatory nasal adhesion repair before definitive cleft palate repair
2016, 2Q, 30	Clipping (occlusion) of cerebral artery, decompressive craniectomy and storage of bone flap in abdominal wall
2015, 3Q, 17	Craniosynostosis with cranial vault reconstruction
2015, 3Q, 27	Moyamoya disease and hemispheric pial synangiosis with craniotomy
2014, 3Q, 23	Le Fort I osteotomy
2013, 3Q, 24	Distraction osteogenesis
2013, 3Q, 25	Fracture of frontal bone with repair and coagulation for hemostasis

AHA Coding Clinic for table ØNU

2021, 3Q, 29	Repair of superior semicircular canal dehiscence
2016, 3Q, 29	Closure of bilateral alveolar clefts
2013, 3Q, 24	Distraction osteogenesis

Head and Facial Bones

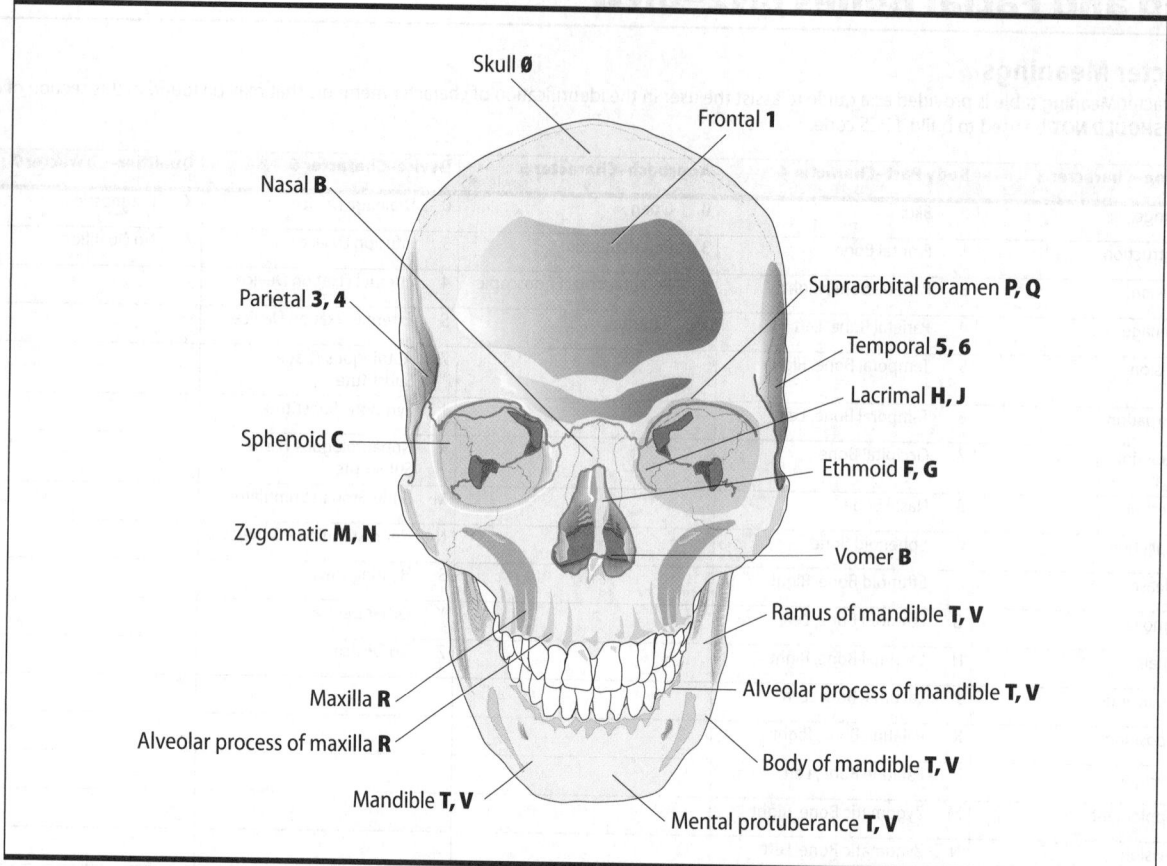

Skull **Ø**

Frontal **1**

Nasal **B**

Supraorbital foramen **P, Q**

Parietal **3, 4**

Temporal **5, 6**

Lacrimal **H, J**

Sphenoid **C**

Ethmoid **F, G**

Zygomatic **M, N**

Vomer **B**

Ramus of mandible **T, V**

Maxilla **R**

Alveolar process of mandible **T, V**

Alveolar process of maxilla **R**

Body of mandible **T, V**

Mandible **T, V**

Mental protuberance **T, V**

Skull Bones

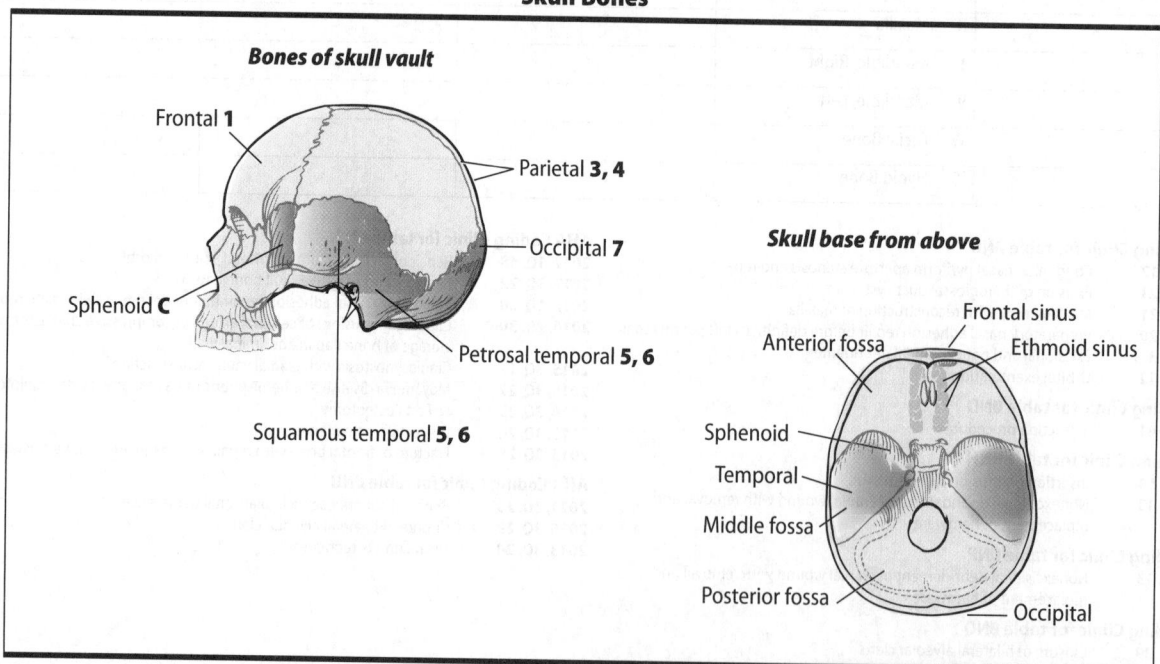

Bones of skull vault

Frontal **1**

Parietal **3, 4**

Occipital **7**

Sphenoid **C**

Petrosal temporal **5, 6**

Squamous temporal **5, 6**

Skull base from above

Frontal sinus

Ethmoid sinus

Anterior fossa

Sphenoid

Temporal

Middle fossa

Posterior fossa

Occipital

Ø   **Medical and Surgical**
N   **Head and Facial Bones**
2   **Change**   Definition: Taking out or off a device from a body part and putting back an identical or similar device in or on the same body part without cutting or puncturing the skin or a mucous membrane

                        Explanation: All CHANGE procedures are coded using the approach EXTERNAL

Body Part Character 4	Approach Character 5	Device Character 6	Qualifier Character 7
Ø Skull **B** Nasal Bone Vomer of nasal septum **W** Facial Bone	**X** External	**Ø** Drainage Device **Y** Other Device	**Z** No Qualifier

  Non-OR   All body part, approach, device, and qualifier values

Ø   **Medical and Surgical**
N   **Head and Facial Bones**
5   **Destruction**   Definition: Physical eradication of all or a portion of a body part by the direct use of energy, force, or a destructive agent

                        Explanation: None of the body part is physically taken out

Body Part Character 4	Approach Character 5	Device Character 6	Qualifier Character 7

Ø Skull
1 Frontal Bone
    Zygomatic process of frontal bone
3 Parietal Bone, Right
4 Parietal Bone, Left
5 Temporal Bone, Right
    Mastoid process
    Petrous part of temporal bone
    Tympanic part of temporal bone
    Zygomatic process of temporal bone
6 Temporal Bone, Left
    See 5 Temporal Bone, Right
7 Occipital Bone
    Foramen magnum
B Nasal Bone
    Vomer of nasal septum
C Sphenoid Bone
    Greater wing
    Lesser wing
    Optic foramen
    Pterygoid process
    Sella turcica
F Ethmoid Bone, Right
    Cribriform plate
G Ethmoid Bone, Left
    See F Ethmoid Bone, Right
H Lacrimal Bone, Right
J Lacrimal Bone, Left
K Palatine Bone, Right
L Palatine Bone, Left
M Zygomatic Bone, Right
N Zygomatic Bone, Left
P Orbit, Right
    Bony orbit
    Orbital portion of ethmoid bone
    Orbital portion of frontal bone
    Orbital portion of lacrimal bone
    Orbital portion of maxilla
    Orbital portion of palatine bone
    Orbital portion of sphenoid bone
    Orbital portion of zygomatic bone
Q Orbit, Left
    See P Orbit, Right
R Maxilla
    Alveolar process of maxilla
T Mandible, Right
    Alveolar process of mandible
    Condyloid process
    Mandibular notch
    Mental foramen
V Mandible, Left
    See T Mandible, Right
X Hyoid Bone
	Ø Open
	3 Percutaneous
	4 Percutaneous Endoscopic
		Z No Device	**Z** No Qualifier

NC Noncovered Procedure   **LC** Limited Coverage   **QA** Questionable OB Admit   **NT** New Tech Add-on   ⊞ Combination Member   ♂ Male   ♀ Female

ICD-10-PCS 2023   **523**

Head and Facial Bones

Ø   **Medical and Surgical**
N   **Head and Facial Bones**
8   **Division**   Definition: Cutting into a body part, without draining fluids and/or gases from the body part, in order to separate or transect a body part
                      Explanation: All or a portion of the body part is separated into two or more portions

Body Part Character 4	Approach Character 5	Device Character 6	Qualifier Character 7
Ø Skull	**Ø** Open	**Z** No Device	**Z** No Qualifier
1 Frontal Bone Zygomatic process of frontal bone	**3** Percutaneous **4** Percutaneous Endoscopic		
3 Parietal Bone, Right			
4 Parietal Bone, Left			

5   Temporal Bone, Right
     Mastoid process
     Petrous part of temporal bone
     Tympanic part of temporal bone
     Zygomatic process of temporal bone			

6 Temporal Bone, Left *See 5 Temporal Bone, Right*			
7 Occipital Bone Foramen magnum			
B Nasal Bone Vomer of nasal septum			

C   Sphenoid Bone
     Greater wing
     Lesser wing
     Optic foramen
     Pterygoid process
     Sella turcica			

F Ethmoid Bone, Right Cribriform plate			
G Ethmoid Bone, Left *See F Ethmoid Bone, Right*			
H Lacrimal Bone, Right			
J Lacrimal Bone, Left			
K Palatine Bone, Right			
L Palatine Bone, Left			
M Zygomatic Bone, Right			
N Zygomatic Bone, Left			

P   Orbit, Right
     Bony orbit
     Orbital portion of ethmoid bone
     Orbital portion of frontal bone
     Orbital portion of lacrimal bone
     Orbital portion of maxilla
     Orbital portion of palatine bone
     Orbital portion of sphenoid bone
     Orbital portion of zygomatic bone			

Q Orbit, Left *See P Orbit, Right*			
R Maxilla Alveolar process of maxilla			

T   Mandible, Right
     Alveolar process of mandible
     Condyloid process
     Mandibular notch
     Mental foramen			

V Mandible, Left *See T Mandible, Right*			
X Hyoid Bone			

Non-OR   ØN8B[Ø,3,4]ZZ

Non-OR Procedure   DRG Non-OR Procedure   Valid OR Procedure   HAC Associated Procedure   Combination Only   New/Revised April   New/Revised October

524   ICD-10-PCS 2023

Ø Medical and Surgical
N Head and Facial Bones
9 Drainage   Definition: Taking or letting out fluids and/or gases from a body part

                 Explanation: The qualifier DIAGNOSTIC is used to identify drainage procedures that are biopsies

Body Part Character 4	Approach Character 5	Device Character 6	Qualifier Character 7
Ø Skull	**Ø Open**	**Ø Drainage Device**	**Z No Qualifier**
1 Frontal Bone	**3 Percutaneous**		
Zygomatic process of frontal bone	**4 Percutaneous Endoscopic**		
3 Parietal Bone, Right			
4 Parietal Bone, Left			
5 Temporal Bone, Right			
Mastoid process			
Petrous part of temporal bone			
Tympanic part of temporal bone			
Zygomatic process of temporal bone			
6 Temporal Bone, Left			
See 5 Temporal Bone, Right			
7 Occipital Bone			
Foramen magnum			
B Nasal Bone			
Vomer of nasal septum			
C Sphenoid Bone			
Greater wing			
Lesser wing			
Optic foramen			
Pterygoid process			
Sella turcica			
F Ethmoid Bone, Right			
Cribriform plate			
G Ethmoid Bone, Left			
See F Ethmoid Bone, Right			
H Lacrimal Bone, Right			
J Lacrimal Bone, Left			
K Palatine Bone, Right			
L Palatine Bone, Left			
M Zygomatic Bone, Right			
N Zygomatic Bone, Left			
P Orbit, Right			
Bony orbit			
Orbital portion of ethmoid bone			
Orbital portion of frontal bone			
Orbital portion of lacrimal bone			
Orbital portion of maxilla			
Orbital portion of palatine bone			
Orbital portion of sphenoid bone			
Orbital portion of zygomatic bone			
Q Orbit, Left			
See P Orbit, Right			
R Maxilla			
Alveolar process of maxilla			
T Mandible, Right			
Alveolar process of mandible			
Condyloid process			
Mandibular notch			
Mental foramen			
V Mandible, Left			
See T Mandible, Right			
X Hyoid Bone			

Non-OR   ØN9[Ø,1,3,4,5,6,7,C,F,G,H,J,K,L,M,N,P,Q,X]3ØZ
Non-OR   ØN9[B,R,T,V][Ø,3,4]ØZ

ØN9 Continued on next page

NC Noncovered Procedure   LC Limited Coverage   OA Questionable OB Admit   NT New Tech Add-on   ✛ Combination Member   ♂ Male   ♀ Female

ICD-10-PCS 2023   **525**

Ø   **Medical and Surgical**
N   **Head and Facial Bones**
9   **Drainage**   Definition: Taking or letting out fluids and/or gases from a body part
                        Explanation: The qualifier DIAGNOSTIC is used to identify drainage procedures that are biopsies

Body Part Character 4	Approach Character 5	Device Character 6	Qualifier Character 7
Ø Skull	**Ø** Open	**Z** No Device	**X** Diagnostic
1 Frontal Bone	**3** Percutaneous		**Z** No Qualifier
Zygomatic process of frontal bone	**4** Percutaneous Endoscopic		
3 Parietal Bone, Right			
4 Parietal Bone, Left			
5 Temporal Bone, Right			
Mastoid process			
Petrous part of temporal bone			
Tympanic part of temporal bone			
Zygomatic process of temporal bone			
6 Temporal Bone, Left			
See 5 Temporal Bone, Right			
7 Occipital Bone			
Foramen magnum			
B Nasal Bone			
Vomer of nasal septum			
C Sphenoid Bone			
Greater wing			
Lesser wing			
Optic foramen			
Pterygoid process			
Sella turcica			
F Ethmoid Bone, Right			
Cribriform plate			
G Ethmoid Bone, Left			
See F Ethmoid Bone, Right			
H Lacrimal Bone, Right			
J Lacrimal Bone, Left			
K Palatine Bone, Right			
L Palatine Bone, Left			
M Zygomatic Bone, Right			
N Zygomatic Bone, Left			
P Orbit, Right			
Bony orbit			
Orbital portion of ethmoid bone			
Orbital portion of frontal bone			
Orbital portion of lacrimal bone			
Orbital portion of maxilla			
Orbital portion of palatine bone			
Orbital portion of sphenoid bone			
Orbital portion of zygomatic bone			
Q Orbit, Left			
See P Orbit, Right			
R Maxilla			
Alveolar process of maxilla			
T Mandible, Right			
Alveolar process of mandible			
Condyloid process			
Mandibular notch			
Mental foramen			
V Mandible, Left			
See T Mandible, Right			
X Hyoid Bone			

Non-OR   ØN9[Ø,1,3,4,5,6,7,C,F,G,H,J,K,L,M,N,P,Q,X]3ZZ
Non-OR   ØN9B[Ø,3,4]Z[X,Z]
Non-OR   ØN9[R,T,V][Ø,3,4]ZZ

Non-OR Procedure   DRG Non-OR Procedure   Valid OR Procedure   HAC Associated Procedure   Combination Only   New/Revised April   New/Revised October
526   ICD-10-PCS 2023

ØN9–ØN9

Ø   **Medical and Surgical**
N   **Head and Facial Bones**
B   **Excision**   Definition: Cutting out or off, without replacement, a portion of a body part
                    Explanation: The qualifier DIAGNOSTIC is used to identify excision procedures that are biopsies

Body Part Character 4	Approach Character 5	Device Character 6	Qualifier Character 7
Ø **Skull**	**Ø** Open	**Z** No Device	**X** Diagnostic
1 **Frontal Bone**	**3** Percutaneous		**Z** No Qualifier
Zygomatic process of frontal bone	**4** Percutaneous Endoscopic		
3 **Parietal Bone, Right**			
4 **Parietal Bone, Left**			
5 **Temporal Bone, Right**			
Mastoid process			
Petrous part of temporal bone			
Tympanic part of temporal bone			
Zygomatic process of temporal bone			
6 **Temporal Bone, Left**			
See 5 Temporal Bone, Right			
7 **Occipital Bone**			
Foramen magnum			
B Nasal Bone			
Vomer of nasal septum			
C **Sphenoid Bone**			
Greater wing			
Lesser wing			
Optic foramen			
Pterygoid process			
Sella turcica			
F **Ethmoid Bone, Right**			
Cribriform plate			
G **Ethmoid Bone, Left**			
See F Ethmoid Bone, Right			
H **Lacrimal Bone, Right**			
J **Lacrimal Bone, Left**			
K **Palatine Bone, Right**			
L **Palatine Bone, Left**			
M **Zygomatic Bone, Right**			
N **Zygomatic Bone, Left**			
P **Orbit, Right**			
Bony orbit			
Orbital portion of ethmoid bone			
Orbital portion of frontal bone			
Orbital portion of lacrimal bone			
Orbital portion of maxilla			
Orbital portion of palatine bone			
Orbital portion of sphenoid bone			
Orbital portion of zygomatic bone			
Q **Orbit, Left**			
See P Orbit, Right			
R Maxilla			
Alveolar process of maxilla			
T Mandible, Right			
Alveolar process of mandible			
Condyloid process			
Mandibular notch			
Mental foramen			
V Mandible, Left			
See T Mandible, Right			
X **Hyoid Bone**			

Non-OR   ØNB[B,R,T,V][Ø,3,4]ZX

NC Noncovered Procedure   LC Limited Coverage   QA Questionable OB Admit   NT New Tech Add-on   ⊞ Combination Member   ♂ Male   ♀ Female

ICD-10-PCS 2023   527

Ø   Medical and Surgical
N   Head and Facial Bones
C   Extirpation   Definition: Taking or cutting out solid matter from a body part

Explanation: The solid matter may be an abnormal byproduct of a biological function or a foreign body; it may be imbedded in a body part or in the lumen of a tubular body part. The solid matter may or may not have been previously broken into pieces.

Body Part Character 4	Approach Character 5	Device Character 6	Qualifier Character 7
1 Frontal Bone Zygomatic process of frontal bone	**Ø Open** **3 Percutaneous** **4 Percutaneous Endoscopic**	**Z No Device**	**Z No Qualifier**
3 Parietal Bone, Right			
4 Parietal Bone, Left			
5 Temporal Bone, Right Mastoid process Petrous part of temporal bone Tympanic part of temporal bone Zygomatic process of temporal bone			
6 Temporal Bone, Left *See 5 Temporal Bone, Right*			
7 Occipital Bone Foramen magnum			
B Nasal Bone Vomer of nasal septum			
C Sphenoid Bone Greater wing Lesser wing Optic foramen Pterygoid process Sella turcica			
F Ethmoid Bone, Right Cribriform plate			
G Ethmoid Bone, Left *See F Ethmoid Bone, Right*			
H Lacrimal Bone, Right			
J Lacrimal Bone, Left			
K Palatine Bone, Right			
L Palatine Bone, Left			
M Zygomatic Bone, Right			
N Zygomatic Bone, Left			
P Orbit, Right Bony orbit Orbital portion of ethmoid bone Orbital portion of frontal bone Orbital portion of lacrimal bone Orbital portion of maxilla Orbital portion of palatine bone Orbital portion of sphenoid bone Orbital portion of zygomatic bone			
Q Orbit, Left *See P Orbit, Right*			
R Maxilla Alveolar process of maxilla			
T Mandible, Right Alveolar process of mandible Condyloid process Mandibular notch Mental foramen			
V Mandible, Left *See T Mandible, Right*			
X Hyoid Bone			

Non-OR   ØNC[B,R,T,V][Ø,3,4]ZZ

Ø   **Medical and Surgical**
N   **Head and Facial Bones**
D   **Extraction**   Definition: Pulling or stripping out or off all or a portion of a body part by the use of force
                    Explanation: The qualifier DIAGNOSTIC is used to identify extraction procedures that are biopsies

Body Part Character 4	Approach Character 5	Device Character 6	Qualifier Character 7
Ø Skull	**Ø** Open	**Z** No Device	**Z** No Qualifier
1 **Frontal Bone** Zygomatic process of frontal bone			
3 **Parietal Bone, Right**			
4 **Parietal Bone, Left**			

5 **Temporal Bone, Right**
    Mastoid process
    Petrous part of temporal bone
    Tympanic part of temporal bone
    Zygomatic process of temporal bone			

6 **Temporal Bone, Left** *See 5 Temporal Bone, Right*			
7 **Occipital Bone** Foramen magnum			
B **Nasal Bone** Vomer of nasal septum			

C **Sphenoid Bone**
    Greater wing
    Lesser wing
    Optic foramen
    Pterygoid process
    Sella turcica			

F **Ethmoid Bone, Right** Cribriform plate			
G **Ethmoid Bone, Left** *See F Ethmoid Bone, Right*			
H **Lacrimal Bone, Right**			
J **Lacrimal Bone, Left**			
K **Palatine Bone, Right**			
L **Palatine Bone, Left**			
M **Zygomatic Bone, Right**			
N **Zygomatic Bone, Left**			

P **Orbit, Right**
    Bony orbit
    Orbital portion of ethmoid bone
    Orbital portion of frontal bone
    Orbital portion of lacrimal bone
    Orbital portion of maxilla
    Orbital portion of palatine bone
    Orbital portion of sphenoid bone
    Orbital portion of zygomatic bone			

Q **Orbit, Left** *See P Orbit, Right*			
R **Maxilla** Alveolar process of maxilla			

T **Mandible, Right**
    Alveolar process of mandible
    Condyloid process
    Mandibular notch
    Mental foramen			

V **Mandible, Left** *See T Mandible, Right*			
X **Hyoid Bone**			

Head and Facial Bones

Ø   **Medical and Surgical**
N   **Head and Facial Bones**
H   **Insertion**   Definition: Putting in a nonbiological appliance that monitors, assists, performs, or prevents a physiological function but does not physically take the place of a body part

        Explanation: None

Body Part Character 4	Approach Character 5	Device Character 6	Qualifier Character 7
Ø Skull ⊞	Ø Open	3 Infusion Device 4 Internal Fixation Device 5 External Fixation Device M Bone Growth Stimulator N Neurostimulator Generator	Z No Qualifier
Ø Skull	3 Percutaneous 4 Percutaneous Endoscopic	3 Infusion Device 4 Internal Fixation Device 5 External Fixation Device M Bone Growth Stimulator	Z No Qualifier

1 Frontal Bone
     Zygomatic process of frontal bone
3 Parietal Bone, Right
4 Parietal Bone, Left
7 Occipital Bone
     Foramen magnum
C Sphenoid Bone
     Greater wing
     Lesser wing
     Optic foramen
     Pterygoid process
     Sella turcica
F Ethmoid Bone, Right
     Cribriform plate
G Ethmoid Bone, Left
     See F Ethmoid Bone, Right
H Lacrimal Bone, Right
J Lacrimal Bone, Left
K Palatine Bone, Right
L Palatine Bone, Left
M Zygomatic Bone, Right
N Zygomatic Bone, Left
P Orbit, Right
     Bony orbit
     Orbital portion of ethmoid bone
     Orbital portion of frontal bone
     Orbital portion of lacrimal bone
     Orbital portion of maxilla
     Orbital portion of palatine bone
     Orbital portion of sphenoid bone
     Orbital portion of zygomatic bone
Q Orbit, Left
     See P Orbit, Right
X Hyoid Bone
	Ø Open
	3 Percutaneous
	4 Percutaneous Endoscopic
		4 Internal Fixation Device	Z No Qualifier

5 Temporal Bone, Right
     Mastoid process
     Petrous part of temporal bone
     Tympanic part of temporal bone
     Zygomatic process of temporal bone
6 Temporal Bone, Left
     See 5 Temporal Bone, Right
	Ø Open
	3 Percutaneous
	4 Percutaneous Endoscopic
		4 Internal Fixation Device
		S Hearing Device
			Z No Qualifier

B Nasal Bone Vomer of nasal septum	Ø Open 3 Percutaneous 4 Percutaneous Endoscopic	4 Internal Fixation Device M Bone Growth Stimulator	Z No Qualifier

R Maxilla
     Alveolar process of maxilla
T Mandible, Right
     Alveolar process of mandible
     Condyloid process
     Mandibular notch
     Mental foramen
V Mandible, Left
     See T Mandible, Right
	Ø Open
	3 Percutaneous
	4 Percutaneous Endoscopic
		4 Internal Fixation Device
		5 External Fixation Device
			Z No Qualifier

W Facial Bone	Ø Open 3 Percutaneous 4 Percutaneous Endoscopic	M Bone Growth Stimulator	Z No Qualifier

Non-OR	ØNHØØ5Z
Non-OR	ØNHØ[3,4]5Z
Non-OR	ØNHB[Ø,3,4][4,M]Z

See Appendix L for Procedure Combinations
⊞   ØNHØØNZ

Non-OR Procedure DRG Non-OR Procedure Valid OR Procedure HAC Associated Procedure Combination Only New/Revised April New/Revised October

530   ICD-10-PCS 2023

Ø   **Medical and Surgical**
N   **Head and Facial Bones**
J   **Inspection**   Definition: Visually and/or manually exploring a body part

                Explanation: Visual exploration may be performed with or without optical instrumentation. Manual exploration may be performed directly or through intervening body layers.

Body Part Character 4	Approach Character 5	Device Character 6	Qualifier Character 7
Ø Skull **B** Nasal Bone Vomer of nasal septum **W** Facial Bone	**Ø** Open **3** Percutaneous **4** Percutaneous Endoscopic **X** External	**Z** No Device	**Z** No Qualifier

     Non-OR   ØNJ[Ø,B,W][3,X]ZZ

Ø   **Medical and Surgical**
N   **Head and Facial Bones**
N   **Release**   Definition: Freeing a body part from an abnormal physical constraint by cutting or by the use of force

                Explanation: Some of the restraining tissue may be taken out but none of the body part is taken out

Body Part Character 4	Approach Character 5	Device Character 6	Qualifier Character 7

1   Frontal Bone
     Zygomatic process of frontal bone
3   Parietal Bone, Right
4   Parietal Bone, Left
5   Temporal Bone, Right
     Mastoid process
     Petrous part of temporal bone
     Tympanic part of temporal bone
     Zygomatic process of temporal bone
6   Temporal Bone, Left
     See 5 Temporal Bone, Right
7   Occipital Bone
     Foramen magnum
B   Nasal Bone
     Vomer of nasal septum
C   Sphenoid Bone
     Greater wing
     Lesser wing
     Optic foramen
     Pterygoid process
     Sella turcica
F   Ethmoid Bone, Right
     Cribriform plate
G   Ethmoid Bone, Left
     See F Ethmoid Bone, Right
H   Lacrimal Bone, Right
J   Lacrimal Bone, Left
K   Palatine Bone, Right
L   Palatine Bone, Left
M   Zygomatic Bone, Right
N   Zygomatic Bone, Left
P   Orbit, Right
     Bony orbit
     Orbital portion of ethmoid bone
     Orbital portion of frontal bone
     Orbital portion of lacrimal bone
     Orbital portion of maxilla
     Orbital portion of palatine bone
     Orbital portion of sphenoid bone
     Orbital portion of zygomatic bone
Q   Orbit, Left
     See P Orbit, Right
R   Maxilla
     Alveolar process of maxilla
T   Mandible, Right
     Alveolar process of mandible
     Condyloid process
     Mandibular notch
     Mental foramen
V   Mandible, Left
     See T Mandible, Right
X   Hyoid Bone
	Ø Open
	3 Percutaneous
	4 Percutaneous Endoscopic
		Z No Device	**Z** No Qualifier

     Non-OR   ØNNB[Ø,3,4]ZZ

NC Noncovered Procedure   **LC** Limited Coverage   **QA** Questionable OB Admit   **NT** New Tech Add-on   ⊞ Combination Member   ♂ Male   ♀ Female

ICD-10-PCS 2023   **531**

Ø   **Medical and Surgical**
N   **Head and Facial Bones**
P   **Removal**   Definition: Taking out or off a device from a body part

Explanation: If a device is taken out and a similar device put in without cutting or puncturing the skin or mucous membrane, the procedure is coded to the root operation CHANGE. Otherwise, the procedure for taking out a device is coded to the root operation REMOVAL.

Body Part Character 4	Approach Character 5	Device Character 6	Qualifier Character 7
Ø Skull	Ø Open	Ø Drainage Device 3 Infusion Device 4 Internal Fixation Device 5 External Fixation Device 7 Autologous Tissue Substitute J Synthetic Substitute K Nonautologous Tissue Substitute M Bone Growth Stimulator N Neurostimulator Generator S Hearing Device	Z No Qualifier
Ø Skull	3 Percutaneous 4 Percutaneous Endoscopic	Ø Drainage Device 3 Infusion Device 4 Internal Fixation Device 5 External Fixation Device 7 Autologous Tissue Substitute J Synthetic Substitute K Nonautologous Tissue Substitute M Bone Growth Stimulator S Hearing Device	Z No Qualifier
Ø Skull	X External	Ø Drainage Device 3 Infusion Device 4 Internal Fixation Device 5 External Fixation Device M Bone Growth Stimulator S Hearing Device	Z No Qualifier
B Nasal Bone Vomer of nasal septum W Facial Bone	Ø Open 3 Percutaneous 4 Percutaneous Endoscopic	Ø Drainage Device 4 Internal Fixation Device 7 Autologous Tissue Substitute J Synthetic Substitute K Nonautologous Tissue Substitute M Bone Growth Stimulator	Z No Qualifier
B Nasal Bone Vomer of nasal septum W Facial Bone	X External	Ø Drainage Device 4 Internal Fixation Device M Bone Growth Stimulator	Z No Qualifier

Non-OR   ØNPØ[3,4]5Z
Non-OR   ØNPØX[Ø,3,5]Z
Non-OR   ØNPB[Ø,3,4][Ø,4,7,J,K,M]Z
Non-OR   ØNPBX[Ø,4,M]Z
Non-OR   ØNPWX[Ø,M]Z

Ø   **Medical and Surgical**
N   **Head and Facial Bones**
Q   **Repair**   Definition: Restoring, to the extent possible, a body part to its normal anatomic structure and function

                     Explanation: Used only when the method to accomplish the repair is not one of the other root operations

Body Part Character 4	Approach Character 5	Device Character 6	Qualifier Character 7
Ø **Skull**	**Ø** Open	**Z** No Device	**Z** No Qualifier
1 **Frontal Bone**	**3** Percutaneous		
Zygomatic process of frontal bone	**4** Percutaneous Endoscopic		
3 **Parietal Bone, Right**	**X** External		
4 **Parietal Bone, Left**			
5 **Temporal Bone, Right**			
Mastoid process			
Petrous part of temporal bone			
Tympanic part of temporal bone			
Zygomatic process of temporal bone			
6 **Temporal Bone, Left**			
See 5 Temporal Bone, Right			
7 **Occipital Bone**			
Foramen magnum			
B **Nasal Bone**			
Vomer of nasal septum			
C **Sphenoid Bone**			
Greater wing			
Lesser wing			
Optic foramen			
Pterygoid process			
Sella turcica			
F **Ethmoid Bone, Right**			
Cribriform plate			
G **Ethmoid Bone, Left**			
See F Ethmoid Bone, Right			
H **Lacrimal Bone, Right**			
J **Lacrimal Bone, Left**			
K **Palatine Bone, Right**			
L **Palatine Bone, Left**			
M **Zygomatic Bone, Right**			
N **Zygomatic Bone, Left**			
P **Orbit, Right**			
Bony orbit			
Orbital portion of ethmoid bone			
Orbital portion of frontal bone			
Orbital portion of lacrimal bone			
Orbital portion of maxilla			
Orbital portion of palatine bone			
Orbital portion of sphenoid bone			
Orbital portion of zygomatic bone			
Q **Orbit, Left**			
See P Orbit, Right			
R **Maxilla**			
Alveolar process of maxilla			
T **Mandible, Right**			
Alveolar process of mandible			
Condyloid process			
Mandibular notch			
Mental foramen			
V **Mandible, Left**			
See T Mandible, Right			
X **Hyoid Bone**			

Non-OR   ØNQ[Ø,1,3,4,5,6,7,B,C,F,G,H,J,K,L,M,N,P,Q,R,T,V,X]XZZ

NC Noncovered Procedure   LC Limited Coverage   QA Questionable OB Admit   NT New Tech Add-on   ⊞ Combination Member   ♂ Male   ♀ Female

ICD-10-PCS 2023   **533**

ØNQ–ØNQ

Head and Facial Bones

Ø   Medical and Surgical
N   Head and Facial Bones
R   Replacement   Definition: Putting in or on biological or synthetic material that physically takes the place and/or function of all or a portion of a body part
Explanation: The body part may have been taken out or replaced, or may be taken out, physically eradicated, or rendered nonfunctional during the REPLACEMENT procedure. A REMOVAL procedure is coded for taking out the device used in a previous replacement procedure.

Body Part Character 4	Approach Character 5	Device Character 6	Qualifier Character 7
Ø Skull	**Ø Open**	**7 Autologous Tissue Substitute**	**Z No Qualifier**
1 Frontal Bone	**3 Percutaneous**	**J Synthetic Substitute**	
Zygomatic process of frontal bone	**4 Percutaneous Endoscopic**	**K Nonautologous Tissue Substitute**	
3 Parietal Bone, Right			
4 Parietal Bone, Left			
5 Temporal Bone, Right			
Mastoid process			
Petrous part of temporal bone			
Tympanic part of temporal bone			
Zygomatic process of temporal bone			
6 Temporal Bone, Left			
See 5 Temporal Bone, Right			
7 Occipital Bone			
Foramen magnum			
B Nasal Bone			
Vomer of nasal septum			
C Sphenoid Bone			
Greater wing			
Lesser wing			
Optic foramen			
Pterygoid process			
Sella turcica			
F Ethmoid Bone, Right			
Cribriform plate			
G Ethmoid Bone, Left			
See F Ethmoid Bone, Right			
H Lacrimal Bone, Right			
J Lacrimal Bone, Left			
K Palatine Bone, Right			
L Palatine Bone, Left			
M Zygomatic Bone, Right			
N Zygomatic Bone, Left			
P Orbit, Right			
Bony orbit			
Orbital portion of ethmoid bone			
Orbital portion of frontal bone			
Orbital portion of lacrimal bone			
Orbital portion of maxilla			
Orbital portion of palatine bone			
Orbital portion of sphenoid bone			
Orbital portion of zygomatic bone			
Q Orbit, Left			
See P Orbit, Right			
R Maxilla			
Alveolar process of maxilla			
T Mandible, Right			
Alveolar process of mandible			
Condyloid process			
Mandibular notch			
Mental foramen			
V Mandible, Left			
See T Mandible, Right			
X Hyoid Bone			

Non-OR Procedure   DRG Non-OR Procedure   Valid OR Procedure   HAC Associated Procedure   Combination Only   New/Revised April   New/Revised October

534   ICD-10-PCS 2023

Ø   Medical and Surgical
N   Head and Facial Bones
S   Reposition   Definition: Moving to its normal location, or other suitable location, all or a portion of a body part

           Explanation: The body part is moved to a new location from an abnormal location, or from a normal location where it is not functioning correctly. The body part may or may not be cut out or off to be moved to the new location.

Body Part Character 4	Approach Character 5	Device Character 6	Qualifier Character 7

Ø Skull
R Maxilla
     Alveolar process of maxilla
T Mandible, Right
     Alveolar process of mandible
     Condyloid process
     Mandibular notch
     Mental foramen
V Mandible, Left
     See T Mandible, Right
	Ø Open
	3 Percutaneous
	4 Percutaneous Endoscopic
		4 Internal Fixation Device
		5 External Fixation Device
		Z No Device
			Z No Qualifier

Ø Skull
R Maxilla
     Alveolar process of maxilla
T Mandible, Right
     Alveolar process of mandible
     Condyloid process
     Mandibular notch
     Mental foramen
V Mandible, Left
     See T Mandible, Right
	X External	**Z** No Device	**Z** No Qualifier

1 Frontal Bone
     Zygomatic process of frontal bone
3 Parietal Bone, Right
4 Parietal Bone, Left
5 Temporal Bone, Right
     Mastoid process
     Petrous part of temporal bone
     Tympanic part of temporal bone
     Zygomatic process of temporal bone
6 Temporal Bone, Left
     See 5 Temporal Bone, Right
7 Occipital Bone
     Foramen magnum
B Nasal Bone
     Vomer of nasal septum
C Sphenoid Bone
     Greater wing
     Lesser wing
     Optic foramen
     Pterygoid process
     Sella turcica
F Ethmoid Bone, Right
     Cribriform plate
G Ethmoid Bone, Left
     See F Ethmoid Bone, Right
H Lacrimal Bone, Right
J Lacrimal Bone, Left
K Palatine Bone, Right
L Palatine Bone, Left
M Zygomatic Bone, Right
N Zygomatic Bone, Left
P Orbit, Right
     Bony orbit
     Orbital portion of ethmoid bone
     Orbital portion of frontal bone
     Orbital portion of lacrimal bone
     Orbital portion of maxilla
     Orbital portion of palatine bone
     Orbital portion of sphenoid bone
     Orbital portion of zygomatic bone
Q Orbit, Left
     See P Orbit, Right
X Hyoid Bone
	Ø Open
	3 Percutaneous
	4 Percutaneous Endoscopic
		4 Internal Fixation Device
		Z No Device
			Z No Qualifier

Non-OR   ØNS[R,T,V][3,4][4,5,Z]Z
Non-OR   ØNS[Ø,R,T,V]XZZ
Non-OR   ØNS[B,C,F,G,H,J,K,L,M,N,P,Q,X][3,4][4,Z]Z

ØNS Continued on next page

NC Noncovered Procedure   **LC** Limited Coverage   **QA** Questionable OB Admit   **NT** New Tech Add-on   ⊞ Combination Member   ♂ Male   ♀ Female

Head and Facial Bones *(left margin)*

Ø   Medical and Surgical
N   Head and Facial Bones   *ØNS Continued*
S   Reposition   Definition: Moving to its normal location, or other suitable location, all or a portion of a body part

Explanation: The body part is moved to a new location from an abnormal location, or from a normal location where it is not functioning correctly. The body part may or may not be cut out or off to be moved to the new location.

Body Part Character 4	Approach Character 5	Device Character 6	Qualifier Character 7
1 Frontal Bone Zygomatic process of frontal bone **3 Parietal Bone, Right** **4 Parietal Bone, Left** **5 Temporal Bone, Right** Mastoid process Petrous part of temporal bone Tympanic part of temporal bone Zygomatic process of temporal bone **6 Temporal Bone, Left** *See 5 Temporal Bone, Right* **7 Occipital Bone** Foramen magnum **B Nasal Bone** Vomer of nasal septum **C Sphenoid Bone** Greater wing Lesser wing Optic foramen Pterygoid process Sella turcica **F Ethmoid Bone, Right** Cribriform plate **G Ethmoid Bone, Left** *See F Ethmoid Bone, Right* **H Lacrimal Bone, Right** **J Lacrimal Bone, Left** **K Palatine Bone, Right** **L Palatine Bone, Left** **M Zygomatic Bone, Right** **N Zygomatic Bone, Left** **P Orbit, Right** Bony orbit Orbital portion of ethmoid bone Orbital portion of frontal bone Orbital portion of lacrimal bone Orbital portion of maxilla Orbital portion of palatine bone Orbital portion of sphenoid bone Orbital portion of zygomatic bone **Q Orbit, Left** *See P Orbit, Right* **X Hyoid Bone**	**X** External	**Z** No Device	**Z** No Qualifier

Non-OR   ØNS[1,3,4,5,6,7,B,C,F,G,H,J,K,L,M,N,P,Q,X]XZZ

Ø　**Medical and Surgical**
N　**Head and Facial Bones**
T　**Resection**　　　Definition: Cutting out or off, without replacement, all of a body part
　　　　　　　　　　　Explanation: None

Body Part Character 4	Approach Character 5	Device Character 6	Qualifier Character 7
1　**Frontal Bone** 　　Zygomatic process of frontal bone	Ø　Open	Z　No Device	Z　No Qualifier
3　**Parietal Bone, Right**			
4　**Parietal Bone, Left**			
5　**Temporal Bone, Right** 　　Mastoid process 　　Petrous part of temporal bone 　　Tympanic part of temporal bone 　　Zygomatic process of temporal bone			
6　**Temporal Bone, Left** 　　*See 5 Temporal Bone, Right*			
7　**Occipital Bone** 　　Foramen magnum			
B　**Nasal Bone** 　　Vomer of nasal septum			
C　**Sphenoid Bone** 　　Greater wing 　　Lesser wing 　　Optic foramen 　　Pterygoid process 　　Sella turcica			
F　**Ethmoid Bone, Right** 　　Cribriform plate			
G　**Ethmoid Bone, Left** 　　*See F Ethmoid Bone, Right*			
H　**Lacrimal Bone, Right**			
J　**Lacrimal Bone, Left**			
K　**Palatine Bone, Right**			
L　**Palatine Bone, Left**			
M　**Zygomatic Bone, Right**			
N　**Zygomatic Bone, Left**			
P　**Orbit, Right** 　　Bony orbit 　　Orbital portion of ethmoid bone 　　Orbital portion of frontal bone 　　Orbital portion of lacrimal bone 　　Orbital portion of maxilla 　　Orbital portion of palatine bone 　　Orbital portion of sphenoid bone 　　Orbital portion of zygomatic bone			
Q　**Orbit, Left** 　　*See P Orbit, Right*			
R　**Maxilla** 　　Alveolar process of maxilla			
T　**Mandible, Right** 　　Alveolar process of mandible 　　Condyloid process 　　Mandibular notch 　　Mental foramen			
V　**Mandible, Left** 　　*See T Mandible, Right*			
X　**Hyoid Bone**			

Head and Facial Bones

Ø **Medical and Surgical**
N **Head and Facial Bones**
U **Supplement**   Definition: Putting in or on biological or synthetic material that physically reinforces and/or augments the function of a portion of a body part

        Explanation: The biological material is non-living, or is living and from the same individual. The body part may have been previously replaced, and the SUPPLEMENT procedure is performed to physically reinforce and/or augment the function of the replaced body part.

Body Part Character 4	Approach Character 5	Device Character 6	Qualifier Character 7
Ø Skull	Ø Open	7 Autologous Tissue Substitute	Z No Qualifier
1 Frontal Bone Zygomatic process of frontal bone	3 Percutaneous 4 Percutaneous Endoscopic	J Synthetic Substitute K Nonautologous Tissue Substitute	
3 Parietal Bone, Right			
4 Parietal Bone, Left			

5 Temporal Bone, Right
    Mastoid process
    Petrous part of temporal bone
    Tympanic part of temporal bone
    Zygomatic process of temporal bone			

6 Temporal Bone, Left *See 5 Temporal Bone, Right*			
7 Occipital Bone Foramen magnum			
B Nasal Bone Vomer of nasal septum			

C Sphenoid Bone
    Greater wing
    Lesser wing
    Optic foramen
    Pterygoid process
    Sella turcica			

F Ethmoid Bone, Right Cribriform plate			
G Ethmoid Bone, Left *See F Ethmoid Bone, Right*			
H Lacrimal Bone, Right			
J Lacrimal Bone, Left			
K Palatine Bone, Right			
L Palatine Bone, Left			
M Zygomatic Bone, Right			
N Zygomatic Bone, Left			

P Orbit, Right
    Bony orbit
    Orbital portion of ethmoid bone
    Orbital portion of frontal bone
    Orbital portion of lacrimal bone
    Orbital portion of maxilla
    Orbital portion of palatine bone
    Orbital portion of sphenoid bone
    Orbital portion of zygomatic bone			

Q Orbit, Left *See P Orbit, Right*			
R Maxilla Alveolar process of maxilla			

T Mandible, Right
    Alveolar process of mandible
    Condyloid process
    Mandibular notch
    Mental foramen			

V Mandible, Left *See T Mandible, Right*			
X Hyoid Bone			

Non-OR Procedure   DRG Non-OR Procedure   Valid OR Procedure   HAC Associated Procedure   Combination Only   New/Revised April   New/Revised October

538   ICD-10-PCS 2023

Ø Medical and Surgical
N Head and Facial Bones
W Revision   Definition: Correcting, to the extent possible, a portion of a malfunctioning device or the position of a displaced device

                  Explanation: Revision can include correcting a malfunctioning or displaced device by taking out or putting in components of the device such as a screw or pin

Body Part Character 4	Approach Character 5	Device Character 6	Qualifier Character 7
Ø Skull	Ø Open	Ø Drainage Device 3 Infusion Device 4 Internal Fixation Device 5 External Fixation Device 7 Autologous Tissue Substitute J Synthetic Substitute K Nonautologous Tissue Substitute M Bone Growth Stimulator N Neurostimulator Generator S Hearing Device	Z No Qualifier
Ø Skull	3 Percutaneous 4 Percutaneous Endoscopic X External	Ø Drainage Device 3 Infusion Device 4 Internal Fixation Device 5 External Fixation Device 7 Autologous Tissue Substitute J Synthetic Substitute K Nonautologous Tissue Substitute M Bone Growth Stimulator S Hearing Device	Z No Qualifier
B Nasal Bone Vomer of nasal septum W Facial Bone	Ø Open 3 Percutaneous 4 Percutaneous Endoscopic X External	Ø Drainage Device 4 Internal Fixation Device 7 Autologous Tissue Substitute J Synthetic Substitute K Nonautologous Tissue Substitute M Bone Growth Stimulator	Z No Qualifier

Non-OR   ØNWØX[Ø,3,4,5,7,J,K,M,S]Z
Non-OR   ØNWB[Ø,3,4,X][Ø,4,7,J,K,M]Z
Non-OR   ØNWWX[Ø,4,7,J,K,M]Z

0. Medical and Surgical
N. Head and Facial Bones
W. Revision

Revision: Correcting, to the extent possible, a malfunctioning or the position of a displaced device

Explanation: Includes correcting a malfunctioning or displaced device by taking out or putting in component of the device, such as a screw or pin

Body Part Character 4	Approach Character 5	Device Character 6	Qualifier Character 7
0 Skull	0 Open	0 Drainage Device	Z No Qualifier
		3 Infusion Device	
		4 Internal Fixation Device	
		5 External Fixation Device	
		7 Autologous Tissue Substitute	
		J Synthetic Substitute	
		K Nonautologous Tissue Substitute	
		M Bone Growth Stimulator	
		N Neurostimulator Generator	
		S Hearing Device	
B Nasal Bone	3 Percutaneous	0 Drainage Device	Z No Qualifier
	4 Percutaneous Endoscopic	3 Infusion Device	
	X External	4 Internal Fixation Device	
		5 External Fixation Device	
		7 Autologous Tissue Substitute	
		J Synthetic Substitute	
		K Nonautologous Tissue Substitute	
		M Bone Growth Stimulator	
		S Hearing Device	
W Facial Bone	0 Open	0 Drainage Device	Z No Qualifier
	3 Percutaneous	4 Internal Fixation Device	
	4 Percutaneous Endoscopic	7 Autologous Tissue Substitute	
	X External	J Synthetic Substitute	
		K Nonautologous Tissue Substitute	
		M Bone Growth Stimulator	

Non-OR Procedure   DR Limited Coverage   DR Limited Coverage   QB Questionable OB Admit   HAC Hospital-Acquired Condition   Combination Member   Male   Female

Upper Bones ØP2–ØPW

Character Meanings

This Character Meaning table is provided as a guide to assist the user in the identification of character members that may be found in this section of code tables. It **SHOULD NOT** be used to build a PCS code.

Operation–Character 3	Body Part–Character 4	Approach–Character 5	Device–Character 6	Qualifier–Character 7
2 Change	Ø Sternum	Ø Open	Ø Drainage Device OR Internal Fixation Device, Rigid Plate	X Diagnostic
5 Destruction	1 Ribs, 1 to 2	3 Percutaneous	3 Spinal Stabilization Device, Vertebral Body Tether	Z No Qualifier
8 Division	2 Ribs, 3 or more	4 Percutaneous Endoscopic	4 Internal Fixation Device	
9 Drainage	3 Cervical Vertebra	X External	5 External Fixation Device	
B Excision	4 Thoracic Vertebra		6 Internal Fixation Device, Intramedullary	
C Extirpation	5 Scapula, Right		7 Autologous Tissue Substitute OR Internal Fixation Device, Intramedullary Limb Lengthening	
D Extraction	6 Scapula, Left		8 External Fixation Device, Limb Lengthening	
H Insertion	7 Glenoid Cavity, Right		B External Fixation Device, Monoplanar	
J Inspection	8 Glenoid Cavity, Left		C External Fixation Device, Ring	
N Release	9 Clavicle, Right		D External Fixation Device, Hybrid	
P Removal	B Clavicle, Left		J Synthetic Substitute	
Q Repair	C Humeral Head, Right		K Nonautologous Tissue Substitute	
R Replacement	D Humeral Head, Left		M Bone Growth Stimulator	
S Reposition	F Humeral Shaft, Right		Y Other Device	
T Resection	G Humeral Shaft, Left		Z No Device	
U Supplement	H Radius, Right			
W Revision	J Radius, Left			
	K Ulna, Right			
	L Ulna, Left			
	M Carpal, Right			
	N Carpal, Left			
	P Metacarpal, Right			
	Q Metacarpal, Left			
	R Thumb Phalanx, Right			
	S Thumb Phalanx, Left			
	T Finger Phalanx, Right			
	V Finger Phalanx, Left			
	Y Upper Bone			

AHA Coding Clinic for table ØPB
2015, 3Q, 3-8   Excisional and nonexcisional debridement
2015, 2Q, 34   Decompressive laminectomy
2013, 4Q, 109   Separating conjoined twins
2013, 4Q, 116   Spinal decompression
2013, 3Q, 20   Superior labrum anterior posterior (SLAP) repair and subacromial decompression
2012, 4Q, 101   Rib resection with reconstruction of anterior chest wall
2012, 2Q, 19   Multiple decompressive cervical laminectomies

AHA Coding Clinic for table ØPC
2021, 3Q, 15   Curettage of bilateral humeral head and bone graft placement
2019, 3Q, 19   Removal of sternal wire

AHA Coding Clinic for table ØPD
2017, 4Q, 41   Extraction procedures

AHA Coding Clinic for table ØPH
2020, 1Q, 29   Repair of sternal dehiscence using Sternal Talon® device
2019, 4Q, 34   Intramedullary limb lengthening internal fixation device
2019, 2Q, 40   Decompression of spinal cord and placement of instrumentation
2018, 3Q, 26   Anterior vertebral tethering using Dynesys Tethering System
2017, 2Q, 20   Exchange of intramedullary antibiotic impregnated spacer
2016, 4Q, 117   Placement of magnetic growth rods
2014, 4Q, 28   Removal and replacement of displaced growing rods

AHA Coding Clinic for table ØPP
2019, 3Q, 19   Removal of sternal wire
2017, 2Q, 20   Exchange of intramedullary antibiotic impregnated spacer
2016, 4Q, 117   Placement of magnetic growth rods
2014, 4Q, 28   Removal and replacement of displaced growing rods

AHA Coding Clinic for table ØPR
2018, 4Q, 92   Radial head arthroplasty

AHA Coding Clinic for table ØPS
2021, 4Q, 51-52   Vertebral body tethering
2020, 1Q, 33   Spinal fusion without use of bone graft
2018, 3Q, 26   Anterior vertebral tethering using Dynesys Tethering System
2017, 4Q, 53   New and revised body part values - Ribs
2016, 1Q, 21   Elongation derotation flexion casting
2015, 4Q, 33   Ravitch operation
2015, 2Q, 35   Application of tongs to reduce and stabilize cervical fracture
2014, 4Q, 26   Placement of vertical expandable prosthetic titanium rib (VEPTR)
2014, 4Q, 32   Open reduction internal fixation of fracture with debridement
2014, 3Q, 33   Radial fracture treatment with open reduction internal fixation, and release of carpal ligament

AHA Coding Clinic for table ØPT
2015, 3Q, 26   Thumb arthroplasty with resection of trapezium

AHA Coding Clinic for table ØPU
2021, 3Q, 15   Curettage of bilateral humeral head and bone graft placement
2015, 2Q, 20   Cervical laminoplasty
2013, 4Q, 109   Separating conjoined twins

AHA Coding Clinic for table ØPW
2014, 4Q, 26   Adjustment of VEPTR lengthening mechanism
2014, 4Q, 27   Bilateral lengthening of growing rods

Upper Bones

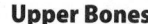

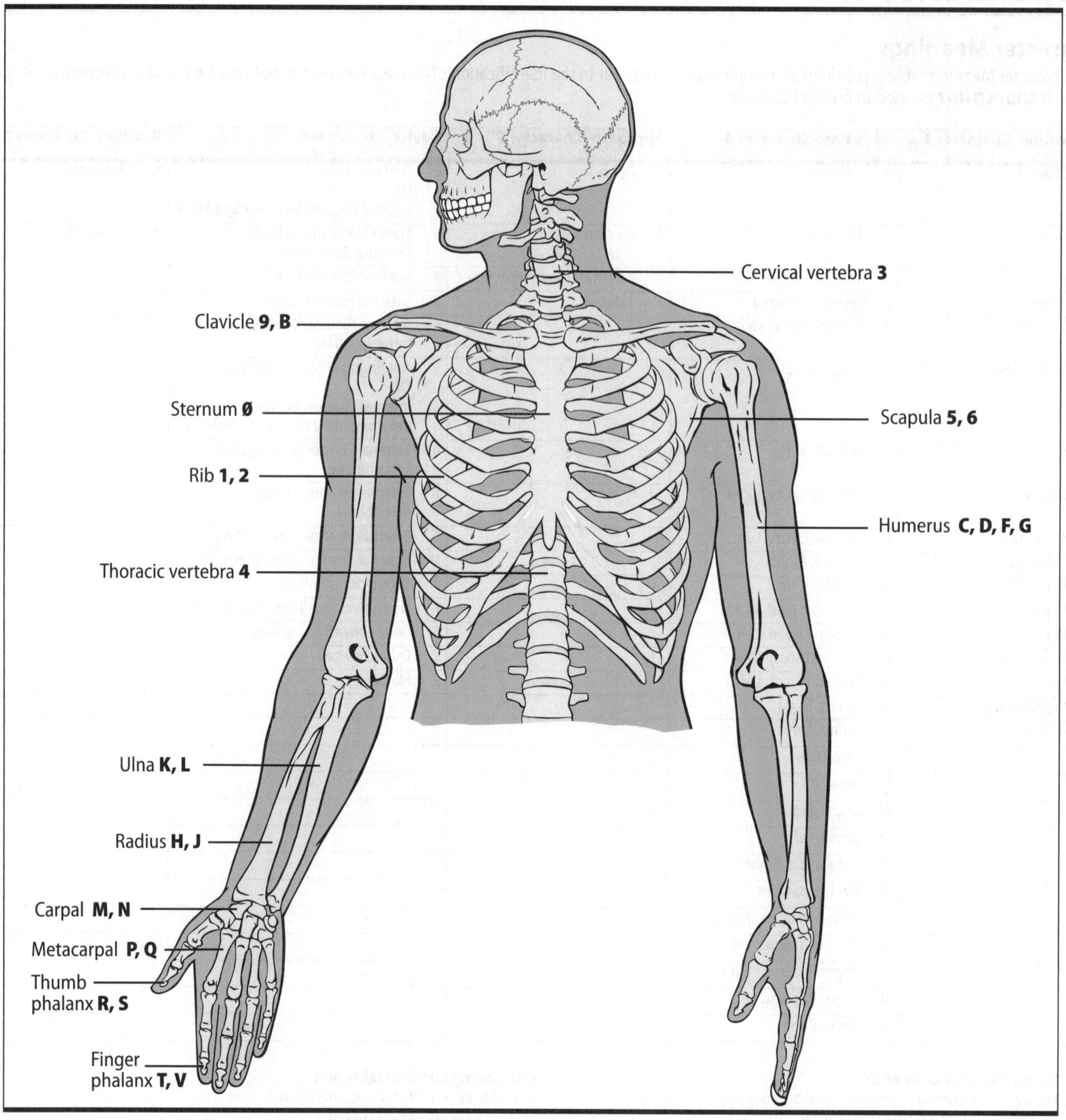

Cervical vertebra **3**

Clavicle **9, B**

Sternum **Ø**

Scapula **5, 6**

Rib **1, 2**

Humerus **C, D, F, G**

Thoracic vertebra **4**

Ulna **K, L**

Radius **H, J**

Carpal **M, N**

Metacarpal **P, Q**

Thumb
phalanx **R, S**

Finger
phalanx **T, V**

Humerus and Scapula

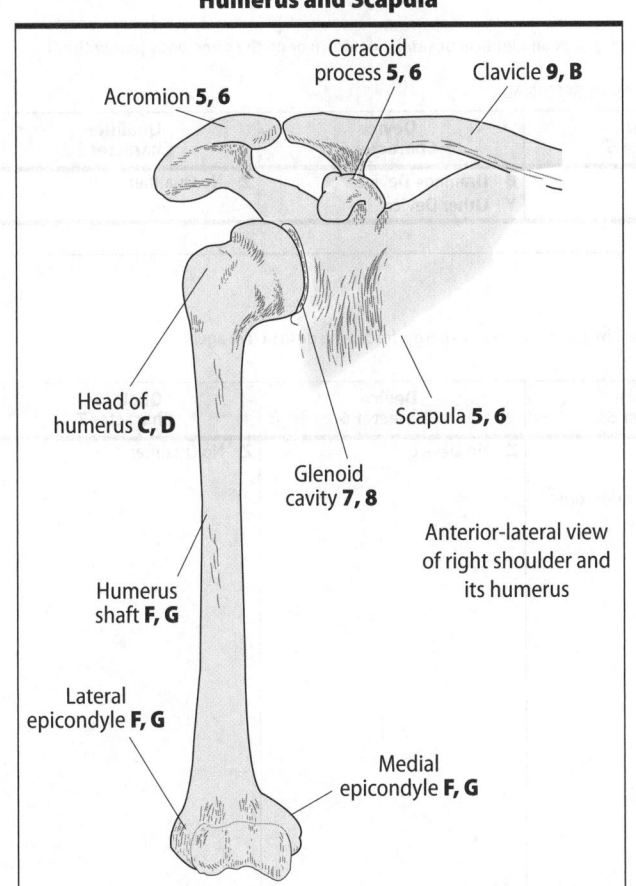

Acromion **5, 6**

Coracoid process **5, 6**

Clavicle **9, B**

Head of humerus **C, D**

Scapula **5, 6**

Glenoid cavity **7, 8**

Anterior-lateral view of right shoulder and its humerus

Humerus shaft **F, G**

Lateral epicondyle **F, G**

Medial epicondyle **F, G**

Radius and Ulna

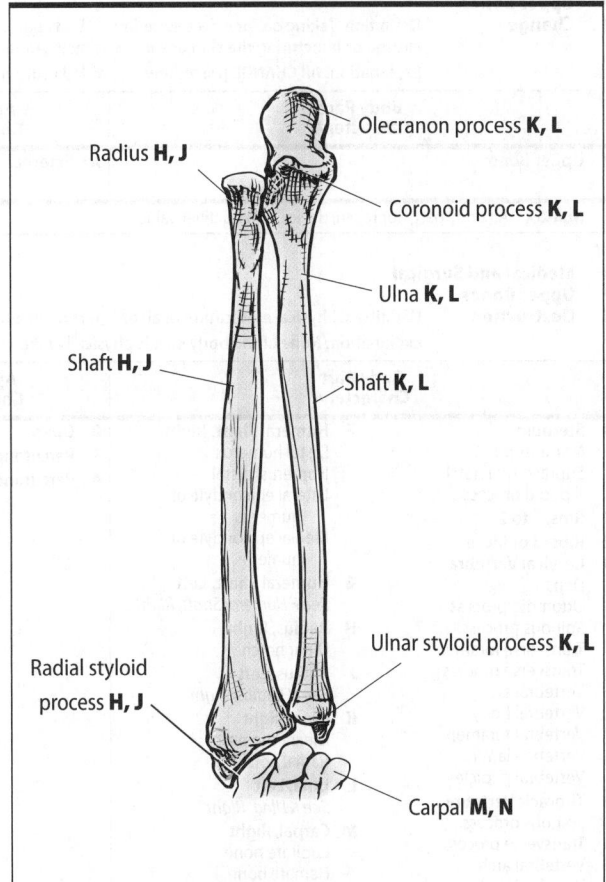

Radius **H, J**

Olecranon process **K, L**

Coronoid process **K, L**

Ulna **K, L**

Shaft **H, J**

Shaft **K, L**

Radial styloid process **H, J**

Ulnar styloid process **K, L**

Carpal **M, N**

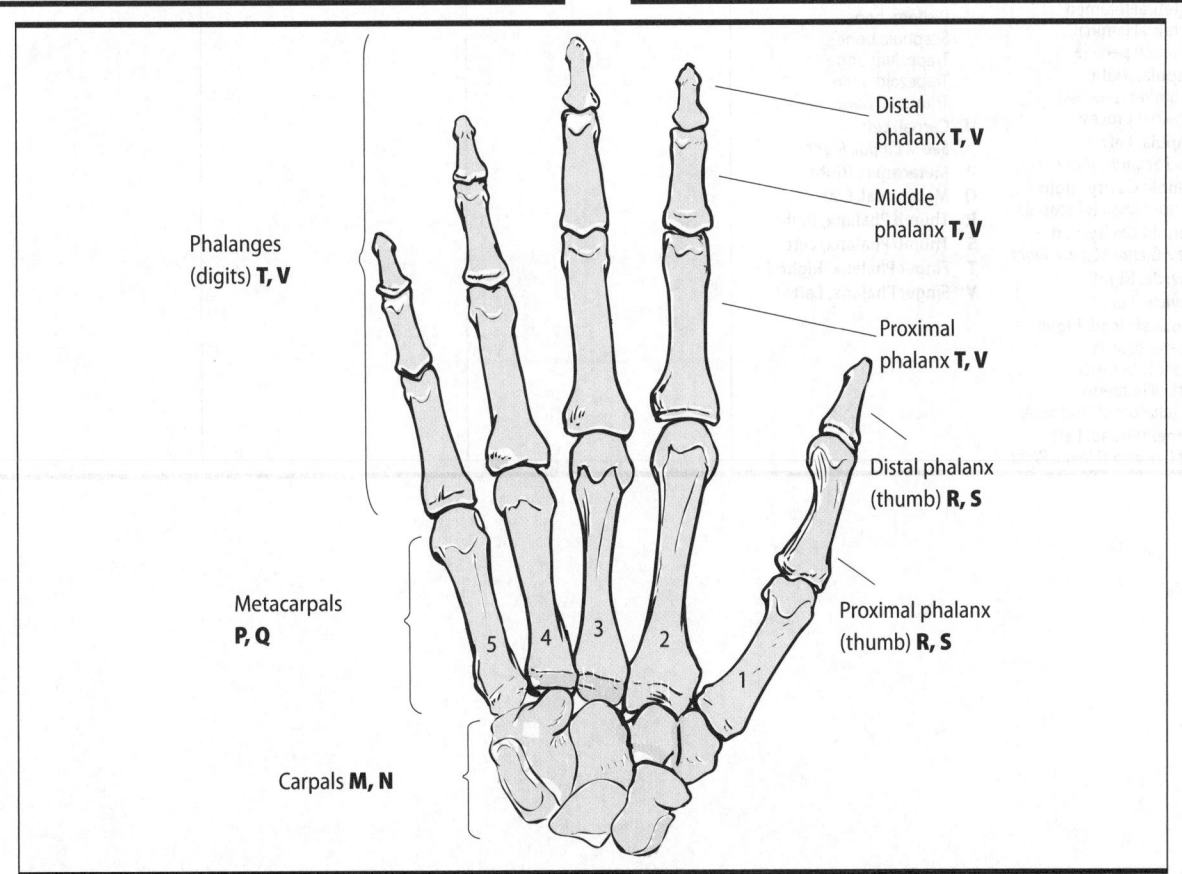

Phalanges (digits) **T, V**

Distal phalanx **T, V**

Middle phalanx **T, V**

Proximal phalanx **T, V**

Distal phalanx (thumb) **R, S**

Proximal phalanx (thumb) **R, S**

Metacarpals **P, Q**

Carpals **M, N**

Ø   Medical and Surgical
P   Upper Bones
2   Change

Definition: Taking out or off a device from a body part and putting back an identical or similar device in or on the same body part without cutting or puncturing the skin or a mucous membrane

Explanation: All CHANGE procedures are coded using the approach EXTERNAL

Body Part Character 4	Approach Character 5	Device Character 6	Qualifier Character 7
Y Upper Bone	**X** External	**Ø** Drainage Device **Y** Other Device	**Z** No Qualifier

Non-OR	All body part, approach, device, and qualifier values

Ø   Medical and Surgical
P   Upper Bones
5   Destruction

Definition: Physical eradication of all or a portion of a body part by the direct use of energy, force, or a destructive agent

Explanation: None of the body part is physically taken out

Body Part Character 4	Approach Character 5	Device Character 6	Qualifier Character 7

Ø   Sternum
    Manubrium
    Suprasternal notch
    Xiphoid process
1   Ribs, 1 to 2
2   Ribs, 3 or More
3   Cervical Vertebra
    Dens
    Odontoid process
    Spinous process
    Transverse foramen
    Transverse process
    Vertebral arch
    Vertebral body
    Vertebral foramen
    Vertebral lamina
    Vertebral pedicle
4   Thoracic Vertebra
    Spinous process
    Transverse process
    Vertebral arch
    Vertebral body
    Vertebral foramen
    Vertebral lamina
    Vertebral pedicle
5   Scapula, Right
    Acromion (process)
    Coracoid process
6   Scapula, Left
    See 5 Scapula, Right
7   Glenoid Cavity, Right
    Glenoid fossa (of scapula)
8   Glenoid Cavity, Left
    See 7 Glenoid Cavity, Right
9   Clavicle, Right
B   Clavicle, Left
C   Humeral Head, Right
    Greater tuberosity
    Lesser tuberosity
    Neck of humerus
      (anatomical)(surgical)
D   Humeral Head, Left
    See C Humeral Head, Right
	F Humeral Shaft, Right
	    Distal humerus
	    Humerus, distal
	    Lateral epicondyle of
	      humerus
	    Medial epicondyle of
	      humerus
	G Humeral Shaft, Left
	    See F Humeral Shaft, Right
	H Radius, Right
	    Ulnar notch
	J Radius, Left
	    See H Radius, Right
	K Ulna, Right
	    Olecranon process
	    Radial notch
	L Ulna, Left
	    See K Ulna, Right
	M Carpal, Right
	    Capitate bone
	    Hamate bone
	    Lunate bone
	    Pisiform bone
	    Scaphoid bone
	    Trapezium bone
	    Trapezoid bone
	    Triquetral bone
	N Carpal, Left
	    See M Carpal, Right
	P Metacarpal, Right
	Q Metacarpal, Left
	R Thumb Phalanx, Right
	S Thumb Phalanx, Left
	T Finger Phalanx, Right
	V Finger Phalanx, Left
		Ø Open
		3 Percutaneous
		4 Percutaneous Endoscopic
			Z No Device	**Z** No Qualifier

Non-OR Procedure   DRG Non-OR Procedure   Valid OR Procedure   HAC Associated Procedure   Combination Only   New/Revised April   New/Revised October

544   ICD-10-PCS 2023

Ø   **Medical and Surgical**
P   **Upper Bones**
8   **Division**   Definition: Cutting into a body part, without draining fluids and/or gases from the body part, in order to separate or transect a body part
                       Explanation: All or a portion of the body part is separated into two or more portions

Body Part Character 4	Approach Character 5	Device Character 6	Qualifier Character 7

Ø   **Sternum**
     Manubrium
     Suprasternal notch
     Xiphoid process
	Ø Open
	3 Percutaneous
	4 Percutaneous Endoscopic
		Z No Device	**Z** No Qualifier

1 **Ribs, 1 to 2**			
2 **Ribs, 3 or More**			

3   **Cervical Vertebra**
     Dens
     Odontoid process
     Spinous process
     Transverse foramen
     Transverse process
     Vertebral arch
     Vertebral body
     Vertebral foramen
     Vertebral lamina
     Vertebral pedicle			

4   **Thoracic Vertebra**
     Spinous process
     Transverse process
     Vertebral arch
     Vertebral body
     Vertebral foramen
     Vertebral lamina
     Vertebral pedicle			

5   **Scapula, Right**
     Acromion (process)
     Coracoid process			

6 **Scapula, Left** *See 5 Scapula, Right*			
7 **Glenoid Cavity, Right** Glenoid fossa (of scapula)			
8 **Glenoid Cavity, Left** *See 7 Glenoid Cavity, Right*			
9 **Clavicle, Right**			
B **Clavicle, Left**			

C   **Humeral Head, Right**
     Greater tuberosity
     Lesser tuberosity
     Neck of humerus (anatomical)(surgical)			

D **Humeral Head, Left** *See C Humeral Head, Right*			

F   **Humeral Shaft, Right**
     Distal humerus
     Humerus, distal
     Lateral epicondyle of humerus
     Medial epicondyle of humerus			

G **Humeral Shaft, Left** *See F Humeral Shaft, Right*			
H **Radius, Right** Ulnar notch			
J **Radius, Left** *See H Radius, Right*			

K   **Ulna, Right**
     Olecranon process
     Radial notch			

L **Ulna, Left** *See K Ulna, Right*			

M   **Carpal, Right**
     Capitate bone
     Hamate bone
     Lunate bone
     Pisiform bone
     Scaphoid bone
     Trapezium bone
     Trapezoid bone
     Triquetral bone			

N **Carpal, Left** *See M Carpal, Right*			
P **Metacarpal, Right**			
Q **Metacarpal, Left**			
R **Thumb Phalanx, Right**			
S **Thumb Phalanx, Left**			
T **Finger Phalanx, Right**			
V **Finger Phalanx, Left**			

NC Noncovered Procedure   **LC** Limited Coverage   **QA** Questionable OB Admit   **NT** New Tech Add-on   ✚ Combination Member   ♂ Male   ♀ Female

Ø   Medical and Surgical
P   Upper Bones
9   Drainage   Definition: Taking or letting out fluids and/or gases from a body part
                           Explanation: The qualifier DIAGNOSTIC is used to identify drainage procedures that are biopsies

Body Part Character 4		Approach Character 5	Device Character 6	Qualifier Character 7
Ø Sternum Manubrium Suprasternal notch Xiphoid process	**D Humeral Head, Left** *See C Humeral Head, Right*	**Ø Open**	**Ø Drainage Device**	**Z No Qualifier**
1 Ribs, 1 to 2	**F Humeral Shaft, Right** Distal humerus Humerus, distal Lateral epicondyle of humerus Medial epicondyle of humerus	**3 Percutaneous**		
2 Ribs, 3 or More		**4 Percutaneous Endoscopic**		
3 Cervical Vertebra Dens Odontoid process Spinous process Transverse foramen Transverse process Vertebral arch Vertebral body Vertebral foramen Vertebral lamina Vertebral pedicle	**G Humeral Shaft, Left** *See F Humeral Shaft, Right*			
	H Radius, Right Ulnar notch			
	J Radius, Left *See H Radius, Right*			
4 Thoracic Vertebra Spinous process Transverse process Vertebral arch Vertebral body Vertebral foramen Vertebral lamina Vertebral pedicle	**K Ulna, Right** Olecranon process Radial notch			
	L Ulna, Left *See K Ulna, Right*			
	M Carpal, Right Capitate bone Hamate bone Lunate bone Pisiform bone Scaphoid bone Trapezium bone Trapezoid bone Triquetral bone			
5 Scapula, Right Acromion (process) Coracoid process				
6 Scapula, Left *See 5 Scapula, Right*	**N Carpal, Left** *See M Carpal, Right*			
7 Glenoid Cavity, Right Glenoid fossa (of scapula)	**P Metacarpal, Right**			
8 Glenoid Cavity, Left *See 7 Glenoid Cavity, Right*	**Q Metacarpal, Left**			
9 Clavicle, Right	**R Thumb Phalanx, Right**			
B Clavicle, Left	**S Thumb Phalanx, Left**			
C Humeral Head, Right Greater tuberosity Lesser tuberosity Neck of humerus (anatomical)(surgical)	**T Finger Phalanx, Right** **V Finger Phalanx, Left**			

Non-OR   ØP9[Ø,1,2,3,4,5,6,7,8,9,B,C,D,F,G,H,J,K,L,M,N,P,Q,R,S,T,V]30Z

ØP9 Continued on next page

Ø	**Medical and Surgical**	
P	**Upper Bones**	**ØP9 Continued**
9	**Drainage**	

Definition: Taking or letting out fluids and/or gases from a body part

Explanation: The qualifier DIAGNOSTIC is used to identify drainage procedures that are biopsies

Body Part Character 4		Approach Character 5	Device Character 6	Qualifier Character 7

Ø **Sternum**
    Manubrium
    Suprasternal notch
    Xiphoid process
1 **Ribs, 1 to 2**
2 **Ribs, 3 or More**
3 **Cervical Vertebra**
    Dens
    Odontoid process
    Spinous process
    Transverse foramen
    Transverse process
    Vertebral arch
    Vertebral body
    Vertebral foramen
    Vertebral lamina
    Vertebral pedicle
4 **Thoracic Vertebra**
    Spinous process
    Transverse process
    Vertebral arch
    Vertebral body
    Vertebral foramen
    Vertebral lamina
    Vertebral pedicle
5 **Scapula, Right**
    Acromion (process)
    Coracoid process
6 **Scapula, Left**
    See 5 Scapula, Right
7 **Glenoid Cavity, Right**
    Glenoid fossa (of scapula)
8 **Glenoid Cavity, Left**
    See 7 Glenoid Cavity, Right
9 **Clavicle, Right**
B **Clavicle, Left**
C **Humeral Head, Right**
    Greater tuberosity
    Lesser tuberosity
    Neck of humerus
      (anatomical)(surgical)
	D **Humeral Head, Left**
	    See C Humeral Head, Right
	F **Humeral Shaft, Right**
	    Distal humerus
	    Humerus, distal
	    Lateral epicondyle of
	      humerus
	    Medial epicondyle of
	      humerus
	G **Humeral Shaft, Left**
	    See F Humeral Shaft, Right
	H **Radius, Right**
	    Ulnar notch
	J **Radius, Left**
	    See H Radius, Right
	K **Ulna, Right**
	    Olecranon process
	    Radial notch
	L **Ulna, Left**
	    See K Ulna, Right
	M **Carpal, Right**
	    Capitate bone
	    Hamate bone
	    Lunate bone
	    Pisiform bone
	    Scaphoid bone
	    Trapezium bone
	    Trapezoid bone
	    Triquetral bone
	N **Carpal, Left**
	    See M Carpal, Right
	P **Metacarpal, Right**
	Q **Metacarpal, Left**
	R **Thumb Phalanx, Right**
	S **Thumb Phalanx, Left**
	T **Finger Phalanx, Right**
	V **Finger Phalanx, Left**
		Ø **Open**
		3 **Percutaneous**
		4 **Percutaneous Endoscopic**
			Z **No Device**	X **Diagnostic**
				Z **No Qualifier**

Non-OR ØP9[Ø,1,2,3,4,5,6,7,8,9,B,C,D,F,G,H,J,K,L,M,N,P,Q,R,S,T,V]3ZZ

NC Noncovered Procedure   **LC** Limited Coverage   **QA** Questionable OB Admit   **NT** New Tech Add-on   ⊞ Combination Member   ♂ Male   ♀ Female

ICD-10-PCS 2023   547

ØP9–ØP9

Upper Bones

Ø   **Medical and Surgical**
P   **Upper Bones**
B   **Excision**   Definition: Cutting out or off, without replacement, a portion of a body part
                      Explanation: The qualifier DIAGNOSTIC is used to identify excision procedures that are biopsies

Body Part Character 4	Approach Character 5	Device Character 6	Qualifier Character 7
Ø Sternum Manubrium Suprasternal notch Xiphoid process	**Ø Open** **3 Percutaneous** **4 Percutaneous Endoscopic**	**Z No Device**	**X Diagnostic** **Z No Qualifier**
1 Ribs, 1 to 2			
2 Ribs, 3 or More			
3 Cervical Vertebra Dens Odontoid process Spinous process Transverse foramen Transverse process Vertebral arch Vertebral body Vertebral foramen Vertebral lamina Vertebral pedicle			
4 Thoracic Vertebra Spinous process Transverse process Vertebral arch Vertebral body Vertebral foramen Vertebral lamina Vertebral pedicle			
5 Scapula, Right Acromion (process) Coracoid process			
6 Scapula, Left *See 5 Scapula, Right*			
7 Glenoid Cavity, Right Glenoid fossa (of scapula)			
8 Glenoid Cavity, Left *See 7 Glenoid Cavity, Right*			
9 Clavicle, Right			
B Clavicle, Left			
C Humeral Head, Right Greater tuberosity Lesser tuberosity Neck of humerus (anatomical)(surgical)			
D Humeral Head, Left *See C Humeral Head, Right*			
F Humeral Shaft, Right Distal humerus Humerus, distal Lateral epicondyle of humerus Medial epicondyle of humerus			
G Humeral Shaft, Left *See F Humeral Shaft, Right*			
H Radius, Right Ulnar notch			
J Radius, Left *See H Radius, Right*			
K Ulna, Right Olecranon process Radial notch			
L Ulna, Left *See K Ulna, Right*			
M Carpal, Right Capitate bone Hamate bone Lunate bone Pisiform bone Scaphoid bone Trapezium bone Trapezoid bone Triquetral bone			
N Carpal, Left *See M Carpal, Right*			
P Metacarpal, Right			
Q Metacarpal, Left			
R Thumb Phalanx, Right			
S Thumb Phalanx, Left			
T Finger Phalanx, Right			
V Finger Phalanx, Left			

Non-OR Procedure   DRG Non-OR Procedure   Valid OR Procedure   HAC Associated Procedure   Combination Only   New/Revised April   New/Revised October

548   ICD-10-PCS 2023

Ø　Medical and Surgical
P　Upper Bones
C　Extirpation　　Definition: Taking or cutting out solid matter from a body part

Explanation: The solid matter may be an abnormal byproduct of a biological function or a foreign body; it may be imbedded in a body part or in the lumen of a tubular body part. The solid matter may or may not have been previously broken into pieces.

Body Part Character 4	Approach Character 5	Device Character 6	Qualifier Character 7
Ø　Sternum 　　Manubrium 　　Suprasternal notch 　　Xiphoid process **1　Ribs, 1 to 2** **2　Ribs, 3 or More** **3　Cervical Vertebra** 　　Dens 　　Odontoid process 　　Spinous process 　　Transverse foramen 　　Transverse process 　　Vertebral arch 　　Vertebral body 　　Vertebral foramen 　　Vertebral lamina 　　Vertebral pedicle **4　Thoracic Vertebra** 　　Spinous process 　　Transverse process 　　Vertebral arch 　　Vertebral body 　　Vertebral foramen 　　Vertebral lamina 　　Vertebral pedicle **5　Scapula, Right** 　　Acromion (process) 　　Coracoid process **6　Scapula, Left** 　　*See 5 Scapula, Right* **7　Glenoid Cavity, Right** 　　Glenoid fossa (of scapula) **8　Glenoid Cavity, Left** 　　*See 7 Glenoid Cavity, Right* **9　Clavicle, Right** **B　Clavicle, Left** **C　Humeral Head, Right** 　　Greater tuberosity 　　Lesser tuberosity 　　Neck of humerus (anatomical)(surgical) **D　Humeral Head, Left** 　　*See C Humeral Head, Right* **F　Humeral Shaft, Right** 　　Distal humerus 　　Humerus, distal 　　Lateral epicondyle of humerus 　　Medial epicondyle of humerus **G　Humeral Shaft, Left** 　　*See F Humeral Shaft, Right* **H　Radius, Right** 　　Ulnar notch **J　Radius, Left** 　　*See H Radius, Right* **K　Ulna, Right** 　　Olecranon process 　　Radial notch **L　Ulna, Left** 　　*See K Ulna, Right* **M　Carpal, Right** 　　Capitate bone 　　Hamate bone 　　Lunate bone 　　Pisiform bone 　　Scaphoid bone 　　Trapezium bone 　　Trapezoid bone 　　Triquetral bone **N　Carpal, Left** 　　*See M Carpal, Right* **P　Metacarpal, Right** **Q　Metacarpal, Left** **R　Thumb Phalanx, Right** **S　Thumb Phalanx, Left** **T　Finger Phalanx, Right** **V　Finger Phalanx, Left**	**Ø　Open** **3　Percutaneous** **4　Percutaneous Endoscopic**	**Z　No Device**	**Z　No Qualifier**

NC Noncovered Procedure　　**LC** Limited Coverage　　**QA** Questionable OB Admit　　**NT** New Tech Add-on　　⊞ Combination Member　　♂ Male　　♀ Female

ICD-10-PCS 2023　　　　　　　　　　　　　　　　　　　　　　　　　　　　　　　　　　　549

ØPC–ØPC

Upper Bones

ØPD–ØPD

Ø   **Medical and Surgical**
P   **Upper Bones**
D   **Extraction**   Definition: Pulling or stripping out or off all or a portion of a body part by the use of force
                              Explanation: The qualifier DIAGNOSTIC is used to identify extraction procedures that are biopsies

Body Part Character 4	Approach Character 5	Device Character 6	Qualifier Character 7

Ø **Sternum**
   Manubrium
   Suprasternal notch
   Xiphoid process
	Ø Open	**Z** No Device	**Z** No Qualifier

1 **Ribs, 1 to 2**			
2 **Ribs, 3 or More**			

3 **Cervical Vertebra**
   Dens
   Odontoid process
   Spinous process
   Transverse foramen
   Transverse process
   Vertebral arch
   Vertebral body
   Vertebral foramen
   Vertebral lamina
   Vertebral pedicle			

4 **Thoracic Vertebra**
   Spinous process
   Transverse process
   Vertebral arch
   Vertebral body
   Vertebral foramen
   Vertebral lamina
   Vertebral pedicle			

5 **Scapula, Right**
   Acromion (process)
   Coracoid process			

6 **Scapula, Left** *See 5 Scapula, Right*			
7 **Glenoid Cavity, Right** Glenoid fossa (of scapula)			
8 **Glenoid Cavity, Left** *See 7 Glenoid Cavity, Right*			
9 **Clavicle, Right**			
B **Clavicle, Left**			

C **Humeral Head, Right**
   Greater tuberosity
   Lesser tuberosity
   Neck of humerus (anatomical)(surgical)			

D **Humeral Head, Left** *See C Humeral Head, Right*			

F **Humeral Shaft, Right**
   Distal humerus
   Humerus, distal
   Lateral epicondyle of humerus
   Medial epicondyle of humerus			

G **Humeral Shaft, Left** *See F Humeral Shaft, Right*			
H **Radius, Right** Ulnar notch			
J **Radius, Left** *See H Radius, Right*			

K **Ulna, Right**
   Olecranon process
   Radial notch			

L **Ulna, Left** *See K Ulna, Right*			

M **Carpal, Right**
   Capitate bone
   Hamate bone
   Lunate bone
   Pisiform bone
   Scaphoid bone
   Trapezium bone
   Trapezoid bone
   Triquetral bone			

N **Carpal, Left** *See M Carpal, Right*			
P **Metacarpal, Right**			
Q **Metacarpal, Left**			
R **Thumb Phalanx, Right**			
S **Thumb Phalanx, Left**			
T **Finger Phalanx, Right**			
V **Finger Phalanx, Left**			

Non-OR Procedure   DRG Non-OR Procedure   Valid OR Procedure   HAC Associated Procedure   Combination Only   New/Revised April   New/Revised October

Ø   **Medical and Surgical**
P   **Upper Bones**
H   **Insertion**   Definition: Putting in a nonbiological appliance that monitors, assists, performs, or prevents a physiological function but does not physically take the place of a body part

                      Explanation: None

Body Part Character 4		Approach Character 5	Device Character 6	Qualifier Character 7
Ø **Sternum** Manubrium Suprasternal notch Xiphoid process		**Ø** Open **3** Percutaneous **4** Percutaneous Endoscopic	**Ø** Internal Fixation Device, Rigid Plate **4** Internal Fixation Device	**Z** No Qualifier
1 **Ribs, 1 to 2** **2** **Ribs, 3 or More** **3** **Cervical Vertebra** Dens Odontoid process Spinous process Transverse foramen Transverse process Vertebral arch Vertebral body Vertebral foramen Vertebral lamina Vertebral pedicle **4** **Thoracic Vertebra** Spinous process Transverse process Vertebral arch Vertebral body Vertebral foramen Vertebral lamina Vertebral pedicle	**5** **Scapula, Right** Acromion (process) Coracoid process **6** **Scapula, Left** *See 5 Scapula, Right* **7** **Glenoid Cavity, Right** Glenoid fossa (of scapula) **8** **Glenoid Cavity, Left** *See 7 Glenoid Cavity, Right* **9** **Clavicle, Right** **B** **Clavicle, Left**	**Ø** Open **3** Percutaneous **4** Percutaneous Endoscopic	**4** Internal Fixation Device	**Z** No Qualifier
C **Humeral Head, Right** Greater tuberosity Lesser tuberosity Neck of humerus (anatomical)(surgical) **D** **Humeral Head, Left** *See C Humeral Head, Right*	**H** **Radius, Right** Ulnar notch **J** **Radius, Left** *See H Radius, Right* **K** **Ulna, Right** Olecranon process Radial notch **L** **Ulna, Left** *See K Ulna, Right*	**Ø** Open **3** Percutaneous **4** Percutaneous Endoscopic	**4** Internal Fixation Device **5** External Fixation Device **6** Internal Fixation Device, Intramedullary **8** External Fixation Device, Limb Lengthening **B** External Fixation Device, Monoplanar **C** External Fixation Device, Ring **D** External Fixation Device, Hybrid	**Z** No Qualifier

F **Humeral Shaft, Right**
 Distal humerus
 Humerus, distal
 Lateral epicondyle of
   humerus
 Medial epicondyle of
   humerus
	G **Humeral Shaft, Left**
	 See F Humeral Shaft, Right
		Ø Open
		 3 Percutaneous
		 4 Percutaneous Endoscopic
			4 Internal Fixation Device
			 5 External Fixation Device
			 6 Internal Fixation Device, Intramedullary
			 7 Internal Fixation Device, Intramedullary Limb Lengthening
			 8 External Fixation Device, Limb Lengthening
			 B External Fixation Device, Monoplanar
			 C External Fixation Device, Ring
			 D External Fixation Device, Hybrid
				Z No Qualifier

M **Carpal, Right** Capitate bone Hamate bone Lunate bone Pisiform bone Scaphoid bone Trapezium bone Trapezoid bone Triquetral bone **N** **Carpal, Left** *See M Carpal, Right*	**P** **Metacarpal, Right** **Q** **Metacarpal, Left** **R** **Thumb Phalanx, Right** **S** **Thumb Phalanx, Left** **T** **Finger Phalanx, Right** **V** **Finger Phalanx, Left**	**Ø** Open **3** Percutaneous **4** Percutaneous Endoscopic	**4** Internal Fixation Device **5** External Fixation Device	**Z** No Qualifier
Y **Upper Bone**		**Ø** Open **3** Percutaneous **4** Percutaneous Endoscopic	**M** Bone Growth Stimulator	**Z** No Qualifier

Non-OR   ØPH[C,D,H,J,K,L][Ø,3,4]8Z
Non-OR   ØPH[F,G][Ø,3,4]8Z

Ø **Medical and Surgical**
P **Upper Bones**
J **Inspection** Definition: Visually and/or manually exploring a body part

Explanation: Visual exploration may be performed with or without optical instrumentation. Manual exploration may be performed directly or through intervening body layers.

Body Part Character 4	Approach Character 5	Device Character 6	Qualifier Character 7
Y Upper Bone	Ø Open 3 Percutaneous 4 Percutaneous Endoscopic X External	Z No Device	Z No Qualifier

Non-OR   ØPJY[3,X]ZZ

Ø **Medical and Surgical**
P **Upper Bones**
N **Release** Definition: Freeing a body part from an abnormal physical constraint by cutting or by the use of force

Explanation: Some of the restraining tissue may be taken out but none of the body part is taken out

Body Part Character 4		Approach Character 5	Device Character 6	Qualifier Character 7

Ø **Sternum**
   Manubrium
   Suprasternal notch
   Xiphoid process
1 **Ribs, 1 to 2**
2 **Ribs, 3 or More**
3 **Cervical Vertebra**
   Dens
   Odontoid process
   Spinous process
   Transverse foramen
   Transverse process
   Vertebral arch
   Vertebral body
   Vertebral foramen
   Vertebral lamina
   Vertebral pedicle
4 **Thoracic Vertebra**
   Spinous process
   Transverse process
   Vertebral arch
   Vertebral body
   Vertebral foramen
   Vertebral lamina
   Vertebral pedicle
5 **Scapula, Right**
   Acromion (process)
   Coracoid process
6 **Scapula, Left**
   See 5 Scapula, Right
7 **Glenoid Cavity, Right**
   Glenoid fossa (of scapula)
8 **Glenoid Cavity, Left**
   See 7 Glenoid Cavity, Right
9 **Clavicle, Right**
B **Clavicle, Left**
C **Humeral Head, Right**
   Greater tuberosity
   Lesser tuberosity
   Neck of humerus
      (anatomical) (surgical)
D **Humeral Head, Left**
   See C Humeral Head, Right
	F **Humeral Shaft, Right**
	   Distal humerus
	   Humerus, distal
	   Lateral epicondyle of
	      humerus
	   Medial epicondyle of
	      humerus
	G **Humeral Shaft, Left**
	   See F Humeral Shaft, Right
	H **Radius, Right**
	   Ulnar notch
	J **Radius, Left**
	   See H Radius, Right
	K **Ulna, Right**
	   Olecranon process
	   Radial notch
	L **Ulna, Left**
	   See K Ulna, Right
	M **Carpal, Right**
	   Capitate bone
	   Hamate bone
	   Lunate bone
	   Pisiform bone
	   Scaphoid bone
	   Trapezium bone
	   Trapezoid bone
	   Triquetral bone
	N **Carpal, Left**
	   See M Carpal, Right
	P **Metacarpal, Right**
	Q **Metacarpal, Left**
	R **Thumb Phalanx, Right**
	S **Thumb Phalanx, Left**
	T **Finger Phalanx, Right**
	V **Finger Phalanx, Left**
		Ø Open
		3 Percutaneous
		4 Percutaneous Endoscopic
			Z No Device	Z No Qualifier

Non-OR Procedure   DRG Non-OR Procedure   Valid OR Procedure   HAC Associated Procedure   Combination Only   New/Revised April   New/Revised October

ØPJ–ØPN

552   ICD-10-PCS 2023

Ø	**Medical and Surgical**
P	**Upper Bones**
P	**Removal**

Definition: Taking out or off a device from a body part

Explanation: If a device is taken out and a similar device put in without cutting or puncturing the skin or mucous membrane, the procedure is coded to the root operation CHANGE. Otherwise, the procedure for taking out a device is coded to the root operation REMOVAL.

Body Part Character 4		Approach Character 5	Device Character 6	Qualifier Character 7

Ø Sternum
  Manubrium
  Suprasternal notch
  Xiphoid process
1 Ribs, 1 to 2
2 Ribs, 3 or More
3 Cervical Vertebra
  Dens
  Odontoid process
  Spinous process
  Transverse foramen
  Transverse process
  Vertebral arch
  Vertebral body
  Vertebral foramen
  Vertebral lamina
  Vertebral pedicle
	4 Thoracic Vertebra
	  Spinous process
	  Transverse process
	  Vertebral arch
	  Vertebral body
	  Vertebral foramen
	  Vertebral lamina
	  Vertebral pedicle
	5 Scapula, Right
	  Acromion (process)
	  Coracoid process
	6 Scapula, Left
	  See 5 Scapula, Right
	7 Glenoid Cavity, Right
	  Glenoid fossa (of scapula)
	8 Glenoid Cavity, Left
	  See 7 Glenoid Cavity, Right
	9 Clavicle, Right
	B Clavicle, Left
		Ø Open
		3 Percutaneous
		4 Percutaneous Endoscopic
			4 Internal Fixation Device
			7 Autologous Tissue Substitute
			J Synthetic Substitute
			K Nonautologous Tissue Substitute
				Z No Qualifier

Ø Sternum
  Manubrium
  Suprasternal notch
  Xiphoid process
1 Ribs, 1 to 2
2 Ribs, 3 or More
3 Cervical Vertebra
  Dens
  Odontoid process
  Spinous process
  Transverse foramen
  Transverse process
  Vertebral arch
  Vertebral body
  Vertebral foramen
  Vertebral lamina
  Vertebral pedicle
	4 Thoracic Vertebra
	  Spinous process
	  Transverse process
	  Vertebral arch
	  Vertebral body
	  Vertebral foramen
	  Vertebral lamina
	  Vertebral pedicle
	5 Scapula, Right
	  Acromion (process)
	  Coracoid process
	6 Scapula, Left
	  See 5 Scapula, Right
	7 Glenoid Cavity, Right
	  Glenoid fossa (of scapula)
	8 Glenoid Cavity, Left
	  See 7 Glenoid Cavity, Right
	9 Clavicle, Right
	B Clavicle, Left
		X External	**4** Internal Fixation Device	**Z** No Qualifier

C Humeral Head, Right
  Greater tuberosity
  Lesser tuberosity
  Neck of humerus
    (anatomical) (surgical)
D Humeral Head, Left
  See C Humeral Head, Right
F Humeral Shaft, Right
  Distal humerus
  Humerus, distal
  Lateral epicondyle of
    humerus
  Medial epicondyle of
    humerus
G Humeral Shaft, Left
  See F Humeral Shaft, Right
H Radius, Right
  Ulnar notch
J Radius, Left
  See H Radius, Right
K Ulna, Right
  Olecranon process
  Radial notch
	L Ulna, Left
	  See K Ulna, Right
	M Carpal, Right
	  Capitate bone
	  Hamate bone
	  Lunate bone
	  Pisiform bone
	  Scaphoid bone
	  Trapezium bone
	  Trapezoid bone
	  Triquetral bone
	N Carpal, Left
	  See M Carpal, Right
	P Metacarpal, Right
	Q Metacarpal, Left
	R Thumb Phalanx, Right
	S Thumb Phalanx, Left
	T Finger Phalanx, Right
	V Finger Phalanx, Left
		Ø Open
		3 Percutaneous
		4 Percutaneous Endoscopic
			4 Internal Fixation Device
			5 External Fixation Device
			7 Autologous Tissue Substitute
			J Synthetic Substitute
			K Nonautologous Tissue Substitute
				Z No Qualifier

Non-OR   ØPP[Ø,1,2,3,4,5,6,7,8,9,B]X4Z

ØPP Continued on next page

NC Noncovered Procedure   **LC** Limited Coverage   **QA** Questionable OB Admit   **NT** New Tech Add-on   ⊞ Combination Member   ♂ Male   ♀ Female

ICD-10-PCS 2023   553

ØPP–ØPP

Ø Medical and Surgical
P Upper Bones

ØPP Continued

P Removal   Definition: Taking out or off a device from a body part

Explanation: If a device is taken out and a similar device put in without cutting or puncturing the skin or mucous membrane, the procedure is coded to the root operation CHANGE. Otherwise, the procedure for taking out a device is coded to the root operation REMOVAL.

Body Part Character 4		Approach Character 5	Device Character 6	Qualifier Character 7

C Humeral Head, Right
  Greater tuberosity
  Lesser tuberosity
  Neck of humerus
    (anatomical) (surgical)
D Humeral Head, Left
  See C Humeral Head, Right
F Humeral Shaft, Right
  Distal humerus
  Humerus, distal
  Lateral epicondyle of
    humerus
  Medial epicondyle of
    humerus
G Humeral Shaft, Left
  See F Humeral Shaft, Right
H Radius, Right
  Ulnar notch
J Radius, Left
  See H Radius, Right
K Ulna, Right
  Olecranon process
Radial notch
	L Ulna, Left
	  See K Ulna, Right
	M Carpal, Right
	  Capitate bone
	  Hamate bone
	  Lunate bone
	  Pisiform bone
	  Scaphoid bone
	  Trapezium bone
	  Trapezoid bone
	  Triquetral bone
	N Carpal, Left
	  See M Carpal, Right
	P Metacarpal, Right
	Q Metacarpal, Left
	R Thumb Phalanx, Right
	S Thumb Phalanx, Left
	T Finger Phalanx, Right
	V Finger Phalanx, Left
		X External	**4** Internal Fixation Device
			5 External Fixation Device
				Z No Qualifier

Y Upper Bone		**Ø** Open **3** Percutaneous **4** Percutaneous Endoscopic **X** External	**Ø** Drainage Device **M** Bone Growth Stimulator	**Z** No Qualifier

Non-OR   ØPP[C,D,F,G,H,J,K,L,M,N,P,Q,R,S,T,V]X[4,5]Z
Non-OR   ØPPY3ØZ
Non-OR   ØPPYX[Ø,M]Z

Non-OR Procedure   DRG Non-OR Procedure   Valid OR Procedure   HAC Associated Procedure   Combination Only   New/Revised April   New/Revised October

554   ICD-10-PCS 2023

Ø   **Medical and Surgical**
P   **Upper Bones**
Q   **Repair**   Definition: Restoring, to the extent possible, a body part to its normal anatomic structure and function
                Explanation: Used only when the method to accomplish the repair is not one of the other root operations

Body Part Character 4		Approach Character 5	Device Character 6	Qualifier Character 7

Ø Sternum
   Manubrium
   Suprasternal notch
   Xiphoid process
1 Ribs, 1 to 2
2 Ribs, 3 or More
3 Cervical Vertebra
   Dens
   Odontoid process
   Spinous process
   Transverse foramen
   Transverse process
   Vertebral arch
   Vertebral body
   Vertebral foramen
   Vertebral lamina
   Vertebral pedicle
4 Thoracic Vertebra
   Spinous process
   Transverse process
   Vertebral arch
   Vertebral body
   Vertebral foramen
   Vertebral lamina
   Vertebral pedicle
5 Scapula, Right
   Acromion (process)
   Coracoid process
6 Scapula, Left
   See 5 Scapula, Right
7 Glenoid Cavity, Right
   Glenoid fossa (of scapula)
8 Glenoid Cavity, Left
   See 7 Glenoid Cavity, Right
9 Clavicle, Right
B Clavicle, Left
C Humeral Head, Right
   Greater tuberosity
   Lesser tuberosity
   Neck of humerus
     (anatomical)(surgical)
D Humeral Head, Left
   See C Humeral Head, Right
	F Humeral Shaft, Right
	   Distal humerus
	   Humerus, distal
	   Lateral epicondyle of
	     humerus
	   Medial epicondyle of
	     humerus
	G Humeral Shaft, Left
	   See F Humeral Shaft, Right
	H Radius, Right
	   Ulnar notch
	J Radius, Left
	   See H Radius, Right
	K Ulna, Right
	   Olecranon process
	   Radial notch
	L Ulna, Left
	   See K Ulna, Right
	M Carpal, Right
	   Capitate bone
	   Hamate bone
	   Lunate bone
	   Pisiform bone
	   Scaphoid bone
	   Trapezium bone
	   Trapezoid bone
	   Triquetral bone
	N Carpal, Left
	   See M Carpal, Right
	P Metacarpal, Right
	Q Metacarpal, Left
	R Thumb Phalanx, Right
	S Thumb Phalanx, Left
	T Finger Phalanx, Right
	V Finger Phalanx, Left
		Ø Open
		3 Percutaneous
		4 Percutaneous Endoscopic
		X External
			Z No Device	**Z** No Qualifier

Non-OR   ØPQ[Ø,1,2,3,4,5,6,7,8,9,B,C,D,F,G,H,J,K,L,M,N,P,Q,R,S,T,V]XZZ

NC Noncovered Procedure   **LC** Limited Coverage   **QA** Questionable OB Admit   **NT** New Tech Add-on   ⊞ Combination Member   ♂ Male   ♀ Female

ICD-10-PCS 2023   555

Upper Bones

Ø   Medical and Surgical
P   Upper Bones
R   Replacement   Definition: Putting in or on biological or synthetic material that physically takes the place and/or function of all or a portion of a body part
Explanation: The body part may have been taken out or replaced, or may be taken out, physically eradicated, or rendered nonfunctional during the REPLACEMENT procedure. A REMOVAL procedure is coded for taking out the device used in a previous replacement procedure.

Body Part Character 4		Approach Character 5	Device Character 6	Qualifier Character 7

Ø Sternum
   Manubrium
   Suprasternal notch
   Xiphoid process
1 Ribs, 1 to 2
2 Ribs, 3 or More
3 Cervical Vertebra
   Dens
   Odontoid process
   Spinous process
   Transverse foramen
   Transverse process
   Vertebral arch
   Vertebral body
   Vertebral foramen
   Vertebral lamina
   Vertebral pedicle
4 Thoracic Vertebra
   Spinous process
   Transverse process
   Vertebral arch
   Vertebral body
   Vertebral foramen
   Vertebral lamina
   Vertebral pedicle
5 Scapula, Right
   Acromion (process)
   Coracoid process
6 Scapula, Left
   See 5 Scapula, Right
7 Glenoid Cavity, Right
   Glenoid fossa (of scapula)
8 Glenoid Cavity, Left
   See 7 Glenoid Cavity, Right
9 Clavicle, Right
B Clavicle, Left
C Humeral Head, Right
   Greater tuberosity
   Lesser tuberosity
   Neck of humerus
      (anatomical)(surgical)
D Humeral Head, Left
   See C Humeral Head, Right
	F Humeral Shaft, Right
	   Distal humerus
	   Humerus, distal
	   Lateral epicondyle of
	      humerus
	   Medial epicondyle of
	      humerus
	G Humeral Shaft, Left
	   See F Humeral Shaft, Right
	H Radius, Right
	   Ulnar notch
	J Radius, Left
	   See H Radius, Right
	K Ulna, Right
	   Olecranon process
	   Radial notch
	L Ulna, Left
	   See K Ulna, Right
	M Carpal, Right
	   Capitate bone
	   Hamate bone
	   Lunate bone
	   Pisiform bone
	   Scaphoid bone
	   Trapezium bone
	   Trapezoid bone
	   Triquetral bone
	N Carpal, Left
	   See M Carpal, Right
	P Metacarpal, Right
	Q Metacarpal, Left
	R Thumb Phalanx, Right
	S Thumb Phalanx, Left
	T Finger Phalanx, Right
	V Finger Phalanx, Left
		Ø Open
		3 Percutaneous
		4 Percutaneous Endoscopic
			7 Autologous Tissue
			   Substitute
			J Synthetic Substitute
			K Nonautologous Tissue
			   Substitute
				Z No Qualifier

Ø   **Medical and Surgical**
P   **Upper Bones**
S   **Reposition**   Definition: Moving to its normal location, or other suitable location, all or a portion of a body part

Explanation: The body part is moved to a new location from an abnormal location, or from a normal location where it is not functioning correctly. The body part may or may not be cut out or off to be moved to the new location.

Body Part Character 4		Approach Character 5	Device Character 6	Qualifier Character 7
Ø **Sternum** Manubrium Suprasternal notch Xiphoid process		**Ø** Open **3** Percutaneous **4** Percutaneous Endoscopic	**Ø** Internal Fixation Device, Rigid Plate **4** Internal Fixation Device **Z** No Device	**Z** No Qualifier
Ø **Sternum** Manubrium Suprasternal notch Xiphoid process		**X** External	**Z** No Device	**Z** No Qualifier
1 **Ribs, 1 to 2** **2** **Ribs, 3 or More** **3** **Cervical Vertebra** ⊞ Dens Odontoid process Spinous process Transverse foramen Transverse process Vertebral arch Vertebral body Vertebral foramen Vertebral lamina Vertebral pedicle	**5** **Scapula, Right** Acromion (process) Coracoid process **6** **Scapula, Left** *See 5 Scapula, Right* **7** **Glenoid Cavity, Right** Glenoid fossa (of scapula) **8** **Glenoid Cavity, Left** *See 7 Glenoid Cavity, Right* **9** **Clavicle, Right** **B** **Clavicle, Left**	**Ø** Open **3** Percutaneous **4** Percutaneous Endoscopic	**4** Internal Fixation Device **Z** No Device	**Z** No Qualifier
1 **Ribs, 1 to 2** **2** **Ribs, 3 or More** **3** **Cervical Vertebra** Dens Odontoid process Spinous process Transverse foramen Transverse process Vertebral arch Vertebral body Vertebral foramen Vertebral lamina Vertebral pedicle	**5** **Scapula, Right** Acromion (process) Coracoid process **6** **Scapula, Left** *See 5 Scapula, Right* **7** **Glenoid Cavity, Right** Glenoid fossa (of scapula) **8** **Glenoid Cavity, Left** *See 7 Glenoid Cavity, Right* **9** **Clavicle, Right** **B** **Clavicle, Left**	**X** External	**Z** No Device	**Z** No Qualifier
4 **Thoracic Vertebra** Spinous process Transverse process Vertebral arch Vertebral body Vertebral foramen Vertebral lamina Vertebral pedicle		**Ø** Open **4** Percutaneous Endoscopic	**3** Spinal Stabilization Device, Vertebral Body Tether **4** Internal Fixation Device **Z** No Device	**Z** No Qualifier
4 **Thoracic Vertebra** ⊞ Spinous process Transverse process Vertebral arch Vertebral body Vertebral foramen Vertebral lamina Vertebral pedicle		**3** Percutaneous	**4** Internal Fixation Device **Z** No Device	**Z** No Qualifier
4 **Thoracic Vertebra** Spinous process Transverse process Vertebral arch Vertebral body Vertebral foramen Vertebral lamina Vertebral pedicle		**X** External	**Z** No Device	**Z** No Qualifier
C **Humeral Head, Right** Greater tuberosity Lesser tuberosity Neck of humerus (anatomical)(surgical) **D** **Humeral Head, Left** *See C Humeral Head, Right* **F** **Humeral Shaft, Right** Distal humerus Humerus, distal Lateral epicondyle of humerus Medial epicondyle of humerus	**G** **Humeral Shaft, Left** *See F Humeral Shaft, Right* **H** **Radius, Right** Ulnar notch **J** **Radius, Left** *See H Radius, Right* **K** **Ulna, Right** Olecranon process Radial notch **L** **Ulna, Left** *See K Ulna, Right*	**Ø** Open **3** Percutaneous **4** Percutaneous Endoscopic	**4** Internal Fixation Device **5** External Fixation Device **6** Internal Fixation Device, Intramedullary **B** External Fixation Device, Monoplanar **C** External Fixation Device, Ring **D** External Fixation Device, Hybrid **Z** No Device	**Z** No Qualifier

Non-OR	ØPSØ[3,4]ZZ
Non-OR	ØPSØXZZ
Non-OR	ØPS[1,2,5,6,7,8,9,B][3,4]ZZ

Non-OR	ØPS[1,2,3,5,6,7,8,9,B]XZZ
Non-OR	ØPS4XZZ
Non-OR	ØPS[C,D,F,G,H,J,K,L][3,4]ZZ

See Appendix L for Procedure Combinations
⊞   ØPS33ZZ
⊞   ØPS43ZZ

ØPS Continued on next page

NC Noncovered Procedure   **LC** Limited Coverage   **QA** Questionable OB Admit   **NT** New Tech Add-on   ⊞ Combination Member   ♂ Male   ♀ Female

Upper Bones

Ø **Medical and Surgical**
P **Upper Bones**
S **Reposition**

ØPS Continued

Definition: Moving to its normal location, or other suitable location, all or a portion of a body part

Explanation: The body part is moved to a new location from an abnormal location, or from a normal location where it is not functioning correctly. The body part may or may not be cut out or off to be moved to the new location.

Body Part Character 4		Approach Character 5	Device Character 6	Qualifier Character 7

C Humeral Head, Right
  Greater tuberosity
  Lesser tuberosity
  Neck of humerus
    (anatomical)(surgical)
D Humeral Head, Left
  See C Humeral Head, Right
F Humeral Shaft, Right
  Distal humerus
  Humerus, distal
  Lateral epicondyle of humerus
  Medial epicondyle of humerus
	G Humeral Shaft, Left
	  See F Humeral Shaft, Right
	H Radius, Right
	  Ulnar notch
	J Radius, Left
	  See H Radius, Right
	K Ulna, Right
	  Olecranon process
	  Radial notch
	L Ulna, Left
	  See K Ulna, Right
		X External	**Z** No Device	**Z** No Qualifier

M Carpal, Right
  Capitate bone
  Hamate bone
  Lunate bone
  Pisiform bone
  Scaphoid bone
  Trapezium bone
  Trapezoid bone
  Triquetral bone
	N Carpal, Left
	  See M Carpal, Right
	P Metacarpal, Right
	Q Metacarpal, Left
	R Thumb Phalanx, Right
	S Thumb Phalanx, Left
	T Finger Phalanx, Right
	V Finger Phalanx, Left
		Ø Open
		3 Percutaneous
		4 Percutaneous Endoscopic
			4 Internal Fixation Device
			5 External Fixation Device
			Z No Device
				Z No Qualifier

M Carpal, Right
  Capitate bone
  Hamate bone
  Lunate bone
  Pisiform bone
  Scaphoid bone
  Trapezium bone
  Trapezoid bone
  Triquetral bone
	N Carpal, Left
	  See M Carpal, Right
	P Metacarpal, Right
	Q Metacarpal, Left
	R Thumb Phalanx, Right
	S Thumb Phalanx, Left
	T Finger Phalanx, Right
	V Finger Phalanx, Left
		X External	**Z** No Device	**Z** No Qualifier

Non-OR ØPS[C,D,F,G,H,J,K,L]XZZ
Non-OR ØPS[M,N,P,Q,R,S,T,V][3,4]ZZ
Non-OR ØPS[M,N,P,Q,R,S,T,V]XZZ

Ø **Medical and Surgical**
P **Upper Bones**
T **Resection**

Definition: Cutting out or off, without replacement, all of a body part

Explanation: None

Body Part Character 4		Approach Character 5	Device Character 6	Qualifier Character 7

Ø Sternum
  Manubrium
  Suprasternal notch
  Xiphoid process
1 Ribs, 1 to 2
2 Ribs, 3 or More
5 Scapula, Right
  Acromion (process)
  Coracoid process
6 Scapula, Left
  See 5 Scapula, Right
7 Glenoid Cavity, Right
  Glenoid fossa (of scapula)
8 Glenoid Cavity, Left
  See 7 Glenoid Cavity, Right
9 Clavicle, Right
B Clavicle, Left
C Humeral Head, Right
  Greater tuberosity
  Lesser tuberosity
  Neck of humerus
    (anatomical) (surgical)
D Humeral Head, Left
  See C Humeral Head, Right
F Humeral Shaft, Right
  Distal humerus
  Humerus, distal
  Lateral epicondyle of humerus
  Medial epicondyle of humerus
	G Humeral Shaft, Left
	  See F Humeral Shaft, Right
	H Radius, Right
	  Ulnar notch
	J Radius, Left
	  See H Radius, Right
	K Ulna, Right
	  Olecranon process
	  Radial notch
	L Ulna, Left
	  See K Ulna, Right
	M Carpal, Right
	  Capitate bone
	  Hamate bone
	  Lunate bone
	  Pisiform bone
	  Scaphoid bone
	  Trapezium bone
	  Trapezoid bone
	  Triquetral bone
	N Carpal, Left
	  See M Carpal, Right
	P Metacarpal, Right
	Q Metacarpal, Left
	R Thumb Phalanx, Right
	S Thumb Phalanx, Left
	T Finger Phalanx, Right
	V Finger Phalanx, Left
		Ø Open	**Z** No Device	**Z** No Qualifier

Ø   Medical and Surgical
P   Upper Bones
U   Supplement   Definition: Putting in or on biological or synthetic material that physically reinforces and/or augments the function of a portion of a body part

Explanation: The biological material is non-living, or is living and from the same individual. The body part may have been previously replaced, and the SUPPLEMENT procedure is performed to physically reinforce and/or augment the function of the replaced body part.

Body Part Character 4		Approach Character 5	Device Character 6	Qualifier Character 7

Ø Sternum
Manubrium
Suprasternal notch
Xiphoid process
1 Ribs, 1 to 2
2 Ribs, 3 or More
3 Cervical Vertebra ⊞
Dens
Odontoid process
Spinous process
Transverse foramen
Transverse process
Vertebral arch
Vertebral body
Vertebral foramen
Vertebral lamina
Vertebral pedicle
4 Thoracic Vertebra ⊞
Spinous process
Transverse process
Vertebral arch
Vertebral body
Vertebral foramen
Vertebral lamina
Vertebral pedicle
5 Scapula, Right
Acromion (process)
Coracoid process
6 Scapula, Left
See 5 Scapula, Right
7 Glenoid Cavity, Right
Glenoid fossa (of scapula)
8 Glenoid Cavity, Left
See 7 Glenoid Cavity, Right
9 Clavicle, Right
B Clavicle, Left
C Humeral Head, Right
Greater tuberosity
Lesser tuberosity
Neck of humerus
  (anatomical) (surgical)
	D Humeral Head, Left
	See C Humeral Head, Right
	F Humeral Shaft, Right
	Distal humerus
	Humerus, distal
	Lateral epicondyle of humerus
	Medial epicondyle of humerus
	G Humeral Shaft, Left
	See F Humeral Shaft, Right
	H Radius, Right
	Ulnar notch
	J Radius, Left
	See H Radius, Right
	K Ulna, Right
	Olecranon process
	Radial notch
	L Ulna, Left
	See K Ulna, Right
	M Carpal, Right
	Capitate bone
	Hamate bone
	Lunate bone
	Pisiform bone
	Scaphoid bone
	Trapezium bone
	Trapezoid bone
	Triquetral bone
	N Carpal, Left
	See M Carpal, Right
	P Metacarpal, Right
	Q Metacarpal, Left
	R Thumb Phalanx, Right
	S Thumb Phalanx, Left
	T Finger Phalanx, Right
	V Finger Phalanx, Left
		Ø Open
		3 Percutaneous
		4 Percutaneous Endoscopic
			**7 Autologous Tissue
			  Substitute**
			J Synthetic Substitute
			**K Nonautologous Tissue
			  Substitute**
				Z No Qualifier

See Appendix L for Procedure Combinations
   ⊞   ØPU[3,4]3JZ

NC Noncovered Procedure   LC Limited Coverage   QA Questionable OB Admit   NT New Tech Add-on   ⊞ Combination Member   ♂ Male   ♀ Female

ICD-10-PCS 2023   **559**

ØPU–ØPU

Ø Medical and Surgical
P Upper Bones
W Revision

Definition: Correcting, to the extent possible, a portion of a malfunctioning device or the position of a displaced device

Explanation: Revision can include correcting a malfunctioning or displaced device by taking out or putting in components of the device such as a screw or pin

Body Part Character 4		Approach Character 5	Device Character 6	Qualifier Character 7
Ø Sternum Manubrium Suprasternal notch Xiphoid process **1 Ribs, 1 to 2** **2 Ribs, 3 or More** **3 Cervical Vertebra** Dens Odontoid process Spinous process Transverse foramen Transverse process Vertebral arch Vertebral body Vertebral foramen Vertebral lamina Vertebral pedicle **4 Thoracic Vertebra** Spinous process Transverse process Vertebral arch Vertebral body Vertebral foramen Vertebral lamina Vertebral pedicle	**5 Scapula, Right** Acromion (process) Coracoid process **6 Scapula, Left** *See 5 Scapula, Right* **7 Glenoid Cavity, Right** Glenoid fossa (of scapula) **8 Glenoid Cavity, Left** *See 7 Glenoid Cavity, Right* **9 Clavicle, Right** **B Clavicle, Left**	**Ø Open** **3 Percutaneous** **4 Percutaneous Endoscopic** **X External**	**4 Internal Fixation Device** **7 Autologous Tissue Substitute** **J Synthetic Substitute** **K Nonautologous Tissue Substitute**	**Z No Qualifier**
C Humeral Head, Right Greater tuberosity Lesser tuberosity Neck of humerus (anatomical)(surgical) **D Humeral Head, Left** *See C Humeral Head, Right* **F Humeral Shaft, Right** Distal humerus Humerus, distal Lateral epicondyle of humerus Medial epicondyle of humerus **G Humeral Shaft, Left** *See F Humeral Shaft, Right* **H Radius, Right** Ulnar notch **J Radius, Left** *See H Radius, Right* **K Ulna, Right** Olecranon process Radial notch	**L Ulna, Left** *See K Ulna, Right* **M Carpal, Right** Capitate bone Hamate bone Lunate bone Pisiform bone Scaphoid bone Trapezium bone Trapezoid bone Triquetral bone **N Carpal, Left** *See M Carpal, Right* **P Metacarpal, Right** **Q Metacarpal, Left** **R Thumb Phalanx, Right** **S Thumb Phalanx, Left** **T Finger Phalanx, Right** **V Finger Phalanx, Left**	**Ø Open** **3 Percutaneous** **4 Percutaneous Endoscopic** **X External**	**4 Internal Fixation Device** **5 External Fixation Device** **7 Autologous Tissue Substitute** **J Synthetic Substitute** **K Nonautologous Tissue Substitute**	**Z No Qualifier**
Y Upper Bone		**Ø Open** **3 Percutaneous** **4 Percutaneous Endoscopic** **X External**	**Ø Drainage Device** **M Bone Growth Stimulator**	**Z No Qualifier**

Non-OR	ØPW[Ø,1,2,3,4,5,6,7,8,9,B]X[4,7,J,K]Z
Non-OR	ØPW[C,D,F,G,H,J,K,L,M,N,P,Q,R,S,T,V]X[4,5,7,J,K]Z
Non-OR	ØPWYX[Ø,M]Z

Lower Bones 0Q2–0QW

Character Meanings

This Character Meaning table is provided as a guide to assist the user in the identification of character members that may be found in this section of code tables. It **SHOULD NOT** be used to build a PCS code.

Operation–Character 3	Body Part–Character 4	Approach–Character 5	Device–Character 6	Qualifier–Character 7
2 Change	0 Lumbar Vertebra	0 Open	0 Drainage Device	2 Sesamoid Bone(s) 1st Toe
5 Destruction	1 Sacrum	3 Percutaneous	3 Spinal Stabilization Device, Vertebral Body Tether	X Diagnostic
8 Division	2 Pelvic Bone, Right	4 Percutaneous Endoscopic	4 Internal Fixation Device	Z No Qualifier
9 Drainage	3 Pelvic Bone, Left	X External	5 External Fixation Device	
B Excision	4 Acetabulum, Right		6 Internal Fixation Device, Intramedullary	
C Extirpation	5 Acetabulum, Left		7 Autologous Tissue Substitute OR Internal Fixation Device, Intramedullary Limb Lengthening	
D Extraction	6 Upper Femur, Right		8 External Fixation Device, Limb Lengthening	
H Insertion	7 Upper Femur, Left		B External Fixation Device, Monoplanar	
J Inspection	8 Femoral Shaft, Right		C External Fixation Device, Ring	
N Release	9 Femoral Shaft, Left		D External Fixation Device, Hybrid	
P Removal	B Lower Femur, Right		J Synthetic Substitute	
Q Repair	C Lower Femur, Left		K Nonautologous Tissue Substitute	
R Replacement	D Patella, Right		M Bone Growth Stimulator	
S Reposition	F Patella, Left		Y Other Device	
T Resection	G Tibia, Right		Z No Device	
U Supplement	H Tibia, Left			
W Revision	J Fibula, Right			
	K Fibula, Left			
	L Tarsal, Right			
	M Tarsal, Left			
	N Metatarsal, Right			
	P Metatarsal, Left			
	Q Toe Phalanx, Right			
	R Toe Phalanx, Left			
	S Coccyx			
	Y Lower Bone			

AHA Coding Clinic for table 0Q8
2018, 1Q, 25	Periacetabular osteotomy for repair of congenital hip dysplasia
2016, 2Q, 31	Periacetabular ostectomy for repair of congenital hip dysplasia

AHA Coding Clinic for table 0Q9
2022, 1Q, 31	Septic arthritis/osteomyelitis of pubic symphysis and aspiration biopsy

AHA Coding Clinic for table 0QB
2021, 4Q, 52-53	Sesamoidectomy of great toe
2021, 2Q, 18	Excision of tibial sesamoid
2020, 2Q, 26	Sacral pressure ulcer with excisional and nonexcisional debridement of same site
2019, 2Q, 19	Cervical spinal fusion, decompression and placement of interfacet stabilization device
2018, 3Q, 17	Excisional debridement of periosteum
2017, 1Q, 23	Reconstruction of mandible using titanium and bone
2016, 3Q, 30	Resection of femur with interposition arthroplasty
2015, 3Q, 3-8	Excisional and nonexcisional debridement
2015, 3Q, 26	Femoral head resection
2015, 2Q, 34	Decompressive laminectomy
2014, 4Q, 25	Femoroacetabular impingement and labral tear with repair
2014, 2Q, 6	Posterior lumbar fusion with discectomy
2013, 4Q, 116	Spinal decompression
2013, 2Q, 39	Ankle fusion, osteotomy, and removal of hardware
2012, 2Q, 19	Multiple decompressive cervical laminectomies

AHA Coding Clinic for table 0QD
2017, 4Q, 41	Extraction procedures

AHA Coding Clinic for table 0QH
2022, 2Q, 19	Limb lengthening surgery
2019, 4Q, 34	Intramedullary limb lengthening internal fixation device
2017, 1Q, 21	Staged scoliosis surgery with iliac fixation and spinal fusion
2016, 3Q, 34	Tibial/fibula epiphysiodesis

AHA Coding Clinic for table 0QP
2020, 4Q, 56	Removal of external fixation device
2017, 4Q, 74-75	Magnetic growth rods
2015, 2Q, 6	Planned implant break

AHA Coding Clinic for table 0QQ
2018, 1Q, 15	Pubic symphysis fusion
2014, 3Q, 24	Repair of lipomyelomeningocele and tethered cord

AHA Coding Clinic for table 0QR
2017, 1Q, 22	Total knee replacement and patellar component
2016, 3Q, 30	Resection of femur with interposition arthroplasty

AHA Coding Clinic for table 0QS
2022, 2Q, 19	Limb lengthening surgery
2021, 4Q, 51-52	Vertebral body tethering
2020, 1Q, 33	Spinal fusion without use of bone graft
2019, 3Q, 26	Open reduction with internal fixation and placement of strut allograft
2018, 1Q, 13	Bilateral cuboid osteotomy for repair of congenital talipes equinovarus
2018, 1Q, 25	Periacetabular osteotomy for repair of congenital hip dysplasia
2016, 3Q, 34	Tibial/fibula epiphysiodesis
2014, 4Q, 29	Rotational osteosynthesis
2014, 4Q, 31	Reposition of femur for correction of valgus and recurvatum deformities

AHA Coding Clinic for table 0QT
2017, 1Q, 22	Chopart amputation of foot
2016, 3Q, 30	Resection of femur with interposition arthroplasty
2015, 3Q, 26	Femoral head resection
2014, 4Q, 29	Rotational osteosynthesis

AHA Coding Clinic for table 0QU
2019, 3Q, 26	Open reduction with internal fixation and placement of strut allograft
2019, 2Q, 35	Kiva® kyphoplasty
2015, 3Q, 18	Total hip replacement with acetabular reconstruction
2014, 4Q, 31	Reposition of femur for correction of valgus and recurvatum deformities
2014, 2Q, 12	Percutaneous vertebroplasty using cement
2013, 2Q, 35	Use of bone void filler in grafting

AHA Coding Clinic for table 0QW
2017, 4Q, 74-75	Magnetic growth rods

Lower Bones

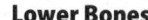

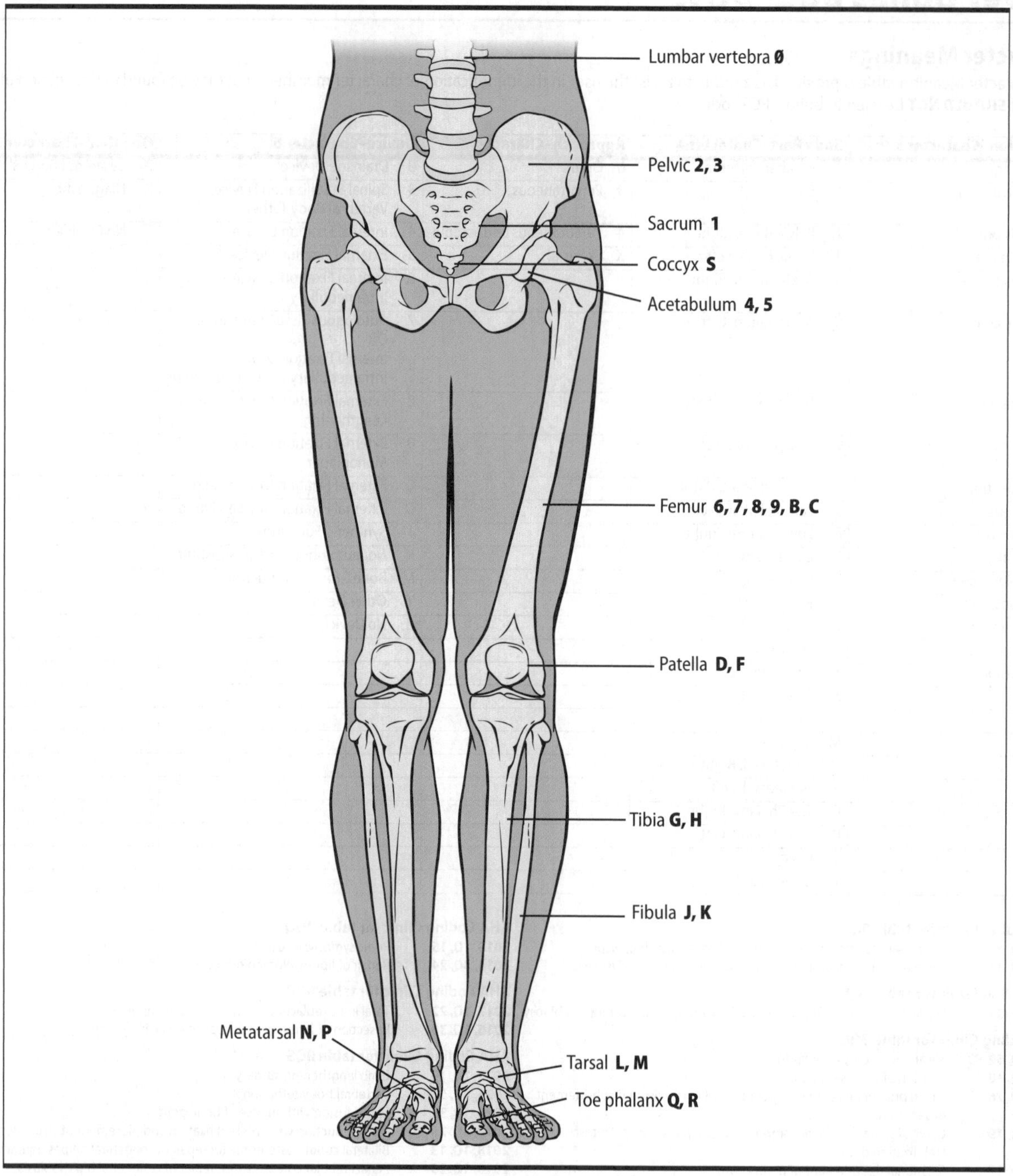

Lumbar vertebra **Ø**

Pelvic **2, 3**

Sacrum **1**

Coccyx **S**

Acetabulum **4, 5**

Femur **6, 7, 8, 9, B, C**

Patella **D, F**

Tibia **G, H**

Fibula **J, K**

Metatarsal **N, P**

Tarsal **L, M**

Toe phalanx **Q, R**

Hip Bone Anatomy

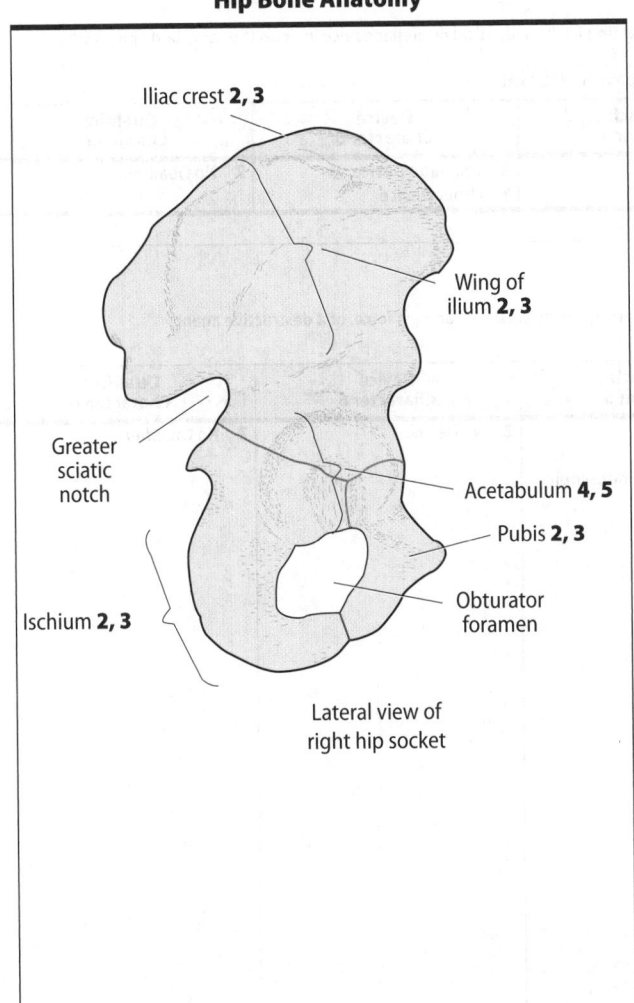

Iliac crest **2, 3**

Wing of ilium **2, 3**

Greater sciatic notch

Acetabulum **4, 5**

Pubis **2, 3**

Obturator foramen

Ischium **2, 3**

Lateral view of right hip socket

Pelvic and Lower Extremity Bones

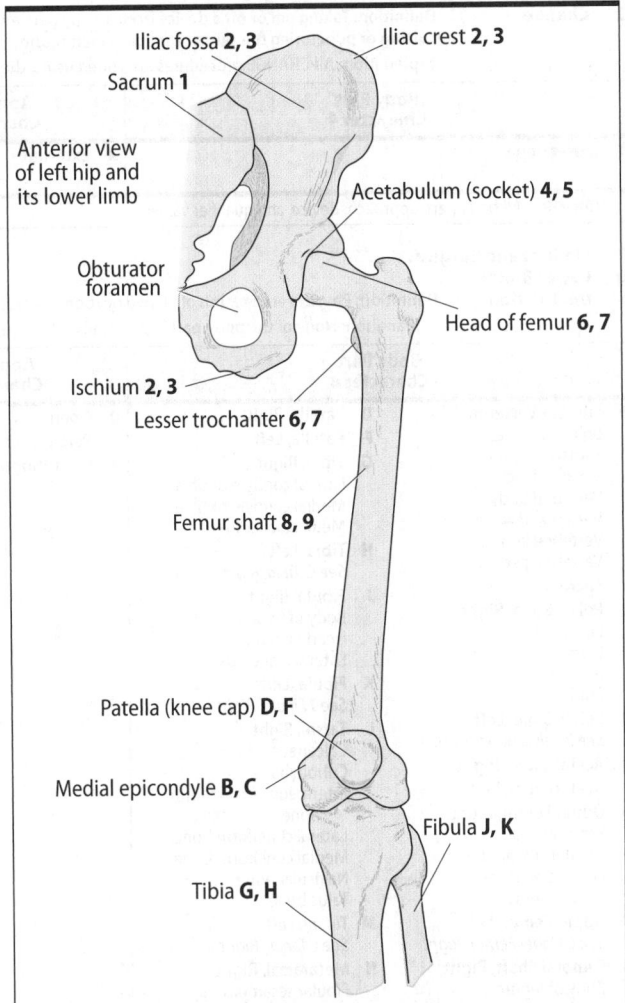

Iliac fossa **2, 3**

Iliac crest **2, 3**

Sacrum **1**

Anterior view of left hip and its lower limb

Acetabulum (socket) **4, 5**

Obturator foramen

Head of femur **6, 7**

Ischium **2, 3**

Lesser trochanter **6, 7**

Femur shaft **8, 9**

Patella (knee cap) **D, F**

Medial epicondyle **B, C**

Fibula **J, K**

Tibia **G, H**

Foot Bones

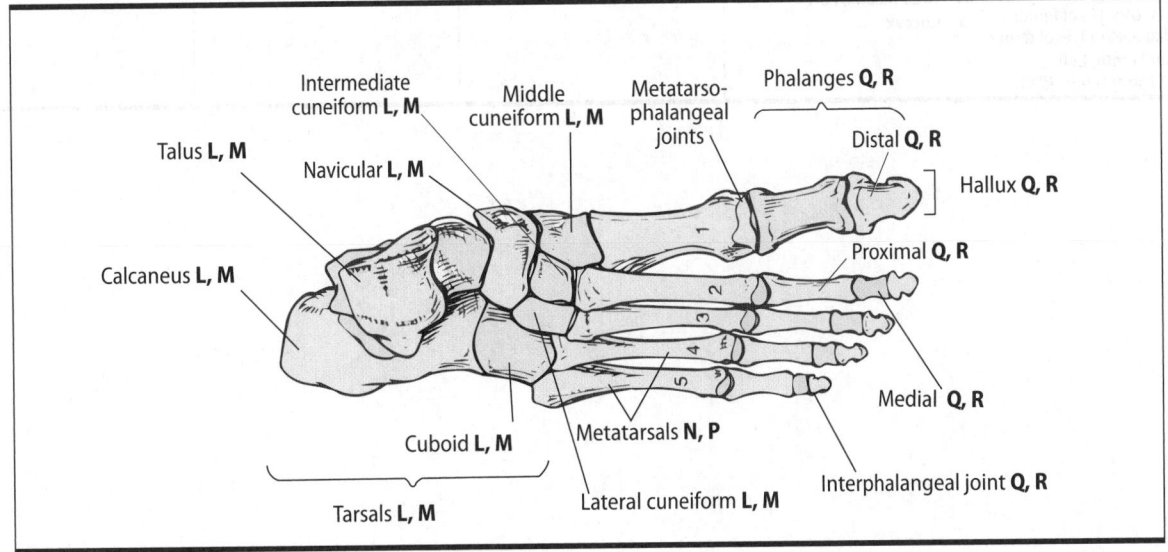

Intermediate cuneiform **L, M**

Middle cuneiform **L, M**

Metatarso-phalangeal joints

Phalanges **Q, R**

Distal **Q, R**

Talus **L, M**

Navicular **L, M**

Hallux **Q, R**

Calcaneus **L, M**

Proximal **Q, R**

Medial **Q, R**

Cuboid **L, M**

Metatarsals **N, P**

Interphalangeal joint **Q, R**

Tarsals **L, M**

Lateral cuneiform **L, M**

Lower Bones

ØQ2–ØQ5   Lower Bones   ICD-10-PCS 2023

Ø Medical and Surgical
Q Lower Bones
2 Change   Definition: Taking out or off a device from a body part and putting back an identical or similar device in or on the same body part without cutting or puncturing the skin or a mucous membrane

       Explanation: All CHANGE procedures are coded using the approach EXTERNAL

Body Part Character 4	Approach Character 5	Device Character 6	Qualifier Character 7
Y Lower Bone	X External	Ø Drainage Device Y Other Device	Z No Qualifier

Non-OR All body part, approach, device, and qualifier values

Ø Medical and Surgical
Q Lower Bones
5 Destruction   Definition: Physical eradication of all or a portion of a body part by the direct use of energy, force, or a destructive agent

       Explanation: None of the body part is physically taken out

Body Part Character 4	Approach Character 5	Device Character 6	Qualifier Character 7

Ø Lumbar Vertebra
  Spinous process
  Transverse process
  Vertebral arch
  Vertebral body
  Vertebral foramen
  Vertebral lamina
  Vertebral pedicle
1 Sacrum
2 Pelvic Bone, Right
  Iliac crest
  Ilium
  Ischium
  Pubis
3 Pelvic Bone, Left
  See 2 Pelvic Bone, Right
4 Acetabulum, Right
5 Acetabulum, Left
6 Upper Femur, Right
  Femoral head
  Greater trochanter
  Lesser trochanter
  Neck of femur
7 Upper Femur, Left
  See 6 Upper Femur, Right
8 Femoral Shaft, Right
  Body of femur
9 Femoral Shaft, Left
  See 8 Femoral Shaft, Right
B Lower Femur, Right
  Lateral condyle of femur
  Lateral epicondyle of femur
  Medial condyle of femur
  Medial epicondyle of femur
C Lower Femur, Left
  See B Lower Femur, Right
 	
D Patella, Right
F Patella, Left
G Tibia, Right
  Lateral condyle of tibia
  Medial condyle of tibia
  Medial malleolus
H Tibia, Left
  See G Tibia, Right
J Fibula, Right
  Body of fibula
  Head of fibula
  Lateral malleolus
K Fibula, Left
  See J Fibula, Right
L Tarsal, Right
  Calcaneus
  Cuboid bone
  Intermediate cuneiform
   bone
  Lateral cuneiform bone
  Medial cuneiform bone
  Navicular bone
  Talus bone
M Tarsal, Left
  See L Tarsal, Right
N Metatarsal, Right
  Fibular sesamoid
  Tibial sesamoid
P Metatarsal, Left
  See N Metatarsal, Right
Q Toe Phalanx, Right
R Toe Phalanx, Left
S Coccyx
	Ø Open
	3 Percutaneous
	4 Percutaneous Endoscopic
		Z No Device	Z No Qualifier

Non-OR Procedure DRG Non-OR Procedure Valid OR Procedure HAC Associated Procedure Combination Only New/Revised April New/Revised October

564   ICD-10-PCS 2023

Lower Bones

Ø   **Medical and Surgical**
Q   **Lower Bones**
8   **Division**   Definition: Cutting into a body part, without draining fluids and/or gases from the body part, in order to separate or transect a body part
                         Explanation: All or a portion of the body part is separated into two or more portions

Body Part Character 4	Approach Character 5	Device Character 6	Qualifier Character 7

Ø **Lumbar Vertebra**
   Spinous process
   Transverse process
   Vertebral arch
   Vertebral body
   Vertebral foramen
   Vertebral lamina
   Vertebral pedicle
1 **Sacrum**
2 **Pelvic Bone, Right**
   Iliac crest
   Ilium
   Ischium
   Pubis
3 **Pelvic Bone, Left**
   See 2 Pelvic Bone, Right
4 **Acetabulum, Right**
5 **Acetabulum, Left**
6 **Upper Femur, Right**
   Femoral head
   Greater trochanter
   Lesser trochanter
   Neck of femur
7 **Upper Femur, Left**
   See 6 Upper Femur, Right
8 **Femoral Shaft, Right**
   Body of femur
9 **Femoral Shaft, Left**
   See 8 Femoral Shaft, Right
B **Lower Femur, Right**
   Lateral condyle of femur
   Lateral epicondyle of femur
   Medial condyle of femur
   Medial epicondyle of femur
C **Lower Femur, Left**
   See B Lower Femur, Right
D **Patella, Right**
F **Patella, Left**
G **Tibia, Right**
   Lateral condyle of tibia
   Medial condyle of tibia
   Medial malleolus
H **Tibia, Left**
   See G Tibia, Right
J **Fibula, Right**
   Body of fibula
   Head of fibula
   Lateral malleolus
K **Fibula, Left**
   See J Fibula, Right
L **Tarsal, Right**
   Calcaneus
   Cuboid bone
   Intermediate cuneiform bone
   Lateral cuneiform bone
   Medial cuneiform bone
   Navicular bone
   Talus bone
M **Tarsal, Left**
   See L Tarsal, Right
N **Metatarsal, Right**
   Fibular sesamoid
   Tibial sesamoid
P **Metatarsal, Left**
   See N Metatarsal, Right
Q **Toe Phalanx, Right**
R **Toe Phalanx, Left**
S **Coccyx**
	Ø Open
	3 Percutaneous
	4 Percutaneous Endoscopic
		Z No Device	**Z** No Qualifier

NC Noncovered Procedure   **LC** Limited Coverage   **QA** Questionable OB Admit   **NT** New Tech Add-on   ⊞ Combination Member   ♂ Male   ♀ Female

ICD-10-PCS 2023   **565**

Ø   Medical and Surgical
Q   Lower Bones
9   Drainage   Definition: Taking or letting out fluids and/or gases from a body part

                 Explanation: The qualifier DIAGNOSTIC is used to identify drainage procedures that are biopsies

Body Part Character 4		Approach Character 5	Device Character 6	Qualifier Character 7

Ø Lumbar Vertebra
  Spinous process
  Transverse process
  Vertebral arch
  Vertebral body
  Vertebral foramen
  Vertebral lamina
  Vertebral pedicle
1 Sacrum
2 Pelvic Bone, Right
  Iliac crest
  Ilium
  Ischium
  Pubis
3 Pelvic Bone, Left
  See 2 Pelvic Bone, Right
4 Acetabulum, Right
5 Acetabulum, Left
6 Upper Femur, Right
  Femoral head
  Greater trochanter
  Lesser trochanter
  Neck of femur
7 Upper Femur, Left
  See 6 Upper Femur, Right
8 Femoral Shaft, Right
  Body of femur
9 Femoral Shaft, Left
  See 8 Femoral Shaft, Right
B Lower Femur, Right
  Lateral condyle of femur
  Lateral epicondyle of femur
  Medial condyle of femur
  Medial epicondyle of femur
	C Lower Femur, Left
	  See B Lower Femur, Right
	D Patella, Right
	F Patella, Left
	G Tibia, Right
	  Lateral condyle of tibia
	  Medial condyle of tibia
	  Medial malleolus
	H Tibia, Left
	  See G Tibia, Right
	J Fibula, Right
	  Body of fibula
	  Head of fibula
	  Lateral malleolus
	K Fibula, Left
	  See J Fibula, Right
	L Tarsal, Right
	  Calcaneus
	  Cuboid bone
	  Intermediate cuneiform bone
	  Lateral cuneiform bone
	  Medial cuneiform bone
	  Navicular bone
	  Talus bone
	M Tarsal, Left
	  See L Tarsal, Right
	N Metatarsal, Right
	  Fibular sesamoid
	  Tibial sesamoid
	P Metatarsal, Left
	  See N Metatarsal, Right
	Q Toe Phalanx, Right
	R Toe Phalanx, Left
	S Coccyx
		Ø Open
		3 Percutaneous
		4 Percutaneous Endoscopic
			Ø Drainage Device	**Z No Qualifier**

Ø Lumbar Vertebra
  Spinous process
  Transverse process
  Vertebral arch
  Vertebral body
  Vertebral foramen
  Vertebral lamina
  Vertebral pedicle
1 Sacrum
2 Pelvic Bone, Right
  Iliac crest
  Ilium
  Ischium
  Pubis
3 Pelvic Bone, Left
  See 2 Pelvic Bone, Right
4 Acetabulum, Right
5 Acetabulum, Left
6 Upper Femur, Right
  Femoral head
  Greater trochanter
  Lesser trochanter
  Neck of femur
7 Upper Femur, Left
  See 6 Upper Femur, Right
8 Femoral Shaft, Right
  Body of femur
9 Femoral Shaft, Left
  See 8 Femoral Shaft, Right
B Lower Femur, Right
  Lateral condyle of femur
  Lateral epicondyle of femur
  Medial condyle of femur
  Medial epicondyle of femur
	C Lower Femur, Left
	  See B Lower Femur, Right
	D Patella, Right
	F Patella, Left
	G Tibia, Right
	  Lateral condyle of tibia
	  Medial condyle of tibia
	  Medial malleolus
	H Tibia, Left
	  See G Tibia, Right
	J Fibula, Right
	  Body of fibula
	  Head of fibula
	  Lateral malleolus
	K Fibula, Left
	  See J Fibula, Right
	L Tarsal, Right
	  Calcaneus
	  Cuboid bone
	  Intermediate cuneiform bone
	  Lateral cuneiform bone
	  Medial cuneiform bone
	  Navicular bone
	  Talus bone
	M Tarsal, Left
	  See L Tarsal, Right
	N Metatarsal, Right
	  Fibular sesamoid
	  Tibial sesamoid
	P Metatarsal, Left
	  See N Metatarsal, Right
	Q Toe Phalanx, Right
	R Toe Phalanx, Left
	S Coccyx
		Ø Open
		3 Percutaneous
		4 Percutaneous Endoscopic
			Z No Device	**X Diagnostic**
				Z No Qualifier

Non-OR   ØQ9[Ø,1,2,3,4,5,6,7,8,9,B,C,D,F,G,H,J,K,L,M,P,Q,R,S]3ØZ
Non-OR   ØQ9[Ø,1,2,3,4,5,6,7,8,9,B,C,D,F,G,H,J,K,L,M,P,Q,R,S]3ZZ

Non-OR Procedure   DRG Non-OR Procedure   Valid OR Procedure   HAC Associated Procedure   Combination Only   New/Revised April   New/Revised October

566   ICD-10-PCS 2023

Ø   **Medical and Surgical**
Q   **Lower Bones**
B   **Excision**   Definition: Cutting out or off, without replacement, a portion of a body part

Explanation: The qualifier DIAGNOSTIC is used to identify excision procedures that are biopsies

Body Part Character 4	Approach Character 5	Device Character 6	Qualifier Character 7

Ø   **Lumbar Vertebra**
   Spinous process
   Transverse process
   Vertebral arch
   Vertebral body
   Vertebral foramen
   Vertebral lamina
   Vertebral pedicle
1   **Sacrum**
2   **Pelvic Bone, Right**
   Iliac crest
   Ilium
   Ischium
   Pubis
3   **Pelvic Bone, Left**
   See 2 Pelvic Bone, Right
4   **Acetabulum, Right**
5   **Acetabulum, Left**
6   **Upper Femur, Right**
   Femoral head
   Greater trochanter
   Lesser trochanter
   Neck of femur
7   **Upper Femur, Left**
   See 6 Upper Femur, Right
8   **Femoral Shaft, Right**
   Body of femur
9   **Femoral Shaft, Left**
   See 8 Femoral Shaft, Right
B   **Lower Femur, Right**
   Lateral condyle of femur
   Lateral epicondyle of femur
   Medial condyle of femur
   Medial epicondyle of femur
C   **Lower Femur, Left**
   See B Lower Femur, Right
D   **Patella, Right**
F   **Patella, Left**
G   **Tibia, Right**
   Lateral condyle of tibia
   Medial condyle of tibia
   Medial malleolus
H   **Tibia, Left**
   See G Tibia, Right
J   **Fibula, Right**
   Body of fibula
   Head of fibula
   Lateral malleolus
K   **Fibula, Left**
   See J Fibula, Right
L   **Tarsal, Right**
   Calcaneus
   Cuboid bone
   Intermediate cuneiform bone
   Lateral cuneiform bone
   Medial cuneiform bone
   Navicular bone
   Talus bone
M   **Tarsal, Left**
   See L Tarsal, Right
Q   **Toe Phalanx, Right**
R   **Toe Phalanx, Left**
S   **Coccyx**
	Ø Open
	3 Percutaneous
	4 Percutaneous Endoscopic
		Z No Device	**X** Diagnostic
			Z No Qualifier

N   **Metatarsal, Right**
   Fibular sesamoid
   Tibial sesamoid
P   **Metatarsal, Left**
   See N Metatarsal, Right
	Ø Open
	3 Percutaneous
	4 Percutaneous Endoscopic
		Z No Device	**2** Sesamoid Bone(s) 1st Toe
			X Diagnostic
			Z No Qualifier

NC Noncovered Procedure   **LC** Limited Coverage   **QA** Questionable OB Admit   **NT** New Tech Add-on   ⊞ Combination Member   ♂ Male   ♀ Female

ICD-10-PCS 2023   567

0QB–0QB

Ø **Medical and Surgical**
Q **Lower Bones**
C **Extirpation** Definition: Taking or cutting out solid matter from a body part

Explanation: The solid matter may be an abnormal byproduct of a biological function or a foreign body; it may be imbedded in a body part or in the lumen of a tubular body part. The solid matter may or may not have been previously broken into pieces.

Body Part Character 4	Approach Character 5	Device Character 6	Qualifier Character 7
Ø Lumbar Vertebra Spinous process Transverse process Vertebral arch Vertebral body Vertebral foramen Vertebral lamina Vertebral pedicle **1 Sacrum** **2 Pelvic Bone, Right** Iliac crest Ilium Ischium Pubis **3 Pelvic Bone, Left** *See 2 Pelvic Bone, Right* **4 Acetabulum, Right** **5 Acetabulum, Left** **6 Upper Femur, Right** Femoral head Greater trochanter Lesser trochanter Neck of femur **7 Upper Femur, Left** *See 6 Upper Femur, Right* **8 Femoral Shaft, Right** Body of femur **9 Femoral Shaft, Left** *See 8 Femoral Shaft, Right* **B Lower Femur, Right** Lateral condyle of femur Lateral epicondyle of femur Medial condyle of femur Medial epicondyle of femur **C Lower Femur, Left** *See B Lower Femur, Right* **D Patella, Right** **F Patella, Left** **G Tibia, Right** Lateral condyle of tibia Medial condyle of tibia Medial malleolus **H Tibia, Left** *See G Tibia, Right* **J Fibula, Right** Body of fibula Head of fibula Lateral malleolus **K Fibula, Left** *See J Fibula, Right* **L Tarsal, Right** Calcaneus Cuboid bone Intermediate cuneiform bone Lateral cuneiform bone Medial cuneiform bone Navicular bone Talus bone **M Tarsal, Left** *See L Tarsal, Right* **N Metatarsal, Right** Fibular sesamoid Tibial sesamoid **P Metatarsal, Left** *See N Metatarsal, Right* **Q Toe Phalanx, Right** **R Toe Phalanx, Left** **S Coccyx**	**Ø Open** **3 Percutaneous** **4 Percutaneous Endoscopic**	**Z No Device**	**Z No Qualifier**

Non-OR Procedure   DRG Non-OR Procedure   Valid OR Procedure   HAC Associated Procedure   Combination Only   New/Revised April   New/Revised October

568   ICD-10-PCS 2023

Ø　Medical and Surgical
Q　Lower Bones
D　Extraction　Definition: Pulling or stripping out or off all or a portion of a body part by the use of force
　　　　　　　　Explanation: The qualifier DIAGNOSTIC is used to identify extraction procedures that are biopsies

Body Part Character 4	Approach Character 5	Device Character 6	Qualifier Character 7
Ø　Lumbar Vertebra	**Ø　Open**	**Z　No Device**	**Z　No Qualifier**
Spinous process			
Transverse process			
Vertebral arch			
Vertebral body			
Vertebral foramen			
Vertebral lamina			
Vertebral pedicle			
1　Sacrum			
2　Pelvic Bone, Right			
Iliac crest			
Ilium			
Ischium			
Pubis			
3　Pelvic Bone, Left			
See 2 Pelvic Bone, Right			
4　Acetabulum, Right			
5　Acetabulum, Left			
6　Upper Femur, Right			
Femoral head			
Greater trochanter			
Lesser trochanter			
Neck of femur			
7　Upper Femur, Left			
See 6 Upper Femur, Right			
8　Femoral Shaft, Right			
Body of femur			
9　Femoral Shaft, Left			
See 8 Femoral Shaft, Right			
B　Lower Femur, Right			
Lateral condyle of femur			
Lateral epicondyle of femur			
Medial condyle of femur			
Medial epicondyle of femur			
C　Lower Femur, Left			
See B Lower Femur, Right			
D　Patella, Right			
F　Patella, Left			
G　Tibia, Right			
Lateral condyle of tibia			
Medial condyle of tibia			
Medial malleolus			
H　Tibia, Left			
See G Tibia, Right			
J　Fibula, Right			
Body of fibula			
Head of fibula			
Lateral malleolus			
K　Fibula, Left			
See J Fibula, Right			
L　Tarsal, Right			
Calcaneus			
Cuboid bone			
Intermediate cuneiform bone			
Lateral cuneiform bone			
Medial cuneiform bone			
Navicular bone			
Talus bone			
M　Tarsal, Left			
See L Tarsal, Right			
N　Metatarsal, Right			
Fibular sesamoid			
Tibial sesamoid			
P　Metatarsal, Left			
See N Metatarsal, Right			
Q　Toe Phalanx, Right			
R　Toe Phalanx, Left			
S　Coccyx			

NC Noncovered Procedure　　**LC** Limited Coverage　　**OA** Questionable OB Admit　　**NT** New Tech Add-on　　✚ Combination Member　　♂ Male　　♀ Female

ICD-10-PCS 2023　　　　　　　　　　　　　　　　　　　　　　　　　　　　　　　　　　　　　　　569

ØQD–ØQD

Ø **Medical and Surgical**
Q **Lower Bones**
H **Insertion**

Definition: Putting in a nonbiological appliance that monitors, assists, performs, or prevents a physiological function but does not physically take the place of a body part

Explanation: None

Body Part Character 4		Approach Character 5	Device Character 6	Qualifier Character 7
Ø Lumbar Vertebra Spinous process Transverse process Vertebral arch Vertebral body Vertebral foramen Vertebral lamina Vertebral pedicle **1** Sacrum **2** Pelvic Bone, Right Iliac crest Ilium Ischium Pubis **3** Pelvic Bone, Left *See 2 Pelvic Bone, Right* **4** Acetabulum, Right **5** Acetabulum, Left	**D** Patella, Right **F** Patella, Left **L** Tarsal, Right Calcaneus Cuboid bone Intermediate cuneiform bone Lateral cuneiform bone Medial cuneiform bone Navicular bone Talus bone **M** Tarsal, Left *See L Tarsal, Right* **N** Metatarsal, Right Fibular sesamoid Tibial sesamoid **P** Metatarsal, Left *See N Metatarsal, Right* **Q** Toe Phalanx, Right **R** Toe Phalanx, Left **S** Coccyx	**Ø** Open **3** Percutaneous **4** Percutaneous Endoscopic	**4** Internal Fixation Device **5** External Fixation Device	**Z** No Qualifier
6 Upper Femur, Right Femoral head Greater trochanter Lesser trochanter Neck of femur **7** Upper Femur, Left *See 6 Upper Femur, Right* **B** Lower Femur, Right Lateral condyle of femur Lateral epicondyle of femur Medial condyle of femur Medial epicondyle of femur	**C** Lower Femur, Left *See B Lower Femur, Right* **J** Fibula, Right Body of fibula Head of fibula Lateral malleolus **K** Fibula, Left *See J Fibula, Right*	**Ø** Open **3** Percutaneous **4** Percutaneous Endoscopic	**4** Internal Fixation Device **5** External Fixation Device **6** Internal Fixation Device, Intramedullary **8** External Fixation Device, Limb Lengthening **B** External Fixation Device, Monoplanar **C** External Fixation Device, Ring **D** External Fixation Device, Hybrid	**Z** No Qualifier
8 Femoral Shaft, Right Body of femur **9** Femoral Shaft, Left *See 8 Femoral Shaft, Right*	**G** Tibia, Right Lateral condyle of tibia Medial condyle of tibia Medial malleolus **H** Tibia, Left *See G Tibia, Right*	**Ø** Open **3** Percutaneous **4** Percutaneous Endoscopic	**4** Internal Fixation Device **5** External Fixation Device **6** Internal Fixation Device, Intramedullary **7** Internal Fixation Device, Intramedullary Limb Lengthening **8** External Fixation Device, Limb Lengthening **B** External Fixation Device, Monoplanar **C** External Fixation Device, Ring **D** External Fixation Device, Hybrid	**Z** No Qualifier
Y Lower Bone		**Ø** Open **3** Percutaneous **4** Percutaneous Endoscopic	**M** Bone Growth Stimulator	**Z** No Qualifier

Non-OR ØQH[6,7,B,C,J,K][Ø,3,4]8Z
Non-OR ØQH[8,9,G,H][Ø,3,4]8Z

Ø **Medical and Surgical**
Q **Lower Bones**
J **Inspection**

Definition: Visually and/or manually exploring a body part

Explanation: Visual exploration may be performed with or without optical instrumentation. Manual exploration may be performed directly or through intervening body layers.

Body Part Character 4	Approach Character 5	Device Character 6	Qualifier Character 7
Y Lower Bone	**Ø** Open **3** Percutaneous **4** Percutaneous Endoscopic **X** External	**Z** No Device	**Z** No Qualifier

Non-OR ØQJY[3,X]ZZ

Non-OR Procedure   DRG Non-OR Procedure   Valid OR Procedure   HAC Associated Procedure   Combination Only   New/Revised April   New/Revised October

Ø Medical and Surgical
Q Lower Bones
N Release   Definition: Freeing a body part from an abnormal physical constraint by cutting or by the use of force

Explanation: Some of the restraining tissue may be taken out but none of the body part is taken out

Body Part Character 4	Approach Character 5	Device Character 6	Qualifier Character 7
Ø Lumbar Vertebra Spinous process Transverse process Vertebral arch Vertebral body Vertebral foramen Vertebral lamina Vertebral pedicle **1 Sacrum** **2 Pelvic Bone, Right** Iliac crest Ilium Ischium Pubis **3 Pelvic Bone, Left** *See 2 Pelvic Bone, Right* **4 Acetabulum, Right** **5 Acetabulum, Left** **6 Upper Femur, Right** Femoral head Greater trochanter Lesser trochanter Neck of femur **7 Upper Femur, Left** *See 6 Upper Femur, Right* **8 Femoral Shaft, Right** Body of femur **9 Femoral Shaft, Left** *See 8 Femoral Shaft, Right* **B Lower Femur, Right** Lateral condyle of femur Lateral epicondyle of femur Medial condyle of femur Medial epicondyle of femur **C Lower Femur, Left** *See B Lower Femur, Right* **D Patella, Right** **F Patella, Left** **G Tibia, Right** Lateral condyle of tibia Medial condyle of tibia Medial malleolus **H Tibia, Left** *See G Tibia, Right* **J Fibula, Right** Body of fibula Head of fibula Lateral malleolus **K Fibula, Left** *See J Fibula, Right* **L Tarsal, Right** Calcaneus Cuboid bone Intermediate cuneiform bone Lateral cuneiform bone Medial cuneiform bone Navicular bone Talus bone **M Tarsal, Left** *See L Tarsal, Right* **N Metatarsal, Right** Fibular sesamoid Tibial sesamoid **P Metatarsal, Left** *See N Metatarsal, Right* **Q Toe Phalanx, Right** **R Toe Phalanx, Left** **S Coccyx**	**Ø Open** **3 Percutaneous** **4 Percutaneous Endoscopic**	**Z No Device**	**Z No Qualifier**

NC Noncovered Procedure   **LC** Limited Coverage   **QA** Questionable OB Admit   **NT** New Tech Add-on   ⊞ Combination Member   ♂ Male   ♀ Female

ICD-10-PCS 2023   571

ØQN–ØQN

Ø **Medical and Surgical**
Q **Lower Bones**
P **Removal**

Definition: Taking out or off a device from a body part

Explanation: If a device is taken out and a similar device put in without cutting or puncturing the skin or mucous membrane, the procedure is coded to the root operation CHANGE. Otherwise, the procedure for taking out a device is coded to the root operation REMOVAL.

Body Part Character 4		Approach Character 5	Device Character 6	Qualifier Character 7
Ø **Lumbar Vertebra** Spinous process Transverse process Vertebral arch Vertebral body Vertebral foramen Vertebral lamina Vertebral pedicle **1** **Sacrum** **2** **Pelvic Bone, Right** Iliac crest Ilium Ischium Pubis **3** **Pelvic Bone, Left** *See 2 Pelvic Bone, Right* **4** **Acetabulum, Right** **5** **Acetabulum, Left** **6** **Upper Femur, Right** Femoral head Greater trochanter Lesser trochanter Neck of femur **7** **Upper Femur, Left** *See 6 Upper Femur, Right* **8** **Femoral Shaft, Right** Body of femur **9** **Femoral Shaft, Left** *See 8 Femoral Shaft, Right* **B** **Lower Femur, Right** Lateral condyle of femur Lateral epicondyle of femur Medial condyle of femur Medial epicondyle of femur	**C** **Lower Femur, Left** *See B Lower Femur, Right* **D** **Patella, Right** **F** **Patella, Left** **G** **Tibia, Right** Lateral condyle of tibia Medial condyle of tibia Medial malleolus **H** **Tibia, Left** *See G Tibia, Right* **J** **Fibula, Right** Body of fibula Head of fibula Lateral malleolus **K** **Fibula, Left** *See J Fibula, Right* **L** **Tarsal, Right** Calcaneus Cuboid bone Intermediate cuneiform bone Lateral cuneiform bone Medial cuneiform bone Navicular bone Talus bone **M** **Tarsal, Left** *See L Tarsal, Right* **N** **Metatarsal, Right** Fibular sesamoid Tibial sesamoid **P** **Metatarsal, Left** *See N Metatarsal, Right* **Q** **Toe Phalanx, Right** **R** **Toe Phalanx, Left** **S** **Coccyx**	**Ø** **Open** **3** **Percutaneous** **4** **Percutaneous Endoscopic**	**4** **Internal Fixation Device** **5** **External Fixation Device** **7** **Autologous Tissue Substitute** **J** **Synthetic Substitute** **K** **Nonautologous Tissue Substitute**	**Z** **No Qualifier**
Ø **Lumbar Vertebra** Spinous process Transverse process Vertebral arch Vertebral body Vertebral foramen Vertebral lamina Vertebral pedicle **1** **Sacrum** **2** **Pelvic Bone, Right** Iliac crest Ilium Ischium Pubis **3** **Pelvic Bone, Left** *See 2 Pelvic Bone, Right* **4** **Acetabulum, Right** **5** **Acetabulum, Left** **6** **Upper Femur, Right** Femoral head Greater trochanter Lesser trochanter Neck of femur **7** **Upper Femur, Left** *See 6 Upper Femur, Right* **8** **Femoral Shaft, Right** Body of femur **9** **Femoral Shaft, Left** *See 8 Femoral Shaft, Right* **B** **Lower Femur, Right** Lateral condyle of femur Lateral epicondyle of femur Medial condyle of femur Medial epicondyle of femur	**C** **Lower Femur, Left** *See B Lower Femur, Right* **D** **Patella, Right** **F** **Patella, Left** **G** **Tibia, Right** Lateral condyle of tibia Medial condyle of tibia Medial malleolus **H** **Tibia, Left** *See G Tibia, Right* **J** **Fibula, Right** Body of fibula Head of fibula Lateral malleolus **K** **Fibula, Left** *See J Fibula, Right* **L** **Tarsal, Right** Calcaneus Cuboid bone Intermediate cuneiform bone Lateral cuneiform bone Medial cuneiform bone Navicular bone Talus bone **M** **Tarsal, Left** *See L Tarsal, Right* **N** **Metatarsal, Right** Fibular sesamoid Tibial sesamoid **P** **Metatarsal, Left** *See N Metatarsal, Right* **Q** **Toe Phalanx, Right** **R** **Toe Phalanx, Left** **S** **Coccyx**	**X** **External**	**4** **Internal Fixation Device** **5** **External Fixation Device**	**Z** **No Qualifier**
Y **Lower Bone**		**Ø** **Open** **3** **Percutaneous** **4** **Percutaneous Endoscopic** **X** **External**	**Ø** **Drainage Device** **M** **Bone Growth Stimulator**	**Z** **No Qualifier**

Non-OR ØQPYX[Ø,M]Z   **Non-OR** ØQPY3ØZ   **Non-OR** ØQP[Ø,1,2,3,4,5,6,7,8,9,B,C,D,F,G,H,J,K,L,M,N,P,Q,R,S]X[4,5]Z

Non-OR Procedure   DRG Non-OR Procedure   Valid OR Procedure   HAC Associated Procedure   Combination Only   New/Revised April   New/Revised October

572

ØQP–ØQP

ICD-10-PCS 2023

Ø   **Medical and Surgical**
Q   **Lower Bones**
Q   **Repair**   Definition: Restoring, to the extent possible, a body part to its normal anatomic structure and function
                    Explanation: Used only when the method to accomplish the repair is not one of the other root operations

Body Part Character 4	Approach Character 5	Device Character 6	Qualifier Character 7

Ø **Lumbar Vertebra**
   Spinous process
   Transverse process
   Vertebral arch
   Vertebral body
   Vertebral foramen
   Vertebral lamina
   Vertebral pedicle
1 **Sacrum**
2 **Pelvic Bone, Right**
   Iliac crest
   Ilium
   Ischium
   Pubis
3 **Pelvic Bone, Left**
   See 2 Pelvic Bone, Right
4 **Acetabulum, Right**
5 **Acetabulum, Left**
6 **Upper Femur, Right**
   Femoral head
   Greater trochanter
   Lesser trochanter
   Neck of femur
7 **Upper Femur, Left**
   See 6 Upper Femur, Right
8 **Femoral Shaft, Right**
   Body of femur
9 **Femoral Shaft, Left**
   See 8 Femoral Shaft, Right
B **Lower Femur, Right**
   Lateral condyle of femur
   Lateral epicondyle of femur
   Medial condyle of femur
   Medial epicondyle of femur
C **Lower Femur, Left**
   See B Lower Femur, Right
D **Patella, Right**
F **Patella, Left**
G **Tibia, Right**
   Lateral condyle of tibia
   Medial condyle of tibia
   Medial malleolus
H **Tibia, Left**
   See G Tibia, Right
J **Fibula, Right**
   Body of fibula
   Head of fibula
   Lateral malleolus
K **Fibula, Left**
   See J Fibula, Right
L **Tarsal, Right**
   Calcaneus
   Cuboid bone
   Intermediate cuneiform bone
   Lateral cuneiform bone
   Medial cuneiform bone
   Navicular bone
   Talus bone
M **Tarsal, Left**
   See L Tarsal, Right
N **Metatarsal, Right**
   Fibular sesamoid
   Tibial sesamoid
P **Metatarsal, Left**
   See N Metatarsal, Right
Q **Toe Phalanx, Right**
R **Toe Phalanx, Left**
S **Coccyx**
	Ø Open
	3 Percutaneous
	4 Percutaneous Endoscopic
	X External
		Z No Device	**Z** No Qualifier

    Non-OR   ØQQ[Ø,1,2,3,4,5,6,7,8,9,B,C,D,F,G,H,J,K,L,M,N,P,Q,R,S]XZZ

NC Noncovered Procedure   **LC** Limited Coverage   **QA** Questionable OB Admit   **NT** New Tech Add-on   ✚ Combination Member   ♂ Male   ♀ Female

ICD-10-PCS 2023   **573**

Lower Bones *(side tab)*

Ø Medical and Surgical
Q Lower Bones
R Replacement Definition: Putting in or on biological or synthetic material that physically takes the place and/or function of all or a portion of a body part
         Explanation: The body part may have been taken out or replaced, or may be taken out, physically eradicated, or rendered nonfunctional during the REPLACEMENT procedure. A REMOVAL procedure is coded for taking out the device used in a previous replacement procedure.

Body Part Character 4	Approach Character 5	Device Character 6	Qualifier Character 7

Ø Lumbar Vertebra
  Spinous process
  Transverse process
  Vertebral arch
  Vertebral body
  Vertebral foramen
  Vertebral lamina
  Vertebral pedicle
1 Sacrum
2 Pelvic Bone, Right
  Iliac crest
  Ilium
  Ischium
  Pubis
3 Pelvic Bone, Left
  See 2 Pelvic Bone, Right
4 Acetabulum, Right
5 Acetabulum, Left
6 Upper Femur, Right
  Femoral head
  Greater trochanter
  Lesser trochanter
  Neck of femur
7 Upper Femur, Left
  See 6 Upper Femur, Right
8 Femoral Shaft, Right
  Body of femur
9 Femoral Shaft, Left
  See 8 Femoral Shaft, Right
B Lower Femur, Right
  Lateral condyle of femur
  Lateral epicondyle of femur
  Medial condyle of femur
  Medial epicondyle of femur
C Lower Femur, Left
  See B Lower Femur, Right
D Patella, Right
F Patella, Left
G Tibia, Right
  Lateral condyle of tibia
  Medial condyle of tibia
  Medial malleolus
H Tibia, Left
  See G Tibia, Right
J Fibula, Right
  Body of fibula
  Head of fibula
  Lateral malleolus
K Fibula, Left
  See J Fibula, Right
L Tarsal, Right
  Calcaneus
  Cuboid bone
  Intermediate cuneiform bone
  Lateral cuneiform bone
  Medial cuneiform bone
  Navicular bone
  Talus bone
M Tarsal, Left
  See L Tarsal, Right
N Metatarsal, Right
  Fibular sesamoid
  Tibial sesamoid
P Metatarsal, Left
  See N Metatarsal, Right
Q Toe Phalanx, Right
R Toe Phalanx, Left
S Coccyx
	Ø Open
	3 Percutaneous
	4 Percutaneous Endoscopic
		7 Autologous Tissue Substitute
		J Synthetic Substitute
		K Nonautologous Tissue Substitute
			Z No Qualifier

Non-OR Procedure   DRG Non-OR Procedure   Valid OR Procedure   HAC Associated Procedure   Combination Only   New/Revised April   New/Revised October

574   ICD-10-PCS 2023

Ø   Medical and Surgical
Q   Lower Bones
S   Reposition   Definition: Moving to its normal location, or other suitable location, all or a portion of a body part

Explanation: The body part is moved to a new location from an abnormal location, or from a normal location where it is not functioning correctly. The body part may or may not be cut out or off to be moved to the new location.

Body Part Character 4		Approach Character 5	Device Character 6	Qualifier Character 7
Ø Lumbar Vertebra Spinous process Transverse process Vertebral arch Vertebral body Vertebral foramen Vertebral lamina Vertebral pedicle		**Ø Open** **4 Percutaneous Endoscopic**	**3 Spinal Stabilization Device, Vertebral Body Tether** **4 Internal Fixation Device** **Z No Device**	**Z No Qualifier**
Ø Lumbar Vertebra ⊞ Spinous process Transverse process Vertebral arch Vertebral body Vertebral foramen Vertebral lamina Vertebral pedicle		**3 Percutaneous**	**4 Internal Fixation Device** **Z No Device**	**Z No Qualifier**
Ø Lumbar Vertebra Spinous process Transverse process Vertebral arch Vertebral body Vertebral foramen Vertebral lamina Vertebral pedicle		**X External**	**Z No Device**	**Z No Qualifier**
1 Sacrum ⊞ **4 Acetabulum, Right** **5 Acetabulum, Left** **S Coccyx** ⊞		**Ø Open** **3 Percutaneous** **4 Percutaneous Endoscopic**	**4 Internal Fixation Device** **Z No Device**	**Z No Qualifier**
1 Sacrum **4 Acetabulum, Right** **5 Acetabulum, Left** **S Coccyx**		**X External**	**Z No Device**	**Z No Qualifier**
2 Pelvic Bone, Right Iliac crest Ilium Ischium Pubis **3 Pelvic Bone, Left** *See 2 Pelvic Bone, Right* **D Patella, Right** **F Patella, Left** **L Tarsal, Right** Calcaneus Cuboid bone Intermediate cuneiform bone Lateral cuneiform bone Medial cuneiform bone Navicular bone Talus bone	**M Tarsal, Left** *See L Tarsal, Right* **Q Toe Phalanx, Right** **R Toe Phalanx, Left**	**Ø Open** **3 Percutaneous** **4 Percutaneous Endoscopic**	**4 Internal Fixation Device** **5 External Fixation Device** **Z No Device**	**Z No Qualifier**
2 Pelvic Bone, Right Iliac crest Ilium Ischium Pubis **3 Pelvic Bone, Left** *See 2 Pelvic Bone, Right* **D Patella, Right** **F Patella, Left** **L Tarsal, Right** Calcaneus Cuboid bone Intermediate cuneiform bone Lateral cuneiform bone Medial cuneiform bone Navicular bone Talus bone	**M Tarsal, Left** *See L Tarsal, Right* **Q Toe Phalanx, Right** **R Toe Phalanx, Left**	**X External**	**Z No Device**	**Z No Qualifier**

		See Appendix L for Procedure Combinations
Non-OR	ØQSØXZZ	
Non-OR	ØQS[4,5][3,4]ZZ	⊞ ØQSØ3ZZ
Non-OR	ØQS[1,4,5,S]XZZ	⊞ ØQS[1,S]3ZZ
Non-OR	ØQS[2,3,D,F,L,M,Q,R][3,4]ZZ	
Non-OR	ØQS[2,3,D,F,L,M,Q,R]XZZ	

ØQS Continued on next page

NC Noncovered Procedure   **LC** Limited Coverage   **QA** Questionable OB Admit   **NT** New Tech Add-on   ⊞ Combination Member   ♂ Male   ♀ Female

Lower Bones

Ø   **Medical and Surgical**
Q   **Lower Bones**
S   **Reposition**

ØQS Continued

Definition: Moving to its normal location, or other suitable location, all or a portion of a body part

Explanation: The body part is moved to a new location from an abnormal location, or from a normal location where it is not functioning correctly. The body part may or may not be cut out or off to be moved to the new location.

Body Part Character 4	Approach Character 5	Device Character 6	Qualifier Character 7

6 Upper Femur, Right
  Femoral head
  Greater trochanter
  Lesser trochanter
  Neck of femur
7 Upper Femur, Left
  See 6 Upper Femur, Right
8 Femoral Shaft, Right
  Body of femur
9 Femoral Shaft, Left
  See 8 Femoral Shaft, Right
B Lower Femur, Right
  Lateral condyle of femur
  Lateral epicondyle of femur
  Medial condyle of femur
  Medial epicondyle of femur
C Lower Femur, Left
  See B Lower Femur, Right
G Tibia, Right
  Lateral condyle of tibia
  Medial condyle of tibia
  Medial malleolus
H Tibia, Left
  See G Tibia, Right
J Fibula, Right
  Body of fibula
  Head of fibula
  Lateral malleolus
K Fibula, Left
  See J Fibula, Right
	Ø Open
	3 Percutaneous
	4 Percutaneous Endoscopic
		4 Internal Fixation Device
		5 External Fixation Device
		6 Internal Fixation Device,
		  Intramedullary
		B External Fixation Device,
		  Monoplanar
		C External Fixation Device, Ring
		D External Fixation Device, Hybrid
		Z No Device
			Z No Qualifier

6 Upper Femur, Right
  Femoral head
  Greater trochanter
  Lesser trochanter
  Neck of femur
7 Upper Femur, Left
  See 6 Upper Femur, Right
8 Femoral Shaft, Right
  Body of femur
9 Femoral Shaft, Left
  See 8 Femoral Shaft, Right
B Lower Femur, Right
  Lateral condyle of femur
  Lateral epicondyle of femur
  Medial condyle of femur
  Medial epicondyle of femur
C Lower Femur, Left
  See B Lower Femur, Right
G Tibia, Right
  Lateral condyle of tibia
  Medial condyle of tibia
  Medial malleolus
H Tibia, Left
  See G Tibia, Right
J Fibula, Right
  Body of fibula
  Head of fibula
  Lateral malleolus
K Fibula, Left
  See J Fibula, Right
	X External	**Z** No Device	**Z** No Qualifier

N Metatarsal, Right
  Fibular sesamoid
  Tibial sesamoid
P Metatarsal, Left
  See N Metatarsal, Right
	Ø Open
	3 Percutaneous
	4 Percutaneous Endoscopic
		4 Internal Fixation Device
		5 External Fixation Device
		Z No Device
			2 Sesamoid Bone(s) 1st Toe
			Z No Qualifier

N Metatarsal, Right
  Fibular sesamoid
  Tibial sesamoid
P Metatarsal, Left
  See N Metatarsal, Right
	X External	**Z** No Device	**2** Sesamoid Bone(s) 1st Toe
			Z No Qualifier

Non-OR   ØQS[6,7,8,9,B,C,G,H,J,K][3,4]ZZ
Non-OR   ØQS[6,7,8,9,B,C,G,H,J,K]XZZ
Non-OR   ØQS[N,P][3,4]Z[2,Z]
Non-OR   ØQS[N,P]XZ[2,Z]

Non-OR Procedure   DRG Non-OR Procedure   Valid OR Procedure   HAC Associated Procedure   Combination Only   New/Revised April   New/Revised October

Ø   **Medical and Surgical**
Q   **Lower Bones**
T   **Resection**   Definition: Cutting out or off, without replacement, all of a body part
                  Explanation: None

Body Part Character 4		Approach Character 5	Device Character 6	Qualifier Character 7
2 Pelvic Bone, Right Iliac crest Ilium Ischium Pubis	**F Patella, Left** **G Tibia, Right** Lateral condyle of tibia Medial condyle of tibia Medial malleolus	Ø Open	Z No Device	Z No Qualifier
3 Pelvic Bone, Left *See 2 Pelvic Bone, Right*	**H Tibia, Left** *See G Tibia, Right*			
4 Acetabulum, Right	**J Fibula, Right** Body of fibula Head of fibula Lateral malleolus			
5 Acetabulum, Left				
6 Upper Femur, Right Femoral head Greater trochanter Lesser trochanter Neck of femur	**K Fibula, Left** *See J Fibula, Right* **L Tarsal, Right** Calcaneus Cuboid bone Intermediate cuneiform bone Lateral cuneiform bone Medial cuneiform bone Navicular bone Talus bone			
7 Upper Femur, Left *See 6 Upper Femur, Right*				
8 Femoral Shaft, Right Body of femur				
9 Femoral Shaft, Left *See 8 Femoral Shaft, Right*	**M Tarsal, Left** *See L Tarsal, Right*			
B Lower Femur, Right Lateral condyle of femur Lateral epicondyle of femur Medial condyle of femur Medial epicondyle of femur	**N Metatarsal, Right** Fibular sesamoid Tibial sesamoid			
C Lower Femur, Left *See B Lower Femur, Right*	**P Metatarsal, Left** *See N Metatarsal, Right* **Q Toe Phalanx, Right**			
D Patella, Right	**R Toe Phalanx, Left** **S Coccyx**			

Ø   **Medical and Surgical**
Q   **Lower Bones**
U   **Supplement**   Definition: Putting in or on biological or synthetic material that physically reinforces and/or augments the function of a portion of a body part
                  Explanation: The biological material is non-living, or is living and from the same individual. The body part may have been previously replaced, and the SUPPLEMENT procedure is performed to physically reinforce and/or augment the function of the replaced body part.

Body Part Character 4		Approach Character 5	Device Character 6	Qualifier Character 7
Ø Lumbar Vertebra ⊞ Spinous process Transverse process Vertebral arch Vertebral body Vertebral foramen Vertebral lamina Vertebral pedicle	**C Lower Femur, Left** *See B Lower Femur, Right* **D Patella, Right** **F Patella, Left** **G Tibia, Right** Lateral condyle of tibia Medial condyle of tibia Medial malleolus	Ø Open 3 Percutaneous 4 Percutaneous Endoscopic	7 Autologous Tissue Substitute J Synthetic Substitute K Nonautologous Tissue Substitute	Z No Qualifier
1 Sacrum ⊞	**H Tibia, Left** *See G Tibia, Right*			
2 Pelvic Bone, Right Iliac crest Ilium Ischium Pubis	**J Fibula, Right** Body of fibula Head of fibula Lateral malleolus			
3 Pelvic Bone, Left *See 2 Pelvic Bone, Right*	**K Fibula, Left** *See J Fibula, Right*			
4 Acetabulum, Right	**L Tarsal, Right** Calcaneus Cuboid bone Intermediate cuneiform bone Lateral cuneiform bone Medial cuneiform bone Navicular bone Talus bone			
5 Acetabulum, Left				
6 Upper Femur, Right Femoral head Greater trochanter Lesser trochanter Neck of femur				
7 Upper Femur, Left *See 6 Upper Femur, Right*	**M Tarsal, Left** *See L Tarsal, Right*			
8 Femoral Shaft, Right Body of femur	**N Metatarsal, Right** Fibular sesamoid Tibial sesamoid			
9 Femoral Shaft, Left *See 8 Femoral Shaft, Right*	**P Metatarsal, Left** *See N Metatarsal, Right*			
B Lower Femur, Right Lateral condyle of femur Lateral epicondyle of femur Medial condyle of femur Medial epicondyle of femur	**Q Toe Phalanx, Right** **R Toe Phalanx, Left** **S Coccyx** ⊞			

See Appendix L for Procedure Combinations
⊞   ØQU[Ø,1,S]3JZ

NC Noncovered Procedure   LC Limited Coverage   QA Questionable OB Admit   NT New Tech Add-on   ⊞ Combination Member   ♂ Male   ♀ Female

Ø   Medical and Surgical
Q   Lower Bones
W   Revision   Definition: Correcting, to the extent possible, a portion of a malfunctioning device or the position of a displaced device

Explanation: Revision can include correcting a malfunctioning or displaced device by taking out or putting in components of the device such as a screw or pin

Body Part Character 4	Approach Character 5	Device Character 6	Qualifier Character 7

Ø Lumbar Vertebra
   Spinous process
   Transverse process
   Vertebral arch
   Vertebral body
   Vertebral foramen
   Vertebral lamina
   Vertebral pedicle
1 Sacrum
4 Acetabulum, Right
5 Acetabulum, Left
S Coccyx
	Ø Open
	3 Percutaneous
	4 Percutaneous Endoscopic
	X External
		4 Internal Fixation Device
		7 Autologous Tissue Substitute
		J Synthetic Substitute
		K Nonautologous Tissue Substitute
			Z No Qualifier

2 Pelvic Bone, Right
   Iliac crest
   Ilium
   Ischium
   Pubis
3 Pelvic Bone, Left
   See 2 Pelvic Bone, Right
6 Upper Femur, Right
   Femoral head
   Greater trochanter
   Lesser trochanter
   Neck of femur
7 Upper Femur, Left
   See 6 Upper Femur, Right
8 Femoral Shaft, Right
   Body of femur
9 Femoral Shaft, Left
   See 8 Femoral Shaft, Right
B Lower Femur, Right
   Lateral condyle of femur
   Lateral epicondyle of femur
   Medial condyle of femur
   Medial epicondyle of femur
C Lower Femur, Left
   See B Lower Femur, Right
D Patella, Right
F Patella, Left
G Tibia, Right
   Lateral condyle of tibia
   Medial condyle of tibia
   Medial malleolus
H Tibia, Left
   See G Tibia, Right
J Fibula, Right
   Body of fibula
   Head of fibula
   Lateral malleolus
K Fibula, Left
   See J Fibula, Right
L Tarsal, Right
   Calcaneus
   Cuboid bone
   Intermediate cuneiform bone
   Lateral cuneiform bone
   Medial cuneiform bone
   Navicular bone
   Talus bone
M Tarsal, Left
   See L Tarsal, Right
N Metatarsal, Right
   Fibular sesamoid
   Tibial sesamoid
P Metatarsal, Left
   See N Metatarsal, Right
Q Toe Phalanx, Right
R Toe Phalanx, Left
	Ø Open
	3 Percutaneous
	4 Percutaneous Endoscopic
	X External
		4 Internal Fixation Device
		5 External Fixation Device
		7 Autologous Tissue Substitute
		J Synthetic Substitute
		K Nonautologous Tissue Substitute
			Z No Qualifier

Y Lower Bone	**Ø** Open **3** Percutaneous **4** Percutaneous Endoscopic **X** External	**Ø** Drainage Device **M** Bone Growth Stimulator	**Z** No Qualifier

Non-OR ØQW[Ø,1,4,5,S]X[4,7,J,K]Z	**Non-OR** ØQWYX[Ø,M]Z
Non-OR ØQW[2,3,6,7,8,9,B,C,D,F,G,H,J,K,L,M,N,P,Q,R]X[4,5,7,J,K]Z	

Non-OR Procedure   DRG Non-OR Procedure   Valid OR Procedure   HAC Associated Procedure   Combination Only   New/Revised April   New/Revised October

578   ICD-10-PCS 2023

Upper Joints ØR2–ØRW

Character Meanings*

This Character Meaning table is provided as a guide to assist the user in the identification of character members that may be found in this section of code tables. It **SHOULD NOT** be used to build a PCS code.

Operation–Character 3	Body Part–Character 4	Approach–Character 5	Device–Character 6	Qualifier–Character 7
2 Change	Ø Occipital-cervical Joint	Ø Open	Ø Drainage Device OR Synthetic Substitute, Reverse Ball and Socket	Ø Anterior Approach, Anterior Column
5 Destruction	1 Cervical Vertebral Joint	3 Percutaneous	3 Infusion Device OR Internal Fixation Device, Sustained Compression	1 Posterior Approach, Posterior Column
9 Drainage	2 Cervical Vertebral Joint, 2 or more	4 Percutaneous Endoscopic	4 Internal Fixation Device	6 Humeral Surface
B Excision	3 Cervical Vertebral Disc	X External	5 External Fixation Device	7 Glenoid Surface
C Extirpation	4 Cervicothoracic Vertebral Joint		7 Autologous Tissue Substitute	J Posterior Approach, Anterior Column
G Fusion	5 Cervicothoracic Vertebral Disc		8 Spacer	X Diagnostic
H Insertion	6 Thoracic Vertebral Joint		A Interbody Fusion Device	Z No Qualifier
J Inspection	7 Thoracic Vertebral Joint, 2 to 7		B Spinal Stabilization Device, Interspinous Process	
N Release	8 Thoracic Vertebral Joint, 8 or more		C Spinal Stabilization Device, Pedicle-Based	
P Removal	9 Thoracic Vertebral Disc		D Spinal Stabilization Device, Facet Replacement	
Q Repair	A Thoracolumbar Vertebral Joint		J Synthetic Substitute	
R Replacement	B Thoracolumbar Vertebral Disc		K Nonautologous Tissue Substitute	
S Reposition	C Temporomandibular Joint, Right		Y Other Device	
T Resection	D Temporomandibular Joint, Left		Z No Device	
U Supplement	E Sternoclavicular Joint, Right			
W Revision	F Sternoclavicular Joint, Left			
	G Acromioclavicular Joint, Right			
	H Acromioclavicular Joint, Left			
	J Shoulder Joint, Right			
	K Shoulder Joint, Left			
	L Elbow Joint, Right			
	M Elbow Joint, Left			
	N Wrist Joint, Right			
	P Wrist Joint, Left			
	Q Carpal Joint, Right			
	R Carpal Joint, Left			
	S Carpometacarpal Joint, Right			
	T Carpometacarpal Joint, Left			
	U Metacarpophalangeal Joint, Right			
	V Metacarpophalangeal Joint, Left			
	W Finger Phalangeal Joint, Right			
	X Finger Phalangeal Joint, Left			
	Y Upper Joint			

* Includes synovial membrane.

AHA Coding Clinic for table ØRB

2019, 3Q, 26	Acromioclavicular joint reconstruction using allograft

AHA Coding Clinic for table ØRG

2021, 4Q, 67	Posterior dynamic distraction
2021, 1Q, 18	Placement of interspinous distraction device (spacer) for decompression
2021, 1Q, 53	Official guidelines for coding and reporting for interbody fusion device B3.10c
2020, 4Q, 56-58	Intramedullary sustained compression joint fusion
2020, 2Q, 27	Spinal fusion with NuVasive® VersaTie®
2020, 1Q, 33	Spinal fusion without use of bone graft
2019, 3Q, 28	Use of VERTE-STACK™ implant with fusion
2019, 3Q, 35	Fusion procedures of the spine (guideline B3.10c)
2019, 2Q, 19	Cervical spinal fusion, decompression and placement of interfacet stabilization device
2019, 1Q, 30	Spinal fusion performed at same level as decompressive laminectomy
2018, 4Q, 43	Joint fusion device value
2018, 1Q, 22	Spinal fusion procedures without bone graft
2017, 4Q, 62	Added and revised device values - Nerve substitutes
2017, 4Q, 76	Radiolucent porous interbody fusion device
2017, 2Q, 23	Decompression of spinal cord and placement of instrumentation
2014, 3Q, 30	Spinal fusion and fixation instrumentation
2014, 2Q, 7	Anterior cervical thoracic fusion with total discectomy
2013, 1Q, 21-23	Spinal fusion of thoracic and lumbar vertebrae
2013, 1Q, 29	Cervical and thoracic spinal fusion

AHA Coding Clinic for table ØRH

2021, 1Q, 18	Placement of interspinous distraction device (spacer) for decompression
2019, 2Q, 40	Decompression of spinal cord and placement of instrumentation
2018, 3Q, 26	Anterior vertebral tethering using Dynesys Tethering System
2017, 2Q, 23	Decompression of spinal cord and placement of instrumentation
2016, 3Q, 32	Rotator cuff repair, tenodesis, decompression, acromioplasty and coracoplasty

AHA Coding Clinic for table ØRN

2019, 1Q, 30	Spinal fusion performed at same level as decompressive laminectomy
2016, 3Q, 32	Rotator cuff repair, tenodesis, decompression, acromioplasty and coracoplasty
2015, 2Q, 22	Arthroscopic subacromial decompression
2015, 2Q, 23	Arthroscopic release of shoulder joint

AHA Coding Clinic for table ØRP

2021, 4Q, 53	Shoulder hemiarthroplasty
2017, 4Q, 107	Total ankle replacement versus revision

AHA Coding Clinic for table ØRQ

2016, 1Q, 30	Thermal capsulorrhaphy of shoulder

AHA Coding Clinic for table ØRR

2018, 4Q, 92	Radial head arthroplasty
2017, 4Q, 107	Total ankle replacement versus revision
2015, 3Q, 14	Endoprosthetic replacement of humerus and tendon reattachment
2015, 1Q, 27	Reverse total shoulder arthroplasty

AHA Coding Clinic for table ØRS

2019, 3Q, 26	Acromioclavicular joint reconstruction using allograft
2018, 3Q, 26	Anterior vertebral tethering using Dynesys Tethering System
2015, 2Q, 35	Application of tongs to reduce and stabilize cervical fracture
2014, 4Q, 32	Open reduction internal fixation of fracture with debridement
2014, 3Q, 33	Radial fracture treatment with open reduction internal fixation, and release of carpal ligament
2013, 2Q, 39	Application of cervical tongs for reduction of cervical fracture

AHA Coding Clinic for table ØRT

2019, 3Q, 26	Acromioclavicular joint reconstruction using allograft
2014, 2Q, 7	Anterior cervical thoracic fusion with total discectomy

AHA Coding Clinic for table ØRU

2019, 3Q, 26	Acromioclavicular joint reconstruction using allograft
2015, 3Q, 26	Thumb arthroplasty with resection of trapezium

AHA Coding Clinic for table ØRW

2021, 4Q, 53	Shoulder hemiarthroplasty
2017, 4Q, 107	Total ankle replacement versus revision

Upper Joints

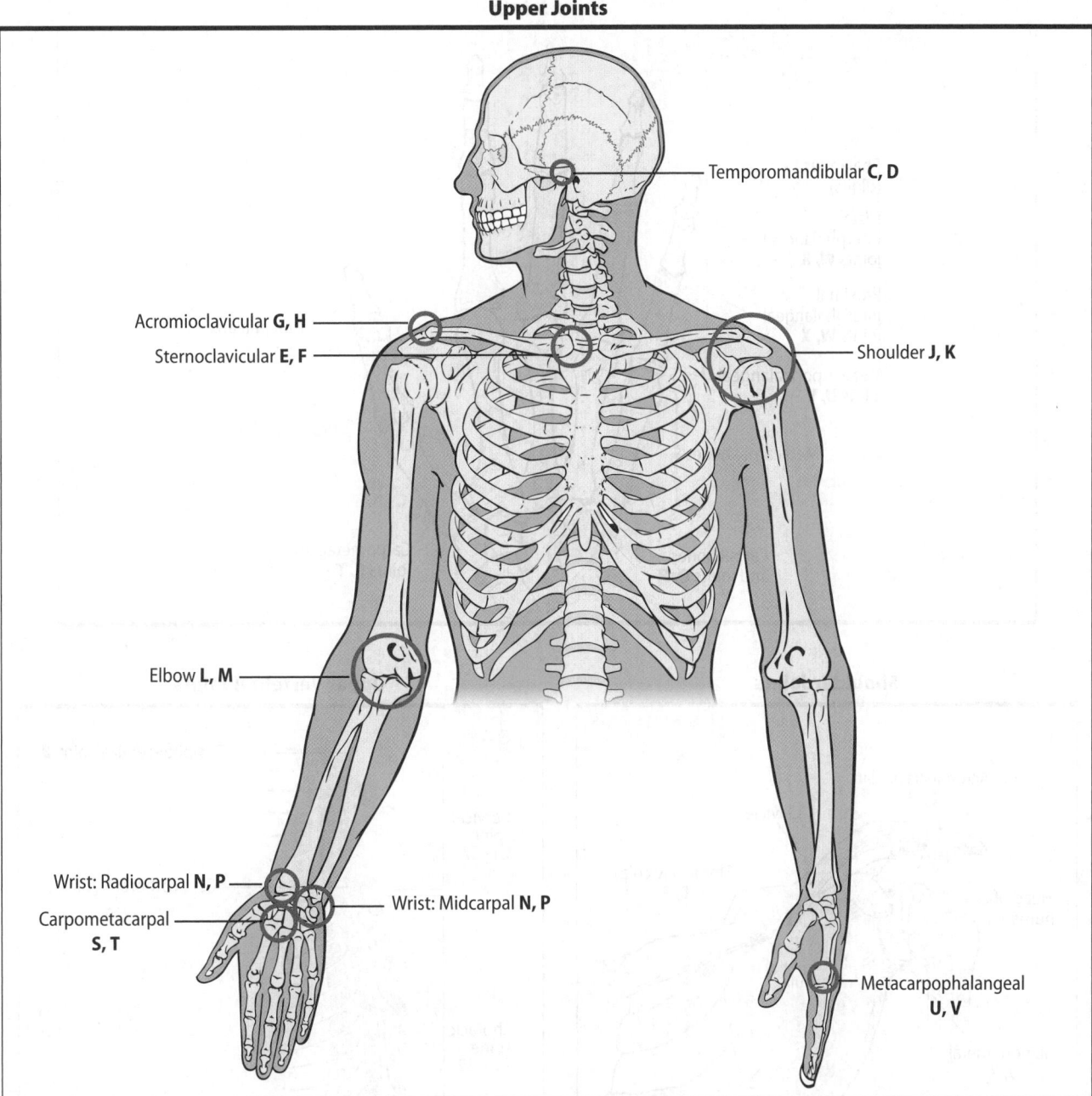

Temporomandibular **C, D**

Acromioclavicular **G, H**

Sternoclavicular **E, F**

Shoulder **J, K**

Elbow **L, M**

Wrist: Radiocarpal **N, P**

Wrist: Midcarpal **N, P**

Carpometacarpal **S, T**

Metacarpophalangeal **U, V**

Hand Joints

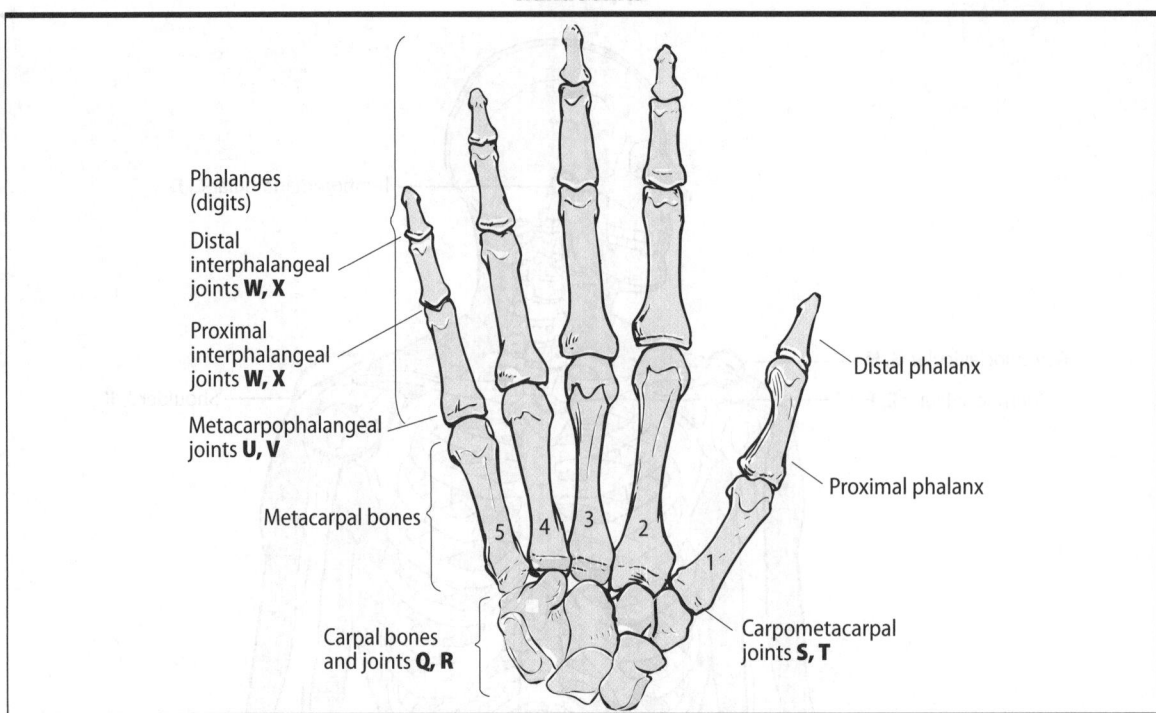

Phalanges (digits)

Distal interphalangeal joints **W, X**

Proximal interphalangeal joints **W, X**

Metacarpophalangeal joints **U, V**

Metacarpal bones

Carpal bones and joints **Q, R**

Distal phalanx

Proximal phalanx

Carpometacarpal joints **S, T**

Shoulder Joints

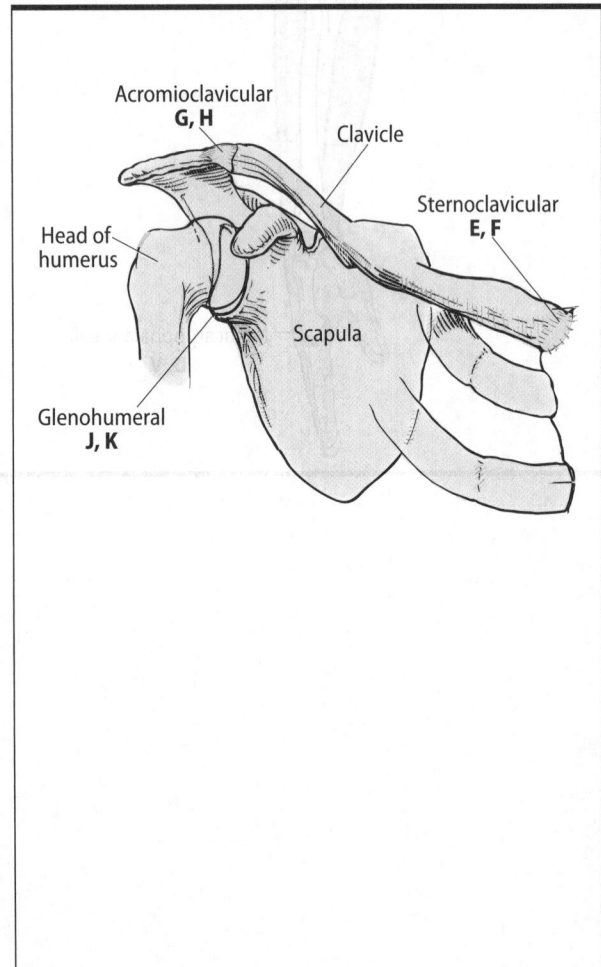

Acromioclavicular **G, H**

Clavicle

Head of humerus

Sternoclavicular **E, F**

Scapula

Glenohumeral **J, K**

Upper Vertebral Joints

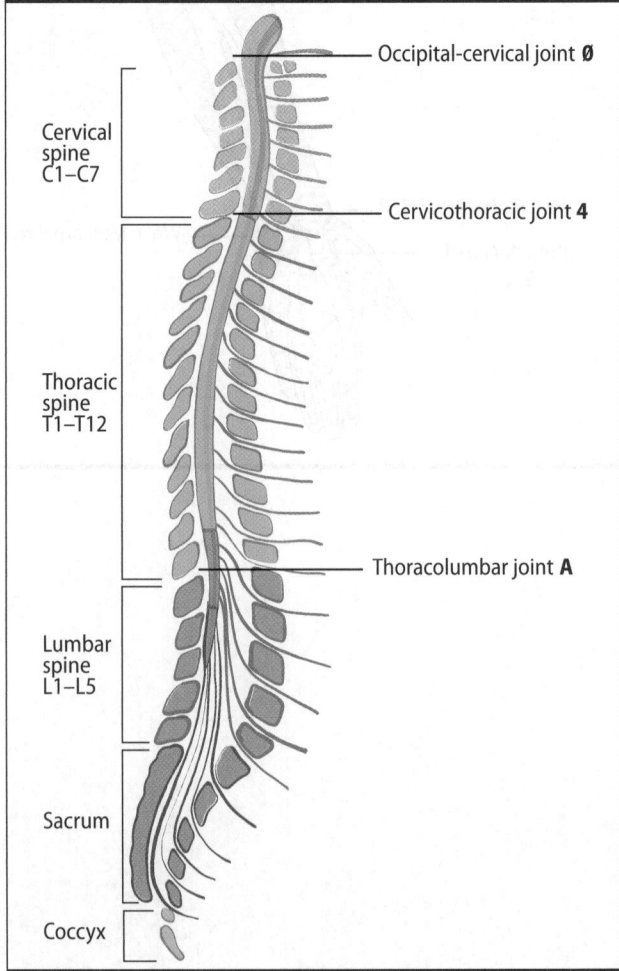

Occipital-cervical joint **Ø**

Cervical spine C1–C7

Cervicothoracic joint **4**

Thoracic spine T1–T12

Thoracolumbar joint **A**

Lumbar spine L1–L5

Sacrum

Coccyx

Ø **Medical and Surgical**
R **Upper Joints**
2 **Change**   Definition: Taking out or off a device from a body part and putting back an identical or similar device in or on the same body part without cutting or puncturing the skin or a mucous membrane
               Explanation: All CHANGE procedures are coded using the approach EXTERNAL

Body Part Character 4	Approach Character 5	Device Character 6	Qualifier Character 7
Y Upper Joint	X External	Ø Drainage Device Y Other Device	Z No Qualifier

Non-OR	All body part, approach, device, and qualifier values

Ø **Medical and Surgical**
R **Upper Joints**
5 **Destruction**   Definition: Physical eradication of all or a portion of a body part by the direct use of energy, force, or a destructive agent
               Explanation: None of the body part is physically taken out

Body Part Character 4	Approach Character 5	Device Character 6	Qualifier Character 7
Ø Occipital-cervical Joint	Ø Open	Z No Device	Z No Qualifier
1 Cervical Vertebral Joint Atlantoaxial joint Cervical facet joint	3 Percutaneous 4 Percutaneous Endoscopic		
3 Cervical Vertebral Disc			
4 Cervicothoracic Vertebral Joint Cervicothoracic facet joint			
5 Cervicothoracic Vertebral Disc			
6 Thoracic Vertebral Joint Costotransverse joint Costovertebral joint Thoracic facet joint			
9 Thoracic Vertebral Disc			
A Thoracolumbar Vertebral Joint Thoracolumbar facet joint			
B Thoracolumbar Vertebral Disc			
C Temporomandibular Joint, Right			
D Temporomandibular Joint, Left			
E Sternoclavicular Joint, Right			
F Sternoclavicular Joint, Left			
G Acromioclavicular Joint, Right			
H Acromioclavicular Joint, Left			
J Shoulder Joint, Right Glenohumeral joint Glenoid ligament (labrum)			
K Shoulder Joint, Left *See J Shoulder Joint, Right*			
L Elbow Joint, Right Distal humerus, involving joint Humeroradial joint Humeroulnar joint Proximal radioulnar joint			
M Elbow Joint, Left *See L Elbow Joint, Right*			
N Wrist Joint, Right Distal radioulnar joint Radiocarpal joint			
P Wrist Joint, Left *See N Wrist Joint, Right*			
Q Carpal Joint, Right Intercarpal joint Midcarpal joint			
R Carpal Joint, Left *See Q Carpal Joint, Right*			
S Carpometacarpal Joint, Right			
T Carpometacarpal Joint, Left			
U Metacarpophalangeal Joint, Right			
V Metacarpophalangeal Joint, Left			
W Finger Phalangeal Joint, Right Interphalangeal (IP) joint			
X Finger Phalangeal Joint, Left *See W Finger Phalangeal Joint, Right*			

Non-OR	ØR5[3,5,9,B][3,4]ZZ

NC Noncovered Procedure   **LC** Limited Coverage   **QA** Questionable OB Admit   **NT** New Tech Add-on   ⊞ Combination Member   ♂ Male   ♀ Female

ICD-10-PCS 2023   583

ØR2-ØR5

Ø   **Medical and Surgical**
R   **Upper Joints**
9   **Drainage**   Definition: Taking or letting out fluids and/or gases from a body part

Explanation: The qualifier DIAGNOSTIC is used to identify drainage procedures that are biopsies

Body Part Character 4		Approach Character 5	Device Character 6	Qualifier Character 7

Ø Occipital-cervical Joint
1 Cervical Vertebral Joint
  Atlantoaxial joint
  Cervical facet joint
3 Cervical Vertebral Disc
4 Cervicothoracic Vertebral Joint
  Cervicothoracic facet joint
5 Cervicothoracic Vertebral Disc
6 Thoracic Vertebral Joint
  Costotransverse joint
  Costovertebral joint
  Thoracic facet joint
9 Thoracic Vertebral Disc
A Thoracolumbar Vertebral Joint
  Thoracolumbar facet joint
B Thoracolumbar Vertebral Disc
C Temporomandibular Joint, Right
D Temporomandibular Joint, Left
E Sternoclavicular Joint, Right
F Sternoclavicular Joint, Left
G Acromioclavicular Joint, Right
H Acromioclavicular Joint, Left
J Shoulder Joint, Right
  Glenohumeral joint
  Glenoid ligament (labrum)
K Shoulder Joint, Left
  See J Shoulder Joint, Right
	L Elbow Joint, Right
	  Distal humerus, involving joint
	  Humeroradial joint
	  Humeroulnar joint
	  Proximal radioulnar joint
	M Elbow Joint, Left
	  See L Elbow Joint, Right
	N Wrist Joint, Right
	  Distal radioulnar joint
	  Radiocarpal joint
	P Wrist Joint, Left
	  See N Wrist Joint, Right
	Q Carpal Joint, Right
	  Intercarpal joint
	  Midcarpal joint
	R Carpal Joint, Left
	  See Q Carpal Joint, Right
	S Carpometacarpal Joint, Right
	T Carpometacarpal Joint, Left
	U Metacarpophalangeal Joint, Right
	V Metacarpophalangeal Joint, Left
	W Finger Phalangeal Joint, Right
	  Interphalangeal (IP) joint
	X Finger Phalangeal Joint, Left
	  See W Finger Phalangeal Joint, Right
		Ø Open
		3 Percutaneous
		4 Percutaneous Endoscopic
			Ø Drainage Device	Z No Qualifier

Ø Occipital-cervical Joint
1 Cervical Vertebral Joint
  Atlantoaxial joint
  Cervical facet joint
3 Cervical Vertebral Disc
4 Cervicothoracic Vertebral Joint
  Cervicothoracic facet joint
5 Cervicothoracic Vertebral Disc
6 Thoracic Vertebral Joint
  Costotransverse joint
  Costovertebral joint
  Thoracic facet joint
9 Thoracic Vertebral Disc
A Thoracolumbar Vertebral Joint
  Thoracolumbar facet joint
B Thoracolumbar Vertebral Disc
C Temporomandibular Joint, Right
D Temporomandibular Joint, Left
E Sternoclavicular Joint, Right
F Sternoclavicular Joint, Left
G Acromioclavicular Joint, Right
H Acromioclavicular Joint, Left
J Shoulder Joint, Right
  Glenohumeral joint
  Glenoid ligament (labrum)
K Shoulder Joint, Left
  See J Shoulder Joint, Right
	L Elbow Joint, Right
	  Distal humerus, involving joint
	  Humeroradial joint
	  Humeroulnar joint
	  Proximal radioulnar joint
	M Elbow Joint, Left
	  See L Elbow Joint, Right
	N Wrist Joint, Right
	  Distal radioulnar joint
	  Radiocarpal joint
	P Wrist Joint, Left
	  See N Wrist Joint, Right
	Q Carpal Joint, Right
	  Intercarpal joint
	  Midcarpal joint
	R Carpal Joint, Left
	  See Q Carpal Joint, Right
	S Carpometacarpal Joint, Right
	T Carpometacarpal Joint, Left
	U Metacarpophalangeal Joint, Right
	V Metacarpophalangeal Joint, Left
	W Finger Phalangeal Joint, Right
	  Interphalangeal (IP) joint
	X Finger Phalangeal Joint, Left
	  See W Finger Phalangeal Joint, Right
		Ø Open
		3 Percutaneous
		4 Percutaneous Endoscopic
			Z No Device	X Diagnostic
				Z No Qualifier

Non-OR	ØR9[Ø,1,3,4,5,6,9,A,B,E,F,G,H,J,K,L,M,N,P,Q,R,S,T,U,V,W,X][3,4]ØZ
Non-OR	ØR9[C,D]3ØZ
Non-OR	ØR9[Ø,1,3,4,5,6,9,A,B,E,F,G,H,J,K,L,M,N,P,Q,R,S,T,U,V,W,X][Ø,3,4]ZX
Non-OR	ØR9[Ø,1,3,4,5,6,9,A,B,E,F,G,H,J,K,L,M,N,P,Q,R,S,T,U,V,W,X][3,4]ZZ
Non-OR	ØR9[C,D]3ZZ

Non-OR Procedure   DRG Non-OR Procedure   Valid OR Procedure   HAC Associated Procedure   Combination Only   New/Revised April   New/Revised October

584   ICD-10-PCS 2023

ØR9–ØR9

Ø   **Medical and Surgical**
R   **Upper Joints**
B   **Excision**   Definition: Cutting out or off, without replacement, a portion of a body part

                               Explanation: The qualifier DIAGNOSTIC is used to identify excision procedures that are biopsies

Body Part Character 4	Approach Character 5	Device Character 6	Qualifier Character 7
Ø **Occipital-cervical Joint**	**Ø** Open	**Z** No Device	**X** Diagnostic
1 **Cervical Vertebral Joint**	**3** Percutaneous		**Z** No Qualifier
Atlantoaxial joint	**4** Percutaneous Endoscopic		
Cervical facet joint			
3 **Cervical Vertebral Disc**			
4 **Cervicothoracic Vertebral Joint**			
Cervicothoracic facet joint			
5 **Cervicothoracic Vertebral Disc**			
6 **Thoracic Vertebral Joint**			
Costotransverse joint			
Costovertebral joint			
Thoracic facet joint			
9 **Thoracic Vertebral Disc**			
A **Thoracolumbar Vertebral Joint**			
Thoracolumbar facet joint			
B **Thoracolumbar Vertebral Disc**			
C **Temporomandibular Joint, Right**			
D **Temporomandibular Joint, Left**			
E **Sternoclavicular Joint, Right**			
F **Sternoclavicular Joint, Left**			
G **Acromioclavicular Joint, Right**			
H **Acromioclavicular Joint, Left**			
J **Shoulder Joint, Right**			
Glenohumeral joint			
Glenoid ligament (labrum)			
K **Shoulder Joint, Left**			
See J Shoulder Joint, Right			
L **Elbow Joint, Right**			
Distal humerus, involving joint			
Humeroradial joint			
Humeroulnar joint			
Proximal radioulnar joint			
M **Elbow Joint, Left**			
See L Elbow Joint, Right			
N **Wrist Joint, Right**			
Distal radioulnar joint			
Radiocarpal joint			
P **Wrist Joint, Left**			
See N Wrist Joint, Right			
Q **Carpal Joint, Right**			
Intercarpal joint			
Midcarpal joint			
R **Carpal Joint, Left**			
See Q Carpal Joint, Right			
S **Carpometacarpal Joint, Right**			
T **Carpometacarpal Joint, Left**			
U **Metacarpophalangeal Joint, Right**			
V **Metacarpophalangeal Joint, Left**			
W **Finger Phalangeal Joint, Right**			
Interphalangeal (IP) joint			
X **Finger Phalangeal Joint, Left**			
See W Finger Phalangeal Joint, Right			

Non-OR   ØRB[Ø,1,3,4,5,6,9,A,B,E,F,G,H,J,K,L,M,N,P,Q,R,S,T,U,V,W,X][Ø,3,4]ZX

NC Noncovered Procedure   **LC** Limited Coverage   **QA** Questionable OB Admit   **NT** New Tech Add-on   ⊞ Combination Member   ♂ Male   ♀ Female

ICD-10-PCS 2023   **585**

ØRB–ØRB

Ø　**Medical and Surgical**
R　**Upper Joints**
C　**Extirpation**　　　Definition: Taking or cutting out solid matter from a body part

Explanation: The solid matter may be an abnormal byproduct of a biological function or a foreign body; it may be imbedded in a body part or in the lumen of a tubular body part. The solid matter may or may not have been previously broken into pieces.

Body Part Character 4	Approach Character 5	Device Character 6	Qualifier Character 7
Ø　Occipital-cervical Joint	Ø　Open	Z　No Device	Z　No Qualifier
1　Cervical Vertebral Joint 　　Atlantoaxial joint 　　Cervical facet joint	3　Percutaneous 4　Percutaneous Endoscopic		
3　Cervical Vertebral Disc			
4　Cervicothoracic Vertebral Joint 　　Cervicothoracic facet joint			
5　Cervicothoracic Vertebral Disc			
6　Thoracic Vertebral Joint 　　Costotransverse joint 　　Costovertebral joint 　　Thoracic facet joint			
9　Thoracic Vertebral Disc			
A　Thoracolumbar Vertebral Joint 　　Thoracolumbar facet joint			
B　Thoracolumbar Vertebral Disc			
C　Temporomandibular Joint, Right			
D　Temporomandibular Joint, Left			
E　Sternoclavicular Joint, Right			
F　Sternoclavicular Joint, Left			
G　Acromioclavicular Joint, Right			
H　Acromioclavicular Joint, Left			
J　Shoulder Joint, Right 　　Glenohumeral joint 　　Glenoid ligament (labrum)			
K　Shoulder Joint, Left 　　*See J Shoulder Joint, Right*			
L　Elbow Joint, Right 　　Distal humerus, involving joint 　　Humeroradial joint 　　Humeroulnar joint 　　Proximal radioulnar joint			
M　Elbow Joint, Left 　　*See L Elbow Joint, Right*			
N　Wrist Joint, Right 　　Distal radioulnar joint 　　Radiocarpal joint			
P　Wrist Joint, Left 　　*See N Wrist Joint, Right*			
Q　Carpal Joint, Right 　　Intercarpal joint 　　Midcarpal joint			
R　Carpal Joint, Left 　　*See Q Carpal Joint, Right*			
S　Carpometacarpal Joint, Right			
T　Carpometacarpal Joint, Left			
U　Metacarpophalangeal Joint, Right			
V　Metacarpophalangeal Joint, Left			
W　Finger Phalangeal Joint, Right 　　Interphalangeal (IP) joint			
X　Finger Phalangeal Joint, Left 　　*See W Finger Phalangeal Joint, Right*			

Ø   **Medical and Surgical**
R   **Upper Joints**
G   **Fusion**   Definition: Joining together portions of an articular body part rendering the articular body part immobile
               Explanation: The body part is joined together by fixation device, bone graft, or other means

Body Part Character 4		Approach Character 5	Device Character 6	Qualifier Character 7

Ø Occipital-cervical Joint
1 Cervical Vertebral Joint
   Atlantoaxial joint
   Cervical facet joint
2 Cervical Vertebral Joints, 2 or more
   Cervical facet joint
4 Cervicothoracic Vertebral Joint
   Cervicothoracic facet joint
6 Thoracic Vertebral Joint
   Costotransverse joint
   Costovertebral joint
   Thoracic facet joint
7 Thoracic Vertebral Joints, 2 to 7   ⊞
8 Thoracic Vertebral Joints, 8 or more
A Thoracolumbar Vertebral Joint
   Thoracolumbar facet joint
		Ø Open
		3 Percutaneous
		4 Percutaneous Endoscopic
			7 Autologous Tissue Substitute
			J Synthetic Substitute
			K Nonautologous Tissue Substitute
				Ø Anterior Approach, Anterior Column
				1 Posterior Approach, Posterior Column
				J Posterior Approach, Anterior Column

Ø Occipital-cervical Joint
1 Cervical Vertebral Joint
   Atlantoaxial joint
   Cervical facet joint
2 Cervical Vertebral Joints, 2 or more
   Cervical facet joint
4 Cervicothoracic Vertebral Joint
   Cervicothoracic facet joint
6 Thoracic Vertebral Joint
   Costotransverse joint
   Costovertebral joint
   Thoracic facet joint
7 Thoracic Vertebral Joints, 2 to 7   ⊞
8 Thoracic Vertebral Joints, 8 or more
A Thoracolumbar Vertebral Joint
   Thoracolumbar facet joint
		Ø Open
		3 Percutaneous
		4 Percutaneous Endoscopic
			A Interbody Fusion Device	Ø Anterior Approach, Anterior Column
				J Posterior Approach, Anterior Column

C Temporomandibular Joint, Right
D Temporomandibular Joint, Left
E Sternoclavicular Joint, Right
F Sternoclavicular Joint, Left
G Acromioclavicular Joint, Right
H Acromioclavicular Joint, Left
J Shoulder Joint, Right
   Glenohumeral joint
   Glenoid ligament (labrum)
K Shoulder Joint, Left
   See J Shoulder Joint, Right
		Ø Open
		3 Percutaneous
		4 Percutaneous Endoscopic
			4 Internal Fixation Device
			7 Autologous Tissue Substitute
			J Synthetic Substitute
			K Nonautologous Tissue Substitute
				Z No Qualifier

L Elbow Joint, Right
   Distal humerus, involving joint
   Humeroradial joint
   Humeroulnar joint
   Proximal radioulnar joint
M Elbow Joint, Left
   See L Elbow Joint, Right
N Wrist Joint, Right
   Distal radioulnar joint
   Radiocarpal joint
P Wrist Joint, Left
   See N Wrist Joint, Right
Q Carpal Joint, Right
   Intercarpal joint
   Midcarpal joint
	R Carpal Joint, Left
	   See Q Carpal Joint, Right
	S Carpometacarpal Joint, Right
	T Carpometacarpal Joint, Left
	U Metacarpophalangeal Joint, Right
	V Metacarpophalangeal Joint, Left
	W Finger Phalangeal Joint, Right
	   Interphalangeal (IP) joint
	X Finger Phalangeal Joint, Left
	   See W Finger Phalangeal Joint, Right
		Ø Open
		3 Percutaneous
		4 Percutaneous Endoscopic
			3 Internal Fixation Device, Sustained Compression
			4 Internal Fixation Device
			5 External Fixation Device
			7 Autologous Tissue Substitute
			J Synthetic Substitute
			K Nonautologous Tissue Substitute
				Z No Qualifier

HAC   ØRG[Ø,1,2,4,6,7,8,A][Ø,3,4][7,J,K][Ø,1,J] when reported with SDx K68.11 or
         T81.4Ø–T81.49, T84.6Ø-T84.619, T84.63-T84.7 with 7th character A
HAC   ØRG[Ø,1,2,4,6,7,8,A][Ø,3,4]A[Ø,J] when reported with SDx K68.11 or T81.4Ø–T81.49,
         T84.6Ø-T84.619, T84.63-T84.7 with 7th character A
HAC   ØRG[E,F,G,H,J,K][Ø,3,4][4,7,J,K]Z when reported with SDx K68.11 or T81.4Ø–T81.49,
         T84.6Ø-T84.619, T84.63-T84.7 with 7th character A
HAC   ØRG[L,M][Ø,3,4][3,4,5,7,J,K]Z when reported with SDx K68.11 or T81.4Ø–T81.49,
         T84.6Ø-T84.619, T84.63-T84.7 with 7th character A

See Appendix L for Procedure Combinations
⊞   ØRG7[Ø,3,4][7,J,K][Ø,1,J]
⊞   ØRG7[Ø,3,4]A[Ø,J]

NC Noncovered Procedure   **LC** Limited Coverage   **QA** Questionable OB Admit   **NT** New Tech Add-on   ⊞ Combination Member   ♂ Male   ♀ Female

ICD-10-PCS 2023   587

ØRG–ØRG

Ø   Medical and Surgical
R   Upper Joints
H   Insertion   Definition: Putting in a nonbiological appliance that monitors, assists, performs, or prevents a physiological function but does not physically take the place of a body part

Explanation: None

Body Part Character 4	Approach Character 5	Device Character 6	Qualifier Character 7
Ø Occipital-cervical Joint 1 Cervical Vertebral Joint 　Atlantoaxial joint 　Cervical facet joint 4 Cervicothoracic Vertebral Joint 　Cervicothoracic facet joint 6 Thoracic Vertebral Joint 　Costotransverse joint 　Costovertebral joint 　Thoracic facet joint A Thoracolumbar Vertebral Joint 　Thoracolumbar facet joint	Ø Open 3 Percutaneous 4 Percutaneous Endoscopic	3 Infusion Device 4 Internal Fixation Device 8 Spacer B Spinal Stabilization Device, 　Interspinous Process C Spinal Stabilization Device, 　Pedicle-Based D Spinal Stabilization Device, 　Facet Replacement	Z No Qualifier
3 Cervical Vertebral Disc 5 Cervicothoracic Vertebral Disc 9 Thoracic Vertebral Disc B Thoracolumbar Vertebral Disc	Ø Open 3 Percutaneous 4 Percutaneous Endoscopic	3 Infusion Device	Z No Qualifier
C Temporomandibular Joint, Right D Temporomandibular Joint, Left E Sternoclavicular Joint, Right F Sternoclavicular Joint, Left G Acromioclavicular Joint, Right H Acromioclavicular Joint, Left J Shoulder Joint, Right 　Glenohumeral joint 　Glenoid ligament (labrum) K Shoulder Joint, Left 　*See J Shoulder Joint, Right*	Ø Open 3 Percutaneous 4 Percutaneous Endoscopic	3 Infusion Device 4 Internal Fixation Device 8 Spacer	Z No Qualifier
L Elbow Joint, Right 　Distal humerus, involving joint 　Humeroradial joint 　Humeroulnar joint 　Proximal radioulnar joint M Elbow Joint, Left 　*See L Elbow Joint, Right* N Wrist Joint, Right 　Distal radioulnar joint 　Radiocarpal joint P Wrist Joint, Left 　*See N Wrist Joint, Right* Q Carpal Joint, Right 　Intercarpal joint 　Midcarpal joint R Carpal Joint, Left 　*See Q Carpal Joint, Right* S Carpometacarpal Joint, Right T Carpometacarpal Joint, Left U Metacarpophalangeal Joint, Right V Metacarpophalangeal Joint, Left W Finger Phalangeal Joint, Right 　Interphalangeal (IP) joint X Finger Phalangeal Joint, Left 　*See W Finger Phalangeal Joint, Right*	Ø Open 3 Percutaneous 4 Percutaneous Endoscopic	3 Infusion Device 4 Internal Fixation Device 5 External Fixation Device 8 Spacer	Z No Qualifier

Non-OR	ØRH[Ø,1,4,6,A][Ø,3,4][3,8]Z
Non-OR	ØRH[3,5,9,B][Ø,3,4]3Z
Non-OR	ØRH[C,D][Ø,4]8Z
Non-OR	ØRH[C,D]3[3,8]Z
Non-OR	ØRH[E,F,G,H][Ø,3,4][3,8]Z
Non-OR	ØRH[J,K][Ø,3,4]3Z
Non-OR	ØRH[J,K]38Z
Non-OR	ØRH[L,M,N,P,Q,R,S,T,U,V,W,X][Ø,3,4][3,8]Z

Ø **Medical and Surgical**
R **Upper Joints**
J **Inspection**　　Definition: Visually and/or manually exploring a body part

Explanation: Visual exploration may be performed with or without optical instrumentation. Manual exploration may be performed directly or through intervening body layers.

Body Part Character 4	Approach Character 5	Device Character 6	Qualifier Character 7
Ø **Occipital-cervical Joint** **1** **Cervical Vertebral Joint** 　Atlantoaxial joint 　Cervical facet joint **3** **Cervical Vertebral Disc** **4** **Cervicothoracic Vertebral Joint** 　Cervicothoracic facet joint **5** **Cervicothoracic Vertebral Disc** **6** **Thoracic Vertebral Joint** 　Costotransverse joint 　Costovertebral joint 　Thoracic facet joint **9** **Thoracic Vertebral Disc** **A** **Thoracolumbar Vertebral Joint** 　Thoracolumbar facet joint **B** **Thoracolumbar Vertebral Disc** **C** **Temporomandibular Joint, Right** **D** **Temporomandibular Joint, Left** **E** **Sternoclavicular Joint, Right** **F** **Sternoclavicular Joint, Left** **G** **Acromioclavicular Joint, Right** **H** **Acromioclavicular Joint, Left** **J** **Shoulder Joint, Right** 　Glenohumeral joint 　Glenoid ligament (labrum) **K** **Shoulder Joint, Left** 　*See J Shoulder Joint, Right* **L** **Elbow Joint, Right** 　Distal humerus, involving joint 　Humeroradial joint 　Humeroulnar joint 　Proximal radioulnar joint **M** **Elbow Joint, Left** 　*See L Elbow Joint, Right* **N** **Wrist Joint, Right** 　Distal radioulnar joint 　Radiocarpal joint **P** **Wrist Joint, Left** 　*See N Wrist Joint, Right* **Q** **Carpal Joint, Right** 　Intercarpal joint 　Midcarpal joint **R** **Carpal Joint, Left** 　*See Q Carpal Joint, Right* **S** **Carpometacarpal Joint, Right** **T** **Carpometacarpal Joint, Left** **U** **Metacarpophalangeal Joint, Right** **V** **Metacarpophalangeal Joint, Left** **W** **Finger Phalangeal Joint, Right** 　Interphalangeal (IP) joint **X** **Finger Phalangeal Joint, Left** 　*See W Finger Phalangeal Joint, Right*	**Ø** Open **3** Percutaneous **4** Percutaneous Endoscopic **X** External	**Z** No Device	**Z** No Qualifier

Non-OR　ØRJ[Ø,1,3,4,5,6,9,A,B,C,D,E,F,G,H,J,K,L,M,N,P,Q,R,S,T,U,V,W,X][3,X]ZZ

NC Noncovered Procedure　　**LC** Limited Coverage　　**QA** Questionable OB Admit　　**NT** New Tech Add-on　　✛ Combination Member　　♂ Male　　♀ Female

ICD-10-PCS 2023　　　　　　　　　　　　　　　　　　　　　　　　　　　　　　　　　　　　　　589

Upper Joints

Ø   **Medical and Surgical**
R   **Upper Joints**
N   **Release**   Definition: Freeing a body part from an abnormal physical constraint by cutting or by the use of force
               Explanation: Some of the restraining tissue may be taken out but none of the body part is taken out

Body Part Character 4	Approach Character 5	Device Character 6	Qualifier Character 7
Ø Occipital-cervical Joint	Ø Open	Z No Device	Z No Qualifier
1 Cervical Vertebral Joint	3 Percutaneous		
Atlantoaxial joint	4 Percutaneous Endoscopic		
Cervical facet joint	X External		
3 Cervical Vertebral Disc			
4 Cervicothoracic Vertebral Joint			
Cervicothoracic facet joint			
5 Cervicothoracic Vertebral Disc			
6 Thoracic Vertebral Joint			
Costotransverse joint			
Costovertebral joint			
Thoracic facet joint			
9 Thoracic Vertebral Disc			
A Thoracolumbar Vertebral Joint			
Thoracolumbar facet joint			
B Thoracolumbar Vertebral Disc			
C Temporomandibular Joint, Right			
D Temporomandibular Joint, Left			
E Sternoclavicular Joint, Right			
F Sternoclavicular Joint, Left			
G Acromioclavicular Joint, Right			
H Acromioclavicular Joint, Left			
J Shoulder Joint, Right			
Glenohumeral joint			
Glenoid ligament (labrum)			
K Shoulder Joint, Left			
See J Shoulder Joint, Right			
L Elbow Joint, Right			
Distal humerus, involving joint			
Humeroradial joint			
Humeroulnar joint			
Proximal radioulnar joint			
M Elbow Joint, Left			
See L Elbow Joint, Right			
N Wrist Joint, Right			
Distal radioulnar joint			
Radiocarpal joint			
P Wrist Joint, Left			
See N Wrist Joint, Right			
Q Carpal Joint, Right			
Intercarpal joint			
Midcarpal joint			
R Carpal Joint, Left			
See Q Carpal Joint, Right			
S Carpometacarpal Joint, Right			
T Carpometacarpal Joint, Left			
U Metacarpophalangeal Joint, Right			
V Metacarpophalangeal Joint, Left			
W Finger Phalangeal Joint, Right			
Interphalangeal (IP) joint			
X Finger Phalangeal Joint, Left			
See W Finger Phalangeal Joint, Right			

Non-OR   ØRN[Ø,1,3,4,5,6,9,A,B,C,D,E,F,G,H,J,K,L,M,N,P,Q,R,S,T,U,V,W,X]XZZ

Non-OR Procedure   DRG Non-OR Procedure   Valid OR Procedure   HAC Associated Procedure   Combination Only   New/Revised April   New/Revised October

Ø Medical and Surgical
R Upper Joints
P Removal

Definition: Taking out or off a device from a body part

Explanation: If a device is taken out and a similar device put in without cutting or puncturing the skin or mucous membrane, the procedure is coded to the root operation CHANGE. Otherwise, the procedure for taking out the device is coded to the root operation REMOVAL.

Body Part Character 4	Approach Character 5	Device Character 6	Qualifier Character 7

Ø Occipital-cervical Joint
1 Cervical Vertebral Joint
  Atlantoaxial joint
  Cervical facet joint
4 Cervicothoracic Vertebral Joint
  Cervicothoracic facet joint
6 Thoracic Vertebral Joint
  Costotransverse joint
  Costovertebral joint
  Thoracic facet joint
A Thoracolumbar Vertebral Joint
  Thoracolumbar facet joint
	Ø Open
	3 Percutaneous
	4 Percutaneous Endoscopic
		Ø Drainage Device
		3 Infusion Device
		4 Internal Fixation Device
		7 Autologous Tissue Substitute
		8 Spacer
		A Interbody Fusion Device
		J Synthetic Substitute
		K Nonautologous Tissue Substitute
			Z No Qualifier

Ø Occipital-cervical Joint
1 Cervical Vertebral Joint
  Atlantoaxial joint
  Cervical facet joint
4 Cervicothoracic Vertebral Joint
  Cervicothoracic facet joint
6 Thoracic Vertebral Joint
  Costotransverse joint
  Costovertebral joint
  Thoracic facet joint
A Thoracolumbar Vertebral Joint
  Thoracolumbar facet joint
	X External	**Ø Drainage Device**
		3 Infusion Device
		4 Internal Fixation Device
			Z No Qualifier

3 Cervical Vertebral Disc **5 Cervicothoracic Vertebral Disc** **9 Thoracic Vertebral Disc** **B Thoracolumbar Vertebral Disc**	**Ø Open** **3 Percutaneous** **4 Percutaneous Endoscopic**	**Ø Drainage Device** **3 Infusion Device** **7 Autologous Tissue Substitute** **J Synthetic Substitute** **K Nonautologous Tissue Substitute**	**Z No Qualifier**
3 Cervical Vertebral Disc **5 Cervicothoracic Vertebral Disc** **9 Thoracic Vertebral Disc** **B Thoracolumbar Vertebral Disc**	**X External**	**Ø Drainage Device** **3 Infusion Device**	**Z No Qualifier**
C Temporomandibular Joint, Right **D Temporomandibular Joint, Left** **E Sternoclavicular Joint, Right** **F Sternoclavicular Joint, Left** **G Acromioclavicular Joint, Right** **H Acromioclavicular Joint, Left**	**Ø Open** **3 Percutaneous** **4 Percutaneous Endoscopic**	**Ø Drainage Device** **3 Infusion Device** **4 Internal Fixation Device** **7 Autologous Tissue Substitute** **8 Spacer** **J Synthetic Substitute** **K Nonautologous Tissue Substitute**	**Z No Qualifier**
C Temporomandibular Joint, Right **D Temporomandibular Joint, Left** **E Sternoclavicular Joint, Right** **F Sternoclavicular Joint, Left** **G Acromioclavicular Joint, Right** **H Acromioclavicular Joint, Left**	**X External**	**Ø Drainage Device** **3 Infusion Device** **4 Internal Fixation Device**	**Z No Qualifier**

J Shoulder Joint, Right
  Glenohumeral joint
  Glenoid ligament (labrum)
K Shoulder Joint, Left
  See J Shoulder Joint, Right
	Ø Open
	3 Percutaneous
	4 Percutaneous Endoscopic
		Ø Drainage Device
		3 Infusion Device
		4 Internal Fixation Device
		7 Autologous Tissue Substitute
		8 Spacer
		K Nonautologous Tissue Substitute
			Z No Qualifier

J Shoulder Joint, Right
  Glenohumeral joint
  Glenoid ligament (labrum)
K Shoulder Joint, Left
  See J Shoulder Joint, Right
	Ø Open
	3 Percutaneous
	4 Percutaneous Endoscopic
		J Synthetic Substitute	**6 Humeral Surface**
			7 Glenoid Surface
			Z No Qualifier

J Shoulder Joint, Right
  Glenohumeral joint
  Glenoid ligament (labrum)
K Shoulder Joint, Left
  See J Shoulder Joint, Right
	X External	**Ø Drainage Device**
		3 Infusion Device
		4 Internal Fixation Device
			Z No Qualifier

Non-OR ØRP[Ø,1,4,6,A]3[Ø,3,8]Z	**Non-OR** ØRP[C,D,E,F,G,H][Ø,4]8Z
Non-OR ØRP[Ø,1,4,6,A][Ø,4]8Z	**Non-OR** ØRP[C,D]X[Ø,3]Z
Non-OR ØRP[Ø,1,4,6,A]X[Ø,3,4]Z	**Non-OR** ØRP[E,F,G,H,J,K]X[Ø,3,4]Z
Non-OR ØRP[3,5,9,B]3[Ø,3]Z	**Non-OR** ØRP[J,K]3[Ø,3,8]Z
Non-OR ØRP[3,5,9,B]X[Ø,3]Z	**Non-OR** ØRP[J,K]X[Ø,3,4]Z
Non-OR ØRP[C,D,E,F,G,H]3[Ø,3,8]Z	

ØRP Continued on next page

NC Noncovered Procedure   **LC** Limited Coverage   **QA** Questionable OB Admit   **NT** New Tech Add-on   ⊞ Combination Member   ♂ Male   ♀ Female

ICD-10-PCS 2023   591

ØRP–ØRP

Ø Medical and Surgical
R Upper Joints
P Removal

ØRP Continued

Definition: Taking out or off a device from a body part

Explanation: If a device is taken out and a similar device put in without cutting or puncturing the skin or mucous membrane, the procedure is coded to the root operation CHANGE. Otherwise, the procedure for taking out the device is coded to the root operation REMOVAL.

Body Part Character 4	Approach Character 5	Device Character 6	Qualifier Character 7
L Elbow Joint, Right Distal humerus, involving joint Humeroradial joint Humeroulnar joint Proximal radioulnar joint **M Elbow Joint, Left** *See L Elbow Joint, Right* **N Wrist Joint, Right** Distal radioulnar joint Radiocarpal joint **P Wrist Joint, Left** *See N Wrist Joint, Right* **Q Carpal Joint, Right** Intercarpal joint Midcarpal joint **R Carpal Joint, Left** *See Q Carpal Joint, Right* **S Carpometacarpal Joint, Right** **T Carpometacarpal Joint, Left** **U Metacarpophalangeal Joint, Right** **V Metacarpophalangeal Joint, Left** **W Finger Phalangeal Joint, Right** Interphalangeal (IP) joint **X Finger Phalangeal Joint, Left** *See W Finger Phalangeal Joint, Right*	**Ø Open** **3 Percutaneous** **4 Percutaneous Endoscopic**	**Ø Drainage Device** **3 Infusion Device** **4 Internal Fixation Device** **5 External Fixation Device** **7 Autologous Tissue Substitute** **8 Spacer** **J Synthetic Substitute** **K Nonautologous Tissue Substitute**	**Z No Qualifier**
L Elbow Joint, Right Distal humerus, involving joint Humeroradial joint Humeroulnar joint Proximal radioulnar joint **M Elbow Joint, Left** *See L Elbow Joint, Right* **N Wrist Joint, Right** Distal radioulnar joint Radiocarpal joint **P Wrist Joint, Left** *See N Wrist Joint, Right* **Q Carpal Joint, Right** Intercarpal joint Midcarpal joint **R Carpal Joint, Left** *See Q Carpal Joint, Right* **S Carpometacarpal Joint, Right** **T Carpometacarpal Joint, Left** **U Metacarpophalangeal Joint, Right** **V Metacarpophalangeal Joint, Left** **W Finger Phalangeal Joint, Right** Interphalangeal (IP) joint **X Finger Phalangeal Joint, Left** *See W Finger Phalangeal Joint, Right*	**X External**	**Ø Drainage Device** **3 Infusion Device** **4 Internal Fixation Device** **5 External Fixation Device**	**Z No Qualifier**

Non-OR	ØRP[L,M,N,P,Q,R,S,T,U,V,W,X]3[Ø,3,8]Z
Non-OR	ØRP[L,M,N,P,Q,R,S,T,U,V,W,X][Ø,4]8Z
Non-OR	ØRP[L,M,N,P,Q,R,S,T,U,V,W,X]X[Ø,3,4,5]Z

Ø   **Medical and Surgical**
R   **Upper Joints**
Q   **Repair**   Definition: Restoring, to the extent possible, a body part to its normal anatomic structure and function
                       Explanation: Used only when the method to accomplish the repair is not one of the other root operations

Body Part Character 4	Approach Character 5	Device Character 6	Qualifier Character 7

Ø Occipital-cervical Joint
1 Cervical Vertebral Joint
    Atlantoaxial joint
    Cervical facet joint
3 Cervical Vertebral Disc
4 Cervicothoracic Vertebral Joint
    Cervicothoracic facet joint
5 Cervicothoracic Vertebral Disc
6 Thoracic Vertebral Joint
    Costotransverse joint
    Costovertebral joint
    Thoracic facet joint
9 Thoracic Vertebral Disc
A Thoracolumbar Vertebral Joint
    Thoracolumbar facet joint
B Thoracolumbar Vertebral Disc
C Temporomandibular Joint, Right
D Temporomandibular Joint, Left
E Sternoclavicular Joint, Right
F Sternoclavicular Joint, Left
G Acromioclavicular Joint, Right
H Acromioclavicular Joint, Left
J Shoulder Joint, Right
    Glenohumeral joint
    Glenoid ligament (labrum)
K Shoulder Joint, Left
    See J Shoulder Joint, Right
L Elbow Joint, Right
    Distal humerus, involving joint
    Humeroradial joint
    Humeroulnar joint
    Proximal radioulnar joint
M Elbow Joint, Left
    See L Elbow Joint, Right
N Wrist Joint, Right
    Distal radioulnar joint
    Radiocarpal joint
P Wrist Joint, Left
    See N Wrist Joint, Right
Q Carpal Joint, Right
    Intercarpal joint
    Midcarpal joint
R Carpal Joint, Left
    See Q Carpal Joint, Right
S Carpometacarpal Joint, Right
T Carpometacarpal Joint, Left
U Metacarpophalangeal Joint, Right
V Metacarpophalangeal Joint, Left
W Finger Phalangeal Joint, Right
    Interphalangeal (IP) joint
X Finger Phalangeal Joint, Left
    See W Finger Phalangeal Joint, Right
	Ø Open
	3 Percutaneous
	4 Percutaneous Endoscopic
	X External
		Z No Device	**Z** No Qualifier

Non-OR   ØRQ[Ø,1,3,4,5,6,9,A,B,C,D,E,F,G,H,J,K,L,M,N,P,Q,R,S,T,U,V,W,X]XZZ
HAC   ØRQ[E,F,G,H,J,K,L,M][Ø,3,4]ZZ when reported with SDx K68.11 or T81.4Ø–T81.49, T84.6Ø-T84.619, T84.63-T84.7 with 7th character A

NC Noncovered Procedure   **LC** Limited Coverage   **QA** Questionable OB Admit   **NT** New Tech Add-on   ⊞ Combination Member   ♂Male   ♀Female

ICD-10-PCS 2023   **593**

ØRQ–ØRQ

Ø   Medical and Surgical
R   Upper Joints
R   Replacement   Definition: Putting in or on biological or synthetic material that physically takes the place and/or function of all or a portion of a body part
                        Explanation: The body part may have been taken out or replaced, or may be taken out, physically eradicated, or rendered nonfunctional during the REPLACEMENT procedure. A REMOVAL procedure is coded for taking out the device used in a previous replacement procedure.

Body Part Character 4	Approach Character 5	Device Character 6	Qualifier Character 7

Ø   Occipital-cervical Joint
1   Cervical Vertebral Joint
    Atlantoaxial joint
    Cervical facet joint
3   Cervical Vertebral Disc
4   Cervicothoracic Vertebral Joint
    Cervicothoracic facet joint
5   Cervicothoracic Vertebral Disc
6   Thoracic Vertebral Joint
    Costotransverse joint
    Costovertebral joint
    Thoracic facet joint
9   Thoracic Vertebral Disc
A   Thoracolumbar Vertebral Joint
    Thoracolumbar facet joint
B   Thoracolumbar Vertebral Disc
C   Temporomandibular Joint, Right
D   Temporomandibular Joint, Left
E   Sternoclavicular Joint, Right
F   Sternoclavicular Joint, Left
G   Acromioclavicular Joint, Right
H   Acromioclavicular Joint, Left
L   Elbow Joint, Right
    Distal humerus, involving joint
    Humeroradial joint
    Humeroulnar joint
    Proximal radioulnar joint
M   Elbow Joint, Left
    See L Elbow Joint, Right
N   Wrist Joint, Right
    Distal radioulnar joint
    Radiocarpal joint
P   Wrist Joint, Left
    See N Wrist Joint, Right
Q   Carpal Joint, Right
    Intercarpal joint
    Midcarpal joint
R   Carpal Joint, Left
    See Q Carpal Joint, Right
S   Carpometacarpal Joint, Right
T   Carpometacarpal Joint, Left
U   Metacarpophalangeal Joint, Right
V   Metacarpophalangeal Joint, Left
W   Finger Phalangeal Joint, Right
    Interphalangeal (IP) joint
X   Finger Phalangeal Joint, Left
    See W Finger Phalangeal Joint, Right
	Ø Open	7 Autologous Tissue Substitute
		J Synthetic Substitute
		K Nonautologous Tissue Substitute
			Z No Qualifier

J   Shoulder Joint, Right
    Glenohumeral joint
    Glenoid ligament (labrum)
K   Shoulder Joint, Left
    See J Shoulder Joint, Right
	Ø Open	Ø Synthetic Substitute, Reverse Ball and Socket
		7 Autologous Tissue Substitute
		K Nonautologous Tissue Substitute
			Z No Qualifier

J   Shoulder Joint, Right
    Glenohumeral joint
    Glenoid ligament (labrum)
K   Shoulder Joint, Left
    See J Shoulder Joint, Right
	Ø Open	J Synthetic Substitute	6 Humeral Surface
			7 Glenoid Surface
			Z No Qualifier

Non-OR Procedure   DRG Non-OR Procedure   Valid OR Procedure   HAC Associated Procedure   Combination Only   New/Revised April   New/Revised October

594   ICD-10-PCS 2023

ØRR–ØRR

Ø   **Medical and Surgical**
R   **Upper Joints**
S   **Reposition**   Definition: Moving to its normal location, or other suitable location, all or a portion of a body part

Explanation: The body part is moved to a new location from an abnormal location, or from a normal location where it is not functioning correctly. The body part may or may not be cut out or off to be moved to the new location.

Body Part Character 4	Approach Character 5	Device Character 6	Qualifier Character 7
Ø **Occipital-cervical Joint**	Ø Open	4 Internal Fixation Device	Z No Qualifier

1 **Cervical Vertebral Joint**
   Atlantoaxial joint
   Cervical facet joint
	3 Percutaneous
	4 Percutaneous Endoscopic
	X External
		Z No Device	

4 **Cervicothoracic Vertebral Joint** Cervicothoracic facet joint			

6 **Thoracic Vertebral Joint**
   Costotransverse joint
   Costovertebral joint
   Thoracic facet joint			

A **Thoracolumbar Vertebral Joint** Thoracolumbar facet joint			
C **Temporomandibular Joint, Right**			
D **Temporomandibular Joint, Left**			
E **Sternoclavicular Joint, Right**			
F **Sternoclavicular Joint, Left**			
G **Acromioclavicular Joint, Right**			
H **Acromioclavicular Joint, Left**			

J **Shoulder Joint, Right**
   Glenohumeral joint
   Glenoid ligament (labrum)			

K **Shoulder Joint, Left** *See J Shoulder Joint, Right*			

L **Elbow Joint, Right**
   Distal humerus, involving joint
   Humeroradial joint
   Humeroulnar joint
   Proximal radioulnar joint
	Ø Open
	3 Percutaneous
	4 Percutaneous Endoscopic
	X External
		4 Internal Fixation Device
		5 External Fixation Device
		Z No Device
			Z No Qualifier

M **Elbow Joint, Left** *See L Elbow Joint, Right*			

N **Wrist Joint, Right**
   Distal radioulnar joint
   Radiocarpal joint			

P **Wrist Joint, Left** *See N Wrist Joint, Right*			

Q **Carpal Joint, Right**
   Intercarpal joint
   Midcarpal joint			

R **Carpal Joint, Left** *See Q Carpal Joint, Right*			
S **Carpometacarpal Joint, Right**			
T **Carpometacarpal Joint, Left**			
U **Metacarpophalangeal Joint, Right**			
V **Metacarpophalangeal Joint, Left**			
W **Finger Phalangeal Joint, Right** Interphalangeal (IP) joint			
X **Finger Phalangeal Joint, Left** *See W Finger Phalangeal Joint, Right*			

Non-OR   ØRS[Ø,1,4,6,A,C,D,E,F,G,H,J,K][3,4,X][4,Z]Z
Non-OR   ØRS[L,M,N,P,Q,R,S,T,U,V,W,X][3,4,X][4,5,Z]Z

NC Noncovered Procedure   LC Limited Coverage   QA Questionable OB Admit   NT New Tech Add-on   ⊞ Combination Member   ♂ Male   ♀ Female

ICD-10-PCS 2023   595

ØRS–ØRS

Ø Medical and Surgical
R Upper Joints
T Resection   Definition: Cutting out or off, without replacement, all of a body part
                          Explanation: None

Body Part Character 4	Approach Character 5	Device Character 6	Qualifier Character 7
3 Cervical Vertebral Disc	**Ø** Open	**Z** No Device	**Z** No Qualifier
4 Cervicothoracic Vertebral Joint			
Cervicothoracic facet joint			
5 Cervicothoracic Vertebral Disc			
9 Thoracic Vertebral Disc			
B Thoracolumbar Vertebral Disc			
C Temporomandibular Joint, Right			
D Temporomandibular Joint, Left			
E Sternoclavicular Joint, Right			
F Sternoclavicular Joint, Left			
G Acromioclavicular Joint, Right			
H Acromioclavicular Joint, Left			
J Shoulder Joint, Right			
Glenohumeral joint			
Glenoid ligament (labrum)			
K Shoulder Joint, Left			
See J Shoulder Joint, Right			
L Elbow Joint, Right			
Distal humerus, involving joint			
Humeroradial joint			
Humeroulnar joint			
Proximal radioulnar joint			
M Elbow Joint, Left			
See L Elbow Joint, Right			
N Wrist Joint, Right			
Distal radioulnar joint			
Radiocarpal joint			
P Wrist Joint, Left			
See N Wrist Joint, Right			
Q Carpal Joint, Right			
Intercarpal joint			
Midcarpal joint			
R Carpal Joint, Left			
See Q Carpal Joint, Right			
S Carpometacarpal Joint, Right			
T Carpometacarpal Joint, Left			
U Metacarpophalangeal Joint, Right			
V Metacarpophalangeal Joint, Left			
W Finger Phalangeal Joint, Right			
Interphalangeal (IP) joint			
X Finger Phalangeal Joint, Left			
See W Finger Phalangeal Joint, Right			

Ø   Medical and Surgical
R   Upper Joints
U   Supplement   Definition: Putting in or on biological or synthetic material that physically reinforces and/or augments the function of a portion of a body part

Explanation: The biological material is non-living, or is living and from the same individual. The body part may have been previously replaced, and the SUPPLEMENT procedure is performed to physically reinforce and/or augment the function of the replaced body part.

Body Part Character 4	Approach Character 5	Device Character 6	Qualifier Character 7
Ø Occipital-cervical Joint	Ø Open	7 Autologous Tissue Substitute	Z No Qualifier

1   Cervical Vertebral Joint
     Atlantoaxial joint
     Cervical facet joint
	3 Percutaneous
	4 Percutaneous Endoscopic
		J Synthetic Substitute
		K Nonautologous Tissue
		     Substitute	

3 Cervical Vertebral Disc			
4 Cervicothoracic Vertebral Joint Cervicothoracic facet joint			
5 Cervicothoracic Vertebral Disc			

6   Thoracic Vertebral Joint
     Costotransverse joint
     Costovertebral joint
     Thoracic facet joint			

9 Thoracic Vertebral Disc			
A Thoracolumbar Vertebral Joint Thoracolumbar facet joint			
B Thoracolumbar Vertebral Disc			
C Temporomandibular Joint, Right			
D Temporomandibular Joint, Left			
E Sternoclavicular Joint, Right			
F Sternoclavicular Joint, Left			
G Acromioclavicular Joint, Right			
H Acromioclavicular Joint, Left			

J   Shoulder Joint, Right
     Glenohumeral joint
     Glenoid ligament (labrum)			

K Shoulder Joint, Left *See J Shoulder Joint, Right*			

L   Elbow Joint, Right
     Distal humerus, involving joint
     Humeroradial joint
     Humeroulnar joint
     Proximal radioulnar joint			

M Elbow Joint, Left *See L Elbow Joint, Right*			

N   Wrist Joint, Right
     Distal radioulnar joint
     Radiocarpal joint			

P Wrist Joint, Left *See N Wrist Joint, Right*			

Q   Carpal Joint, Right
     Intercarpal joint
     Midcarpal joint			

R Carpal Joint, Left *See Q Carpal Joint, Right*			
S Carpometacarpal Joint, Right			
T Carpometacarpal Joint, Left			
U Metacarpophalangeal Joint, Right			
V Metacarpophalangeal Joint, Left			
W Finger Phalangeal Joint, Right Interphalangeal (IP) joint			
X Finger Phalangeal Joint, Left *See W Finger Phalangeal Joint, Right*			

HAC   ØRU[E,F,G,H,J,K,L,M][Ø,3,4][7,J,K]Z when reported with SDx K68.11 or T81.4Ø–T81.49, T84.6Ø-T84.619, T84.63-T84.7 with 7th character A

NC Noncovered Procedure   **LC** Limited Coverage   **QA** Questionable OB Admit   **NT** New Tech Add-on   ⊞ Combination Member   ♂ Male   ♀ Female

ICD-10-PCS 2023   597

ØRU–ØRU

Ø **Medical and Surgical**
R **Upper Joints**
W **Revision**   Definition: Correcting, to the extent possible, a portion of a malfunctioning device or the position of a displaced device

Explanation: Revision can include correcting a malfunctioning or displaced device by taking out or putting in components of the device such as a screw or pin

Body Part Character 4	Approach Character 5	Device Character 6	Qualifier Character 7
Ø Occipital-cervical Joint 1 Cervical Vertebral Joint Atlantoaxial joint Cervical facet joint 4 Cervicothoracic Vertebral Joint Cervicothoracic facet joint 6 Thoracic Vertebral Joint Costotransverse joint Costovertebral joint Thoracic facet joint A Thoracolumbar Vertebral Joint Thoracolumbar facet joint	Ø Open 3 Percutaneous 4 Percutaneous Endoscopic X External	Ø Drainage Device 3 Infusion Device 4 Internal Fixation Device 7 Autologous Tissue Substitute 8 Spacer A Interbody Fusion Device J Synthetic Substitute K Nonautologous Tissue Substitute	Z No Qualifier
3 Cervical Vertebral Disc 5 Cervicothoracic Vertebral Disc 9 Thoracic Vertebral Disc B Thoracolumbar Vertebral Disc	Ø Open 3 Percutaneous 4 Percutaneous Endoscopic X External	Ø Drainage Device 3 Infusion Device 7 Autologous Tissue Substitute J Synthetic Substitute K Nonautologous Tissue Substitute	Z No Qualifier
C Temporomandibular Joint, Right D Temporomandibular Joint, Left E Sternoclavicular Joint, Right F Sternoclavicular Joint, Left G Acromioclavicular Joint, Right H Acromioclavicular Joint, Left	Ø Open 3 Percutaneous 4 Percutaneous Endoscopic X External	Ø Drainage Device 3 Infusion Device 4 Internal Fixation Device 7 Autologous Tissue Substitute 8 Spacer J Synthetic Substitute K Nonautologous Tissue Substitute	Z No Qualifier
J Shoulder Joint, Right Glenohumeral joint Glenoid ligament (labrum) K Shoulder Joint, Left *See J Shoulder Joint, Right*	Ø Open 3 Percutaneous 4 Percutaneous Endoscopic X External	Ø Drainage Device 3 Infusion Device 4 Internal Fixation Device 7 Autologous Tissue Substitute 8 Spacer J Synthetic Substitute K Nonautologous Tissue Substitute	Z No Qualifier
J Shoulder Joint, Right Glenohumeral joint Glenoid ligament (labrum) K Shoulder Joint, Left *See J Shoulder Joint, Right*	Ø Open 3 Percutaneous 4 Percutaneous Endoscopic X External	J Synthetic Substitute	6 Humeral Surface 7 Glenoid Surface Z No Qualifier
L Elbow Joint, Right Distal humerus, involving joint Humeroradial joint Humeroulnar joint Proximal radioulnar joint M Elbow Joint, Left *See L Elbow Joint, Right* N Wrist Joint, Right Distal radioulnar joint Radiocarpal joint P Wrist Joint, Left *See N Wrist Joint, Right* Q Carpal Joint, Right Intercarpal joint Midcarpal joint R Carpal Joint, Left *See Q Carpal Joint, Right* S Carpometacarpal Joint, Right T Carpometacarpal Joint, Left U Metacarpophalangeal Joint, Right V Metacarpophalangeal Joint, Left W Finger Phalangeal Joint, Right Interphalangeal (IP) joint X Finger Phalangeal Joint, Left *See W Finger Phalangeal Joint, Right*	Ø Open 3 Percutaneous 4 Percutaneous Endoscopic X External	Ø Drainage Device 3 Infusion Device 4 Internal Fixation Device 5 External Fixation Device 7 Autologous Tissue Substitute 8 Spacer J Synthetic Substitute K Nonautologous Tissue Substitute	Z No Qualifier

Non-OR	ØRW[Ø,1,4,6,A]X[Ø,3,4,7,8,A,J,K]Z
Non-OR	ØRW[3,5,9,B]X[Ø,3,7,J,K]Z
Non-OR	ØRW[C,D,E,F,G,H]X[Ø,3,4,7,8,J,K]Z
Non-OR	ØRW[J,K]X[Ø,3,4,7,8,J,K]Z
Non-OR	ØRW[J,K]XJ[6,7,Z]
Non-OR	ØRW[L,M,N,P,Q,R,S,T,U,V,W,X]X[Ø,3,4,5,7,8,J,K]Z

Non-OR Procedure   DRG Non-OR Procedure   Valid OR Procedure   HAC Associated Procedure   Combination Only   New/Revised April   New/Revised October

598

ICD-10-PCS 2023

Lower Joints ØS2–ØSW

Character Meanings*

This Character Meaning table is provided as a guide to assist the user in the identification of character members that may be found in this section of code tables. It **SHOULD NOT** be used to build a PCS code.

Operation–Character 3	Body Part–Character 4	Approach–Character 5	Device–Character 6	Qualifier–Character 7
2 Change	Ø Lumbar Vertebral Joint	Ø Open	Ø Drainage Device OR Synthetic Substitute, Polyethylene	Ø Anterior Approach, Anterior Column
5 Destruction	1 Lumbar Vertebral Joint, 2 or more	3 Percutaneous	1 Synthetic Substitute, Metal	1 Posterior Approach, Posterior Column
9 Drainage	2 Lumbar Vertebral Disc	4 Percutaneous Endoscopic	2 Synthetic Substitute, Metal on Polyethylene	9 Cemented
B Excision	3 Lumbosacral Joint	X External	3 Infusion Device OR Internal Fixation Device, Sustained Compression OR Synthetic Substitute, Ceramic	A Uncemented
C Extirpation	4 Lumbosacral Disc		4 Internal Fixation Device OR Synthetic Substitute, Ceramic on Polyethylene	C Patellar Surface
G Fusion	5 Sacrococcygeal Joint		5 External Fixation Device	J Posterior Approach, Anterior Column
H Insertion	6 Coccygeal Joint		6 Synthetic Substitute, Oxidized Zirconium on Polyethylene	X Diagnostic
J Inspection	7 Sacroiliac Joint, Right		7 Autologous Tissue Substitute	Z No Qualifier
N Release	8 Sacroiliac Joint, Left		8 Spacer	
P Removal	9 Hip Joint, Right		9 Liner	
Q Repair	A Hip Joint, Acetabular Surface, Right		A Interbody Fusion Device	
R Replacement	B Hip Joint, Left		B Resurfacing Device OR Spinal Stabilization Device, Interspinous Process	
S Reposition	C Knee Joint, Right		C Spinal Stabilization Device, Pedicle-Based	
T Resection	D Knee Joint, Left		D Spinal Stabilization Device, Facet Replacement	
U Supplement	E Hip Joint, Acetabular Surface, Left		E Articulating Spacer	
W Revision	F Ankle Joint, Right		J Synthetic Substitute	
	G Ankle Joint, Left		K Nonautologous Tissue Substitute	
	H Tarsal Joint, Right		L Synthetic Substitute, Unicondylar Medial	
	J Tarsal Joint, Left		M Synthetic Substitute, Unicondylar Lateral	
	K Tarsometatarsal Joint, Right		N Synthetic Substitute, Patellofemoral	
	L Tarsometatarsal Joint, Left		Y Other Device	
	M Metatarsal-Phalangeal Joint, Right		Z No Device	
	N Metatarsal-Phalangeal Joint, Left			
	P Toe Phalangeal Joint, Right			
	Q Toe Phalangeal Joint, Left			
	R Hip Joint, Femoral Surface, Right			
	S Hip Joint, Femoral Surface, Left			
	T Knee Joint, Femoral Surface, Right			
	U Knee Joint, Femoral Surface, Left			
	V Knee Joint, Tibial Surface, Right			
	W Knee Joint, Tibial Surface, Left			
	Y Lower Joint			

* Includes synovial membrane.

AHA Coding Clinic for table 0S9

2018, 2Q, 17	Arthroscopic drainage of knee and nonexcisional debridement
2017, 1Q, 50	Dry aspiration of ankle joint

AHA Coding Clinic for table 0SB

2017, 4Q, 76	Radiolucent porous interbody fusion device
2016, 2Q, 16	Decompressive laminectomy/foraminotomy and lumbar discectomy
2016, 1Q, 20	Metatarsophalangeal joint resection arthroplasty
2015, 1Q, 34	Arthroscopic meniscectomy with debridement and abrasion chondroplasty
2014, 2Q, 6	Posterior lumbar fusion with discectomy

AHA Coding Clinic for table 0SG

2022, 2Q, 23	Sacroiliac joint fusion
2021, 4Q, 67	Posterior dynamic distraction
2021, 3Q, 24	Mid-foot fusion with bone graft
2021, 3Q, 25	Placement of X-Spine Axle Cage
2021, 1Q, 18	Placement of interspinous distraction device (spacer) for decompression
2021, 1Q, 53	Official guidelines for coding and reporting for interbody fusion device B3.10c
2020, 4Q, 56-58	Intramedullary sustained compression joint fusion
2020, 2Q, 27	Spinal fusion with NuVasive® VersaTie®
2020, 1Q, 33	Spinal fusion without use of bone graft
2019, 3Q, 35	Fusion procedures of the spine (guideline B3.10c)
2019, 1Q, 30	Spinal fusion performed at same level as decompressive laminectomy
2018, 4Q, 43	Joint fusion device value
2018, 1Q, 22	Spinal fusion procedures without bone graft
2017, 4Q, 76	Radiolucent porous interbody fusion device
2017, 2Q, 23	Decompression of spinal cord and placement of instrumentation
2014, 3Q, 30	Spinal fusion and fixation instrumentation
2014, 3Q, 36	Lumbar interbody fusion of two vertebral levels
2014, 2Q, 6	Posterior lumbar fusion with discectomy
2013, 3Q, 25	360-degree spinal fusion
2013, 2Q, 39	Ankle fusion, osteotomy, and removal of hardware
2013, 1Q, 21-23	Spinal fusion of thoracic and lumbar vertebrae

AHA Coding Clinic for table 0SH

2021, 3Q, 25	Placement of X-Spine Axle Cage
2021, 1Q, 18	Placement of interspinous distraction device (spacer) for decompression
2017, 2Q, 23	Decompression of spinal cord and placement of instrumentation

AHA Coding Clinic for table 0SJ

2017, 1Q, 50	Dry aspiration of ankle joint

AHA Coding Clinic for table 0SN

2020, 2Q, 26	Arthroscopic manipulation and nonexcisional debridement of knee joint
2019, 1Q, 30	Spinal fusion performed at same level as decompressive laminectomy

AHA Coding Clinic for table 0SP

2021, 3Q, 25	Revision total knee arthroplasty
2021, 1Q, 17	Revision of ankle arthroplasty with placement of tibial insert
2018, 4Q, 43	Articulating spacer for hip and knee joint
2018, 2Q, 16	Exchange of tibial polyethylene component with stabilizing insert (tibial tray)
2017, 4Q, 107	Total ankle replacement versus revision
2016, 4Q, 110-112	Removal and revision of hip and knee devices
2015, 2Q, 18	Total knee revision
2015, 2Q, 19	Revision of femoral head and acetabular liner
2013, 2Q, 39	Ankle fusion, osteotomy, and removal of hardware

AHA Coding Clinic for table 0SQ

2014, 4Q, 25	Femoroacetabular impingement and labral tear with repair

AHA Coding Clinic for table 0SR

2022, 1Q, 39	Provisional total hip arthroplasty
2021, 3Q, 25	Revision total knee arthroplasty
2021, 1Q, 17	Revision of ankle arthroplasty with placement of tibial insert
2020, 3Q, 33	Total hip arthroplasty using dual mobility components
2018, 4Q, 43	Articulating spacer for hip and knee joint
2018, 2Q, 16	Exchange of tibial polyethylene component with stabilizing insert (tibial tray)
2017, 4Q, 38-39	Oxidized zirconium on polyethylene bearing surface
2017, 4Q, 107	Total ankle replacement versus revision
2017, 1Q, 22	Total knee replacement and patellar component
2016, 4Q, 110-111	Partial (unicondylar) knee replacement
2016, 4Q, 111-112	Removal and revision of hip and knee devices
2016, 3Q, 35	Use of cemented versus uncemented qualifier for joint replacement
2015, 3Q, 18	Total hip replacement with acetabular reconstruction
2015, 2Q, 18	Total knee revision
2015, 2Q, 19	Revision of femoral head and acetabular liner

AHA Coding Clinic for table 0SS

2022, 2Q, 22	Ankle distraction procedure
2016, 2Q, 31	Periacetabular ostectomy for repair of congenital hip dysplasia

AHA Coding Clinic for table 0ST

2016, 1Q, 20	Metatarsophalangeal joint resection arthroplasty
2014, 4Q, 29	Rotational osteosynthesis

AHA Coding Clinic for table 0SU

2022, 1Q, 47	Matrix-induced autologous chondrocyte implantation
2021, 1Q, 17	Revision of ankle arthroplasty with placement of tibial insert
2018, 2Q, 16	Exchange of tibial polyethylene component with stabilizing insert (tibial tray)
2016, 4Q, 111	Removal and revision of hip and knee devices
2015, 2Q, 19	Revision of femoral head and acetabular liner

AHA Coding Clinic for table 0SW

2017, 4Q, 107	Total ankle replacement versus revision
2016, 4Q, 110-112	Removal and revision of hip and knee devices
2015, 2Q, 18	Total knee revision
2015, 2Q, 19	Revision of femoral head and acetabular liner

Lower Joints

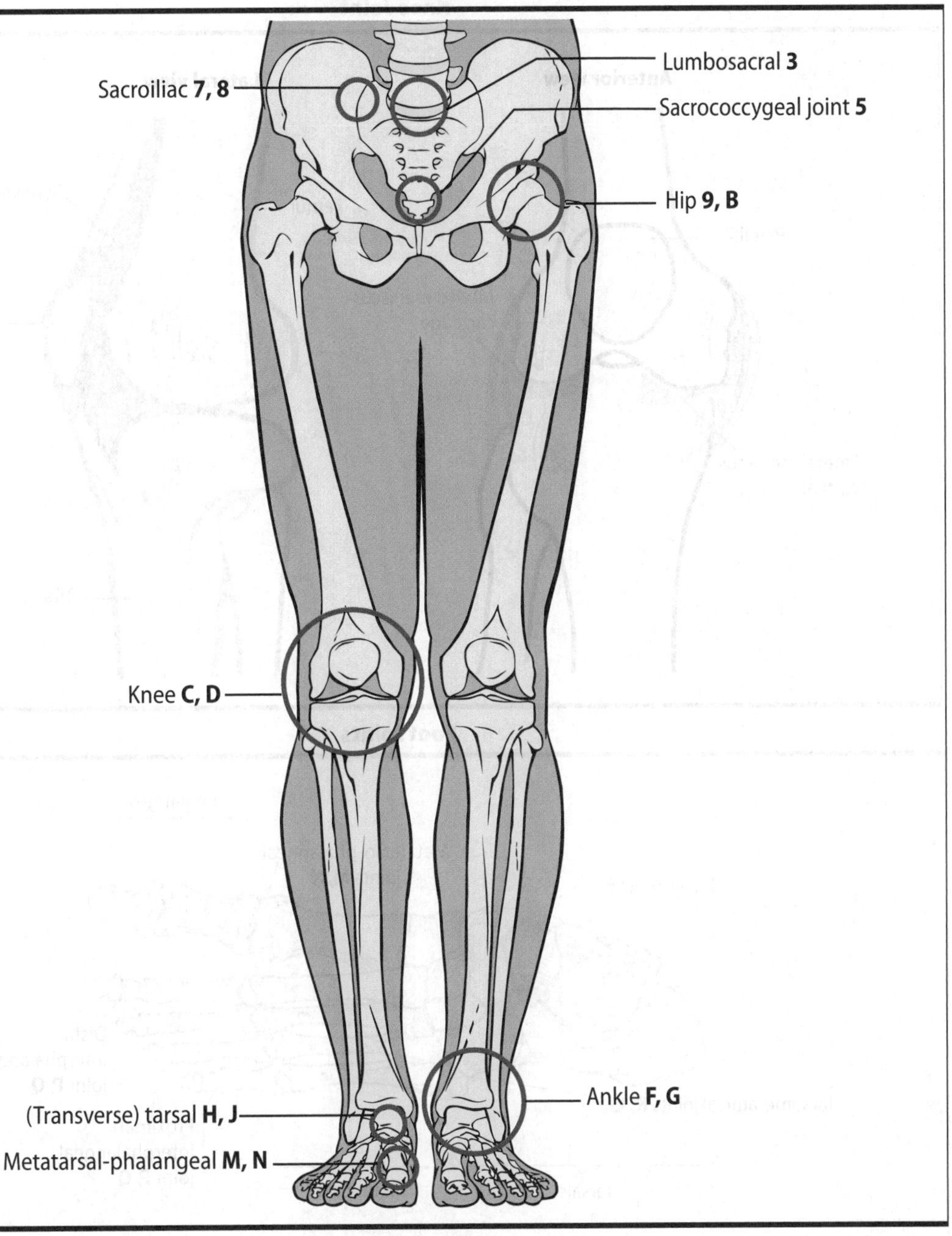

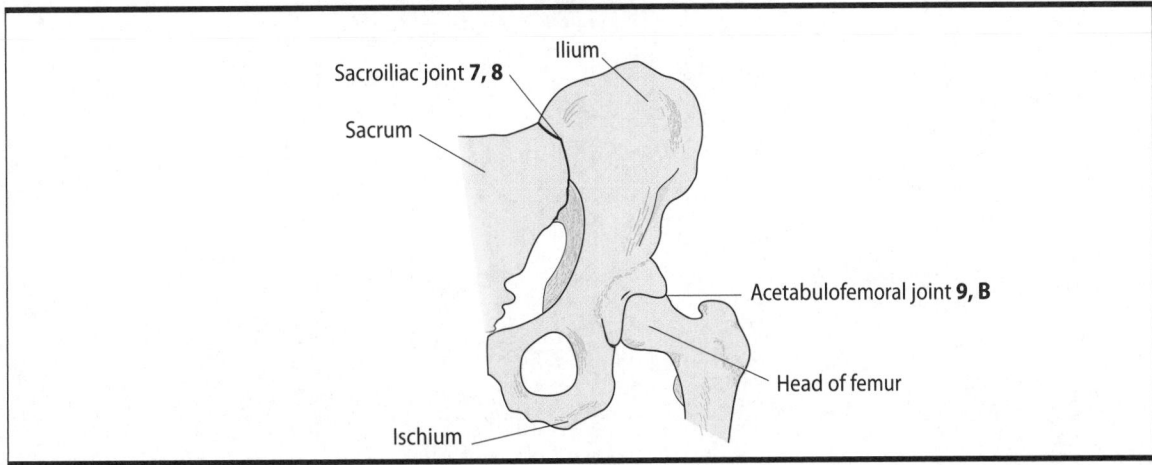

Sacroiliac **7, 8**

Lumbosacral **3**

Sacrococcygeal joint **5**

Hip **9, B**

Knee **C, D**

(Transverse) tarsal **H, J**

Metatarsal-phalangeal **M, N**

Ankle **F, G**

Hip Joint

Sacroiliac joint **7, 8**

Ilium

Sacrum

Acetabulofemoral joint **9, B**

Head of femur

Ischium

Knee Joint

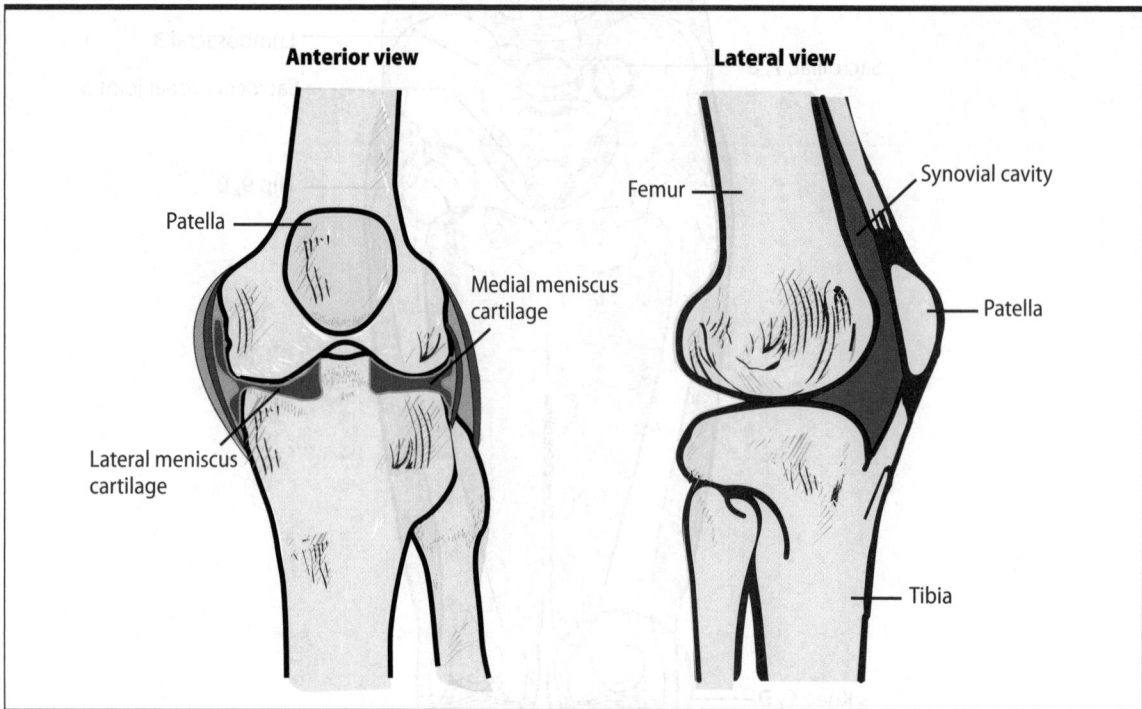

Anterior view

Patella

Medial meniscus cartilage

Lateral meniscus cartilage

Lateral view

Femur

Synovial cavity

Patella

Tibia

Foot Joints

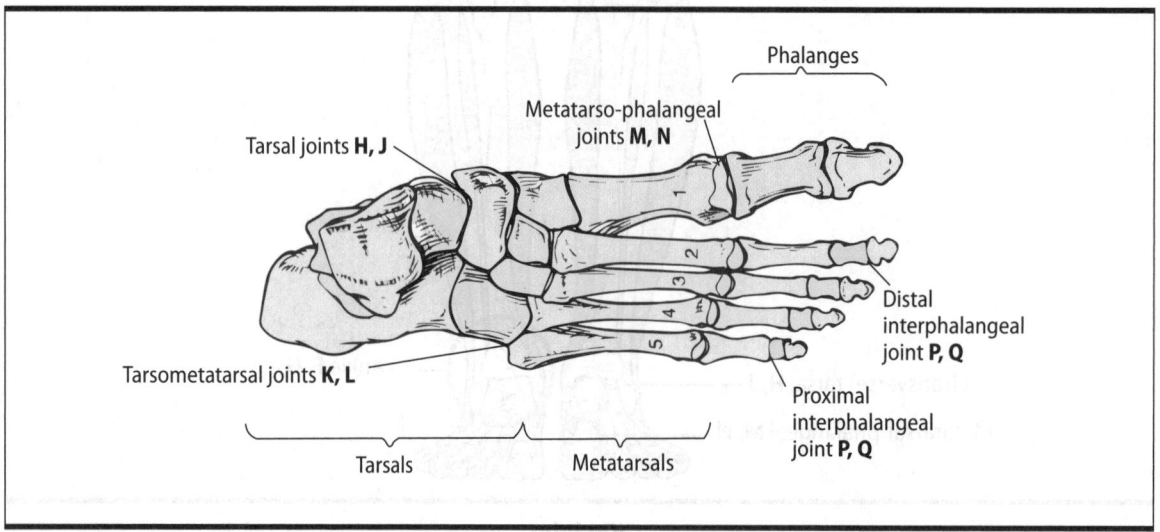

Phalanges

Metatarso-phalangeal joints **M, N**

Tarsal joints **H, J**

Tarsometatarsal joints **K, L**

Distal interphalangeal joint **P, Q**

Proximal interphalangeal joint **P, Q**

Tarsals

Metatarsals

Ø Medical and Surgical
S Lower Joints
2 Change

Definition: Taking out or off a device from a body part and putting back an identical or similar device in or on the same body part without cutting or puncturing the skin or a mucous membrane

Explanation: All CHANGE procedures are coded using the approach EXTERNAL

Body Part Character 4	Approach Character 5	Device Character 6	Qualifier Character 7
Y Lower Joint	X External	Ø Drainage Device Y Other Device	Z No Qualifier

Non-OR	All body part, approach, device, and qualifier values

Ø Medical and Surgical
S Lower Joints
5 Destruction

Definition: Physical eradication of all or a portion of a body part by the direct use of energy, force, or a destructive agent

Explanation: None of the body part is physically taken out

Body Part Character 4	Approach Character 5	Device Character 6	Qualifier Character 7

Ø **Lumbar Vertebral Joint**
    Lumbar facet joint
2 **Lumbar Vertebral Disc**
3 **Lumbosacral Joint**
    Lumbosacral facet joint
4 **Lumbosacral Disc**
5 **Sacrococcygeal Joint**
    Sacrococcygeal symphysis
6 **Coccygeal Joint**
7 **Sacroiliac Joint, Right**
8 **Sacroiliac Joint, Left**
9 **Hip Joint, Right**
    Acetabulofemoral joint
B **Hip Joint, Left**
    See 9 Hip Joint, Right
C **Knee Joint, Right**
    Femoropatellar joint
    Femorotibial joint
    Lateral meniscus
    Medial meniscus
    Patellofemoral joint
    Tibiofemoral joint
D **Knee Joint, Left**
    See C Knee Joint, Right
F **Ankle Joint, Right**
    Inferior tibiofibular joint
    Talocrural joint
G **Ankle Joint, Left**
    See F Ankle Joint, Right
H **Tarsal Joint, Right**
    Calcaneocuboid joint
    Cuboideonavicular joint
    Cuneonavicular joint
    Intercuneiform joint
    Subtalar (talocalcaneal) joint
    Talocalcaneal (subtalar) joint
    Talocalcaneonavicular joint
J **Tarsal Joint, Left**
    See H Tarsal Joint, Right
K **Tarsometatarsal Joint, Right**
L **Tarsometatarsal Joint, Left**
M **Metatarsal-Phalangeal Joint, Right**
    Metatarsophalangeal (MTP) joint
N **Metatarsal-Phalangeal Joint, Left**
    See M Metatarsal-Phalangeal Joint, Right
P **Toe Phalangeal Joint, Right**
    Interphalangeal (IP) joint
Q **Toe Phalangeal Joint, Left**
    See P Toe Phalangeal Joint, Right
	Ø Open
	3 Percutaneous
	4 Percutaneous Endoscopic
		Z No Device	Z No Qualifier

NC Noncovered Procedure   LC Limited Coverage   QA Questionable OB Admit   NT New Tech Add-on   ⊞ Combination Member   ♂ Male   ♀ Female

ICD-10-PCS 2023   603

Ø   Medical and Surgical
S   Lower Joints
9   Drainage   Definition: Taking or letting out fluids and/or gases from a body part
                  Explanation: The qualifier DIAGNOSTIC is used to identify drainage procedures that are biopsies

Body Part Character 4		Approach Character 5	Device Character 6	Qualifier Character 7

Ø Lumbar Vertebral Joint
  Lumbar facet joint
2 Lumbar Vertebral Disc
3 Lumbosacral Joint
  Lumbosacral facet joint
4 Lumbosacral Disc
5 Sacrococcygeal Joint
  Sacrococcygeal symphysis
6 Coccygeal Joint
7 Sacroiliac Joint, Right
8 Sacroiliac Joint, Left
9 Hip Joint, Right
  Acetabulofemoral joint
B Hip Joint, Left
  See 9 Hip Joint, Right
C Knee Joint, Right
  Femoropatellar joint
  Femorotibial joint
  Lateral meniscus
  Medial meniscus
  Patellofemoral joint
  Tibiofemoral joint
D Knee Joint, Left
  See C Knee Joint, Right
F Ankle Joint, Right
  Inferior tibiofibular joint
  Talocrural joint
G Ankle Joint, Left
  See F Ankle Joint, Right
	H Tarsal Joint, Right
	  Calcaneocuboid joint
	  Cuboideonavicular joint
	  Cuneonavicular joint
	  Intercuneiform joint
	  Subtalar (talocalcaneal) joint
	  Talocalcaneal (subtalar)
	    joint
	  Talocalcaneonavicular joint
	J Tarsal Joint, Left
	  See H Tarsal Joint, Right
	K Tarsometatarsal Joint,
	  Right
	L Tarsometatarsal Joint, Left
	M Metatarsal-Phalangeal
	  Joint, Right
	  Metatarsophalangeal (MTP)
	    joint
	N Metatarsal-Phalangeal
	  Joint, Left
	  *See M Metatarsal-Phalangeal
	    Joint, Right*
	P Toe Phalangeal Joint, Right
	  Interphalangeal (IP) joint
	Q Toe Phalangeal Joint, Left
	  *See P Toe Phalangeal Joint,
	    Right*
		Ø Open
		3 Percutaneous
		4 Percutaneous Endoscopic
			Ø Drainage Device	**Z** No Qualifier

Ø Lumbar Vertebral Joint
  Lumbar facet joint
2 Lumbar Vertebral Disc
3 Lumbosacral Joint
  Lumbosacral facet joint
4 Lumbosacral Disc
5 Sacrococcygeal Joint
  Sacrococcygeal symphysis
6 Coccygeal Joint
7 Sacroiliac Joint, Right
8 Sacroiliac Joint, Left
9 Hip Joint, Right
  Acetabulofemoral joint
B Hip Joint, Left
  See 9 Hip Joint, Right
C Knee Joint, Right
  Femoropatellar joint
  Femorotibial joint
  Lateral meniscus
  Medial meniscus
  Patellofemoral joint
  Tibiofemoral joint
D Knee Joint, Left
  See C Knee Joint, Right
F Ankle Joint, Right
  Inferior tibiofibular joint
  Talocrural joint
G Ankle Joint, Left
  See F Ankle Joint, Right
	H Tarsal Joint, Right
	  Calcaneocuboid joint
	  Cuboideonavicular joint
	  Cuneonavicular joint
	  Intercuneiform joint
	  Subtalar (talocalcaneal) joint
	  Talocalcaneal (subtalar)
	    joint
	  Talocalcaneonavicular joint
	J Tarsal Joint, Left
	  See H Tarsal Joint, Right
	K Tarsometatarsal Joint,
	  Right
	L Tarsometatarsal Joint, Left
	M Metatarsal-Phalangeal
	  Joint, Right
	  Metatarsophalangeal (MTP)
	    joint
	N Metatarsal-Phalangeal
	  Joint, Left
	  *See M Metatarsal-Phalangeal
	    Joint, Right*
	P Toe Phalangeal Joint, Right
	  Interphalangeal (IP) joint
	Q Toe Phalangeal Joint, Left
	  *See P Toe Phalangeal Joint,
	    Right*
		Ø Open
		3 Percutaneous
		4 Percutaneous Endoscopic
			Z No Device	**X** Diagnostic
				Z No Qualifier

Non-OR	ØS9[Ø,2,3,4,5,6,7,8,9,B,C,D,F,G,H,J,K,L,M,N,P,Q][3,4]ØZ
Non-OR	ØS9[Ø,2,3,4,5,6,7,8,9,B,C,D,F,G,H,J,K,L,M,N,P,Q][Ø,3,4]ZX
Non-OR	ØS9[Ø,2,3,4,5,6,7,8,9,B,C,D,F,G,H,J,K,L,M,N,P,Q][3,4]ZZ

Non-OR Procedure   DRG Non-OR Procedure   Valid OR Procedure   HAC Associated Procedure   Combination Only   New/Revised April   New/Revised October

604   **ICD-10-PCS 2023**

Ø **Medical and Surgical**
S **Lower Joints**
B **Excision**   Definition: Cutting out or off, without replacement, a portion of a body part
                   Explanation: The qualifier DIAGNOSTIC is used to identify excision procedures that are biopsies

Body Part Character 4	Approach Character 5	Device Character 6	Qualifier Character 7

Ø Lumbar Vertebral Joint
   Lumbar facet joint
2 Lumbar Vertebral Disc
3 Lumbosacral Joint
   Lumbosacral facet joint
4 Lumbosacral Disc
5 Sacrococcygeal Joint
   Sacrococcygeal symphysis
6 Coccygeal Joint
7 Sacroiliac Joint, Right
8 Sacroiliac Joint, Left
9 Hip Joint, Right
   Acetabulofemoral joint
B Hip Joint, Left
   See 9 Hip Joint, Right
C Knee Joint, Right
   Femoropatellar joint
   Femorotibial joint
   Lateral meniscus
   Medial meniscus
   Patellofemoral joint
   Tibiofemoral joint
D Knee Joint, Left
   See C Knee Joint, Right
F Ankle Joint, Right
   Inferior tibiofibular joint
   Talocrural joint
G Ankle Joint, Left
   See F Ankle Joint, Right
H Tarsal Joint, Right
   Calcaneocuboid joint
   Cuboideonavicular joint
   Cuneonavicular joint
   Intercuneiform joint
   Subtalar (talocalcaneal) joint
   Talocalcaneal (subtalar) joint
   Talocalcaneonavicular joint
J Tarsal Joint, Left
   See H Tarsal Joint, Right
K Tarsometatarsal Joint, Right
L Tarsometatarsal Joint, Left
M Metatarsal-Phalangeal Joint, Right
   Metatarsophalangeal (MTP) joint
N Metatarsal-Phalangeal Joint, Left
   See M Metatarsal-Phalangeal Joint, Right
P Toe Phalangeal Joint, Right
   Interphalangeal (IP) joint
Q Toe Phalangeal Joint, Left
   See P Toe Phalangeal Joint, Right
	Ø Open
	3 Percutaneous
	4 Percutaneous Endoscopic
		Z No Device	**X** Diagnostic
			Z No Qualifier

Non-OR ØSB[Ø,2,3,4,5,6,7,8,9,B,C,D,F,G,H,J,K,L,M,N,P,Q][Ø,3,4]ZX

Ø   Medical and Surgical
S   Lower Joints
C   Extirpation   Definition: Taking or cutting out solid matter from a body part

Explanation: The solid matter may be an abnormal byproduct of a biological function or a foreign body; it may be imbedded in a body part or in the lumen of a tubular body part. The solid matter may or may not have been previously broken into pieces.

Body Part Character 4	Approach Character 5	Device Character 6	Qualifier Character 7

Ø   Lumbar Vertebral Joint
    Lumbar facet joint
2   Lumbar Vertebral Disc
3   Lumbosacral Joint
    Lumbosacral facet joint
4   Lumbosacral Disc
5   Sacrococcygeal Joint
    Sacrococcygeal symphysis
6   Coccygeal Joint
7   Sacroiliac Joint, Right
8   Sacroiliac Joint, Left
9   Hip Joint, Right
    Acetabulofemoral joint
B   Hip Joint, Left
    See 9 Hip Joint, Right
C   Knee Joint, Right
    Femoropatellar joint
    Femorotibial joint
    Lateral meniscus
    Medial meniscus
    Patellofemoral joint
    Tibiofemoral joint
D   Knee Joint, Left
    See C Knee Joint, Right
F   Ankle Joint, Right
    Inferior tibiofibular joint
    Talocrural joint
G   Ankle Joint, Left
    See F Ankle Joint, Right
H   Tarsal Joint, Right
    Calcaneocuboid joint
    Cuboideonavicular joint
    Cuneonavicular joint
    Intercuneiform joint
    Subtalar (talocalcaneal) joint
    Talocalcaneal (subtalar) joint
    Talocalcaneonavicular joint
J   Tarsal Joint, Left
    See H Tarsal Joint, Right
K   Tarsometatarsal Joint, Right
L   Tarsometatarsal Joint, Left
M   Metatarsal-Phalangeal Joint, Right
    Metatarsophalangeal (MTP) joint
N   Metatarsal-Phalangeal Joint, Left
    See M Metatarsal-Phalangeal Joint, Right
P   Toe Phalangeal Joint, Right
    Interphalangeal (IP) joint
Q   Toe Phalangeal Joint, Left
    See P Toe Phalangeal Joint, Right
	Ø Open
	3 Percutaneous
	4 Percutaneous Endoscopic
		Z No Device	**Z No Qualifier**

Ø   **Medical and Surgical**
S   **Lower Joints**
G   **Fusion**   Definition: Joining together portions of an articular body part rendering the articular body part immobile
                 Explanation: The body part is joined together by fixation device, bone graft, or other means

Body Part Character 4	Approach Character 5	Device Character 6	Qualifier Character 7
Ø Lumbar Vertebral Joint Lumbar facet joint **1 Lumbar Vertebral Joints, 2 or more** ⊞ **3 Lumbosacral Joint** Lumbosacral facet joint	**Ø Open** **3 Percutaneous** **4 Percutaneous Endoscopic**	**7 Autologous Tissue Substitute** **J Synthetic Substitute** **K Nonautologous Tissue Substitute**	**Ø Anterior Approach, Anterior Column** **1 Posterior Approach, Posterior Column** **J Posterior Approach, Anterior Column**
Ø Lumbar Vertebral Joint Lumbar facet joint **1 Lumbar Vertebral Joints, 2 or more** ⊞ **3 Lumbosacral Joint** Lumbosacral facet joint	**Ø Open** **3 Percutaneous** **4 Percutaneous Endoscopic**	**A Interbody Fusion Device**	**Ø Anterior Approach, Anterior Column** **J Posterior Approach, Anterior Column**
5 Sacrococcygeal Joint Sacrococcygeal symphysis **6 Coccygeal Joint** **7 Sacroiliac Joint, Right** **8 Sacroiliac Joint, Left**	**Ø Open** **3 Percutaneous** **4 Percutaneous Endoscopic**	**4 Internal Fixation Device** **7 Autologous Tissue Substitute** **J Synthetic Substitute** **K Nonautologous Tissue Substitute**	**Z No Qualifier**
9 Hip Joint, Right Acetabulofemoral joint **B Hip Joint, Left** *See 9 Hip Joint, Right* **C Knee Joint, Right** Femoropatellar joint Femorotibial joint Lateral meniscus Medial meniscus Patellofemoral joint Tibiofemoral joint **D Knee Joint, Left** *See C Knee Joint, Right* **F Ankle Joint, Right** Inferior tibiofibular joint Talocrural joint **G Ankle Joint, Left** *See F Ankle Joint, Right* **H Tarsal Joint, Right** Calcaneocuboid joint Cuboideonavicular joint Cuneonavicular joint Intercuneiform joint Subtalar (talocalcaneal) joint Talocalcaneal (subtalar) joint Talocalcaneonavicular joint **J Tarsal Joint, Left** *See H Tarsal Joint, Right* **K Tarsometatarsal Joint, Right** **L Tarsometatarsal Joint, Left** **M Metatarsal-Phalangeal Joint, Right** Metatarsophalangeal (MTP) joint **N Metatarsal-Phalangeal Joint, Left** *See M Metatarsal-Phalangeal Joint, Right* **P Toe Phalangeal Joint, Right** Interphalangeal (IP) joint **Q Toe Phalangeal Joint, Left** *See P Toe Phalangeal Joint, Right*	**Ø Open** **3 Percutaneous** **4 Percutaneous Endoscopic**	**3 Internal Fixation Device, Sustained Compression** **4 Internal Fixation Device** **5 External Fixation Device** **7 Autologous Tissue Substitute** **J Synthetic Substitute** **K Nonautologous Tissue Substitute**	**Z No Qualifier**

HAC   ØSG[Ø,1,3][Ø,3,4][7,J,K][Ø,1,J] when reported with SDx K68.11 or T81.40–
        T81.49, T84.60-T84.619, T84.63-T84.7 with 7th character A

HAC   ØSG[Ø,1,3][Ø,3,4]A[Ø,J] when reported with SDx K68.11 or T81.40–T81.49,
        T84.60-T84.619, T84.63-T84.7 with 7th character A

HAC   ØSG[7,8][Ø,3,4][4,7,J,K]Z when reported with SDx K68.11 or T81.40–T81.49,
        T84.60-T84.619, T84.63-T84.7 with 7th character A

See Appendix L for Procedure Combinations
⊞   ØSG1[Ø,3,4][7,J,K][Ø,1,J]
⊞   ØSG1[Ø,3,4]A[Ø,J]

NC Noncovered Procedure   **LC** Limited Coverage   **OA** Questionable OB Admit   **NT** New Tech Add-on   ⊞ Combination Member   ♂ Male   ♀ Female

ICD-10-PCS 2023   607

ØSG–ØSG

Ø   **Medical and Surgical**
S   **Lower Joints**
H   **Insertion**   Definition: Putting in a nonbiological appliance that monitors, assists, performs, or prevents a physiological function but does not physically take the place of a body part

                         Explanation: None

Body Part Character 4	Approach Character 5	Device Character 6	Qualifier Character 7
Ø Lumbar Vertebral Joint Lumbar facet joint **3 Lumbosacral Joint** Lumbosacral facet joint	**Ø** Open **3** Percutaneous **4** Percutaneous Endoscopic	**3** Infusion Device **4** Internal Fixation Device **8** Spacer **B** Spinal Stabilization Device, Interspinous Process **C** Spinal Stabilization Device, Pedicle-Based **D** Spinal Stabilization Device, Facet Replacement	**Z** No Qualifier
2 Lumbar Vertebral Disc **4 Lumbosacral Disc**	**Ø** Open **3** Percutaneous **4** Percutaneous Endoscopic	**3** Infusion Device **8** Spacer	**Z** No Qualifier
5 Sacrococcygeal Joint Sacrococcygeal symphysis **6 Coccygeal Joint** **7 Sacroiliac Joint, Right** **8 Sacroiliac Joint, Left**	**Ø** Open **3** Percutaneous **4** Percutaneous Endoscopic	**3** Infusion Device **4** Internal Fixation Device **8** Spacer	**Z** No Qualifier
9 Hip Joint, Right Acetabulofemoral joint **B Hip Joint, Left** *See 9 Hip Joint, Right* **C Knee Joint, Right** Femoropatellar joint Femorotibial joint Lateral meniscus Medial meniscus Patellofemoral joint Tibiofemoral joint **D Knee Joint, Left** *See C Knee Joint, Right* **F Ankle Joint, Right** Inferior tibiofibular joint Talocrural joint **G Ankle Joint, Left** *See F Ankle Joint, Right* **H Tarsal Joint, Right** Calcaneocuboid joint Cuboideonavicular joint Cuneonavicular joint Intercuneiform joint Subtalar (talocalcaneal) joint Talocalcaneal (subtalar) joint Talocalcaneonavicular joint **J Tarsal Joint, Left** *See H Tarsal Joint, Right* **K Tarsometatarsal Joint, Right** **L Tarsometatarsal Joint, Left** **M Metatarsal-Phalangeal Joint, Right** Metatarsophalangeal (MTP) joint **N Metatarsal-Phalangeal Joint, Left** *See M Metatarsal-Phalangeal Joint, Right* **P Toe Phalangeal Joint, Right** Interphalangeal (IP) joint **Q Toe Phalangeal Joint, Left** *See P Toe Phalangeal Joint, Right*	**Ø** Open **3** Percutaneous **4** Percutaneous Endoscopic	**3** Infusion Device **4** Internal Fixation Device **5** External Fixation Device **8** Spacer	**Z** No Qualifier

Non-OR	ØSH[Ø,3][Ø,3,4][3,8]Z
Non-OR	ØSH[2,4][Ø,3,4][3,8]Z
Non-OR	ØSH[5,6,7,8][Ø,3,4][3,8]Z
Non-OR	ØSH[9,B,C,D][Ø,3,4]3Z
Non-OR	ØSH[9,B,C,D][3,4]8Z
Non-OR	ØSH[F,G,H,J,K,L,M,N,P,Q][Ø,3,4][3,8]Z

Non-OR Procedure   DRG Non-OR Procedure   Valid OR Procedure   HAC Associated Procedure   Combination Only   New/Revised April   New/Revised October

608   ICD-10-PCS 2023

ØSH–ØSH

Ø   **Medical and Surgical**
S   **Lower Joints**
J   **Inspection**   Definition: Visually and/or manually exploring a body part
     Explanation: Visual exploration may be performed with or without optical instrumentation. Manual exploration may be performed directly or through intervening body layers.

Body Part Character 4		Approach Character 5	Device Character 6	Qualifier Character 7

Ø Lumbar Vertebral Joint
  Lumbar facet joint
2 Lumbar Vertebral Disc
3 Lumbosacral Joint
  Lumbosacral facet joint
4 Lumbosacral Disc
5 Sacrococcygeal Joint
  Sacrococcygeal symphysis
6 Coccygeal Joint
7 Sacroiliac Joint, Right
8 Sacroiliac Joint, Left
9 Hip Joint, Right
  Acetabulofemoral joint
B Hip Joint, Left
  See 9 Hip Joint, Right
C Knee Joint, Right
  Femoropatellar joint
  Femorotibial joint
  Lateral meniscus
  Medial meniscus
  Patellofemoral joint
  Tibiofemoral joint
D Knee Joint, Left
  See C Knee Joint, Right
F Ankle Joint, Right
  Inferior tibiofibular joint
  Talocrural joint
G Ankle Joint, Left
  See F Ankle Joint, Right
	H Tarsal Joint, Right
	  Calcaneocuboid joint
	  Cuboideonavicular joint
	  Cuneonavicular joint
	  Intercuneiform joint
	  Subtalar (talocalcaneal) joint
	  Talocalcaneal (subtalar)
	    joint
	  Talocalcaneonavicular joint
	J Tarsal Joint, Left
	  See H Tarsal Joint, Right
	K Tarsometatarsal Joint,
	  Right
	L Tarsometatarsal Joint, Left
	M Metatarsal-Phalangeal
	  Joint, Right
	  Metatarsophalangeal (MTP)
	    joint
	N Metatarsal-Phalangeal
	  Joint, Left
	  *See M Metatarsal-Phalangeal
	    Joint, Right*
	P Toe Phalangeal Joint, Right
	  Interphalangeal (IP) joint
	Q Toe Phalangeal Joint, Left
	  *See P Toe Phalangeal Joint,
	    Right*
		Ø Open
		3 Percutaneous
		4 Percutaneous Endoscopic
		X External
			Z No Device	Z No Qualifier

Non-OR   ØSJ[Ø,2,3,4,5,6,7,8,9,B,C,D,F,G,H,J,K,L,M,N,P,Q][3,X]ZZ

Ø   **Medical and Surgical**
S   **Lower Joints**
N   **Release**   Definition: Freeing a body part from an abnormal physical constraint by cutting or by the use of force
     Explanation: Some of the restraining tissue may be taken out but none of the body part is taken out

Body Part Character 4		Approach Character 5	Device Character 6	Qualifier Character 7

Ø Lumbar Vertebral Joint
  Lumbar facet joint
2 Lumbar Vertebral Disc
3 Lumbosacral Joint
  Lumbosacral facet joint
4 Lumbosacral Disc
5 Sacrococcygeal Joint
  Sacrococcygeal symphysis
6 Coccygeal Joint
7 Sacroiliac Joint, Right
8 Sacroiliac Joint, Left
9 Hip Joint, Right
  Acetabulofemoral joint
B Hip Joint, Left
  See 9 Hip Joint, Right
C Knee Joint, Right
  Femoropatellar joint
  Femorotibial joint
  Lateral meniscus
  Medial meniscus
  Patellofemoral joint
  Tibiofemoral joint
D Knee Joint, Left
  See C Knee Joint, Right
F Ankle Joint, Right
  Inferior tibiofibular joint
  Talocrural joint
G Ankle Joint, Left
  See F Ankle Joint, Right
	H Tarsal Joint, Right
	  Calcaneocuboid joint
	  Cuboideonavicular joint
	  Cuneonavicular joint
	  Intercuneiform joint
	  Subtalar (talocalcaneal) joint
	  Talocalcaneal (subtalar)
	    joint
	  Talocalcaneonavicular joint
	J Tarsal Joint, Left
	  See H Tarsal Joint, Right
	K Tarsometatarsal Joint,
	  Right
	L Tarsometatarsal Joint, Left
	M Metatarsal-Phalangeal
	  Joint, Right
	  Metatarsophalangeal (MTP)
	    joint
	N Metatarsal-Phalangeal
	  Joint, Left
	  *See M Metatarsal-Phalangeal
	    Joint, Right*
	P Toe Phalangeal Joint, Right
	  Interphalangeal (IP) joint
	Q Toe Phalangeal Joint, Left
	  *See P Toe Phalangeal Joint,
	    Right*
		Ø Open
		3 Percutaneous
		4 Percutaneous Endoscopic
		X External
			Z No Device	Z No Qualifier

Non-OR   ØSN[Ø,2,3,4,5,6,7,8,9,B,C,D,F,G,H,J,K,L,M,N,P,Q]XZZ

NC Noncovered Procedure   LC Limited Coverage   QA Questionable OB Admit   NT New Tech Add-on   ⊞ Combination Member   ♂ Male   ♀ Female

ICD-10-PCS 2023   609

ØSJ–ØSN

Ø   Medical and Surgical
S   Lower Joints
P   Removal   Definition: Taking out or off a device from a body part

Explanation: If a device is taken out and a similar device put in without cutting or puncturing the skin or mucous membrane, the procedure is coded to the root operation CHANGE. Otherwise, the procedure for taking out the device is coded to the root operation REMOVAL.

Body Part Character 4	Approach Character 5	Device Character 6	Qualifier Character 7
Ø Lumbar Vertebral Joint Lumbar facet joint **3** Lumbosacral Joint Lumbosacral facet joint	**Ø** Open **3** Percutaneous **4** Percutaneous Endoscopic	**Ø** Drainage Device **3** Infusion Device **4** Internal Fixation Device **7** Autologous Tissue Substitute **8** Spacer **A** Interbody Fusion Device **J** Synthetic Substitute **K** Nonautologous Tissue Substitute	**Z** No Qualifier
Ø Lumbar Vertebral Joint Lumbar facet joint **3** Lumbosacral Joint Lumbosacral facet joint	**X** External	**Ø** Drainage Device **3** Infusion Device **4** Internal Fixation Device	**Z** No Qualifier
2 Lumbar Vertebral Disc **4** Lumbosacral Disc	**Ø** Open **3** Percutaneous **4** Percutaneous Endoscopic	**Ø** Drainage Device **3** Infusion Device **7** Autologous Tissue Substitute **J** Synthetic Substitute **K** Nonautologous Tissue Substitute	**Z** No Qualifier
2 Lumbar Vertebral Disc **4** Lumbosacral Disc	**X** External	**Ø** Drainage Device **3** Infusion Device	**Z** No Qualifier
5 Sacrococcygeal Joint Sacrococcygeal symphysis **6** Coccygeal Joint **7** Sacroiliac Joint, Right **8** Sacroiliac Joint, Left	**Ø** Open **3** Percutaneous **4** Percutaneous Endoscopic	**Ø** Drainage Device **3** Infusion Device **4** Internal Fixation Device **7** Autologous Tissue Substitute **8** Spacer **J** Synthetic Substitute **K** Nonautologous Tissue Substitute	**Z** No Qualifier
5 Sacrococcygeal Joint Sacrococcygeal symphysis **6** Coccygeal Joint **7** Sacroiliac Joint, Right **8** Sacroiliac Joint, Left	**X** External	**Ø** Drainage Device **3** Infusion Device **4** Internal Fixation Device	**Z** No Qualifier
9 Hip Joint, Right ⊞ Acetabulofemoral joint **B** Hip Joint, Left ⊞ See 9 Hip Joint, Right	**Ø** Open	**Ø** Drainage Device **3** Infusion Device **4** Internal Fixation Device **5** External Fixation Device **7** Autologous Tissue Substitute **8** Spacer **9** Liner **B** Resurfacing Device **E** Articulating Spacer **J** Synthetic Substitute **K** Nonautologous Tissue Substitute	**Z** No Qualifier
9 Hip Joint, Right ⊞ Acetabulofemoral joint **B** Hip Joint, Left ⊞ See 9 Hip Joint, Right	**3** Percutaneous **4** Percutaneous Endoscopic	**Ø** Drainage Device **3** Infusion Device **4** Internal Fixation Device **5** External Fixation Device **7** Autologous Tissue Substitute **8** Spacer **J** Synthetic Substitute **K** Nonautologous Tissue Substitute	**Z** No Qualifier
9 Hip Joint, Right Acetabulofemoral joint **B** Hip Joint, Left See 9 Hip Joint, Right	**X** External	**Ø** Drainage Device **3** Infusion Device **4** Internal Fixation Device **5** External Fixation Device	**Z** No Qualifier

Non-OR ØSP[Ø,3][Ø,3,4]8Z	**See Appendix L for Procedure Combinations**
Non-OR ØSP[Ø,3]3[Ø,3]Z	**Combo-only** ØSP[9,B]48Z
Non-OR ØSP[Ø,3]X[Ø,3,4]Z	⊞ ØSP[9,B]Ø[8,9,B,E,J]Z
Non-OR ØSP[2,4]3[Ø,3]Z	⊞ ØSP[9,B]4JZ
Non-OR ØSP[2,4]X[Ø,3]Z	
Non-OR ØSP[5,6,7,8][Ø,3,4]8Z	
Non-OR ØSP[5,6,7,8]3[Ø,3]Z	
Non-OR ØSP[5,6,7,8]X[Ø,3,4]Z	
Non-OR ØSP[9,B]3[Ø,3,8]Z	
Non-OR ØSP[9,B]X[Ø,3,4,5]Z	

ØSP Continued on next page

ØSP Continued

Ø   Medical and Surgical
S   Lower Joints
P   Removal

Definition: Taking out or off a device from a body part

Explanation: If a device is taken out and a similar device put in without cutting or puncturing the skin or mucous membrane, the procedure is coded to the root operation CHANGE. Otherwise, the procedure for taking out the device is coded to the root operation REMOVAL.

Body Part Character 4	Approach Character 5	Device Character 6	Qualifier Character 7

A   Hip Joint, Acetabular Surface, Right ⊞
E   Hip Joint, Acetabular Surface, Left ⊞
R   Hip Joint, Femoral Surface, Right ⊞
S   Hip Joint, Femoral Surface, Left ⊞
T   Knee Joint, Femoral Surface, Right ⊞
     Femoropatellar joint
     Patellofemoral joint
U   Knee Joint, Femoral Surface, Left ⊞
     See T Knee Joint, Femoral Surface, Right
V   Knee Joint, Tibial Surface, Right ⊞
     Femorotibial joint
     Tibiofemoral joint
W   Knee Joint, Tibial Surface, Left ⊞
     See V Knee Joint, Tibial Surface, Right
	Ø Open
	3 Percutaneous
	4 Percutaneous Endoscopic
		J Synthetic Substitute	Z No Qualifier

C   Knee Joint, Right ⊞
     Femoropatellar joint
     Femorotibial joint
     Lateral meniscus
     Medial meniscus
     Patellofemoral joint
     Tibiofemoral joint
D   Knee Joint, Left ⊞
     See C Knee Joint, Right
	Ø Open	Ø Drainage Device
		3 Infusion Device
		4 Internal Fixation Device
		5 External Fixation Device
		7 Autologous Tissue Substitute
		8 Spacer
		9 Liner
		E Articulating Spacer
		K Nonautologous Tissue Substitute
		L Synthetic Substitute, Unicondylar Medial
		M Synthetic Substitute, Unicondylar Lateral
		N Synthetic Substitute, Patellofemoral
			Z No Qualifier

C   Knee Joint, Right ⊞
     Femoropatellar joint
     Femorotibial joint
     Lateral meniscus
     Medial meniscus
     Patellofemoral joint
     Tibiofemoral joint
D   Knee Joint, Left ⊞
     See C Knee Joint, Right
	Ø Open	J Synthetic Substitute	C Patellar Surface
			Z No Qualifier

C   Knee Joint, Right ⊞
     Femoropatellar joint
     Femorotibial joint
     Lateral meniscus
     Medial meniscus
     Patellofemoral joint
     Tibiofemoral joint
D   Knee Joint, Left ⊞
     See C Knee Joint, Right
	3 Percutaneous
	4 Percutaneous Endoscopic
		Ø Drainage Device
		3 Infusion Device
		4 Internal Fixation Device
		5 External Fixation Device
		7 Autologous Tissue Substitute
		8 Spacer
		K Nonautologous Tissue Substitute
		L Synthetic Substitute, Unicondylar Medial
		M Synthetic Substitute, Unicondylar Lateral
		N Synthetic Substitute, Patellofemoral
			Z No Qualifier

C   Knee Joint, Right ⊞
     Femoropatellar joint
     Femorotibial joint
     Lateral meniscus
     Medial meniscus
     Patellofemoral joint
     Tibiofemoral joint
D   Knee Joint, Left ⊞
     See C Knee Joint, Right
	3 Percutaneous
	4 Percutaneous Endoscopic
		J Synthetic Substitute	C Patellar Surface
			Z No Qualifier

Non-OR	ØSP[C,D]3[Ø,3]Z

See Appendix L for Procedure Combinations

Combo-only	ØSP[C,D][3,4]8Z	⊞	ØSP[C,D]ØJ[C,Z]
⊞	ØSP[A,E,R,S,T,U,V,W][Ø,4]JZ	⊞	ØSP[C,D]4[L,M,N]Z
⊞	ØSP[C,D]Ø[8,9,E,L,M,N]Z	⊞	ØSP[C,D]4J[C,Z]

ØSP Continued on next page

NC Noncovered Procedure   LC Limited Coverage   QA Questionable OB Admit   NT New Tech Add-on   ⊞ Combination Member   ♂ Male   ♀ Female

ICD-10-PCS 2023   611

ØSP–ØSP

Lower Joints *(side tab)*

Ø   **Medical and Surgical**
S   **Lower Joints**
P   **Removal**

ØSP Continued

Definition: Taking out or off a device from a body part

Explanation: If a device is taken out and a similar device put in without cutting or puncturing the skin or mucous membrane, the procedure is coded to the root operation CHANGE. Otherwise, the procedure for taking out the device is coded to the root operation REMOVAL.

Body Part Character 4	Approach Character 5	Device Character 6	Qualifier Character 7

C   Knee Joint, Right
    Femoropatellar joint
    Femorotibial joint
    Lateral meniscus
    Medial meniscus
    Patellofemoral joint
    Tibiofemoral joint
D   Knee Joint, Left
    See C Knee Joint, Right
	X External	Ø Drainage Device
		3 Infusion Device
		4 Internal Fixation Device
		5 External Fixation Device
			Z No Qualifier

F   Ankle Joint, Right
    Inferior tibiofibular joint
    Talocrural joint
G   Ankle Joint, Left
    See F Ankle Joint, Right
H   Tarsal Joint, Right
    Calcaneocuboid joint
    Cuboideonavicular joint
    Cuneonavicular joint
    Intercuneiform joint
    Subtalar (talocalcaneal) joint
    Talocalcaneal (subtalar) joint
    Talocalcaneonavicular joint
J   Tarsal Joint, Left
    See H Tarsal Joint, Right
K   Tarsometatarsal Joint, Right
L   Tarsometatarsal Joint, Left
M   Metatarsal-Phalangeal Joint, Right
    Metatarsophalangeal (MTP) joint
N   Metatarsal-Phalangeal Joint, Left
    See M Metatarsal-Phalangeal Joint,
    Right
P   Toe Phalangeal Joint, Right
    Interphalangeal (IP) joint
Q   Toe Phalangeal Joint, Left
    See P Toe Phalangeal Joint, Right
	Ø Open
	3 Percutaneous
	4 Percutaneous Endoscopic
		Ø Drainage Device
		3 Infusion Device
		4 Internal Fixation Device
		5 External Fixation Device
		7 Autologous Tissue Substitute
		8 Spacer
		J Synthetic Substitute
		K Nonautologous Tissue Substitute
			Z No Qualifier

F   Ankle Joint, Right
    Inferior tibiofibular joint
    Talocrural joint
G   Ankle Joint, Left
    See F Ankle Joint, Right
H   Tarsal Joint, Right
    Calcaneocuboid joint
    Cuboideonavicular joint
    Cuneonavicular joint
    Intercuneiform joint
    Subtalar (talocalcaneal) joint
    Talocalcaneal (subtalar) joint
    Talocalcaneonavicular joint
J   Tarsal Joint, Left
    See H Tarsal Joint, Right
K   Tarsometatarsal Joint, Right
L   Tarsometatarsal Joint, Left
M   Metatarsal-Phalangeal Joint, Right
    Metatarsophalangeal (MTP) joint
N   Metatarsal-Phalangeal Joint, Left
    See M Metatarsal-Phalangeal Joint,
    Right
P   Toe Phalangeal Joint, Right
    Interphalangeal (IP) joint
Q   Toe Phalangeal Joint, Left
    See P Toe Phalangeal Joint, Right
	X External	Ø Drainage Device
		3 Infusion Device
		4 Internal Fixation Device
		5 External Fixation Device
			Z No Qualifier

Non-OR	ØSP[C,D]X[Ø,3,4,5]Z
Non-OR	ØSP[F,G,H,J,K,L,M,N,P,Q]3[Ø,3,8]Z
Non-OR	ØSP[F,G,H,J,K,L,M,N,P,Q][Ø,4]8Z
Non-OR	ØSP[F,G,H,J,K,L,M,N,P,Q]X[Ø,3,4,5]Z

Non-OR Procedure   DRG Non-OR Procedure   Valid OR Procedure   HAC Associated Procedure   Combination Only   New/Revised April   New/Revised October

ØSP–ØSP *(side tab)*

612   ICD-10-PCS 2023

Ø   **Medical and Surgical**
S   **Lower Joints**
Q   **Repair**   Definition: Restoring, to the extent possible, a body part to its normal anatomic structure and function
                            Explanation: Used only when the method to accomplish the repair is not one of the other root operations

Body Part Character 4	Approach Character 5	Device Character 6	Qualifier Character 7

Ø **Lumbar Vertebral Joint**
    Lumbar facet joint
2 **Lumbar Vertebral Disc**
3 **Lumbosacral Joint**
    Lumbosacral facet joint
4 **Lumbosacral Disc**
5 **Sacrococcygeal Joint**
    Sacrococcygeal symphysis
6 **Coccygeal Joint**
7 **Sacroiliac Joint, Right**
8 **Sacroiliac Joint, Left**
9 **Hip Joint, Right**
    Acetabulofemoral joint
B **Hip Joint, Left**
    See 9 Hip Joint, Right
C **Knee Joint, Right**
    Femoropatellar joint
    Femorotibial joint
    Lateral meniscus
    Medial meniscus
    Patellofemoral joint
    Tibiofemoral joint
D **Knee Joint, Left**
    See C Knee Joint, Right
F **Ankle Joint, Right**
    Inferior tibiofibular joint
    Talocrural joint
G **Ankle Joint, Left**
    See F Ankle Joint, Right
H **Tarsal Joint, Right**
    Calcaneocuboid joint
    Cuboideonavicular joint
    Cuneonavicular joint
    Intercuneiform joint
    Subtalar (talocalcaneal) joint
    Talocalcaneal (subtalar) joint
    Talocalcaneonavicular joint
J **Tarsal Joint, Left**
    See H Tarsal Joint, Right
K **Tarsometatarsal Joint, Right**
L **Tarsometatarsal Joint, Left**
M **Metatarsal-Phalangeal Joint, Right**
    Metatarsophalangeal (MTP) joint
N **Metatarsal-Phalangeal Joint, Left**
    See M Metatarsal-Phalangeal Joint, Right
P **Toe Phalangeal Joint, Right**
    Interphalangeal (IP) joint
Q **Toe Phalangeal Joint, Left**
    See P Toe Phalangeal Joint, Right
	Ø Open
	3 Percutaneous
	4 Percutaneous Endoscopic
	X External
		Z No Device	**Z** No Qualifier

Non-OR   ØSQ[Ø,2,3,4,5,6,7,8,9,B,C,D,F,G,H,J,K,L,M,N,P,Q]XZZ

Ø **Medical and Surgical**
S **Lower Joints**
R **Replacement** Definition: Putting in or on biological or synthetic material that physically takes the place and/or function of all or a portion of a body part
Explanation: The body part may have been taken out or replaced, or may be taken out, physically eradicated, or rendered nonfunctional during the REPLACEMENT procedure. A REMOVAL procedure is coded for taking out the device used in a previous replacement procedure.

Body Part Character 4	Approach Character 5	Device Character 6	Qualifier Character 7
Ø **Lumbar Vertebral Joint** Lumbar facet joint **2** **Lumbar Vertebral Disc** [NC] **3** **Lumbosacral Joint** Lumbosacral facet joint **4** **Lumbosacral Disc** [NC] **5** **Sacrococcygeal Joint** Sacrococcygeal symphysis **6** **Coccygeal Joint** **7** **Sacroiliac Joint, Right** **8** **Sacroiliac Joint, Left** **H** **Tarsal Joint, Right** Calcaneocuboid joint Cuboideonavicular joint Cuneonavicular joint Intercuneiform joint Subtalar (talocalcaneal) joint Talocalcaneal (subtalar) joint Talocalcaneonavicular joint **J** **Tarsal Joint, Left** *See H Tarsal Joint, Right* **K** **Tarsometatarsal Joint, Right** **L** **Tarsometatarsal Joint, Left** **M** **Metatarsal-Phalangeal Joint, Right** Metatarsophalangeal (MTP) joint **N** **Metatarsal-Phalangeal Joint, Left** *See M Metatarsal-Phalangeal Joint, Right* **P** **Toe Phalangeal Joint, Right** Interphalangeal (IP) joint **Q** **Toe Phalangeal Joint, Left** *See P Toe Phalangeal Joint, Right*	**Ø** Open	**7** Autologous Tissue Substitute **J** Synthetic Substitute **K** Nonautologous Tissue Substitute	**Z** No Qualifier
9 **Hip Joint, Right** ⊞ Acetabulofemoral joint **B** **Hip Joint, Left** ⊞ *See 9 Hip Joint, Right*	**Ø** Open	**1** Synthetic Substitute, Metal **2** Synthetic Substitute, Metal on Polyethylene **3** Synthetic Substitute, Ceramic **4** Synthetic Substitute, Ceramic on Polyethylene **6** Synthetic Substitute, Oxidized Zirconium on Polyethylene **J** Synthetic Substitute	**9** Cemented **A** Uncemented **Z** No Qualifier
9 **Hip Joint, Right** ⊞ Acetabulofemoral joint **B** **Hip Joint, Left** ⊞ *See 9 Hip Joint, Right*	**Ø** Open	**7** Autologous Tissue Substitute **E** Articulating Spacer **K** Nonautologous Tissue Substitute	**Z** No Qualifier
A **Hip Joint, Acetabular Surface, Right** ⊞ **E** **Hip Joint, Acetabular Surface, Left** ⊞	**Ø** Open	**Ø** Synthetic Substitute, Polyethylene **1** Synthetic Substitute, Metal **3** Synthetic Substitute, Ceramic **J** Synthetic Substitute	**9** Cemented **A** Uncemented **Z** No Qualifier
A **Hip Joint, Acetabular Surface, Right** **E** **Hip Joint, Acetabular Surface, Left**	**Ø** Open	**7** Autologous Tissue Substitute **K** Nonautologous Tissue Substitute	**Z** No Qualifier

HAC ØSR[9,B]Ø[1,2,3,4,6,J][9,A,Z] when reported with SDx of I26.Ø2-I26.Ø9, I26.92-I26.99, or I82.4Ø1-I82.4Z9

HAC ØSR[9,B]Ø[7,E,K]Z when reported with SDx of I26.Ø2-I26.Ø9, I26.92-I26.99, or I82.4Ø1-I82.4Z9

HAC ØSR[A,E]Ø[Ø,1,3,J][9,A,Z] when reported with SDx of I26.Ø2-I26.Ø9, I26.92-I26.99, or I82.4Ø1-I82.4Z9

HAC ØSR[A,E]Ø[7,K]Z when reported with SDx of I26.Ø2-I26.Ø9, I26.92-I26.99, or I82.4Ø1-I82.4Z9

NC ØSR[2,4]ØJZ when beneficiary age is over 6Ø

See Appendix L for Procedure Combinations
⊞ ØSR[9,B]Ø[1,2,3,4,6,J][9,A,Z]
⊞ ØSR[9,B]ØEZ
⊞ ØSR[A,E]Ø[Ø,1,3,J][9,A,Z]

ØSR Continued on next page

Ø	**Medical and Surgical**
S	**Lower Joints**
R	**Replacement**

ØSR Continued

Definition: Putting in or on biological or synthetic material that physically takes the place and/or function of all or a portion of a body part

Explanation: The body part may have been taken out or replaced, or may be taken out, physically eradicated, or rendered nonfunctional during the REPLACEMENT procedure. A REMOVAL procedure is coded for taking out the device used in a previous replacement procedure.

Body Part Character 4	Approach Character 5	Device Character 6	Qualifier Character 7
C Knee Joint, Right ⊞ Femoropatellar joint Femorotibial joint Lateral meniscus Medial meniscus Patellofemoral joint Tibiofemoral joint **D Knee Joint, Left** ⊞ *See C Knee Joint, Right*	Ø Open	6 Synthetic Substitute, Oxidized Zirconium on Polyethylene J Synthetic Substitute L Synthetic Substitute, Unicondylar Medial M Synthetic Substitute, Unicondylar Lateral N Synthetic Substitute, Patellofemoral	9 Cemented A Uncemented Z No Qualifier
C Knee Joint, Right ⊞ Femoropatellar joint Femorotibial joint Lateral meniscus Medial meniscus Patellofemoral joint Tibiofemoral joint **D Knee Joint, Left** ⊞ *See C Knee Joint, Right*	Ø Open	7 Autologous Tissue Substitute E Articulating Spacer K Nonautologous Tissue Substitute	Z No Qualifier
F Ankle Joint, Right Inferior tibiofibular joint Talocrural joint **G Ankle Joint, Left** *See F Ankle Joint, Right* **T Knee Joint, Femoral Surface, Right** Femoropatellar joint Patellofemoral joint **U Knee Joint, Femoral Surface, Left** *See T Knee Joint, Femoral Surface, Right* **V Knee Joint, Tibial Surface, Right** Femorotibial joint Tibiofemoral joint **W Knee Joint, Tibial Surface, Left** *See V Knee Joint, Tibial Surface, Right*	Ø Open	7 Autologous Tissue Substitute K Nonautologous Tissue Substitute	Z No Qualifier
F Ankle Joint, Right Inferior tibiofibular joint Talocrural joint **G Ankle Joint, Left** *See F Ankle Joint, Right* **T Knee Joint, Femoral Surface, Right** ⊞ Femoropatellar joint Patellofemoral joint **U Knee Joint, Femoral Surface, Left** ⊞ *See T Knee Joint, Femoral Surface, Right* **V Knee Joint, Tibial Surface, Right** ⊞ Femorotibial joint Tibiofemoral joint **W Knee Joint, Tibial Surface, Left** ⊞ *See V Knee Joint, Tibial Surface, Right*	Ø Open	J Synthetic Substitute	9 Cemented A Uncemented Z No Qualifier
R Hip Joint, Femoral Surface, Right ⊞ **S Hip Joint, Femoral Surface, Left** ⊞	Ø Open	1 Synthetic Substitute, Metal 3 Synthetic Substitute, Ceramic J Synthetic Substitute	9 Cemented A Uncemented Z No Qualifier
R Hip Joint, Femoral Surface, Right **S Hip Joint, Femoral Surface, Left**	Ø Open	7 Autologous Tissue Substitute K Nonautologous Tissue Substitute	Z No Qualifier

HAC ØSR[C,D]Ø[6,J,L,M,N][9,A,Z] when reported with SDx of I26.Ø2-I26.Ø9, I26.92-I26.99 or I82.4Ø1-I82.4Z9

HAC ØSR[C,D]Ø[7,E,K]Z when reported with SDx of I26.Ø2-I26.Ø9, I26.92-I26.99 or I82.4Ø1-I82.4Z9

HAC ØSR[T,U,V,W]Ø[7,K]Z when reported with SDx of I26.Ø2-I26.Ø9, I26.92-I26.99 or I82.4Ø1-I82.4Z9

HAC ØSR[T,U,V,W]ØJ[9,A,Z] when reported with SDx of I26.Ø2-I26.Ø9, I26.92-I26.99 or I82.4Ø1-I82.4Z9

HAC ØSR[R,S]Ø[1,3,J][9,A,Z] when reported with SDx of I26.Ø2-I26.Ø9, I26.92-I26.99, or I82.4Ø1-I82.4Z9

HAC ØSR[R,S]Ø[7,K]Z when reported with SDx of I26.Ø2-I26.Ø9, I26.92-I26.99, or I82.4Ø1-I82.4Z9

See Appendix L for Procedure Combinations
⊞ ØSR[C,D]Ø[6,J,L,M,N][9,A,Z]
⊞ ØSR[C,D]ØEZ
⊞ ØSR[T,U,V,W]ØJ[9,A,Z]
⊞ ØSR[R,S]Ø[1,3,J][9,A,Z]

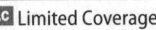 Noncovered Procedure   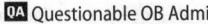 Limited Coverage   **ᴏᴀ** Questionable OB Admit   **ɴᴛ** New Tech Add-on   ⊞ Combination Member   ♂ Male   ♀ Female

ICD-10-PCS 2023   615

Ø Medical and Surgical
S Lower Joints
S Reposition Definition: Moving to its normal location, or other suitable location, all or a portion of a body part

Explanation: The body part is moved to a new location from an abnormal location, or from a normal location where it is not functioning correctly. The body part may or may not be cut out or off to be moved to the new location.

Body Part Character 4	Approach Character 5	Device Character 6	Qualifier Character 7
Ø Lumbar Vertebral Joint Lumbar facet joint **3** Lumbosacral Joint Lumbosacral facet joint **5** Sacrococcygeal Joint Sacrococcygeal symphysis **6** Coccygeal Joint **7** Sacroiliac Joint, Right **8** Sacroiliac Joint, Left	**Ø** Open **3** Percutaneous **4** Percutaneous Endoscopic **X** External	**4** Internal Fixation Device **Z** No Device	**Z** No Qualifier
9 Hip Joint, Right Acetabulofemoral joint **B** Hip Joint, Left *See 9 Hip Joint, Right* **C** Knee Joint, Right Femoropatellar joint Femorotibial joint Lateral meniscus Medial meniscus Patellofemoral joint Tibiofemoral joint **D** Knee Joint, Left *See C Knee Joint, Right* **F** Ankle Joint, Right Inferior tibiofibular joint Talocrural joint **G** Ankle Joint, Left *See F Ankle Joint, Right* **H** Tarsal Joint, Right Calcaneocuboid joint Cuboideonavicular joint Cuneonavicular joint Intercuneiform joint Subtalar (talocalcaneal) joint Talocalcaneal (subtalar) joint Talocalcaneonavicular joint **J** Tarsal Joint, Left *See H Tarsal Joint, Right* **K** Tarsometatarsal Joint, Right **L** Tarsometatarsal Joint, Left **M** Metatarsal-Phalangeal Joint, Right Metatarsophalangeal (MTP) joint **N** Metatarsal-Phalangeal Joint, Left *See M Metatarsal-Phalangeal Joint, Right* **P** Toe Phalangeal Joint, Right Interphalangeal (IP) joint **Q** Toe Phalangeal Joint, Left *See P Toe Phalangeal Joint, Right*	**Ø** Open **3** Percutaneous **4** Percutaneous Endoscopic **X** External	**4** Internal Fixation Device **5** External Fixation Device **Z** No Device	**Z** No Qualifier

Non-OR ØSS[Ø,3,5,6,][3,4,X][4,Z]Z
Non-OR ØSS[7,8]3ZZ
Non-OR ØSS[7,8][4,X][4,Z]Z
Non-OR ØSS[9,B]3ZZ
Non-OR ØSS[9,B][3,4,X]5Z
Non-OR ØSS[9,B][4,X][4,Z]Z
Non-OR ØSS[C,D,F,G,H,J,K,L,M,N,P,Q][3,4,X][4,5,Z]Z

Ø   Medical and Surgical
S   Lower Joints
T   Resection   Definition: Cutting out or off, without replacement, all of a body part
           Explanation: None

Body Part Character 4	Approach Character 5	Device Character 6	Qualifier Character 7
2 **Lumbar Vertebral Disc**	**Ø** Open	**Z** No Device	**Z** No Qualifier
4 **Lumbosacral Disc**			
5 **Sacrococcygeal Joint** Sacrococcygeal symphysis			
6 **Coccygeal Joint**			
7 **Sacroiliac Joint, Right**			
8 **Sacroiliac Joint, Left**			
9 **Hip Joint, Right** Acetabulofemoral joint			
B **Hip Joint, Left** *See 9 Hip Joint, Right*			

C   **Knee Joint, Right**
     Femoropatellar joint
     Femorotibial joint
     Lateral meniscus
     Medial meniscus
     Patellofemoral joint
     Tibiofemoral joint			

D **Knee Joint, Left** *See C Knee Joint, Right*			

F   **Ankle Joint, Right**
     Inferior tibiofibular joint
     Talocrural joint			

G **Ankle Joint, Left** *See F Ankle Joint, Right*			

H   **Tarsal Joint, Right**
     Calcaneocuboid joint
     Cuboideonavicular joint
     Cuneonavicular joint
     Intercuneiform joint
     Subtalar (talocalcaneal) joint
     Talocalcaneal (subtalar) joint
     Talocalcaneonavicular joint			

J **Tarsal Joint, Left** *See H Tarsal Joint, Right*			
K **Tarsometatarsal Joint, Right**			
L **Tarsometatarsal Joint, Left**			
M **Metatarsal-Phalangeal Joint, Right** Metatarsophalangeal (MTP) joint			
N **Metatarsal-Phalangeal Joint, Left** *See M Metatarsal-Phalangeal Joint, Right*			
P **Toe Phalangeal Joint, Right** Interphalangeal (IP) joint			
Q **Toe Phalangeal Joint, Left** *See P Toe Phalangeal Joint, Right*			

NC Noncovered Procedure   **LC** Limited Coverage   **QA** Questionable OB Admit   **NT** New Tech Add-on   **⊞** Combination Member   ♂ Male   ♀ Female

ICD-10-PCS 2023   617

Ø   Medical and Surgical
S   Lower Joints
U   Supplement

Definition: Putting in or on biological or synthetic material that physically reinforces and/or augments the function of a portion of a body part
Explanation: The biological material is non-living, or is living and from the same individual. The body part may have been previously replaced, and the SUPPLEMENT procedure is performed to physically reinforce and/or augment the function of the replaced body part.

Body Part Character 4	Approach Character 5	Device Character 6	Qualifier Character 7
Ø Lumbar Vertebral Joint Lumbar facet joint **2 Lumbar Vertebral Disc** **3 Lumbosacral Joint** Lumbosacral facet joint **4 Lumbosacral Disc** **5 Sacrococcygeal Joint** Sacrococcygeal symphysis **6 Coccygeal Joint** **7 Sacroiliac Joint, Right** **8 Sacroiliac Joint, Left** **F Ankle Joint, Right** Inferior tibiofibular joint Talocrural joint **G Ankle Joint, Left** *See F Ankle Joint, Right* **H Tarsal Joint, Right** Calcaneocuboid joint Cuboideonavicular joint Cuneonavicular joint Intercuneiform joint Subtalar (talocalcaneal) joint Talocalcaneal (subtalar) joint Talocalcaneonavicular joint **J Tarsal Joint, Left** *See H Tarsal Joint, Right* **K Tarsometatarsal Joint, Right** **L Tarsometatarsal Joint, Left** **M Metatarsal-Phalangeal Joint, Right** Metatarsophalangeal (MTP) joint **N Metatarsal-Phalangeal Joint, Left** *See M Metatarsal-Phalangeal Joint, Right* **P Toe Phalangeal Joint, Right** Interphalangeal (IP) joint **Q Toe Phalangeal Joint, Left** *See P Toe Phalangeal Joint, Right*	**Ø Open** **3 Percutaneous** **4 Percutaneous Endoscopic**	**7 Autologous Tissue Substitute** **J Synthetic Substitute** **K Nonautologous Tissue Substitute**	**Z No Qualifier**
9 Hip Joint, Right ⊞ Acetabulofemoral joint **B Hip Joint, Left** ⊞ *See 9 Hip Joint, Right*	**Ø Open**	**7 Autologous Tissue Substitute** **9 Liner** **B Resurfacing Device** **J Synthetic Substitute** **K Nonautologous Tissue Substitute**	**Z No Qualifier**
9 Hip Joint, Right Acetabulofemoral joint **B Hip Joint, Left** *See 9 Hip Joint, Right*	**3 Percutaneous** **4 Percutaneous Endoscopic**	**7 Autologous Tissue Substitute** **J Synthetic Substitute** **K Nonautologous Tissue Substitute**	**Z No Qualifier**
A Hip Joint, Acetabular Surface, Right ⊞ **E Hip Joint, Acetabular Surface, Left** ⊞ **R Hip Joint, Femoral Surface, Right** ⊞ **S Hip Joint, Femoral Surface, Left** ⊞	**Ø Open**	**9 Liner** **B Resurfacing Device**	**Z No Qualifier**
C Knee Joint, Right Femoropatellar joint Femorotibial joint Lateral meniscus Medial meniscus Patellofemoral joint Tibiofemoral joint **D Knee Joint, Left** *See C Knee Joint, Right*	**Ø Open**	**7 Autologous Tissue Substitute** **J Synthetic Substitute** **K Nonautologous Tissue Substitute**	**Z No Qualifier**
C Knee Joint, Right Femoropatellar joint Femorotibial joint Lateral meniscus Medial meniscus Patellofemoral joint Tibiofemoral joint **D Knee Joint, Left** *See C Knee Joint, Right*	**Ø Open**	**9 Liner**	**C Patellar Surface** **Z No Qualifier**

HAC   ØSU[9,B]ØBZ when reported with SDx of I26.Ø2-I26.Ø9,
       I26.92-I26.99, or I82.4Ø1-I82.4Z9
HAC   ØSU[A,E,R,S]ØBZ when reported with SDx of I26.Ø2-I26.Ø9,
       I26.92-I26.99, or I82.4Ø1-I82.4Z9

See Appendix L for Procedure Combinations
⊞   ØSU[9,B]Ø9Z
⊞   ØSU[A,E,R,S]Ø9Z

ØSU Continued on next page

Non-OR Procedure   DRG Non-OR Procedure   Valid OR Procedure   HAC Associated Procedure   Combination Only   New/Revised April   New/Revised October

ØSU Continued

Ø **Medical and Surgical**
S **Lower Joints**
U **Supplement**

Definition: Putting in or on biological or synthetic material that physically reinforces and/or augments the function of a portion of a body part
Explanation: The biological material is non-living, or is living and from the same individual. The body part may have been previously replaced, and the SUPPLEMENT procedure is performed to physically reinforce and/or augment the function of the replaced body part.

Body Part Character 4	Approach Character 5	Device Character 6	Qualifier Character 7

C **Knee Joint, Right**
  Femoropatellar joint
  Femorotibial joint
  Lateral meniscus
  Medial meniscus
  Patellofemoral joint
  Tibiofemoral joint
D **Knee Joint, Left**
  See C Knee Joint, Right
	3 Percutaneous
	4 Percutaneous Endoscopic
		7 Autologous Tissue Substitute
		J Synthetic Substitute
		K Nonautologous Tissue Substitute
			Z No Qualifier

T **Knee Joint, Femoral Surface, Right**
  Femoropatellar joint
  Patellofemoral joint
U **Knee Joint, Femoral Surface, Left**
  See T Knee Joint, Femoral Surface, Right
V **Knee Joint, Tibial Surface, Right** ⊞
  Femorotibial joint
  Tibiofemoral joint
W **Knee Joint, Tibial Surface, Left** ⊞
  See V Knee Joint, Tibial Surface, Right
	Ø Open	9 Liner	Z No Qualifier

See Appendix L for Procedure Combinations
⊞   ØSU[V,W]Ø9Z

NC Noncovered Procedure   LC Limited Coverage   QA Questionable OB Admit   NT New Tech Add-on   ⊞ Combination Member   ♂ Male   ♀ Female

ICD-10-PCS 2023   619

Ø Medical and Surgical
S Lower Joints
W Revision   Definition: Correcting, to the extent possible, a portion of a malfunctioning device or the position of a displaced device

Explanation: Revision can include correcting a malfunctioning or displaced device by taking out or putting in components of the device such as a screw or pin

Body Part Character 4	Approach Character 5	Device Character 6	Qualifier Character 7
Ø Lumbar Vertebral Joint Lumbar facet joint **3 Lumbosacral Joint** Lumbosacral facet joint	**Ø** Open **3** Percutaneous **4** Percutaneous Endoscopic **X** External	**Ø** Drainage Device **3** Infusion Device **4** Internal Fixation Device **7** Autologous Tissue Substitute **8** Spacer **A** Interbody Fusion Device **J** Synthetic Substitute **K** Nonautologous Tissue Substitute	**Z** No Qualifier
2 Lumbar Vertebral Disc **4 Lumbosacral Disc**	**Ø** Open **3** Percutaneous **4** Percutaneous Endoscopic **X** External	**Ø** Drainage Device **3** Infusion Device **7** Autologous Tissue Substitute **J** Synthetic Substitute **K** Nonautologous Tissue Substitute	**Z** No Qualifier
5 Sacrococcygeal Joint Sacrococcygeal symphysis **6 Coccygeal Joint** **7 Sacroiliac Joint, Right** **8 Sacroiliac Joint, Left**	**Ø** Open **3** Percutaneous **4** Percutaneous Endoscopic **X** External	**Ø** Drainage Device **3** Infusion Device **4** Internal Fixation Device **7** Autologous Tissue Substitute **8** Spacer **J** Synthetic Substitute **K** Nonautologous Tissue Substitute	**Z** No Qualifier
9 Hip Joint, Right Acetabulofemoral joint **B Hip Joint, Left** *See 9 Hip Joint, Right*	**Ø** Open	**Ø** Drainage Device **3** Infusion Device **4** Internal Fixation Device **5** External Fixation Device **7** Autologous Tissue Substitute **8** Spacer **9** Liner **B** Resurfacing Device **J** Synthetic Substitute **K** Nonautologous Tissue Substitute	**Z** No Qualifier
9 Hip Joint, Right Acetabulofemoral joint **B Hip Joint, Left** *See 9 Hip Joint, Right*	**3** Percutaneous **4** Percutaneous Endoscopic **X** External	**Ø** Drainage Device **3** Infusion Device **4** Internal Fixation Device **5** External Fixation Device **7** Autologous Tissue Substitute **8** Spacer **J** Synthetic Substitute **K** Nonautologous Tissue Substitute	**Z** No Qualifier
A Hip Joint, Acetabular Surface, Right **E Hip Joint, Acetabular Surface, Left** **R Hip Joint, Femoral Surface, Right** **S Hip Joint, Femoral Surface, Left** **T Knee Joint, Femoral Surface, Right** Femoropatellar joint Patellofemoral joint **U Knee Joint, Femoral Surface, Left** *See T Knee Joint, Femoral Surface, Right* **V Knee Joint, Tibial Surface, Right** Femorotibial joint Tibiofemoral joint **W Knee Joint, Tibial Surface, Left** *See V Knee Joint, Tibial Surface, Right*	**Ø** Open **3** Percutaneous **4** Percutaneous Endoscopic **X** External	**J** Synthetic Substitute	**Z** No Qualifier
C Knee Joint, Right Femoropatellar joint Femorotibial joint Lateral meniscus Medial meniscus Patellofemoral joint Tibiofemoral joint **D Knee Joint, Left** *See C Knee Joint, Right*	**Ø** Open	**Ø** Drainage Device **3** Infusion Device **4** Internal Fixation Device **5** External Fixation Device **7** Autologous Tissue Substitute **8** Spacer **9** Liner **K** Nonautologous Tissue Substitute	**Z** No Qualifier

Non-OR   ØSW[Ø,3]X[Ø,3,4,7,8,A,J,K]Z
Non-OR   ØSW[2,4]X[Ø,3,7,J,K]Z
Non-OR   ØSW[5,6,7,8]X[Ø,3,4,7,8,J,K]Z
Non-OR   ØSW[9,B]X[Ø,3,4,5,7,8,J,K]Z
Non-OR   ØSW[A,E,R,S,T,U,V,W]XJZ

ØSW Continued on next page

Non-OR Procedure   DRG Non-OR Procedure   Valid OR Procedure   HAC Associated Procedure   Combination Only   New/Revised April   New/Revised October

620   ICD-10-PCS 2023

Ø   **Medical and Surgical**
S   **Lower Joints**
W   **Revision**

ØSW Continued

Definition: Correcting, to the extent possible, a portion of a malfunctioning device or the position of a displaced device

Explanation: Revision can include correcting a malfunctioning or displaced device by taking out or putting in components of the device such as a screw or pin

Body Part Character 4	Approach Character 5	Device Character 6	Qualifier Character 7

C   **Knee Joint, Right**
   Femoropatellar joint
   Femorotibial joint
   Lateral meniscus
   Medial meniscus
   Patellofemoral joint
   Tibiofemoral joint
D   **Knee Joint, Left**
   See C Knee Joint, Right
	Ø Open	**J** Synthetic Substitute	**C** Patellar Surface
			Z No Qualifier

C   **Knee Joint, Right**
   Femoropatellar joint
   Femorotibial joint
   Lateral meniscus
   Medial meniscus
   Patellofemoral joint
   Tibiofemoral joint
D   **Knee Joint, Left**
   See C Knee Joint, Right
	3 Percutaneous
	4 Percutaneous Endoscopic
	X External
		Ø Drainage Device
		3 Infusion Device
		4 Internal Fixation Device
		5 External Fixation Device
		7 Autologous Tissue Substitute
		8 Spacer
		K Nonautologous Tissue Substitute
			Z No Qualifier

C   **Knee Joint, Right**
   Femoropatellar joint
   Femorotibial joint
   Lateral meniscus
   Medial meniscus
   Patellofemoral joint
   Tibiofemoral joint
D   **Knee Joint, Left**
   See C Knee Joint, Right
	3 Percutaneous
	4 Percutaneous Endoscopic
	X External
		J Synthetic Substitute	**C** Patellar Surface
			Z No Qualifier

F   **Ankle Joint, Right**
   Inferior tibiofibular joint
   Talocrural joint
G   **Ankle Joint, Left**
   See F Ankle Joint, Right
H   **Tarsal Joint, Right**
   Calcaneocuboid joint
   Cuboideonavicular joint
   Cuneonavicular joint
   Intercuneiform joint
   Subtalar (talocalcaneal) joint
   Talocalcaneal (subtalar) joint
   Talocalcaneonavicular joint
J   **Tarsal Joint, Left**
   See H Tarsal Joint, Right
K   **Tarsometatarsal Joint, Right**
L   **Tarsometatarsal Joint, Left**
M   **Metatarsal-Phalangeal Joint, Right**
   Metatarsophalangeal (MTP) joint
N   **Metatarsal-Phalangeal Joint, Left**
   See M Metatarsal-Phalangeal Joint, Right
P   **Toe Phalangeal Joint, Right**
   Interphalangeal (IP) joint
Q   **Toe Phalangeal Joint, Left**
   See P Toe Phalangeal Joint, Right
	Ø Open
	3 Percutaneous
	4 Percutaneous Endoscopic
	X External
		Ø Drainage Device
		3 Infusion Device
		4 Internal Fixation Device
		5 External Fixation Device
		7 Autologous Tissue Substitute
		8 Spacer
		J Synthetic Substitute
		K Nonautologous Tissue Substitute
			Z No Qualifier

Non-OR   ØSW[C,D]X[Ø,3,4,5,7,8,K]Z
Non-OR   ØSW[C,D]XJ[C,Z]
Non-OR   ØSW[F,G,H,J,K,L,M,N,P,Q]X[Ø,3,4,5,7,8,J,K]Z

NC Noncovered Procedure   **LC** Limited Coverage   **QA** Questionable OB Admit   **NT** New Tech Add-on   ⊞ Combination Member   ♂ Male   ♀ Female

ICD-10-PCS 2023   621

ØSW–ØSW

B   **Medical and Surgical**
S   **Lower Joints**
W   **Revision**   Definition: Correcting, to the extent possible, a malfunctioning or displaced device

Explanation: Revision can include correcting a malfunctioning or displaced device by taking out or putting in a portion of the device such as a screw or pin

0SW Continued

Body Part — Character 4	Approach — Character 5	Device — Character 6	Qualifier — Character 7
C Knee Joint, Right D Knee Joint, Left	0 Open	J Synthetic Substitute	C Patellar Surface Z No Qualifier

Urinary System ØT1–ØTY

Character Meanings

This Character Meaning table is provided as a guide to assist the user in the identification of character members that may be found in this section of code tables. It **SHOULD NOT** be used to build a PCS code.

Operation–Character 3	Body Part–Character 4	Approach–Character 5	Device–Character 6	Qualifier–Character 7
1　Bypass	Ø　Kidney, Right	Ø　Open	Ø　Drainage Device	Ø　Allogeneic
2　Change	1　Kidney, Left	3　Percutaneous	1　Radioactive Element	1　Syngeneic
5　Destruction	2　Kidneys, Bilateral	4　Percutaneous Endoscopic	2　Monitoring Device	2　Zooplastic
7　Dilation	3　Kidney Pelvis, Right	7　Via Natural or Artificial Opening	3　Infusion Device	3　Kidney Pelvis, Right
8　Division	4　Kidney Pelvis, Left	8　Via Natural or Artificial Opening Endoscopic	7　Autologous Tissue Substitute	4　Kidney Pelvis, Left
9　Drainage	5　Kidney	X　External	C　Extraluminal Device	6　Ureter, Right
B　Excision	6　Ureter, Right		D　Intraluminal Device	7　Ureter, Left
C　Extirpation	7　Ureter, Left		J　Synthetic Substitute	8　Colon
D　Extraction	8　Ureters, Bilateral		K　Nonautologous Tissue Substitute	9　Colocutaneous
F　Fragmentation	9　Ureter		L　Artificial Sphincter	A　Ileum
H　Insertion	B　Bladder		M　Stimulator Lead	B　Bladder
J　Inspection	C　Bladder Neck		Y　Other Device	C　Ileocutaneous
L　Occlusion	D　Urethra		Z　No Device	D　Cutaneous
M　Reattachment				X　Diagnostic
N　Release				Z　No Qualifier
P　Removal				
Q　Repair				
R　Replacement				
S　Reposition				
T　Resection				
U　Supplement				
V　Restriction				
W　Revision				
Y　Transplantation				

AHA Coding Clinic for table ØT1
2017, 3Q, 20　　Creation of Indiana pouch
2017, 3Q, 21　　Augmentation cystoplasty with Indiana pouch and continent urinary diversion
2017, 1Q, 37　　Perineal urethrostomy
2015, 3Q, 34　　Redo urinary diversion surgery via left ureteral reimplantation

AHA Coding Clinic for table ØT7
2019, 2Q, 16　　Reimplantation of ureters with insertion of tubes
2017, 4Q, 111　Exchange of ureteral stent
2016, 2Q, 27　　Exchange of ureteral stents
2015, 2Q, 8　　Urinary calculi fragmentation and evacuation
2013, 4Q, 123　Urolift® procedure

AHA Coding Clinic for table ØT9
2017, 3Q, 19　　Ureteral stent placement for urinary leakage
2017, 3Q, 20　　Creation of Indiana pouch
2017, 3Q, 21　　Augmentation cystoplasty with Indiana pouch and continent urinary diversion

AHA Coding Clinic for table ØTB
2016, 1Q, 19　　Biopsy of neobladder malignancy
2015, 3Q, 34　　Excision of Mitrofanoff polyp
2014, 2Q, 8　　Ileoscopy with excision of polyp of Ileal loop urinary diversion

AHA Coding Clinic for table ØTC
2019, 3Q, 4　　Evacuation of clots from bladder dome
2016, 3Q, 23　　Ureteral stone migrating into bladder
2015, 2Q, 7　　Urinary calculi fragmentation and evacuation
2015, 2Q, 8　　Urinary calculi fragmentation and evacuation
2013, 4Q, 122　Laser lithotripsy with removal of fragments

AHA Coding Clinic for table ØTF
2015, 2Q, 7　　Urinary calculi fragmentation and evacuation
2013, 4Q, 122　Extracorporeal shock wave lithotripsy
2013, 4Q, 122　Laser lithotripsy with removal of fragments

AHA Coding Clinic for table ØTH
2020, 4Q, 43-44　Insertion of radioactive element
2019, 2Q, 16　　Reimplantation of ureters with insertion of tubes

AHA Coding Clinic for table ØTP
2017, 4Q, 111　Exchange of ureteral stent
2016, 2Q, 27　　Exchange of ureteral stents

AHA Coding Clinic for table ØTQ
2018, 2Q, 27　　Dismembered pyeloplasty
2017, 1Q, 37　　Perineal urethrostomy

AHA Coding Clinic for table ØTR
2017, 3Q, 20　　Creation of Indiana pouch

AHA Coding Clinic for table ØTS
2019, 1Q, 29　　Young-Dees-Leadbetter bladder neck reconstruction
2018, 2Q, 27　　Dismembered pyeloplasty
2017, 1Q, 36　　Dismembered pyeloplasty
2016, 1Q, 15　　Pubovaginal sling placement

AHA Coding Clinic for table ØTT
2014, 3Q, 16　　Hand-assisted laparoscopy nephroureterectomy

AHA Coding Clinic for table ØTU
2019, 1Q, 29　　Young-Dees-Leadbetter bladder neck reconstruction
2017, 3Q, 21　　Augmentation cystoplasty with Indiana pouch and continent urinary diversion

AHA Coding Clinic for table ØTV
2015, 2Q, 11　　Cystourethroscopic Deflux® injection

Urinary System

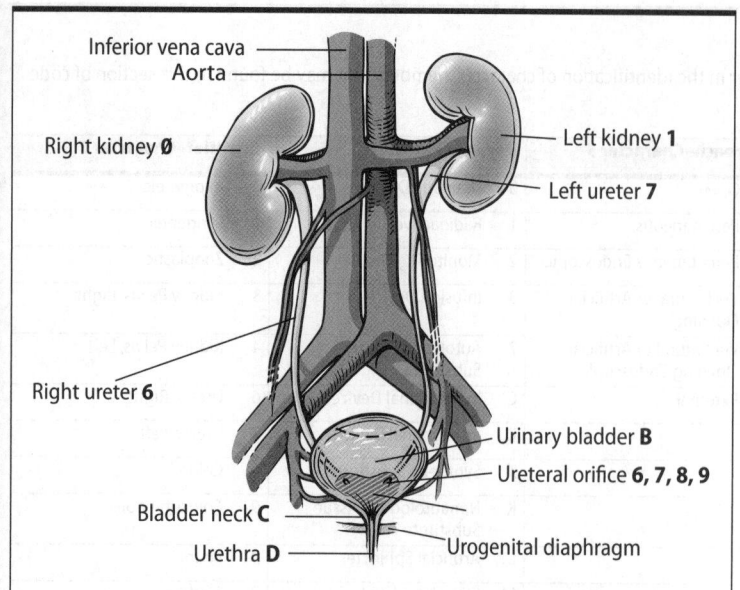

- Inferior vena cava
- Aorta
- Right kidney **Ø**
- Right ureter **6**
- Left kidney **1**
- Left ureter **7**
- Urinary bladder **B**
- Ureteral orifice **6, 7, 8, 9**
- Bladder neck **C**
- Urethra **D**
- Urogenital diaphragm

Kidney

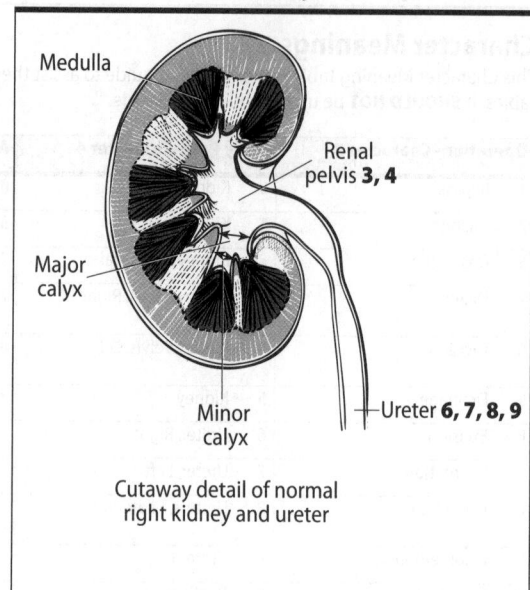

- Medulla
- Renal pelvis **3, 4**
- Major calyx
- Minor calyx
- Ureter **6, 7, 8, 9**

Cutaway detail of normal right kidney and ureter

Bladder

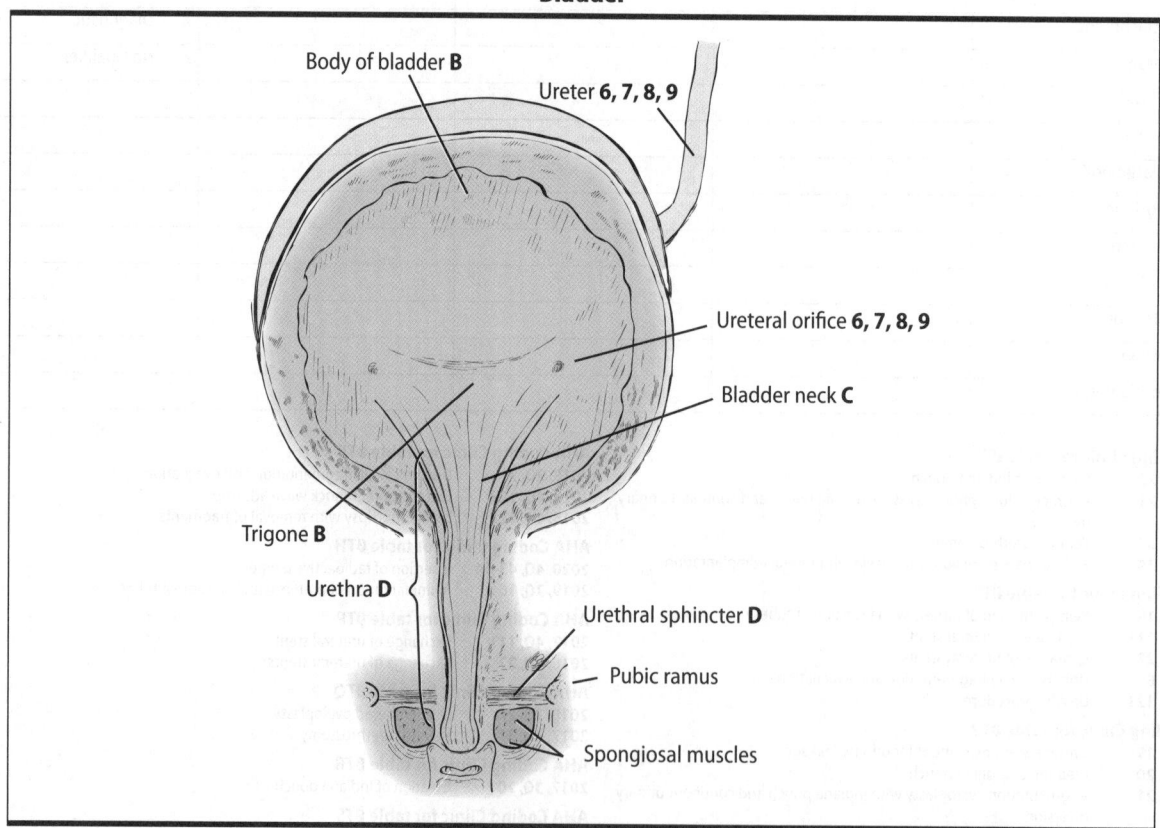

- Body of bladder **B**
- Ureter **6, 7, 8, 9**
- Ureteral orifice **6, 7, 8, 9**
- Bladder neck **C**
- Trigone **B**
- Urethra **D**
- Urethral sphincter **D**
- Pubic ramus
- Spongiosal muscles

Ø   **Medical and Surgical**
T   **Urinary System**
1   **Bypass**   Definition: Altering the route of passage of the contents of a tubular body part

           Explanation: Rerouting contents of a body part to a downstream area of the normal route, to a similar route and body part, or to an abnormal route and dissimilar body part. Includes one or more anastomoses, with or without the use of a device.

Body Part Character 4	Approach Character 5	Device Character 6	Qualifier Character 7

3 **Kidney Pelvis, Right**
  Ureteropelvic junction (UPJ)
4 **Kidney Pelvis, Left**
  See 3 Kidney Pelvis, Right
	Ø Open
	4 Percutaneous Endoscopic
		7 Autologous Tissue Substitute
		J Synthetic Substitute
		K Nonautologous Tissue Substitute
		Z No Device
			3 Kidney Pelvis, Right
			4 Kidney Pelvis, Left
			6 Ureter, Right
			7 Ureter, Left
			8 Colon
			9 Colocutaneous
			A Ileum
			B Bladder
			C Ileocutaneous
			D Cutaneous

3 **Kidney Pelvis, Right**
  Ureteropelvic junction (UPJ)
4 **Kidney Pelvis, Left**
  See 3 Kidney Pelvis, Right
	3 Percutaneous	J Synthetic Substitute	D Cutaneous

6 **Ureter, Right**
  Ureteral orifice
  Ureterovesical orifice
7 **Ureter, Left**
  See 6 Ureter, Right
8 **Ureters, Bilateral**
  See 6 Ureter, Right
	Ø Open
	4 Percutaneous Endoscopic
		7 Autologous Tissue Substitute
		J Synthetic Substitute
		K Nonautologous Tissue Substitute
		Z No Device
			6 Ureter, Right
			7 Ureter, Left
			8 Colon
			9 Colocutaneous
			A Ileum
			B Bladder
			C Ileocutaneous
			D Cutaneous

6 **Ureter, Right**
  Ureteral orifice
  Ureterovesical orifice
7 **Ureter, Left**
  See 6 Ureter, Right
8 **Ureters, Bilateral**
  See 6 Ureter, Right
	3 Percutaneous	J Synthetic Substitute	D Cutaneous

B **Bladder** Trigone of bladder	Ø Open 4 Percutaneous Endoscopic	7 Autologous Tissue Substitute J Synthetic Substitute K Nonautologous Tissue Substitute Z No Device	9 Colocutaneous C Ileocutaneous D Cutaneous
B **Bladder** Trigone of bladder	3 Percutaneous	J Synthetic Substitute	D Cutaneous

Ø   **Medical and Surgical**
T   **Urinary System**
2   **Change**   Definition: Taking out or off a device from a body part and putting back an identical or similar device in or on the same body part without cutting or puncturing the skin or a mucous membrane

           Explanation: All CHANGE procedures are coded using the approach EXTERNAL

Body Part Character 4	Approach Character 5	Device Character 6	Qualifier Character 7

5 **Kidney**
  Renal calyx
  Renal capsule
  Renal cortex
  Renal segment
9 **Ureter**
  Ureteral orifice
  Ureterovesical orifice
B **Bladder**
  Trigone of bladder
D **Urethra**
  Bulbourethral (Cowper's) gland
  Cowper's (bulbourethral) gland
  External urethral sphincter
  Internal urethral sphincter
  Membranous urethra
  Penile urethra
  Prostatic urethra
	X External	Ø Drainage Device
		Y Other Device
			Z No Qualifier

Non-OR   All body part, approach, device, and qualifier values

NC Noncovered Procedure   LC Limited Coverage   QA Questionable OB Admit   NT New Tech Add-on   ⊞ Combination Member   ♂ Male   ♀ Female

ICD-10-PCS 2023   625

ØT1–ØT2

Urinary System

Ø   **Medical and Surgical**
T   **Urinary System**
5   **Destruction**   Definition: Physical eradication of all or a portion of a body part by the direct use of energy, force, or a destructive agent

Explanation: None of the body part is physically taken out

Body Part Character 4	Approach Character 5	Device Character 6	Qualifier Character 7

Ø **Kidney, Right**
   Renal calyx
   Renal capsule
   Renal cortex
   Renal segment
1 **Kidney, Left**
   See Ø Kidney, Right
3 **Kidney Pelvis, Right**
   Ureteropelvic junction (UPJ)
4 **Kidney Pelvis, Left**
   See 3 Kidney Pelvis, Right
6 **Ureter, Right**
   Ureteral orifice
   Ureterovesical orifice
7 **Ureter, Left**
   See 6 Ureter, Right
B **Bladder**
   Trigone of bladder
C **Bladder Neck**
	Ø Open
	3 Percutaneous
	4 Percutaneous Endoscopic
	7 Via Natural or Artificial Opening
	8 Via Natural or Artificial Opening
	   Endoscopic
		Z No Device	Z No Qualifier

D **Urethra**
   Bulbourethral (Cowper's) gland
   Cowper's (bulbourethral) gland
   External urethral sphincter
   Internal urethral sphincter
   Membranous urethra
   Penile urethra
   Prostatic urethra
	Ø Open
	3 Percutaneous
	4 Percutaneous Endoscopic
	7 Via Natural or Artificial Opening
	8 Via Natural or Artificial Opening
	   Endoscopic
	X External
		Z No Device	Z No Qualifier

Non-OR   ØT5D[Ø,3,4,7,8,X]ZZ

Ø   **Medical and Surgical**
T   **Urinary System**
7   **Dilation**   Definition: Expanding an orifice or the lumen of a tubular body part

Explanation: The orifice can be a natural orifice or an artificially created orifice. Accomplished by stretching a tubular body part using intraluminal pressure or by cutting part of the orifice or wall of the tubular body part.

Body Part Character 4	Approach Character 5	Device Character 6	Qualifier Character 7

3 **Kidney Pelvis, Right**
   Ureteropelvic junction (UPJ)
4 **Kidney Pelvis, Left**
   See 3 Kidney Pelvis, Right
6 **Ureter, Right**
   Ureteral orifice
   Ureterovesical orifice
7 **Ureter, Left**
   See 6 Ureter, Right
8 **Ureters, Bilateral**
   See 6 Ureter, Right
B **Bladder**
   Trigone of bladder
C **Bladder Neck**
D **Urethra**
   Bulbourethral (Cowper's) gland
   Cowper's (bulbourethral) gland
   External urethral sphincter
   Internal urethral sphincter
   Membranous urethra
   Penile urethra
   Prostatic urethra
	Ø Open
	3 Percutaneous
	4 Percutaneous Endoscopic
	7 Via Natural or Artificial Opening
	8 Via Natural or Artificial Opening
	   Endoscopic
		D Intraluminal Device
		Z No Device
			Z No Qualifier

Non-OR   ØT7[6,7,8][Ø,3,4,7]DZ   Non-OR   ØT7B7[D,Z]Z   Non-OR   ØT7[C,D][7,8][D,Z]Z
Non-OR   ØT7[6,7,8]7ZZ   Non-OR   ØT7C[Ø,3,4]ZZ
Non-OR   ØT788ZZ   Non-OR   ØT7[C,D][Ø,3,4]DZ

Ø   **Medical and Surgical**
T   **Urinary System**
8   **Division**   Definition: Cutting into a body part, without draining fluids and/or gases from the body part, in order to separate or transect a body part

Explanation: All or a portion of the body part is separated into two or more portions

Body Part Character 4	Approach Character 5	Device Character 6	Qualifier Character 7

2 **Kidneys, Bilateral**
   Renal calyx
   Renal capsule
   Renal cortex
   Renal segment
C **Bladder Neck**
	Ø Open
	3 Percutaneous
	4 Percutaneous Endoscopic
		Z No Device	Z No Qualifier

Non-OR Procedure   DRG Non-OR Procedure   Valid OR Procedure   HAC Associated Procedure   Combination Only   New/Revised April   New/Revised October

626   ICD-10-PCS 2023

0   Medical and Surgical
T   Urinary System
9   Drainage   Definition: Taking or letting out fluids and/or gases from a body part
                          Explanation: The qualifier DIAGNOSTIC is used to identify drainage procedures that are biopsies

Body Part Character 4	Approach Character 5	Device Character 6	Qualifier Character 7
0 Kidney, Right Renal calyx Renal capsule Renal cortex Renal segment **1 Kidney, Left** *See 0 Kidney, Right* **3 Kidney Pelvis, Right** Ureteropelvic junction (UPJ) **4 Kidney Pelvis, Left** *See 3 Kidney Pelvis, Right* **6 Ureter, Right** Ureteral orifice Ureterovesical orifice **7 Ureter, Left** *See 6 Ureter, Right* **8 Ureters, Bilateral** *See 6 Ureter, Right* **B Bladder** Trigone of bladder **C Bladder Neck**	**0 Open** **3 Percutaneous** **4 Percutaneous Endoscopic** **7 Via Natural or Artificial Opening** **8 Via Natural or Artificial Opening** **Endoscopic**	**0 Drainage Device**	**Z No Qualifier**
0 Kidney, Right Renal calyx Renal capsule Renal cortex Renal segment **1 Kidney, Left** *See 0 Kidney, Right* **3 Kidney Pelvis, Right** Ureteropelvic junction (UPJ) **4 Kidney Pelvis, Left** *See 3 Kidney Pelvis, Right* **6 Ureter, Right** Ureteral orifice Ureterovesical orifice **7 Ureter, Left** *See 6 Ureter, Right* **8 Ureters, Bilateral** *See 6 Ureter, Right* **B Bladder** Trigone of bladder **C Bladder Neck**	**0 Open** **3 Percutaneous** **4 Percutaneous Endoscopic** **7 Via Natural or Artificial Opening** **8 Via Natural or Artificial Opening** **Endoscopic**	**Z No Device**	**X Diagnostic** **Z No Qualifier**
D Urethra Bulbourethral (Cowper's) gland Cowper's (bulbourethral) gland External urethral sphincter Internal urethral sphincter Membranous urethra Penile urethra Prostatic urethra	**0 Open** **3 Percutaneous** **4 Percutaneous Endoscopic** **7 Via Natural or Artificial Opening** **8 Via Natural or Artificial Opening** **Endoscopic** **X External**	**0 Drainage Device**	**Z No Qualifier**
D Urethra Bulbourethral (Cowper's) gland Cowper's (bulbourethral) gland External urethral sphincter Internal urethral sphincter Membranous urethra Penile urethra Prostatic urethra	**0 Open** **3 Percutaneous** **4 Percutaneous Endoscopic** **7 Via Natural or Artificial Opening** **8 Via Natural or Artificial Opening** **Endoscopic** **X External**	**Z No Device**	**X Diagnostic** **Z No Qualifier**

Non-OR	0T9[0,1,3,4]30Z
Non-OR	0T9[6,7,8][0,3,4,7,8]0Z
Non-OR	0T9[B,C][3,4,7,8]0Z
Non-OR	0T9[0,1,3,4,6,7,8][3,4,7,8]ZX
Non-OR	0T9[0,1,3,4][3,4]ZZ
Non-OR	0T9[6,7,8]3ZZ
Non-OR	0T9[B,C][3,4,7,8]ZZ
Non-OR	0T9D30Z
Non-OR	0T9D[0,3,4,7,8,X]ZX
Non-OR	0T9D3ZZ

NC Noncovered Procedure   LC Limited Coverage   QA Questionable OB Admit   NT New Tech Add-on   ⊞ Combination Member   ♂ Male   ♀ Female

ICD-10-PCS 2023   627

Urinary System

Ø Medical and Surgical
T Urinary System
B Excision

Definition: Cutting out or off, without replacement, a portion of a body part

Explanation: The qualifier DIAGNOSTIC is used to identify excision procedures that are biopsies

Body Part Character 4	Approach Character 5	Device Character 6	Qualifier Character 7
Ø Kidney, Right Renal calyx Renal capsule Renal cortex Renal segment **1** Kidney, Left *See Ø Kidney, Right* **3** Kidney Pelvis, Right Ureteropelvic junction (UPJ) **4** Kidney Pelvis, Left *See 3 Kidney Pelvis, Right* **6** Ureter, Right Ureteral orifice Ureterovesical orifice **7** Ureter, Left *See 6 Ureter, Right* **B** Bladder Trigone of bladder **C** Bladder Neck	**Ø** Open **3** Percutaneous **4** Percutaneous Endoscopic **7** Via Natural or Artificial Opening **8** Via Natural or Artificial Opening Endoscopic	**Z** No Device	**X** Diagnostic **Z** No Qualifier
D Urethra Bulbourethral (Cowper's) gland Cowper's (bulbourethral) gland External urethral sphincter Internal urethral sphincter Membranous urethra Penile urethra Prostatic urethra	**Ø** Open **3** Percutaneous **4** Percutaneous Endoscopic **7** Via Natural or Artificial Opening **8** Via Natural or Artificial Opening Endoscopic **X** External	**Z** No Device	**X** Diagnostic **Z** No Qualifier

Non-OR   ØTB[Ø,1,3,4,6,7][3,4,7,8]ZX
Non-OR   ØTBD[Ø,3,4,7,8,X]ZX

Ø Medical and Surgical
T Urinary System
C Extirpation

Definition: Taking or cutting out solid matter from a body part

Explanation: The solid matter may be an abnormal byproduct of a biological function or a foreign body; it may be imbedded in a body part or in the lumen of a tubular body part. The solid matter may or may not have been previously broken into pieces.

Body Part Character 4	Approach Character 5	Device Character 6	Qualifier Character 7
Ø Kidney, Right Renal calyx Renal capsule Renal cortex Renal segment **1** Kidney, Left *See Ø Kidney, Right* **3** Kidney Pelvis, Right Ureteropelvic junction (UPJ) **4** Kidney Pelvis, Left *See 3 Kidney Pelvis, Right* **6** Ureter, Right Ureteral orifice Ureterovesical orifice **7** Ureter, Left *See 6 Ureter, Right* **B** Bladder Trigone of bladder **C** Bladder Neck	**Ø** Open **3** Percutaneous **4** Percutaneous Endoscopic **7** Via Natural or Artificial Opening **8** Via Natural or Artificial Opening Endoscopic	**Z** No Device	**Z** No Qualifier
D Urethra Bulbourethral (Cowper's) gland Cowper's (bulbourethral) gland External urethral sphincter Internal urethral sphincter Membranous urethra Penile urethra Prostatic urethra	**Ø** Open **3** Percutaneous **4** Percutaneous Endoscopic **7** Via Natural or Artificial Opening **8** Via Natural or Artificial Opening Endoscopic **X** External	**Z** No Device	**Z** No Qualifier

Non-OR   ØTC[Ø,1,3,4,6,7]8ZZ
Non-OR   ØTC[B,C][7,8]ZZ
Non-OR   ØTCD[7,8,X]ZZ

Non-OR Procedure   DRG Non-OR Procedure   Valid OR Procedure   HAC Associated Procedure   Combination Only   New/Revised April   New/Revised October

Ø   Medical and Surgical
T   Urinary System
D   Extraction   Definition: Pulling or stripping out or off all or a portion of a body part by the use of force

       Explanation: The qualifier DIAGNOSTIC is used to identify extraction procedures that are biopsies

Body Part Character 4	Approach Character 5	Device Character 6	Qualifier Character 7

Ø Kidney, Right
   Renal calyx
   Renal capsule
   Renal cortex
   Renal segment
1 Kidney, Left
   See Ø Kidney, Right
	Ø Open
	3 Percutaneous
	4 Percutaneous Endoscopic
		Z No Device	**Z** No Qualifier

Ø   Medical and Surgical
T   Urinary System
F   Fragmentation   Definition: Breaking solid matter in a body part into pieces

       Explanation: Physical force (e.g., manual, ultrasonic) applied directly or indirectly is used to break the solid matter into pieces. The solid matter may be an abnormal byproduct of a biological function or a foreign body. The pieces of solid matter are not taken out.

Body Part Character 4	Approach Character 5	Device Character 6	Qualifier Character 7

3 Kidney Pelvis, Right
   Ureteropelvic junction (UPJ)
4 Kidney Pelvis, Left
   See 3 Kidney Pelvis, Right
6 Ureter, Right
   Ureteral orifice
   Ureterovesical orifice
7 Ureter, Left
   See 6 Ureter, Right
B Bladder
   Trigone of bladder
C Bladder Neck
D Urethra   `NC`
   Bulbourethral (Cowper's) gland
   Cowper's (bulbourethral) gland
   External urethral sphincter
   Internal urethral sphincter
   Membranous urethra
   Penile urethra
   Prostatic urethra
	Ø Open
	3 Percutaneous
	4 Percutaneous Endoscopic
	7 Via Natural or Artificial Opening
	8 Via Natural or Artificial Opening
	   Endoscopic
	X External
		Z No Device	**Z** No Qualifier

Non-OR	ØTF[3,4][Ø,7,8]ZZ
Non-OR	ØTF[6,7,B,C,D][Ø,3,4,7,8]ZZ
Non-OR	ØTF[3,4,6,7,B,C,D]XZZ
NC	ØTFDXZZ

`NC` Noncovered Procedure   `LC` Limited Coverage   `QA` Questionable OB Admit   `NT` New Tech Add-on   ⊞ Combination Member   ♂ Male   ♀ Female

ICD-10-PCS 2023   **629**

Urinary System

Ø   **Medical and Surgical**
T   **Urinary System**
H   **Insertion**   Definition: Putting in a nonbiological appliance that monitors, assists, performs, or prevents a physiological function but does not physically
                          take the place of a body part
                          Explanation: None

Body Part Character 4	Approach Character 5	Device Character 6	Qualifier Character 7

5 Kidney
   Renal calyx
   Renal capsule
   Renal cortex
   Renal segment
	Ø Open
	3 Percutaneous
	4 Percutaneous Endoscopic
	7 Via Natural or Artificial Opening
	8 Via Natural or Artificial Opening
	    Endoscopic
		1 Radioactive Element
		2 Monitoring Device
		3 Infusion Device
		Y Other Device
			Z No Qualifier

9 Ureter
   Ureteral orifice
   Ureterovesical orifice
	Ø Open
	3 Percutaneous
	4 Percutaneous Endoscopic
	7 Via Natural or Artificial Opening
	8 Via Natural or Artificial Opening
	    Endoscopic
		1 Radioactive Element
		2 Monitoring Device
		3 Infusion Device
		M Stimulator Lead
		Y Other Device
			Z No Qualifier

B Bladder   **NC**
   Trigone of bladder
	Ø Open
	3 Percutaneous
	4 Percutaneous Endoscopic
	7 Via Natural or Artificial Opening
	8 Via Natural or Artificial Opening
	    Endoscopic
		1 Radioactive Element
		2 Monitoring Device
		3 Infusion Device
		L Artificial Sphincter
		M Stimulator Lead
		Y Other Device
			Z No Qualifier

C Bladder Neck	**Ø** Open **3** Percutaneous **4** Percutaneous Endoscopic **7** Via Natural or Artificial Opening **8** Via Natural or Artificial Opening Endoscopic	**L** Artificial Sphincter	**Z** No Qualifier

D Urethra
   Bulbourethral (Cowper's) gland
   Cowper's (bulbourethral) gland
   External urethral sphincter
   Internal urethral sphincter
   Membranous urethra
   Penile urethra
   Prostatic urethra
	Ø Open
	3 Percutaneous
	4 Percutaneous Endoscopic
	7 Via Natural or Artificial Opening
	8 Via Natural or Artificial Opening
	    Endoscopic
		1 Radioactive Element
		2 Monitoring Device
		3 Infusion Device
		L Artificial Sphincter
		Y Other Device
			Z No Qualifier

D Urethra
   Bulbourethral (Cowper's) gland
   Cowper's (bulbourethral) gland
   External urethral sphincter
   Internal urethral sphincter
   Membranous urethra
   Penile urethra
   Prostatic urethra
	X External	**2** Monitoring Device
		3 Infusion Device
		L Artificial Sphincter
			Z No Qualifier

Non-OR ØTH5Ø3Z		**Non-OR** ØTHB3[1,3,Y]Z	
Non-OR ØTH53[1,3,Y]Z		**Non-OR** ØTHB4[3,Y]Z	
Non-OR ØTH54[3,Y]Z		**Non-OR** ØTHB7[1,2,3,Y]Z	
Non-OR ØTH57[1,2,3,Y]Z		**Non-OR** ØTHB8[2,3]Z	
Non-OR ØTH58[2,3]Z		**Non-OR** ØTHDØ3Z	
Non-OR ØTH9Ø3Z		**Non-OR** ØTHD3[1,3,Y]Z	
Non-OR ØTH93[1,3,Y]Z		**Non-OR** ØTHD4[3,Y]Z	
Non-OR ØTH94[3,Y]Z		**Non-OR** ØTHD7[1,2,3,Y]Z	
Non-OR ØTH97[1,2,3,Y]Z		**Non-OR** ØTHD8[2,3,Y]Z	
Non-OR ØTH98[2,3]Z		**Non-OR** ØTHDX3Z	
Non-OR ØTHBØ3Z		**NC** ØTHB[Ø,3,4,7,8]MZ	

Non-OR Procedure   DRG Non-OR Procedure   Valid OR Procedure   HAC Associated Procedure   Combination Only   New/Revised April   New/Revised October

630   ICD-10-PCS 2023

Ø   Medical and Surgical
T   Urinary System
J   Inspection   Definition: Visually and/or manually exploring a body part

Explanation: Visual exploration may be performed with or without optical instrumentation. Manual exploration may be performed directly or through intervening body layers.

Body Part Character 4	Approach Character 5	Device Character 6	Qualifier Character 7
5 Kidney Renal calyx Renal capsule Renal cortex Renal segment **9 Ureter** Ureteral orifice Ureterovesical orifice **B Bladder** Trigone of bladder **D Urethra** Bulbourethral (Cowper's) gland Cowper's (bulbourethral) gland External urethral sphincter Internal urethral sphincter Membranous urethra Penile urethra Prostatic urethra	**Ø** Open **3** Percutaneous **4** Percutaneous Endoscopic **7** Via Natural or Artificial Opening **8** Via Natural or Artificial Opening Endoscopic **X** External	**Z** No Device	**Z** No Qualifier

Non-OR   ØTJ[5,9,D][3,4,7,8,X]ZZ
Non-OR   ØTJB[3,7,8,X]ZZ

Ø   Medical and Surgical
T   Urinary System
L   Occlusion   Definition: Completely closing an orifice or the lumen of a tubular body part

Explanation: The orifice can be a natural orifice or an artificially created orifice

Body Part Character 4	Approach Character 5	Device Character 6	Qualifier Character 7
3 Kidney Pelvis, Right Ureteropelvic junction (UPJ) **4 Kidney Pelvis, Left** *See 3 Kidney Pelvis, Right* **6 Ureter, Right** Ureteral orifice Ureterovesical orifice **7 Ureter, Left** *See 6 Ureter, Right* **B Bladder** Trigone of bladder **C Bladder Neck**	**Ø** Open **3** Percutaneous **4** Percutaneous Endoscopic	**C** Extraluminal Device **D** Intraluminal Device **Z** No Device	**Z** No Qualifier
3 Kidney Pelvis, Right Ureteropelvic junction (UPJ) **4 Kidney Pelvis, Left** *See 3 Kidney Pelvis, Right* **6 Ureter, Right** Ureteral orifice Ureterovesical orifice **7 Ureter, Left** *See 6 Ureter, Right* **B Bladder** Trigone of bladder **C Bladder Neck**	**7** Via Natural or Artificial Opening **8** Via Natural or Artificial Opening Endoscopic	**D** Intraluminal Device **Z** No Device	**Z** No Qualifier
D Urethra Bulbourethral (Cowper's) gland Cowper's (bulbourethral) gland External urethral sphincter Internal urethral sphincter Membranous urethra Penile urethra Prostatic urethra	**Ø** Open **3** Percutaneous **4** Percutaneous Endoscopic **X** External	**C** Extraluminal Device **D** Intraluminal Device **Z** No Device	**Z** No Qualifier
D Urethra Bulbourethral (Cowper's) gland Cowper's (bulbourethral) gland External urethral sphincter Internal urethral sphincter Membranous urethra Penile urethra Prostatic urethra	**7** Via Natural or Artificial Opening **8** Via Natural or Artificial Opening Endoscopic	**D** Intraluminal Device **Z** No Device	**Z** No Qualifier

NC Noncovered Procedure   **LC** Limited Coverage   **OA** Questionable OB Admit   **NT** New Tech Add-on   ⊞ Combination Member   ♂ Male   ♀ Female

ICD-10-PCS 2023   **631**

ØTJ–ØTL

Ø Medical and Surgical
T Urinary System
M Reattachment   Definition: Putting back in or on all or a portion of a separated body part to its normal location or other suitable location
                     Explanation: Vascular circulation and nervous pathways may or may not be reestablished

Body Part Character 4	Approach Character 5	Device Character 6	Qualifier Character 7
Ø Kidney, Right Renal calyx Renal capsule Renal cortex Renal segment **1 Kidney, Left** *See Ø Kidney, Right* **2 Kidneys, Bilateral** *See Ø Kidney, Right* **3 Kidney Pelvis, Right** Ureteropelvic junction (UPJ) **4 Kidney Pelvis, Left** *See 3 Kidney Pelvis, Right* **6 Ureter, Right** Ureteral orifice Ureterovesical orifice **7 Ureter, Left** *See 6 Ureter, Right* **8 Ureters, Bilateral** *See 6 Ureter, Right* **B Bladder** Trigone of bladder **C Bladder Neck** **D Urethra** Bulbourethral (Cowper's) gland Cowper's (bulbourethral) gland External urethral sphincter Internal urethral sphincter Membranous urethra Penile urethra Prostatic urethra	**Ø Open** **4 Percutaneous Endoscopic**	**Z No Device**	**Z No Qualifier**

Ø Medical and Surgical
T Urinary System
N Release   Definition: Freeing a body part from an abnormal physical constraint by cutting or by the use of force
                  Explanation: Some of the restraining tissue may be taken out but none of the body part is taken out

Body Part Character 4	Approach Character 5	Device Character 6	Qualifier Character 7
Ø Kidney, Right Renal calyx Renal capsule Renal cortex Renal segment **1 Kidney, Left** *See Ø Kidney, Right* **3 Kidney Pelvis, Right** Ureteropelvic junction (UPJ) **4 Kidney Pelvis, Left** *See 3 Kidney Pelvis, Right* **6 Ureter, Right** Ureteral orifice Ureterovesical orifice **7 Ureter, Left** *See 6 Ureter, Right* **B Bladder** Trigone of bladder **C Bladder Neck**	**Ø Open** **3 Percutaneous** **4 Percutaneous Endoscopic** **7 Via Natural or Artificial Opening** **8 Via Natural or Artificial Opening Endoscopic**	**Z No Device**	**Z No Qualifier**
D Urethra Bulbourethral (Cowper's) gland Cowper's (bulbourethral) gland External urethral sphincter Internal urethral sphincter Membranous urethra Penile urethra Prostatic urethra	**Ø Open** **3 Percutaneous** **4 Percutaneous Endoscopic** **7 Via Natural or Artificial Opening** **8 Via Natural or Artificial Opening Endoscopic** **X External**	**Z No Device**	**Z No Qualifier**

Non-OR Procedure   DRG Non-OR Procedure   Valid OR Procedure   HAC Associated Procedure   Combination Only   New/Revised April   New/Revised October

Ø Medical and Surgical
T Urinary System
P Removal   Definition: Taking out or off a device from a body part

Explanation: If a device is taken out and a similar device put in without cutting or puncturing the skin or mucous membrane, the procedure is coded to the root operation CHANGE. Otherwise, the procedure for taking out the device is coded to the root operation REMOVAL.

Body Part Character 4	Approach Character 5	Device Character 6	Qualifier Character 7
5 Kidney Renal calyx Renal capsule Renal cortex Renal segment	Ø Open 3 Percutaneous 4 Percutaneous Endoscopic 7 Via Natural or Artificial Opening 8 Via Natural or Artificial Opening Endoscopic	Ø Drainage Device 2 Monitoring Device 3 Infusion Device 7 Autologous Tissue Substitute C Extraluminal Device D Intraluminal Device J Synthetic Substitute K Nonautologous Tissue Substitute Y Other Device	Z No Qualifier
5 Kidney Renal calyx Renal capsule Renal cortex Renal segment	X External	Ø Drainage Device 2 Monitoring Device 3 Infusion Device D Intraluminal Device	Z No Qualifier
9 Ureter Ureteral orifice Ureterovesical orifice	Ø Open 3 Percutaneous 4 Percutaneous Endoscopic 7 Via Natural or Artificial Opening 8 Via Natural or Artificial Opening Endoscopic	Ø Drainage Device 2 Monitoring Device 3 Infusion Device 7 Autologous Tissue Substitute C Extraluminal Device D Intraluminal Device J Synthetic Substitute K Nonautologous Tissue Substitute M Stimulator Lead Y Other Device	Z No Qualifier
9 Ureter Ureteral orifice Ureterovesical orifice	X External	Ø Drainage Device 2 Monitoring Device 3 Infusion Device D Intraluminal Device M Stimulator Lead	Z No Qualifier
B Bladder NC Trigone of bladder	Ø Open 3 Percutaneous 4 Percutaneous Endoscopic 7 Via Natural or Artificial Opening 8 Via Natural or Artificial Opening Endoscopic	Ø Drainage Device 2 Monitoring Device 3 Infusion Device 7 Autologous Tissue Substitute C Extraluminal Device D Intraluminal Device J Synthetic Substitute K Nonautologous Tissue Substitute L Artificial Sphincter M Stimulator Lead Y Other Device	Z No Qualifier
B Bladder Trigone of bladder	X External	Ø Drainage Device 2 Monitoring Device 3 Infusion Device D Intraluminal Device L Artificial Sphincter M Stimulator Lead	Z No Qualifier
D Urethra Bulbourethral (Cowper's) gland Cowper's (bulbourethral) gland External urethral sphincter Internal urethral sphincter Membranous urethra Penile urethra Prostatic urethra	Ø Open 3 Percutaneous 4 Percutaneous Endoscopic 7 Via Natural or Artificial Opening 8 Via Natural or Artificial Opening Endoscopic	Ø Drainage Device 2 Monitoring Device 3 Infusion Device 7 Autologous Tissue Substitute C Extraluminal Device D Intraluminal Device J Synthetic Substitute K Nonautologous Tissue Substitute L Artificial Sphincter Y Other Device	Z No Qualifier
D Urethra Bulbourethral (Cowper's) gland Cowper's (bulbourethral) gland External urethral sphincter Internal urethral sphincter Membranous urethra Penile urethra Prostatic urethra	X External	Ø Drainage Device 2 Monitoring Device 3 Infusion Device D Intraluminal Device L Artificial Sphincter	Z No Qualifier

Non-OR ØTP5[3,4,7]YZ	**Non-OR** ØTP9[7,8][Ø,2,3,D]Z	**Non-OR** ØTPB[7,8][Ø,2,3,D]Z	**Non-OR** ØTPD[7,8][Ø,2,3,D,Y]Z
Non-OR ØTP5[7,8][Ø,2,3,D]Z	**Non-OR** ØTP9X[Ø,2,3,D]Z	**Non-OR** ØTPBX[Ø,2,3,D,L]Z	**Non-OR** ØTPDX[Ø,2,3,D]Z
Non-OR ØTP5X[Ø,2,3,D]Z	**Non-OR** ØTPB[3,4,7]YZ	**Non-OR** ØTPD[3,4]YZ	**NC** ØTPB[Ø,3,4,7,8]MZ
Non-OR ØTP9[3,4,7]YZ			

NC Noncovered Procedure   LC Limited Coverage   QA Questionable OB Admit   NT New Tech Add-on   ⊞ Combination Member   ♂ Male   ♀ Female

Ø Medical and Surgical
T Urinary System
Q Repair   Definition: Restoring, to the extent possible, a body part to its normal anatomic structure and function
          Explanation: Used only when the method to accomplish the repair is not one of the other root operations

Body Part Character 4	Approach Character 5	Device Character 6	Qualifier Character 7
Ø Kidney, Right Renal calyx Renal capsule Renal cortex Renal segment **1 Kidney, Left** *See Ø Kidney, Right* **3 Kidney Pelvis, Right** Ureteropelvic junction (UPJ) **4 Kidney Pelvis, Left** *See 3 Kidney Pelvis, Right* **6 Ureter, Right** Ureteral orifice Ureterovesical orifice **7 Ureter, Left** *See 6 Ureter, Right* **B Bladder** ⊞ Trigone of bladder **C Bladder Neck**	**Ø Open** **3 Percutaneous** **4 Percutaneous Endoscopic** **7 Via Natural or Artificial Opening** **8 Via Natural or Artificial Opening Endoscopic**	**Z No Device**	**Z No Qualifier**
D Urethra Bulbourethral (Cowper's) gland Cowper's (bulbourethral) gland External urethral sphincter Internal urethral sphincter Membranous urethra Penile urethra Prostatic urethra	**Ø Open** **3 Percutaneous** **4 Percutaneous Endoscopic** **7 Via Natural or Artificial Opening** **8 Via Natural or Artificial Opening Endoscopic** **X External**	**Z No Device**	**Z No Qualifier**

See Appendix L for Procedure Combinations
⊞   ØTQB[Ø,3,4]ZZ

Ø Medical and Surgical
T Urinary System
R Replacement   Definition: Putting in or on biological or synthetic material that physically takes the place and/or function of all or a portion of a body part
          Explanation: The body part may have been taken out or replaced, or may be taken out, physically eradicated, or rendered nonfunctional during the REPLACEMENT procedure. A REMOVAL procedure is coded for taking out the device used in a previous replacement procedure.

Body Part Character 4	Approach Character 5	Device Character 6	Qualifier Character 7
3 Kidney Pelvis, Right Ureteropelvic junction (UPJ) **4 Kidney Pelvis, Left** *See 3 Kidney Pelvis, Right* **6 Ureter, Right** Ureteral orifice Ureterovesical orifice **7 Ureter, Left** *See 6 Ureter, Right* **B Bladder** Trigone of bladder **C Bladder Neck**	**Ø Open** **4 Percutaneous Endoscopic** **7 Via Natural or Artificial Opening** **8 Via Natural or Artificial Opening Endoscopic**	**7 Autologous Tissue Substitute** **J Synthetic Substitute** **K Nonautologous Tissue Substitute**	**Z No Qualifier**
D Urethra Bulbourethral (Cowper's) gland Cowper's (bulbourethral) gland External urethral sphincter Internal urethral sphincter Membranous urethra Penile urethra Prostatic urethra	**Ø Open** **4 Percutaneous Endoscopic** **7 Via Natural or Artificial Opening** **8 Via Natural or Artificial Opening Endoscopic** **X External**	**7 Autologous Tissue Substitute** **J Synthetic Substitute** **K Nonautologous Tissue Substitute**	**Z No Qualifier**

Ø   **Medical and Surgical**
T   **Urinary System**
S   **Reposition**   Definition: Moving to its normal location, or other suitable location, all or a portion of a body part

Explanation: The body part is moved to a new location from an abnormal location, or from a normal location where it is not functioning correctly. The body part may or may not be cut out or off to be moved to the new location.

Body Part Character 4	Approach Character 5	Device Character 6	Qualifier Character 7

Ø **Kidney, Right**
   Renal calyx
   Renal capsule
   Renal cortex
   Renal segment
1 **Kidney, Left**
   See Ø Kidney, Right
2 **Kidneys, Bilateral**
   See Ø Kidney, Right
3 **Kidney Pelvis, Right**
   Ureteropelvic junction (UPJ)
4 **Kidney Pelvis, Left**
   See 3 Kidney Pelvis, Right
6 **Ureter, Right**
   Ureteral orifice
   Ureterovesical orifice
7 **Ureter, Left**
   See 6 Ureter, Right
8 **Ureters, Bilateral**
   See 6 Ureter, Right
B **Bladder**
   Trigone of bladder
C **Bladder Neck**
D **Urethra**
   Bulbourethral (Cowper's) gland
   Cowper's (bulbourethral) gland
   External urethral sphincter
   Internal urethral sphincter
   Membranous urethra
   Penile urethra
   Prostatic urethra
	Ø Open
	4 Percutaneous Endoscopic
		Z No Device	**Z** No Qualifier

Ø   **Medical and Surgical**
T   **Urinary System**
T   **Resection**   Definition: Cutting out or off, without replacement, all of a body part

Explanation: None

Body Part Character 4	Approach Character 5	Device Character 6	Qualifier Character 7

Ø **Kidney, Right**
   Renal calyx
   Renal capsule
   Renal cortex
   Renal segment
1 **Kidney, Left**
   See Ø Kidney, Right
2 **Kidneys, Bilateral**
   See Ø Kidney, Right
	Ø Open
	4 Percutaneous Endoscopic
		Z No Device	**Z** No Qualifier

3 **Kidney Pelvis, Right**
   Ureteropelvic junction (UPJ)
4 **Kidney Pelvis, Left**
   See 3 Kidney Pelvis, Right
6 **Ureter, Right**
   Ureteral orifice
   Ureterovesical orifice
7 **Ureter, Left**
   See 6 Ureter, Right
B **Bladder** ⊞
   Trigone of bladder
C **Bladder Neck**
D **Urethra**
   Bulbourethral (Cowper's) gland
   Cowper's (bulbourethral) gland
   External urethral sphincter
   Internal urethral sphincter
   Membranous urethra
   Penile urethra
   Prostatic urethra
	Ø Open
	4 Percutaneous Endoscopic
	7 Via Natural or Artificial Opening
	8 Via Natural or Artificial Opening Endoscopic
		Z No Device	**Z** No Qualifier

Non-OR   ØTTD[4,7,8]ZZ

See Appendix L for Procedure Combinations
Combo-only   ØTTDØZZ
⊞   ØTTBØZZ

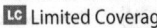

NC Noncovered Procedure   LC Limited Coverage   QA Questionable OB Admit   NT New Tech Add-on   ⊞ Combination Member   ♂ Male   ♀ Female

ICD-10-PCS 2023   635

Urinary System (side tab)

Ø   **Medical and Surgical**
T   **Urinary System**
U   **Supplement**   Definition: Putting in or on biological or synthetic material that physically reinforces and/or augments the function of a portion of a body part

Explanation: The biological material is non-living, or is living and from the same individual. The body part may have been previously replaced, and the SUPPLEMENT procedure is performed to physically reinforce and/or augment the function of the replaced body part.

Body Part Character 4	Approach Character 5	Device Character 6	Qualifier Character 7
3 Kidney Pelvis, Right Ureteropelvic junction (UPJ) **4** Kidney Pelvis, Left *See 3 Kidney Pelvis, Right* **6** Ureter, Right Ureteral orifice Ureterovesical orifice **7** Ureter, Left *See 6 Ureter, Right* **B** Bladder Trigone of bladder **C** Bladder Neck	**Ø** Open **4** Percutaneous Endoscopic **7** Via Natural or Artificial Opening **8** Via Natural or Artificial Opening Endoscopic	**7** Autologous Tissue Substitute **J** Synthetic Substitute **K** Nonautologous Tissue Substitute	**Z** No Qualifier
D Urethra Bulbourethral (Cowper's) gland Cowper's (bulbourethral) gland External urethral sphincter Internal urethral sphincter Membranous urethra Penile urethra Prostatic urethra	**Ø** Open **4** Percutaneous Endoscopic **7** Via Natural or Artificial Opening **8** Via Natural or Artificial Opening Endoscopic **X** External	**7** Autologous Tissue Substitute **J** Synthetic Substitute **K** Nonautologous Tissue Substitute	**Z** No Qualifier

Ø   **Medical and Surgical**
T   **Urinary System**
V   **Restriction**   Definition: Partially closing an orifice or the lumen of a tubular body part

Explanation: The orifice can be a natural orifice or an artificially created orifice

Body Part Character 4	Approach Character 5	Device Character 6	Qualifier Character 7
3 Kidney Pelvis, Right Ureteropelvic junction (UPJ) **4** Kidney Pelvis, Left *See 3 Kidney Pelvis, Right* **6** Ureter, Right Ureteral orifice Ureterovesical orifice **7** Ureter, Left *See 6 Ureter, Right* **B** Bladder Trigone of bladder **C** Bladder Neck	**Ø** Open **3** Percutaneous **4** Percutaneous Endoscopic	**C** Extraluminal Device **D** Intraluminal Device **Z** No Device	**Z** No Qualifier
3 Kidney Pelvis, Right Ureteropelvic junction (UPJ) **4** Kidney Pelvis, Left *See 3 Kidney Pelvis, Right* **6** Ureter, Right Ureteral orifice Ureterovesical orifice **7** Ureter, Left *See 6 Ureter, Right* **B** Bladder Trigone of bladder **C** Bladder Neck	**7** Via Natural or Artificial Opening **8** Via Natural or Artificial Opening Endoscopic	**D** Intraluminal Device **Z** No Device	**Z** No Qualifier
D Urethra Bulbourethral (Cowper's) gland Cowper's (bulbourethral) gland External urethral sphincter Internal urethral sphincter Membranous urethra Penile urethra Prostatic urethra	**Ø** Open **3** Percutaneous **4** Percutaneous Endoscopic	**C** Extraluminal Device **D** Intraluminal Device **Z** No Device	**Z** No Qualifier
D Urethra Bulbourethral (Cowper's) gland Cowper's (bulbourethral) gland External urethral sphincter Internal urethral sphincter Membranous urethra Penile urethra Prostatic urethra	**7** Via Natural or Artificial Opening **8** Via Natural or Artificial Opening Endoscopic	**D** Intraluminal Device **Z** No Device	**Z** No Qualifier
D Urethra Bulbourethral (Cowper's) gland Cowper's (bulbourethral) gland External urethral sphincter Internal urethral sphincter Membranous urethra Penile urethra Prostatic urethra	**X** External	**Z** No Device	**Z** No Qualifier

Non-OR Procedure   DRG Non-OR Procedure   Valid OR Procedure   HAC Associated Procedure   Combination Only   New/Revised April   New/Revised October

636   ICD-10-PCS 2023

Ø   **Medical and Surgical**
T   **Urinary System**
W   **Revision**   Definition: Correcting, to the extent possible, a portion of a malfunctioning device or the position of a displaced device

Explanation: Revision can include correcting a malfunctioning or displaced device by taking out or putting in components of the device such as a screw or pin

Body Part Character 4	Approach Character 5	Device Character 6	Qualifier Character 7
5 Kidney Renal calyx Renal capsule Renal cortex Renal segment	**Ø** Open **3** Percutaneous **4** Percutaneous Endoscopic **7** Via Natural or Artificial Opening **8** Via Natural or Artificial Opening Endoscopic	**Ø** Drainage Device **2** Monitoring Device **3** Infusion Device **7** Autologous Tissue Substitute **C** Extraluminal Device **D** Intraluminal Device **J** Synthetic Substitute **K** Nonautologous Tissue Substitute **Y** Other Device	**Z** No Qualifier
5 Kidney Renal calyx Renal capsule Renal cortex Renal segment	**X** External	**Ø** Drainage Device **2** Monitoring Device **3** Infusion Device **7** Autologous Tissue Substitute **C** Extraluminal Device **D** Intraluminal Device **J** Synthetic Substitute **K** Nonautologous Tissue Substitute	**Z** No Qualifier
9 Ureter Ureteral orifice Ureterovesical orifice	**Ø** Open **3** Percutaneous **4** Percutaneous Endoscopic **7** Via Natural or Artificial Opening **8** Via Natural or Artificial Opening Endoscopic	**Ø** Drainage Device **2** Monitoring Device **3** Infusion Device **7** Autologous Tissue Substitute **C** Extraluminal Device **D** Intraluminal Device **J** Synthetic Substitute **K** Nonautologous Tissue Substitute **M** Stimulator Lead **Y** Other Device	**Z** No Qualifier
9 Ureter Ureteral orifice Ureterovesical orifice	**X** External	**Ø** Drainage Device **2** Monitoring Device **3** Infusion Device **7** Autologous Tissue Substitute **C** Extraluminal Device **D** Intraluminal Device **J** Synthetic Substitute **K** Nonautologous Tissue Substitute **M** Stimulator Lead	**Z** No Qualifier
B Bladder Trigone of bladder	**Ø** Open **3** Percutaneous **4** Percutaneous Endoscopic **7** Via Natural or Artificial Opening **8** Via Natural or Artificial Opening Endoscopic	**Ø** Drainage Device **2** Monitoring Device **3** Infusion Device **7** Autologous Tissue Substitute **C** Extraluminal Device **D** Intraluminal Device **J** Synthetic Substitute **K** Nonautologous Tissue Substitute **L** Artificial Sphincter **M** Stimulator Lead **Y** Other Device	**Z** No Qualifier
B Bladder Trigone of bladder	**X** External	**Ø** Drainage Device **2** Monitoring Device **3** Infusion Device **7** Autologous Tissue Substitute **C** Extraluminal Device **D** Intraluminal Device **J** Synthetic Substitute **K** Nonautologous Tissue Substitute **L** Artificial Sphincter **M** Stimulator Lead	**Z** No Qualifier

Non-OR ØTW5[3,4,7]YZ		**Non-OR** ØTW9X[Ø,2,3,7,C,D,J,K,M]Z	
Non-OR ØTW5X[Ø,2,3,7,C,D,J,K]Z		**Non-OR** ØTWB[3,4,7]YZ	
Non-OR ØTW9[3,4,7]YZ		**Non-OR** ØTWBX[Ø,2,3,7,C,D,J,K,L,M]Z	

ØTW Continued on next page

NC Noncovered Procedure   **LC** Limited Coverage   **QA** Questionable OB Admit   **NT** New Tech Add-on   ⊞ Combination Member   ♂ Male   ♀ Female

ICD-10-PCS 2023   **637**

ØTW–ØTW

Ø Medical and Surgical
T Urinary System
W Revision

ØTW Continued

Definition: Correcting, to the extent possible, a portion of a malfunctioning device or the position of a displaced device

Explanation: Revision can include correcting a malfunctioning or displaced device by taking out or putting in components of the device such as a screw or pin

Body Part Character 4	Approach Character 5	Device Character 6	Qualifier Character 7
D Urethra Bulbourethral (Cowper's) gland Cowper's (bulbourethral) gland External urethral sphincter Internal urethral sphincter Membranous urethra Penile urethra Prostatic urethra	**Ø** Open **3** Percutaneous **4** Percutaneous Endoscopic **7** Via Natural or Artificial Opening **8** Via Natural or Artificial Opening Endoscopic	**Ø** Drainage Device **2** Monitoring Device **3** Infusion Device **7** Autologous Tissue Substitute **C** Extraluminal Device **D** Intraluminal Device **J** Synthetic Substitute **K** Nonautologous Tissue Substitute **L** Artificial Sphincter **Y** Other Device	**Z** No Qualifier
D Urethra Bulbourethral (Cowper's) gland Cowper's (bulbourethral) gland External urethral sphincter Internal urethral sphincter Membranous urethra Penile urethra Prostatic urethra	**X** External	**Ø** Drainage Device **2** Monitoring Device **3** Infusion Device **7** Autologous Tissue Substitute **C** Extraluminal Device **D** Intraluminal Device **J** Synthetic Substitute **K** Nonautologous Tissue Substitute **L** Artificial Sphincter	**Z** No Qualifier

Non-OR   ØTWD[3,4,7,8]YZ
Non-OR   ØTWDX[Ø,2,3,7,C,D,J,K,L]Z

Ø Medical and Surgical
T Urinary System
Y Transplantation

Definition: Putting in or on all or a portion of a living body part taken from another individual or animal to physically take the place and/or function of all or a portion of a similar body part

Explanation: The native body part may or may not be taken out, and the transplanted body part may take over all or a portion of its function

Body Part Character 4	Approach Character 5	Device Character 6	Qualifier Character 7
Ø Kidney, Right LC ⊞ Renal calyx Renal capsule Renal cortex Renal segment **1 Kidney, Left** LC ⊞ *See Ø Kidney, Right*	**Ø** Open	**Z** No Device	**Ø** Allogeneic **1** Syngeneic **2** Zooplastic

LC   ØTY[Ø,1]ØZ[Ø,1,2]   **See Appendix L for Procedure Combinations**
                                            ⊞   ØTY[Ø,1]ØZ[Ø,1,2]

Female Reproductive System ØU1–ØUY

Character Meanings

This Character Meaning table is provided as a guide to assist the user in the identification of character members that may be found in this section of code tables. It **SHOULD NOT** be used to build a PCS code.

Operation–Character 3		Body Part–Character 4		Approach–Character 5		Device–Character 6		Qualifier–Character 7	
1	Bypass	Ø	Ovary, Right	Ø	Open	Ø	Drainage Device	Ø	Allogeneic
2	Change	1	Ovary, Left	3	Percutaneous	1	Radioactive Element	1	Syngeneic
5	Destruction	2	Ovaries, Bilateral	4	Percutaneous Endoscopic	3	Infusion Device	2	Zooplastic
7	Dilation	3	Ovary	7	Via Natural or Artificial Opening	7	Autologous Tissue Substitute	5	Fallopian Tube, Right
8	Division	4	Uterine Supporting Structure	8	Via Natural or Artificial Opening Endoscopic	C	Extraluminal Device	6	Fallopian Tube, Left
9	Drainage	5	Fallopian Tube, Right	F	Via Natural or Artificial Opening With Percutaneous Endoscopic Assistance	D	Intraluminal Device	9	Uterus
B	Excision	6	Fallopian Tube, Left	X	External	G	Intraluminal Device, Pessary	L	Supracervical
C	Extirpation	7	Fallopian Tubes, Bilateral			H	Contraceptive Device	X	Diagnostic
D	Extraction	8	Fallopian Tube			J	Synthetic Substitute	Z	No Qualifier
F	Fragmentation	9	Uterus			K	Nonautologous Tissue Substitute		
H	Insertion	B	Endometrium			Y	Other Device		
J	Inspection	C	Cervix			Z	No Device		
L	Occlusion	D	Uterus and Cervix						
M	Reattachment	F	Cul-de-sac						
N	Release	G	Vagina						
P	Removal	H	Vagina and Cul-de-sac						
Q	Repair	J	Clitoris						
S	Reposition	K	Hymen						
T	Resection	L	Vestibular Gland						
U	Supplement	M	Vulva						
V	Restriction	N	Ova						
W	Revision								
Y	Transplantation								

AHA Coding Clinic for table ØU5
2015, 3Q, 31 Tubal ligation for sterilization

AHA Coding Clinic for table ØU7
2020, 2Q, 30 Duhrssen cervical incision

AHA Coding Clinic for table ØU9
2016, 4Q, 58 Longitudinal vaginal septum

AHA Coding Clinic for table ØUB
2018, 1Q, 23 Tubal ligation procedure
2015, 3Q, 31 Laparoscopic partial salpingectomy for ectopic pregnancy
2015, 3Q, 31 Tubal ligation for sterilization
2014, 4Q, 16 Excision of multiple uterine fibroids
2014, 3Q, 12 Excision of skin tag from labia majora

AHA Coding Clinic for table ØUC
2015, 3Q, 30 Removal of cervical cerclage
2013, 2Q, 38 Evacuation of clot post-partum

AHA Coding Clinic for table ØUH
2020, 4Q, 43-44 Insertion of radioactive element
2018, 1Q, 25 Intrauterine brachytherapy & placement of tandems & ovoids
2013, 2Q, 34 Placement of intrauterine device via open approach

AHA Coding Clinic for table ØUJ
2015, 1Q, 33 Robotic-assisted laparoscopic hysterectomy converted to open procedure

AHA Coding Clinic for table ØUL
2018, 1Q, 23 Tubal ligation procedure
2015, 3Q, 31 Tubal ligation for sterilization

AHA Coding Clinic for table ØUQ
2020, 4Q, 59-60 Extraction of ectopic products of conception
2014, 4Q, 18 Obstetrical periurethral laceration
2013, 4Q, 120 Repair of clitoral obstetric laceration

AHA Coding Clinic for table ØUS
2016, 1Q, 9 Anteversion of retroverted pregnant uterus

AHA Coding Clinic for table ØUT
2022, 1Q, 21 Gravid hysterectomy due to placenta increta
2017, 4Q, 68 New qualifier values - Supracervical hysterectomy
2015, 1Q, 33 Robotic-assisted laparoscopic hysterectomy converted to open procedure
2013, 3Q, 28 Total hysterectomy
2013, 1Q, 24 Excision versus Resection of remaining ovarian remnant following previous excision

AHA Coding Clinic for table ØUV
2015, 3Q, 30 Insertion of cervical cerclage

AHA Coding Clinic for table ØUY
2018, 4Q, 40 Uterus transplant

Female Reproductive System

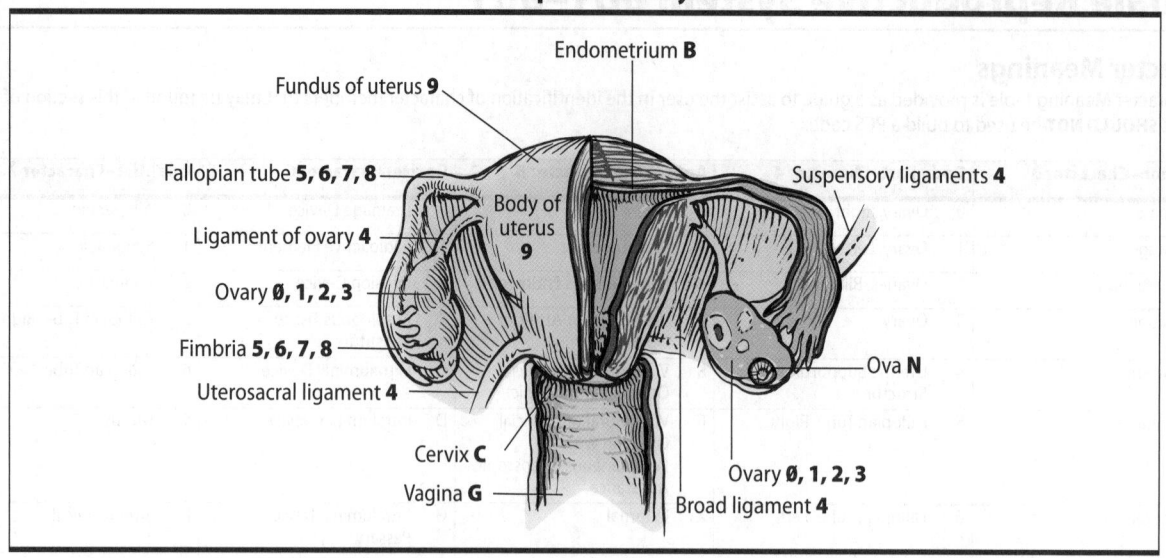

- Fundus of uterus **9**
- Endometrium **B**
- Fallopian tube **5, 6, 7, 8**
- Body of uterus **9**
- Suspensory ligaments **4**
- Ligament of ovary **4**
- Ovary **Ø, 1, 2, 3**
- Fimbria **5, 6, 7, 8**
- Ova **N**
- Uterosacral ligament **4**
- Cervix **C**
- Ovary **Ø, 1, 2, 3**
- Vagina **G**
- Broad ligament **4**

Female Internal/External Structures

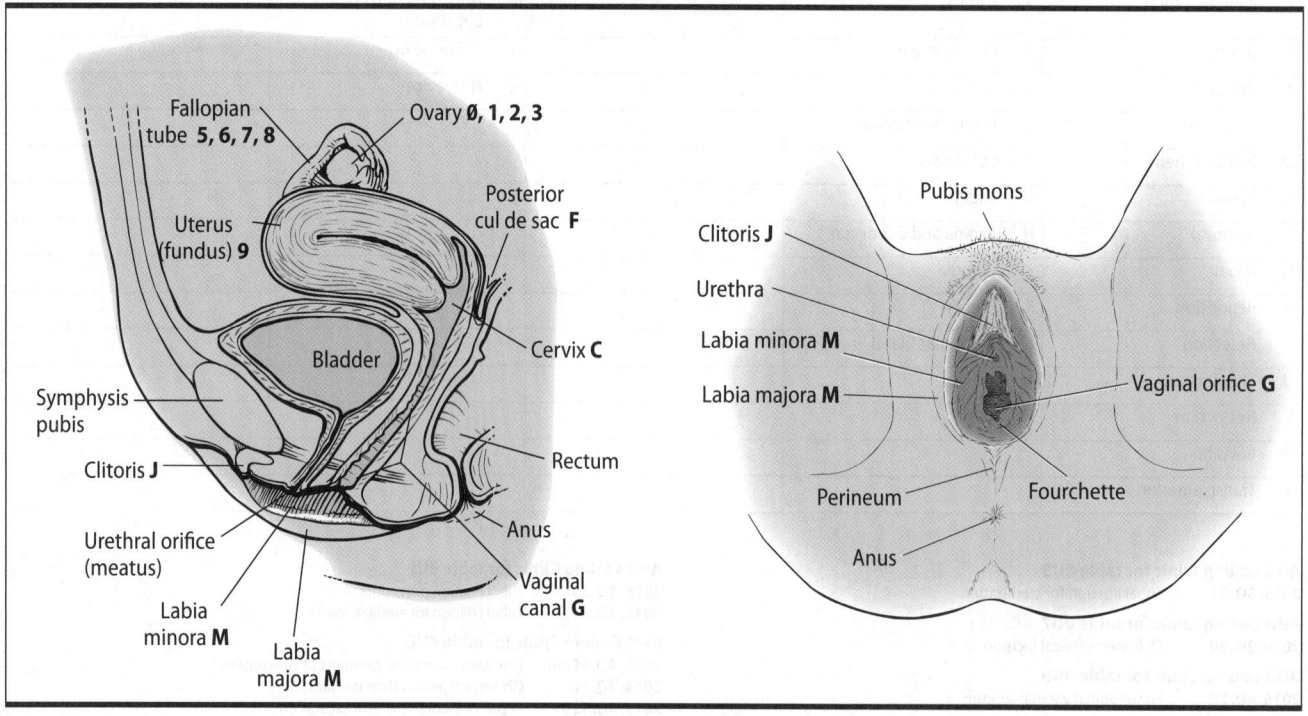

- Fallopian tube **5, 6, 7, 8**
- Ovary **Ø, 1, 2, 3**
- Posterior cul de sac **F**
- Uterus (fundus) **9**
- Cervix **C**
- Bladder
- Symphysis pubis
- Clitoris **J**
- Rectum
- Urethral orifice (meatus)
- Anus
- Labia minora **M**
- Vaginal canal **G**
- Labia majora **M**

- Pubis mons
- Clitoris **J**
- Urethra
- Labia minora **M**
- Labia majora **M**
- Vaginal orifice **G**
- Perineum
- Fourchette
- Anus

Female Reproductive System

Ø   **Medical and Surgical**
U   **Female Reproductive System**
1   **Bypass**   Definition: Altering the route of passage of the contents of a tubular body part

               Explanation: Rerouting contents of a body part to a downstream area of the normal route, to a similar route and body part, or to an abnormal route and dissimilar body part. Includes one or more anastomoses, with or without the use of a device.

Body Part Character 4	Approach Character 5	Device Character 6	Qualifier Character 7

5   Fallopian Tube, Right   ♀
     Oviduct
     Salpinx
     Uterine tube
6   Fallopian Tube, Left   ♀
     See 5 Fallopian Tube, Right
	Ø Open
	4 Percutaneous Endoscopic
		7 Autologous Tissue Substitute
		J Synthetic Substitute
		K Nonautologous Tissue Substitute
		Z No Device
			5 Fallopian Tube, Right
			6 Fallopian Tube, Left
			9 Uterus

     ♀   All body part, approach, device, and qualifier values

Ø   **Medical and Surgical**
U   **Female Reproductive System**
2   **Change**   Definition: Taking out or off a device from a body part and putting back an identical or similar device in or on the same body part without cutting or puncturing the skin or a mucous membrane

               Explanation: All CHANGE procedures are coded using the approach EXTERNAL

Body Part Character 4	Approach Character 5	Device Character 6	Qualifier Character 7

3   Ovary   ♀
8   Fallopian Tube   ♀
M   Vulva   ♀
     Labia majora
     Labia minora
	X External	Ø Drainage Device
		Y Other Device
			Z No Qualifier

D Uterus and Cervix ♀	X External	Ø Drainage Device H Contraceptive Device Y Other Device	Z No Qualifier
H Vagina and Cul-de-sac ♀	X External	Ø Drainage Device G Intraluminal Device, Pessary Y Other Device	Z No Qualifier

     Non-OR   All body part, approach, device, and qualifier values   ♀   All body part, approach, device, and qualifier values

NC Noncovered Procedure   **LC** Limited Coverage   **QA** Questionable OB Admit   **NT** New Tech Add-on   ⊞ Combination Member   ♂ Male   ♀ Female

ICD-10-PCS 2023   641

Female Reproductive System

Ø　**Medical and Surgical**
U　**Female Reproductive System**
5　**Destruction**　　Definition: Physical eradication of all or a portion of a body part by the direct use of energy, force, or a destructive agent
　　　　　　　　　　Explanation: None of the body part is physically taken out

Body Part Character 4		Approach Character 5	Device Character 6	Qualifier Character 7
Ø Ovary, Right ♀ 1 Ovary, Left ♀ 2 Ovaries, Bilateral ♀ 4 Uterine Supporting Structure ♀ 　Broad ligament 　Infundibulopelvic ligament 　Ovarian ligament 　Round ligament of uterus		Ø Open 3 Percutaneous 4 Percutaneous Endoscopic 8 Via Natural or Artificial Opening 　Endoscopic	Z No Device	Z No Qualifier
5 Fallopian Tube, Right ♀ 　Oviduct 　Salpinx 　Uterine tube 6 Fallopian Tube, Left ♀ 　*See 5 Fallopian Tube, Right* 7 Fallopian Tubes, Bilateral ᴺᶜ♀ 9 Uterus ♀ 　Fundus uteri 　Myometrium 　Perimetrium 　Uterine cornu B Endometrium ♀ C Cervix ♀ F Cul-de-sac ♀		Ø Open 3 Percutaneous 4 Percutaneous Endoscopic 7 Via Natural or Artificial Opening 8 Via Natural or Artificial Opening 　Endoscopic	Z No Device	Z No Qualifier
G Vagina ♀ K Hymen ♀		Ø Open 3 Percutaneous 4 Percutaneous Endoscopic 7 Via Natural or Artificial Opening 8 Via Natural or Artificial Opening 　Endoscopic X External	Z No Device	Z No Qualifier
J Clitoris ♀ L Vestibular Gland ♀ 　Bartholin's (greater vestibular) gland 　Greater vestibular (Bartholin's) gland 　Paraurethral (Skene's) gland 　Skene's (paraurethral) gland M Vulva ♀ 　Labia majora 　Labia minora		Ø Open X External	Z No Device	Z No Qualifier

ᴺᶜ　ØU57[Ø,3,4,7,8]ZZ with principal or secondary diagnosis of Z3Ø.2　　　　♀　All body part, approach, device, and qualifier values

Ø   **Medical and Surgical**
U   **Female Reproductive System**
7   **Dilation**   Definition: Expanding an orifice or the lumen of a tubular body part

                       Explanation: The orifice can be a natural orifice or an artificially created orifice. Accomplished by stretching a tubular body part using intraluminal pressure or by cutting part of the orifice or wall of the tubular body part.

Body Part Character 4	Approach Character 5	Device Character 6	Qualifier Character 7

5 Fallopian Tube, Right ♀
    Oviduct
    Salpinx
    Uterine tube
6 Fallopian Tube, Left ♀
    See 5 Fallopian Tube, Right
7 Fallopian Tubes, Bilateral ♀
9 Uterus ♀
    Fundus uteri
    Myometrium
    Perimetrium
    Uterine cornu
C Cervix ♀
G Vagina ♀
	Ø Open
	3 Percutaneous
	4 Percutaneous Endoscopic
	7 Via Natural or Artificial Opening
	8 Via Natural or Artificial Opening
	    Endoscopic
		D Intraluminal Device
		Z No Device
			Z No Qualifier

K Hymen ♀	**Ø** Open **3** Percutaneous **4** Percutaneous Endoscopic **7** Via Natural or Artificial Opening **8** Via Natural or Artificial Opening Endoscopic **X** External	**D** Intraluminal Device **Z** No Device	**Z** No Qualifier

Non-OR   ØU7C[Ø,3,4,7,8][D,Z]Z   ♀   All body part, approach, device, and qualifier values
Non-OR   ØU7G[7,8][D,Z]Z

Ø   **Medical and Surgical**
U   **Female Reproductive System**
8   **Division**   Definition: Cutting into a body part, without draining fluids and/or gases from the body part, in order to separate or transect a body part

                       Explanation: All or a portion of the body part is separated into two or more portions

Body Part Character 4	Approach Character 5	Device Character 6	Qualifier Character 7

Ø Ovary, Right ♀
1 Ovary, Left ♀
2 Ovaries, Bilateral ♀
4 Uterine Supporting Structure ♀
    Broad ligament
    Infundibulopelvic ligament
    Ovarian ligament
    Round ligament of uterus
	Ø Open ·
	3 Percutaneous
	4 Percutaneous Endoscopic
		Z No Device	**Z** No Qualifier

K Hymen ♀	**7** Via Natural or Artificial Opening **8** Via Natural or Artificial Opening Endoscopic **X** External	**Z** No Device	**Z** No Qualifier

Non-OR   ØU8K[7,8,X]ZZ   ♀   All body part, approach, device, and qualifier values

Female Reproductive System

0   **Medical and Surgical**
U   **Female Reproductive System**
9   **Drainage**   Definition: Taking or letting out fluids and/or gases from a body part
                         Explanation: The qualifier DIAGNOSTIC is used to identify drainage procedures that are biopsies

Body Part Character 4	Approach Character 5	Device Character 6	Qualifier Character 7
0 Ovary, Right ♀ **1** Ovary, Left ♀ **2** Ovaries, Bilateral ♀	**0** Open **3** Percutaneous **4** Percutaneous Endoscopic **8** Via Natural or Artificial Opening Endoscopic	**0** Drainage Device	**Z** No Qualifier
0 Ovary, Right ♀ **1** Ovary, Left ♀ **2** Ovaries, Bilateral ♀	**0** Open **3** Percutaneous **4** Percutaneous Endoscopic **8** Via Natural or Artificial Opening Endoscopic	**Z** No Device	**X** Diagnostic **Z** No Qualifier
0 Ovary, Right ♀ **1** Ovary, Left ♀ **2** Ovaries, Bilateral ♀	**X** External	**Z** No Device	**Z** No Qualifier

4 Uterine Supporting Structure ♀
  Broad ligament
  Infundibulopelvic ligament
  Ovarian ligament
  Round ligament of uterus
	0 Open
	3 Percutaneous
	4 Percutaneous Endoscopic
	8 Via Natural or Artificial Opening Endoscopic
		0 Drainage Device	**Z** No Qualifier

4 Uterine Supporting Structure ♀
  Broad ligament
  Infundibulopelvic ligament
  Ovarian ligament
  Round ligament of uterus
	0 Open
	3 Percutaneous
	4 Percutaneous Endoscopic
	8 Via Natural or Artificial Opening Endoscopic
		Z No Device	**X** Diagnostic
			Z No Qualifier

5 Fallopian Tube, Right ♀
  Oviduct
  Salpinx
  Uterine tube
6 Fallopian Tube, Left ♀
  See 5 Fallopian Tube, Right
7 Fallopian Tubes, Bilateral ♀
9 Uterus ♀
  Fundus uteri
  Myometrium
  Perimetrium
  Uterine cornu
C Cervix ♀
F Cul-de-sac ♀
	0 Open
	3 Percutaneous
	4 Percutaneous Endoscopic
	7 Via Natural or Artificial Opening
	8 Via Natural or Artificial Opening Endoscopic
		0 Drainage Device	**Z** No Qualifier

5 Fallopian Tube, Right ♀
  Oviduct
  Salpinx
  Uterine tube
6 Fallopian Tube, Left ♀
  See 5 Fallopian Tube, Right
7 Fallopian Tubes, Bilateral ♀
9 Uterus ♀
  Fundus uteri
  Myometrium
  Perimetrium
  Uterine cornu
C Cervix ♀
F Cul-de-sac ♀
	0 Open
	3 Percutaneous
	4 Percutaneous Endoscopic
	7 Via Natural or Artificial Opening
	8 Via Natural or Artificial Opening Endoscopic
		Z No Device	**X** Diagnostic
			Z No Qualifier

Non-OR 0U9[0,1,2][3,8]0Z		**Non-OR** 0U9[5,6,7,9,C]30Z
Non-OR 0U9[0,1,2][3,8]ZZ		**Non-OR** 0U9F[3,4]0Z
Non-OR 0U9[0,1,2]8ZX		**Non-OR** 0U9[5,6,7][3,4,7,8]ZZ
Non-OR 0U94[3,8]0Z		**Non-OR** 0U9[9,C]3ZZ
Non-OR 0U94[3,8]ZZ		**Non-OR** 0U9F[3,4]ZZ
Non-OR 0U948ZX		♀ All body part, approach, device, and qualifier values

0U9 Continued on next page

Non-OR Procedure   DRG Non-OR Procedure   Valid OR Procedure   HAC Associated Procedure   Combination Only   New/Revised April   New/Revised October

644   ICD-10-PCS 2023

Ø	**Medical and Surgical**			
U	**Female Reproductive System**			
9	**Drainage**	Definition: Taking or letting out fluids and/or gases from a body part		

ØU9 Continued

Explanation: The qualifier DIAGNOSTIC is used to identify drainage procedures that are biopsies

Body Part Character 4	Approach Character 5	Device Character 6	Qualifier Character 7
G Vagina ♀ **K** Hymen ♀	**Ø** Open **3** Percutaneous **4** Percutaneous Endoscopic **7** Via Natural or Artificial Opening **8** Via Natural or Artificial Opening Endoscopic **X** External	**Ø** Drainage Device	**Z** No Qualifier
G Vagina ♀ **K** Hymen ♀	**Ø** Open **3** Percutaneous **4** Percutaneous Endoscopic **7** Via Natural or Artificial Opening **8** Via Natural or Artificial Opening Endoscopic **X** External	**Z** No Device	**X** Diagnostic **Z** No Qualifier

J Clitoris ♀
L Vestibular Gland ♀
    Bartholin's (greater vestibular) gland
    Greater vestibular (Bartholin's) gland
    Paraurethral (Skene's) gland
    Skene's (paraurethral) gland
M Vulva ♀
    Labia majora
    Labia minora
	Ø Open
	X External
		Ø Drainage Device	**Z** No Qualifier

J Clitoris ♀
L Vestibular Gland ♀
    Bartholin's (greater vestibular) gland
    Greater vestibular (Bartholin's) gland
    Paraurethral (Skene's) gland
    Skene's (paraurethral) gland
M Vulva ♀
    Labia majora
    Labia minora
	Ø Open
	X External
		Z No Device	**X** Diagnostic
			Z No Qualifier

Non-OR	ØU9G3ØZ	Non-OR	ØU9L[Ø,X]ØZ
Non-OR	ØU9K[Ø,3,4,7,8,X]ØZ	Non-OR	ØU9L[Ø,X]Z[X,Z]
Non-OR	ØU9G3ZZ	♀	All body part, approach, device, and qualifier values
Non-OR	ØU9K[Ø,3,4,7,8,X]ZZ		

NC Noncovered Procedure   **LC** Limited Coverage   **QA** Questionable OB Admit   **NT** New Tech Add-on   ⊞ Combination Member   ♂ Male   ♀ Female

ICD-10-PCS 2023   645

Female Reproductive System

Ø   **Medical and Surgical**
U   **Female Reproductive System**
B   **Excision**   Definition: Cutting out or off, without replacement, a portion of a body part

                         Explanation: The qualifier DIAGNOSTIC is used to identify excision procedures that are biopsies

Body Part — Character 4	Approach — Character 5	Device — Character 6	Qualifier — Character 7

Ø Ovary, Right ♀
 1 Ovary, Left ♀
 2 Ovaries, Bilateral ♀
 4 Uterine Supporting Structure ♀
    Broad ligament
    Infundibulopelvic ligament
    Ovarian ligament
    Round ligament of uterus
 5 Fallopian Tube, Right ♀
    Oviduct
    Salpinx
    Uterine tube
 6 Fallopian Tube, Left ♀
    See 5 Fallopian Tube, Right
 7 Fallopian Tubes, Bilateral ♀
 9 Uterus ♀
    Fundus uteri
    Myometrium
    Perimetrium
    Uterine cornu
 C Cervix ♀
 F Cul-de-sac ♀
	Ø Open
	 3 Percutaneous
	 4 Percutaneous Endoscopic
	 7 Via Natural or Artificial Opening
	 8 Via Natural or Artificial Opening Endoscopic
		Z No Device	**X** Diagnostic
			 Z No Qualifier

G Vagina ♀ **K** Hymen ♀	**Ø** Open **3** Percutaneous **4** Percutaneous Endoscopic **7** Via Natural or Artificial Opening **8** Via Natural or Artificial Opening Endoscopic **X** External	**Z** No Device	**X** Diagnostic **Z** No Qualifier

J Clitoris ♀
 L Vestibular Gland ♀
    Bartholin's (greater vestibular) gland
    Greater vestibular (Bartholin's) gland
    Paraurethral (Skene's) gland
    Skene's (paraurethral) gland
 M Vulva ♀
    Labia majora
    Labia minora
	Ø Open
	 X External
		Z No Device	**X** Diagnostic
			 Z No Qualifier

♀   All body part, approach, device, and qualifier values

Non-OR Procedure   DRG Non-OR Procedure   Valid OR Procedure   HAC Associated Procedure   Combination Only   New/Revised April   New/Revised October

646   ICD-10-PCS 2023

Ø   **Medical and Surgical**
U   **Female Reproductive System**
C   **Extirpation**   Definition: Taking or cutting out solid matter from a body part

Explanation: The solid matter may be an abnormal byproduct of a biological function or a foreign body; it may be imbedded in a body part or in the lumen of a tubular body part. The solid matter may or may not have been previously broken into pieces.

Body Part Character 4	Approach Character 5	Device Character 6	Qualifier Character 7

Ø Ovary, Right ♀
1 Ovary, Left ♀
2 Ovaries, Bilateral ♀
4 Uterine Supporting Structure ♀
    Broad ligament
    Infundibulopelvic ligament
    Ovarian ligament
    Round ligament of uterus
	Ø Open
	3 Percutaneous
	4 Percutaneous Endoscopic
	8 Via Natural or Artificial Opening
	    Endoscopic
		Z No Device	Z No Qualifier

5 Fallopian Tube, Right ♀
    Oviduct
    Salpinx
    Uterine tube
6 Fallopian Tube, Left ♀
    See 5 Fallopian Tube, Right
7 Fallopian Tubes, Bilateral ♀
9 Uterus ♀
    Fundus uteri
    Myometrium
    Perimetrium
    Uterine cornu
B Endometrium ♀
C Cervix ♀
F Cul-de-sac ♀
	Ø Open
	3 Percutaneous
	4 Percutaneous Endoscopic
	7 Via Natural or Artificial Opening
	8 Via Natural or Artificial Opening
	    Endoscopic
		Z No Device	Z No Qualifier

G Vagina ♀ K Hymen ♀	Ø Open 3 Percutaneous 4 Percutaneous Endoscopic 7 Via Natural or Artificial Opening 8 Via Natural or Artificial Opening Endoscopic X External	Z No Device	Z No Qualifier

J Clitoris ♀
L Vestibular Gland ♀
    Bartholin's (greater vestibular) gland
    Greater vestibular (Bartholin's) gland
    Paraurethral (Skene's) gland
    Skene's (paraurethral) gland
M Vulva ♀
    Labia majora
    Labia minora
	Ø Open
	X External
		Z No Device	Z No Qualifier

Non-OR   ØUC9[7,8]ZZ
Non-OR   ØUCG[7,8,X]ZZ
Non-OR   ØUCK[Ø,3,4,7,8,X]ZZ

Non-OR   ØUCMXZZ
♀   All body part, approach, device, and qualifier values

Ø   **Medical and Surgical**
U   **Female Reproductive System**
D   **Extraction**   Definition: Pulling or stripping out or off all or a portion of a body part by the use of force

Explanation: The qualifier DIAGNOSTIC is used to identify extraction procedures that are biopsies

Body Part Character 4	Approach Character 5	Device Character 6	Qualifier Character 7
B Endometrium ♀	7 Via Natural or Artificial Opening 8 Via Natural or Artificial Opening Endoscopic	Z No Device	X Diagnostic Z No Qualifier
N Ova ♀	Ø Open 3 Percutaneous 4 Percutaneous Endoscopic	Z No Device	Z No Qualifier

♀   All body part, approach, device, and qualifier values

NC Noncovered Procedure   LC Limited Coverage   QA Questionable OB Admit   NT New Tech Add-on   ⊞ Combination Member   ♂ Male   ♀ Female

ICD-10-PCS 2023   647

ØUC–ØUD

Female Reproductive System *(side tab)*

Ø   Medical and Surgical
U   Female Reproductive System
F   Fragmentation   Definition: Breaking solid matter in a body part into pieces

Explanation: Physical force (e.g., manual, ultrasonic) applied directly or indirectly is used to break the solid matter into pieces. The solid matter may be an abnormal byproduct of a biological function or a foreign body. The pieces of solid matter are not taken out.

Body Part Character 4	Approach Character 5	Device Character 6	Qualifier Character 7

5 Fallopian Tube, Right   NC ♀
   Oviduct
   Salpinx
   Uterine tube
6 Fallopian Tube, Left   NC ♀
   See 5 Fallopian Tube, Right
7 Fallopian Tubes, Bilateral   NC ♀
9 Uterus   NC ♀
   Fundus uteri
   Myometrium
   Perimetrium
   Uterine cornu
	0 Open
	3 Percutaneous
	4 Percutaneous Endoscopic
	7 Via Natural or Artificial Opening
	8 Via Natural or Artificial Opening
	   Endoscopic
	X External
		Z No Device	Z No Qualifier

Non-OR ØUF[5,6,7,9]XZZ	♀	All body part, approach, device, and qualifier values
NC ØUF[5,6,7,9]XZZ		

Ø   Medical and Surgical
U   Female Reproductive System
H   Insertion   Definition: Putting in a nonbiological appliance that monitors, assists, performs, or prevents a physiological function but does not physically take the place of a body part

Explanation: None

Body Part Character 4	Approach Character 5	Device Character 6	Qualifier Character 7
3 Ovary ♀	0 Open 3 Percutaneous 4 Percutaneous Endoscopic	1 Radioactive Element 3 Infusion Device Y Other Device	Z No Qualifier
3 Ovary ♀	7 Via Natural or Artificial Opening 8 Via Natural or Artificial Opening Endoscopic	1 Radioactive Element Y Other Device	Z No Qualifier
8 Fallopian Tube ♀ D Uterus and Cervix ♀ H Vagina and Cul-de-sac ♀	0 Open 3 Percutaneous 4 Percutaneous Endoscopic 7 Via Natural or Artificial Opening 8 Via Natural or Artificial Opening Endoscopic	3 Infusion Device Y Other Device	Z No Qualifier

9 Uterus   ♀
   Fundus uteri
   Myometrium
   Perimetrium
   Uterine cornu
	0 Open
	7 Via Natural or Artificial Opening
	8 Via Natural or Artificial Opening
	   Endoscopic
		1 Radioactive Element
		H Contraceptive Device
			Z No Qualifier

C Cervix ♀	0 Open 3 Percutaneous 4 Percutaneous Endoscopic	1 Radioactive Element	Z No Qualifier
C Cervix ♀	7 Via Natural or Artificial Opening 8 Via Natural or Artificial Opening Endoscopic	1 Radioactive Element H Contraceptive Device	Z No Qualifier
F Cul-de-sac ♀	7 Via Natural or Artificial Opening 8 Via Natural or Artificial Opening Endoscopic	G Intraluminal Device, Pessary	Z No Qualifier
G Vagina ♀	0 Open 3 Percutaneous 4 Percutaneous Endoscopic X External	1 Radioactive Element	Z No Qualifier
G Vagina ♀	7 Via Natural or Artificial Opening 8 Via Natural or Artificial Opening Endoscopic	1 Radioactive Element G Intraluminal Device, Pessary	Z No Qualifier

Non-OR ØUH3[Ø,4][3,Y]Z	**Non-OR** ØUH9[Ø,7,8][1,H]Z
Non-OR ØUH33[1,3,Y]Z	**Non-OR** ØUHC[7,8]HZ
Non-OR ØUH3[7,8][1,Y]Z	**Non-OR** ØUHF[7,8]HZ
Non-OR ØUH[8,D][Ø,3,4,7,8][3,Y]Z	**Non-OR** ØUHG[7,8]HZ
Non-OR ØUHH[3,4]YZ	♀ All body part, approach, device, and qualifier values
Non-OR ØUHH[7,8][3,Y]Z	

Non-OR Procedure   DRG Non-OR Procedure   Valid OR Procedure   HAC Associated Procedure   Combination Only   New/Revised April   *New/Revised October*

648   ICD-10-PCS 2023

Ø   **Medical and Surgical**
U   **Female Reproductive System**
J   **Inspection**   Definition: Visually and/or manually exploring a body part

Explanation: Visual exploration may be performed with or without optical instrumentation. Manual exploration may be performed directly or through intervening body layers.

Body Part Character 4	Approach Character 5	Device Character 6	Qualifier Character 7
3 Ovary ♀	**Ø** Open **3** Percutaneous **4** Percutaneous Endoscopic **8** Via Natural or Artificial Opening Endoscopic **X** External	**Z** No Device	**Z** No Qualifier
8 Fallopian Tube ♀ **D** Uterus and Cervix ♀ **H** Vagina and Cul-de-sac ♀	**Ø** Open **3** Percutaneous **4** Percutaneous Endoscopic **7** Via Natural or Artificial Opening **8** Via Natural or Artificial Opening Endoscopic **X** External	**Z** No Device	**Z** No Qualifier
M Vulva ♀ Labia majora Labia minora	**Ø** Open **X** External	**Z** No Device	**Z** No Qualifier

Non-OR ØUJ3[3,8,X]ZZ		**Non-OR** ØUJMXZZ	
Non-OR ØUJ[8,D,H][3,7,8,X]ZZ		♀ All body part, approach, device, and qualifier values	

Ø   **Medical and Surgical**
U   **Female Reproductive System**
L   **Occlusion**   Definition: Completely closing an orifice or the lumen of a tubular body part

Explanation: The orifice can be a natural orifice or an artificially created orifice

Body Part Character 4	Approach Character 5	Device Character 6	Qualifier Character 7
5 Fallopian Tube, Right ♀ Oviduct Salpinx Uterine tube **6** Fallopian Tube, Left ♀ *See 5 Fallopian Tube, Right* **7** Fallopian Tubes, Bilateral NC ♀	**Ø** Open **3** Percutaneous **4** Percutaneous Endoscopic	**C** Extraluminal Device **D** Intraluminal Device **Z** No Device	**Z** No Qualifier
5 Fallopian Tube, Right ♀ Oviduct Salpinx Uterine tube **6** Fallopian Tube, Left ♀ *See 5 Fallopian Tube, Right* **7** Fallopian Tubes, Bilateral NC ♀	**7** Via Natural or Artificial Opening **8** Via Natural or Artificial Opening Endoscopic	**D** Intraluminal Device **Z** No Device	**Z** No Qualifier
F Cul-de-sac ♀ **G** Vagina ♀	**7** Via Natural or Artificial Opening **8** Via Natural or Artificial Opening Endoscopic	**D** Intraluminal Device **Z** No Device	**Z** No Qualifier

NC ØUL7[Ø,3,4][C,D,Z]Z with principal or secondary diagnosis of Z3Ø.2		♀ All body part, approach, device, and qualifier values
NC ØUL7[7,8][D,Z]Z with principal or secondary diagnosis of Z3Ø.2		

NC Noncovered Procedure   LC Limited Coverage   QA Questionable OB Admit   NT New Tech Add-on   ⊞ Combination Member   ♂ Male   ♀ Female

ICD-10-PCS 2023   649

Ø Medical and Surgical
U Female Reproductive System
M Reattachment Definition: Putting back in or on all or a portion of a separated body part to its normal location or other suitable location
Explanation: Vascular circulation and nervous pathways may or may not be reestablished

Body Part Character 4		Approach Character 5	Device Character 6	Qualifier Character 7

Ø **Ovary, Right** ♀
1 **Ovary, Left** ♀
2 **Ovaries, Bilateral** ♀
4 **Uterine Supporting Structure** ♀
   Broad ligament
   Infundibulopelvic ligament
   Ovarian ligament
   Round ligament of uterus
5 **Fallopian Tube, Right** ♀
   Oviduct
   Salpinx
   Uterine tube
6 **Fallopian Tube, Left** ♀
   See 5 Fallopian Tube, Right
7 **Fallopian Tubes, Bilateral** ♀
9 **Uterus** ♀
   Fundus uteri
   Myometrium
   Perimetrium
   Uterine cornu
C **Cervix** ♀
F **Cul-de-sac** ♀
G **Vagina** ♀
		Ø **Open**
		4 **Percutaneous Endoscopic**
			Z **No Device**	**Z** **No Qualifier**

J **Clitoris** ♀
M **Vulva** ♀
   Labia majora
   Labia minora
		X **External**	**Z** **No Device**	**Z** **No Qualifier**

K **Hymen** ♀		**Ø** **Open** **4** **Percutaneous Endoscopic** **X** **External**	**Z** **No Device**	**Z** **No Qualifier**

♀   All body part, approach, device, and qualifier values

Ø   Medical and Surgical
U   Female Reproductive System
N   Release   Definition: Freeing a body part from an abnormal physical constraint by cutting or by the use of force
                                Explanation: Some of the restraining tissue may be taken out but none of the body part is taken out

Body Part Character 4	Approach Character 5	Device Character 6	Qualifier Character 7

Ø   **Ovary, Right** ♀
1   **Ovary, Left** ♀
2   **Ovaries, Bilateral** ♀
4   **Uterine Supporting Structure** ♀
     Broad ligament
     Infundibulopelvic ligament
     Ovarian ligament
     Round ligament of uterus
	Ø **Open**
	3 **Percutaneous**
	4 **Percutaneous Endoscopic**
	8 **Via Natural or Artificial Opening
	     Endoscopic**
		Z **No Device**	Z **No Qualifier**

5   **Fallopian Tube, Right** ♀
     Oviduct
     Salpinx
     Uterine tube
6   **Fallopian Tube, Left** ♀
     See 5 Fallopian Tube, Right
7   **Fallopian Tubes, Bilateral** ♀
9   **Uterus** ♀
     Fundus uteri
     Myometrium
     Perimetrium
     Uterine cornu
C   **Cervix** ♀
F   **Cul-de-sac** ♀
	Ø **Open**
	3 **Percutaneous**
	4 **Percutaneous Endoscopic**
	7 **Via Natural or Artificial Opening**
	8 **Via Natural or Artificial Opening
	     Endoscopic**
		Z **No Device**	Z **No Qualifier**

G **Vagina** ♀ K **Hymen** ♀	Ø **Open** 3 **Percutaneous** 4 **Percutaneous Endoscopic** 7 **Via Natural or Artificial Opening** 8 **Via Natural or Artificial Opening Endoscopic** X **External**	Z **No Device**	Z **No Qualifier**

J   **Clitoris** ♀
L   **Vestibular Gland** ♀
     Bartholin's (greater vestibular) gland
     Greater vestibular (Bartholin's) gland
     Paraurethral (Skene's) gland
     Skene's (paraurethral) gland
M   **Vulva** ♀
     Labia majora
     Labia minora
	Ø **Open**
	X **External**
		Z **No Device**	Z **No Qualifier**

     ♀   All body part, approach, device, and qualifier values

Female Reproductive System

Ø   **Medical and Surgical**
U   **Female Reproductive System**
P   **Removal**   Definition: Taking out or off a device from a body part

       Explanation: If a device is taken out and a similar device put in without cutting or puncturing the skin or mucous membrane, the procedure is coded to the root operation CHANGE. Otherwise, the procedure for taking out the device is coded to the root operation REMOVAL.

Body Part Character 4		Approach Character 5	Device Character 6	Qualifier Character 7
3 Ovary	♀	Ø Open 3 Percutaneous 4 Percutaneous Endoscopic	Ø Drainage Device 3 Infusion Device Y Other Device	Z No Qualifier
3 Ovary	♀	7 Via Natural or Artificial Opening 8 Via Natural or Artificial Opening Endoscopic	Y Other Device	Z No Qualifier
3 Ovary	♀	X External	Ø Drainage Device 3 Infusion Device	Z No Qualifier
8 Fallopian Tube	♀	Ø Open 3 Percutaneous 4 Percutaneous Endoscopic 7 Via Natural or Artificial Opening 8 Via Natural or Artificial Opening Endoscopic	Ø Drainage Device 3 Infusion Device 7 Autologous Tissue Substitute C Extraluminal Device D Intraluminal Device J Synthetic Substitute K Nonautologous Tissue Substitute Y Other Device	Z No Qualifier
8 Fallopian Tube	♀	X External	Ø Drainage Device 3 Infusion Device D Intraluminal Device	Z No Qualifier
D Uterus and Cervix	♀	Ø Open 3 Percutaneous 4 Percutaneous Endoscopic 7 Via Natural or Artificial Opening 8 Via Natural or Artificial Opening Endoscopic	Ø Drainage Device 1 Radioactive Element 3 Infusion Device 7 Autologous Tissue Substitute C Extraluminal Device D Intraluminal Device H Contraceptive Device J Synthetic Substitute K Nonautologous Tissue Substitute Y Other Device	Z No Qualifier
D Uterus and Cervix	♀	X External	Ø Drainage Device 3 Infusion Device D Intraluminal Device H Contraceptive Device	Z No Qualifier
H Vagina and Cul-de-sac	♀	Ø Open 3 Percutaneous 4 Percutaneous Endoscopic 7 Via Natural or Artificial Opening 8 Via Natural or Artificial Opening Endoscopic	Ø Drainage Device 1 Radioactive Element 3 Infusion Device 7 Autologous Tissue Substitute D Intraluminal Device J Synthetic Substitute K Nonautologous Tissue Substitute Y Other Device	Z No Qualifier
H Vagina and Cul-de-sac	♀	X External	Ø Drainage Device 1 Radioactive Element 3 Infusion Device D Intraluminal Device	Z No Qualifier

M Vulva
  Labia majora
  Labia minora
	♀	Ø Open	Ø Drainage Device
			7 Autologous Tissue Substitute
			J Synthetic Substitute
			K Nonautologous Tissue Substitute
				Z No Qualifier

M Vulva
  Labia majora
  Labia minora
	♀	X External	Ø Drainage Device	Z No Qualifier

Non-OR	ØUP3[3,4]YZ		Non-OR	ØUPD[7,8][Ø,3,C,D,H,Y]Z
Non-OR	ØUP3[7,8]YZ		Non-OR	ØUPDX[Ø,3,D,H]Z
Non-OR	ØUP3X[Ø,3]Z		Non-OR	ØUPH[3,4]YZ
Non-OR	ØUP8[3,4]YZ		Non-OR	ØUPH[7,8][Ø,3,D,Y]Z
Non-OR	ØUP8[7,8][Ø,3,D,Y]Z		Non-OR	ØUPHX[Ø,1,3,D]Z
Non-OR	ØUP8X[Ø,3,D]Z		Non-OR	ØUPMXØZ
Non-OR	ØUPD[3,4][C,Y]Z		♀	All body part, approach, device, and qualifier values

Non-OR Procedure   DRG Non-OR Procedure   Valid OR Procedure   HAC Associated Procedure   Combination Only   New/Revised April   New/Revised October

652   ICD-10-PCS 2023

Ø   **Medical and Surgical**
U   **Female Reproductive System**
Q   **Repair**   Definition: Restoring, to the extent possible, a body part to its normal anatomic structure and function

            Explanation: Used only when the method to accomplish the repair is not one of the other root operations

Body Part Character 4	Approach Character 5	Device Character 6	Qualifier Character 7

Ø Ovary, Right ♀
1 Ovary, Left ♀
2 Ovaries, Bilateral ♀
4 Uterine Supporting Structure ♀
    Broad ligament
    Infundibulopelvic ligament
    Ovarian ligament
    Round ligament of uterus
	Ø Open
	3 Percutaneous
	4 Percutaneous Endoscopic
	8 Via Natural or Artificial Opening
	    Endoscopic
		Z No Device	**Z** No Qualifier

5 Fallopian Tube, Right ♀
    Oviduct
    Salpinx
    Uterine tube
6 Fallopian Tube, Left ♀
    See 5 Fallopian Tube, Right
7 Fallopian Tubes, Bilateral ♀
9 Uterus ♀
    Fundus uteri
    Myometrium
    Perimetrium
    Uterine cornu
C Cervix ♀
F Cul-de-sac ♀
	Ø Open
	3 Percutaneous
	4 Percutaneous Endoscopic
	7 Via Natural or Artificial Opening
	8 Via Natural or Artificial Opening
	    Endoscopic
		Z No Device	**Z** No Qualifier

G Vagina ♀ **K** Hymen ♀	**Ø** Open **3** Percutaneous **4** Percutaneous Endoscopic **7** Via Natural or Artificial Opening **8** Via Natural or Artificial Opening Endoscopic **X** External	**Z** No Device	**Z** No Qualifier

J Clitoris ♀
L Vestibular Gland ♀
    Bartholin's (greater vestibular) gland
    Greater vestibular (Bartholin's) gland
    Paraurethral (Skene's) gland
    Skene's (paraurethral) gland
M Vulva ♀
    Labia majora
    Labia minora
	Ø Open
	X External
		Z No Device	**Z** No Qualifier

Non-OR   ØUQG[7,X]ZZ
Non-OR   ØUQKXZZ
Non-OR   ØUQMXZZ
♀   All body part, approach, device, and qualifier values

Ø   **Medical and Surgical**
U   **Female Reproductive System**
S   **Reposition**   Definition: Moving to its normal location, or other suitable location, all or a portion of a body part

            Explanation: The body part is moved to a new location from an abnormal location, or from a normal location where it is not functioning correctly. The body part may or may not be cut out or off to be moved to the new location.

Body Part Character 4	Approach Character 5	Device Character 6	Qualifier Character 7

Ø Ovary, Right ♀
1 Ovary, Left ♀
2 Ovaries, Bilateral ♀
4 Uterine Supporting Structure ♀
    Broad ligament
    Infundibulopelvic ligament
    Ovarian ligament
    Round ligament of uterus
5 Fallopian Tube, Right ♀
    Oviduct
    Salpinx
    Uterine tube
6 Fallopian Tube, Left ♀
    See 5 Fallopian Tube, Right
7 Fallopian Tubes, Bilateral ♀
C Cervix ♀
F Cul-de-sac ♀
	Ø Open
	4 Percutaneous Endoscopic
	8 Via Natural or Artificial Opening
	    Endoscopic
		Z No Device	**Z** No Qualifier

9 Uterus ♀
    Fundus uteri
    Myometrium
    Perimetrium
    Uterine cornu
G Vagina ♀
	Ø Open
	4 Percutaneous Endoscopic
	7 Via Natural or Artificial Opening
	8 Via Natural or Artificial Opening
	    Endoscopic
	X External
		Z No Device	**Z** No Qualifier

Non-OR   ØUS9XZZ
♀   All body part, approach, device, and qualifier values

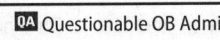

NC Noncovered Procedure   **LC** Limited Coverage   **QA** Questionable OB Admit   **NT** New Tech Add-on   ⊞ Combination Member   ♂ Male   ♀ Female

Ø Medical and Surgical
U Female Reproductive System
T Resection   Definition: Cutting out or off, without replacement, all of a body part
                         Explanation: None

Body Part Character 4	Approach Character 5	Device Character 6	Qualifier Character 7

Ø Ovary, Right ♀
1 Ovary, Left ♀
2 Ovaries, Bilateral ⊞♀
5 Fallopian Tube, Right ♀
   Oviduct
   Salpinx
   Uterine tube
6 Fallopian Tube, Left ♀
   See 5 Fallopian Tube, Right
7 Fallopian Tubes, Bilateral ⊞♀
	Ø Open
	4 Percutaneous Endoscopic
	7 Via Natural or Artificial Opening
	8 Via Natural or Artificial Opening
	   Endoscopic
	F Via Natural or Artificial Opening
	   With Percutaneous Endoscopic
	   Assistance
		Z No Device	**Z** No Qualifier

4 Uterine Supporting Structure ⊞♀
   Broad ligament
   Infundibulopelvic ligament
   Ovarian ligament
   Round ligament of uterus
C Cervix ⊞♀
F Cul-de-sac ♀
G Vagina ⊞♀
	Ø Open
	4 Percutaneous Endoscopic
	7 Via Natural or Artificial Opening
	8 Via Natural or Artificial Opening
	   Endoscopic
		Z No Device	**Z** No Qualifier

9 Uterus ⊞♀
   Fundus uteri
   Myometrium
   Perimetrium
   Uterine cornu
	Ø Open
	4 Percutaneous Endoscopic
	7 Via Natural or Artificial Opening
	8 Via Natural or Artificial Opening
	   Endoscopic
	F Via Natural or Artificial Opening
	   With Percutaneous Endoscopic
	   Assistance
		Z No Device	**L** Supracervical
			Z No Qualifier

J Clitoris ♀
L Vestibular Gland ♀
   Bartholin's (greater vestibular)
     gland
   Greater vestibular (Bartholin's)
     gland
   Paraurethral (Skene's) gland
   Skene's (paraurethral) gland
M Vulva ⊞♀
   Labia majora
   Labia minora
	Ø Open
	X External
		Z No Device	**Z** No Qualifier

K Hymen ♀	**Ø** Open **4** Percutaneous Endoscopic **7** Via Natural or Artificial Opening **8** Via Natural or Artificial Opening Endoscopic **X** External	**Z** No Device	**Z** No Device

♀ All body part, approach, device, and qualifier values

See Appendix L for Procedure Combinations
⊞ ØUT[2,7]ØZZ
⊞ ØUT[4,C][Ø,4,7,8]ZZ
⊞ ØUTGØZZ
⊞ ØUT9[Ø,4,7,8,F]ZZ
⊞ ØUTM[Ø,X]ZZ

Ø   **Medical and Surgical**
U   **Female Reproductive System**
U   **Supplement**   Definition: Putting in or on biological or synthetic material that physically reinforces and/or augments the function of a portion of a body part

                      Explanation: The biological material is non-living, or is living and from the same individual. The body part may have been previously replaced, and the SUPPLEMENT procedure is performed to physically reinforce and/or augment the function of the replaced body part.

Body Part Character 4	Approach Character 5	Device Character 6	Qualifier Character 7

4 **Uterine Supporting Structure** ♀
   Broad ligament
   Infundibulopelvic ligament
   Ovarian ligament
   Round ligament of uterus
	Ø Open
	4 Percutaneous Endoscopic
		7 Autologous Tissue Substitute
		J Synthetic Substitute
		K Nonautologous Tissue Substitute
			Z No Qualifier

5 **Fallopian Tube, Right** ♀
   Oviduct
   Salpinx
   Uterine tube
6 **Fallopian Tube, Left** ♀
   See 5 Fallopian Tube, Right
7 **Fallopian Tubes, Bilateral** ♀
F **Cul-de-sac** ♀
	Ø Open
	4 Percutaneous Endoscopic
	7 Via Natural or Artificial Opening
	8 Via Natural or Artificial Opening
	   Endoscopic
		7 Autologous Tissue Substitute
		J Synthetic Substitute
		K Nonautologous Tissue Substitute
			Z No Qualifier

G **Vagina** ♀ **K** **Hymen** ♀	**Ø** Open **4** Percutaneous Endoscopic **7** Via Natural or Artificial Opening **8** Via Natural or Artificial Opening Endoscopic **X** External	**7** Autologous Tissue Substitute **J** Synthetic Substitute **K** Nonautologous Tissue Substitute	**Z** No Qualifier

J **Clitoris** ♀
M **Vulva** ♀
   Labia majora
   Labia minora
	Ø Open
	X External
		7 Autologous Tissue Substitute
		J Synthetic Substitute
		K Nonautologous Tissue Substitute
			Z No Qualifier

   ♀   All body part, approach, device, and qualifier values

Ø   **Medical and Surgical**
U   **Female Reproductive System**
V   **Restriction**   Definition: Partially closing an orifice or the lumen of a tubular body part

                      Explanation: The orifice can be a natural orifice or an artificially created orifice

Body Part Character 4	Approach Character 5	Device Character 6	Qualifier Character 7
C **Cervix** ♀	**Ø** Open **3** Percutaneous **4** Percutaneous Endoscopic	**C** Extraluminal Device **D** Intraluminal Device **Z** No Device	**Z** No Qualifier
C **Cervix** ♀	**7** Via Natural or Artificial Opening **8** Via Natural or Artificial Opening Endoscopic	**D** Intraluminal Device **Z** No Device	**Z** No Qualifier

   ♀   All body part, approach, device, and qualifier values

Female Reproductive System

Ø   **Medical and Surgical**
U   **Female Reproductive System**
W   **Revision**   Definition: Correcting, to the extent possible, a portion of a malfunctioning device or the position of a displaced device
          Explanation: Revision can include correcting a malfunctioning or displaced device by taking out or putting in components of the device such as a screw or pin

Body Part Character 4	Approach Character 5	Device Character 6	Qualifier Character 7
3 Ovary ♀	Ø Open 3 Percutaneous 4 Percutaneous Endoscopic	Ø Drainage Device 3 Infusion Device Y Other Device	Z No Qualifier
3 Ovary ♀	7 Via Natural or Artificial Opening 8 Via Natural or Artificial Opening Endoscopic	Y Other Device	Z No Qualifier
3 Ovary ♀	X External	Ø Drainage Device 3 Infusion Device	Z No Qualifier
8 Fallopian Tube ♀	Ø Open 3 Percutaneous 4 Percutaneous Endoscopic 7 Via Natural or Artificial Opening 8 Via Natural or Artificial Opening Endoscopic	Ø Drainage Device 3 Infusion Device 7 Autologous Tissue Substitute C Extraluminal Device D Intraluminal Device J Synthetic Substitute K Nonautologous Tissue Substitute Y Other Device	Z No Qualifier
8 Fallopian Tube ♀	X External	Ø Drainage Device 3 Infusion Device 7 Autologous Tissue Substitute C Extraluminal Device D Intraluminal Device J Synthetic Substitute K Nonautologous Tissue Substitute	Z No Qualifier
D Uterus and Cervix ♀	Ø Open 3 Percutaneous 4 Percutaneous Endoscopic 7 Via Natural or Artificial Opening 8 Via Natural or Artificial Opening Endoscopic	Ø Drainage Device 1 Radioactive Element 3 Infusion Device 7 Autologous Tissue Substitute C Extraluminal Device D Intraluminal Device H Contraceptive Device J Synthetic Substitute K Nonautologous Tissue Substitute Y Other Device	Z No Qualifier
D Uterus and Cervix ♀	X External	Ø Drainage Device 3 Infusion Device 7 Autologous Tissue Substitute C Extraluminal Device D Intraluminal Device H Contraceptive Device J Synthetic Substitute K Nonautologous Tissue Substitute	Z No Qualifier
H Vagina and Cul-de-sac ♀	Ø Open 3 Percutaneous 4 Percutaneous Endoscopic 7 Via Natural or Artificial Opening 8 Via Natural or Artificial Opening Endoscopic	Ø Drainage Device 1 Radioactive Element 3 Infusion Device 7 Autologous Tissue Substitute D Intraluminal Device J Synthetic Substitute K Nonautologous Tissue Substitute Y Other Device	Z No Qualifier
H Vagina and Cul-de-sac ♀	X External	Ø Drainage Device 3 Infusion Device 7 Autologous Tissue Substitute D Intraluminal Device J Synthetic Substitute K Nonautologous Tissue Substitute	Z No Qualifier

M Vulva ♀
  Labia majora
  Labia minora
	Ø Open
	X External
		Ø Drainage Device
		7 Autologous Tissue Substitute
		J Synthetic Substitute
		K Nonautologous Tissue Substitute
			Z No Qualifier

Non-OR ØUW3[3,4]YZ		**Non-OR** ØUWDX[Ø,3,7,C,D,H,J,K]Z	
Non-OR ØUW3[7,8]YZ		**Non-OR** ØUWH[3,4,7,8]YZ	
Non-OR ØUW3X[Ø,3]Z		**Non-OR** ØUWHX[Ø,3,7,D,J,K]Z	
Non-OR ØUW8[3,4,7,8]YZ		**Non-OR** ØUWMX[Ø,7,J,K]Z	
Non-OR ØUW8X[Ø,3,7,C,D,J,K]Z		♀ All body part, approach, device, and qualifier values	
Non-OR ØUWD[3,4,7,8]YZ			

Ø　**Medical and Surgical**
U　**Female Reproductive System**
Y　**Transplantation**　Definition: Putting in or on all or a portion of a living body part taken from another individual or animal to physically take the place and/or function of all or a portion of a similar body part

Explanation: The native body part may or may not be taken out, and the transplanted body part may take over all or a portion of its function

Body Part Character 4		Approach Character 5	Device Character 6	Qualifier Character 7
Ø　Ovary, Right	♀	Ø　Open	Z　No Device	Ø　Allogeneic
1　Ovary, Left	♀			1　Syngeneic
9　Uterus	♀			2　Zooplastic
♀　　All body part, approach, device, and qualifier values				

NC Noncovered Procedure　　**LC** Limited Coverage　　**QA** Questionable OB Admit　　**NT** New Tech Add-on　　⊞ Combination Member　　♂ Male　　♀ Female

ICD-10-PCS 2023　　　　　　　　　　　　　　　　　　　　　　　　　　　　　　　　　　657

ØUY–ØUY

Male Reproductive System ØV1–ØVX

Character Meanings

This Character Meaning table is provided as a guide to assist the user in the identification of character members that may be found in this section of code tables. It **SHOULD NOT** be used to build a PCS code.

Operation–Character 3	Body Part–Character 4	Approach–Character 5	Device–Character 6	Qualifier–Character 7
1 Bypass	Ø Prostate	Ø Open	Ø Drainage Device	Ø Allogeneic
2 Change	1 Seminal Vesicle, Right	3 Percutaneous	1 Radioactive Element	1 Syngeneic
5 Destruction	2 Seminal Vesicle, Left	4 Percutaneous Endoscopic	3 Infusion Device	2 Zooplastic
7 Dilation	3 Seminal Vesicles, Bilateral	7 Via Natural or Artificial Opening	7 Autologous Tissue Substitute	3 Laser Interstitial Thermal Therapy
9 Drainage	4 Prostate and Seminal Vesicles	8 Via Natural or Artificial Opening Endoscopic	C Extraluminal Device	D Urethra
B Excision	5 Scrotum	X External	D Intraluminal Device	J Epididymis, Right
C Extirpation	6 Tunica Vaginalis, Right		J Synthetic Substitute	K Epididymis, Left
H Insertion	7 Tunica Vaginalis, Left		K Nonautologous Tissue Substitute	N Vas Deferens, Right
J Inspection	8 Scrotum and Tunica Vaginalis		Y Other Device	P Vas Deferens, Left
L Occlusion	9 Testis, Right		Z No Device	S Penis
M Reattachment	B Testis, Left			X Diagnostic
N Release	C Testes, Bilateral			Z No Qualifier
P Removal	D Testis			
Q Repair	F Spermatic Cord, Right			
R Replacement	G Spermatic Cord, Left			
S Reposition	H Spermatic Cords, Bilateral			
T Resection	J Epididymis, Right			
U Supplement	K Epididymis, Left			
W Revision	L Epididymis, Bilateral			
X Transfer	M Epididymis and Spermatic Cord			
Y Transplantation	N Vas Deferens, Right			
	P Vas Deferens, Left			
	Q Vas Deferens, Bilateral			
	R Vas Deferens			
	S Penis			
	T Prepuce			

AHA Coding Clinic for table ØV1
2018, 3Q, 12   Al-Ghorab distal penile shunt surgery

AHA Coding Clinic for table ØV9
2018, 3Q, 12   Al-Ghorab distal penile shunt surgery

AHA Coding Clinic for table ØVB
2020, 1Q, 31   Repair of buried penis
2019, 3Q, 18   Radical prostatectomy and lymph node dissection with biopsy of neurovascular bundle
2016, 1Q, 23   Transurethral resection of ejaculatory ducts
2014, 4Q, 33   Radical prostatectomy

AHA Coding Clinic for table ØVH
2020, 4Q, 43-44   Insertion of radioactive element

AHA Coding Clinic for table ØVP
2016, 2Q, 28   Removal of multi-component inflatable penile prosthesis with placement of new malleable device

AHA Coding Clinic for table ØVQ
2018, 3Q, 12   Al-Ghorab distal penile shunt surgery

AHA Coding Clinic for table ØVT
2020, 4Q, 99   Robotic-assisted prostatectomy with extension of incision for specimen removal
2019, 3Q, 18   Radical prostatectomy and lymph node dissection with biopsy of neurovascular bundle
2014, 4Q, 33   Radical prostatectomy

AHA Coding Clinic for table ØVU
2020, 1Q, 31   Repair of buried penis
2016, 2Q, 28   Removal of multi-component inflatable penile prosthesis with placement of new malleable device
2015, 3Q, 25   Placement of inflatable penile prosthesis

AHA Coding Clinic for table ØVX
2018, 4Q, 40   Transfer of prepuce

AHA Coding Clinic for table ØVY
2020, 4Q, 58   Male reproductive organ transplant

Male Reproductive System

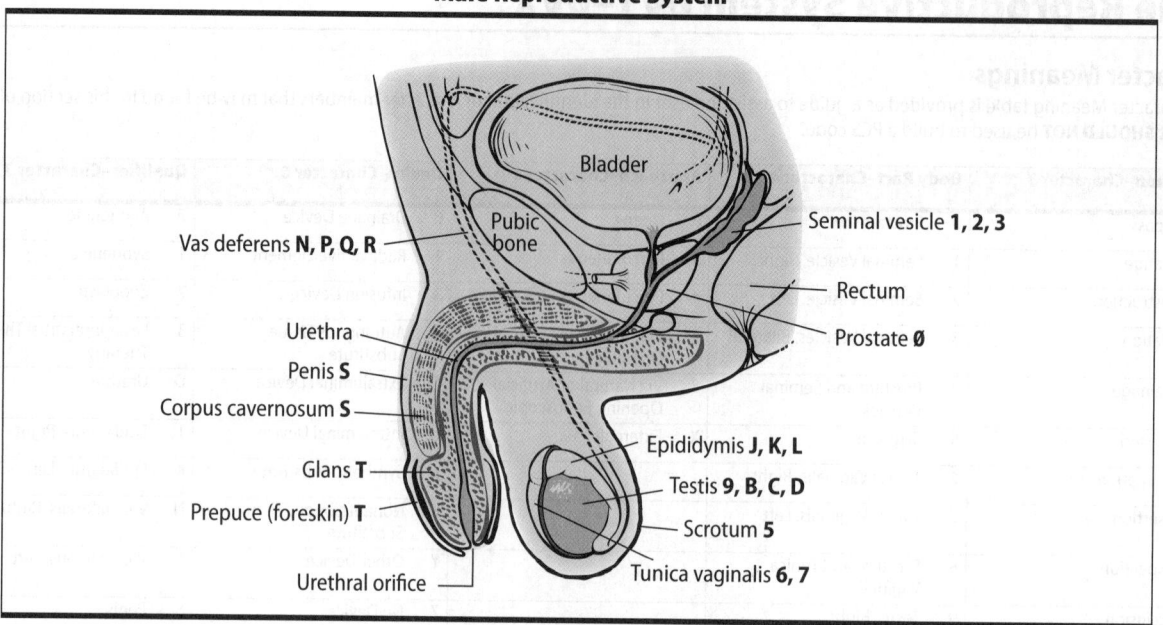

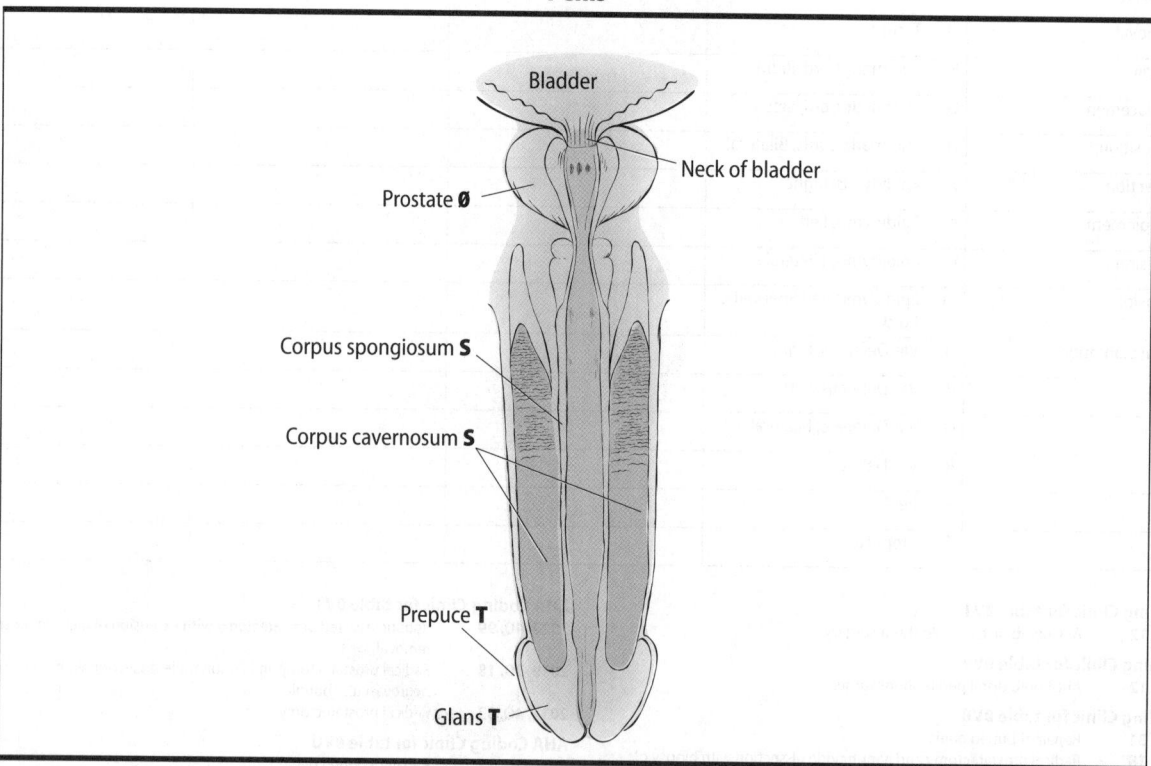

Ø   **Medical and Surgical**
V   **Male Reproductive System**
1   **Bypass**   Definition: Altering the route of passage of the contents of a tubular body part
                        Explanation: Rerouting contents of a body part to a downstream area of the normal route, to a similar route and body part, or to an abnormal route and dissimilar body part. Includes one or more anastomoses, with or without the use of a device.

Body Part Character 4	Approach Character 5	Device Character 6	Qualifier Character 7

N   Vas Deferens, Right   ♂
     Ductus deferens
     Ejaculatory duct
P   Vas Deferens, Left   ♂
     See N Vas Deferens, Right
Q   Vas Deferens, Bilateral   ♂
     See N Vas Deferens, Right
	Ø Open
	4 Percutaneous Endoscopic
		7 Autologous Tissue Substitute
		J Synthetic Substitute
		K Nonautologous Tissue Substitute
		Z No Device
			J Epididymis, Right
			K Epididymis, Left
			N Vas Deferens, Right
			P Vas Deferens, Left

     ♂   All body part, approach, device, and qualifier values

Ø   **Medical and Surgical**
V   **Male Reproductive System**
2   **Change**   Definition: Taking out or off a device from a body part and putting back an identical or similar device in or on the same body part without cutting or puncturing the skin or a mucous membrane
                        Explanation: All CHANGE procedures are coded using the approach EXTERNAL

Body Part Character 4	Approach Character 5	Device Character 6	Qualifier Character 7

4   Prostate and Seminal Vesicles   ♂
8   Scrotum and Tunica Vaginalis   ♂
D   Testis   ♂
M   Epididymis and Spermatic Cord   ♂
R   Vas Deferens   ♂
     Ductus deferens
     Ejaculatory duct
S   Penis   ♂
     Corpus cavernosum
     Corpus spongiosum
	X External	Ø Drainage Device
		Y Other Device
			Z No Qualifier

   Non-OR   All body part, approach, device, and qualifier values   ♂   All body part, approach, device, and qualifier values

Ø   **Medical and Surgical**
V   **Male Reproductive System**
5   **Destruction**   Definition: Physical eradication of all or a portion of a body part by the direct use of energy, force, or a destructive agent
                        Explanation: None of the body part is physically taken out

Body Part Character 4	Approach Character 5	Device Character 6	Qualifier Character 7
Ø Prostate ♂	Ø Open 3 Percutaneous 4 Percutaneous Endoscopic	Z No Device	3 Laser Interstitial Thermal Therapy Z No Qualifier
Ø Prostate ♂	7 Via Natural or Artificial Opening 8 Via Natural or Artificial Opening Endoscopic	Z No Device	Z No Qualifier
1 Seminal Vesicle, Right ♂ 2 Seminal Vesicle, Left ♂ 3 Seminal Vesicles, Bilateral ♂ 6 Tunica Vaginalis, Right ♂ 7 Tunica Vaginalis, Left ♂ 9 Testis, Right ♂ B Testis, Left ♂ C Testes, Bilateral ♂	Ø Open 3 Percutaneous 4 Percutaneous Endoscopic	Z No Device	Z No Qualifier

5   Scrotum   ♂
S   Penis   ♂
     Corpus cavernosum
     Corpus spongiosum
T   Prepuce   ♂
     Foreskin
     Glans penis
	Ø Open
	3 Percutaneous
	4 Percutaneous Endoscopic
	X External
		Z No Device	Z No Qualifier

F   Spermatic Cord, Right   ♂
G   Spermatic Cord, Left   ♂
H   Spermatic Cords, Bilateral   ♂
J   Epididymis, Right   ♂
K   Epididymis, Left   ♂
L   Epididymis, Bilateral   ♂
N   Vas Deferens, Right   **NC** ♂
     Ductus deferens
     Ejaculatory duct
P   Vas Deferens, Left   **NC** ♂
     See N Vas Deferens, Right
Q   Vas Deferens, Bilateral   **NC** ♂
     See N Vas Deferens, Right
	Ø Open
	3 Percutaneous
	4 Percutaneous Endoscopic
	8 Via Natural or Artificial Opening Endoscopic
		Z No Device	Z No Qualifier

   Non-OR   ØV55[Ø,3,4,X]ZZ   **NC**   ØV5[N,P,Q][Ø,3,4]ZZ with principal or secondary diagnosis of Z30.2
   Non-OR   ØV5[N,P,Q][Ø,3,4,8]ZZ   ♂   All body part, approach, device, and qualifier values

---

NC Noncovered Procedure   **LC** Limited Coverage   **QA** Questionable OB Admit   **NT** New Tech Add-on   ✚ Combination Member   ♂ Male   ♀ Female

0   **Medical and Surgical**
V   **Male Reproductive System**
7   **Dilation**   Definition: Expanding an orifice or the lumen of a tubular body part

Explanation: The orifice can be a natural orifice or an artificially created orifice. Accomplished by stretching a tubular body part using intraluminal pressure or by cutting part of the orifice or wall of the tubular body part.

Body Part Character 4	Approach Character 5	Device Character 6	Qualifier Character 7
N Vas Deferens, Right ♂ Ductus deferens Ejaculatory duct **P** Vas Deferens, Left ♂ *See N Vas Deferens, Right* **Q** Vas Deferens, Bilateral ♂ *See N Vas Deferens, Right*	**0** Open **3** Percutaneous **4** Percutaneous Endoscopic	**D** Intraluminal Device **Z** No Device	**Z** No Qualifier

♂   All body part, approach, device, and qualifier values

0   **Medical and Surgical**
V   **Male Reproductive System**
9   **Drainage**   Definition: Taking or letting out fluids and/or gases from a body part

Explanation: The qualifier DIAGNOSTIC is used to identify drainage procedures that are biopsies

Body Part Character 4	Approach Character 5	Device Character 6	Qualifier Character 7
0 Prostate ♂	**0** Open **3** Percutaneous **4** Percutaneous Endoscopic **7** Via Natural or Artificial Opening **8** Via Natural or Artificial Opening Endoscopic	**0** Drainage Device	**Z** No Qualifier
0 Prostate ♂	**0** Open **3** Percutaneous **4** Percutaneous Endoscopic **7** Via Natural or Artificial Opening **8** Via Natural or Artificial Opening Endoscopic	**Z** No Device	**X** Diagnostic **Z** No Qualifier
1 Seminal Vesicle, Right ♂ **2** Seminal Vesicle, Left ♂ **3** Seminal Vesicles, Bilateral ♂ **6** Tunica Vaginalis, Right ♂ **7** Tunica Vaginalis, Left ♂ **9** Testis, Right ♂ **B** Testis, Left ♂ **C** Testes, Bilateral ♂ **F** Spermatic Cord, Right ♂ **G** Spermatic Cord, Left ♂ **H** Spermatic Cords, Bilateral ♂ **J** Epididymis, Right ♂ **K** Epididymis, Left ♂ **L** Epididymis, Bilateral ♂ **N** Vas Deferens, Right ♂ Ductus deferens Ejaculatory duct **P** Vas Deferens, Left ♂ *See N Vas Deferens, Right* **Q** Vas Deferens, Bilateral ♂ *See N Vas Deferens, Right*	**0** Open **3** Percutaneous **4** Percutaneous Endoscopic	**0** Drainage Device	**Z** No Qualifier

Non-OR 0V90[3,4]0Z	**Non-OR** 0V9[6,7,F,G,H,N,P,Q][0,3,4]0Z
Non-OR 0V90[3,4]Z[X,Z]	**Non-OR** 0V9[J,K,L]30Z
Non-OR 0V90[7,8]ZX	♂ All body part, approach, device, and qualifier values
Non-OR 0V9[1,2,3,9,B,C][3,4]0Z	

0V9 Continued on next page

Non-OR Procedure   DRG Non-OR Procedure   Valid OR Procedure   HAC Associated Procedure   Combination Only   New/Revised April   New/Revised October

662   ICD-10-PCS 2023

0   **Medical and Surgical**
V   **Male Reproductive System**
9   **Drainage**   Definition: Taking or letting out fluids and/or gases from a body part

Explanation: The qualifier DIAGNOSTIC is used to identify drainage procedures that are biopsies

Body Part Character 4	Approach Character 5	Device Character 6	Qualifier Character 7

1 Seminal Vesicle, Right ♂
2 Seminal Vesicle, Left ♂
3 Seminal Vesicles, Bilateral ♂
6 Tunica Vaginalis, Right ♂
7 Tunica Vaginalis, Left ♂
9 Testis, Right ♂
B Testis, Left ♂
C Testes, Bilateral ♂
F Spermatic Cord, Right ♂
G Spermatic Cord, Left ♂
H Spermatic Cords, Bilateral ♂
J Epididymis, Right ♂
K Epididymis, Left ♂
L Epididymis, Bilateral ♂
N Vas Deferens, Right ♂
    Ductus deferens
    Ejaculatory duct
P Vas Deferens, Left ♂
    See N Vas Deferens, Right
Q Vas Deferens, Bilateral ♂
    See N Vas Deferens, Right
	0 Open
	3 Percutaneous
	4 Percutaneous Endoscopic
		Z No Device	**X** Diagnostic
			Z No Qualifier

5 Scrotum ♂
S Penis ♂
    Corpus cavernosum
    Corpus spongiosum
T Prepuce ♂
    Foreskin
    Glans penis
	0 Open
	3 Percutaneous
	4 Percutaneous Endoscopic
	X External
		0 Drainage Device	**Z** No Qualifier

5 Scrotum ♂
S Penis ♂
    Corpus cavernosum
    Corpus spongiosum
T Prepuce ♂
    Foreskin
    Glans penis
	0 Open
	3 Percutaneous
	4 Percutaneous Endoscopic
	X External
		Z No Device	**X** Diagnostic
			Z No Qualifier

Non-OR	0V9[1,2,3,9,B,C][3,4]Z[X,Z]	**Non-OR**	0V9[S,T]30Z
Non-OR	0V9[6,7,F,G,H,J,K,L,N,P,Q][0,3,4]ZX	**Non-OR**	0V950ZX
Non-OR	0V9[6,7,F,G,H,N,P,Q][0,3,4]ZZ	**Non-OR**	0V95[3,4,X]Z[X,Z]
Non-OR	0V9[J,K,L]3ZZ	**Non-OR**	0V9[S,T]3ZZ
Non-OR	0V95[0,3,4,X]0Z	♂	All body part, approach, device, and qualifier values

NC Noncovered Procedure   LC Limited Coverage   QA Questionable OB Admit   NT New Tech Add-on   ⊞ Combination Member   ♂ Male   ♀ Female

ICD-10-PCS 2023   663

Ø   Medical and Surgical
V   Male Reproductive System
B   Excision   Definition: Cutting out or off, without replacement, a portion of a body part
                 Explanation: The qualifier DIAGNOSTIC is used to identify excision procedures that are biopsies

Body Part Character 4	Approach Character 5	Device Character 6	Qualifier Character 7
Ø Prostate ♂	Ø Open 3 Percutaneous 4 Percutaneous Endoscopic 7 Via Natural or Artificial Opening 8 Via Natural or Artificial Opening Endoscopic	Z No Device	X Diagnostic Z No Qualifier
1 Seminal Vesicle, Right ♂ 2 Seminal Vesicle, Left ♂ 3 Seminal Vesicles, Bilateral ♂ 6 Tunica Vaginalis, Right ♂ 7 Tunica Vaginalis, Left ♂ 9 Testis, Right ♂ B Testis, Left ♂ C Testes, Bilateral ♂	Ø Open 3 Percutaneous 4 Percutaneous Endoscopic	Z No Device	X Diagnostic Z No Qualifier

5 Scrotum ♂
S Penis ♂
   Corpus cavernosum
   Corpus spongiosum
T Prepuce ♂
   Foreskin
   Glans penis
	Ø Open
	3 Percutaneous
	4 Percutaneous Endoscopic
	X External
		Z No Device	X Diagnostic
			Z No Qualifier

F Spermatic Cord, Right ♂
G Spermatic Cord, Left ♂
H Spermatic Cords, Bilateral ♂
J Epididymis, Right ♂
K Epididymis, Left ♂
L Epididymis, Bilateral ♂
N Vas Deferens, Right NC ♂
   Ductus deferens
   Ejaculatory duct
P Vas Deferens, Left NC ♂
   See N Vas Deferens, Right
Q Vas Deferens, Bilateral NC ♂
   See N Vas Deferens, Right
	Ø Open
	3 Percutaneous
	4 Percutaneous Endoscopic
	8 Via Natural or Artificial Opening
	   Endoscopic
		Z No Device	X Diagnostic
			Z No Qualifier

Non-OR ØVBØ[3,4,7,8]ZX	**Non-OR** ØVB[F,G,H,J,K,L][Ø,3,4,8]ZX
Non-OR ØVB[1,2,3,9,B,C][3,4]ZX	**Non-OR** ØVB[N,P,Q][Ø,3,4,8]Z[X,Z]
Non-OR ØVB[6,7][Ø,3,4]ZX	**NC** ØVB[N,P,Q][Ø,3,4]ZZ with principal or secondary diagnosis of Z30.2
Non-OR ØVB5ØZX	♂ All body part, approach, device, and qualifier values
Non-OR ØVB5[3,4,X]Z[X,Z]	

Ø   Medical and Surgical
V   Male Reproductive System
C   Extirpation   Definition: Taking or cutting out solid matter from a body part

Explanation: The solid matter may be an abnormal byproduct of a biological function or a foreign body; it may be imbedded in a body part or in the lumen of a tubular body part. The solid matter may or may not have been previously broken into pieces.

Body Part Character 4	Approach Character 5	Device Character 6	Qualifier Character 7
Ø Prostate ♂	**Ø** Open **3** Percutaneous **4** Percutaneous Endoscopic **7** Via Natural or Artificial Opening **8** Via Natural or Artificial Opening Endoscopic	**Z** No Device	**Z** No Qualifier

1   Seminal Vesicle, Right   ♂
2   Seminal Vesicle, Left   ♂
3   Seminal Vesicles, Bilateral   ♂
6   Tunica Vaginalis, Right   ♂
7   Tunica Vaginalis, Left   ♂
9   Testis, Right   ♂
B   Testis, Left   ♂
C   Testes, Bilateral   ♂
F   Spermatic Cord, Right   ♂
G   Spermatic Cord, Left   ♂
H   Spermatic Cords, Bilateral   ♂
J   Epididymis, Right   ♂
K   Epididymis, Left   ♂
L   Epididymis, Bilateral   ♂
N   Vas Deferens, Right   ♂
     Ductus deferens
     Ejaculatory duct
P   Vas Deferens, Left   ♂
     See N Vas Deferens, Right
Q   Vas Deferens, Bilateral   ♂
     See N Vas Deferens, Right
	Ø Open
	3 Percutaneous
	4 Percutaneous Endoscopic
		Z No Device	**Z** No Qualifier

5   Scrotum   ♂
S   Penis   ♂
     Corpus cavernosum
     Corpus spongiosum
T   Prepuce   ♂
     Foreskin
     Glans penis
	Ø Open
	3 Percutaneous
	4 Percutaneous Endoscopic
	X External
		Z No Device	**Z** No Qualifier

Non-OR ØVC[6,7,N,P,Q][Ø,3,4]ZZ	**Non-OR** ØVCSXZZ
Non-OR ØVC5[3,4,X]ZZ	♂ All body part, approach, device, and qualifier values

NC Noncovered Procedure   **LC** Limited Coverage   **OA** Questionable OB Admit   **NT** New Tech Add-on   ⊞ Combination Member   ♂ Male   ♀ Female

ICD-10-PCS 2023   665

Ø   **Medical and Surgical**
V   **Male Reproductive System**
H   **Insertion**   Definition: Putting in a nonbiological appliance that monitors, assists, performs, or prevents a physiological function but does not physically take the place of a body part
                       Explanation: None

Body Part Character 4	Approach Character 5	Device Character 6	Qualifier Character 7
Ø Prostate ♂	**Ø** Open **3** Percutaneous **4** Percutaneous Endoscopic **7** Via Natural or Artificial Opening **8** Via Natural or Artificial Opening Endoscopic	**1** Radioactive Element	**Z** No Qualifier

4 Prostate and Seminal Vesicles ♂
8 Scrotum and Tunica Vaginalis ♂
M Epididymis and Spermatic Cord ♂
R Vas Deferens ♂
    Ductus deferens
    Ejaculatory duct
	Ø Open
	3 Percutaneous
	4 Percutaneous Endoscopic
	7 Via Natural or Artificial Opening
	8 Via Natural or Artificial Opening Endoscopic
		3 Infusion Device
		Y Other Device
			Z No Qualifier

D Testis ♂	**Ø** Open **3** Percutaneous **4** Percutaneous Endoscopic **7** Via Natural or Artificial Opening **8** Via Natural or Artificial Opening Endoscopic	**1** Radioactive Element **3** Infusion Device **Y** Other Device	**Z** No Qualifier

S Penis ♂
    Corpus cavernosum
    Corpus spongiosum
	Ø Open
	3 Percutaneous
	4 Percutaneous Endoscopic
		3 Infusion Device
		Y Other Device
			Z No Qualifier

S Penis ♂
    Corpus cavernosum
    Corpus spongiosum
	7 Via Natural or Artificial Opening
	8 Via Natural or Artificial Opening Endoscopic
		Y Other Device	**Z** No Qualifier

S Penis ♂
    Corpus cavernosum
    Corpus spongiosum
	X External	**3** Infusion Device	**Z** No Qualifier

Non-OR   ØVH[4,8,M,R][Ø,3,4,7,8][3,Y]Z
Non-OR   ØVHD[Ø,3,4,7,8][1,3,Y]Z
Non-OR   ØVHS[Ø,3,4][3,Y]Z
Non-OR   ØVHS[7,8]YZ

Non-OR   ØVHSX3Z
♂   All body part, approach, device, and qualifier values

Ø   **Medical and Surgical**
V   **Male Reproductive System**
J   **Inspection**   Definition: Visually and/or manually exploring a body part
                       Explanation: Visual exploration may be performed with or without optical instrumentation. Manual exploration may be performed directly or through intervening body layers.

Body Part Character 4	Approach Character 5	Device Character 6	Qualifier Character 7

4 Prostate and Seminal Vesicles ♂
8 Scrotum and Tunica Vaginalis ♂
D Testis ♂
M Epididymis and Spermatic Cord ♂
R Vas Deferens ♂
    Ductus deferens
    Ejaculatory duct
S Penis ♂
    Corpus cavernosum
    Corpus spongiosum
	Ø Open
	3 Percutaneous
	4 Percutaneous Endoscopic
	X External
		Z No Device	**Z** No Qualifier

Non-OR   ØVJ[4,D,M,R][3,X]ZZ
Non-OR   ØVJ8[Ø,3,4,X]ZZ
Non-OR   ØVJS[3,4,X]ZZ

♂   All body part, approach, device, and qualifier values

Non-OR Procedure   DRG Non-OR Procedure   Valid OR Procedure   HAC Associated Procedure   Combination Only   New/Revised April   New/Revised October

666   ICD-10-PCS 2023

Ø   **Medical and Surgical**
V   **Male Reproductive System**
L   **Occlusion**   Definition: Completely closing an orifice or the lumen of a tubular body part

Explanation: The orifice can be a natural orifice or an artificially created orifice

Body Part Character 4	Approach Character 5	Device Character 6	Qualifier Character 7

F Spermatic Cord, Right NC ♂
G Spermatic Cord, Left NC ♂
H Spermatic Cords, Bilateral NC ♂
N Vas Deferens, Right NC ♂
   Ductus deferens
   Ejaculatory duct
P Vas Deferens, Left NC ♂
   See N Vas Deferens, Right
Q Vas Deferens, Bilateral NC ♂
   See N Vas Deferens, Right
	Ø Open
	3 Percutaneous
	4 Percutaneous Endoscopic
	8 Via Natural or Artificial Opening Endoscopic
		C Extraluminal Device
		D Intraluminal Device
		Z No Device
			Z No Qualifier

Non-OR ØVL[F,G,H][Ø,3,4,8][C,D,Z]Z **Non-OR** ØVL[N,P,Q][Ø,3,4,8][C,Z]Z		NC ØVL[F,G,H][Ø,3,4][C,D,Z]Z with principal or secondary diagnosis of Z30.2 NC ØVL[N,P,Q][Ø,3,4][C,Z]Z with principal or secondary diagnosis of Z30.2 ♂ All body part, approach, device, and qualifier values	

Ø   **Medical and Surgical**
V   **Male Reproductive System**
M   **Reattachment**   Definition: Putting back in or on all or a portion of a separated body part to its normal location or other suitable location

Explanation: Vascular circulation and nervous pathways may or may not be reestablished

Body Part Character 4	Approach Character 5	Device Character 6	Qualifier Character 7

5 Scrotum ♂
S Penis ♂
   Corpus cavernosum
   Corpus spongiosum
	X External	**Z** No Device	**Z** No Qualifier

6 Tunica Vaginalis, Right ♂ **7** Tunica Vaginalis, Left ♂ **9** Testis, Right ♂ **B** Testis, Left ♂ **C** Testes, Bilateral ♂ **F** Spermatic Cord, Right ♂ **G** Spermatic Cord, Left ♂ **H** Spermatic Cords, Bilateral ♂	**Ø** Open **4** Percutaneous Endoscopic	**Z** No Device	**Z** No Qualifier

♂ All body part, approach, device, and qualifier values	

NC Noncovered Procedure   LC Limited Coverage   OA Questionable OB Admit   NT New Tech Add-on   ⊞ Combination Member   ♂ Male   ♀ Female

ICD-10-PCS 2023   667

ØVL–ØVM

Ø   Medical and Surgical
V   Male Reproductive System
N   Release   Definition: Freeing a body part from an abnormal physical constraint by cutting or by the use of force
                       Explanation: Some of the restraining tissue may be taken out but none of the body part is taken out

Body Part Character 4	Approach Character 5	Device Character 6	Qualifier Character 7
Ø Prostate ♂	Ø Open 3 Percutaneous 4 Percutaneous Endoscopic 7 Via Natural or Artificial Opening 8 Via Natural or Artificial Opening Endoscopic	Z No Device	Z No Qualifier
1 Seminal Vesicle, Right ♂ 2 Seminal Vesicle, Left ♂ 3 Seminal Vesicles, Bilateral ♂ 6 Tunica Vaginalis, Right ♂ 7 Tunica Vaginalis, Left ♂ 9 Testis, Right ♂ B Testis, Left ♂ C Testes, Bilateral ♂	Ø Open 3 Percutaneous 4 Percutaneous Endoscopic	Z No Device	Z No Qualifier

5   Scrotum   ♂
S   Penis   ♂
     Corpus cavernosum
     Corpus spongiosum
T   Prepuce   ♂
     Foreskin
     Glans penis
	Ø Open
	3 Percutaneous
	4 Percutaneous Endoscopic
	X External
		Z No Device	Z No Qualifier

F   Spermatic Cord, Right   ♂
G   Spermatic Cord, Left   ♂
H   Spermatic Cords, Bilateral   ♂
J   Epididymis, Right   ♂
K   Epididymis, Left   ♂
L   Epididymis, Bilateral   ♂
N   Vas Deferens, Right   ♂
     Ductus deferens
     Ejaculatory duct
P   Vas Deferens, Left   ♂
     See N Vas Deferens, Right
Q   Vas Deferens, Bilateral   ♂
     See N Vas Deferens, Right
	Ø Open
	3 Percutaneous
	4 Percutaneous Endoscopic
	8 Via Natural or Artificial Opening
	     Endoscopic
		Z No Device	Z No Qualifier

Non-OR ØVN[9,B,C][Ø,3,4]ZZ		♂ All body part, approach, device, and qualifier values	
Non-OR ØVNT[Ø,3,4,X]ZZ			

Ø   Medical and Surgical
V   Male Reproductive System
P   Removal   Definition: Taking out or off a device from a body part

Explanation: If a device is taken out and a similar device put in without cutting or puncturing the skin or mucous membrane, the procedure is coded to the root operation CHANGE. Otherwise, the procedure for taking out the device is coded to the root operation REMOVAL.

Body Part Character 4	Approach Character 5	Device Character 6	Qualifier Character 7
4 Prostate and Seminal Vesicles ♂	Ø Open 3 Percutaneous 4 Percutaneous Endoscopic 7 Via Natural or Artificial Opening 8 Via Natural or Artificial Opening Endoscopic	Ø Drainage Device 1 Radioactive Element 3 Infusion Device 7 Autologous Tissue Substitute J Synthetic Substitute K Nonautologous Tissue Substitute Y Other Device	Z No Qualifier
4 Prostate and Seminal Vesicles ♂	X External	Ø Drainage Device 1 Radioactive Element 3 Infusion Device	Z No Qualifier

8 Scrotum and Tunica Vaginalis ♂
D Testis ♂
S Penis ♂
  Corpus cavernosum
  Corpus spongiosum
	Ø Open
	3 Percutaneous
	4 Percutaneous Endoscopic
	7 Via Natural or Artificial Opening
	8 Via Natural or Artificial Opening Endoscopic
		Ø Drainage Device
		3 Infusion Device
		7 Autologous Tissue Substitute
		J Synthetic Substitute
		K Nonautologous Tissue Substitute
		Y Other Device
			Z No Qualifier

8 Scrotum and Tunica Vaginalis ♂
D Testis ♂
S Penis ♂
  Corpus cavernosum
  Corpus spongiosum
	X External	Ø Drainage Device
		3 Infusion Device
			Z No Qualifier

M Epididymis and Spermatic Cord ♂	Ø Open 3 Percutaneous 4 Percutaneous Endoscopic 7 Via Natural or Artificial Opening 8 Via Natural or Artificial Opening Endoscopic	Ø Drainage Device 3 Infusion Device 7 Autologous Tissue Substitute C Extraluminal Device J Synthetic Substitute K Nonautologous Tissue Substitute Y Other Device	Z No Qualifier
M Epididymis and Spermatic Cord ♂	X External	Ø Drainage Device 3 Infusion Device	Z No Qualifier

R Vas Deferens ♂
  Ductus deferens
  Ejaculatory duct
	Ø Open
	3 Percutaneous
	4 Percutaneous Endoscopic
	7 Via Natural or Artificial Opening
	8 Via Natural or Artificial Opening Endoscopic
		Ø Drainage Device
		3 Infusion Device
		7 Autologous Tissue Substitute
		C Extraluminal Device
		D Intraluminal Device
		J Synthetic Substitute
		K Nonautologous Tissue Substitute
		Y Other Device
			Z No Qualifier

R Vas Deferens ♂
  Ductus deferens
  Ejaculatory duct
	X External	Ø Drainage Device
		3 Infusion Device
		D Intraluminal Device
			Z No Qualifier

Non-OR ØVP4[3,4]YZ	**Non-OR** ØVPM[3,4]YZ
Non-OR ØVP4[7,8][Ø,3,Y]Z	**Non-OR** ØVPM[7,8][Ø,3,Y]Z
Non-OR ØVP4X[Ø,1,3]Z	**Non-OR** ØVPMX[Ø,3]Z
Non-OR ØVP8[Ø,3,4,7,8][Ø,3,7,J,K,Y]Z	**Non-OR** ØVPR[Ø,3,4][Ø,3,7,C,J,K,Y]Z
Non-OR ØVP[D,S][3,4]YZ	**Non-OR** ØVPR[7,8][Ø,3,7,C,D,J,K,Y]Z
Non-OR ØVP[D,S][7,8][Ø,3,Y]Z	**Non-OR** ØVPRX[Ø,3,D]Z
Non-OR ØVP[8,D,S]X[Ø,3]Z	♂ All body part, approach, device, and qualifier values

NC Noncovered Procedure   **LC** Limited Coverage   **OA** Questionable OB Admit   **NT** New Tech Add-on   ⊞ Combination Member   ♂ Male   ♀ Female

ICD-10-PCS 2023   **669**

ØVP–ØVP

Ø   **Medical and Surgical**
V   **Male Reproductive System**
Q   **Repair**   Definition: Restoring, to the extent possible, a body part to its normal anatomic structure and function

         Explanation: Used only when the method to accomplish the repair is not one of the other root operations

Body Part Character 4		Approach Character 5	Device Character 6	Qualifier Character 7
Ø Prostate ♂		Ø Open 3 Percutaneous 4 Percutaneous Endoscopic 7 Via Natural or Artificial Opening 8 Via Natural or Artificial Opening Endoscopic	Z No Device	Z No Qualifier
1 Seminal Vesicle, Right ♂ 2 Seminal Vesicle, Left ♂ 3 Seminal Vesicles, Bilateral ♂ 6 Tunica Vaginalis, Right ♂ 7 Tunica Vaginalis, Left ♂ 9 Testis, Right ♂ B Testis, Left ♂ C Testes, Bilateral ♂		Ø Open 3 Percutaneous 4 Percutaneous Endoscopic	Z No Device	Z No Qualifier

5   Scrotum   ♂
S   Penis   ♂
      Corpus cavernosum
      Corpus spongiosum
T   Prepuce   ♂
      Foreskin
      Glans penis
		Ø Open
		3 Percutaneous
		4 Percutaneous Endoscopic
		X External
			Z No Device	Z No Qualifier

F   Spermatic Cord, Right   ♂
G   Spermatic Cord, Left   ♂
H   Spermatic Cords, Bilateral   ♂
J   Epididymis, Right   ♂
K   Epididymis, Left   ♂
L   Epididymis, Bilateral   ♂
N   Vas Deferens, Right   ♂
      Ductus deferens
      Ejaculatory duct
P   Vas Deferens, Left   ♂
      See N Vas Deferens, Right
Q   Vas Deferens, Bilateral   ♂
      See N Vas Deferens, Right
		Ø Open
		3 Percutaneous
		4 Percutaneous Endoscopic
		8 Via Natural or Artificial Opening
		      Endoscopic
			Z No Device	Z No Qualifier

Non-OR   ØVQ[6,7][Ø,3,4]ZZ   ♂   All body part, approach, device, and qualifier values
Non-OR   ØVQ5[Ø,3,4,X]ZZ

Ø   **Medical and Surgical**
V   **Male Reproductive System**
R   **Replacement**   Definition: Putting in or on biological or synthetic material that physically takes the place and/or function of all or a portion of a body part

         Explanation: The body part may have been taken out or replaced, or may be taken out, physically eradicated, or rendered nonfunctional during the REPLACEMENT procedure. A REMOVAL procedure is coded for taking out the device used in a previous replacement procedure.

Body Part Character 4		Approach Character 5	Device Character 6	Qualifier Character 7
9 Testis, Right ♂ B Testis, Left ♂ C Testes, Bilateral ♂		Ø Open	J Synthetic Substitute	Z No Qualifier

♂   All body part, approach, device, and qualifier values

Ø   **Medical and Surgical**
V   **Male Reproductive System**
S   **Reposition**   Definition: Moving to its normal location, or other suitable location, all or a portion of a body part

         Explanation: The body part is moved to a new location from an abnormal location, or from a normal location where it is not functioning correctly. The body part may or may not be cut out or off to be moved to the new location.

Body Part Character 4		Approach Character 5	Device Character 6	Qualifier Character 7
9 Testis, Right ♂ B Testis, Left ♂ C Testes, Bilateral ♂ F Spermatic Cord, Right ♂ G Spermatic Cord, Left ♂ H Spermatic Cords, Bilateral ♂		Ø Open 3 Percutaneous 4 Percutaneous Endoscopic 8 Via Natural or Artificial Opening Endoscopic	Z No Device	Z No Qualifier

♂   All body part, approach, device, and qualifier values

Non-OR Procedure   DRG Non-OR Procedure   Valid OR Procedure   HAC Associated Procedure   Combination Only   New/Revised April   New/Revised October

670   ICD-10-PCS 2023

Ø   **Medical and Surgical**
V   **Male Reproductive System**
T   **Resection**   Definition: Cutting out or off, without replacement, all of a body part
                      Explanation: None

Body Part Character 4	Approach Character 5	Device Character 6	Qualifier Character 7
Ø Prostate ⊞♂	**Ø** Open **4** Percutaneous Endoscopic **7** Via Natural or Artificial Opening **8** Via Natural or Artificial Opening Endoscopic	**Z** No Device	**Z** No Qualifier

1 Seminal Vesicle, Right   ♂
2 Seminal Vesicle, Left   ♂
3 Seminal Vesicles, Bilateral   ⊞♂
6 Tunica Vaginalis, Right   ♂
7 Tunica Vaginalis, Left   ♂
9 Testis, Right   ♂
B Testis, Left   ♂
C Testes, Bilateral   ♂
F Spermatic Cord, Right   ♂
G Spermatic Cord, Left   ♂
H Spermatic Cords, Bilateral   ♂
J Epididymis, Right   ♂
K Epididymis, Left   ♂
L Epididymis, Bilateral   ♂
N Vas Deferens, Right   NC♂
     Ductus deferens
     Ejaculatory duct
P Vas Deferens, Left   NC♂
     See N Vas Deferens, Right
Q Vas Deferens, Bilateral   NC♂
     See N Vas Deferens, Right
	Ø Open
	4 Percutaneous Endoscopic
		Z No Device	**Z** No Qualifier

5 Scrotum   ♂
S Penis   ♂
     Corpus cavernosum
     Corpus spongiosum
T Prepuce   ♂
     Foreskin
     Glans penis
	Ø Open
	4 Percutaneous Endoscopic
	X External
		Z No Device	**Z** No Qualifier

Non-OR ØVT[N,P,Q][Ø,4]ZZ	**See Appendix L for Procedure Combinations**
Non-OR ØVT[5,T][Ø,4,X]ZZ	⊞ ØVTØ[Ø,4,7,8]ZZ
NC ØVT[N,P,Q][Ø,4]ZZ with principal or secondary diagnosis of Z3Ø.2	⊞ ØVT3[Ø,4]ZZ
♂ All body part, approach, device, and qualifier values	

NC Noncovered Procedure   **LC** Limited Coverage   **QA** Questionable OB Admit   **NT** New Tech Add-on   ⊞ Combination Member   ♂ Male   ♀ Female

ICD-10-PCS 2023   671

Male Reproductive System

Ø **Medical and Surgical**
V **Male Reproductive System**
U **Supplement** Definition: Putting in or on biological or synthetic material that physically reinforces and/or augments the function of a portion of a body part
Explanation: The biological material is non-living, or is living and from the same individual. The body part may have been previously replaced, and the SUPPLEMENT procedure is performed to physically reinforce and/or augment the function of the replaced body part.

Body Part Character 4	Approach Character 5	Device Character 6	Qualifier Character 7
1 Seminal Vesicle, Right ♂ **2** Seminal Vesicle, Left ♂ **3** Seminal Vesicles, Bilateral ♂ **6** Tunica Vaginalis, Right ♂ **7** Tunica Vaginalis, Left ♂ **F** Spermatic Cord, Right ♂ **G** Spermatic Cord, Left ♂ **H** Spermatic Cords, Bilateral ♂ **J** Epididymis, Right ♂ **K** Epididymis, Left ♂ **L** Epididymis, Bilateral ♂ **N** Vas Deferens, Right ♂ Ductus deferens Ejaculatory duct **P** Vas Deferens, Left ♂ *See N Vas Deferens, Right* **Q** Vas Deferens, Bilateral ♂ *See N Vas Deferens, Right*	**Ø** Open **4** Percutaneous Endoscopic **8** Via Natural or Artificial Opening Endoscopic	**7** Autologous Tissue Substitute **J** Synthetic Substitute **K** Nonautologous Tissue Substitute	**Z** No Qualifier
5 Scrotum ♂ **S** Penis ♂ Corpus cavernosum Corpus spongiosum **T** Prepuce ♂ Foreskin Glans penis	**Ø** Open **4** Percutaneous Endoscopic **X** External	**7** Autologous Tissue Substitute **J** Synthetic Substitute **K** Nonautologous Tissue Substitute	**Z** No Qualifier
9 Testis, Right ♂ **B** Testis, Left ♂ **C** Testes, Bilateral ♂	**Ø** Open	**7** Autologous Tissue Substitute **J** Synthetic Substitute **K** Nonautologous Tissue Substitute	**Z** No Qualifier

Non-OR	ØVUSX[7,J,K]Z	♂	All body part, approach, device, and qualifier values

Non-OR Procedure   DRG Non-OR Procedure   Valid OR Procedure   HAC Associated Procedure   Combination Only   New/Revised April   New/Revised October

672

ICD-10-PCS 2023

Ø Medical and Surgical
V Male Reproductive System
W Revision   Definition: Correcting, to the extent possible, a portion of a malfunctioning device or the position of a displaced device
                 Explanation: Revision can include correcting a malfunctioning or displaced device by taking out or putting in components of the device such as a screw or pin

Body Part Character 4	Approach Character 5	Device Character 6	Qualifier Character 7

4 Prostate and Seminal Vesicles ♂
8 Scrotum and Tunica Vaginalis ♂
D Testis ♂
S Penis ♂
   Corpus cavernosum
   Corpus spongiosum
	Ø Open
	3 Percutaneous
	4 Percutaneous Endoscopic
	7 Via Natural or Artificial Opening
	8 Via Natural or Artificial Opening
	   Endoscopic
		Ø Drainage Device
		3 Infusion Device
		7 Autologous Tissue Substitute
		J Synthetic Substitute
		K Nonautologous Tissue Substitute
		Y Other Device
			Z No Qualifier

4 Prostate and Seminal Vesicles ♂
8 Scrotum and Tunica Vaginalis ♂
D Testis ♂
S Penis ♂
   Corpus cavernosum
   Corpus spongiosum
	X External	**Ø** Drainage Device
		3 Infusion Device
		7 Autologous Tissue Substitute
		J Synthetic Substitute
		K Nonautologous Tissue Substitute
			Z No Qualifier

M Epididymis and Spermatic Cord ♂	**Ø** Open **3** Percutaneous **4** Percutaneous Endoscopic **7** Via Natural or Artificial Opening **8** Via Natural or Artificial Opening Endoscopic	**Ø** Drainage Device **3** Infusion Device **7** Autologous Tissue Substitute **C** Extraluminal Device **J** Synthetic Substitute **K** Nonautologous Tissue Substitute **Y** Other Device	**Z** No Qualifier
M Epididymis and Spermatic Cord ♂	**X** External	**Ø** Drainage Device **3** Infusion Device **7** Autologous Tissue Substitute **C** Extraluminal Device **J** Synthetic Substitute **K** Nonautologous Tissue Substitute	**Z** No Qualifier

R Vas Deferens ♂
   Ductus deferens
   Ejaculatory duct
	Ø Open
	3 Percutaneous
	4 Percutaneous Endoscopic
	7 Via Natural or Artificial Opening
	8 Via Natural or Artificial Opening
	   Endoscopic
		Ø Drainage Device
		3 Infusion Device
		7 Autologous Tissue Substitute
		C Extraluminal Device
		D Intraluminal Device
		J Synthetic Substitute
		K Nonautologous Tissue Substitute
		Y Other Device
			Z No Qualifier

R Vas Deferens ♂
   Ductus deferens
   Ejaculatory duct
	X External	**Ø** Drainage Device
		3 Infusion Device
		7 Autologous Tissue Substitute
		C Extraluminal Device
		D Intraluminal Device
		J Synthetic Substitute
		K Nonautologous Tissue Substitute
			Z No Qualifier

Non-OR	ØVW[4,D,S][3,4,7,8]YZ	**Non-OR**	ØVWMX[Ø,3,7,C,J,K]Z
Non-OR	ØVW8[Ø,3,4,7,8][Ø,3,7,J,K,Y]Z	**Non-OR**	ØVWR[Ø,3,4,7,8][Ø,3,7,C,D,J,K,Y]Z
Non-OR	ØVW[4,8,D,S]X[Ø,3,7,J,K]Z	**Non-OR**	ØVWRX[Ø,3,7,C,D,J,K]Z
Non-OR	ØVWM[3,4,7,8]YZ	♂	All body part, approach, device, and qualifier values

NC Noncovered Procedure   **LC** Limited Coverage   **QA** Questionable OB Admit   **NT** New Tech Add-on   ⊞ Combination Member   ♂ Male   ♀ Female

ICD-10-PCS 2023   673

Ø **Medical and Surgical**
V **Male Reproductive System**
X **Transfer**   Definition: Moving, without taking out, all or a portion of a body part to another location to take over the function of all or a portion of a body part

Explanation: The body part transferred remains connected to its vascular and nervous supply

Body Part Character 4	Approach Character 5	Device Character 6	Qualifier Character 7

T Prepuce
  Foreskin
  Glans penis
	Ø Open
	X External
		Z No Device	D Urethra
			S Penis

Ø **Medical and Surgical**
V **Male Reproductive System**
Y **Transplantation**   Definition: Putting in or on all or a portion of a living body part taken from another individual or animal to physically take the place and/or function of all or a portion of a similar body part

Explanation: The native body part may or may not be taken out, and the transplanted body part may take over all or a portion of its function

Body Part Character 4	Approach Character 5	Device Character 6	Qualifier Character 7

5 Scrotum ♂
S Penis ♂
  Corpus cavernosum
  Corpus spongiosum
	Ø Open	Z No Device	Ø Allogeneic
			1 Syngeneic
			2 Zooplastic

♂   All body part, approach, device, and qualifier values

Anatomical Regions, General ØWØ–ØWY

Character Meanings

This Character Meaning table is provided as a guide to assist the user in the identification of character members that may be found in this section of code tables. It **SHOULD NOT** be used to build a PCS code.

Operation–Character 3	Body Region–Character 4	Approach–Character 5	Device–Character 6	Qualifier–Character 7
Ø Alteration	Ø Head	Ø Open	Ø Drainage Device	Ø Vagina OR Allogeneic
1 Bypass	1 Cranial Cavity	3 Percutaneous	1 Radioactive Element	1 Penis OR Syngeneic
2 Change	2 Face	4 Percutaneous Endoscopic	3 Infusion Device	2 Stoma
3 Control	3 Oral Cavity and Throat	7 Via Natural or Artificial Opening	7 Autologous Tissue Substitute	4 Cutaneous
4 Creation	4 Upper Jaw	8 Via Natural or Artificial Opening Endoscopic	J Synthetic Substitute	6 Bladder
8 Division	5 Lower Jaw	X External	K Nonautologous Tissue Substitute	9 Pleural Cavity, Right
9 Drainage	6 Neck		Y Other Device	B Pleural Cavity, Left
B Excision	8 Chest Wall		Z No Device	G Peritoneal Cavity
C Extirpation	9 Pleural Cavity, Right			J Pelvic Cavity
F Fragmentation	B Pleural Cavity, Left			W Upper Vein
H Insertion	C Mediastinum			X Diagnostic
J Inspection	D Pericardial Cavity			Y Lower Vein
M Reattachment	F Abdominal Wall			Z No Qualifier
P Removal	G Peritoneal Cavity			
Q Repair	H Retroperitoneum			
U Supplement	J Pelvic Cavity			
W Revision	K Upper Back			
Y Transplantation	L Lower Back			
	M Perineum, Male			
	N Perineum, Female			
	P Gastrointestinal Tract			
	Q Respiratory Tract			
	R Genitourinary Tract			

AHA Coding Clinic for table ØWØ
2015, 1Q, 31   Bilateral browpexy

AHA Coding Clinic for table ØW1
2020, 4Q, 55   Insertion of subcutaneous pump system for ascites drainage
2018, 4Q, 41-42 Anatomical regions bypass qualifiers
2015, 2Q, 36   Insertion of infusion device into peritoneal cavity
2013, 4Q, 126-127 Creation of percutaneous cutaneoperitoneal fistula

AHA Coding Clinic for table ØW3
2021, 3Q, 26   Cavoatrial junction tear with repair and relief of cardiac tamponade
2019, 3Q, 4   Evacuation of subdural hematoma and control of bleeding artery
2018, 4Q, 38   Control of epistaxis
2018, 1Q, 19   Argon plasma coagulation of duodenal arteriovenous malformation
2018, 1Q, 19   Control of epistaxis via silver nitrate cauterization
2017, 4Q, 57-58 Added approach values - Transorifice esophageal vein banding
2017, 4Q, 105   Control of gastrointestinal bleeding
2017, 4Q, 106   Control of bleeding of external naris using suture
2017, 4Q, 106   Nasal packing for epistaxis
2016, 4Q, 99-100 Root operation Control
2014, 4Q, 44   Bakri balloon for control of postpartum hemorrhage
2013, 3Q, 23   Control of intraoperative bleeding

AHA Coding Clinic for table ØW4
2019, 4Q, 30   Transfer large intestine to vagina
2016, 4Q, 101   Root operation Creation

AHA Coding Clinic for table ØW9
2021, 3Q, 17   Incision and drainage of retropharyngeal space abscess
2021, 3Q, 21   Drainage of midline neck abscess
2021, 3Q, 26   Cavoatrial junction tear with repair and relief of cardiac tamponade
2020, 4Q, 56   Transvaginal drainage of pelvis
2017, 3Q, 12   Therapeutic and diagnostic paracentesis
2017, 2Q, 16   Incision and drainage of floor of mouth

AHA Coding Clinic for table ØWB
2021, 3Q, 21   Excision of thyroglossal duct cyst
2019, 1Q, 27   Excision of pelvic sidewall mass
2017, 2Q, 16   Excision of floor of mouth
2016, 1Q, 21   Excision of urachal mass
2013, 4Q, 119   Excision of inclusion cyst of perineum

AHA Coding Clinic for table ØWC
2022, 1Q, 42   Removal of fat necrosis from retroperitoneum and space of Retzius
2019, 4Q, 35   Extirpation of jaw
2017, 2Q, 16   Excision of floor of mouth

AHA Coding Clinic for table ØWH
2021, 2Q, 14   Peritoneal dialysis catheter placement
2019, 4Q, 43   Unidirectional source brachytherapy
2018, 1Q, 25   Intrauterine brachytherapy & placement of tandems & ovoids
2017, 4Q, 104   Intrauterine brachytherapy & placement of tandems & ovoids
2016, 2Q, 14   Insertion of peritoneal totally implantable venous access device
2015, 2Q, 36   Insertion of infusion device into peritoneal cavity

AHA Coding Clinic for table ØWJ
2021, 2Q, 19   Electromagnetic stealth guided ventriculoperitoneal shunt insertion with endoscopy
2019, 1Q, 3-8   Whipple procedure
2019, 1Q, 25   Laparoscopic appendectomy converted to open procedure
2018, 3Q, 29   Decommissioning of left ventricular assist device with exploration of mediastinum
2016, 4Q, 58   Longitudinal vaginal septum
2013, 2Q, 36   Insertion of ventriculoperitoneal shunt with laparoscopic assistance

AHA Coding Clinic for table ØWP
2021, 2Q, 14   Removal of peritoneal dialysis catheter

AHA Coding Clinic for table ØWQ
2017, 4Q, 106   Control of bleeding of external naris using suture
2017, 3Q, 8   Removal of silo and closure of gastroschisis
2016, 3Q, 3-7   Stoma creation & takedown procedures
2014, 4Q, 38   Abdominoplasty and abdominal wall plication for hernia repair
2014, 3Q, 28   Ileostomy takedown and parastomal hernia repair

AHA Coding Clinic for table ØWU
2017, 3Q, 8   First stage of gastroschisis repair with silo placement
2016, 3Q, 40   Omentoplasty
2015, 2Q, 29   Placement of Ioban™ antimicrobial drape over surgical wound
2014, 4Q, 39   Abdominal component release with placement of mesh for hernia repair
2012, 4Q, 101   Rib resection with reconstruction of anterior chest wall

AHA Coding Clinic for table ØWW
2015, 2Q, 9   Revision of ventriculoperitoneal (VP) shunt

AHA Coding Clinic for table ØWY
2016, 4Q, 112-113 Transplantation

Ø   **Medical and Surgical**
W   **Anatomical Regions, General**
Ø   **Alteration**   Definition: Modifying the anatomic structure of a body part without affecting the function of the body part
                     Explanation: Principal purpose is to improve appearance

Body Part Character 4	Approach Character 5	Device Character 6	Qualifier Character 7

Ø   Head
2   Face
4   Upper Jaw
5   Lower Jaw
6   Neck
     Parapharyngeal space
     Retropharyngeal space
8   Chest Wall
F   Abdominal Wall
K   Upper Back
L   Lower Back
M   Perineum, Male   ♂
N   Perineum, Female   ♀
	Ø Open
	3 Percutaneous
	4 Percutaneous Endoscopic
		7 Autologous Tissue Substitute
		J Synthetic Substitute
		K Nonautologous Tissue Substitute
		Z No Device
			Z No Qualifier

     ♂   ØWØM[Ø,3,4][7,J,K,Z]Z
     ♀   ØWØN[Ø,3,4][7,J,K,Z]Z

Ø   **Medical and Surgical**
W   **Anatomical Regions, General**
1   **Bypass**   Definition: Altering the route of passage of the contents of a tubular body part
                 Explanation: Rerouting contents of a body part to a downstream area of the normal route, to a similar route and body part, or to an abnormal route and dissimilar body part. Includes one or more anastomoses, with or without the use of a device.

Body Part Character 4	Approach Character 5	Device Character 6	Qualifier Character 7
1 Cranial Cavity	**Ø** Open	**J** Synthetic Substitute	**9** Pleural Cavity, Right **B** Pleural Cavity, Left **G** Peritoneal Cavity **J** Pelvic Cavity
9 Pleural Cavity, Right **B** Pleural Cavity, Left **J** Pelvic Cavity Retropubic space	**Ø** Open **3** Percutaneous **4** Percutaneous Endoscopic	**J** Synthetic Substitute	**4** Cutaneous **9** Pleural Cavity, Right **B** Pleural Cavity, Left **G** Peritoneal Cavity **J** Pelvic Cavity **W** Upper Vein **Y** Lower Vein
G Peritoneal Cavity Abdominal cavity	**Ø** Open **3** Percutaneous **4** Percutaneous Endoscopic	**J** Synthetic Substitute	**4** Cutaneous **6** Bladder **9** Pleural Cavity, Right **B** Pleural Cavity, Left **G** Peritoneal Cavity **J** Pelvic Cavity **W** Upper Vein **Y** Lower Vein

Non-OR	ØW1[9,B][Ø,3,4]J[4,G,W,Y]
Non-OR	ØW1J[Ø,3,4]J[4,W,Y]
Non-OR	ØW1G[Ø,3,4]J[9,B,G,J]

Non-OR Procedure   DRG Non-OR Procedure   Valid OR Procedure   HAC Associated Procedure   Combination Only   New/Revised April   New/Revised October

676   ICD-10-PCS 2023

Ø Medical and Surgical
W Anatomical Regions, General
2 Change   Definition: Taking out or off a device from a body part and putting back an identical or similar device in or on the same body part without cutting or puncturing the skin or a mucous membrane
           Explanation: All CHANGE procedures are coded using the approach EXTERNAL

Body Part Character 4	Approach Character 5	Device Character 6	Qualifier Character 7
Ø Head	**X** External	**Ø** Drainage Device	**Z** No Qualifier
1 Cranial Cavity		**Y** Other Device	
2 Face			
4 Upper Jaw			
5 Lower Jaw			
6 Neck			
Parapharyngeal space			
Retropharyngeal space			
8 Chest Wall			
9 Pleural Cavity, Right			
B Pleural Cavity, Left			
C Mediastinum			
Mediastinal cavity			
Mediastinal space			
D Pericardial Cavity			
F Abdominal Wall			
G Peritoneal Cavity			
Abdominal cavity			
H Retroperitoneum			
Retroperitoneal cavity			
Retroperitoneal space			
J Pelvic Cavity			
Retropubic space			
K Upper Back			
L Lower Back			
M Perineum, Male ♂			
N Perineum, Female ♀			

Non-OR	All body part, approach, device, and qualifier values	♂ ØW2MX[Ø,Y]Z
		♀ ØW2NX[Ø,Y]Z

NC Noncovered Procedure   **LC** Limited Coverage   **QA** Questionable OB Admit   **NT** New Tech Add-on   ⊞ Combination Member   ♂ Male   ♀ Female

ICD-10-PCS 2023   **677**

Ø   Medical and Surgical
W   Anatomical Regions, General
3   Control   Definition: Stopping, or attempting to stop, postprocedural or other acute bleeding
                         Explanation: None

Body Part Character 4	Approach Character 5	Device Character 6	Qualifier Character 7

Ø Head
1 Cranial Cavity
2 Face
4 Upper Jaw
5 Lower Jaw
6 Neck
  Parapharyngeal space
  Retropharyngeal space
8 Chest Wall
9 Pleural Cavity, Right
B Pleural Cavity, Left
C Mediastinum
  Mediastinal cavity
  Mediastinal space
D Pericardial Cavity
F Abdominal Wall
G Peritoneal Cavity
  Abdominal cavity
H Retroperitoneum
  Retroperitoneal cavity
  Retroperitoneal space
J Pelvic Cavity
  Retropubic space
K Upper Back
L Lower Back
M Perineum, Male   ♂
N Perineum, Female   ♀
	Ø Open
	3 Percutaneous
	4 Percutaneous Endoscopic
		Z No Device	Z No Qualifier

3 Oral Cavity and Throat	Ø Open 3 Percutaneous 4 Percutaneous Endoscopic 7 Via Natural or Artificial Opening 8 Via Natural or Artificial Opening Endoscopic X External	Z No Device	Z No Qualifier
P Gastrointestinal Tract Q Respiratory Tract R Genitourinary Tract	Ø Open 3 Percutaneous 4 Percutaneous Endoscopic 7 Via Natural or Artificial Opening 8 Via Natural or Artificial Opening Endoscopic	Z No Device	Z No Qualifier

Non-OR   ØW3P8ZZ

♂   ØW3M[Ø,3,4]ZZ
♀   ØW3N[Ø,3,4]ZZ

Ø   Medical and Surgical
W   Anatomical Regions, General
4   Creation   Definition: Putting in or on biological or synthetic material to form a new body part that to the extent possible replicates the anatomic structure or function of an absent body part
                         Explanation: Used for gender reassignment surgery and corrective procedures in individuals with congenital anomalies

Body Part Character 4	Approach Character 5	Device Character 6	Qualifier Character 7
M Perineum, Male ♂	Ø Open	7 Autologous Tissue Substitute J Synthetic Substitute K Nonautologous Tissue Substitute	Ø Vagina
N Perineum, Female ♀	Ø Open	7 Autologous Tissue Substitute J Synthetic Substitute K Nonautologous Tissue Substitute	1 Penis

♂   ØW4MØ[7,J,K]Ø
♀   ØW4NØ[7,J,K]1

Ø   Medical and Surgical
W   Anatomical Regions, General
8   Division   Definition: Cutting into a body part, without draining fluids and/or gases from the body part, in order to separate or transect a body part
                         Explanation: All or a portion of the body part is separated into two or more portions

Body Part Character 4	Approach Character 5	Device Character 6	Qualifier Character 7
N Perineum, Female ♀	X External	Z No Device	Z No Qualifier

Non-OR   ØW8NXZZ

♀   ØW8NXZZ

Non-OR Procedure   DRG Non-OR Procedure   Valid OR Procedure   HAC Associated Procedure   Combination Only   New/Revised April   New/Revised October

678   ICD-10-PCS 2023

Ø   **Medical and Surgical**
W   **Anatomical Regions, General**
9   **Drainage**   Definition: Taking or letting out fluids and/or gases from a body part
                  Explanation: The qualifier DIAGNOSTIC is used to identify drainage procedures that are biopsies

Body Part Character 4	Approach Character 5	Device Character 6	Qualifier Character 7

Ø Head
1 Cranial Cavity
2 Face
3 Oral Cavity and Throat
4 Upper Jaw
5 Lower Jaw
8 Chest Wall
9 Pleural Cavity, Right
B Pleural Cavity, Left
C Mediastinum
    Mediastinal cavity
    Mediastinal space
D Pericardial Cavity
F Abdominal Wall
G Peritoneal Cavity
    Abdominal cavity
H Retroperitoneum
    Retroperitoneal cavity
    Retroperitoneal space
K Upper Back
L Lower Back
M Perineum, Male   ♂
N Perineum, Female   ♀
	Ø Open
	3 Percutaneous
	4 Percutaneous Endoscopic
		Ø Drainage Device	Z No Qualifier

Ø Head
1 Cranial Cavity
2 Face
3 Oral Cavity and Throat
4 Upper Jaw
5 Lower Jaw
8 Chest Wall
9 Pleural Cavity, Right
B Pleural Cavity, Left
C Mediastinum
    Mediastinal cavity
    Mediastinal space
D Pericardial Cavity
F Abdominal Wall
G Peritoneal Cavity
    Abdominal cavity
H Retroperitoneum
    Retroperitoneal cavity
    Retroperitoneal space
K Upper Back
L Lower Back
M Perineum, Male   ♂
N Perineum, Female   ♀
	Ø Open
	3 Percutaneous
	4 Percutaneous Endoscopic
		Z No Device	X Diagnostic
			Z No Qualifier

6 Neck
    Parapharyngeal space
    Retropharyngeal space
J Pelvic Cavity
    Retropubic space
	Ø Open
	3 Percutaneous
	4 Percutaneous Endoscopic
	7 Via Natural or Artificial Opening
	8 Via Natural or Artificial Opening
	    Endoscopic
		Ø Drainage Device	Z No Qualifier

6 Neck
    Parapharyngeal space
    Retropharyngeal space
J Pelvic Cavity
    Retropubic space
	Ø Open
	3 Percutaneous
	4 Percutaneous Endoscopic
	7 Via Natural or Artificial Opening
	8 Via Natural or Artificial Opening
	    Endoscopic
		Z No Device	X Diagnostic
			Z No Qualifier

Non-OR	ØW9[Ø,8,9,B,K,L,M]ØØZ	**Non-OR**	ØW9J[3,7,8]ØZ
Non-OR	ØW9[Ø,1,2,3,4,5,8,9,B,C,D,F,G,H,K,L,M,N]3ØZ	**Non-OR**	ØW96[Ø,3,4]ZX
Non-OR	ØW9[Ø,1,8,F,K,L,M]4ØZ	**Non-OR**	ØW9J[3,7,8]Z[X,Z]
Non-OR	ØW9[Ø,2,3,4,5,8,9,B,K,L,M,N]ØZX	**Non-OR**	ØW963ZZ
Non-OR	ØW9[Ø,1,2,3,4,5,8,9,B,C,D,G,K,L,M,N]3ZX	♂	ØW9M[Ø,3,4]ØZ
Non-OR	ØW9[Ø,1,2,3,4,5,8,C,K,L,M,N]4ZX	♂	ØW9M[Ø,3,4]Z[X,Z]
Non-OR	ØW9[Ø,8,9,B,K,L,M]ØZZ	♀	ØW9N[Ø,3,4]ØZ
Non-OR	ØW9[Ø,1,2,3,4,5,8,9,B,C,D,F,G,H,K,L,M,N]3ZZ	♀	ØW9N[Ø,3]Z[X,Z]
Non-OR	ØW9[Ø,1,8,F,K,L,M]4ZZ	♀	ØW9N4ZZ
Non-OR	ØW963ØZ		

🅝🅒 Noncovered Procedure   🅛🅒 Limited Coverage   🅠🅐 Questionable OB Admit   🅝🅣 New Tech Add-on   ⊞ Combination Member   ♂ Male   ♀ Female

ICD-10-PCS 2023   679

Ø   **Medical and Surgical**
W   **Anatomical Regions, General**
B   **Excision**   Definition: Cutting out or off, without replacement, a portion of a body part
                     Explanation: The qualifier DIAGNOSTIC is used to identify excision procedures that are biopsies

Body Part Character 4	Approach Character 5	Device Character 6	Qualifier Character 7
Ø Head 2 Face 3 Oral Cavity and Throat 4 Upper Jaw 5 Lower Jaw 8 Chest Wall K Upper Back L Lower Back M Perineum, Male ♂ N Perineum, Female ♀	Ø Open 3 Percutaneous 4 Percutaneous Endoscopic X External	Z No Device	X Diagnostic Z No Qualifier

6   Neck
      Parapharyngeal space
      Retropharyngeal space
F   Abdominal Wall
	Ø Open
	3 Percutaneous
	4 Percutaneous Endoscopic
		Z No Device	X Diagnostic
			Z No Qualifier

6   Neck
      Parapharyngeal space
      Retropharyngeal space
F   Abdominal Wall
	X External	Z No Device	2 Stoma
			X Diagnostic
			Z No Qualifier

C   Mediastinum
      Mediastinal cavity
      Mediastinal space
H   Retroperitoneum
      Retroperitoneal cavity
      Retroperitoneal space
	Ø Open
	3 Percutaneous
	4 Percutaneous Endoscopic
		Z No Device	X Diagnostic
			Z No Qualifier

Non-OR ØWB[Ø,2,4,5,8,K,L,M][Ø,3,4,X]ZX			
Non-OR ØWB6[Ø,3,4]ZX		♂ ØWBM[Ø,3,4,X]Z[X,Z]	
Non-OR ØWB6XZX		♀ ØWBN[Ø,3,4,X]Z[X,Z]	
Non-OR ØWBH[3,4]ZX			

Ø   **Medical and Surgical**
W   **Anatomical Regions, General**
C   **Extirpation**   Definition: Taking or cutting out solid matter from a body part
                     Explanation: The solid matter may be an abnormal byproduct of a biological function or a foreign body; it may be imbedded in a body part or in the lumen of a tubular body part. The solid matter may or may not have been previously broken into pieces.

Body Part Character 4	Approach Character 5	Device Character 6	Qualifier Character 7

1   Cranial Cavity
3   Oral Cavity and Throat
9   Pleural Cavity, Right
B   Pleural Cavity, Left
C   Mediastinum
      Mediastinal cavity
      Mediastinal space
D   Pericardial Cavity
G   Peritoneal Cavity
      Abdominal cavity
H   Retroperitoneum
      Retroperitoneal cavity
      Retroperitoneal space
J   Pelvic Cavity
      Retropubic space
	Ø Open
	3 Percutaneous
	4 Percutaneous Endoscopic
	X External
		Z No Device	Z No Qualifier

4 Upper Jaw 5 Lower Jaw	Ø Open 3 Percutaneous 4 Percutaneous Endoscopic	Z No Device	Z No Qualifier
P Gastrointestinal Tract Q Respiratory Tract R Genitourinary Tract	Ø Open 3 Percutaneous 4 Percutaneous Endoscopic 7 Via Natural or Artificial Opening 8 Via Natural or Artificial Opening Endoscopic X External	Z No Device	Z No Qualifier

Non-OR   ØWC[1,3]XZZ
Non-OR   ØWC[9,B][Ø,3,4,X]ZZ
Non-OR   ØWC[C,D,G,H,J]XZZ
Non-OR   ØWC[4,5]3ZZ
Non-OR   ØWC[P,R][7,8,X]ZZ
Non-OR   ØWCQ[Ø,3,4,X]ZZ

Ø   Medical and Surgical
W   Anatomical Regions, General
F   Fragmentation   Definition: Breaking solid matter in a body part into pieces

Explanation: Physical force (e.g., manual, ultrasonic) applied directly or indirectly is used to break the solid matter into pieces. The solid matter may be an abnormal byproduct of a biological function or a foreign body. The pieces of solid matter are not taken out.

Body Part Character 4	Approach Character 5	Device Character 6	Qualifier Character 7

1 Cranial Cavity NC
3 Oral Cavity and Throat NC
9 Pleural Cavity, Right NC
B Pleural Cavity, Left NC
C Mediastinum NC
   Mediastinal cavity
   Mediastinal space
D Pericardial Cavity
G Peritoneal Cavity NC
   Abdominal cavity
J Pelvic Cavity NC
   Retropubic space
	Ø Open
	3 Percutaneous
	4 Percutaneous Endoscopic
	X External
		Z No Device	Z No Qualifier

P Gastrointestinal Tract NC Q Respiratory Tract NC R Genitourinary Tract	Ø Open 3 Percutaneous 4 Percutaneous Endoscopic 7 Via Natural or Artificial Opening 8 Via Natural or Artificial Opening Endoscopic X External	Z No Device	Z No Qualifier

Non-OR	ØWF[1,3,9,B,C,G]XZZ		
Non-OR	ØWFJ[Ø,3,4,X]ZZ	**NC** ØWF[1,3,9,B,C,G,J]XZZ	
Non-OR	ØWFP[Ø,3,4,7,8,X]ZZ	**NC** ØWF[P,Q]XZZ	
Non-OR	ØWFQXZZ		
Non-OR	ØWFR[Ø,3,4,7,8,X]ZZ		

Ø   Medical and Surgical
W   Anatomical Regions, General
H   Insertion   Definition: Putting in a nonbiological appliance that monitors, assists, performs, or prevents a physiological function but does not physically take the place of a body part

Explanation: None

Body Part Character 4	Approach Character 5	Device Character 6	Qualifier Character 7

Ø Head
1 Cranial Cavity
2 Face
3 Oral Cavity and Throat
4 Upper Jaw
5 Lower Jaw
6 Neck
   Parapharyngeal space
   Retropharyngeal space
8 Chest Wall
9 Pleural Cavity, Right
B Pleural Cavity, Left
C Mediastinum
   Mediastinal cavity
   Mediastinal space
D Pericardial Cavity
F Abdominal Wall
G Peritoneal Cavity
   Abdominal cavity
H Retroperitoneum
   Retroperitoneal cavity
   Retroperitoneal space
J Pelvic Cavity
   Retropubic space
K Upper Back
L Lower Back
M Perineum, Male
N Perineum, Female ♀
	Ø Open
	3 Percutaneous
	4 Percutaneous Endoscopic
		1 Radioactive Element
		3 Infusion Device
		Y Other Device
			Z No Qualifier

P Gastrointestinal Tract Q Respiratory Tract R Genitourinary Tract	Ø Open 3 Percutaneous 4 Percutaneous Endoscopic 7 Via Natural or Artificial Opening 8 Via Natural or Artificial Opening Endoscopic	1 Radioactive Element 3 Infusion Device Y Other Device	Z No Qualifier

DRG Non-OR	ØWH[Ø,2,4,5,6,K,L,M][Ø,3,4][3,Y]Z	Non-OR	ØWHP[3,4,7,8][3,Y]Z
Non-OR	ØWH1[Ø,3,4]3Z	Non-OR	ØWHQ[Ø,7,8][3,Y]Z
Non-OR	ØWH[8,9,B][Ø,3,4][3,Y]Z	Non-OR	ØWHR[Ø,3,4,7,8][3,Y]Z
Non-OR	ØWHPØYZ	♀	ØWHN[Ø,3,4][3,Y]Z

NC Noncovered Procedure   **LC** Limited Coverage   **QA** Questionable OB Admit   **NT** New Tech Add-on   ⊞ Combination Member   ♂ Male   ♀ Female

Ø   Medical and Surgical
W   Anatomical Regions, General
J   Inspection   Definition: Visually and/or manually exploring a body part

Explanation: Visual exploration may be performed with or without optical instrumentation. Manual exploration may be performed directly or through intervening body layers.

Body Part Character 4	Approach Character 5	Device Character 6	Qualifier Character 7

Ø Head
2 Face
3 Oral Cavity and Throat
4 Upper Jaw
5 Lower Jaw
6 Neck
   Parapharyngeal space
   Retropharyngeal space
8 Chest Wall
F Abdominal Wall
K Upper Back
L Lower Back
M Perineum, Male ♂
N Perineum, Female ♀
	Ø Open
	3 Percutaneous
	4 Percutaneous Endoscopic
	X External
		Z No Device	Z No Qualifier

1 Cranial Cavity
9 Pleural Cavity, Right
B Pleural Cavity, Left
C Mediastinum
   Mediastinal cavity
   Mediastinal space
D Pericardial Cavity
G Peritoneal Cavity
   Abdominal cavity
H Retroperitoneum
   Retroperitoneal cavity
   Retroperitoneal space
J Pelvic Cavity
   Retropubic space
	Ø Open
	3 Percutaneous
	4 Percutaneous Endoscopic
		Z No Device	Z No Qualifier

P Gastrointestinal Tract Q Respiratory Tract R Genitourinary Tract	Ø Open 3 Percutaneous 4 Percutaneous Endoscopic 7 Via Natural or Artificial Opening 8 Via Natural or Artificial Opening Endoscopic	Z No Device	Z No Qualifier

DRG Non-OR	ØWJ[Ø,2,4,5,K,L]ØZZ		♂	ØWJM[Ø,3,4,X]ZZ
DRG Non-OR	ØWJM[Ø,4]ZZ		♀	ØWJN[Ø,3,4,X]ZZ
Non-OR	ØWJ3ØZZ			
Non-OR	ØWJ[Ø,2,3,4,5,6,8,F,K,L,M,N][3,X]ZZ			
Non-OR	ØWJ[Ø,2,3,4,5,K,L]4ZZ			
Non-OR	ØWJDØZZ			
Non-OR	ØWJ[1,9,B,C,D,G,H,J]3ZZ			
Non-OR	ØWJ[P,Q,R][3,7,8]ZZ			

Ø   Medical and Surgical
W   Anatomical Regions, General
M   Reattachment   Definition: Putting back in or on all or a portion of a separated body part to its normal location or other suitable location

Explanation: Vascular circulation and nervous pathways may or may not be reestablished

Body Part Character 4	Approach Character 5	Device Character 6	Qualifier Character 7

2 Face
4 Upper Jaw
5 Lower Jaw
6 Neck
   Parapharyngeal space
   Retropharyngeal space
8 Chest Wall
F Abdominal Wall
K Upper Back
L Lower Back
M Perineum, Male ♂
N Perineum, Female ♀
	Ø Open	Z No Device	Z No Qualifier

♂	ØWMMØZZ
♀	ØWMNØZZ

Non-OR Procedure   DRG Non-OR Procedure   Valid OR Procedure   HAC Associated Procedure   Combination Only   New/Revised April   New/Revised October

Ø   Medical and Surgical
W   Anatomical Regions, General
P   Removal   Definition: Taking out or off a device from a body part

Explanation: If a device is taken out and a similar device put in without cutting or puncturing the skin or mucous membrane, the procedure is coded to the root operation CHANGE. Otherwise, the procedure for taking out the device is coded to the root operation REMOVAL.

Body Part Character 4	Approach Character 5	Device Character 6	Qualifier Character 7

Ø   Head
2   Face
4   Upper Jaw
5   Lower Jaw
6   Neck
    Parapharyngeal space
    Retropharyngeal space
8   Chest Wall
C   Mediastinum
    Mediastinal cavity
    Mediastinal space
F   Abdominal Wall
K   Upper Back
L   Lower Back
M   Perineum, Male   ♂
N   Perineum, Female   ♀
	Ø Open
	3 Percutaneous
	4 Percutaneous Endoscopic
	X External
		Ø Drainage Device
		1 Radioactive Element
		3 Infusion Device
		7 Autologous Tissue Substitute
		J Synthetic Substitute
		K Nonautologous Tissue Substitute
		Y Other Device
			Z No Qualifier

1   Cranial Cavity
9   Pleural Cavity, Right
B   Pleural Cavity, Left
G   Peritoneal Cavity
    Abdominal cavity
J   Pelvic Cavity
    Retropubic space
	Ø Open
	3 Percutaneous
	4 Percutaneous Endoscopic
		Ø Drainage Device
		1 Radioactive Element
		3 Infusion Device
		J Synthetic Substitute
		Y Other Device
			Z No Qualifier

1   Cranial Cavity
9   Pleural Cavity, Right
B   Pleural Cavity, Left
G   Peritoneal Cavity
    Abdominal cavity
J   Pelvic Cavity
    Retropubic space
	X External	Ø Drainage Device
		1 Radioactive Element
		3 Infusion Device
			Z No Qualifier

D   Pericardial Cavity
H   Retroperitoneum
    Retroperitoneal cavity
    Retroperitoneal space
	Ø Open
	3 Percutaneous
	4 Percutaneous Endoscopic
		Ø Drainage Device
		1 Radioactive Element
		3 Infusion Device
		Y Other Device
			Z No Qualifier

D   Pericardial Cavity
H   Retroperitoneum
    Retroperitoneal cavity
    Retroperitoneal space
	X External	Ø Drainage Device
		1 Radioactive Element
		3 Infusion Device
			Z No Qualifier

P Gastrointestinal Tract Q Respiratory Tract R Genitourinary Tract	Ø Open 3 Percutaneous 4 Percutaneous Endoscopic 7 Via Natural or Artificial Opening 8 Via Natural or Artificial Opening Endoscopic X External	1 Radioactive Element 3 Infusion Device Y Other Device	Z No Qualifier

Non-OR	ØWP[Ø,2,4,5,6,8][Ø,3,4,X][Ø,1,3,7,J,K,Y]Z	♂	ØWPM[Ø,3,4,X][Ø,1,3,7,J,K,Y]Z
Non-OR	ØWP[C,F]X[Ø,1,3,7,J,K,Y]Z	♀	ØWPN[Ø,3,4,X][Ø,1,3,7,J,K,Y]Z
Non-OR	ØWP[K,L][Ø,3,4,X][Ø,1,3,7,J,K,Y]Z		
Non-OR	ØWPM[Ø,3,4][Ø,1,3,J,Y]Z		
Non-OR	ØWPMX[Ø,1,3,Y]Z		
Non-OR	ØWPNX[Ø,1,3,7,J,K,Y]Z		
Non-OR	ØWP1[Ø,3,4]3Z		
Non-OR	ØWP[9,B,J][Ø,3,4][Ø,1,3,J,Y]Z		
Non-OR	ØWP[1,9,B,G,J]X[Ø,1,3]Z		
Non-OR	ØWP[D,H]X[Ø,1,3]Z		
Non-OR	ØWPP[3,4,7,8,X][1,3,Y]Z		
Non-OR	ØWPQ73Z		
Non-OR	ØWPQ8[3,Y]Z		
Non-OR	ØWPQ[Ø,X][1,3,Y]Z		
Non-OR	ØWPR[Ø,3,4,7,8,X][1,3,Y]Z		

NC Noncovered Procedure   **LC** Limited Coverage   **QA** Questionable OB Admit   **NT** New Tech Add-on   ➕ Combination Member   ♂ Male   ♀ Female

ICD-10-PCS 2023   **683**

Ø **Medical and Surgical**
W **Anatomical Regions, General**
Q **Repair**   Definition: Restoring, to the extent possible, a body part to its normal anatomic structure and function
                       Explanation: Used only when the method to accomplish the repair is not one of the other root operations

Body Part Character 4	Approach Character 5	Device Character 6	Qualifier Character 7
Ø Head **2** Face **3** Oral Cavity and Throat **4** Upper Jaw **5** Lower Jaw **8** Chest Wall **K** Upper Back **L** Lower Back **M** Perineum, Male ♂ **N** Perineum, Female ♀	**Ø** Open **3** Percutaneous **4** Percutaneous Endoscopic **X** External	**Z** No Device	**Z** No Qualifier

6 Neck
   Parapharyngeal space
   Retropharyngeal space
F Abdominal Wall
	Ø Open
	3 Percutaneous
	4 Percutaneous Endoscopic
		Z No Device	**Z** No Qualifier

6 Neck
   Parapharyngeal space
   Retropharyngeal space
F Abdominal Wall   ⊞
	X External	**Z** No Device	**2** Stoma
			Z No Qualifier

C Mediastinum
   Mediastinal cavity
   Mediastinal space
	Ø Open
	3 Percutaneous
	4 Percutaneous Endoscopic
		Z No Device	**Z** No Qualifier

Non-OR   ØWQNXZZ
♂   ØWQM[Ø,3,4,X]ZZ
♀   ØWQN[Ø,3,4,X]ZZ

See Appendix L for Procedure Combinations
  ⊞   ØWQFXZ[2,Z]

Ø **Medical and Surgical**
W **Anatomical Regions, General**
U **Supplement**   Definition: Putting in or on biological or synthetic material that physically reinforces and/or augments the function of a portion of a body part
                      Explanation: The biological material is non-living, or is living and from the same individual. The body part may have been previously replaced, and the SUPPLEMENT procedure is performed to physically reinforce and/or augment the function of the replaced body part.

Body Part Character 4	Approach Character 5	Device Character 6	Qualifier Character 7

Ø Head
2 Face
4 Upper Jaw
5 Lower Jaw
6 Neck
   Parapharyngeal space
   Retropharyngeal space
8 Chest Wall
C Mediastinum
   Mediastinal cavity
   Mediastinal space
F Abdominal Wall
K Upper Back
L Lower Back
M Perineum, Male   ♂
N Perineum, Female   ♀
	Ø Open
	4 Percutaneous Endoscopic
		7 Autologous Tissue Substitute
		J Synthetic Substitute
		K Nonautologous Tissue Substitute
			Z No Qualifier

♂   ØWUM[Ø,4][7,J,K]Z
♀   ØWUN[Ø,4][7,J,K]Z

Ø   Medical and Surgical
W   Anatomical Regions, General
W   Revision   Definition: Correcting, to the extent possible, a portion of a malfunctioning device or the position of a displaced device

          Explanation: Revision can include correcting a malfunctioning or displaced device by taking out or putting in components of the device such as a screw or pin

Body Part Character 4	Approach Character 5	Device Character 6	Qualifier Character 7

Ø Head
2 Face
4 Upper Jaw
5 Lower Jaw
6 Neck
   Parapharyngeal space
   Retropharyngeal space
8 Chest Wall
C Mediastinum
   Mediastinal cavity
   Mediastinal space
F Abdominal Wall
K Upper Back
L Lower Back
M Perineum, Male   ♂
N Perineum, Female   ♀
	Ø Open
	3 Percutaneous
	4 Percutaneous Endoscopic
	X External
		Ø Drainage Device
		1 Radioactive Element
		3 Infusion Device
		7 Autologous Tissue Substitute
		J Synthetic Substitute
		K Nonautologous Tissue Substitute
		Y Other Device
			Z No Qualifier

1 Cranial Cavity
9 Pleural Cavity, Right
B Pleural Cavity, Left
G Peritoneal Cavity
   Abdominal cavity
J Pelvic Cavity
   Retropubic space
	Ø Open
	3 Percutaneous
	4 Percutaneous Endoscopic
	X External
		Ø Drainage Device
		1 Radioactive Element
		3 Infusion Device
		J Synthetic Substitute
		Y Other Device
			Z No Qualifier

D Pericardial Cavity
H Retroperitoneum
   Retroperitoneal cavity
   Retroperitoneal space
	Ø Open
	3 Percutaneous
	4 Percutaneous Endoscopic
	X External
		Ø Drainage Device
		1 Radioactive Element
		3 Infusion Device
		Y Other Device
			Z No Qualifier

P Gastrointestinal Tract Q Respiratory Tract R Genitourinary Tract	Ø Open 3 Percutaneous 4 Percutaneous Endoscopic 7 Via Natural or Artificial Opening 8 Via Natural or Artificial Opening Endoscopic X External	1 Radioactive Element 3 Infusion Device Y Other Device	Z No Qualifier

DRG Non-OR	ØWW[Ø,2,4,5,6,K,L][Ø,3,4][Ø,1,3,7,J,K,Y]Z	♂	ØWWM[Ø,3,4,X][Ø,1,3,7,K,Y]Z
DRG Non-OR	ØWWM[Ø,3,4][Ø,1,3,J,Y]Z	♀	ØWWN[Ø,3,4,X][Ø,1,3,7,K,Y]Z
Non-OR	ØWW[Ø,2,4,5,6,C,F,K,L,M,N]X[Ø,1,3,7,J,K,Y]Z		
Non-OR	ØWW8[Ø,3,4,X][Ø,1,3,7,J,K,Y]Z		
Non-OR	ØWW[1,G,J]X[Ø,1,3,J,Y]Z		
Non-OR	ØWW[9,B][Ø,3,4,X][Ø,1,3,J,Y]Z		
Non-OR	ØWW[D,H]X[Ø,1,Y]Z		
Non-OR	ØWWP[3,4,7,8,X][1,3,Y]Z		
Non-OR	ØWWQ[Ø,X][1,3,Y]Z		
Non-OR	ØWWR[Ø,3,4,7,8,X][1,3,Y]Z		

Ø   Medical and Surgical
W   Anatomical Regions, General
Y   Transplantation   Definition: Putting in or on all or a portion of a living body part taken from another individual or animal to physically take the place and/or function of all or a portion of a similar body part

          Explanation: The native body part may or may not be taken out, and the transplanted body part may take over all or a portion of its function

Body Part Character 4	Approach Character 5	Device Character 6	Qualifier Character 7
2 Face	Ø Open	Z No Device	Ø Allogeneic 1 Syngeneic

NC Noncovered Procedure   **LC** Limited Coverage   **QA** Questionable OB Admit   **NT** New Tech Add-on   ⊞ Combination Member   ♂ Male   ♀ Female

ICD-10-PCS 2023   685

Anatomical Regions, Upper Extremities ØXØ–ØXY

Character Meanings

This Character Meaning table is provided as a guide to assist the user in the identification of character members that may be found in this section of code tables. It **SHOULD NOT** be used to build a PCS code.

Operation–Character 3		Body Part–Character 4		Approach–Character 5		Device–Character 6		Qualifier–Character 7	
Ø	Alteration	Ø	Forequarter, Right	Ø	Open	Ø	Drainage Device	Ø	Allogeneic OR Complete
2	Change	1	Forequarter, Left	3	Percutaneous	1	Radioactive Element	1	High OR Syngeneic
3	Control	2	Shoulder Region, Right	4	Percutaneous Endoscopic	3	Infusion Device	2	Mid
6	Detachment	3	Shoulder Region, Left	X	External	7	Autologous Tissue Substitute	3	Low
9	Drainage	4	Axilla, Right			J	Synthetic Substitute	4	Complete 1st Ray
B	Excision	5	Axilla, Left			K	Nonautologous Tissue Substitute	5	Complete 2nd Ray
H	Insertion	6	Upper Extremity, Right			Y	Other Device	6	Complete 3rd Ray
J	Inspection	7	Upper Extremity, Left			Z	No Device	7	Complete 4th Ray
M	Reattachment	8	Upper Arm, Right					8	Complete 5th Ray
P	Removal	9	Upper Arm, Left					9	Partial 1st Ray
Q	Repair	B	Elbow Region, Right					B	Partial 2nd Ray
R	Replacement	C	Elbow Region, Left					C	Partial 3rd Ray
U	Supplement	D	Lower Arm, Right					D	Partial 4th Ray
W	Revision	F	Lower Arm, Left					F	Partial 5th Ray
X	Transfer	G	Wrist Region, Right					L	Thumb, Right
Y	Transplantation	H	Wrist Region, Left					M	Thumb, Left
		J	Hand, Right					N	Toe, Right
		K	Hand, Left					P	Toe, Left
		L	Thumb, Right					X	Diagnostic
		M	Thumb, Left					Z	No Qualifier
		N	Index Finger, Right						
		P	Index Finger, Left						
		Q	Middle Finger, Right						
		R	Middle Finger, Left						
		S	Ring Finger, Right						
		T	Ring Finger, Left						
		V	Little Finger, Right						
		W	Little Finger, Left						

AHA Coding Clinic for table ØX3
2016, 4Q, 99	Root operation Control
2015, 1Q, 35	Evacuation of hematoma for control of postprocedural bleeding
2013, 3Q, 23	Control of intraoperative bleeding

AHA Coding Clinic for table ØX6
2017, 2Q, 3-4	Qualifiers for the root operation detachment
2017, 2Q, 18	Removal of polydactyl digits
2017, 1Q, 52	Further distal phalangeal amputation
2016, 3Q, 33	Traumatic amputation of fingers with further revision amputation

AHA Coding Clinic for table ØXH
2017, 2Q, 20	Exchange of intramedullary antibiotic impregnated spacer

AHA Coding Clinic for table ØXP
2017, 2Q, 20	Exchange of intramedullary antibiotic impregnated spacer

AHA Coding Clinic for table ØXY
2016, 4Q, 112-113	Transplantation

Detachment Qualifier Descriptions

Qualifier Definition	Upper Arm	Lower Arm
1 **High:** Amputation at the proximal portion of the shaft of the:	Humerus	Radius/Ulna
2 **Mid:** Amputation at the middle portion of the shaft of the:	Humerus	Radius/Ulna
3 **Low:** Amputation at the distal portion of the shaft of the:	Humerus	Radius/Ulna

Qualifier Definition	Hand
Ø Complete 1st through 5th Rays Ray: digit of hand or foot with corresponding metacarpus or metatarsus	Through carpo-metacarpal joint, **Wrist**
4 Complete 1st Ray	Through carpo-metacarpal joint, **Thumb**
5 Complete 2nd Ray	Through carpo-metacarpal joint, **Index Finger**
6 Complete 3rd Ray	Through carpo-metacarpal joint, **Middle Finger**
7 Complete 4th Ray	Through carpo-metacarpal joint, **Ring Finger**
8 Complete 5th Ray	Through carpo-metacarpal joint, **Little Finger**
9 Partial 1st Ray	Anywhere along shaft or head of metacarpal bone, **Thumb**
B Partial 2nd Ray	Anywhere along shaft or head of metacarpal bone, **Index Finger**
C Partial 3rd Ray	Anywhere along shaft or head of metacarpal bone, **Middle Finger**
D Partial 4th Ray	Anywhere along shaft or head of metacarpal bone, **Ring Finger**
F Partial 5th Ray	Anywhere along shaft or head of metacarpal bone, **Little Finger**

Qualifier Definition	Thumb/Finger
Ø Complete	At the metacarpophalangeal joint
1 High	Anywhere along the proximal phalanx
2 Mid	Through the proximal interphalangeal joint or anywhere along the middle phalanx
3 Low	Through the distal interphalangeal joint or anywhere along the distal phalanx

Ø   **Medical and Surgical**
X   **Anatomical Regions, Upper Extremities**
Ø   **Alteration**   Definition: Modifying the anatomic structure of a body part without affecting the function of the body part
                              Explanation: Principal purpose is to improve appearance

Body Part Character 4	Approach Character 5	Device Character 6	Qualifier Character 7
2 Shoulder Region, Right	Ø Open	7 Autologous Tissue Substitute	Z No Qualifier
3 Shoulder Region, Left	3 Percutaneous	J Synthetic Substitute	
4 Axilla, Right	4 Percutaneous Endoscopic	K Nonautologous Tissue Substitute	
5 Axilla, Left		Z No Device	
6 Upper Extremity, Right			
7 Upper Extremity, Left			
8 Upper Arm, Right			
9 Upper Arm, Left			
B Elbow Region, Right			
C Elbow Region, Left			
D Lower Arm, Right			
F Lower Arm, Left			
G Wrist Region, Right			
H Wrist Region, Left			

Ø   **Medical and Surgical**
X   **Anatomical Regions, Upper Extremities**
2   **Change**   Definition: Taking out or off a device from a body part and putting back an identical or similar device in or on the same body part without cutting or puncturing the skin or a mucous membrane
                          Explanation: All CHANGE procedures are coded using the approach EXTERNAL

Body Part Character 4	Approach Character 5	Device Character 6	Qualifier Character 7
6 Upper Extremity, Right	X External	Ø Drainage Device	Z No Qualifier
7 Upper Extremity, Left		Y Other Device	

Non-OR   All body part, approach, device, and qualifier values

Ø   **Medical and Surgical**
X   **Anatomical Regions, Upper Extremities**
3   **Control**   Definition: Stopping, or attempting to stop, postprocedural or other acute bleeding
                          Explanation: None

Body Part Character 4	Approach Character 5	Device Character 6	Qualifier Character 7
2 Shoulder Region, Right	Ø Open	Z No Device	Z No Qualifier
3 Shoulder Region, Left	3 Percutaneous		
4 Axilla, Right	4 Percutaneous Endoscopic		
5 Axilla, Left			
6 Upper Extremity, Right			
7 Upper Extremity, Left			
8 Upper Arm, Right			
9 Upper Arm, Left			
B Elbow Region, Right			
C Elbow Region, Left			
D Lower Arm, Right			
F Lower Arm, Left			
G Wrist Region, Right			
H Wrist Region, Left			
J Hand, Right			
K Hand, Left			

Anatomical Regions, Upper Extremities

Ø   Medical and Surgical
X   Anatomical Regions, Upper Extremities
6   Detachment   Definition: Cutting off all or a portion of the upper or lower extremities
                             Explanation: The body part value is the site of the detachment, with a qualifier if applicable to further specify the level where the extremity was detached

Body Part Character 4	Approach Character 5	Device Character 6	Qualifier Character 7
Ø Forequarter, Right 1 Forequarter, Left 2 Shoulder Region, Right 3 Shoulder Region, Left B Elbow Region, Right C Elbow Region, Left	Ø Open	Z No Device	Z No Qualifier
8 Upper Arm, Right 9 Upper Arm, Left D Lower Arm, Right F Lower Arm, Left	Ø Open	Z No Device	1 High 2 Mid 3 Low
J Hand, Right K Hand, Left	Ø Open	Z No Device	Ø Complete 4 Complete 1st Ray 5 Complete 2nd Ray 6 Complete 3rd Ray 7 Complete 4th Ray 8 Complete 5th Ray 9 Partial 1st Ray B Partial 2nd Ray C Partial 3rd Ray D Partial 4th Ray F Partial 5th Ray
L Thumb, Right M Thumb, Left N Index Finger, Right P Index Finger, Left Q Middle Finger, Right R Middle Finger, Left S Ring Finger, Right T Ring Finger, Left V Little Finger, Right W Little Finger, Left	Ø Open	Z No Device	Ø Complete 1 High 2 Mid 3 Low

Ø Medical and Surgical
X Anatomical Regions, Upper Extremities
9 Drainage   Definition: Taking or letting out fluids and/or gases from a body part

                 Explanation: The qualifier DIAGNOSTIC is used to identify drainage procedures that are biopsies

Body Part Character 4	Approach Character 5	Device Character 6	Qualifier Character 7
2 Shoulder Region, Right 3 Shoulder Region, Left 4 Axilla, Right 5 Axilla, Left 6 Upper Extremity, Right 7 Upper Extremity, Left 8 Upper Arm, Right 9 Upper Arm, Left B Elbow Region, Right C Elbow Region, Left D Lower Arm, Right F Lower Arm, Left G Wrist Region, Right H Wrist Region, Left J Hand, Right K Hand, Left	Ø Open 3 Percutaneous 4 Percutaneous Endoscopic	Ø Drainage Device	Z No Qualifier
2 Shoulder Region, Right 3 Shoulder Region, Left 4 Axilla, Right 5 Axilla, Left 6 Upper Extremity, Right 7 Upper Extremity, Left 8 Upper Arm, Right 9 Upper Arm, Left B Elbow Region, Right C Elbow Region, Left D Lower Arm, Right F Lower Arm, Left G Wrist Region, Right H Wrist Region, Left J Hand, Right K Hand, Left	Ø Open 3 Percutaneous 4 Percutaneous Endoscopic	Z No Device	X Diagnostic Z No Qualifier

Non-OR   All body part, approach, device, and qualifier values

Ø Medical and Surgical
X Anatomical Regions, Upper Extremities
B Excision   Definition: Cutting out or off, without replacement, a portion of a body part

                 Explanation: The qualifier DIAGNOSTIC is used to identify excision procedures that are biopsies

Body Part Character 4	Approach Character 5	Device Character 6	Qualifier Character 7
2 Shoulder Region, Right 3 Shoulder Region, Left 4 Axilla, Right 5 Axilla, Left 6 Upper Extremity, Right 7 Upper Extremity, Left 8 Upper Arm, Right 9 Upper Arm, Left B Elbow Region, Right C Elbow Region, Left D Lower Arm, Right F Lower Arm, Left G Wrist Region, Right H Wrist Region, Left J Hand, Right K Hand, Left	Ø Open 3 Percutaneous 4 Percutaneous Endoscopic	Z No Device	X Diagnostic Z No Qualifier

Non-OR   ØXB[2,3,4,5,6,7,8,9,B,C,D,F,G,H,J,K][Ø,3,4]ZX

NC Noncovered Procedure   LC Limited Coverage   QA Questionable OB Admit   COM New Tech Add-on   ⊞ Combination Member   ♂ Male   ♀ Female

ICD-10-PCS 2023   691

Ø   Medical and Surgical
X   Anatomical Regions, Upper Extremities
H   Insertion   Definition: Putting in a nonbiological appliance that monitors, assists, performs, or prevents a physiological function but does not physically take the place of a body part

                          Explanation: None

Body Part Character 4	Approach Character 5	Device Character 6	Qualifier Character 7
2 Shoulder Region, Right 3 Shoulder Region, Left 4 Axilla, Right 5 Axilla, Left 6 Upper Extremity, Right 7 Upper Extremity, Left 8 Upper Arm, Right 9 Upper Arm, Left B Elbow Region, Right C Elbow Region, Left D Lower Arm, Right F Lower Arm, Left G Wrist Region, Right H Wrist Region, Left J Hand, Right K Hand, Left	0 Open 3 Percutaneous 4 Percutaneous Endoscopic	1 Radioactive Element 3 Infusion Device Y Other Device	Z No Qualifier

DRG Non-OR   ØXH[2,3,4,5,6,7,8,9,B,C,D,F,G,H,J,K][Ø,3,4][3,Y]Z

Ø   Medical and Surgical
X   Anatomical Regions, Upper Extremities
J   Inspection   Definition: Visually and/or manually exploring a body part

                          Explanation: Visual exploration may be performed with or without optical instrumentation. Manual exploration may be performed directly or through intervening body layers.

Body Part Character 4	Approach Character 5	Device Character 6	Qualifier Character 7
2 Shoulder Region, Right 3 Shoulder Region, Left 4 Axilla, Right 5 Axilla, Left 6 Upper Extremity, Right 7 Upper Extremity, Left 8 Upper Arm, Right 9 Upper Arm, Left B Elbow Region, Right C Elbow Region, Left D Lower Arm, Right F Lower Arm, Left G Wrist Region, Right H Wrist Region, Left J Hand, Right K Hand, Left	0 Open 3 Percutaneous 4 Percutaneous Endoscopic X External	Z No Device	Z No Qualifier

DRG Non-OR   ØXJ[2,3,4,5,6,7,8,9,B,C,D,F,G,H,J,K]ØZZ
Non-OR   ØXJ[2,3,4,5,6,7,8,9,B,C,D,F,G,H][3,4,X]ZZ
Non-OR   ØXJ[J,K][3,X]ZZ

Ø **Medical and Surgical**
X **Anatomical Regions, Upper Extremities**
M **Reattachment**   Definition: Putting back in or on all or a portion of a separated body part to its normal location or other suitable location
　　　　　　　　　　　Explanation: Vascular circulation and nervous pathways may or may not be reestablished

Body Part Character 4	Approach Character 5	Device Character 6	Qualifier Character 7
Ø Forequarter, Right	Ø Open	Z No Device	Z No Qualifier
1 Forequarter, Left			
2 Shoulder Region, Right			
3 Shoulder Region, Left			
4 Axilla, Right			
5 Axilla, Left			
6 Upper Extremity, Right			
7 Upper Extremity, Left			
8 Upper Arm, Right			
9 Upper Arm, Left			
B Elbow Region, Right			
C Elbow Region, Left			
D Lower Arm, Right			
F Lower Arm, Left			
G Wrist Region, Right			
H Wrist Region, Left			
J Hand, Right			
K Hand, Left			
L Thumb, Right			
M Thumb, Left			
N Index Finger, Right			
P Index Finger, Left			
Q Middle Finger, Right			
R Middle Finger, Left			
S Ring Finger, Right			
T Ring Finger, Left			
V Little Finger, Right			
W Little Finger, Left			

Ø **Medical and Surgical**
X **Anatomical Regions, Upper Extremities**
P **Removal**   Definition: Taking out or off a device from a body part
　　　　　　　Explanation: If a device is taken out and a similar device put in without cutting or puncturing the skin or mucous membrane, the procedure is
　　　　　　　coded to the root operation CHANGE. Otherwise, the procedure for taking out the device is coded to the root operation REMOVAL.

Body Part Character 4	Approach Character 5	Device Character 6	Qualifier Character 7
6 Upper Extremity, Right	Ø Open	Ø Drainage Device	Z No Qualifier
7 Upper Extremity, Left	3 Percutaneous	1 Radioactive Element	
	4 Percutaneous Endoscopic	3 Infusion Device	
	X External	7 Autologous Tissue Substitute	
		J Synthetic Substitute	
		K Nonautologous Tissue Substitute	
		Y Other Device	

Non-OR   All body part, approach, device, and qualifier values

NC Noncovered Procedure   **LC** Limited Coverage   **QA** Questionable OB Admit   **COM** New Tech Add-on   ✚ Combination Member   ♂ Male   ♀ Female

ICD-10-PCS 2023   **693**

Anatomical Regions, Upper Extremities *(left margin)*

Ø   **Medical and Surgical**
X   **Anatomical Regions, Upper Extremities**
Q   **Repair**   Definition: Restoring, to the extent possible, a body part to its normal anatomic structure and function

                        Explanation: Used only when the method to accomplish the repair is not one of the other root operations

Body Part Character 4	Approach Character 5	Device Character 6	Qualifier Character 7
2 Shoulder Region, Right	Ø Open	Z No Device	Z No Qualifier
3 Shoulder Region, Left	3 Percutaneous		
4 Axilla, Right	4 Percutaneous Endoscopic		
5 Axilla, Left	X External		
6 Upper Extremity, Right			
7 Upper Extremity, Left			
8 Upper Arm, Right			
9 Upper Arm, Left			
B Elbow Region, Right			
C Elbow Region, Left			
D Lower Arm, Right			
F Lower Arm, Left			
G Wrist Region, Right			
H Wrist Region, Left			
J Hand, Right			
K Hand, Left			
L Thumb, Right			
M Thumb, Left			
N Index Finger, Right			
P Index Finger, Left			
Q Middle Finger, Right			
R Middle Finger, Left			
S Ring Finger, Right			
T Ring Finger, Left			
V Little Finger, Right			
W Little Finger, Left			

Ø   **Medical and Surgical**
X   **Anatomical Regions, Upper Extremities**
R   **Replacement**   Definition: Putting in or on biological or synthetic material that physically takes the place and/or function of all or a portion of a body part

                        Explanation: The body part may have been taken out or replaced, or may be taken out, physically eradicated, or rendered nonfunctional during the REPLACEMENT procedure. A REMOVAL procedure is coded for taking out the device used in a previous replacement procedure.

Body Part Character 4	Approach Character 5	Device Character 6	Qualifier Character 7
L Thumb, Right	Ø Open	7 Autologous Tissue Substitute	N Toe, Right
M Thumb, Left	4 Percutaneous Endoscopic		P Toe, Left

Ø   **Medical and Surgical**
X   **Anatomical Regions, Upper Extremities**
U   **Supplement**   Definition: Putting in or on biological or synthetic material that physically reinforces and/or augments the function of a portion of a body part
                Explanation: The biological material is non-living, or is living and from the same individual. The body part may have been previously replaced, and the SUPPLEMENT procedure is performed to physically reinforce and/or augment the function of the replaced body part.

Body Part Character 4	Approach Character 5	Device Character 6	Qualifier Character 7
2 Shoulder Region, Right	Ø Open	7 Autologous Tissue Substitute	Z No Qualifier
3 Shoulder Region, Left	4 Percutaneous Endoscopic	J Synthetic Substitute	
4 Axilla, Right		K Nonautologous Tissue Substitute	
5 Axilla, Left			
6 Upper Extremity, Right			
7 Upper Extremity, Left			
8 Upper Arm, Right			
9 Upper Arm, Left			
B Elbow Region, Right			
C Elbow Region, Left			
D Lower Arm, Right			
F Lower Arm, Left			
G Wrist Region, Right			
H Wrist Region, Left			
J Hand, Right			
K Hand, Left			
L Thumb, Right			
M Thumb, Left			
N Index Finger, Right			
P Index Finger, Left			
Q Middle Finger, Right			
R Middle Finger, Left			
S Ring Finger, Right			
T Ring Finger, Left			
V Little Finger, Right			
W Little Finger, Left			

NC Noncovered Procedure   **LC** Limited Coverage   **QA** Questionable OB Admit   **COM** New Tech Add-on   ⊞ Combination Member   ♂ Male   ♀ Female

ICD-10-PCS 2023   695

ØXU–ØXU

Ø **Medical and Surgical**
X **Anatomical Regions, Upper Extremities**
W **Revision**   Definition: Correcting, to the extent possible, a portion of a malfunctioning device or the position of a displaced device

Explanation: Revision can include correcting a malfunctioning or displaced device by taking out or putting in components of the device such as a screw or pin

Body Part Character 4	Approach Character 5	Device Character 6	Qualifier Character 7
6 Upper Extremity, Right 7 Upper Extremity, Left	Ø Open 3 Percutaneous 4 Percutaneous Endoscopic X External	Ø Drainage Device 3 Infusion Device 7 Autologous Tissue Substitute J Synthetic Substitute K Nonautologous Tissue Substitute Y Other Device	Z No Qualifier

DRG Non-OR   ØXW[6,7][Ø,3,4][Ø,3,7,J,K,Y]Z
Non-OR   ØXW[6,7]X[Ø,3,7,J,K,Y]Z

Ø **Medical and Surgical**
X **Anatomical Regions, Upper Extremities**
X **Transfer**   Definition: Moving, without taking out, all or a portion of a body part to another location to take over the function of all or a portion of a body part

Explanation: The body part transferred remains connected to its vascular and nervous supply

Body Part Character 4	Approach Character 5	Device Character 6	Qualifier Character 7
N Index Finger, Right	Ø Open	Z No Device	L Thumb, Right
P Index Finger, Left	Ø Open	Z No Device	M Thumb, Left

Ø **Medical and Surgical**
X **Anatomical Regions, Upper Extremities**
Y **Transplantation**   Definition: Putting in or on all or a portion of a living body part taken from another individual or animal to physically take the place and/or function of all or a portion of a similar body part

Explanation: The native body part may or may not be taken out, and the transplanted body part may take over all or a portion of its function

Body Part Character 4	Approach Character 5	Device Character 6	Qualifier Character 7
J Hand, Right K Hand, Left	Ø Open	Z No Device	Ø Allogeneic 1 Syngeneic

Anatomical Regions, Lower Extremities ØYØ–ØYW

Character Meanings

This Character Meaning table is provided as a guide to assist the user in the identification of character members that may be found in this section of code tables. It **SHOULD NOT** be used to build a PCS code.

Operation–Character 3	Body Part–Character 4	Approach–Character 5	Device–Character 6	Qualifier–Character 7
Ø Alteration	Ø Buttock, Right	Ø Open	Ø Drainage Device	Ø Complete
2 Change	1 Buttock, Left	3 Percutaneous	1 Radioactive Element	1 High
3 Control	2 Hindquarter, Right	4 Percutaneous Endoscopic	3 Infusion Device	2 Mid
6 Detachment	3 Hindquarter, Left	X External	7 Autologous Tissue Substitute	3 Low
9 Drainage	4 Hindquarter, Bilateral		J Synthetic Substitute	4 Complete 1st Ray
B Excision	5 Inguinal Region, Right		K Nonautologous Tissue Substitute	5 Complete 2nd Ray
H Insertion	6 Inguinal Region, Left		Y Other Device	6 Complete 3rd Ray
J Inspection	7 Femoral Region, Right		Z No Device	7 Complete 4th Ray
M Reattachment	8 Femoral Region, Left			8 Complete 5th Ray
P Removal	9 Lower Extremity, Right			9 Partial 1st Ray
Q Repair	A Inguinal Region, Bilateral			B Partial 2nd Ray
U Supplement	B Lower Extremity, Left			C Partial 3rd Ray
W Revision	C Upper Leg, Right			D Partial 4th Ray
	D Upper Leg, Left			F Partial 5th Ray
	E Femoral Region, Bilateral			X Diagnostic
	F Knee Region, Right			Z No Qualifier
	G Knee Region, Left			
	H Lower Leg, Right			
	J Lower Leg, Left			
	K Ankle Region, Right			
	L Ankle Region, Left			
	M Foot, Right			
	N Foot, Left			
	P 1st Toe, Right			
	Q 1st Toe, Left			
	R 2nd Toe, Right			
	S 2nd Toe, Left			
	T 3rd Toe, Right			
	U 3rd Toe, Left			
	V 4th Toe, Right			
	W 4th Toe, Left			
	X 5th Toe, Right			
	Y 5th Toe, Left			

AHA Coding Clinic for table ØY3

2016, 4Q, 99	Root operation Control
2013, 3Q, 23	Control of intraoperative bleeding

AHA Coding Clinic for table ØY6

2019, 2Q, 17	Cryoamputation of lower leg
2017, 2Q, 3-4	Qualifiers for the root operation detachment
2017, 1Q, 22	Chopart amputation of foot
2015, 2Q, 28	Partial amputation of hallux at interphalangeal Joint
2015, 1Q, 28	Mid-foot amputation

AHA Coding Clinic for table ØY9

2015, 1Q, 22	Incision and drainage of abscess of femoropopliteal bypass site
2015, 1Q, 22	Incision and drainage of groin abscess

Detachment Qualifier Descriptions

Qualifier Definition		Upper Leg	Lower Leg
1	**High:** Amputation at the proximal portion of the shaft of the:	Femur	Tibia/Fibula
2	**Mid:** Amputation at the middle portion of the shaft of the:	Femur	Tibia/Fibula
3	**Low:** Amputation at the distal portion of the shaft of the:	Femur	Tibia/Fibula

Qualifier Definition		Foot
Ø	Complete 1st through 5th Rays Ray: digit of hand or foot with corresponding metacarpus or metatarsus	Through tarso-metatarsal Joint, **Ankle**
4	Complete 1st Ray	Through tarso-metatarsal joint, **Great Toe**
5	Complete 2nd Ray	Through tarso-metatarsal joint, **2nd Toe**
6	Complete 3rd Ray	Through tarso-metatarsal joint, **3rd Toe**
7	Complete 4th Ray	Through tarso-metatarsal joint, **4th Toe**
8	Complete 5th Ray	Through tarso-metatarsal joint, **Little Toe**
9	Partial 1st Ray	Anywhere along shaft or head of metatarsal bone, **Great Toe**
B	Partial 2nd Ray	Anywhere along shaft or head of metatarsal bone, **2nd Toe**
C	Partial 3rd Ray	Anywhere along shaft or head of metatarsal bone, **3rd Toe**
D	Partial 4th Ray	Anywhere along shaft or head of metatarsal bone, **4th Toe**
F	Partial 5th Ray	Anywhere along shaft or head of metatarsal bone, **Little Toe**

Qualifier Definition	Toe
Ø Complete	At the metatarsal-phalangeal joint
1 High	Anywhere along the proximal phalanx
2 Mid	Through the proximal interphalangeal joint or anywhere along the middle phalanx
3 Low	Through the distal interphalangeal joint or anywhere along the distal phalanx

Ø   **Medical and Surgical**
Y   **Anatomical Regions, Lower Extremities**
Ø   **Alteration**   Definition: Modifying the anatomic structure of a body part without affecting the function of the body part
                       Explanation: Principal purpose is to improve appearance

Body Part Character 4	Approach Character 5	Device Character 6	Qualifier Character 7
Ø Buttock, Right 1 Buttock, Left 9 Lower Extremity, Right B Lower Extremity, Left C Upper Leg, Right D Upper Leg, Left F Knee Region, Right G Knee Region, Left H Lower Leg, Right J Lower Leg, Left K Ankle Region, Right L Ankle Region, Left	Ø Open 3 Percutaneous 4 Percutaneous Endoscopic	7 Autologous Tissue Substitute J Synthetic Substitute K Nonautologous Tissue Substitute Z No Device	Z No Qualifier

Ø   **Medical and Surgical**
Y   **Anatomical Regions, Lower Extremities**
2   **Change**   Definition: Taking out or off a device from a body part and putting back an identical or similar device in or on the same body part without
                       cutting or puncturing the skin or a mucous membrane
                       Explanation: All CHANGE procedures are coded using the approach EXTERNAL

Body Part Character 4	Approach Character 5	Device Character 6	Qualifier Character 7
9 Lower Extremity, Right B Lower Extremity, Left	X External	Ø Drainage Device Y Other Device	Z No Qualifier

Non-OR   All body part, approach, device, and qualifier values

Ø   **Medical and Surgical**
Y   **Anatomical Regions, Lower Extremities**
3   **Control**   Definition: Stopping, or attempting to stop, postprocedural or other acute bleeding
                       Explanation: None

Body Part Character 4	Approach Character 5	Device Character 6	Qualifier Character 7

Ø   Buttock, Right
1   Buttock, Left
5   Inguinal Region, Right
     Inguinal canal
     Inguinal triangle
6   Inguinal Region, Left
     See 5 Inguinal Region, Right
7   Femoral Region, Right
8   Femoral Region, Left
9   Lower Extremity, Right
B   Lower Extremity, Left
C   Upper Leg, Right
D   Upper Leg, Left
F   Knee Region, Right
G   Knee Region, Left
H   Lower Leg, Right
J   Lower Leg, Left
K   Ankle Region, Right
L   Ankle Region, Left
M   Foot, Right
N   Foot, Left
	Ø Open
	3 Percutaneous
	4 Percutaneous Endoscopic
		Z No Device	Z No Qualifier

Anatomical Regions, Lower Extremities

ØYØ–ØY3

NC Noncovered Procedure   **LC** Limited Coverage   **QA** Questionable OB Admit   **COM** New Tech Add-on   ⊞ Combination Member   ♂ Male   ♀ Female

ICD-10-PCS 2023   **699**

Anatomical Regions, Lower Extremities (side tab)

Ø   **Medical and Surgical**
Y   **Anatomical Regions, Lower Extremities**
6   **Detachment**   Definition: Cutting off all or a portion of the upper or lower extremities

                      Explanation: The body part value is the site of the detachment, with a qualifier if applicable to further specify the level where the extremity was detached

Body Part Character 4	Approach Character 5	Device Character 6	Qualifier Character 7
2 Hindquarter, Right 3 Hindquarter, Left 4 Hindquarter, Bilateral 7 Femoral Region, Right 8 Femoral Region, Left F Knee Region, Right G Knee Region, Left	Ø Open	Z No Device	Z No Qualifier
C Upper Leg, Right D Upper Leg, Left H Lower Leg, Right J Lower Leg, Left	Ø Open	Z No Device	1 High 2 Mid 3 Low
M Foot, Right N Foot, Left	Ø Open	Z No Device	Ø Complete 4 Complete 1st Ray 5 Complete 2nd Ray 6 Complete 3rd Ray 7 Complete 4th Ray 8 Complete 5th Ray 9 Partial 1st Ray B Partial 2nd Ray C Partial 3rd Ray D Partial 4th Ray F Partial 5th Ray

P 1st Toe, Right
     Hallux
Q 1st Toe, Left
     See 1st Toe, Right
R 2nd Toe, Right
S 2nd Toe, Left
T 3rd Toe, Right
U 3rd Toe, Left
V 4th Toe, Right
W 4th Toe, Left
X 5th Toe, Right
Y 5th Toe, Left
	Ø Open	Z No Device	Ø Complete
			1 High
			2 Mid
			3 Low

Anatomical Regions, Lower Extremities

0 Medical and Surgical
Y Anatomical Regions, Lower Extremities
9 Drainage   Definition: Taking or letting out fluids and/or gases from a body part

Explanation: The qualifier DIAGNOSTIC is used to identify drainage procedures that are biopsies

Body Part Character 4	Approach Character 5	Device Character 6	Qualifier Character 7

0 Buttock, Right
1 Buttock, Left
5 Inguinal Region, Right
  Inguinal canal
  Inguinal triangle
6 Inguinal Region, Left
  See 5 Inguinal Region, Right
7 Femoral Region, Right
8 Femoral Region, Left
9 Lower Extremity, Right
B Lower Extremity, Left
C Upper Leg, Right
D Upper Leg, Left
F Knee Region, Right
G Knee Region, Left
H Lower Leg, Right
J Lower Leg, Left
K Ankle Region, Right
L Ankle Region, Left
M Foot, Right
N Foot, Left
	0 Open
	3 Percutaneous
	4 Percutaneous Endoscopic
		0 Drainage Device	Z No Qualifier

0 Buttock, Right
1 Buttock, Left
5 Inguinal Region, Right
  Inguinal canal
  Inguinal triangle
6 Inguinal Region, Left
  See 5 Inguinal Region, Right
7 Femoral Region, Right
8 Femoral Region, Left
9 Lower Extremity, Right
B Lower Extremity, Left
C Upper Leg, Right
D Upper Leg, Left
F Knee Region, Right
G Knee Region, Left
H Lower Leg, Right
J Lower Leg, Left
K Ankle Region, Right
L Ankle Region, Left
M Foot, Right
N Foot, Left
	0 Open
	3 Percutaneous
	4 Percutaneous Endoscopic
		Z No Device	X Diagnostic
			Z No Qualifier

Non-OR   0Y9[0,1,7,8,9,B,C,D,F,G,H,J,K,L,M,N][0,3,4]0Z
Non-OR   0Y9[5,6]30Z
Non-OR   0Y9[0,1,7,8,9,B,C,D,F,G,H,J,K,L,M,N][0,3,4]Z[X,Z]
Non-OR   0Y9[5,6]3ZZ

NC Noncovered Procedure   LC Limited Coverage   QA Questionable OB Admit   COM New Tech Add-on   ⊞ Combination Member   ♂ Male   ♀ Female

ICD-10-PCS 2023   701

Ø   Medical and Surgical
Y   Anatomical Regions, Lower Extremities
B   Excision   Definition: Cutting out or off, without replacement, a portion of a body part

Explanation: The qualifier DIAGNOSTIC is used to identify excision procedures that are biopsies

Body Part Character 4	Approach Character 5	Device Character 6	Qualifier Character 7
Ø Buttock, Right	Ø Open	Z No Device	X Diagnostic
1 Buttock, Left	3 Percutaneous		Z No Qualifier

5   Inguinal Region, Right
    Inguinal canal
    Inguinal triangle
	4 Percutaneous Endoscopic		

6 Inguinal Region, Left *See 5 Inguinal Region, Right*			
7 Femoral Region, Right			
8 Femoral Region, Left			
9 Lower Extremity, Right			
B Lower Extremity, Left			
C Upper Leg, Right			
D Upper Leg, Left			
F Knee Region, Right			
G Knee Region, Left			
H Lower Leg, Right			
J Lower Leg, Left			
K Ankle Region, Right			
L Ankle Region, Left			
M Foot, Right			
N Foot, Left			

Non-OR   ØYB[Ø,1,9,B,C,D,F,G,H,J,K,L,M,N][Ø,3,4]ZX

Ø   Medical and Surgical
Y   Anatomical Regions, Lower Extremities
H   Insertion   Definition: Putting in a nonbiological appliance that monitors, assists, performs, or prevents a physiological function but does not physically take the place of a body part

Explanation: None

Body Part Character 4	Approach Character 5	Device Character 6	Qualifier Character 7
Ø Buttock, Right	Ø Open	1 Radioactive Element	Z No Qualifier
1 Buttock, Left	3 Percutaneous	3 Infusion Device	

5   Inguinal Region, Right
    Inguinal canal
    Inguinal triangle
	4 Percutaneous Endoscopic	Y Other Device	

6 Inguinal Region, Left *See 5 Inguinal Region, Right*			
7 Femoral Region, Right			
8 Femoral Region, Left			
9 Lower Extremity, Right			
B Lower Extremity, Left			
C Upper Leg, Right			
D Upper Leg, Left			
F Knee Region, Right			
G Knee Region, Left			
H Lower Leg, Right			
J Lower Leg, Left			
K Ankle Region, Right			
L Ankle Region, Left			
M Foot, Right			
N Foot, Left			

DRG Non-OR   ØYH[Ø,1,5,6,7,8,9,B,C,D,F,G,H,J,K,L,M,N][Ø,3,4][3,Y]Z

Non-OR Procedure   DRG Non-OR Procedure   Valid OR Procedure   HAC Associated Procedure   Combination Only   New/Revised GREEN

Ø   **Medical and Surgical**
Y   **Anatomical Regions, Lower Extremities**
J   **Inspection**   Definition: Visually and/or manually exploring a body part

                       Explanation: Visual exploration may be performed with or without optical instrumentation. Manual exploration may be performed directly or through intervening body layers.

Body Part Character 4	Approach Character 5	Device Character 6	Qualifier Character 7

Ø   Buttock, Right
1   Buttock, Left
5   Inguinal Region, Right
     Inguinal canal
     Inguinal triangle
6   Inguinal Region, Left
     See 5 Inguinal Region, Right
7   Femoral Region, Right
8   Femoral Region, Left
9   Lower Extremity, Right
A   Inguinal Region, Bilateral
     See 5 Inguinal Region, Right
B   Lower Extremity, Left
C   Upper Leg, Right
D   Upper Leg, Left
E   Femoral Region, Bilateral
F   Knee Region, Right
G   Knee Region, Left
H   Lower Leg, Right
J   Lower Leg, Left
K   Ankle Region, Right
L   Ankle Region, Left
M   Foot, Right
N   Foot, Left
	Ø Open
	3 Percutaneous
	4 Percutaneous Endoscopic
	X External
		Z No Device	Z No Qualifier

DRG Non-OR	ØYJ[Ø,1,8,9,B,C,D,E,F,G,H,J,K,L,M,N]ØZZ
Non-OR	ØYJ[Ø,1,9,B,C,D,F,G,H,J,K,L,M,N][3,4,X]ZZ
Non-OR	ØYJ[5,6,7,8,A,E][3,X]ZZ

Ø   **Medical and Surgical**
Y   **Anatomical Regions, Lower Extremities**
M   **Reattachment**   Definition: Putting back in or on all or a portion of a separated body part to its normal location or other suitable location
           Explanation: Vascular circulation and nervous pathways may or may not be reestablished

Body Part Character 4	Approach Character 5	Device Character 6	Qualifier Character 7

Ø Buttock, Right
1 Buttock, Left
2 Hindquarter, Right
3 Hindquarter, Left
4 Hindquarter, Bilateral
5 Inguinal Region, Right
    Inguinal canal
    Inguinal triangle
6 Inguinal Region, Left
    See 5 Inguinal Region, Right
7 Femoral Region, Right
8 Femoral Region, Left
9 Lower Extremity, Right
B Lower Extremity, Left
C Upper Leg, Right
D Upper Leg, Left
F Knee Region, Right
G Knee Region, Left
H Lower Leg, Right
J Lower Leg, Left
K Ankle Region, Right
L Ankle Region, Left
M Foot, Right
N Foot, Left
P 1st Toe, Right
    Hallux
Q 1st Toe, Left
    See 1st Toe, Right
R 2nd Toe, Right
S 2nd Toe, Left
T 3rd Toe, Right
U 3rd Toe, Left
V 4th Toe, Right
W 4th Toe, Left
X 5th Toe, Right
Y 5th Toe, Left
	Ø Open	**Z** No Device	**Z** No Qualifier

Ø   **Medical and Surgical**
Y   **Anatomical Regions, Lower Extremities**
P   **Removal**   Definition: Taking out or off a device from a body part
           Explanation: If a device is taken out and a similar device put in without cutting or puncturing the skin or mucous membrane, the procedure is coded to the root operation CHANGE. Otherwise, the procedure for taking out the device is coded to the root operation REMOVAL.

Body Part Character 4	Approach Character 5	Device Character 6	Qualifier Character 7
9 Lower Extremity, Right **B** Lower Extremity, Left	**Ø** Open **3** Percutaneous **4** Percutaneous Endoscopic **X** External	**Ø** Drainage Device **1** Radioactive Element **3** Infusion Device **7** Autologous Tissue Substitute **J** Synthetic Substitute **K** Nonautologous Tissue Substitute **Y** Other Device	**Z** No Qualifier

     Non-OR   All body part, approach, device, and qualifier values

---

Non-OR Procedure   DRG Non-OR Procedure   Valid OR Procedure   HAC Associated Procedure   Combination Only   New/Revised GREEN

Ø **Medical and Surgical**
Y **Anatomical Regions, Lower Extremities**
Q **Repair**　　Definition: Restoring, to the extent possible, a body part to its normal anatomic structure and function
　　　　　　　Explanation: Used only when the method to accomplish the repair is not one of the other root operations

Body Part Character 4	Approach Character 5	Device Character 6	Qualifier Character 7
Ø Buttock, Right	Ø Open	Z No Device	Z No Qualifier
1 Buttock, Left	3 Percutaneous		
5 Inguinal Region, Right	4 Percutaneous Endoscopic		
Inguinal canal	X External		
Inguinal triangle			
6 Inguinal Region, Left			
See 5 Inguinal Region, Right			
7 Femoral Region, Right			
8 Femoral Region, Left			
9 Lower Extremity, Right			
A Inguinal Region, Bilateral			
See 5 Inguinal Region, Right			
B Lower Extremity, Left			
C Upper Leg, Right			
D Upper Leg, Left			
E Femoral Region, Bilateral			
F Knee Region, Right			
G Knee Region, Left			
H Lower Leg, Right			
J Lower Leg, Left			
K Ankle Region, Right			
L Ankle Region, Left			
M Foot, Right			
N Foot, Left			
P 1st Toe, Right			
Hallux			
Q 1st Toe, Left			
See 1st Toe, Right			
R 2nd Toe, Right			
S 2nd Toe, Left			
T 3rd Toe, Right			
U 3rd Toe, Left			
V 4th Toe, Right			
W 4th Toe, Left			
X 5th Toe, Right			
Y 5th Toe, Left			

Non-OR　　ØYQ[5,6,7,8,A,E]XZZ

Anatomical Regions, Lower Extremities *(left margin)*

Ø Medical and Surgical
Y Anatomical Regions, Lower Extremities
U Supplement   Definition: Putting in or on biological or synthetic material that physically reinforces and/or augments the function of a portion of a body part

        Explanation: The biological material is non-living, or is living and from the same individual. The body part may have been previously replaced, and the SUPPLEMENT procedure is performed to physically reinforce and/or augment the function of the replaced body part.

Body Part Character 4	Approach Character 5	Device Character 6	Qualifier Character 7

Ø Buttock, Right
1 Buttock, Left
5 Inguinal Region, Right
   Inguinal canal
   Inguinal triangle
6 Inguinal Region, Left
   See 5 Inguinal Region, Right
7 Femoral Region, Right
8 Femoral Region, Left
9 Lower Extremity, Right
A Inguinal Region, Bilateral
   See 5 Inguinal Region, Right
B Lower Extremity, Left
C Upper Leg, Right
D Upper Leg, Left
E Femoral Region, Bilateral
F Knee Region, Right
G Knee Region, Left
H Lower Leg, Right
J Lower Leg, Left
K Ankle Region, Right
L Ankle Region, Left
M Foot, Right
N Foot, Left
P 1st Toe, Right
   Hallux
Q 1st Toe, Left
   See 1st Toe, Right
R 2nd Toe, Right
S 2nd Toe, Left
T 3rd Toe, Right
U 3rd Toe, Left
V 4th Toe, Right
W 4th Toe, Left
X 5th Toe, Right
Y 5th Toe, Left
	Ø Open
	4 Percutaneous Endoscopic
		7 Autologous Tissue Substitute
		J Synthetic Substitute
		K Nonautologous Tissue Substitute
			Z No Qualifier

Ø Medical and Surgical
Y Anatomical Regions, Lower Extremities
W Revision   Definition: Correcting, to the extent possible, a portion of a malfunctioning device or the position of a displaced device

        Explanation: Revision can include correcting a malfunctioning or displaced device by taking out or putting in components of the device such as a screw or pin

Body Part Character 4	Approach Character 5	Device Character 6	Qualifier Character 7
9 Lower Extremity, Right B Lower Extremity, Left	Ø Open 3 Percutaneous 4 Percutaneous Endoscopic X External	Ø Drainage Device 3 Infusion Device 7 Autologous Tissue Substitute J Synthetic Substitute K Nonautologous Tissue Substitute Y Other Device	Z No Qualifier

DRG Non-OR   ØYW[9,B][Ø,3,4][Ø,3,7,J,K,Y]Z
Non-OR   ØYW[9,B]X[Ø,3,7,J,K,Y]Z

Non-OR Procedure   DRG Non-OR Procedure   Valid OR Procedure   HAC Associated Procedure   Combination Only   New/Revised GREEN

Obstetrics 102–10Y

Character Meanings

This Character Meaning table is provided as a guide to assist the user in the identification of character members that may be found in this section of code tables. It **SHOULD NOT** be used to build a PCS code.

0: Pregnancy

Operation–Character 3	Body Part–Character 4	Approach–Character 5	Device–Character 6	Qualifier–Character 7
2 Change	0 Products of Conception	0 Open	3 Monitoring Electrode	0 High
9 Drainage	1 Products of Conception, Retained	3 Percutaneous	Y Other Device	1 Low
A Abortion	2 Products of Conception, Ectopic	4 Percutaneous Endoscopic	Z No Device	2 Extraperitoneal
D Extraction		7 Via Natural or Artificial Opening		3 Low Forceps
E Delivery		8 Via Natural or Artificial Opening Endoscopic		4 Mid Forceps
H Insertion		X External		5 High Forceps
J Inspection				6 Vacuum
P Removal				7 Internal Version
Q Repair				8 Other
S Reposition				9 Fetal Blood OR Manual
T Resection				A Fetal Cerebrospinal Fluid
Y Transplantation				B Fetal Fluid, Other
				C Amniotic Fluid, Therapeutic
				D Fluid, Other
				E Nervous System
				F Cardiovascular System
				G Lymphatics & Hemic
				H Eye
				J Ear, Nose & Sinus
				K Respiratory System
				L Mouth & Throat
				M Gastrointestinal System
				N Hepatobiliary & Pancreas
				P Endocrine System
				Q Skin
				R Musculoskeletal System
				S Urinary System
				T Female Reproductive System
				U Amniotic Fluid, Diagnostic
				V Male Reproductive System
				W Laminaria
				X Abortifacient
				Y Other Body System
				Z No Qualifier

AHA Coding Clinic for table 109
2014, 3Q, 12   Fetoscopic laser photocoagulation and laser microseptostomy for twin-twin transfusion syndrome
2014, 2Q, 9   Pitocin administration to augment labor

AHA Coding Clinic for table 10A
2022, 1Q, 21   Gravid hysterectomy due to placenta increta
2022, 1Q, 41   Intrauterine Cook balloon placement for ectopic pregnancy

AHA Coding Clinic for table 10D
2022, 1Q, 19   Spontaneous abortion with retained placenta of Twin B
2021, 1Q, 52   Removal of ectopic pregnancy via laparotomy
2020, 4Q, 59-60   Extraction of ectopic products of conception
2018, 4Q, 49-51   Revised qualifier values for root operation "extraction" (cesarean delivery)
2018, 2Q, 17   High transverse cesarean section
2016, 1Q, 9   Vaginal delivery assisted by vacuum and low forceps extraction
2014, 4Q, 43   Cesarean delivery assisted by vacuum extraction
2014, 4Q, 43   Vacuum dilation and curettage for blighted ovum

AHA Coding Clinic for table 10E
2017, 3Q, 5   Delivery of placenta
2016, 2Q, 34   Assisted vaginal delivery
2014, 4Q, 17   RH (D) alloimmunization (sensitization)
2014, 2Q, 9   Pitocin administration to augment labor

AHA Coding Clinic for table 10H
2013, 2Q, 36   Intrauterine pressure monitor

AHA Coding Clinic for table 10Q
2021, 2Q, 21   Ex Utero intrapartum treatment procedure
2014, 3Q, 12   Fetoscopic laser photocoagulation and laser microseptostomy for twin-twin transfusion syndrome

AHA Coding Clinic for table 10T
2020, 3Q, 47   Removal of ectopic cornual pregnancy
2015, 3Q, 31   Laparoscopic partial salpingectomy for ectopic pregnancy

Obstetrics

1 Obstetrics
Ø Pregnancy
2 Change Definition: Taking out or off a device from a body part and putting back an identical or similar device in or on the same body part without cutting or puncturing the skin or a mucous membrane
Explanation: None

Body Part Character 4		Approach Character 5	Device Character 6	Qualifier Character 7
Ø Products of Conception	♀	7 Via Natural or Artificial Opening	3 Monitoring Electrode Y Other Device	Z No Qualifier

Non-OR	All body part, approach, device, and qualifier values	♀	All body part, approach, device, and qualifier values

1 Obstetrics
Ø Pregnancy
9 Drainage Definition: Taking or letting out fluids and/or gases from a body part
Explanation: None

Body Part Character 4		Approach Character 5	Device Character 6	Qualifier Character 7
Ø Products of Conception	♀	Ø Open 3 Percutaneous 4 Percutaneous Endoscopic 7 Via Natural or Artificial Opening 8 Via Natural or Artificial Opening Endoscopic	Z No Device	9 Fetal Blood A Fetal Cerebrospinal Fluid B Fetal Fluid, Other C Amniotic Fluid, Therapeutic D Fluid, Other U Amniotic Fluid, Diagnostic

Non-OR	All body part, approach, device, and qualifier values	♀	All body part, approach, device, and qualifier values

1 Obstetrics
Ø Pregnancy
A Abortion Definition: Artificially terminating a pregnancy
Explanation: None

Body Part Character 4		Approach Character 5	Device Character 6	Qualifier Character 7
Ø Products of Conception	♀	Ø Open 3 Percutaneous 4 Percutaneous Endoscopic 8 Via Natural or Artificial Opening Endoscopic	Z No Device	Z No Qualifier
Ø Products of Conception	♀	7 Via Natural or Artificial Opening	Z No Device	6 Vacuum W Laminaria X Abortifacient Z No Qualifier

Non-OR	10A07Z[6,W,X]	♀	All body part, approach, device, and qualifier values

1 Obstetrics
Ø Pregnancy
D Extraction Definition: Pulling or stripping out or off all or a portion of a body part by the use of force
Explanation: None

Body Part Character 4		Approach Character 5	Device Character 6	Qualifier Character 7
Ø Products of Conception	`0A` ♀	Ø Open	Z No Device	Ø High 1 Low 2 Extraperitoneal
Ø Products of Conception	`0A` ♀	7 Via Natural or Artificial Opening	Z No Device	3 Low Forceps 4 Mid Forceps 5 High Forceps 6 Vacuum 7 Internal Version 8 Other
1 Products of Conception, Retained	♀	7 Via Natural or Artificial Opening 8 Via Natural or Artificial Opening Endoscopic	Z No Device	9 Manual Z No Qualifier
2 Products of Conception, Ectopic	♀	Ø Open 4 Percutaneous Endoscopic 7 Via Natural or Artificial Opening 8 Via Natural or Artificial Opening Endoscopic	Z No Device	Z No Qualifier

DRG Non-OR `0A`	10D07Z[3,4,5,6,7,8] 10D00Z[0,1,2] except when a corresponding SDX of Z37.0-Z37.9 is also reported	♀	All body part, approach, device, and qualifier values
`0A`	10D07Z[3,4,5,7] except when a corresponding SDX of Z37.0-Z37.9 is also reported		

1   Obstetrics
Ø   Pregnancy
E   Delivery   Definition: Assisting the passage of the products of conception from the genital canal
                Explanation: None

Body Part Character 4	Approach Character 5	Device Character 6	Qualifier Character 7
Ø Products of Conception **QA**♀	X External	Z No Device	Z No Qualifier

DRG Non-OR	10E0XZZ	♀	All body part, approach, device, and qualifier values
QA	10E0XZZ except when a corresponding SDX of Z37.0-Z37.9 is also reported		

1   Obstetrics
Ø   Pregnancy
H   Insertion   Definition: Putting in a nonbiological appliance that monitors, assists, performs, or prevents a physiological function but does not physically take the place of a body part
                Explanation: None

Body Part Character 4	Approach Character 5	Device Character 6	Qualifier Character 7
Ø Products of Conception ♀	0 Open 7 Via Natural or Artificial Opening	3 Monitoring Electrode Y Other Device	Z No Qualifier

Non-OR	All body part, approach, device, and qualifier values	♀	All body part, approach, device, and qualifier values

1   Obstetrics
Ø   Pregnancy
J   Inspection   Definition: Visually and/or manually exploring a body part
                Explanation: Visual exploration may be performed with or without optical instrumentation. Manual exploration may be performed directly or through intervening body layers.

Body Part Character 4	Approach Character 5	Device Character 6	Qualifier Character 7
Ø Products of Conception ♀ 1 Products of Conception, Retained ♀ 2 Products of Conception, Ectopic ♀	0 Open 3 Percutaneous 4 Percutaneous Endoscopic 7 Via Natural or Artificial Opening 8 Via Natural or Artificial Opening Endoscopic X External	Z No Device	Z No Qualifier

Non-OR	All body part, approach, device, and qualifier values	♀	All body part, approach, device, and qualifier values

1   Obstetrics
Ø   Pregnancy
P   Removal   Definition: Taking out or off a device from a body part, region or orifice
                Explanation: If a device is taken out and a similar device put in without cutting or puncturing the skin or mucous membrane, the procedure is coded to the root operation CHANGE. Otherwise, the procedure for taking out a device is coded to the root operation REMOVAL.

Body Part Character 4	Approach Character 5	Device Character 6	Qualifier Character 7
Ø Products of Conception ♀	0 Open 7 Via Natural or Artificial Opening	3 Monitoring Electrode Y Other Device	Z No Qualifier

Non-OR	All body part, approach, device, and qualifier values	♀	All body part, approach, device, and qualifier values

1   Obstetrics
Ø   Pregnancy
Q   Repair   Definition: Restoring, to the extent possible, a body part to its normal anatomic structure and function
                Explanation: Used only when the method to accomplish the repair is not one of the other root operations

Body Part Character 4	Approach Character 5	Device Character 6	Qualifier Character 7
Ø Products of Conception ♀	0 Open 3 Percutaneous 4 Percutaneous Endoscopic 7 Via Natural or Artificial Opening 8 Via Natural or Artificial Opening Endoscopic	Y Other Device Z No Device	E Nervous System F Cardiovascular System G Lymphatics and Hemic H Eye J Ear, Nose and Sinus K Respiratory System L Mouth and Throat M Gastrointestinal System N Hepatobiliary and Pancreas P Endocrine System Q Skin R Musculoskeletal System S Urinary System T Female Reproductive System V Male Reproductive System Y Other Body System

Non-OR	All body part, approach, device, and qualifier values	♀	All body part, approach, device, and qualifier values

---

NC Noncovered Procedure   **LC** Limited Coverage   **QA** Questionable OB Admit   **NT** New Tech Add-on   ⊞ Combination Member   ♂ Male   ♀ Female

1   Obstetrics
0   Pregnancy
S   Reposition   Definition: Moving to its normal location, or other suitable location, all or a portion of a body part

Explanation: The body part is moved to a new location from an abnormal location, or from a normal location where it is not functioning correctly. The body part may or may not be cut out or off to be moved to the new location.

Body Part Character 4	Approach Character 5	Device Character 6	Qualifier Character 7
0 Products of Conception ♀	7 Via Natural or Artificial Opening X External	Z No Device	Z No Qualifier
2 Products of Conception, Ectopic ♀	0 Open 3 Percutaneous 4 Percutaneous Endoscopic 7 Via Natural or Artificial Opening 8 Via Natural or Artificial Opening Endoscopic	Z No Device	Z No Qualifier

Non-OR	10S0[7,X]ZZ	♀	All body part, approach, device, and qualifier values

1   Obstetrics
0   Pregnancy
T   Resection   Definition: Cutting out or off, without replacement, all of a body part

Explanation: None

Body Part Character 4	Approach Character 5	Device Character 6	Qualifier Character 7
2 Products of Conception, Ectopic ♀	0 Open 3 Percutaneous 4 Percutaneous Endoscopic 7 Via Natural or Artificial Opening 8 Via Natural or Artificial Opening Endoscopic	Z No Device	Z No Qualifier

♀	All body part, approach, device, and qualifier values

1   Obstetrics
0   Pregnancy
Y   Transplantation   Definition: Putting in or on all or a portion of a living body part taken from another individual or animal to physically take the place and/or function of all or a portion of a similar body part

Explanation: The native body part may or may not be taken out, and the transplanted body part may take over all or a portion of its function

Body Part Character 4	Approach Character 5	Device Character 6	Qualifier Character 7
0 Products of Conception ♀	3 Percutaneous 4 Percutaneous Endoscopic 7 Via Natural or Artificial Opening	Z No Device	E Nervous System F Cardiovascular System G Lymphatics and Hemic H Eye J Ear, Nose and Sinus K Respiratory System L Mouth and Throat M Gastrointestinal System N Hepatobiliary and Pancreas P Endocrine System Q Skin R Musculoskeletal System S Urinary System T Female Reproductive System V Male Reproductive System Y Other Body System

Non-OR	All body part, approach, device, and qualifier values	♀	All body part, approach, device, and qualifier values

Non-OR Procedure   DRG Non-OR Procedure   Valid OR Procedure   HAC Associated Procedure   Combination Only   New/Revised April   New/Revised October

710   ICD-10-PCS 2023

Placement 2WØ–2Y5

AHA Coding Clinic for table 2W6

2015, 2Q, 35	Application of tongs to reduce and stabilize cervical fracture
2013, 2Q, 39	Application of cervical tongs for reduction of cervical fracture

AHA Coding Clinic for table 2Y4

2018, 4Q, 38	Control of epistaxis
2017, 4Q, 106	Nasal packing for epistaxis

2   Placement
W   Anatomical Regions
Ø   Change   Definition: Taking out or off a device from a body part and putting back an identical or similar device in or on the same body part without cutting or puncturing the skin or a mucous membrane

Body Region Character 4	Approach Character 5	Device Character 6	Qualifier Character 7
Ø Head	**X** External	**Ø** Traction Apparatus	**Z** No Qualifier
2 Neck		**1** Splint	
3 Abdominal Wall		**2** Cast	
4 Chest Wall		**3** Brace	
5 Back		**4** Bandage	
6 Inguinal Region, Right		**5** Packing Material	
7 Inguinal Region, Left		**6** Pressure Dressing	
8 Upper Extremity, Right		**7** Intermittent Pressure Device	
9 Upper Extremity, Left		**Y** Other Device	
A Upper Arm, Right			
B Upper Arm, Left			
C Lower Arm, Right			
D Lower Arm, Left			
E Hand, Right			
F Hand, Left			
G Thumb, Right			
H Thumb, Left			
J Finger, Right			
K Finger, Left			
L Lower Extremity, Right			
M Lower Extremity, Left			
N Upper Leg, Right			
P Upper Leg, Left			
Q Lower Leg, Right			
R Lower Leg, Left			
S Foot, Right			
T Foot, Left			
U Toe, Right			
V Toe, Left			
1 Face	**X** External	**Ø** Traction Apparatus	**Z** No Qualifier
		1 Splint	
		2 Cast	
		3 Brace	
		4 Bandage	
		5 Packing Material	
		6 Pressure Dressing	
		7 Intermittent Pressure Device	
		9 Wire	
		Y Other Device	

NC Noncovered Procedure   **LC** Limited Coverage   **QA** Questionable OB Admit   **NT** New Tech Add-on   ⊞ Combination Member   ♂ Male   ♀ Female

ICD-10-PCS 2023   711

2WØ–2WØ

2　Placement
W　Anatomical Regions
1　Compression　　Definition: Putting pressure on a body region

Body Region Character 4	Approach Character 5	Device Character 6	Qualifier Character 7
0 Head 1 Face 2 Neck 3 Abdominal Wall 4 Chest Wall 5 Back 6 Inguinal Region, Right 7 Inguinal Region, Left 8 Upper Extremity, Right 9 Upper Extremity, Left A Upper Arm, Right B Upper Arm, Left C Lower Arm, Right D Lower Arm, Left E Hand, Right F Hand, Left G Thumb, Right H Thumb, Left J Finger, Right K Finger, Left L Lower Extremity, Right M Lower Extremity, Left N Upper Leg, Right P Upper Leg, Left Q Lower Leg, Right R Lower Leg, Left S Foot, Right T Foot, Left U Toe, Right V Toe, Left	X External	6 Pressure Dressing 7 Intermittent Pressure Device	Z No Qualifier

2　Placement
W　Anatomical Regions
2　Dressing　　Definition: Putting material on a body region for protection

Body Region Character 4	Approach Character 5	Device Character 6	Qualifier Character 7
0 Head 1 Face 2 Neck 3 Abdominal Wall 4 Chest Wall 5 Back 6 Inguinal Region, Right 7 Inguinal Region, Left 8 Upper Extremity, Right 9 Upper Extremity, Left A Upper Arm, Right B Upper Arm, Left C Lower Arm, Right D Lower Arm, Left E Hand, Right F Hand, Left G Thumb, Right H Thumb, Left J Finger, Right K Finger, Left L Lower Extremity, Right M Lower Extremity, Left N Upper Leg, Right P Upper Leg, Left Q Lower Leg, Right R Lower Leg, Left S Foot, Right T Foot, Left U Toe, Right V Toe, Left	X External	4 Bandage	Z No Qualifier

Non-OR Procedure　　DRG Non-OR Procedure　　Valid OR Procedure　　HAC Associated Procedure　　Combination Only　　New/Revised April　　New/Revised October

2   Placement
W   Anatomical Regions
3   Immobilization   Definition: Limiting or preventing motion of a body region

Body Region Character 4	Approach Character 5	Device Character 6	Qualifier Character 7
Ø Head 2 Neck 3 Abdominal Wall 4 Chest Wall 5 Back 6 Inguinal Region, Right 7 Inguinal Region, Left 8 Upper Extremity, Right 9 Upper Extremity, Left A Upper Arm, Right B Upper Arm, Left C Lower Arm, Right D Lower Arm, Left E Hand, Right F Hand, Left G Thumb, Right H Thumb, Left J Finger, Right K Finger, Left L Lower Extremity, Right M Lower Extremity, Left N Upper Leg, Right P Upper Leg, Left Q Lower Leg, Right R Lower Leg, Left S Foot, Right T Foot, Left U Toe, Right V Toe, Left	X External	1 Splint 2 Cast 3 Brace Y Other Device	Z No Qualifier
1 Face	X External	1 Splint 2 Cast 3 Brace 9 Wire Y Other Device	Z No Qualifier

2   Placement
W   Anatomical Regions
4   Packing   Definition: Putting material in a body region or orifice

Body Region Character 4	Approach Character 5	Device Character 6	Qualifier Character 7
Ø Head 1 Face 2 Neck 3 Abdominal Wall 4 Chest Wall 5 Back 6 Inguinal Region, Right 7 Inguinal Region, Left 8 Upper Extremity, Right 9 Upper Extremity, Left A Upper Arm, Right B Upper Arm, Left C Lower Arm, Right D Lower Arm, Left E Hand, Right F Hand, Left G Thumb, Right H Thumb, Left J Finger, Right K Finger, Left L Lower Extremity, Right M Lower Extremity, Left N Upper Leg, Right P Upper Leg, Left Q Lower Leg, Right R Lower Leg, Left S Foot, Right T Foot, Left U Toe, Right V Toe, Left	X External	5 Packing Material	Z No Qualifier

NC Noncovered Procedure   **LC** Limited Coverage   **QA** Questionable OB Admit   **NT** New Tech Add-on   ⊞ Combination Member   ♂ Male   ♀ Female

ICD-10-PCS 2023   713

2W3–2W4

2　Placement
W　Anatomical Regions
5　Removal　　Definition: Taking out or off a device from a body part

Body Region Character 4	Approach Character 5	Device Character 6	Qualifier Character 7
0　Head 2　Neck 3　Abdominal Wall 4　Chest Wall 5　Back 6　Inguinal Region, Right 7　Inguinal Region, Left 8　Upper Extremity, Right 9　Upper Extremity, Left A　Upper Arm, Right B　Upper Arm, Left C　Lower Arm, Right D　Lower Arm, Left E　Hand, Right F　Hand, Left G　Thumb, Right H　Thumb, Left J　Finger, Right K　Finger, Left L　Lower Extremity, Right M　Lower Extremity, Left N　Upper Leg, Right P　Upper Leg, Left Q　Lower Leg, Right R　Lower Leg, Left S　Foot, Right T　Foot, Left U　Toe, Right V　Toe, Left	X　External	0　Traction Apparatus 1　Splint 2　Cast 3　Brace 4　Bandage 5　Packing Material 6　Pressure Dressing 7　Intermittent Pressure Device Y　Other Device	Z　No Qualifier
1　Face	X　External	0　Traction Apparatus 1　Splint 2　Cast 3　Brace 4　Bandage 5　Packing Material 6　Pressure Dressing 7　Intermittent Pressure Device 9　Wire Y　Other Device	Z　No Qualifier

Non-OR Procedure　　DRG Non-OR Procedure　　Valid OR Procedure　　HAC Associated Procedure　　Combination Only　　New/Revised April　　New/Revised October

714

ICD-10-PCS 2023

2   Placement
W   Anatomical Regions
6   Traction   Definition: Exerting a pulling force on a body region in a distal direction

Body Region Character 4	Approach Character 5	Device Character 6	Qualifier Character 7
0 Head	X External	0 Traction Apparatus	Z No Qualifier
1 Face		Z No Device	
2 Neck			
3 Abdominal Wall			
4 Chest Wall			
5 Back			
6 Inguinal Region, Right			
7 Inguinal Region, Left			
8 Upper Extremity, Right			
9 Upper Extremity, Left			
A Upper Arm, Right			
B Upper Arm, Left			
C Lower Arm, Right			
D Lower Arm, Left			
E Hand, Right			
F Hand, Left			
G Thumb, Right			
H Thumb, Left			
J Finger, Right			
K Finger, Left			
L Lower Extremity, Right			
M Lower Extremity, Left			
N Upper Leg, Right			
P Upper Leg, Left			
Q Lower Leg, Right			
R Lower Leg, Left			
S Foot, Right			
T Foot, Left			
U Toe, Right			
V Toe, Left			

2   Placement
Y   Anatomical Orifices
0   Change   Definition: Taking out or off a device from a body part and putting back an identical or similar device in or on the same body part without cutting or puncturing the skin or a mucous membrane

Body Region Character 4	Approach Character 5	Device Character 6	Qualifier Character 7
0 Mouth and Pharynx	X External	5 Packing Material	Z No Qualifier
1 Nasal			
2 Ear			
3 Anorectal			
4 Female Genital Tract ♀			
5 Urethra			

♀   2Y04X5Z

2   Placement
Y   Anatomical Orifices
4   Packing   Definition: Putting material in a body region or orifice

Body Region Character 4	Approach Character 5	Device Character 6	Qualifier Character 7
0 Mouth and Pharynx 1 Nasal 2 Ear 3 Anorectal 4 Female Genital Tract ♀ 5 Urethra	X External	5 Packing Material	Z No Qualifier

♀   2Y44X5Z

2   Placement
Y   Anatomical Orifices
5   Removal   Definition: Taking out or off a device from a body part

Body Region Character 4	Approach Character 5	Device Character 6	Qualifier Character 7
0 Mouth and Pharynx 1 Nasal 2 Ear 3 Anorectal 4 Female Genital Tract ♀ 5 Urethra	X External	5 Packing Material	Z No Qualifier

♀   2Y54X5Z

Non-OR Procedure   DRG Non-OR Procedure   Valid OR Procedure   HAC Associated Procedure   Combination Only   New/Revised April   New/Revised October

716   ICD-10-PCS 2023

2Y4–2Y5

Administration 3Ø2–3E1

AHA Coding Clinic for table 3Ø2

2021, 4Q, 54	Nonautologous pathogen reduced cryoprecipitated fibrinogen complex
2020, 4Q, 60-61	Transfusion stem cell progenitor cells
2019, 4Q, 35	Transfusion of blood products
2019, 4Q, 36	T-cell depleted hematopoietic stem cells for transplantation
2016, 4Q, 113	Bone marrow and stem cell transfusion (Transplantation)

AHA Coding Clinic for table 3EØ

2022, 1Q, 8	Other monoclonal antibody
2021, 4Q, 54-55	Antineoplastic monoclonal antibody
2021, 4Q, 110	New/revised frequently asked questions regarding ICD-10-CM/PCS coding for COVID-19
2021, 1Q, 49	Frequently asked questions regarding ICD-10-CM and ICD-10-PCS coding for COVID-19
2020, 4Q, 49-50	Intravascular ultrasound assisted thrombolysis
2020, 4Q, 95	Frequently asked questions regarding ICD-10-PCS coding for COVID-19
2020, 3Q, 17-21	New procedure codes for introduction or infusion of therapeutics
2019, 4Q, 36-37	Hyperthermic antineoplastic chemotherapy
2018, 3Q, 7	Coronary brachytherapy with angioplasty
2018, 1Q, 8	Placement of bone morphogenetic protein & spinal fusion surgery
2017, 2Q, 14	Infusion of tPA into pleural cavity
2017, 1Q, 37	Injection of glue into enteric fistula tract
2016, 4Q, 113-114	Substances applied to cranial cavity and brain
2016, 3Q, 29	Closure of bilateral alveolar clefts
2016, 1Q, 20	Metatarsophalangeal joint resection arthroplasty

AHA Coding Clinic for table 3EØ (Continued)

2015, 3Q, 24	Esophagogastroduodenoscopy with epinephrine injection for control of bleeding
2015, 3Q, 29	Placement of adhesion barrier
2015, 2Q, 29	Insertion of nasogastric tube for drainage and feeding
2015, 2Q, 31	Thoracoscopic talc pleurodesis
2015, 1Q, 31	Intrathecal chemotherapy
2015, 1Q, 38	Chemoembolization of the hepatic artery
2014, 4Q, 16	Administration of RH (D) immunoglobulin
2014, 4Q, 17	RH (D) alloimmunization (sensitization)
2014, 4Q, 19	Ultrasound accelerated thrombolysis
2014, 4Q, 34	Resection of brain malignancy with implantation of chemotherapeutic wafer
2014, 4Q, 38	Placement of saline and Sepralfilm solution into abdominal cavity
2014, 3Q, 26	Coil embolization of gastroduodenal artery with chemoembolization of hepatic artery
2014, 2Q, 8	Medical induction of labor with Cervidil tampon insertion
2014, 2Q, 10	Prophylactic Neulasta injection for infection prevention
2013, 4Q, 124	Administration of tPA for stroke treatment prior to transfer
2013, 1Q, 27	Injection of sclerosing agent into an esophageal varix

AHA Coding Clinic for table 3E1

2021, 4Q, 55	Laparoscopic irrigation of peritoneal cavity
2019, 4Q, 38	Irrigation of joint using irrigating substance
2017, 3Q, 14	Bronchoscopy with suctioning and washings for removal of mucus plug

3　Administration
Ø　Circulatory
2　Transfusion　　Definition: Putting in blood or blood products

Body System/Region Character 4	Approach Character 5	Substance Character 6	Qualifier Character 7
3　Peripheral Vein　NC 4　Central Vein　NC	3　Percutaneous	A　Stem Cells, Embryonic	Z　No Qualifier
3　Peripheral Vein 4　Central Vein	3　Percutaneous	C　Hematopoietic Stem/Progenitor Cells, Genetically Modified	Ø　Autologous
3　Peripheral Vein 4　Central Vein	3　Percutaneous	D　Pathogen Reduced Cryoprecipitated Fibrinogen Complex　NT	1　Nonautologous
3　Peripheral Vein　NC 4　Central Vein　NC	3　Percutaneous	G　Bone Marrow X　Stem Cells, Cord Blood Y　Stem Cells, Hematopoietic	Ø　Autologous 2　Allogeneic, Related 3　Allogeneic, Unrelated 4　Allogeneic, Unspecified
3　Peripheral Vein 4　Central Vein	3　Percutaneous	H　Whole Blood J　Serum Albumin K　Frozen Plasma L　Fresh Plasma M　Plasma Cryoprecipitate N　Red Blood Cells P　Frozen Red Cells Q　White Cells R　Platelets S　Globulin T　Fibrinogen V　Antihemophilic Factors W　Factor IX	Ø　Autologous 1　Nonautologous
3　Peripheral Vein 4　Central Vein	3　Percutaneous	U　Stem Cells, T-cell Depleted Hematopoietic	2　Allogeneic, Related 3　Allogeneic, Unrelated 4　Allogeneic, Unspecified
7　Products of Conception,♀ 　　Circulatory	3　Percutaneous 7　Via Natural or Artificial Opening	H　Whole Blood J　Serum Albumin K　Frozen Plasma L　Fresh Plasma M　Plasma Cryoprecipitate N　Red Blood Cells P　Frozen Red Cells Q　White Cells R　Platelets S　Globulin T　Fibrinogen V　Antihemophilic Factors W　Factor IX	1　Nonautologous
8　Vein	3　Percutaneous	B　4-Factor Prothrombin Complex Concentrate	1　Nonautologous

DRG Non-OR　3Ø2[3,4]3AZ
DRG Non-OR　3Ø2[3,4]3CØ
DRG Non-OR　3Ø2[3,4]3[G,X,Y][Ø,2,3,4]
DRG Non-OR　3Ø2[3,4]3U[2,3,4]

NC　3Ø2[3,4]3AZ Only when reported with PDx or SDx of C91.00, C92.00, C92.10, C92.11, C92.40, C92.50, C92.60, C92.A0, C93.00, C94.00, C95.00
NC　3Ø2[3,4]3[G,Y]Ø Only when reported with PDx or SDx of C91.00, C92.00, C92.10, C92.11, C92.40, C92.50, C92.60, C92.A0, C93.00, C94.00, C95.00
NT　3Ø2[3,4]3D1 for Intercept® (PRCFC) in combination with dx code D62, D65, D68.2, D68.4, or D68.9
♀　3Ø27[3,7][H,J,K,L,M,N,P,Q,R,S,T,V,W]1

NC Noncovered Procedure　　**LC** Limited Coverage　　**QA** Questionable OB Admit　　**NT** New Tech Add-on　　✛ Combination Member　　♂ Male　　♀ Female

3   Administration
C   Indwelling Device
1   Irrigation   Definition: Putting in or on a cleansing substance

Body System/Region Character 4	Approach Character 5	Substance Character 6	Qualifier Character 7
Z None	X External	8 Irrigating Substance	Z No Qualifier

3   Administration
E   Physiological Systems and Anatomical Regions
0   Introduction   Definition: Putting in or on a therapeutic, diagnostic, nutritional, physiological, or prophylactic substance except blood or blood products

Body System/Region Character 4	Approach Character 5	Substance Character 6	Qualifier Character 7
0 Skin and Mucous Membranes	X External	0 Antineoplastic	5 Other Antineoplastic M Monoclonal Antibody
0 Skin and Mucous Membranes	X External	2 Anti-infective	8 Oxazolidinones 9 Other Anti-infective
0 Skin and Mucous Membranes	X External	3 Anti-inflammatory 4 Serum, Toxoid and Vaccine B Anesthetic Agent K Other Diagnostic Substance M Pigment N Analgesics, Hypnotics, Sedatives T Destructive Agent	Z No Qualifier
0 Skin and Mucous Membranes	X External	G Other Therapeutic Substance	C Other Substance
1 Subcutaneous Tissue	0 Open	2 Anti-infective	A Anti-Infective Envelope
1 Subcutaneous Tissue	3 Percutaneous	0 Antineoplastic	5 Other Antineoplastic M Monoclonal Antibody
1 Subcutaneous Tissue	3 Percutaneous	2 Anti-infective	8 Oxazolidinones 9 Other Anti-infective A Anti-Infective Envelope
1 Subcutaneous Tissue	3 Percutaneous	3 Anti-inflammatory 6 Nutritional Substance 7 Electrolytic and Water Balance Substance B Anesthetic Agent H Radioactive Substance K Other Diagnostic Substance N Analgesics, Hypnotics, Sedatives T Destructive Agent	Z No Qualifier
1 Subcutaneous Tissue	3 Percutaneous	4 Serum, Toxoid and Vaccine	0 Influenza Vaccine Z No Qualifier
1 Subcutaneous Tissue	3 Percutaneous	G Other Therapeutic Substance	C Other Substance
1 Subcutaneous Tissue	3 Percutaneous	V Hormone	G Insulin J Other Hormone
2 Muscle	3 Percutaneous	0 Antineoplastic	5 Other Antineoplastic M Monoclonal Antibody
2 Muscle	3 Percutaneous	2 Anti-infective	8 Oxazolidinones 9 Other Anti-infective
2 Muscle	3 Percutaneous	3 Anti-inflammatory 6 Nutritional Substance 7 Electrolytic and Water Balance Substance B Anesthetic Agent H Radioactive Substance K Other Diagnostic Substance N Analgesics, Hypnotics, Sedatives T Destructive Agent	Z No Qualifier
2 Muscle	3 Percutaneous	4 Serum, Toxoid and Vaccine	0 Influenza Vaccine Z No Qualifier
2 Muscle	3 Percutaneous	G Other Therapeutic Substance	C Other Substance
3 Peripheral Vein	0 Open	0 Antineoplastic	2 High-dose Interleukin-2 3 Low-dose Interleukin-2 5 Other Antineoplastic M Monoclonal Antibody P Clofarabine
3 Peripheral Vein	0 Open	1 Thrombolytic	6 Recombinant Human- activated Protein C 7 Other Thrombolytic
3 Peripheral Vein	0 Open	2 Anti-infective	8 Oxazolidinones 9 Other Anti-infective

DRG Non-OR   3E03002
DRG Non-OR   3E03017

3E0 Continued on next page

Non-OR Procedure   DRG Non-OR Procedure   Valid OR Procedure   HAC Associated Procedure   Combination Only   New/Revised April   New/Revised October

718   ICD-10-PCS 2023

3C1-3E0

3E0 Continued

3   **Administration**
E   **Physiological Systems and Anatomical Regions**
0   **Introduction**   Definition: Putting in or on a therapeutic, diagnostic, nutritional, physiological, or prophylactic substance except blood or blood products

Body System/Region Character 4	Approach Character 5	Substance Character 6	Qualifier Character 7
3 Peripheral Vein	0 Open	3 Anti-inflammatory 4 Serum, Toxoid and Vaccine 6 Nutritional Substance 7 Electrolytic and Water Balance Substance F Intracirculatory Anesthetic H Radioactive Substance K Other Diagnostic Substance N Analgesics, Hypnotics, Sedatives P Platelet Inhibitor R Antiarrhythmic T Destructive Agent X Vasopressor	Z No Qualifier
3 Peripheral Vein	0 Open	G Other Therapeutic Substance	C Other Substance N Blood Brain Barrier Disruption
3 Peripheral Vein	0 Open	U Pancreatic Islet Cells	0 Autologous 1 Nonautologous
3 Peripheral Vein	0 Open	V Hormone	G Insulin H Human B-type Natriuretic Peptide J Other Hormone
3 Peripheral Vein	0 Open	W Immunotherapeutic	K Immunostimulator L Immunosuppressive
3 Peripheral Vein	3 Percutaneous	0 Antineoplastic	2 High-dose Interleukin-2 3 Low-dose Interleukin-2 5 Other Antineoplastic M Monoclonal Antibody P Clofarabine
3 Peripheral Vein	3 Percutaneous	1 Thrombolytic	6 Recombinant Human- activated Protein C 7 Other Thrombolytic
3 Peripheral Vein	3 Percutaneous	2 Anti-infective	8 Oxazolidinones 9 Other Anti-infective
3 Peripheral Vein	3 Percutaneous	3 Anti-inflammatory 4 Serum, Toxoid and Vaccine 6 Nutritional Substance 7 Electrolytic and Water Balance Substance F Intracirculatory Anesthetic H Radioactive Substance K Other Diagnostic Substance N Analgesics, Hypnotics, Sedatives P Platelet Inhibitor R Antiarrhythmic T Destructive Agent X Vasopressor	Z No Qualifier
3 Peripheral Vein	3 Percutaneous	G Other Therapeutic Substance	C Other Substance N Blood Brain Barrier Disruption Q Glucarpidase R Other Therapeutic Monoclonal Antibody
3 Peripheral Vein	3 Percutaneous	U Pancreatic Islet Cells	0 Autologous 1 Nonautologous
3 Peripheral Vein	3 Percutaneous	V Hormone	G Insulin H Human B-type Natriuretic Peptide J Other Hormone
3 Peripheral Vein	3 Percutaneous	W Immunotherapeutic	K Immunostimulator L Immunosuppressive
4 Central Vein	0 Open	0 Antineoplastic	2 High-dose Interleukin-2 3 Low-dose Interleukin-2 5 Other Antineoplastic M Monoclonal Antibody P Clofarabine
4 Central Vein	0 Open	1 Thrombolytic	6 Recombinant Human- activated Protein C 7 Other Thrombolytic

Valid OR 3E030TZ		**DRG Non-OR** 3E033U[0,1]	
DRG Non-OR 3E030U[0,1]		**DRG Non-OR** 3E04002	
DRG Non-OR 3E03302		**DRG Non-OR** 3E04017	
DRG Non-OR 3E03317			

3E0 Continued on next page

NC Noncovered Procedure   **LC** Limited Coverage   **OA** Questionable OB Admit   **NT** New Tech Add-on   ⊞ Combination Member   ♂ Male   ♀ Female

Administration

3   Administration
E   Physiological Systems and Anatomical Regions
Ø   Introduction   Definition: Putting in or on a therapeutic, diagnostic, nutritional, physiological, or prophylactic substance except blood or blood products

3EØ Continued

Body System/Region Character 4	Approach Character 5	Substance Character 6	Qualifier Character 7
4 Central Vein	**Ø** Open	**2** Anti-infective	**8** Oxazolidinones **9** Other Anti-infective
4 Central Vein	**Ø** Open	**3** Anti-inflammatory **4** Serum, Toxoid and Vaccine **6** Nutritional Substance **7** Electrolytic and Water Balance Substance **F** Intracirculatory Anesthetic **H** Radioactive Substance **K** Other Diagnostic Substance **N** Analgesics, Hypnotics, Sedatives **P** Platelet Inhibitor **R** Antiarrhythmic **T** Destructive Agent **X** Vasopressor	**Z** No Qualifier
4 Central Vein	**Ø** Open	**G** Other Therapeutic Substance	**C** Other Substance **N** Blood Brain Barrier Disruption
4 Central Vein	**Ø** Open	**V** Hormone	**G** Insulin **H** Human B-type Natriuretic Peptide **J** Other Hormone
4 Central Vein	**Ø** Open	**W** Immunotherapeutic	**K** Immunostimulator **L** Immunosuppressive
4 Central Vein	**3** Percutaneous	**Ø** Antineoplastic	**2** High-dose Interleukin-2 **3** Low-dose Interleukin-2 **5** Other Antineoplastic **M** Monoclonal Antibody **P** Clofarabine
4 Central Vein	**3** Percutaneous	**1** Thrombolytic	**6** Recombinant Human- activated Protein C **7** Other Thrombolytic
4 Central Vein	**3** Percutaneous	**2** Anti-infective	**8** Oxazolidinones **9** Other Anti-infective
4 Central Vein	**3** Percutaneous	**3** Anti-inflammatory **4** Serum, Toxoid and Vaccine **6** Nutritional Substance **7** Electrolytic and Water Balance Substance **F** Intracirculatory Anesthetic **H** Radioactive Substance **K** Other Diagnostic Substance **N** Analgesics, Hypnotics, Sedatives **P** Platelet Inhibitor **R** Antiarrhythmic **T** Destructive Agent **X** Vasopressor	**Z** No Qualifier
4 Central Vein	**3** Percutaneous	**G** Other Therapeutic Substance	**C** Other Substance **N** Blood Brain Barrier Disruption **Q** Glucarpidase **R** Other Therapeutic Monoclonal Antibody
4 Central Vein	**3** Percutaneous	**V** Hormone	**G** Insulin **H** Human B-type Natriuretic Peptide **J** Other Hormone
4 Central Vein	**3** Percutaneous	**W** Immunotherapeutic	**K** Immunostimulator **L** Immunosuppressive
5 Peripheral Artery **6** Central Artery	**Ø** Open **3** Percutaneous	**Ø** Antineoplastic	**2** High-dose Interleukin-2 **3** Low-dose Interleukin-2 **5** Other Antineoplastic **M** Monoclonal Antibody **P** Clofarabine
5 Peripheral Artery **6** Central Artery	**Ø** Open **3** Percutaneous	**1** Thrombolytic	**6** Recombinant Human- activated Protein C **7** Other Thrombolytic
5 Peripheral Artery **6** Central Artery	**Ø** Open **3** Percutaneous	**2** Anti-infective	**8** Oxazolidinones **9** Other Anti-infective

Valid OR   3EØ40TZ   DRG Non-OR   3EØ[5,6][Ø,3]02
DRG Non-OR   3EØ43Ø2   DRG Non-OR   3EØ[5,6][Ø,3]17
DRG Non-OR   3EØ4317

3EØ Continued on next page

Non-OR Procedure   DRG Non-OR Procedure   Valid OR Procedure   HAC Associated Procedure   Combination Only   New/Revised April   New/Revised October

3   **Administration**
E   **Physiological Systems and Anatomical Regions**
0   **Introduction**   Definition: Putting in or on a therapeutic, diagnostic, nutritional, physiological, or prophylactic substance except blood or blood products

Body System/Region Character 4	Approach Character 5	Substance Character 6	Qualifier Character 7
5 Peripheral Artery 6 Central Artery	0 Open 3 Percutaneous	3 Anti-inflammatory 4 Serum, Toxoid and Vaccine 6 Nutritional Substance 7 Electrolytic and Water Balance Substance F Intracirculatory Anesthetic H Radioactive Substance K Other Diagnostic Substance N Analgesics, Hypnotics, Sedatives P Platelet Inhibitor R Antiarrhythmic T Destructive Agent X Vasopressor	Z No Qualifier
5 Peripheral Artery 6 Central Artery	0 Open 3 Percutaneous	G Other Therapeutic Substance	C Other Substance N Blood Brain Barrier Disruption
5 Peripheral Artery 6 Central Artery	0 Open 3 Percutaneous	V Hormone	G Insulin H Human B-type Natriuretic Peptide J Other Hormone
5 Peripheral Artery 6 Central Artery	0 Open 3 Percutaneous	W Immunotherapeutic	K Immunostimulator L Immunosuppressive
7 Coronary Artery 8 Heart	0 Open 3 Percutaneous	1 Thrombolytic	6 Recombinant Human- activated Protein C 7 Other Thrombolytic
7 Coronary Artery 8 Heart	0 Open 3 Percutaneous	G Other Therapeutic Substance	C Other Substance
7 Coronary Artery 8 Heart	0 Open 3 Percutaneous	K Other Diagnostic Substance P Platelet Inhibitor	Z No Qualifier
7 Coronary Artery 8 Heart	4 Percutaneous Endoscopic	G Other Therapeutic Substance	C Other Substance
9 Nose	3 Percutaneous 7 Via Natural or Artificial Opening X External	0 Antineoplastic	5 Other Antineoplastic M Monoclonal Antibody
9 Nose	3 Percutaneous 7 Via Natural or Artificial Opening X External	2 Anti-infective	8 Oxazolidinones 9 Other Anti-infective
9 Nose	3 Percutaneous 7 Via Natural or Artificial Opening X External	3 Anti-inflammatory 4 Serum, Toxoid and Vaccine B Anesthetic Agent H Radioactive Substance K Other Diagnostic Substance N Analgesics, Hypnotics, Sedatives T Destructive Agent	Z No Qualifier
9 Nose	3 Percutaneous 7 Via Natural or Artificial Opening X External	G Other Therapeutic Substance	C Other Substance
A Bone Marrow	3 Percutaneous	0 Antineoplastic	5 Other Antineoplastic M Monoclonal Antibody
A Bone Marrow	3 Percutaneous	G Other Therapeutic Substance	C Other Substance
B Ear	3 Percutaneous 7 Via Natural or Artificial Opening X External	0 Antineoplastic	4 Liquid Brachytherapy Radioisotope 5 Other Antineoplastic M Monoclonal Antibody
B Ear	3 Percutaneous 7 Via Natural or Artificial Opening X External	2 Anti-infective	8 Oxazolidinones 9 Other Anti-infective
B Ear	3 Percutaneous 7 Via Natural or Artificial Opening X External	3 Anti-inflammatory B Anesthetic Agent H Radioactive Substance K Other Diagnostic Substance N Analgesics, Hypnotics, Sedatives T Destructive Agent	Z No Qualifier
B Ear	3 Percutaneous 7 Via Natural or Artificial Opening X External	G Other Therapeutic Substance	C Other Substance

DRG Non-OR   3E08[0,3]17

3E0 Continued on next page

NC Noncovered Procedure   **LC** Limited Coverage   **QA** Questionable OB Admit   **NT** New Tech Add-on   ⊞ Combination Member   ♂ Male   ♀ Female

ICD-10-PCS 2023   **721**

Administration

3   **Administration**
E   **Physiological Systems and Anatomical Regions**
Ø   **Introduction**   Definition: Putting in or on a therapeutic, diagnostic, nutritional, physiological, or prophylactic substance except blood or blood products

3EØ Continued

Body System/Region Character 4	Approach Character 5	Substance Character 6	Qualifier Character 7
C Eye	**3** Percutaneous **7** Via Natural or Artificial Opening **X** External	**Ø** Antineoplastic	**4** Liquid Brachytherapy Radioisotope **5** Other Antineoplastic **M** Monoclonal Antibody
C Eye	**3** Percutaneous **7** Via Natural or Artificial Opening **X** External	**2** Anti-infective	**8** Oxazolidinones **9** Other Anti-infective
C Eye	**3** Percutaneous **7** Via Natural or Artificial Opening **X** External	**3** Anti-inflammatory **B** Anesthetic Agent **H** Radioactive Substance **K** Other Diagnostic Substance **M** Pigment **N** Analgesics, Hypnotics, Sedatives **T** Destructive Agent	**Z** No Qualifier
C Eye	**3** Percutaneous **7** Via Natural or Artificial Opening **X** External	**G** Other Therapeutic Substance	**C** Other Substance
C Eye	**3** Percutaneous **7** Via Natural or Artificial Opening **X** External	**S** Gas	**F** Other Gas
D Mouth and Pharynx	**3** Percutaneous **7** Via Natural or Artificial Opening **X** External	**Ø** Antineoplastic	**4** Liquid Brachytherapy Radioisotope **5** Other Antineoplastic **M** Monoclonal Antibody
D Mouth and Pharynx	**3** Percutaneous **7** Via Natural or Artificial Opening **X** External	**2** Anti-infective	**8** Oxazolidinones **9** Other Anti-infective
D Mouth and Pharynx	**3** Percutaneous **7** Via Natural or Artificial Opening **X** External	**3** Anti-inflammatory **4** Serum, Toxoid and Vaccine **6** Nutritional Substance **7** Electrolytic and Water Balance Substance **B** Anesthetic Agent **H** Radioactive Substance **K** Other Diagnostic Substance **N** Analgesics, Hypnotics, Sedatives **R** Antiarrhythmic **T** Destructive Agent	**Z** No Qualifier
D Mouth and Pharynx	**3** Percutaneous **7** Via Natural or Artificial Opening **X** External	**G** Other Therapeutic Substance	**C** Other Substance
E Products of Conception ♀ **G** Upper GI **H** Lower GI **K** Genitourinary Tract **N** Male Reproductive ♂	**3** Percutaneous **7** Via Natural or Artificial Opening **8** Via Natural or Artificial Opening Endoscopic	**Ø** Antineoplastic	**4** Liquid Brachytherapy Radioisotope **5** Other Antineoplastic **M** Monoclonal Antibody
E Products of Conception ♀ **G** Upper GI **H** Lower GI **K** Genitourinary Tract **N** Male Reproductive ♂	**3** Percutaneous **7** Via Natural or Artificial Opening **8** Via Natural or Artificial Opening Endoscopic	**2** Anti-infective	**8** Oxazolidinones **9** Other Anti-infective
E Products of Conception ♀ **G** Upper GI **H** Lower GI **K** Genitourinary Tract **N** Male Reproductive ♂	**3** Percutaneous **7** Via Natural or Artificial Opening **8** Via Natural or Artificial Opening Endoscopic	**3** Anti-inflammatory **6** Nutritional Substance **7** Electrolytic and Water Balance Substance **B** Anesthetic Agent **H** Radioactive Substance **K** Other Diagnostic Substance **N** Analgesics, Hypnotics, Sedatives **T** Destructive Agent	**Z** No Qualifier
E Products of Conception ♀ **G** Upper GI **H** Lower GI **K** Genitourinary Tract **N** Male Reproductive ♂	**3** Percutaneous **7** Via Natural or Artificial Opening **8** Via Natural or Artificial Opening Endoscopic	**G** Other Therapeutic Substance	**C** Other Substance

♂   All approach, substance, and qualifier values for body system/region (character 4) with this icon
♀   All approach, substance, and qualifier values for body system/region (character 4) with this icon

3EØ Continued on next page

Non-OR Procedure   DRG Non-OR Procedure   Valid OR Procedure   HAC Associated Procedure   Combination Only   New/Revised April   New/Revised October

722   ICD-10-PCS 2023

3   **Administration**
E   **Physiological Systems and Anatomical Regions**
0   **Introduction**   Definition: Putting in or on a therapeutic, diagnostic, nutritional, physiological, or prophylactic substance except blood or blood products

Body System/Region Character 4		Approach Character 5		Substance Character 6		Qualifier Character 7	
E G H K N	Products of Conception ♀ Upper GI Lower GI Genitourinary Tract Male Reproductive ♂	3 7 8	Percutaneous Via Natural or Artificial Opening Via Natural or Artificial Opening Endoscopic	S	Gas	F	Other Gas
E G H K N	Products of Conception ♀ Upper GI Lower GI Genitourinary Tract Male Reproductive ♂	4	Percutaneous Endoscopic	G	Other Therapeutic Substance	C	Other Substance
F	Respiratory Tract	3 7 8	Percutaneous Via Natural or Artificial Opening Via Natural or Artificial Opening Endoscopic	0	Antineoplastic	4 5 M	Liquid Brachytherapy Radioisotope Other Antineoplastic Monoclonal Antibody
F	Respiratory Tract	3 7 8	Percutaneous Via Natural or Artificial Opening Via Natural or Artificial Opening Endoscopic	2	Anti-infective	8 9	Oxazolidinones Other Anti-infective
F	Respiratory Tract	3 7 8	Percutaneous Via Natural or Artificial Opening Via Natural or Artificial Opening Endoscopic	3 6 7 B H K N T	Anti-inflammatory Nutritional Substance Electrolytic and Water Balance Substance Anesthetic Agent Radioactive Substance Other Diagnostic Substance Analgesics, Hypnotics, Sedatives Destructive Agent	Z	No Qualifier
F	Respiratory Tract	3 7 8	Percutaneous Via Natural or Artificial Opening Via Natural or Artificial Opening Endoscopic	G	Other Therapeutic Substance	C	Other Substance
F	Respiratory Tract	3 7 8	Percutaneous Via Natural or Artificial Opening Via Natural or Artificial Opening Endoscopic	S	Gas	D F	Nitric Oxide Other Gas
F	Respiratory Tract	4	Percutaneous Endoscopic	G	Other Therapeutic Substance	C	Other Substance
J	Biliary and Pancreatic Tract	3 7 8	Percutaneous Via Natural or Artificial Opening Via Natural or Artificial Opening Endoscopic	0	Antineoplastic	4 5 M	Liquid Brachytherapy Radioisotope Other Antineoplastic Monoclonal Antibody
J	Biliary and Pancreatic Tract	3 7 8	Percutaneous Via Natural or Artificial Opening Via Natural or Artificial Opening Endoscopic	2	Anti-infective	8 9	Oxazolidinones Other Anti-infective
J	Biliary and Pancreatic Tract	3 7 8	Percutaneous Via Natural or Artificial Opening Via Natural or Artificial Opening Endoscopic	3 6 7 B H K N T	Anti-inflammatory Nutritional Substance Electrolytic and Water Balance Substance Anesthetic Agent Radioactive Substance Other Diagnostic Substance Analgesics, Hypnotics, Sedatives Destructive Agent	Z	No Qualifier
J	Biliary and Pancreatic Tract	3 7 8	Percutaneous Via Natural or Artificial Opening Via Natural or Artificial Opening Endoscopic	G	Other Therapeutic Substance	C	Other Substance
J	Biliary and Pancreatic Tract	3 7 8	Percutaneous Via Natural or Artificial Opening Via Natural or Artificial Opening Endoscopic	S	Gas	F	Other Gas

♂   All approach, substance, and qualifier values for body system/region (character 4) with this icon
♀   All approach, substance, and qualifier values for body system/region (character 4) with this icon

3E0 Continued on next page

3 Administration
E Physiological Systems and Anatomical Regions
0 Introduction   Definition: Putting in or on a therapeutic, diagnostic, nutritional, physiological, or prophylactic substance except blood or blood products

Body System/Region Character 4		Approach Character 5		Substance Character 6		Qualifier Character 7	
J	Biliary and Pancreatic Tract	3	Percutaneous	U	Pancreatic Islet Cells	0	Autologous
		7	Via Natural or Artificial Opening			1	Nonautologous
		8	Via Natural or Artificial Opening Endoscopic				
J	Biliary and Pancreatic Tract	4	Percutaneous Endoscopic	G	Other Therapeutic Substance	C	Other Substance
L	Pleural Cavity	0	Open	5	Adhesion Barrier	Z	No Qualifier
L	Pleural Cavity	3	Percutaneous	0	Antineoplastic	4	Liquid Brachytherapy Radioisotope
						5	Other Antineoplastic
						M	Monoclonal Antibody
L	Pleural Cavity	3	Percutaneous	2	Anti-infective	8	Oxazolidinones
						9	Other Anti-infective
L	Pleural Cavity	3	Percutaneous	3	Anti-inflammatory	Z	No Qualifier
				5	Adhesion Barrier		
				6	Nutritional Substance		
				7	Electrolytic and Water Balance Substance		
				B	Anesthetic Agent		
				H	Radioactive Substance		
				K	Other Diagnostic Substance		
				N	Analgesics, Hypnotics, Sedatives		
				T	Destructive Agent		
L	Pleural Cavity	3	Percutaneous	G	Other Therapeutic Substance	C	Other Substance
L	Pleural Cavity	3	Percutaneous	S	Gas	F	Other Gas
L	Pleural Cavity	4	Percutaneous Endoscopic	5	Adhesion Barrier	Z	No Qualifier
L	Pleural Cavity	4	Percutaneous Endoscopic	G	Other Therapeutic Substance	C	Other Substance
L	Pleural Cavity	7	Via Natural or Artificial Opening	0	Antineoplastic	4	Liquid Brachytherapy Radioisotope
						5	Other Antineoplastic
						M	Monoclonal Antibody
L	Pleural Cavity	7	Via Natural or Artificial Opening	S	Gas	F	Other Gas
M	Peritoneal Cavity	0	Open	5	Adhesion Barrier	Z	No Qualifier
M	Peritoneal Cavity	3	Percutaneous	0	Antineoplastic	4	Liquid Brachytherapy Radioisotope
						5	Other Antineoplastic
						M	Monoclonal Antibody
						Y	Hyperthermic
M	Peritoneal Cavity	3	Percutaneous	2	Anti-infective	8	Oxazolidinones
						9	Other Anti-infective
M	Peritoneal Cavity	3	Percutaneous	3	Anti-inflammatory	Z	No Qualifier
				5	Adhesion Barrier		
				6	Nutritional Substance		
				7	Electrolytic and Water Balance Substance		
				B	Anesthetic Agent		
				H	Radioactive Substance		
				K	Other Diagnostic Substance		
				N	Analgesics, Hypnotics, Sedatives		
				T	Destructive Agent		
M	Peritoneal Cavity	3	Percutaneous	G	Other Therapeutic Substance	C	Other Substance
M	Peritoneal Cavity	3	Percutaneous	S	Gas	F	Other Gas
M	Peritoneal Cavity	4	Percutaneous Endoscopic	5	Adhesion Barrier	Z	No Qualifier
M	Peritoneal Cavity	4	Percutaneous Endoscopic	G	Other Therapeutic Substance	C	Other Substance
M	Peritoneal Cavity	7	Via Natural or Artificial Opening	0	Antineoplastic	4	Liquid Brachytherapy Radioisotope
						5	Other Antineoplastic
						M	Monoclonal Antibody
M	Peritoneal Cavity	7	Via Natural or Artificial Opening	S	Gas	F	Other Gas
P	Female Reproductive ♀	0	Open	5	Adhesion Barrier	Z	No Qualifier
P	Female Reproductive ♀	3	Percutaneous	0	Antineoplastic	4	Liquid Brachytherapy Radioisotope
						5	Other Antineoplastic
						M	Monoclonal Antibody
P	Female Reproductive ♀	3	Percutaneous	2	Anti-infective	8	Oxazolidinones
						9	Other Anti-infective

Valid OR   3E0L4GC
DRG Non-OR   3E0J[3,7,8]U[0,1]
♀   All approach, substance, and qualifier values for body system/region (character 4) with this icon

3E0 Continued on next page

Non-OR Procedure   DRG Non-OR Procedure   Valid OR Procedure   HAC Associated Procedure   Combination Only   New/Revised April   New/Revised October

724   ICD-10-PCS 2023

3 Administration
E Physiological Systems and Anatomical Regions
0 Introduction Definition: Putting in or on a therapeutic, diagnostic, nutritional, physiological, or prophylactic substance except blood or blood products

Body System/Region Character 4		Approach Character 5	Substance Character 6	Qualifier Character 7
P Female Reproductive	♀	3 Percutaneous	3 Anti-inflammatory 5 Adhesion Barrier 6 Nutritional Substance 7 Electrolytic and Water Balance Substance B Anesthetic Agent H Radioactive Substance K Other Diagnostic Substance L Sperm N Analgesics, Hypnotics, Sedatives T Destructive Agent V Hormone	Z No Qualifier
P Female Reproductive	♀	3 Percutaneous	G Other Therapeutic Substance	C Other Substance
P Female Reproductive	♀	3 Percutaneous	Q Fertilized Ovum	0 Autologous 1 Nonautologous
P Female Reproductive	♀	3 Percutaneous	S Gas	F Other Gas
P Female Reproductive	♀	4 Percutaneous Endoscopic	5 Adhesion Barrier	Z No Qualifier
P Female Reproductive	♀	4 Percutaneous Endoscopic	G Other Therapeutic Substance	C Other Substance
P Female Reproductive	♀	7 Via Natural or Artificial Opening	0 Antineoplastic	4 Liquid Brachytherapy Radioisotope 5 Other Antineoplastic M Monoclonal Antibody
P Female Reproductive	♀	7 Via Natural or Artificial Opening	2 Anti-infective	8 Oxazolidinones 9 Other Anti-infective
P Female Reproductive	♀	7 Via Natural or Artificial Opening	3 Anti-inflammatory 6 Nutritional Substance 7 Electrolytic and Water Balance Substance B Anesthetic Agent H Radioactive Substance K Other Diagnostic Substance L Sperm N Analgesics, Hypnotics, Sedatives T Destructive Agent V Hormone	Z No Qualifier
P Female Reproductive	♀	7 Via Natural or Artificial Opening	G Other Therapeutic Substance	C Other Substance
P Female Reproductive	♀	7 Via Natural or Artificial Opening	Q Fertilized Ovum	0 Autologous 1 Nonautologous
P Female Reproductive	♀	7 Via Natural or Artificial Opening	S Gas	F Other Gas
P Female Reproductive	♀	8 Via Natural or Artificial Opening Endoscopic	0 Antineoplastic	4 Liquid Brachytherapy Radioisotope 5 Other Antineoplastic M Monoclonal Antibody
P Female Reproductive	♀	8 Via Natural or Artificial Opening Endoscopic	2 Anti-infective	8 Oxazolidinones 9 Other Anit-infective
P Female Reproductive	♀	8 Via Natural or Artificial Opening Endoscopic	3 Anti-inflammatory 6 Nutritional Substance 7 Electrolytic and Water Balance Substance B Anesthetic Agent H Radioactive Substance K Other Diagnostic Substance N Analgesics, Hypnotics, Sedatives T Destructive Agent	Z No Qualifier
P Female Reproductive	♀	8 Via Natural or Artificial Opening Endoscopic	G Other Therapeutic Substance	C Other Substance
P Female Reproductive	♀	8 Via Natural or Artificial Opening Endoscopic	S Gas	F Other Gas
Q Cranial Cavity and Brain		0 Open 3 Percutaneous	0 Antineoplastic	4 Liquid Brachytherapy Radioisotope 5 Other Antineoplastic M Monoclonal Antibody
Q Cranial Cavity and Brain		0 Open 3 Percutaneous	2 Anti-infective	8 Oxazolidinones 9 Other Anti-infective

Valid OR	3E0P3Q[0,1]
Valid OR	3E0P7Q[0,1]
DRG Non-OR	3E0Q[0,3]05
♀	All approach, substance, and qualifier values for body system/region (character 4) with this icon

3E0 Continued on next page

NC Noncovered Procedure   **LC** Limited Coverage   **QA** Questionable OB Admit   **NT** New Tech Add-on   ⊞ Combination Member   ♂ Male   ♀ Female

ICD-10-PCS 2023   **725**

3   Administration
E   Physiological Systems and Anatomical Regions
Ø   Introduction   Definition: Putting in or on a therapeutic, diagnostic, nutritional, physiological, or prophylactic substance except blood or blood products

3EØ Continued

Body System/Region Character 4	Approach Character 5	Substance Character 6	Qualifier Character 7
Q Cranial Cavity and Brain	Ø Open 3 Percutaneous	3 Anti-inflammatory 6 Nutritional Substance 7 Electrolytic and Water Balance Substance A Stem Cells, Embryonic B Anesthetic Agent H Radioactive Substance K Other Diagnostic Substance N Analgesics, Hypnotics, Sedatives T Destructive Agent	Z No Qualifier
Q Cranial Cavity and Brain	Ø Open 3 Percutaneous	E Stem Cells, Somatic	Ø Autologous 1 Nonautologous
Q Cranial Cavity and Brain	Ø Open 3 Percutaneous	G Other Therapeutic Substance	C Other Substance
Q Cranial Cavity and Brain	Ø Open 3 Percutaneous	S Gas	F Other Gas
Q Cranial Cavity and Brain	7 Via Natural or Artificial Opening	Ø Antineoplastic	4 Liquid Brachytherapy Radioisotope 5 Other Antineoplastic M Monoclonal Antibody
Q Cranial Cavity and Brain	7 Via Natural or Artificial Opening	S Gas	F Other Gas
R Spinal Canal	Ø Open	A Stem Cells, Embryonic	Z No Qualifier
R Spinal Canal	Ø Open	E Stem Cells, Somatic	Ø Autologous 1 Nonautologous
R Spinal Canal	3 Percutaneous	Ø Antineoplastic	2 High-dose Interleukin-2 3 Low-dose Interleukin-2 4 Liquid Brachytherapy Radioisotope 5 Other Antineoplastic M Monoclonal Antibody
R Spinal Canal	3 Percutaneous	2 Anti-infective	8 Oxazolidinones 9 Other Anti-infective
R Spinal Canal	3 Percutaneous	3 Anti-inflammatory 6 Nutritional Substance 7 Electrolytic and Water Balance Substance A Stem Cells, Embryonic B Anesthetic Agent H Radioactive Substance K Other Diagnostic Substance N Analgesics, Hypnotics, Sedatives T Destructive Agent	Z No Qualifier
R Spinal Canal	3 Percutaneous	E Stem Cells, Somatic	Ø Autologous 1 Nonautologous
R Spinal Canal	3 Percutaneous	G Other Therapeutic Substance	C Other Substance
R Spinal Canal	3 Percutaneous	S Gas	F Other Gas
R Spinal Canal	7 Via Natural or Artificial Opening	S Gas	F Other Gas
S Epidural Space	3 Percutaneous	Ø Antineoplastic	2 High-dose Interleukin-2 3 Low-dose Interleukin-2 4 Liquid Brachytherapy Radioisotope 5 Other Antineoplastic M Monoclonal Antibody
S Epidural Space	3 Percutaneous	2 Anti-infective	8 Oxazolidinones 9 Other Anti-infective
S Epidural Space	3 Percutaneous	3 Anti-inflammatory 6 Nutritional Substance 7 Electrolytic and Water Balance Substance B Anesthetic Agent H Radioactive Substance K Other Diagnostic Substance N Analgesics, Hypnotics, Sedatives T Destructive Agent	Z No Qualifier

DRG Non-OR	3E0Q705
DRG Non-OR	3E0R302
DRG Non-OR	3E0S302

3EØ Continued on next page

Non-OR Procedure   DRG Non-OR Procedure   Valid OR Procedure   HAC Associated Procedure   Combination Only   New/Revised April   New/Revised October

726   ICD-10-PCS 2023

3 Administration
E Physiological Systems and Anatomical Regions
Ø Introduction   Definition: Putting in or on a therapeutic, diagnostic, nutritional, physiological, or prophylactic substance except blood or blood products

3EØ Continued

Body System/Region Character 4	Approach Character 5	Substance Character 6	Qualifier Character 7
S Epidural Space	**3** Percutaneous	**G** Other Therapeutic Substance	**C** Other Substance
S Epidural Space	**3** Percutaneous	**S** Gas	**F** Other Gas
S Epidural Space	**7** Via Natural or Artificial Opening	**S** Gas	**F** Other Gas
T Peripheral Nerves and Plexi **X** Cranial Nerves	**3** Percutaneous	**3** Anti-inflammatory **B** Anesthetic Agent **T** Destructive Agent	**Z** No Qualifier
T Peripheral Nerves and Plexi **X** Cranial Nerves	**3** Percutaneous	**G** Other Therapeutic Substance	**C** Other Substance
U Joints	**Ø** Open	**2** Anti-infective	**8** Oxazolidinones **9** Other Anti-infective
U Joints	**Ø** Open	**G** Other Therapeutic Substance	**B** Recombinant Bone Morphogenetic Protein
U Joints	**3** Percutaneous	**Ø** Antineoplastic	**4** Liquid Brachytherapy Radioisotope **5** Other Antineoplastic **M** Monoclonal Antibody
U Joints	**3** Percutaneous	**2** Anti-infective	**8** Oxazolidinones **9** Other Anti-infective
U Joints	**3** Percutaneous	**3** Anti-inflammatory **6** Nutritional Substance **7** Electrolytic and Water Balance Substance **B** Anesthetic Agent **H** Radioactive Substance **K** Other Diagnostic Substance **N** Analgesics, Hypnotics, Sedatives **T** Destructive Agent	**Z** No Qualifier
U Joints	**3** Percutaneous	**G** Other Therapeutic Substance	**B** Recombinant Bone Morphogenetic Protein **C** Other Substance
U Joints	**3** Percutaneous	**S** Gas	**F** Other Gas
U Joints	**4** Percutaneous Endoscopic	**G** Other Therapeutic Substance	**C** Other Substance
V Bones	**Ø** Open	**G** Other Therapeutic Substance	**B** Recombinant Bone Morphogenetic Protein **C** Other Substance
V Bones	**3** Percutaneous	**Ø** Antineoplastic	**5** Other Antineoplastic **M** Monoclonal Antibody
V Bones	**3** Percutaneous	**2** Anti-infective	**8** Oxazolidinones **9** Other Anti-infective
V Bones	**3** Percutaneous	**3** Anti-inflammatory **6** Nutritional Substance **7** Electrolytic and Water Balance Substance **B** Anesthetic Agent **H** Radioactive Substance **K** Other Diagnostic Substance **N** Analgesics, Hypnotics, Sedatives **T** Destructive Agent	**Z** No Qualifier
V Bones	**3** Percutaneous	**G** Other Therapeutic Substance	**B** Recombinant Bone Morphogenetic Protein **C** Other Substance
V Bones	**4** Percutaneous Endoscopic	**G** Other Therapeutic Substance	**C** Other Substance
W Lymphatics	**3** Percutaneous	**Ø** Antineoplastic	**5** Other Antineoplastic **M** Monoclonal Antibody
W Lymphatics	**3** Percutaneous	**2** Anti-infective	**8** Oxazolidinones **9** Other Anti-infective
W Lymphatics	**3** Percutaneous	**3** Anti-inflammatory **6** Nutritional Substance **7** Electrolytic and Water Balance Substance **B** Anesthetic Agent **H** Radioactive Substance **K** Other Diagnostic Substance **N** Analgesics, Hypnotics, Sedatives **T** Destructive Agent	**Z** No Qualifier
W Lymphatics	**3** Percutaneous	**G** Other Therapeutic Substance	**C** Other Substance

3EØ Continued on next page

NC Noncovered Procedure   **LC** Limited Coverage   **QA** Questionable OB Admit   **NT** New Tech Add-on   ⊞ Combination Member   ♂ Male   ♀ Female

ICD-10-PCS 2023   727

3EØ–3EØ

3   Administration
E   Physiological Systems and Anatomical Regions
Ø   Introduction   Definition: Putting in or on a therapeutic, diagnostic, nutritional, physiological, or prophylactic substance except blood or blood products

3EØ Continued

Body System/Region Character 4		Approach Character 5		Substance Character 6		Qualifier Character 7	
Y	Pericardial Cavity	3	Percutaneous	Ø	Antineoplastic	4 5 M	Liquid Brachytherapy Radioisotope Other Antineoplastic Monoclonal Antibody
Y	Pericardial Cavity	3	Percutaneous	2	Anti-infective	8 9	Oxazolidinones Other Anti-infective
Y	Pericardial Cavity	3	Percutaneous	3 6 7 B H K N T	Anti-inflammatory Nutritional Substance Electrolytic and Water Balance Substance Anesthetic Agent Radioactive Substance Other Diagnostic Substance Analgesics, Hypnotics, Sedatives Destructive Agent	Z	No Qualifier
Y	Pericardial Cavity	3	Percutaneous	G	Other Therapeutic Substance	C	Other Substance
Y	Pericardial Cavity	3	Percutaneous	S	Gas	F	Other Gas
Y	Pericardial Cavity	4	Percutaneous Endoscopic	G	Other Therapeutic Substance	C	Other Substance
Y	Pericardial Cavity	7	Via Natural or Artificial Opening	Ø	Antineoplastic	4 5 M	Liquid Brachytherapy Radioisotope Other Antineoplastic Monoclonal Antibody
Y	Pericardial Cavity	7	Via Natural or Artificial Opening	S	Gas	F	Other Gas

3   Administration
E   Physiological Systems and Anatomical Regions
1   Irrigation   Definition: Putting in or on a cleansing substance

Body System/Region Character 4		Approach Character 5		Substance Character 6		Qualifier Character 7	
Ø C	Skin and Mucous Membranes Eye	3 X	Percutaneous External	8	Irrigating Substance	X Z	Diagnostic No Qualifier
9 B F G H J K N P	Nose Ear Respiratory Tract Upper GI Lower GI Biliary and Pancreatic Tract Genitourinary Tract Male Reproductive ♂ Female Reproductive ♀	3 7 8	Percutaneous Via Natural or Artificial Opening Via Natural or Artificial Opening Endoscopic	8	Irrigating Substance	X Z	Diagnostic No Qualifier
L Q R S Y	Pleural Cavity Cranial Cavity and Brain Spinal Canal Epidural Space Pericardial Cavity	3	Percutaneous	8	Irrigating Substance	X Z	Diagnostic No Qualifier
M	Peritoneal Cavity	3	Percutaneous	8	Irrigating Substance	X Z	Diagnostic No Qualifier
M	Peritoneal Cavity	3	Percutaneous	9	Dialysate	Z	No Qualifier
M	Peritoneal Cavity	4	Percutaneous Endoscopic	8	Irrigating Substance	X Z	Diagnostic No Qualifier
U	Joints	3 4	Percutaneous Percutaneous Endoscopic	8	Irrigating Substance	X Z	Diagnostic No Qualifier

♂   3E1N[3,7,8]8[X,Z]
♀   3E1P[3,7,8]8[X,Z]

Non-OR Procedure   DRG Non-OR Procedure   Valid OR Procedure   HAC Associated Procedure   Combination Only   New/Revised April   New/Revised October

728   ICD-10-PCS 2023

Measurement and Monitoring 4A0–4B0

AHA Coding Clinic for table 4A0

2022, 1Q, 46	Internal cardioversion
2020, 4Q, 62	Measurement of intracranial arterial flow
2020, 4Q, 62	Percutaneous endoscopic measurement of portal venous pressure
2020, 4Q, 63	Intercompartmental pressure measurement
2019, 3Q, 32	Endomyocardial biopsy and right heart catheterization
2018, 1Q, 12	Percutaneous balloon valvuloplasty & cardiac catheterization with ventriculogram
2016, 3Q, 37	Fractional flow reserve
2015, 3Q, 29	Approach value for esophageal electrophysiology study

AHA Coding Clinic for table 4B0

2021, 4Q, 55-56	Measurement of flow in a cerebral fluid shunt

AHA Coding Clinic for table 4A1

2019, 4Q, 38-39	Intraoperative fluorescence lymphatic mapping using Indocyanine green dye
2016, 4Q, 114	Fluorescence vascular angiography
2016, 2Q, 29	Decompressive craniectomy with cryopreservation and storage of bone flap
2016, 2Q, 33	Monitoring of arterial pressure & pulse
2015, 3Q, 35	Swan Ganz catheterization
2015, 2Q, 14	Intraoperative EMG monitoring via endotracheal tube
2015, 1Q, 26	Intraoperative monitoring using Sentio MMG®
2014, 4Q, 28	Removal and replacement of displaced growing rods

4   **Measurement and Monitoring**
A   **Physiological Systems**
0   **Measurement**   Definition: Determining the level of a physiological or physical function at a point in time

Body System Character 4	Approach Character 5	Function/Device Character 6	Qualifier Character 7
0 Central Nervous	0 Open	2 Conductivity 4 Electrical Activity B Pressure	Z No Qualifier
0 Central Nervous	3 Percutaneous 7 Via Natural or Artificial Opening 8 Via Natural or Artificial Opening Endoscopic	4 Electrical Activity	Z No Qualifier
0 Central Nervous	3 Percutaneous 7 Via Natural or Artificial Opening 8 Via Natural or Artificial Opening Endoscopic	B Pressure K Temperature R Saturation	D Intracranial
0 Central Nervous	X External	2 Conductivity 4 Electrical Activity	Z No Qualifier
1 Peripheral Nervous	0 Open 3 Percutaneous 7 Via Natural or Artificial Opening 8 Via Natural or Artificial Opening Endoscopic X External	2 Conductivity	9 Sensory B Motor
1 Peripheral Nervous	0 Open 3 Percutaneous 7 Via Natural or Artificial Opening 8 Via Natural or Artificial Opening Endoscopic X External	4 Electrical Activity	Z No Qualifier
2 Cardiac	0 Open 3 Percutaneous 7 Via Natural or Artificial Opening 8 Via Natural or Artificial Opening Endoscopic	4 Electrical Activity 9 Output C Rate F Rhythm H Sound P Action Currents	Z No Qualifier
2 Cardiac	0 Open 3 Percutaneous 7 Via Natural or Artificial Opening 8 Via Natural or Artificial Opening Endoscopic	N Sampling and Pressure	6 Right Heart 7 Left Heart 8 Bilateral
2 Cardiac	X External	4 Electrical Activity	A Guidance Z No Qualifier
2 Cardiac	X External	9 Output C Rate F Rhythm H Sound P Action Currents	Z No Qualifier
2 Cardiac	X External	M Total Activity	4 Stress
3 Arterial	0 Open 3 Percutaneous	5 Flow J Pulse	1 Peripheral 3 Pulmonary C Coronary
3 Arterial	0 Open 3 Percutaneous	B Pressure	1 Peripheral 3 Pulmonary C Coronary F Other Thoracic

DRG Non-OR	4A02[3,7,8]FZ
DRG Non-OR	4A02[0,3,7,8]N[6,7,8]

4A0 Continued on next page

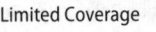 **Noncovered Procedure**   **LC** Limited Coverage   **QA** Questionable OB Admit   **NT** New Tech Add-on   ⊞ Combination Member   ♂ Male   ♀ Female

4   Measurement and Monitoring
A   Physiological Systems
0   Measurement   Definition: Determining the level of a physiological or physical function at a point in time

Body System Character 4	Approach Character 5	Function/Device Character 6	Qualifier Character 7
3 Arterial	0 Open 3 Percutaneous	H Sound R Saturation	1 Peripheral
3 Arterial	X External	5 Flow	1 Peripheral D Intracranial
3 Arterial	X External	B Pressure H Sound J Pulse R Saturation	1 Peripheral
4 Venous	0 Open 3 Percutaneous	5 Flow B Pressure J Pulse	0 Central 1 Peripheral 2 Portal 3 Pulmonary
4 Venous	0 Open 3 Percutaneous	R Saturation	1 Peripheral
4 Venous	4 Percutaneous Endoscopic	B Pressure	2 Portal
4 Venous	X External	5 Flow B Pressure J Pulse R Saturation	1 Peripheral
5 Circulatory	X External	L Volume	Z No Qualifier
6 Lymphatic	0 Open 3 Percutaneous 7 Via Natural or Artificial Opening 8 Via Natural or Artificial Opening Endoscopic	5 Flow B Pressure	Z No Qualifier
7 Visual	X External	0 Acuity 7 Mobility B Pressure	Z No Qualifier
8 Olfactory	X External	0 Acuity	Z No Qualifier
9 Respiratory	7 Via Natural or Artificial Opening 8 Via Natural or Artificial Opening Endoscopic X External	1 Capacity 5 Flow C Rate D Resistance L Volume M Total Activity	Z No Qualifier
B Gastrointestinal	7 Via Natural or Artificial Opening 8 Via Natural or Artificial Opening Endoscopic	8 Motility B Pressure G Secretion	Z No Qualifier
C Biliary	3 Percutaneous 4 Percutaneous Endoscopic 7 Via Natural or Artificial Opening 8 Via Natural or Artificial Opening Endoscopic	5 Flow B Pressure	Z No Qualifier
D Urinary	7 Via Natural or Artificial Opening 8 Via Natural or Artificial Opening Endoscopic	3 Contractility 5 Flow B Pressure D Resistance L Volume	Z No Qualifier
F Musculoskeletal	3 Percutaneous	3 Contractility	Z No Qualifier
F Musculoskeletal	3 Percutaneous	B Pressure	E Compartment
F Musculoskeletal	X External	3 Contractility	Z No Qualifier
H Products of Conception, ♀ Cardiac	7 Via Natural or Artificial Opening 8 Via Natural or Artificial Opening Endoscopic X External	4 Electrical Activity C Rate F Rhythm H Sound	Z No Qualifier
J Products of Conception, ♀ Nervous	7 Via Natural or Artificial Opening 8 Via Natural or Artificial Opening Endoscopic X External	2 Conductivity 4 Electrical Activity B Pressure	Z No Qualifier
Z None	7 Via Natural or Artificial Opening	6 Metabolism K Temperature	Z No Qualifier
Z None	X External	6 Metabolism K Temperature Q Sleep	Z No Qualifier

Valid OR	4A060[5,B]Z	♀	4A0H[7,8,X][4,C,F,H]Z
Valid OR	4A0C4[5,B]Z	♀	4A0J[7,8,X][2,4,B]Z

Non-OR Procedure   DRG Non-OR Procedure   Valid OR Procedure   HAC Associated Procedure   Combination Only   New/Revised April   New/Revised October

730   ICD-10-PCS 2023

4   Measurement and Monitoring
A   Physiological Systems
1   Monitoring   Definition: Determining the level of a physiological or physical function repetitively over a period of time

Body System Character 4	Approach Character 5	Function/Device Character 6	Qualifier Character 7
Ø Central Nervous	Ø Open	2 Conductivity B Pressure	Z No Qualifier
Ø Central Nervous	Ø Open	4 Electrical Activity	G Intraoperative Z No Qualifier
Ø Central Nervous	3 Percutaneous 7 Via Natural or Artificial Opening 8 Via Natural or Artificial Opening Endoscopic	4 Electrical Activity	G Intraoperative Z No Qualifier
Ø Central Nervous	3 Percutaneous 7 Via Natural or Artificial Opening 8 Via Natural or Artificial Opening Endoscopic	B Pressure K Temperature R Saturation	D Intracranial
Ø Central Nervous	X External	2 Conductivity	Z No Qualifier
Ø Central Nervous	X External	4 Electrical Activity	G Intraoperative Z No Qualifier
1 Peripheral Nervous	Ø Open 3 Percutaneous 7 Via Natural or Artificial Opening 8 Via Natural or Artificial Opening Endoscopic X External	2 Conductivity	9 Sensory B Motor
1 Peripheral Nervous	Ø Open 3 Percutaneous 7 Via Natural or Artificial Opening 8 Via Natural or Artificial Opening Endoscopic X External	4 Electrical Activity	G Intraoperative Z No Qualifier
2 Cardiac	Ø Open 3 Percutaneous 7 Via Natural or Artificial Opening 8 Via Natural or Artificial Opening Endoscopic	4 Electrical Activity 9 Output C Rate F Rhythm H Sound	Z No Qualifier
2 Cardiac	X External	4 Electrical Activity	5 Ambulatory Z No Qualifier
2 Cardiac	X External	9 Output C Rate F Rhythm H Sound	Z No Qualifier
2 Cardiac	X External	M Total Activity	4 Stress
2 Cardiac	X External	S Vascular Perfusion	H Indocyanine Green Dye
3 Arterial	Ø Open 3 Percutaneous	5 Flow B Pressure J Pulse	1 Peripheral 3 Pulmonary C Coronary
3 Arterial	Ø Open 3 Percutaneous	H Sound R Saturation	1 Peripheral
3 Arterial	X External	5 Flow B Pressure H Sound J Pulse R Saturation	1 Peripheral
4 Venous	Ø Open 3 Percutaneous	5 Flow B Pressure J Pulse	Ø Central 1 Peripheral 2 Portal 3 Pulmonary
4 Venous	Ø Open 3 Percutaneous	R Saturation	Ø Central 2 Portal 3 Pulmonary
4 Venous	X External	5 Flow B Pressure J Pulse	1 Peripheral
6 Lymphatic	Ø Open 3 Percutaneous 7 Via Natural or Artificial Opening 8 Via Natural or Artificial Opening Endoscopic	5 Flow	H Indocyanine Green Dye Z No Qualifier

Valid OR   4A1605Z

4A1 Continued on next page

NC Noncovered Procedure   LC Limited Coverage   QA Questionable OB Admit   NT New Tech Add-on   ⊞ Combination Member   ♂ Male   ♀ Female

ICD-10-PCS 2023   731

4   Measurement and Monitoring
A   Physiological Systems
1   Monitoring   Definition: Determining the level of a physiological or physical function repetitively over a period of time

4A1 Continued

Body System Character 4		Approach Character 5		Function/Device Character 6		Qualifier Character 7	
6	Lymphatic	Ø 3 7 8	Open Percutaneous Via Natural or Artificial Opening Via Natural or Artificial Opening Endoscopic	B	Pressure	Z	No Qualifier
9	Respiratory	7 X	Via Natural or Artificial Opening External	1 5 C D L	Capacity Flow Rate Resistance Volume	Z	No Qualifier
B	Gastrointestinal	7 8	Via Natural or Artificial Opening Via Natural or Artificial Opening Endoscopic	8 B G	Motility Pressure Secretion	Z	No Qualifier
B	Gastrointestinal	X	External	S	Vascular Perfusion	H	Indocyanine Green Dye
D	Urinary	7 8	Via Natural or Artificial Opening Via Natural or Artificial Opening Endoscopic	3 5 B D L	Contractility Flow Pressure Resistance Volume	Z	No Qualifier
G	Skin and Breast	X	External	S	Vascular Perfusion	H	Indocyanine Green Dye
H	Products of Conception, ♀ Cardiac	7 8 X	Via Natural or Artificial Opening Via Natural or Artificial Opening Endoscopic External	4 C F H	Electrical Activity Rate Rhythm Sound	Z	No Qualifier
J	Products of Conception, ♀ Nervous	7 8 X	Via Natural or Artificial Opening Via Natural or Artificial Opening Endoscopic External	2 4 B	Conductivity Electrical Activity Pressure	Z	No Qualifier
Z	None	7	Via Natural or Artificial Opening	K	Temperature	Z	No Qualifier
Z	None	X	External	K Q	Temperature Sleep	Z	No Qualifier

Valid OR   4A16ØBZ
♀   4A1H[7,8,X][4,C,F,H]Z
♀   4A1J[7,8,X][2,4,B]Z

4   Measurement and Monitoring
B   Physiological Devices
Ø   Measurement   Definition: Determining the level of a physiological or physical function at a point in time

Body System Character 4		Approach Character 5		Function/Device Character 6		Qualifier Character 7	
Ø	Central Nervous	X	External	V	Stimulator	Z	No Qualifier
Ø	Central Nervous	X	External	W	Cerebrospinal Fluid Shunt	Ø	Wireless Sensor
1 F	Peripheral Nervous Musculoskeletal	X	External	V	Stimulator	Z	No Qualifier
2	Cardiac	X	External	S T	Pacemaker Defibrillator	Z	No Qualifier
9	Respiratory	X	External	S	Pacemaker	Z	No Qualifier

Extracorporeal or Systemic Assistance and Performance 5A0–5A2

AHA Coding Clinic for table 5A0

2021, 2Q, 12	Repositioning of displaced intra-aortic balloon pump
2020, 4Q, 64-65	Ventilatory assistance by high flow or high velocity nasal cannula devices
2020, 1Q, 10	Intermittent use of continuous positive airway pressure
2018, 2Q, 3-5	Intra-aortic balloon pump
2017, 4Q, 43-44	Insertion of external heart assist devices
2017, 3Q, 18	Intra-aortic balloon pump removal
2017, 1Q, 10-11	External heart assist device
2017, 1Q, 29	Newborn resuscitation using positive pressure ventilation
2017, 1Q, 29	Newborn noninvasive ventilation
2016, 4Q, 137-139	Heart assist device systems
2014, 4Q, 9	Mechanical ventilation
2014, 3Q, 19	Ablation of ventricular tachycardia with Impella® support
2013, 3Q, 18	Heart transplant surgery

AHA Coding Clinic for table 5A1

2022, 2Q, 25	Temporary-permanent pacemaker placement
2021, 4Q, 56	Automated chest compression
2019, 4Q, 39-41	Intraoperative extracorporeal membrane oxygenation
2019, 3Q, 19	Insertion of left ventricular catheter
2019, 3Q, 20	Removal and revision of ECMO component
2019, 3Q, 21	Exchange of extracorporeal membrane oxygenation component (oxygenator)

AHA Coding Clinic for table 5A1 (Continued)

2019, 2Q, 36	Veno-arterial extracorporeal membrane oxygenation via sternotomy
2019, 3Q, 22	Extracorporeal membrane oxygenation and Centrimag™ pump
2019, 3Q, 22	Extracorporeal membrane oxygenation transfers
2018, 4Q, 52-54	Percutaneous extracorporeal membrane oxygenation
2018, 1Q, 13	Mechanical ventilation using patient's equipment
2017, 4Q, 71-73	Hemodialysis and renal replacement therapy
2017, 3Q, 7	Senning procedure (arterial switch)
2017, 1Q, 19	Norwood Sano procedure
2016, 1Q, 27	Aortocoronary bypass graft utilizing Y-graft
2016, 1Q, 28	Extracorporeal liver assist device
2016, 1Q, 29	Duration of hemodialysis
2015, 4Q, 22-24	Congenital heart corrective procedures
2014, 4Q, 3-10	Mechanical ventilation
2014, 4Q, 11-15	Sequencing of mechanical ventilation with other procedures
2014, 3Q, 16	Repair of Tetralogy of Fallot
2014, 3Q, 20	MAZE procedure performed with coronary artery bypass graft
2014, 1Q, 10	Repair of thoracic aortic aneurysm & coronary artery bypass graft
2013, 3Q, 18	Heart transplant surgery

AHA Coding Clinic for table 5A2

2022, 1Q, 46	Internal cardioversion

5   **Extracorporeal or Systemic Assistance and Performance**
A   **Physiological Systems**
Ø   **Assistance**   Definition: Taking over a portion of a physiological function by extracorporeal means

Body System Character 4	Duration Character 5	Function Character 6	Qualifier Character 7
2 Cardiac	1 Intermittent	1 Output	Ø Balloon Pump 5 Pulsatile Compression 6 Other Pump D Impeller Pump
2 Cardiac	2 Continuous	1 Output	Ø Balloon Pump 5 Pulsatile Compression 6 Other Pump D Impeller Pump
2 Cardiac	2 Continuous	2 Oxygenation	C Supersaturated
5 Circulatory	1 Intermittent 2 Continuous	2 Oxygenation	1 Hyperbaric
9 Respiratory	2 Continuous	Ø Filtration	Z No Qualifier
9 Respiratory	3 Less than 24 Consecutive Hours 4 24-96 Consecutive Hours 5 Greater than 96 Consecutive Hours	5 Ventilation	7 Continuous Positive Airway Pressure 8 Intermittent Positive Airway Pressure 9 Continuous Negative Airway Pressure A High Nasal Flow/Velocity B Intermittent Negative Airway Pressure Z No Qualifier

Valid OR	5A0211[Ø,6,D]
Valid OR	5A0221[Ø,6,D]

NC Noncovered Procedure   **LC** Limited Coverage   **QA** Questionable OB Admit   **NT** New Tech Add-on   **⊞** Combination Member   ♂ Male   ♀ Female

ICD-10-PCS 2023   **733**

5　Extracorporeal or Systemic Assistance and Performance
A　Physiological Systems
1　Performance　　Definition: Completely taking over a physiological function by extracorporeal means

Body System Character 4	Duration Character 5	Function Character 6	Qualifier Character 7
2　Cardiac	Ø　Single	1　Output	2　Manual
2　Cardiac	1　Intermittent	3　Pacing	Z　No Qualifier
2　Cardiac	2　Continuous	1　Output	J　Automated Z　No Qualifier
2　Cardiac	2　Continuous	3　Pacing	Z　No Qualifier
5　Circulatory	2　Continuous A　Intraoperative	2　Oxygenation	F　Membrane, Central G　Membrane, Peripheral Veno-arterial H　Membrane, Peripheral Veno-venous
9　Respiratory	Ø　Single	5　Ventilation	4　Nonmechanical
9　Respiratory	3　Less than 24 Consecutive Hours 4　24-96 Consecutive Hours 5　Greater than 96 Consecutive Hours	5　Ventilation	Z　No Qualifier
C　Biliary	Ø　Single 6　Multiple	Ø　Filtration	Z　No Qualifier
D　Urinary	7　Intermittent, Less than 6 Hours per day 8　Prolonged Intermittent, 6-18 Hours per day 9　Continuous, Greater than 18 Hours per day	Ø　Filtration	Z　No Qualifier

Valid OR　5A1522F
DRG Non-OR　5A1522[G,H]
DRG Non-OR　5A19[3,4]5Z
DRG Non-OR　5A1955Z Length of stay must be > 4 consecutive days.
DRG Non-OR　5A1D[7,8,9]ØZ

5　Extracorporeal or Systemic Assistance and Performance
A　Physiological Systems
2　Restoration　　Definition: Returning, or attempting to return, a physiological function to its original state by extracorporeal means

Body System Character 4	Duration Character 5	Function Character 6	Qualifier Character 7
2　Cardiac	Ø　Single	4　Rhythm	Z　No Qualifier

Extracorporeal or Systemic Therapies 6AØ–6AB

AHA Coding Clinic for table 6A4
2019, 2Q, 17   Cryoamputation of lower leg

AHA Coding Clinic for table 6A5
2022, 1Q, 48   Umbilical cord blood sampling

AHA Coding Clinic for table 6A7
2014, 4Q, 19   Ultrasound accelerated thrombolysis

AHA Coding Clinic for table 6AB
2016, 4Q, 115   Donor organ perfusion

6   **Extracorporeal or Systemic Therapies**
A   **Physiological Systems**
Ø   **Atmospheric Control**   Definition: Extracorporeal control of atmospheric pressure and composition

Body System Character 4	Duration Character 5	Qualifier Character 6	Qualifier Character 7
Z None	Ø Single 1 Multiple	Z No Qualifier	Z No Qualifier

6   **Extracorporeal or Systemic Therapies**
A   **Physiological Systems**
1   **Decompression**   Definition: Extracorporeal elimination of undissolved gas from body fluids

Body System Character 4	Duration Character 5	Qualifier Character 6	Qualifier Character 7
5 Circulatory	Ø Single 1 Multiple	Z No Qualifier	Z No Qualifier

6   **Extracorporeal or Systemic Therapies**
A   **Physiological Systems**
2   **Electromagnetic Therapy**   Definition: Extracorporeal treatment by electromagnetic rays

Body System Character 4	Duration Character 5	Qualifier Character 6	Qualifier Character 7
1 Urinary 2 Central Nervous	Ø Single 1 Multiple	Z No Qualifier	Z No Qualifier

6   **Extracorporeal or Systemic Therapies**
A   **Physiological Systems**
3   **Hyperthermia**   Definition: Extracorporeal raising of body temperature

Body System Character 4	Duration Character 5	Qualifier Character 6	Qualifier Character 7
Z None	Ø Single 1 Multiple	Z No Qualifier	Z No Qualifier

6   **Extracorporeal or Systemic Therapies**
A   **Physiological Systems**
4   **Hypothermia**   Definition: Extracorporeal lowering of body temperature

Body System Character 4	Duration Character 5	Qualifier Character 6	Qualifier Character 7
Z None	Ø Single 1 Multiple	Z No Qualifier	Z No Qualifier

6   **Extracorporeal or Systemic Therapies**
A   **Physiological Systems**
5   **Pheresis**   Definition: Extracorporeal separation of blood products

Body System Character 4	Duration Character 5	Qualifier Character 6	Qualifier Character 7
5 Circulatory	Ø Single 1 Multiple	Z No Qualifier	Ø Erythrocytes 1 Leukocytes 2 Platelets 3 Plasma T Stem Cells, Cord Blood V Stem Cells, Hematopoietic

NC Noncovered Procedure   **LC** Limited Coverage   **QA** Questionable OB Admit   **NT** New Tech Add-on   ⊞ Combination Member   ♂ Male   ♀ Female

ICD-10-PCS 2023   **735**

Extracorporeal or Systemic Therapies

6   **Extracorporeal or Systemic Therapies**
A   **Physiological Systems**
6   **Phototherapy**   Definition: Extracorporeal treatment by light rays

Body System Character 4	Duration Character 5	Qualifier Character 6	Qualifier Character 7
Ø Skin 5 Circulatory	Ø Single 1 Multiple	Z No Qualifier	Z No Qualifier

6   **Extracorporeal or Systemic Therapies**
A   **Physiological Systems**
7   **Ultrasound Therapy**   Definition: Extracorporeal treatment by ultrasound

Body System Character 4	Duration Character 5	Qualifier Character 6	Qualifier Character 7
5 Circulatory	Ø Single 1 Multiple	Z No Qualifier	4 Head and Neck Vessels 5 Heart 6 Peripheral Vessels 7 Other Vessels Z No Qualifier

6   **Extracorporeal or Systemic Therapies**
A   **Physiological Systems**
8   **Ultraviolet Light Therapy**   Definition: Extracorporeal treatment by ultraviolet light

Body System Character 4	Duration Character 5	Qualifier Character 6	Qualifier Character 7
Ø Skin	Ø Single 1 Multiple	Z No Qualifier	Z No Qualifier

6   **Extracorporeal or Systemic Therapies**
A   **Physiological Systems**
9   **Shock Wave Therapy**   Definition: Extracorporeal treatment by shock waves

Body System Character 4	Duration Character 5	Qualifier Character 6	Qualifier Character 7
3 Musculoskeletal	Ø Single 1 Multiple	Z No Qualifier	Z No Qualifier

6   **Extracorporeal or Systemic Therapies**
A   **Physiological Systems**
B   **Perfusion**   Definition: Extracorporeal treatment by diffusion of therapeutic fluid

Body System Character 4	Duration Character 5	Qualifier Character 6	Qualifier Character 7
5 Circulatory B Respiratory System F Hepatobiliary System and Pancreas T Urinary System	Ø Single	B Donor Organ	Z No Qualifier

Non-OR Procedure   DRG Non-OR Procedure   Valid OR Procedure   HAC Associated Procedure   Combination Only   New/Revised April   New/Revised October

736   ICD-10-PCS 2023

Osteopathic 7W0

7　Osteopathic
W　Anatomical Regions
0　Treatment　　Definition: Manual treatment to eliminate or alleviate somatic dysfunction and related disorders

Body Region Character 4	Approach Character 5	Method Character 6	Qualifier Character 7
0　Head	X　External	0　Articulatory-Raising	Z　None
1　Cervical		1　Fascial Release	
2　Thoracic		2　General Mobilization	
3　Lumbar		3　High Velocity-Low Amplitude	
4　Sacrum		4　Indirect	
5　Pelvis		5　Low Velocity-High Amplitude	
6　Lower Extremities		6　Lymphatic Pump	
7　Upper Extremities		7　Muscle Energy-Isometric	
8　Rib Cage		8　Muscle Energy-Isotonic	
9　Abdomen		9　Other Method	

NC Noncovered Procedure　　LC Limited Coverage　　QA Questionable OB Admit　　NT New Tech Add-on　　✚ Combination Member　　♂ Male　　♀ Female

ICD-10-PCS 2023　　　　　　　　　　　　　　　　　　　　　　　　　　　　　737

Other Procedures 8C0–8E0

AHA Coding Clinic for table 8E0

2021, 4Q, 49	Division of liver for staged hepatectomy
2021, 2Q, 19	Electromagnetic stealth guided ventriculoperitoneal shunt insertion with endoscopy
2020, 4Q, 53	Bypass pancreatic duct to stomach
2020, 4Q, 65-66	Near infrared spectroscopy for tissue viability assessment
2020, 4Q, 99	Robotic-assisted prostatectomy with extension of incision for specimen removal
2020, 4Q, 100	Robotic-assisted sigmoid colectomy with extension of incision for specimen removal
2019, 4Q, 41-42	Intraoperative fluorescence guidance
2019, 1Q, 30	Laparoscopic-assisted rectopexy with manual reduction of prolapse
2015, 1Q, 33	Robotic-assisted laparoscopic hysterectomy converted to open procedure
2014, 4Q, 33	Radical prostatectomy

8　Other Procedures
C　Indwelling Device
0　Other Procedures　Definition: Methodologies which attempt to remediate or cure a disorder or disease

Body Region Character 4	Approach Character 5	Method Character 6	Qualifier Character 7
1　Nervous System	X　External	6　Collection	J　Cerebrospinal Fluid L　Other Fluid
2　Circulatory System	X　External	6　Collection	K　Blood L　Other Fluid

8　Other Procedures
E　Physiological Systems and Anatomical Regions
0　Other Procedures　Definition: Methodologies which attempt to remediate or cure a disorder or disease

Body Region Character 4	Approach Character 5	Method Character 6	Qualifier Character 7
1　Nervous System U　Female Reproductive System　♀	X　External	Y　Other Method	7　Examination
2　Circulatory System	3　Percutaneous X　External	D　Near Infrared Spectroscopy	Z　No Qualifier
9　Head and Neck Region	0　Open	C　Robotic Assisted Procedure	Z　No Qualifier
9　Head and Neck Region	0　Open	E　Fluorescence Guided Procedure	M　Aminolevulinic Acid Z　No Qualifier
9　Head and Neck Region	3　Percutaneous 4　Percutaneous Endoscopic 7　Via Natural or Artificial Opening 8　Via Natural or Artificial Opening Endoscopic	C　Robotic Assisted Procedure E　Fluorescence Guided Procedure	Z　No Qualifier
9　Head and Neck Region	X　External	B　Computer Assisted Procedure	F　With Fluoroscopy G　With Computerized Tomography H　With Magnetic Resonance Imaging Z　No Qualifier
9　Head and Neck Region	X　External	C　Robotic Assisted Procedure	Z　No Qualifier
9　Head and Neck Region	X　External	Y　Other Method	8　Suture Removal
H　Integumentary System and Breast	3　Percutaneous	0　Acupuncture	0　Anesthesia Z　No Qualifier
H　Integumentary System and Breast　♀	X　External	6　Collection	2　Breast Milk
H　Integumentary System and Breast	X　External	Y　Other Method	9　Piercing
K　Musculoskeletal System	X　External	1　Therapeutic Massage	Z　No Qualifier
K　Musculoskeletal System	X　External	Y　Other Method	7　Examination
V　Male Reproductive System　♂	X　External	1　Therapeutic Massage	C　Prostate D　Rectum
V　Male Reproductive System　♂	X　External	6　Collection	3　Sperm
W　Trunk Region	0　Open 3　Percutaneous 4　Percutaneous Endoscopic 7　Via Natural or Artificial Opening 8　Via Natural or Artificial Opening Endoscopic	C　Robotic Assisted Procedure E　Fluorescence Guided Procedure	Z　No Qualifier
W　Trunk Region	X　External	B　Computer Assisted Procedure	F　With Fluoroscopy G　With Computerized Tomography H　With Magnetic Resonance Imaging Z　No Qualifier
W　Trunk Region	X　External	C　Robotic Assisted Procedure	Z　No Qualifier
W　Trunk Region	X　External	Y　Other Method	8　Suture Removal
X　Upper Extremity Y　Lower Extremity	0　Open 3　Percutaneous 4　Percutaneous Endoscopic	C　Robotic Assisted Procedure E　Fluorescence Guided Procedure	Z　No Qualifier

♂	8E0VX1C	♀	8E0UXY7
♂	8E0VX63	♀	8E0HX62

8E0 Continued on next page

NC Noncovered Procedure　**LC** Limited Coverage　**QA** Questionable OB Admit　**NT** New Tech Add-on　⊞ Combination Member　♂ Male　♀ Female

8   Other Procedures
E   Physiological Systems and Anatomical Regions
0   Other Procedures   Definition: Methodologies which attempt to remediate or cure a disorder or disease

Body Region Character 4	Approach Character 5	Method Character 6	Qualifier Character 7
X Upper Extremity Y Lower Extremity	X External	B Computer Assisted Procedure	F With Fluoroscopy G With Computerized Tomography H With Magnetic Resonance Imaging Z No Qualifier
X Upper Extremity Y Lower Extremity	X External	C Robotic Assisted Procedure	Z No Qualifier
X Upper Extremity Y Lower Extremity	X External	Y Other Method	8 Suture Removal
Z None	X External	Y Other Method	1 In Vitro Fertilization 4 Yoga Therapy 5 Meditation 6 Isolation

Chiropractic 9WB

9 **Chiropractic**
W **Anatomical Regions**
B **Manipulation** Definition: Manual procedure that involves a directed thrust to move a joint past the physiological range of motion, without exceeding the anatomical limit

Body Region Character 4	Approach Character 5	Method Character 6	Qualifier Character 7
Ø Head 1 Cervical 2 Thoracic 3 Lumbar 4 Sacrum 5 Pelvis 6 Lower Extremities 7 Upper Extremities 8 Rib Cage 9 Abdomen	X External	B Non-Manual C Indirect Visceral D Extra-Articular F Direct Visceral G Long Lever Specific Contact H Short Lever Specific Contact J Long and Short Lever Specific Contact K Mechanically Assisted L Other Method	Z None

Chiropractic 9WB

9   Chiropractic
W   Anatomical Regions
B   Manipulation: Manual procedure that involves a directed thrust to move a joint past the physiological range of motion, without exceeding the anatomical limit

Body Region Character 4	Approach Character 5	Method Character 6	Qualifier Character 7
0 Head	X External	B Non-Manual	Z None
1 Cervical		C Indirect Visceral	
2 Thoracic		D Extra-Articular	
3 Lumbar		F Direct Visceral	
4 Sacrum		G Long Lever Specific Contact	
5 Pelvis		H Short Lever Specific Contact	
6 Lower Extremities		J Long and Short Lever Specific	
7 Upper Extremities		Contact	
8 Rib Cage		K Mechanically Assisted	
9 Abdomen		L Other Method	

Imaging BØØ–BY4

AHA Coding Clinic for table B21

2018, 1Q, 12	Percutaneous balloon valvuloplasty & cardiac catheterization with ventriculogram
2016, 3Q, 36	Type of contrast medium for angiography (high osmolar, low osmolar, and other)

AHA Coding Clinic for table B41

2015, 3Q, 9	Aborted endovascular stenting of superficial femoral artery

AHA Coding Clinic for table B51

2015, 4Q, 30	Vascular access devices

AHA Coding Clinic for table BF1

2021, 4Q, 57	Fluoroscopic guidance of hepatobiliary sites

AHA Coding Clinic for table BF4

2014, 3Q, 15	Drainage of pancreatic pseudocyst
2020, 4Q, 66	Other imaging type

AHA Coding Clinic for table BF5

2020, 4Q, 66	Other imaging type
2020, 4Q, 66-67	Fluorescence imaging of hepatobiliary system

AHA Coding Clinic for table BW5

2020, 4Q, 66	Other imaging type
2020, 4Q, 68	Bacterial autofluorescence detection

Contrast Agents

High Osmolar (Ø)	Low Osmolar (1)	Other Contrast (Y)
cholografin meglumine	hexabrix	iodixanol
conray	iohexol	iotrolan
cysto-conray II	iomeprol	isovist
cystografin	iomeron	visipaque
cystografin-dilute	iopamidol	
diatrizoate	iopromide	
gastrografin	ioversol	
hypaque	ioxaglate	
iothalamate	ioxilan	
isopaque	isovue	
md-76r	omnipaque	
metrizoate	optiray	
reno-dip	oxilan	
sinografin	ultravist	

B   **Imaging**
Ø   **Central Nervous System**
Ø   **Plain Radiography**   Definition: Planar display of an image developed from the capture of external ionizing radiation on photographic or photoconductive plate

Body Part Character 4	Contrast Character 5	Qualifier Character 6	Qualifier Character 7
B Spinal Cord	**Ø** High Osmolar **1** Low Osmolar **Y** Other Contrast **Z** None	**Z** None	**Z** None

B   **Imaging**
Ø   **Central Nervous System**
1   **Fluoroscopy**   Definition: Single plane or bi-plane real time display of an image developed from the capture of external ionizing radiation on a fluorescent screen. The image may also be stored by either digital or analog means.

Body Part Character 4	Contrast Character 5	Qualifier Character 6	Qualifier Character 7
B Spinal Cord	**Ø** High Osmolar **1** Low Osmolar **Y** Other Contrast **Z** None	**Z** None	**Z** None

NC Noncovered Procedure   **LC** Limited Coverage   **QA** Questionable OB Admit   **NT** New Tech Add-on   ⊞ Combination Member   ♂ Male   ♀ Female

ICD-10-PCS 2023   **743**

B   **Imaging**
Ø   **Central Nervous System**
2   **Computerized Tomography (CT Scan)**   Definition: Computer reformatted digital display of multiplanar images developed from the capture of multiple exposures of external ionizing radiation

Body Part Character 4	Contrast Character 5	Qualifier Character 6	Qualifier Character 7
Ø Brain 7 Cisterna 8 Cerebral Ventricle(s) 9 Sella Turcica/Pituitary Gland B Spinal Cord	Ø High Osmolar 1 Low Osmolar Y Other Contrast	Ø Unenhanced and Enhanced Z None	Z None
Ø Brain 7 Cisterna 8 Cerebral Ventricle(s) 9 Sella Turcica/Pituitary Gland B Spinal Cord	Z None	Z None	Z None

B   **Imaging**
Ø   **Central Nervous System**
3   **Magnetic Resonance Imaging (MRI)**   Definition: Computer reformatted digital display of multiplanar images developed from the capture of radio-frequency signals emitted by nuclei in a body site excited within a magnetic field

Body Part Character 4	Contrast Character 5	Qualifier Character 6	Qualifier Character 7
Ø Brain 9 Sella Turcica/Pituitary Gland B Spinal Cord C Acoustic Nerves	Y Other Contrast	Ø Unenhanced and Enhanced Z None	Z None
Ø Brain 9 Sella Turcica/Pituitary Gland B Spinal Cord C Acoustic Nerves	Z None	Z None	Z None

B   **Imaging**
Ø   **Central Nervous System**
4   **Ultrasonography**   Definition: Real time display of images of anatomy or flow information developed from the capture of reflected and attenuated high frequency sound waves

Body Part Character 4	Contrast Character 5	Qualifier Character 6	Qualifier Character 7
Ø Brain B Spinal Cord	Z None	Z None	Z None

B   **Imaging**
2   **Heart**
Ø   **Plain Radiography**   Definition: Planar display of an image developed from the capture of external ionizing radiation on photographic or photoconductive plate

Body Part Character 4	Contrast Character 5	Qualifier Character 6	Qualifier Character 7
Ø Coronary Artery, Single 1 Coronary Arteries, Multiple 2 Coronary Artery Bypass Graft, Single 3 Coronary Artery Bypass Grafts, Multiple 4 Heart, Right 5 Heart, Left 6 Heart, Right and Left 7 Internal Mammary Bypass Graft, Right 8 Internal Mammary Bypass Graft, Left F Bypass Graft, Other	Ø High Osmolar 1 Low Osmolar Y Other Contrast	Z None	Z None

DRG Non-OR   All body part, contrast, and qualifier values

Non-OR Procedure   DRG Non-OR Procedure   Valid OR Procedure   HAC Associated Procedure   Combination Only   New/Revised April   New/Revised October

B   **Imaging**
2   **Heart**
1   **Fluoroscopy**   Definition: Single plane or bi-plane real time display of an image developed from the capture of external ionizing radiation on a fluorescent screen. The image may also be stored by either digital or analog means.

Body Part Character 4	Contrast Character 5	Qualifier Character 6	Qualifier Character 7
0 Coronary Artery, Single 1 Coronary Arteries, Multiple 2 Coronary Artery Bypass Graft, Single 3 Coronary Artery Bypass Grafts, Multiple	0 High Osmolar 1 Low Osmolar Y Other Contrast	1 Laser	0 Intraoperative
0 Coronary Artery, Single 1 Coronary Arteries, Multiple 2 Coronary Artery Bypass Graft, Single 3 Coronary Artery Bypass Grafts, Multiple	0 High Osmolar 1 Low Osmolar Y Other Contrast	Z None	Z None
4 Heart, Right 5 Heart, Left 6 Heart, Right and Left 7 Internal Mammary Bypass Graft, Right 8 Internal Mammary Bypass Graft, Left F Bypass Graft, Other	0 High Osmolar 1 Low Osmolar Y Other Contrast	Z None	Z None

DRG Non-OR   B21[0,1,2,3][0,1,Y]ZZ
DRG Non-OR   B21[4,5,6,7,8,F][0,1,Y]ZZ

B   **Imaging**
2   **Heart**
2   **Computerized Tomography (CT Scan)**   Definition: Computer reformatted digital display of multiplanar images developed from the capture of multiple exposures of external ionizing radiation

Body Part Character 4	Contrast Character 5	Qualifier Character 6	Qualifier Character 7
1 Coronary Arteries, Multiple 3 Coronary Artery Bypass Grafts, Multiple 6 Heart, Right and Left	0 High Osmolar 1 Low Osmolar Y Other Contrast	0 Unenhanced and Enhanced Z None	Z None
1 Coronary Arteries, Multiple 3 Coronary Artery Bypass Grafts, Multiple 6 Heart, Right and Left	Z None	2 Intravascular Optical Coherence Z None	Z None

B   **Imaging**
2   **Heart**
3   **Magnetic Resonance Imaging (MRI)**   Definition: Computer reformatted digital display of multiplanar images developed from the capture of radio-frequency signals emitted by nuclei in a body site excited within a magnetic field

Body Part Character 4	Contrast Character 5	Qualifier Character 6	Qualifier Character 7
1 Coronary Arteries, Multiple 3 Coronary Artery Bypass Grafts, Multiple 6 Heart, Right and Left	Y Other Contrast	0 Unenhanced and Enhanced Z None	Z None
1 Coronary Arteries, Multiple 3 Coronary Artery Bypass Grafts, Multiple 6 Heart, Right and Left	Z None	Z None	Z None

NC Noncovered Procedure   **LC** Limited Coverage   **QA** Questionable OB Admit   **NT** New Tech Add-on   ⊞ Combination Member   ♂ Male   ♀ Female

ICD-10-PCS 2023   **745**

B   Imaging
2   Heart
4   Ultrasonography   Definition: Real time display of images of anatomy or flow information developed from the capture of reflected and attenuated high frequency sound waves

Body Part Character 4	Contrast Character 5	Qualifier Character 6	Qualifier Character 7
Ø Coronary Artery, Single 1 Coronary Arteries, Multiple 4 Heart, Right 5 Heart, Left 6 Heart, Right and Left B Heart with Aorta C Pericardium D Pediatric Heart	Y Other Contrast	Z None	Z None
Ø Coronary Artery, Single 1 Coronary Arteries, Multiple 4 Heart, Right 5 Heart, Left 6 Heart, Right and Left B Heart with Aorta C Pericardium D Pediatric Heart	Z None	Z None	3 Intravascular 4 Transesophageal Z None

B   Imaging
3   Upper Arteries
Ø   Plain Radiography   Definition: Planar display of an image developed from the capture of external ionizing radiation on photographic or photoconductive plate

Body Part Character 4	Contrast Character 5	Qualifier Character 6	Qualifier Character 7
Ø Thoracic Aorta 1 Brachiocephalic-Subclavian Artery, Right 2 Subclavian Artery, Left 3 Common Carotid Artery, Right 4 Common Carotid Artery, Left 5 Common Carotid Arteries, Bilateral 6 Internal Carotid Artery, Right 7 Internal Carotid Artery, Left 8 Internal Carotid Arteries, Bilateral 9 External Carotid Artery, Right B External Carotid Artery, Left C External Carotid Arteries, Bilateral D Vertebral Artery, Right F Vertebral Artery, Left G Vertebral Arteries, Bilateral H Upper Extremity Arteries, Right J Upper Extremity Arteries, Left K Upper Extremity Arteries, Bilateral L Intercostal and Bronchial Arteries M Spinal Arteries N Upper Arteries, Other P Thoraco-Abdominal Aorta Q Cervico-Cerebral Arch R Intracranial Arteries S Pulmonary Artery, Right T Pulmonary Artery, Left	Ø High Osmolar 1 Low Osmolar Y Other Contrast Z None	Z None	Z None

B   Imaging
3   Upper Arteries
1   Fluoroscopy   Definition: Single plane or bi-plane real time display of an image developed from the capture of external ionizing radiation on a fluorescent screen. The image may also be stored by either digital or analog means.

Body Part Character 4	Contrast Character 5	Qualifier Character 6	Qualifier Character 7
Ø Thoracic Aorta 1 Brachiocephalic-Subclavian Artery, Right 2 Subclavian Artery, Left 3 Common Carotid Artery, Right 4 Common Carotid Artery, Left 5 Common Carotid Arteries, Bilateral 6 Internal Carotid Artery, Right 7 Internal Carotid Artery, Left 8 Internal Carotid Arteries, Bilateral 9 External Carotid Artery, Right B External Carotid Artery, Left C External Carotid Arteries, Bilateral D Vertebral Artery, Right F Vertebral Artery, Left G Vertebral Arteries, Bilateral H Upper Extremity Arteries, Right J Upper Extremity Arteries, Left K Upper Extremity Arteries, Bilateral L Intercostal and Bronchial Arteries M Spinal Arteries N Upper Arteries, Other P Thoraco-Abdominal Aorta Q Cervico-Cerebral Arch R Intracranial Arteries S Pulmonary Artery, Right T Pulmonary Artery, Left U Pulmonary Trunk	Ø High Osmolar 1 Low Osmolar Y Other Contrast	1 Laser	Ø Intraoperative
Ø Thoracic Aorta 1 Brachiocephalic-Subclavian Artery, Right 2 Subclavian Artery, Left 3 Common Carotid Artery, Right 4 Common Carotid Artery, Left 5 Common Carotid Arteries, Bilateral 6 Internal Carotid Artery, Right 7 Internal Carotid Artery, Left 8 Internal Carotid Arteries, Bilateral 9 External Carotid Artery, Right B External Carotid Artery, Left C External Carotid Arteries, Bilateral D Vertebral Artery, Right F Vertebral Artery, Left G Vertebral Arteries, Bilateral H Upper Extremity Arteries, Right J Upper Extremity Arteries, Left K Upper Extremity Arteries, Bilateral L Intercostal and Bronchial Arteries M Spinal Arteries N Upper Arteries, Other P Thoraco-Abdominal Aorta Q Cervico-Cerebral Arch R Intracranial Arteries S Pulmonary Artery, Right T Pulmonary Artery, Left U Pulmonary Trunk	Ø High Osmolar 1 Low Osmolar Y Other Contrast	Z None	Z None

B31 Continued on next page

NC Noncovered Procedure   **LC** Limited Coverage   **QA** Questionable OB Admit   **NT** New Tech Add-on   ⊞ Combination Member   ♂ Male   ♀ Female

ICD-10-PCS 2023   747

B   **Imaging**
3   **Upper Arteries**
1   **Fluoroscopy**   Definition: Single plane or bi-plane real time display of an image developed from the capture of external ionizing radiation on a fluorescent screen. The image may also be stored by either digital or analog means.

B31 Continued

Body Part Character 4	Contrast Character 5	Qualifier Character 6	Qualifier Character 7
Ø Thoracic Aorta	**Z** None	**Z** None	**Z** None
1 Brachiocephalic-Subclavian Artery, Right			
2 Subclavian Artery, Left			
3 Common Carotid Artery, Right			
4 Common Carotid Artery, Left			
5 Common Carotid Arteries, Bilateral			
6 Internal Carotid Artery, Right			
7 Internal Carotid Artery, Left			
8 Internal Carotid Arteries, Bilateral			
9 External Carotid Artery, Right			
B External Carotid Artery, Left			
C External Carotid Arteries, Bilateral			
D Vertebral Artery, Right			
F Vertebral Artery, Left			
G Vertebral Arteries, Bilateral			
H Upper Extremity Arteries, Right			
J Upper Extremity Arteries, Left			
K Upper Extremity Arteries, Bilateral			
L Intercostal and Bronchial Arteries			
M Spinal Arteries			
N Upper Arteries, Other			
P Thoraco-Abdominal Aorta			
Q Cervico-Cerebral Arch			
R Intracranial Arteries			
S Pulmonary Artery, Right			
T Pulmonary Artery, Left			
U Pulmonary Trunk			

B   **Imaging**
3   **Upper Arteries**
2   **Computerized Tomography (CT Scan)**   Definition: Computer reformatted digital display of multiplanar images developed from the capture of multiple exposures of external ionizing radiation

Body Part Character 4	Contrast Character 5	Qualifier Character 6	Qualifier Character 7
Ø Thoracic Aorta	**Ø** High Osmolar	**Z** None	**Z** None
5 Common Carotid Arteries, Bilateral	**1** Low Osmolar		
8 Internal Carotid Arteries, Bilateral	**Y** Other Contrast		
G Vertebral Arteries, Bilateral			
R Intracranial Arteries			
S Pulmonary Artery, Right			
T Pulmonary Artery, Left			
Ø Thoracic Aorta	**Z** None	**2** Intravascular Optical Coherence	**Z** None
5 Common Carotid Arteries, Bilateral		**Z** None	
8 Internal Carotid Arteries, Bilateral			
G Vertebral Arteries, Bilateral			
R Intracranial Arteries			
S Pulmonary Artery, Right			
T Pulmonary Artery, Left			

Non-OR Procedure   DRG Non-OR Procedure   Valid OR Procedure   HAC Associated Procedure   Combination Only   New/Revised April   New/Revised October

748   ICD-10-PCS 2023

B   **Imaging**
3   **Upper Arteries**
3   **Magnetic Resonance Imaging (MRI)**   Definition: Computer reformatted digital display of multiplanar images developed from the capture of radio-frequency signals emitted by nuclei in a body site excited within a magnetic field

Body Part Character 4	Contrast Character 5	Qualifier Character 6	Qualifier Character 7
Ø Thoracic Aorta 5 Common Carotid Arteries, Bilateral 8 Internal Carotid Arteries, Bilateral G Vertebral Arteries, Bilateral H Upper Extremity Arteries, Right J Upper Extremity Arteries, Left K Upper Extremity Arteries, Bilateral M Spinal Arteries Q Cervico-Cerebral Arch R Intracranial Arteries	Y Other Contrast	Ø Unenhanced and Enhanced Z None	Z None
Ø Thoracic Aorta 5 Common Carotid Arteries, Bilateral 8 Internal Carotid Arteries, Bilateral G Vertebral Arteries, Bilateral H Upper Extremity Arteries, Right J Upper Extremity Arteries, Left K Upper Extremity Arteries, Bilateral M Spinal Arteries Q Cervico-Cerebral Arch R Intracranial Arteries	Z None	Z None	Z None

B   **Imaging**
3   **Upper Arteries**
4   **Ultrasonography**   Definition: Real time display of images of anatomy or flow information developed from the capture of reflected and attenuated high frequency sound waves

Body Part Character 4	Contrast Character 5	Qualifier Character 6	Qualifier Character 7
Ø Thoracic Aorta 1 Brachiocephalic-Subclavian Artery, Right 2 Subclavian Artery, Left 3 Common Carotid Artery, Right 4 Common Carotid Artery, Left 5 Common Carotid Arteries, Bilateral 6 Internal Carotid Artery, Right 7 Internal Carotid Artery, Left 8 Internal Carotid Arteries, Bilateral H Upper Extremity Arteries, Right J Upper Extremity Arteries, Left K Upper Extremity Arteries, Bilateral R Intracranial Arteries S Pulmonary Artery, Right T Pulmonary Artery, Left V Ophthalmic Arteries	Z None	Z None	3 Intravascular Z None

B   **Imaging**
4   **Lower Arteries**
Ø   **Plain Radiography**   Definition: Planar display of an image developed from the capture of external ionizing radiation on photographic or photoconductive plate

Body Part Character 4	Contrast Character 5	Qualifier Character 6	Qualifier Character 7
Ø Abdominal Aorta 2 Hepatic Artery 3 Splenic Arteries 4 Superior Mesenteric Artery 5 Inferior Mesenteric Artery 6 Renal Artery, Right 7 Renal Artery, Left 8 Renal Arteries, Bilateral 9 Lumbar Arteries B Intra-Abdominal Arteries, Other C Pelvic Arteries D Aorta and Bilateral Lower Extremity Arteries F Lower Extremity Arteries, Right G Lower Extremity Arteries, Left J Lower Arteries, Other M Renal Artery Transplant	Ø High Osmolar 1 Low Osmolar Y Other Contrast	Z None	Z None

NC Noncovered Procedure   LC Limited Coverage   QA Questionable OB Admit   NT New Tech Add-on   ⊞ Combination Member   ♂Male   ♀Female

ICD-10-PCS 2023   749

B **Imaging**
4 **Lower Arteries**
1 **Fluoroscopy** Definition: Single plane or bi-plane real time display of an image developed from the capture of external ionizing radiation on a fluorescent screen. The image may also be stored by either digital or analog means.

Body Part Character 4	Contrast Character 5	Qualifier Character 6	Qualifier Character 7
0 Abdominal Aorta **2** Hepatic Artery **3** Splenic Arteries **4** Superior Mesenteric Artery **5** Inferior Mesenteric Artery **6** Renal Artery, Right **7** Renal Artery, Left **8** Renal Arteries, Bilateral **9** Lumbar Arteries **B** Intra-Abdominal Arteries, Other **C** Pelvic Arteries **D** Aorta and Bilateral Lower Extremity Arteries **F** Lower Extremity Arteries, Right **G** Lower Extremity Arteries, Left **J** Lower Arteries, Other	**0** High Osmolar **1** Low Osmolar **Y** Other Contrast	**1** Laser	**0** Intraoperative
0 Abdominal Aorta **2** Hepatic Artery **3** Splenic Arteries **4** Superior Mesenteric Artery **5** Inferior Mesenteric Artery **6** Renal Artery, Right **7** Renal Artery, Left **8** Renal Arteries, Bilateral **9** Lumbar Arteries **B** Intra-Abdominal Arteries, Other **C** Pelvic Arteries **D** Aorta and Bilateral Lower Extremity Arteries **F** Lower Extremity Arteries, Right **G** Lower Extremity Arteries, Left **J** Lower Arteries, Other	**0** High Osmolar **1** Low Osmolar **Y** Other Contrast	**Z** None	**Z** None
0 Abdominal Aorta **2** Hepatic Artery **3** Splenic Arteries **4** Superior Mesenteric Artery **5** Inferior Mesenteric Artery **6** Renal Artery, Right **7** Renal Artery, Left **8** Renal Arteries, Bilateral **9** Lumbar Arteries **B** Intra-Abdominal Arteries, Other **C** Pelvic Arteries **D** Aorta and Bilateral Lower Extremity Arteries **F** Lower Extremity Arteries, Right **G** Lower Extremity Arteries, Left **J** Lower Arteries, Other	**Z** None	**Z** None	**Z** None

B   **Imaging**
4   **Lower Arteries**
2   **Computerized Tomography (CT Scan)** Definition: Computer reformatted digital display of multiplanar images developed from the capture of multiple exposures of external ionizing radiation

Body Part Character 4	Contrast Character 5	Qualifier Character 6	Qualifier Character 7
Ø Abdominal Aorta 1 Celiac Artery 4 Superior Mesenteric Artery 8 Renal Arteries, Bilateral C Pelvic Arteries F Lower Extremity Arteries, Right G Lower Extremity Arteries, Left H Lower Extremity Arteries, Bilateral M Renal Artery Transplant	Ø High Osmolar 1 Low Osmolar Y Other Contrast	Z None	Z None
Ø Abdominal Aorta 1 Celiac Artery 4 Superior Mesenteric Artery 8 Renal Arteries, Bilateral C Pelvic Arteries F Lower Extremity Arteries, Right G Lower Extremity Arteries, Left H Lower Extremity Arteries, Bilateral M Renal Artery Transplant	Z None	2 Intravascular Optical Coherence Z None	Z None

B   **Imaging**
4   **Lower Arteries**
3   **Magnetic Resonance Imaging (MRI)** Definition: Computer reformatted digital display of multiplanar images developed from the capture of radio-frequency signals emitted by nuclei in a body site excited within a magnetic field

Body Part Character 4	Contrast Character 5	Qualifier Character 6	Qualifier Character 7
Ø Abdominal Aorta 1 Celiac Artery 4 Superior Mesenteric Artery 8 Renal Arteries, Bilateral C Pelvic Arteries F Lower Extremity Arteries, Right G Lower Extremity Arteries, Left H Lower Extremity Arteries, Bilateral	Y Other Contrast	Ø Unenhanced and Enhanced Z None	Z None
Ø Abdominal Aorta 1 Celiac Artery 4 Superior Mesenteric Artery 8 Renal Arteries, Bilateral C Pelvic Arteries F Lower Extremity Arteries, Right G Lower Extremity Arteries, Left H Lower Extremity Arteries, Bilateral	Z None	Z None	Z None

B   **Imaging**
4   **Lower Arteries**
4   **Ultrasonography** Definition: Real time display of images of anatomy or flow information developed from the capture of reflected and attenuated high frequency sound waves

Body Part Character 4	Contrast Character 5	Qualifier Character 6	Qualifier Character 7
Ø Abdominal Aorta 4 Superior Mesenteric Artery 5 Inferior Mesenteric Artery 6 Renal Artery, Right 7 Renal Artery, Left 8 Renal Arteries, Bilateral B Intra-Abdominal Arteries, Other F Lower Extremity Arteries, Right G Lower Extremity Arteries, Left H Lower Extremity Arteries, Bilateral K Celiac and Mesenteric Arteries L Femoral Artery N Penile Arteries	Z None	Z None	3 Intravascular Z None

NC Noncovered Procedure   **LC** Limited Coverage   **QA** Questionable OB Admit   **NT** New Tech Add-on   ⊞ Combination Member   ♂ Male   ♀ Female

ICD-10-PCS 2023   751

B   Imaging
5   Veins
0   Plain Radiography Definition: Planar display of an image developed from the capture of external ionizing radiation on photographic or photoconductive plate

Body Part Character 4	Contrast Character 5	Qualifier Character 6	Qualifier Character 7
0 Epidural Veins	0 High Osmolar	Z None	Z None
1 Cerebral and Cerebellar Veins	1 Low Osmolar		
2 Intracranial Sinuses	Y Other Contrast		
3 Jugular Veins, Right			
4 Jugular Veins, Left			
5 Jugular Veins, Bilateral			
6 Subclavian Vein, Right			
7 Subclavian Vein, Left			
8 Superior Vena Cava			
9 Inferior Vena Cava			
B Lower Extremity Veins, Right			
C Lower Extremity Veins, Left			
D Lower Extremity Veins, Bilateral			
F Pelvic (Iliac) Veins, Right			
G Pelvic (Iliac) Veins, Left			
H Pelvic (Iliac) Veins, Bilateral			
J Renal Vein, Right			
K Renal Vein, Left			
L Renal Veins, Bilateral			
M Upper Extremity Veins, Right			
N Upper Extremity Veins, Left			
P Upper Extremity Veins, Bilateral			
Q Pulmonary Vein, Right			
R Pulmonary Vein, Left			
S Pulmonary Veins, Bilateral			
T Portal and Splanchnic Veins			
V Veins, Other			
W Dialysis Shunt/Fistula			

B   Imaging
5   Veins
1   Fluoroscopy Definition: Single plane or bi-plane real time display of an image developed from the capture of external ionizing radiation on a fluorescent screen. The image may also be stored by either digital or analog means.

Body Part Character 4	Contrast Character 5	Qualifier Character 6	Qualifier Character 7
0 Epidural Veins	0 High Osmolar	Z None	A Guidance
1 Cerebral and Cerebellar Veins	1 Low Osmolar		Z None
2 Intracranial Sinuses	Y Other Contrast		
3 Jugular Veins, Right	Z None		
4 Jugular Veins, Left			
5 Jugular Veins, Bilateral			
6 Subclavian Vein, Right			
7 Subclavian Vein, Left			
8 Superior Vena Cava			
9 Inferior Vena Cava			
B Lower Extremity Veins, Right			
C Lower Extremity Veins, Left			
D Lower Extremity Veins, Bilateral			
F Pelvic (Iliac) Veins, Right			
G Pelvic (Iliac) Veins, Left			
H Pelvic (Iliac) Veins, Bilateral			
J Renal Vein, Right			
K Renal Vein, Left			
L Renal Veins, Bilateral			
M Upper Extremity Veins, Right			
N Upper Extremity Veins, Left			
P Upper Extremity Veins, Bilateral			
Q Pulmonary Vein, Right			
R Pulmonary Vein, Left			
S Pulmonary Veins, Bilateral			
T Portal and Splanchnic Veins			
V Veins, Other			
W Dialysis Shunt/Fistula			

Non-OR Procedure   DRG Non-OR Procedure   Valid OR Procedure   HAC Associated Procedure   Combination Only   New/Revised April   New/Revised October

752   ICD-10-PCS 2023

B50–B51

B Imaging
5 Veins
2 **Computerized Tomography (CT Scan)** Definition: Computer reformatted digital display of multiplanar images developed from the capture of multiple exposures of external ionizing radiation

Body Part Character 4	Contrast Character 5	Qualifier Character 6	Qualifier Character 7
2 Intracranial Sinuses 8 Superior Vena Cava 9 Inferior Vena Cava F Pelvic (Iliac) Veins, Right G Pelvic (Iliac) Veins, Left H Pelvic (Iliac) Veins, Bilateral J Renal Vein, Right K Renal Vein, Left L Renal Veins, Bilateral Q Pulmonary Vein, Right R Pulmonary Vein, Left S Pulmonary Veins, Bilateral T Portal and Splanchnic Veins	Ø High Osmolar 1 Low Osmolar Y Other Contrast	Ø Unenhanced and Enhanced Z None	Z None
2 Intracranial Sinuses 8 Superior Vena Cava 9 Inferior Vena Cava F Pelvic (Iliac) Veins, Right G Pelvic (Iliac) Veins, Left H Pelvic (Iliac) Veins, Bilateral J Renal Vein, Right K Renal Vein, Left L Renal Veins, Bilateral Q Pulmonary Vein, Right R Pulmonary Vein, Left S Pulmonary Veins, Bilateral T Portal and Splanchnic Veins	Z None	2 Intravascular Optical Coherence Z None	Z None

B Imaging
5 Veins
3 **Magnetic Resonance Imaging (MRI)** Definition: Computer reformatted digital display of multiplanar images developed from the capture of radio-frequency signals emitted by nuclei in a body site excited within a magnetic field

Body Part Character 4	Contrast Character 5	Qualifier Character 6	Qualifier Character 7
1 Cerebral and Cerebellar Veins 2 Intracranial Sinuses 5 Jugular Veins, Bilateral 8 Superior Vena Cava 9 Inferior Vena Cava B Lower Extremity Veins, Right C Lower Extremity Veins, Left D Lower Extremity Veins, Bilateral H Pelvic (Iliac) Veins, Bilateral L Renal Veins, Bilateral M Upper Extremity Veins, Right N Upper Extremity Veins, Left P Upper Extremity Veins, Bilateral S Pulmonary Veins, Bilateral T Portal and Splanchnic Veins V Veins, Other	Y Other Contrast	Ø Unenhanced and Enhanced Z None	Z None
1 Cerebral and Cerebellar Veins 2 Intracranial Sinuses 5 Jugular Veins, Bilateral 8 Superior Vena Cava 9 Inferior Vena Cava B Lower Extremity Veins, Right C Lower Extremity Veins, Left D Lower Extremity Veins, Bilateral H Pelvic (Iliac) Veins, Bilateral L Renal Veins, Bilateral M Upper Extremity Veins, Right N Upper Extremity Veins, Left P Upper Extremity Veins, Bilateral S Pulmonary Veins, Bilateral T Portal and Splanchnic Veins V Veins, Other	Z None	Z None	Z None

B   **Imaging**
5   **Veins**
4   **Ultrasonography**   Definition: Real time display of images of anatomy or flow information developed from the capture of reflected and attenuated high frequency sound waves

Body Part Character 4	Contrast Character 5	Qualifier Character 6	Qualifier Character 7
3 Jugular Veins, Right 4 Jugular Veins, Left 6 Subclavian Vein, Right 7 Subclavian Vein, Left 8 Superior Vena Cava 9 Inferior Vena Cava B Lower Extremity Veins, Right C Lower Extremity Veins, Left D Lower Extremity Veins, Bilateral J Renal Vein, Right K Renal Vein, Left L Renal Veins, Bilateral M Upper Extremity Veins, Right N Upper Extremity Veins, Left P Upper Extremity Veins, Bilateral T Portal and Splanchnic Veins	Z None	Z None	3 Intravascular A Guidance Z None

B   **Imaging**
7   **Lymphatic System**
Ø   **Plain Radiography**   Definition: Planar display of an image developed from the capture of external ionizing radiation on photographic or photoconductive plate

Body Part Character 4	Contrast Character 5	Qualifier Character 6	Qualifier Character 7

Ø Abdominal/Retroperitoneal
   Lymphatics, Unilateral
1 Abdominal/Retroperitoneal
   Lymphatics, Bilateral
4 Lymphatics, Head and Neck
5 Upper Extremity Lymphatics, Right
6 Upper Extremity Lymphatics, Left
7 Upper Extremity Lymphatics,
   Bilateral
8 Lower Extremity Lymphatics, Right
9 Lower Extremity Lymphatics, Left
B Lower Extremity Lymphatics,
   Bilateral
C Lymphatics, Pelvic
	Ø High Osmolar
	1 Low Osmolar
	Y Other Contrast
		Z None	Z None

B   **Imaging**
8   **Eye**
Ø   **Plain Radiography**   Definition: Planar display of an image developed from the capture of external ionizing radiation on photographic or photoconductive plate

Body Part Character 4	Contrast Character 5	Qualifier Character 6	Qualifier Character 7
Ø Lacrimal Duct, Right 1 Lacrimal Duct, Left 2 Lacrimal Ducts, Bilateral	Ø High Osmolar 1 Low Osmolar Y Other Contrast	Z None	Z None
3 Optic Foramina, Right 4 Optic Foramina, Left 5 Eye, Right 6 Eye, Left 7 Eyes, Bilateral	Z None	Z None	Z None

B   **Imaging**
8   **Eye**
2   **Computerized Tomography (CT Scan)**   Definition: Computer reformatted digital display of multiplanar images developed from the capture of multiple exposures of external ionizing radiation

Body Part Character 4	Contrast Character 5	Qualifier Character 6	Qualifier Character 7
5 Eye, Right 6 Eye, Left 7 Eyes, Bilateral	Ø High Osmolar 1 Low Osmolar Y Other Contrast	Ø Unenhanced and Enhanced Z None	Z None
5 Eye, Right 6 Eye, Left 7 Eyes, Bilateral	Z None	Z None	Z None

---

Non-OR Procedure   DRG Non-OR Procedure   Valid OR Procedure   HAC Associated Procedure   Combination Only   New/Revised April   New/Revised October

754   ICD-10-PCS 2023

B   **Imaging**
8   **Eye**
3   **Magnetic Resonance Imaging (MRI)**   Definition: Computer reformatted digital display of multiplanar images developed from the capture of radio-frequency signals emitted by nuclei in a body site excited within a magnetic field

Body Part Character 4	Contrast Character 5	Qualifier Character 6	Qualifier Character 7
5 Eye, Right 6 Eye, Left 7 Eyes, Bilateral	Y Other Contrast	Ø Unenhanced and Enhanced Z None	Z None
5 Eye, Right 6 Eye, Left 7 Eyes, Bilateral	Z None	Z None	Z None

B   **Imaging**
8   **Eye**
4   **Ultrasonography**   Definition: Real time display of images of anatomy or flow information developed from the capture of reflected and attenuated high frequency sound waves

Body Part Character 4	Contrast Character 5	Qualifier Character 6	Qualifier Character 7
5 Eye, Right 6 Eye, Left 7 Eyes, Bilateral	Z None	Z None	Z None

B   **Imaging**
9   **Ear, Nose, Mouth and Throat**
Ø   **Plain Radiography**   Definition: Planar display of an image developed from the capture of external ionizing radiation on photographic or photoconductive plate

Body Part Character 4	Contrast Character 5	Qualifier Character 6	Qualifier Character 7
2 Paranasal Sinuses F Nasopharynx/Oropharynx H Mastoids	Z None	Z None	Z None
4 Parotid Gland, Right 5 Parotid Gland, Left 6 Parotid Glands, Bilateral 7 Submandibular Gland, Right 8 Submandibular Gland, Left 9 Submandibular Glands, Bilateral B Salivary Gland, Right C Salivary Gland, Left D Salivary Glands, Bilateral	Ø High Osmolar 1 Low Osmolar Y Other Contrast	Z None	Z None

B   **Imaging**
9   **Ear, Nose, Mouth and Throat**
1   **Fluoroscopy**   Definition: Single plane or bi-plane real time display of an image developed from the capture of external ionizing radiation on a fluorescent screen. The image may also be stored by either digital or analog means.

Body Part Character 4	Contrast Character 5	Qualifier Character 6	Qualifier Character 7
G Pharynx and Epiglottis J Larynx	Y Other Contrast Z None	Z None	Z None

B   **Imaging**
9   **Ear, Nose, Mouth and Throat**
2   **Computerized Tomography (CT Scan)**   Definition: Computer reformatted digital display of multiplanar images developed from the capture of multiple exposures of external ionizing radiation

Body Part Character 4	Contrast Character 5	Qualifier Character 6	Qualifier Character 7
Ø Ear 2 Paranasal Sinuses 6 Parotid Glands, Bilateral 9 Submandibular Glands, Bilateral D Salivary Glands, Bilateral F Nasopharynx/Oropharynx J Larynx	Ø High Osmolar 1 Low Osmolar Y Other Contrast	Ø Unenhanced and Enhanced Z None	Z None
Ø Ear 2 Paranasal Sinuses 6 Parotid Glands, Bilateral 9 Submandibular Glands, Bilateral D Salivary Glands, Bilateral F Nasopharynx/Oropharynx J Larynx	Z None	Z None	Z None

---

NC Noncovered Procedure   **LC** Limited Coverage   **QA** Questionable OB Admit   **NT** New Tech Add-on   ⊞ Combination Member   ♂ Male   ♀ Female

ICD-10-PCS 2023   **755**

B   Imaging
9   Ear, Nose, Mouth and Throat
3   Magnetic Resonance Imaging (MRI)   Definition: Computer reformatted digital display of multiplanar images developed from the capture of radio-frequency signals emitted by nuclei in a body site excited within a magnetic field

Body Part Character 4	Contrast Character 5	Qualifier Character 6	Qualifier Character 7
Ø Ear 2 Paranasal Sinuses 6 Parotid Glands, Bilateral 9 Submandibular Glands, Bilateral D Salivary Glands, Bilateral F Nasopharynx/Oropharynx J Larynx	Y Other Contrast	Ø Unenhanced and Enhanced Z None	Z None
Ø Ear 2 Paranasal Sinuses 6 Parotid Glands, Bilateral 9 Submandibular Glands, Bilateral D Salivary Glands, Bilateral F Nasopharynx/Oropharynx J Larynx	Z None	Z None	Z None

B   Imaging
B   Respiratory System
Ø   Plain Radiography   Definition: Planar display of an image developed from the capture of external ionizing radiation on photographic or photoconductive plate

Body Part Character 4	Contrast Character 5	Qualifier Character 6	Qualifier Character 7
7 Tracheobronchial Tree, Right 8 Tracheobronchial Tree, Left 9 Tracheobronchial Trees, Bilateral	Y Other Contrast	Z None	Z None
D Upper Airways	Z None	Z None	Z None

B   Imaging
B   Respiratory System
1   Fluoroscopy   Definition: Single plane or bi-plane real time display of an image developed from the capture of external ionizing radiation on a fluorescent screen. The image may also be stored by either digital or analog means.

Body Part Character 4	Contrast Character 5	Qualifier Character 6	Qualifier Character 7
2 Lung, Right 3 Lung, Left 4 Lungs, Bilateral 6 Diaphragm C Mediastinum D Upper Airways	Z None	Z None	Z None
7 Tracheobronchial Tree, Right 8 Tracheobronchial Tree, Left 9 Tracheobronchial Trees, Bilateral	Y Other Contrast	Z None	Z None

B   Imaging
B   Respiratory System
2   Computerized Tomography (CT Scan)   Definition: Computer reformatted digital display of multiplanar images developed from the capture of multiple exposures of external ionizing radiation

Body Part Character 4	Contrast Character 5	Qualifier Character 6	Qualifier Character 7
4 Lungs, Bilateral 7 Tracheobronchial Tree, Right 8 Tracheobronchial Tree, Left 9 Tracheobronchial Trees, Bilateral F Trachea/Airways	Ø High Osmolar 1 Low Osmolar Y Other Contrast	Ø Unenhanced and Enhanced Z None	Z None
4 Lungs, Bilateral 7 Tracheobronchial Tree, Right 8 Tracheobronchial Tree, Left 9 Tracheobronchial Trees, Bilateral F Trachea/Airways	Z None	Z None	Z None

B   **Imaging**
B   **Respiratory System**
3   **Magnetic Resonance Imaging (MRI)**   Definition: Computer reformatted digital display of multiplanar images developed from the capture of radio-frequency signals emitted by nuclei in a body site excited within a magnetic field

Body Part Character 4	Contrast Character 5	Qualifier Character 6	Qualifier Character 7
4 Lungs, Bilateral	**Z** None	**3** Hyperpolarized Xenon 129 (Xe-129)	**Z** None
G Lung Apices	**Y** Other Contrast	**Ø** Unenhanced and Enhanced **Z** None	**Z** None
G Lung Apices	**Z** None	**Z** None	**Z** None

B   **Imaging**
B   **Respiratory System**
4   **Ultrasonography**   Definition: Real time display of images of anatomy or flow information developed from the capture of reflected and attenuated high frequency sound waves

Body Part Character 4	Contrast Character 5	Qualifier Character 6	Qualifier Character 7
B Pleura C Mediastinum	**Z** None	**Z** None	**Z** None

B   **Imaging**
D   **Gastrointestinal System**
1   **Fluoroscopy**   Definition: Single plane or bi-plane real time display of an image developed from the capture of external ionizing radiation on a fluorescent screen. The image may also be stored by either digital or analog means.

Body Part Character 4	Contrast Character 5	Qualifier Character 6	Qualifier Character 7
1 Esophagus 2 Stomach 3 Small Bowel 4 Colon 5 Upper GI 6 Upper GI and Small Bowel 9 Duodenum B Mouth/Oropharynx	**Y** Other Contrast **Z** None	**Z** None	**Z** None

B   **Imaging**
D   **Gastrointestinal System**
2   **Computerized Tomography (CT Scan)**   Definition: Computer reformatted digital display of multiplanar images developed from the capture of multiple exposures of external ionizing radiation

Body Part Character 4	Contrast Character 5	Qualifier Character 6	Qualifier Character 7
4 Colon	**Ø** High Osmolar **1** Low Osmolar **Y** Other Contrast	**Ø** Unenhanced and Enhanced **Z** None	**Z** None
4 Colon	**Z** None	**Z** None	**Z** None

B   **Imaging**
D   **Gastrointestinal System**
4   **Ultrasonography**   Definition: Real time display of images of anatomy or flow information developed from the capture of reflected and attenuated high frequency sound waves

Body Part Character 4	Contrast Character 5	Qualifier Character 6	Qualifier Character 7
1 Esophagus 2 Stomach 7 Gastrointestinal Tract 8 Appendix 9 Duodenum C Rectum	**Z** None	**Z** None	**Z** None

B   **Imaging**
F   **Hepatobiliary System and Pancreas**
Ø   **Plain Radiography**   Definition: Planar display of an image developed from the capture of external ionizing radiation on photographic or photoconductive plate

Body Part Character 4	Contrast Character 5	Qualifier Character 6	Qualifier Character 7
Ø Bile Ducts 3 Gallbladder and Bile Ducts C Hepatobiliary System, All	**Ø** High Osmolar **1** Low Osmolar **Y** Other Contrast	**Z** None	**Z** None

NC Noncovered Procedure   LC Limited Coverage   QA Questionable OB Admit   NT New Tech Add-on   ⊞ Combination Member   ♂ Male   ♀ Female

ICD-10-PCS 2023   757

B   **Imaging**
F   **Hepatobiliary System and Pancreas**
1   **Fluoroscopy**   Definition: Single plane or bi-plane real time display of an image developed from the capture of external ionizing radiation on a fluorescent screen. The image may also be stored by either digital or analog means.

Body Part Character 4	Contrast Character 5	Qualifier Character 6	Qualifier Character 7
0 Bile Ducts 1 Biliary and Pancreatic Ducts 2 Gallbladder 3 Gallbladder and Bile Ducts 4 Gallbladder, Bile Ducts and Pancreatic Ducts 8 Pancreatic Ducts	0 High Osmolar 1 Low Osmolar Y Other Contrast	Z None	Z None
5 Liver	0 High Osmolar 1 Low Osmolar Y Other Contrast	Z None	Z None
5 Liver	Z None	Z None	A Guidance

B   **Imaging**
F   **Hepatobiliary System and Pancreas**
2   **Computerized Tomography (CT Scan)**   Definition: Computer reformatted digital display of multiplanar images developed from the capture of multiple exposures of external ionizing radiation

Body Part Character 4	Contrast Character 5	Qualifier Character 6	Qualifier Character 7
5 Liver 6 Liver and Spleen 7 Pancreas C Hepatobiliary System, All	0 High Osmolar 1 Low Osmolar Y Other Contrast	0 Unenhanced and Enhanced Z None	Z None
5 Liver 6 Liver and Spleen 7 Pancreas C Hepatobiliary System, All	Z None	Z None	Z None

B   **Imaging**
F   **Hepatobiliary System and Pancreas**
3   **Magnetic Resonance Imaging (MRI)**   Definition: Computer reformatted digital display of multiplanar images developed from the capture of radio-frequency signals emitted by nuclei in a body site excited within a magnetic field

Body Part Character 4	Contrast Character 5	Qualifier Character 6	Qualifier Character 7
5 Liver 6 Liver and Spleen 7 Pancreas	Y Other Contrast	0 Unenhanced and Enhanced Z None	Z None
5 Liver 6 Liver and Spleen 7 Pancreas	Z None	Z None	Z None

B   **Imaging**
F   **Hepatobiliary System and Pancreas**
4   **Ultrasonography**   Definition: Real time display of images of anatomy or flow information developed from the capture of reflected and attenuated high frequency sound waves

Body Part Character 4	Contrast Character 5	Qualifier Character 6	Qualifier Character 7
0 Bile Ducts 2 Gallbladder 3 Gallbladder and Bile Ducts 5 Liver 6 Liver and Spleen 7 Pancreas C Hepatobiliary System, All	Z None	Z None	Z None

B   **Imaging**
F   **Hepatobiliary System and Pancreas**
5   **Other Imaging**   Definition: Other specified modality for visualizing a body part

Body Part Character 4	Contrast Character 5	Qualifier Character 6	Qualifier Character 7
0 Bile Ducts 2 Gallbladder 3 Gallbladder and Bile Ducts 5 Liver 6 Liver and Spleen 7 Pancreas C Hepatobiliary System, All	2 Fluorescing Agent	0 Indocyanine Green Dye Z None	0 Intraoperative Z None

Non-OR Procedure   DRG Non-OR Procedure   Valid OR Procedure   HAC Associated Procedure   Combination Only   New/Revised April   New/Revised October

758   ICD-10-PCS 2023

B   Imaging
G   Endocrine System
2   Computerized Tomography (CT Scan)   Definition: Computer reformatted digital display of multiplanar images developed from the capture of multiple exposures of external ionizing radiation

Body Part Character 4	Contrast Character 5	Qualifier Character 6	Qualifier Character 7
2 Adrenal Glands, Bilateral 3 Parathyroid Glands 4 Thyroid Gland	Ø High Osmolar 1 Low Osmolar Y Other Contrast	Ø Unenhanced and Enhanced Z None	Z None
2 Adrenal Glands, Bilateral 3 Parathyroid Glands 4 Thyroid Gland	Z None	Z None	Z None

B   Imaging
G   Endocrine System
3   Magnetic Resonance Imaging (MRI)   Definition: Computer reformatted digital display of multiplanar images developed from the capture of radio-frequency signals emitted by nuclei in a body site excited within a magnetic field

Body Part Character 4	Contrast Character 5	Qualifier Character 6	Qualifier Character 7
2 Adrenal Glands, Bilateral 3 Parathyroid Glands 4 Thyroid Gland	Y Other Contrast	Ø Unenhanced and Enhanced Z None	Z None
2 Adrenal Glands, Bilateral 3 Parathyroid Glands 4 Thyroid Gland	Z None	Z None	Z None

B   Imaging
G   Endocrine System
4   Ultrasonography   Definition: Real time display of images of anatomy or flow information developed from the capture of reflected and attenuated high frequency sound waves

Body Part Character 4	Contrast Character 5	Qualifier Character 6	Qualifier Character 7
Ø Adrenal Gland, Right 1 Adrenal Gland, Left 2 Adrenal Glands, Bilateral 3 Parathyroid Glands 4 Thyroid Gland	Z None	Z None	Z None

B   Imaging
H   Skin, Subcutaneous Tissue and Breast
Ø   Plain Radiography   Definition: Planar display of an image developed from the capture of external ionizing radiation on photographic or photoconductive plate

Body Part Character 4	Contrast Character 5	Qualifier Character 6	Qualifier Character 7
Ø Breast, Right 1 Breast, Left 2 Breasts, Bilateral	Z None	Z None	Z None
3 Single Mammary Duct, Right 4 Single Mammary Duct, Left 5 Multiple Mammary Ducts, Right 6 Multiple Mammary Ducts, Left	Ø High Osmolar 1 Low Osmolar Y Other Contrast Z None	Z None	Z None

NC Noncovered Procedure   **LC** Limited Coverage   **QA** Questionable OB Admit   **NT** New Tech Add-on   ⊞ Combination Member   ♂ Male   ♀ Female

ICD-10-PCS 2023   759

B   **Imaging**
H   **Skin, Subcutaneous Tissue and Breast**
3   **Magnetic Resonance Imaging (MRI)**   Definition: Computer reformatted digital display of multiplanar images developed from the capture of radio-frequency signals emitted by nuclei in a body site excited within a magnetic field

Body Part Character 4	Contrast Character 5	Qualifier Character 6	Qualifier Character 7
Ø Breast, Right 1 Breast, Left 2 Breasts, Bilateral D Subcutaneous Tissue, Head/Neck F Subcutaneous Tissue, Upper Extremity G Subcutaneous Tissue, Thorax H Subcutaneous Tissue, Abdomen and Pelvis J Subcutaneous Tissue, Lower Extremity	Y Other Contrast	Ø Unenhanced and Enhanced Z None	Z None
Ø Breast, Right 1 Breast, Left 2 Breasts, Bilateral D Subcutaneous Tissue, Head/Neck F Subcutaneous Tissue, Upper Extremity G Subcutaneous Tissue, Thorax H Subcutaneous Tissue, Abdomen and Pelvis J Subcutaneous Tissue, Lower Extremity	Z None	Z None	Z None

B   **Imaging**
H   **Skin, Subcutaneous Tissue and Breast**
4   **Ultrasonography**   Definition: Real time display of images of anatomy or flow information developed from the capture of reflected and attenuated high frequency sound waves

Body Part Character 4	Contrast Character 5	Qualifier Character 6	Qualifier Character 7
Ø Breast, Right 1 Breast, Left 2 Breasts, Bilateral 7 Extremity, Upper 8 Extremity, Lower 9 Abdominal Wall B Chest Wall C Head and Neck	Z None	Z None	Z None

B   **Imaging**
L   **Connective Tissue**
3   **Magnetic Resonance Imaging (MRI)**   Definition: Computer reformatted digital display of multiplanar images developed from the capture of radio-frequency signals emitted by nuclei in a body site excited within a magnetic field

Body Part Character 4	Contrast Character 5	Qualifier Character 6	Qualifier Character 7
Ø Connective Tissue, Upper Extremity 1 Connective Tissue, Lower Extremity 2 Tendons, Upper Extremity 3 Tendons, Lower Extremity	Y Other Contrast	Ø Unenhanced and Enhanced Z None	Z None
Ø Connective Tissue, Upper Extremity 1 Connective Tissue, Lower Extremity 2 Tendons, Upper Extremity 3 Tendons, Lower Extremity	Z None	Z None	Z None

B   **Imaging**
L   **Connective Tissue**
4   **Ultrasonography**   Definition: Real time display of images of anatomy or flow information developed from the capture of reflected and attenuated high frequency sound waves

Body Part Character 4	Contrast Character 5	Qualifier Character 6	Qualifier Character 7
Ø Connective Tissue, Upper Extremity 1 Connective Tissue, Lower Extremity 2 Tendons, Upper Extremity 3 Tendons, Lower Extremity	Z None	Z None	Z None

Non-OR Procedure   DRG Non-OR Procedure   Valid OR Procedure   HAC Associated Procedure   Combination Only   New/Revised April   New/Revised October

760   ICD-10-PCS 2023

B   **Imaging**
N   **Skull and Facial Bones**
Ø   **Plain Radiography**   Definition: Planar display of an image developed from the capture of external ionizing radiation on photographic or photoconductive plate

Body Part Character 4	Contrast Character 5	Qualifier Character 6	Qualifier Character 7
Ø Skull 1 Orbit, Right 2 Orbit, Left 3 Orbits, Bilateral 4 Nasal Bones 5 Facial Bones 6 Mandible B Zygomatic Arch, Right C Zygomatic Arch, Left D Zygomatic Arches, Bilateral G Tooth, Single H Teeth, Multiple J Teeth, All	Z None	Z None	Z None
7 Temporomandibular Joint, Right 8 Temporomandibular Joint, Left 9 Temporomandibular Joints, Bilateral	Ø High Osmolar 1 Low Osmolar Y Other Contrast Z None	Z None	Z None

B   **Imaging**
N   **Skull and Facial Bones**
1   **Fluoroscopy**   Definition: Single plane or bi-plane real time display of an image developed from the capture of external ionizing radiation on a fluorescent screen. The image may also be stored by either digital or analog means.

Body Part Character 4	Contrast Character 5	Qualifier Character 6	Qualifier Character 7
7 Temporomandibular Joint, Right 8 Temporomandibular Joint, Left 9 Temporomandibular Joints, Bilateral	Ø High Osmolar 1 Low Osmolar Y Other Contrast Z None	Z None	Z None

B   **Imaging**
N   **Skull and Facial Bones**
2   **Computerized Tomography (CT Scan)**   Definition: Computer reformatted digital display of multiplanar images developed from the capture of multiple exposures of external ionizing radiation

Body Part Character 4	Contrast Character 5	Qualifier Character 6	Qualifier Character 7
Ø Skull 3 Orbits, Bilateral 5 Facial Bones 6 Mandible 9 Temporomandibular Joints, Bilateral F Temporal Bones	Ø High Osmolar 1 Low Osmolar Y Other Contrast Z None	Z None	Z None

B   **Imaging**
N   **Skull and Facial Bones**
3   **Magnetic Resonance Imaging (MRI)**   Definition: Computer reformatted digital display of multiplanar images developed from the capture of radio-frequency signals emitted by nuclei in a body site excited within a magnetic field

Body Part Character 4	Contrast Character 5	Qualifier Character 6	Qualifier Character 7
9 Temporomandibular Joints, Bilateral	Y Other Contrast Z None	Z None	Z None

NC Noncovered Procedure   **LC** Limited Coverage   **QA** Questionable OB Admit   **NT** New Tech Add-on   ⊞ Combination Member   ♂ Male   ♀ Female

ICD-10-PCS 2023   761

B   **Imaging**
P   **Non-Axial Upper Bones**
0   **Plain Radiography**   Definition: Planar display of an image developed from the capture of external ionizing radiation on photographic or photoconductive plate

Body Part Character 4	Contrast Character 5	Qualifier Character 6	Qualifier Character 7
0 Sternoclavicular Joint, Right 1 Sternoclavicular Joint, Left 2 Sternoclavicular Joints, Bilateral 3 Acromioclavicular Joints, Bilateral 4 Clavicle, Right 5 Clavicle, Left 6 Scapula, Right 7 Scapula, Left A Humerus, Right B Humerus, Left E Upper Arm, Right F Upper Arm, Left J Forearm, Right K Forearm, Left N Hand, Right P Hand, Left R Finger(s), Right S Finger(s), Left X Ribs, Right Y Ribs, Left	Z None	Z None	Z None
8 Shoulder, Right 9 Shoulder, Left C Hand/Finger Joint, Right D Hand/Finger Joint, Left G Elbow, Right H Elbow, Left L Wrist, Right M Wrist, Left	0 High Osmolar 1 Low Osmolar Y Other Contrast Z None	Z None	Z None

B   **Imaging**
P   **Non-Axial Upper Bones**
1   **Fluoroscopy**   Definition: Single plane or bi-plane real time display of an image developed from the capture of external ionizing radiation on a fluorescent screen. The image may also be stored by either digital or analog means.

Body Part Character 4	Contrast Character 5	Qualifier Character 6	Qualifier Character 7
0 Sternoclavicular Joint, Right 1 Sternoclavicular Joint, Left 2 Sternoclavicular Joints, Bilateral 3 Acromioclavicular Joints, Bilateral 4 Clavicle, Right 5 Clavicle, Left 6 Scapula, Right 7 Scapula, Left A Humerus, Right B Humerus, Left E Upper Arm, Right F Upper Arm, Left J Forearm, Right K Forearm, Left N Hand, Right P Hand, Left R Finger(s), Right S Finger(s), Left X Ribs, Right Y Ribs, Left	Z None	Z None	Z None
8 Shoulder, Right 9 Shoulder, Left L Wrist, Right M Wrist, Left	0 High Osmolar 1 Low Osmolar Y Other Contrast Z None	Z None	Z None
C Hand/Finger Joint, Right D Hand/Finger Joint, Left G Elbow, Right H Elbow, Left	0 High Osmolar 1 Low Osmolar Y Other Contrast	Z None	Z None

Non-OR Procedure   DRG Non-OR Procedure   Valid OR Procedure   HAC Associated Procedure   Combination Only   New/Revised April   New/Revised October

762   ICD-10-PCS 2023

B　Imaging
P　Non-Axial Upper Bones
2　Computerized Tomography (CT Scan) Definition: Computer reformatted digital display of multiplanar images developed from the capture of multiple exposures of external ionizing radiation

Body Part Character 4	Contrast Character 5	Qualifier Character 6	Qualifier Character 7
0 Sternoclavicular Joint, Right **1** Sternoclavicular Joint, Left **W** Thorax	**0** High Osmolar **1** Low Osmolar **Y** Other Contrast	**Z** None	**Z** None
2 Sternoclavicular Joints, Bilateral **3** Acromioclavicular Joints, Bilateral **4** Clavicle, Right **5** Clavicle, Left **6** Scapula, Right **7** Scapula, Left **8** Shoulder, Right **9** Shoulder, Left **A** Humerus, Right **B** Humerus, Left **E** Upper Arm, Right **F** Upper Arm, Left **G** Elbow, Right **H** Elbow, Left **J** Forearm, Right **K** Forearm, Left **L** Wrist, Right **M** Wrist, Left **N** Hand, Right **P** Hand, Left **Q** Hands and Wrists, Bilateral **R** Finger(s), Right **S** Finger(s), Left **T** Upper Extremity, Right **U** Upper Extremity, Left **V** Upper Extremities, Bilateral **X** Ribs, Right **Y** Ribs, Left	**0** High Osmolar **1** Low Osmolar **Y** Other Contrast **Z** None	**Z** None	**Z** None
C Hand/Finger Joint, Right **D** Hand/Finger Joint, Left	**Z** None	**Z** None	**Z** None

B　Imaging
P　Non-Axial Upper Bones
3　Magnetic Resonance Imaging (MRI) Definition: Computer reformatted digital display of multiplanar images developed from the capture of radio-frequency signals emitted by nuclei in a body site excited within a magnetic field

Body Part Character 4	Contrast Character 5	Qualifier Character 6	Qualifier Character 7
8 Shoulder, Right **9** Shoulder, Left **C** Hand/Finger Joint, Right **D** Hand/Finger Joint, Left **E** Upper Arm, Right **F** Upper Arm, Left **G** Elbow, Right **H** Elbow, Left **J** Forearm, Right **K** Forearm, Left **L** Wrist, Right **M** Wrist, Left	**Y** Other Contrast	**0** Unenhanced and Enhanced **Z** None	**Z** None
8 Shoulder, Right **9** Shoulder, Left **C** Hand/Finger Joint, Right **D** Hand/Finger Joint, Left **E** Upper Arm, Right **F** Upper Arm, Left **G** Elbow, Right **H** Elbow, Left **J** Forearm, Right **K** Forearm, Left **L** Wrist, Right **M** Wrist, Left	**Z** None	**Z** None	**Z** None

NC Noncovered Procedure　　**LC** Limited Coverage　　**QA** Questionable OB Admit　　**NT** New Tech Add-on　　⊞ Combination Member　　♂ Male　　♀ Female

ICD-10-PCS 2023　　　　　　　　　　　　　　　　　　　　　　　　　　　　　763

B   **Imaging**
P   **Non-Axial Upper Bones**
4   **Ultrasonography**   Definition: Real time display of images of anatomy or flow information developed from the capture of reflected and attenuated high frequency sound waves

Body Part Character 4	Contrast Character 5	Qualifier Character 6	Qualifier Character 7
8 Shoulder, Right 9 Shoulder, Left G Elbow, Right H Elbow, Left L Wrist, Right M Wrist, Left N Hand, Right P Hand, Left	Z None	Z None	1 Densitometry Z None

B   **Imaging**
Q   **Non-Axial Lower Bones**
0   **Plain Radiography**   Definition: Planar display of an image developed from the capture of external ionizing radiation on photographic or photoconductive plate

Body Part Character 4	Contrast Character 5	Qualifier Character 6	Qualifier Character 7
0 Hip, Right 1 Hip, Left	0 High Osmolar 1 Low Osmolar Y Other Contrast	Z None	Z None
0 Hip, Right 1 Hip, Left	Z None	Z None	1 Densitometry Z None
3 Femur, Right 4 Femur, Left	Z None	Z None	1 Densitometry Z None
7 Knee, Right 8 Knee, Left G Ankle, Right H Ankle, Left	0 High Osmolar 1 Low Osmolar Y Other Contrast Z None	Z None	Z None
D Lower Leg, Right F Lower Leg, Left J Calcaneus, Right K Calcaneus, Left L Foot, Right M Foot, Left P Toe(s), Right Q Toe(s), Left V Patella, Right W Patella, Left	Z None	Z None	Z None
X Foot/Toe Joint, Right Y Foot/Toe Joint, Left	0 High Osmolar 1 Low Osmolar Y Other Contrast	Z None	Z None

B   **Imaging**
Q   **Non-Axial Lower Bones**
1   **Fluoroscopy**   Definition: Single plane or bi-plane real time display of an image developed from the capture of external ionizing radiation on a fluorescent screen. The image may also be stored by either digital or analog means.

Body Part Character 4	Contrast Character 5	Qualifier Character 6	Qualifier Character 7
0 Hip, Right 1 Hip, Left 7 Knee, Right 8 Knee, Left G Ankle, Right H Ankle, Left X Foot/Toe Joint, Right Y Foot/Toe Joint, Left	0 High Osmolar 1 Low Osmolar Y Other Contrast Z None	Z None	Z None
3 Femur, Right 4 Femur, Left D Lower Leg, Right F Lower Leg, Left J Calcaneus, Right K Calcaneus, Left L Foot, Right M Foot, Left P Toe(s), Right Q Toe(s), Left V Patella, Right W Patella, Left	Z None	Z None	Z None

Non-OR Procedure   DRG Non-OR Procedure   Valid OR Procedure   HAC Associated Procedure   Combination Only   New/Revised April   New/Revised October

764   ICD-10-PCS 2023

B   **Imaging**
Q   **Non-Axial Lower Bones**
2   **Computerized Tomography (CT Scan)** Definition: Computer reformatted digital display of multiplanar images developed from the capture of multiple exposures of external ionizing radiation

Body Part Character 4	Contrast Character 5	Qualifier Character 6	Qualifier Character 7
Ø Hip, Right 1 Hip, Left 3 Femur, Right 4 Femur, Left 7 Knee, Right 8 Knee, Left D Lower Leg, Right F Lower Leg, Left G Ankle, Right H Ankle, Left J Calcaneus, Right K Calcaneus, Left L Foot, Right M Foot, Left P Toe(s), Right Q Toe(s), Left R Lower Extremity, Right S Lower Extremity, Left V Patella, Right W Patella, Left X Foot/Toe Joint, Right Y Foot/Toe Joint, Left	Ø High Osmolar 1 Low Osmolar Y Other Contrast Z None	Z None	Z None
B Tibia/Fibula, Right C Tibia/Fibula, Left	Ø High Osmolar 1 Low Osmolar Y Other Contrast	Z None	Z None

B   **Imaging**
Q   **Non-Axial Lower Bones**
3   **Magnetic Resonance Imaging (MRI)** Definition: Computer reformatted digital display of multiplanar images developed from the capture of radio-frequency signals emitted by nuclei in a body site excited within a magnetic field

Body Part Character 4	Contrast Character 5	Qualifier Character 6	Qualifier Character 7
Ø Hip, Right 1 Hip, Left 3 Femur, Right 4 Femur, Left 7 Knee, Right 8 Knee, Left D Lower Leg, Right F Lower Leg, Left G Ankle, Right H Ankle, Left J Calcaneus, Right K Calcaneus, Left L Foot, Right M Foot, Left P Toe(s), Right Q Toe(s), Left V Patella, Right W Patella, Left	Y Other Contrast	Ø Unenhanced and Enhanced Z None	Z None
Ø Hip, Right 1 Hip, Left 3 Femur, Right 4 Femur, Left 7 Knee, Right 8 Knee, Left D Lower Leg, Right F Lower Leg, Left G Ankle, Right H Ankle, Left J Calcaneus, Right K Calcaneus, Left L Foot, Right M Foot, Left P Toe(s), Right Q Toe(s), Left V Patella, Right W Patella, Left	Z None	Z None	Z None

NC Noncovered Procedure   **LC** Limited Coverage   **OA** Questionable OB Admit   **NT** New Tech Add-on   ⊞ Combination Member   ♂ Male   ♀ Female

ICD-10-PCS 2023   765

B　Imaging
Q　Non-Axial Lower Bones
4　Ultrasonography　Definition: Real time display of images of anatomy or flow information developed from the capture of reflected and attenuated high frequency sound waves

Body Part Character 4	Contrast Character 5	Qualifier Character 6	Qualifier Character 7
Ø　Hip, Right 1　Hip, Left 2　Hips, Bilateral 7　Knee, Right 8　Knee, Left 9　Knees, Bilateral	Z　None	Z　None	Z　None

B　Imaging
R　Axial Skeleton, Except Skull and Facial Bones
Ø　Plain Radiography　Definition: Planar display of an image developed from the capture of external ionizing radiation on photographic or photoconductive plate

Body Part Character 4	Contrast Character 5	Qualifier Character 6	Qualifier Character 7
Ø　Cervical Spine 7　Thoracic Spine 9　Lumbar Spine G　Whole Spine	Z　None	Z　None	1　Densitometry Z　None
1　Cervical Disc(s) 2　Thoracic Disc(s) 3　Lumbar Disc(s) 4　Cervical Facet Joint(s) 5　Thoracic Facet Joint(s) 6　Lumbar Facet Joint(s) D　Sacroiliac Joints	Ø　High Osmolar 1　Low Osmolar Y　Other Contrast Z　None	Z　None	Z　None
8　Thoracolumbar Joint B　Lumbosacral Joint C　Pelvis F　Sacrum and Coccyx H　Sternum	Z　None	Z　None	Z　None

B　Imaging
R　Axial Skeleton, Except Skull and Facial Bones
1　Fluoroscopy　Definition: Single plane or bi-plane real time display of an image developed from the capture of external ionizing radiation on a fluorescent screen. The image may also be stored by either digital or analog means.

Body Part Character 4	Contrast Character 5	Qualifier Character 6	Qualifier Character 7
Ø　Cervical Spine 1　Cervical Disc(s) 2　Thoracic Disc(s) 3　Lumbar Disc(s) 4　Cervical Facet Joint(s) 5　Thoracic Facet Joint(s) 6　Lumbar Facet Joint(s) 7　Thoracic Spine 8　Thoracolumbar Joint 9　Lumbar Spine B　Lumbosacral Joint C　Pelvis D　Sacroiliac Joints F　Sacrum and Coccyx G　Whole Spine H　Sternum	Ø　High Osmolar 1　Low Osmolar Y　Other Contrast Z　None	Z　None	Z　None

B　Imaging
R　Axial Skeleton, Except Skull and Facial Bones
2　Computerized Tomography (CT Scan)　Definition: Computer reformatted digital display of multiplanar images developed from the capture of multiple exposures of external ionizing radiation

Body Part Character 4	Contrast Character 5	Qualifier Character 6	Qualifier Character 7
Ø　Cervical Spine 7　Thoracic Spine 9　Lumbar Spine C　Pelvis D　Sacroiliac Joints F　Sacrum and Coccyx	Ø　High Osmolar 1　Low Osmolar Y　Other Contrast Z　None	Z　None	Z　None

Non-OR Procedure　　DRG Non-OR Procedure　　Valid OR Procedure　　HAC Associated Procedure　　Combination Only　　New/Revised April　　New/Revised October

766

ICD-10-PCS 2023

B   Imaging
R   Axial Skeleton, Except Skull and Facial Bones
3   Magnetic Resonance Imaging (MRI)   Definition: Computer reformatted digital display of multiplanar images developed from the capture of radio-frequency
signals emitted by nuclei in a body site excited within a magnetic field

Body Part Character 4	Contrast Character 5	Qualifier Character 6	Qualifier Character 7
Ø Cervical Spine 1 Cervical Disc(s) 2 Thoracic Disc(s) 3 Lumbar Disc(s) 7 Thoracic Spine 9 Lumbar Spine C Pelvis F Sacrum and Coccyx	Y Other Contrast	Ø Unenhanced and Enhanced Z None	Z None
Ø Cervical Spine 1 Cervical Disc(s) 2 Thoracic Disc(s) 3 Lumbar Disc(s) 7 Thoracic Spine 9 Lumbar Spine C Pelvis F Sacrum and Coccyx	Z None	Z None	Z None

B   Imaging
R   Axial Skeleton, Except Skull and Facial Bones
4   Ultrasonography   Definition: Real time display of images of anatomy or flow information developed from the capture of reflected and attenuated high
frequency sound waves

Body Part Character 4	Contrast Character 5	Qualifier Character 6	Qualifier Character 7
Ø Cervical Spine 7 Thoracic Spine 9 Lumbar Spine F Sacrum and Coccyx	Z None	Z None	Z None

B   Imaging
T   Urinary System
Ø   Plain Radiography   Definition: Planar display of an image developed from the capture of external ionizing radiation on photographic or photoconductive plate

Body Part Character 4	Contrast Character 5	Qualifier Character 6	Qualifier Character 7
Ø Bladder 1 Kidney, Right 2 Kidney, Left 3 Kidneys, Bilateral 4 Kidneys, Ureters and Bladder 5 Urethra 6 Ureter, Right 7 Ureter, Left 8 Ureters, Bilateral B Bladder and Urethra C Ileal Diversion Loop	Ø High Osmolar 1 Low Osmolar Y Other Contrast Z None	Z None	Z None

B   Imaging
T   Urinary System
1   Fluoroscopy   Definition: Single plane or bi-plane real time display of an image developed from the capture of external ionizing radiation on a fluorescent
screen. The image may also be stored by either digital or analog means.

Body Part Character 4	Contrast Character 5	Qualifier Character 6	Qualifier Character 7
Ø Bladder 1 Kidney, Right 2 Kidney, Left 3 Kidneys, Bilateral 4 Kidneys, Ureters and Bladder 5 Urethra 6 Ureter, Right 7 Ureter, Left B Bladder and Urethra C Ileal Diversion Loop D Kidney, Ureter and Bladder, Right F Kidney, Ureter and Bladder, Left G Ileal Loop, Ureters and Kidneys	Ø High Osmolar 1 Low Osmolar Y Other Contrast Z None	Z None	Z None

NC Noncovered Procedure   **LC** Limited Coverage   **QA** Questionable OB Admit   **NT** New Tech Add-on   ⊞ Combination Member   ♂ Male   ♀ Female

ICD-10-PCS 2023   767

B   Imaging
T   Urinary System
2   Computerized Tomography (CT Scan) Definition: Computer reformatted digital display of multiplanar images developed from the capture of multiple exposures of external ionizing radiation

Body Part Character 4	Contrast Character 5	Qualifier Character 6	Qualifier Character 7
Ø Bladder 1 Kidney, Right 2 Kidney, Left 3 Kidneys, Bilateral 9 Kidney Transplant	Ø High Osmolar 1 Low Osmolar Y Other Contrast	Ø Unenhanced and Enhanced Z None	Z None
Ø Bladder 1 Kidney, Right 2 Kidney, Left 3 Kidneys, Bilateral 9 Kidney Transplant	Z None	Z None	Z None

B   Imaging
T   Urinary System
3   Magnetic Resonance Imaging (MRI) Definition: Computer reformatted digital display of multiplanar images developed from the capture of radio-frequency signals emitted by nuclei in a body site excited within a magnetic field

Body Part Character 4	Contrast Character 5	Qualifier Character 6	Qualifier Character 7
Ø Bladder 1 Kidney, Right 2 Kidney, Left 3 Kidneys, Bilateral 9 Kidney Transplant	Y Other Contrast	Ø Unenhanced and Enhanced Z None	Z None
Ø Bladder 1 Kidney, Right 2 Kidney, Left 3 Kidneys, Bilateral 9 Kidney Transplant	Z None	Z None	Z None

B   Imaging
T   Urinary System
4   Ultrasonography Definition: Real time display of images of anatomy or flow information developed from the capture of reflected and attenuated high frequency sound waves

Body Part Character 4	Contrast Character 5	Qualifier Character 6	Qualifier Character 7
Ø Bladder 1 Kidney, Right 2 Kidney, Left 3 Kidneys, Bilateral 5 Urethra 6 Ureter, Right 7 Ureter, Left 8 Ureters, Bilateral 9 Kidney Transplant J Kidneys and Bladder	Z None	Z None	Z None

B   Imaging
U   Female Reproductive System
Ø   Plain Radiography Definition: Planar display of an image developed from the capture of external ionizing radiation on photographic or photoconductive plate

Body Part Character 4	Contrast Character 5	Qualifier Character 6	Qualifier Character 7
Ø Fallopian Tube, Right ♀ 1 Fallopian Tube, Left ♀ 2 Fallopian Tubes, Bilateral ♀ 6 Uterus ♀ 8 Uterus and Fallopian Tubes ♀ 9 Vagina ♀	Ø High Osmolar 1 Low Osmolar Y Other Contrast	Z None	Z None
♀ All body part, contrast, and qualifier values			

B   **Imaging**
U   **Female Reproductive System**
1   **Fluoroscopy**   Definition: Single plane or bi-plane real time display of an image developed from the capture of external ionizing radiation on a fluorescent screen. The image may also be stored by either digital or analog means.

Body Part Character 4		Contrast Character 5	Qualifier Character 6	Qualifier Character 7
Ø Fallopian Tube, Right ♀	Ø High Osmolar ♀	Z None	Z None
1 Fallopian Tube, Left ♀	1 Low Osmolar ♀		
2 Fallopian Tubes, Bilateral ♀	Y Other Contrast ♀		
6 Uterus ♀	Z None ♀		
8 Uterus and Fallopian Tubes ♀			
9 Vagina ♀			

    ♀   All body part, contrast, and qualifier values

B   **Imaging**
U   **Female Reproductive System**
3   **Magnetic Resonance Imaging (MRI)**   Definition: Computer reformatted digital display of multiplanar images developed from the capture of radio-frequency signals emitted by nuclei in a body site excited within a magnetic field

Body Part Character 4		Contrast Character 5	Qualifier Character 6	Qualifier Character 7
3 Ovary, Right ♀	Y Other Contrast	Ø Unenhanced and Enhanced	Z None
4 Ovary, Left ♀		Z None	
5 Ovaries, Bilateral ♀			
6 Uterus ♀			
9 Vagina ♀			
B Pregnant Uterus ♀			
C Uterus and Ovaries ♀			
3 Ovary, Right ♀	Z None	Z None	Z None
4 Ovary, Left ♀			
5 Ovaries, Bilateral ♀			
6 Uterus ♀			
9 Vagina ♀			
B Pregnant Uterus ♀			
C Uterus and Ovaries ♀			

    ♀   All body part, contrast, and qualifier values

B   **Imaging**
U   **Female Reproductive System**
4   **Ultrasonography**   Definition: Real time display of images of anatomy or flow information developed from the capture of reflected and attenuated high frequency sound waves

Body Part Character 4		Contrast Character 5	Qualifier Character 6	Qualifier Character 7
Ø Fallopian Tube, Right ♀	Y Other Contrast	Z None	Z None
1 Fallopian Tube, Left ♀	Z None		
2 Fallopian Tubes, Bilateral ♀			
3 Ovary, Right ♀			
4 Ovary, Left ♀			
5 Ovaries, Bilateral ♀			
6 Uterus ♀			
C Uterus and Ovaries ♀			

    ♀   All body part, contrast, and qualifier values

B   **Imaging**
V   **Male Reproductive System**
Ø   **Plain Radiography**   Definition: Planar display of an image developed from the capture of external ionizing radiation on photographic or photoconductive plate

Body Part Character 4		Contrast Character 5	Qualifier Character 6	Qualifier Character 7
Ø Corpora Cavernosa ♂	Ø High Osmolar	Z None	Z None
1 Epididymis, Right ♂	1 Low Osmolar		
2 Epididymis, Left ♂	Y Other Contrast		
3 Prostate ♂			
5 Testicle, Right ♂			
6 Testicle, Left ♂			
8 Vasa Vasorum ♂			

    ♂   All body part, contrast, and qualifier values

NC Noncovered Procedure   **LC** Limited Coverage   **QA** Questionable OB Admit   **NT** New Tech Add-on   ⊞ Combination Member   ♂ Male   ♀ Female

ICD-10-PCS 2023   769

B Imaging
V Male Reproductive System
1 Fluoroscopy Definition: Single plane or bi-plane real time display of an image developed from the capture of external ionizing radiation on a fluorescent screen. The image may also be stored by either digital or analog means.

Body Part Character 4	Contrast Character 5	Qualifier Character 6	Qualifier Character 7
Ø Corpora Cavernosa ♂ 8 Vasa Vasorum ♂	Ø High Osmolar 1 Low Osmolar Y Other Contrast Z None	Z None	Z None

♂ All body part, contrast, and qualifier values

B Imaging
V Male Reproductive System
2 Computerized Tomography (CT Scan) Definition: Computer reformatted digital display of multiplanar images developed from the capture of multiple exposures of external ionizing radiation

Body Part Character 4	Contrast Character 5	Qualifier Character 6	Qualifier Character 7
3 Prostate ♂	Ø High Osmolar 1 Low Osmolar Y Other Contrast	Ø Unenhanced and Enhanced Z None	Z None
3 Prostate ♂	Z None	Z None	Z None

♂ BV23[Ø,Y][Ø,Z]Z   ♂ BV23ZZZ
♂ BV231ØZ

B Imaging
V Male Reproductive System
3 Magnetic Resonance Imaging (MRI) Definition: Computer reformatted digital display of multiplanar images developed from the capture of radio-frequency signals emitted by nuclei in a body site excited within a magnetic field

Body Part Character 4	Contrast Character 5	Qualifier Character 6	Qualifier Character 7
Ø Corpora Cavernosa ♂ 3 Prostate ♂ 4 Scrotum ♂ 5 Testicle, Right ♂ 6 Testicle, Left ♂ 7 Testicles, Bilateral ♂	Y Other Contrast	Ø Unenhanced and Enhanced Z None	Z None
Ø Corpora Cavernosa ♂ 3 Prostate ♂ 4 Scrotum ♂ 5 Testicle, Right ♂ 6 Testicle, Left ♂ 7 Testicles, Bilateral ♂	Z None	Z None	Z None

♂ All body part, contrast, and qualifier values

B Imaging
V Male Reproductive System
4 Ultrasonography Definition: Real time display of images of anatomy or flow information developed from the capture of reflected and attenuated high frequency sound waves

Body Part Character 4	Contrast Character 5	Qualifier Character 6	Qualifier Character 7
4 Scrotum ♂ 9 Prostate and Seminal Vesicles ♂ B Penis ♂	Z None	Z None	Z None

♂ All body part, contrast, and qualifier values

B Imaging
W Anatomical Regions
Ø Plain Radiography Definition: Planar display of an image developed from the capture of external ionizing radiation on photographic or photoconductive plate

Body Part Character 4	Contrast Character 5	Qualifier Character 6	Qualifier Character 7
Ø Abdomen 1 Abdomen and Pelvis 3 Chest B Long Bones, All C Lower Extremity J Upper Extremity K Whole Body L Whole Skeleton M Whole Body, Infant	Z None	Z None	Z None

Non-OR Procedure   DRG Non-OR Procedure   Valid OR Procedure   HAC Associated Procedure   Combination Only   New/Revised April   New/Revised October

B   **Imaging**
W   **Anatomical Regions**
1   **Fluoroscopy**   Definition: Single plane or bi-plane real time display of an image developed from the capture of external ionizing radiation on a fluorescent screen. The image may also be stored by either digital or analog means.

Body Part Character 4	Contrast Character 5	Qualifier Character 6	Qualifier Character 7
1 Abdomen and Pelvis	**Ø** High Osmolar	**Z** None	**Z** None
9 Head and Neck	**1** Low Osmolar		
C Lower Extremity	**Y** Other Contrast		
J Upper Extremity	**Z** None		

B   **Imaging**
W   **Anatomical Regions**
2   **Computerized Tomography (CT Scan)**   Definition: Computer reformatted digital display of multiplanar images developed from the capture of multiple exposures of external ionizing radiation

Body Part Character 4	Contrast Character 5	Qualifier Character 6	Qualifier Character 7
Ø Abdomen	**Ø** High Osmolar	**Ø** Unenhanced and Enhanced	**Z** None
1 Abdomen and Pelvis	**1** Low Osmolar	**Z** None	
4 Chest and Abdomen	**Y** Other Contrast		
5 Chest, Abdomen and Pelvis			
8 Head			
9 Head and Neck			
F Neck			
G Pelvic Region			
Ø Abdomen	**Z** None	**Z** None	**Z** None
1 Abdomen and Pelvis			
4 Chest and Abdomen			
5 Chest, Abdomen and Pelvis			
8 Head			
9 Head and Neck			
F Neck			
G Pelvic Region			

B   **Imaging**
W   **Anatomical Regions**
3   **Magnetic Resonance Imaging (MRI)**   Definition: Computer reformatted digital display of multiplanar images developed from the capture of radio-frequency signals emitted by nuclei in a body site excited within a magnetic field

Body Part Character 4	Contrast Character 5	Qualifier Character 6	Qualifier Character 7
Ø Abdomen	**Y** Other Contrast	**Ø** Unenhanced and Enhanced	**Z** None
8 Head		**Z** None	
F Neck			
G Pelvic Region			
H Retroperitoneum			
P Brachial Plexus			
Ø Abdomen	**Z** None	**Z** None	**Z** None
8 Head			
F Neck			
G Pelvic Region			
H Retroperitoneum			
P Brachial Plexus			
3 Chest	**Y** Other Contrast	**Ø** Unenhanced and Enhanced	**Z** None
		Z None	

B   **Imaging**
W   **Anatomical Regions**
4   **Ultrasonography**   Definition: Real time display of images of anatomy or flow information developed from the capture of reflected and attenuated high frequency sound waves

Body Part Character 4	Contrast Character 5	Qualifier Character 6	Qualifier Character 7
Ø Abdomen	**Z** None	**Z** None	**Z** None
1 Abdomen and Pelvis			
F Neck			
G Pelvic Region			

NC Noncovered Procedure   **LC** Limited Coverage   **QA** Questionable OB Admit   **NT** New Tech Add-on   ⊞ Combination Member   ♂ Male   ♀ Female

ICD-10-PCS 2023   771

B   **Imaging**
W   **Anatomical Regions**
5   **Other Imaging**   **Definition:** Other specified modality for visualizing a body part

Body Part Character 4	Contrast Character 5	Qualifier Character 6	Qualifier Character 7
2 Trunk **9** Head and Neck **C** Lower Extremity **J** Upper Extremity	**Z** None	**1** Bacterial Autofluorescence	**Z** None

B   **Imaging**
Y   **Fetus and Obstetrical**
3   **Magnetic Resonance Imaging (MRI)**   **Definition:** Computer reformatted digital display of multiplanar images developed from the capture of radio-frequency signals emitted by nuclei in a body site excited within a magnetic field

Body Part Character 4	Contrast Character 5	Qualifier Character 6	Qualifier Character 7
0 Fetal Head ♀ **1** Fetal Heart ♀ **2** Fetal Thorax ♀ **3** Fetal Abdomen ♀ **4** Fetal Spine ♀ **5** Fetal Extremities ♀ **6** Whole Fetus ♀	**Y** Other Contrast	**0** Unenhanced and Enhanced **Z** None	**Z** None
0 Fetal Head ♀ **1** Fetal Heart ♀ **2** Fetal Thorax ♀ **3** Fetal Abdomen ♀ **4** Fetal Spine ♀ **5** Fetal Extremities ♀ **6** Whole Fetus ♀	**Z** None	**Z** None	**Z** None

  ♀   BY3[0,1,2,3,5,6]Y[0,Z]Z
  ♀   BY34YZZ
  ♀   BY3[0,1,2,3,4,5,6]ZZZ

B   **Imaging**
Y   **Fetus and Obstetrical**
4   **Ultrasonography**   **Definition:** Real time display of images of anatomy or flow information developed from the capture of reflected and attenuated high frequency sound waves

Body Part Character 4	Contrast Character 5	Qualifier Character 6	Qualifier Character 7
7 Fetal Umbilical Cord ♀ **8** Placenta ♀ **9** First Trimester, Single Fetus ♀ **B** First Trimester, Multiple Gestation ♀ **C** Second Trimester, Single Fetus ♀ **D** Second Trimester, Multiple Gestation ♀ **F** Third Trimester, Single Fetus ♀ **G** Third Trimester, Multiple Gestation ♀	**Z** None	**Z** None	**Z** None

  ♀   All body part, contrast, and qualifier values

Non-OR Procedure   DRG Non-OR Procedure   Valid OR Procedure   HAC Associated Procedure   Combination Only   New/Revised April   New/Revised October

772   ICD-10-PCS 2023

Nuclear Medicine C01–CW7

C   **Nuclear Medicine**
0   **Central Nervous System**
1   **Planar Nuclear Medicine Imaging**   Definition: Introduction of radioactive materials into the body for single plane display of images developed from the capture of radioactive emissions

Body Part Character 4	Radionuclide Character 5	Qualifier Character 6	Qualifier Character 7
0 Brain	1 Technetium 99m (Tc-99m) Y Other Radionuclide	Z None	Z None
5 Cerebrospinal Fluid	D Indium 111 (In-111) Y Other Radionuclide	Z None	Z None
Y Central Nervous System	Y Other Radionuclide	Z None	Z None

C   **Nuclear Medicine**
0   **Central Nervous System**
2   **Tomographic (Tomo) Nuclear Medicine Imaging**   Definition: Introduction of radioactive materials into the body for three dimensional display of images developed from the capture of radioactive emissions

Body Part Character 4	Radionuclide Character 5	Qualifier Character 6	Qualifier Character 7
0 Brain	1 Technetium 99m (Tc-99m) F Iodine 123 (I-123) S Thallium 201 (Tl-201) Y Other Radionuclide	Z None	Z None
5 Cerebrospinal Fluid	D Indium 111 (In-111) Y Other Radionuclide	Z None	Z None
Y Central Nervous System	Y Other Radionuclide	Z None	Z None

C   **Nuclear Medicine**
0   **Central Nervous System**
3   **Positron Emission Tomographic (PET) Imaging**   Definition: Introduction of radioactive materials into the body for three dimensional display of images developed from the simultaneous capture, 180 degrees apart, of radioactive emissions

Body Part Character 4	Radionuclide Character 5	Qualifier Character 6	Qualifier Character 7
0 Brain	B Carbon 11 (C-11) K Fluorine 18 (F-18) M Oxygen 15 (O-15) Y Other Radionuclide	Z None	Z None
Y Central Nervous System	Y Other Radionuclide	Z None	Z None

C   **Nuclear Medicine**
0   **Central Nervous System**
5   **Nonimaging Nuclear Medicine Probe**   Definition: Introduction of radioactive materials into the body for the study of distribution and fate of certain substances by the detection of radioactive emissions; or, alternatively, measurement of absorption of radioactive emissions from an external source

Body Part Character 4	Radionuclide Character 5	Qualifier Character 6	Qualifier Character 7
0 Brain	V Xenon 133 (Xe-133) Y Other Radionuclide	Z None	Z None
Y Central Nervous System	Y Other Radionuclide	Z None	Z None

C   **Nuclear Medicine**
2   **Heart**
1   **Planar Nuclear Medicine Imaging**   Definition: Introduction of radioactive materials into the body for single plane display of images developed from the capture of radioactive emissions

Body Part Character 4	Radionuclide Character 5	Qualifier Character 6	Qualifier Character 7
6 Heart, Right and Left	1 Technetium 99m (Tc-99m) Y Other Radionuclide	Z None	Z None
G Myocardium	1 Technetium 99m (Tc-99m) D Indium 111 (In-111) S Thallium 201 (Tl-201) Y Other Radionuclide Z None	Z None	Z None
Y Heart	Y Other Radionuclide	Z None	Z None

NC Noncovered Procedure   **LC** Limited Coverage   **QA** Questionable OB Admit   **NT** New Tech Add-on   ⊞ Combination Member   ♂ Male   ♀ Female

ICD-10-PCS 2023   773

Nuclear Medicine *(left margin)*

C   Nuclear Medicine
2   Heart
2   Tomographic (Tomo) Nuclear Medicine Imaging   Definition: Introduction of radioactive materials into the body for three dimensional display of images developed from the capture of radioactive emissions

Body Part Character 4	Radionuclide Character 5	Qualifier Character 6	Qualifier Character 7
6 Heart, Right and Left	1 Technetium 99m (Tc-99m) Y Other Radionuclide	Z None	Z None
G Myocardium	1 Technetium 99m (Tc-99m) D Indium 111 (In-111) K Fluorine 18 (F-18) S Thallium 201 (Tl-201) Y Other Radionuclide Z None	Z None	Z None
Y Heart	Y Other Radionuclide	Z None	Z None

C   Nuclear Medicine
2   Heart
3   Positron Emission Tomographic (PET) Imaging   Definition: Introduction of radioactive materials into the body for three dimensional display of images developed from the simultaneous capture, 180 degrees apart, of radioactive emissions

Body Part Character 4	Radionuclide Character 5	Qualifier Character 6	Qualifier Character 7
G Myocardium	K Fluorine 18 (F-18) M Oxygen 15 (O-15) Q Rubidium 82 (Rb-82) R Nitrogen 13 (N-13) Y Other Radionuclide	Z None	Z None
Y Heart	Y Other Radionuclide	Z None	Z None

C   Nuclear Medicine
2   Heart
5   Nonimaging Nuclear Medicine Probe   Definition: Introduction of radioactive materials into the body for the study of distribution and fate of certain substances by the detection of radioactive emissions; or, alternatively, measurement of absorption of radioactive emissions from an external source

Body Part Character 4	Radionuclide Character 5	Qualifier Character 6	Qualifier Character 7
6 Heart, Right and Left	1 Technetium 99m (Tc-99m) Y Other Radionuclide	Z None	Z None
Y Heart	Y Other Radionuclide	Z None	Z None

C   Nuclear Medicine
5   Veins
1   Planar Nuclear Medicine Imaging   Definition: Introduction of radioactive materials into the body for single plane display of images developed from the capture of radioactive emissions

Body Part Character 4	Radionuclide Character 5	Qualifier Character 6	Qualifier Character 7
B Lower Extremity Veins, Right C Lower Extremity Veins, Left D Lower Extremity Veins, Bilateral N Upper Extremity Veins, Right P Upper Extremity Veins, Left Q Upper Extremity Veins, Bilateral R Central Veins	1 Technetium 99m (Tc-99m) Y Other Radionuclide	Z None	Z None
Y Veins	Y Other Radionuclide	Z None	Z None

Non-OR Procedure   DRG Non-OR Procedure   Valid OR Procedure   HAC Associated Procedure   Combination Only   New/Revised April   New/Revised October

774   ICD-10-PCS 2023

C22–C51 *(left margin)*

C   **Nuclear Medicine**
7   **Lymphatic and Hematologic System**
1   **Planar Nuclear Medicine Imaging**   Definition: Introduction of radioactive materials into the body for single plane display of images developed from the capture of radioactive emissions

Body Part Character 4	Radionuclide Character 5	Qualifier Character 6	Qualifier Character 7
Ø Bone Marrow	1 Technetium 99m (Tc-99m) D Indium 111 (In-111) Y Other Radionuclide	Z None	Z None
2 Spleen 5 Lymphatics, Head and Neck D Lymphatics, Pelvic J Lymphatics, Head K Lymphatics, Neck L Lymphatics, Upper Chest M Lymphatics, Trunk N Lymphatics, Upper Extremity P Lymphatics, Lower Extremity	1 Technetium 99m (Tc-99m) Y Other Radionuclide	Z None	Z None
3 Blood	D Indium 111 (In-111) Y Other Radionuclide	Z None	Z None
Y Lymphatic and Hematologic System	Y Other Radionuclide	Z None	Z None

C   **Nuclear Medicine**
7   **Lymphatic and Hematologic System**
2   **Tomographic (Tomo) Nuclear Medicine Imaging**   Definition: Introduction of radioactive materials into the body for three dimensional display of images developed from the capture of radioactive emissions

Body Part Character 4	Radionuclide Character 5	Qualifier Character 6	Qualifier Character 7
2 Spleen	1 Technetium 99m (Tc-99m) Y Other Radionuclide	Z None	Z None
Y Lymphatic and Hematologic System	Y Other Radionuclide	Z None	Z None

C   **Nuclear Medicine**
7   **Lymphatic and Hematologic System**
5   **Nonimaging Nuclear Medicine Probe**   Definition: Introduction of radioactive materials into the body for the study of distribution and fate of certain substances by the detection of radioactive emissions; or, alternatively, measurement of absorption of radioactive emissions from an external source

Body Part Character 4	Radionuclide Character 5	Qualifier Character 6	Qualifier Character 7
5 Lymphatics, Head and Neck D Lymphatics, Pelvic J Lymphatics, Head K Lymphatics, Neck L Lymphatics, Upper Chest M Lymphatics, Trunk N Lymphatics, Upper Extremity P Lymphatics, Lower Extremity	1 Technetium 99m (Tc-99m) Y Other Radionuclide	Z None	Z None
Y Lymphatic and Hematologic System	Y Other Radionuclide	Z None	Z None

C   **Nuclear Medicine**
7   **Lymphatic and Hematologic System**
6   **Nonimaging Nuclear Medicine Assay**   Definition: Introduction of radioactive materials into the body for the study of body fluids and blood elements, by the detection of radioactive emissions

Body Part Character 4	Radionuclide Character 5	Qualifier Character 6	Qualifier Character 7
3 Blood	1 Technetium 99m (Tc-99m) 7 Cobalt 58 (Co-58) C Cobalt 57 (Co-57) D Indium 111 (In-111) H Iodine 125 (I-125) W Chromium (Cr-51) Y Other Radionuclide	Z None	Z None
Y Lymphatic and Hematologic System	Y Other Radionuclide	Z None	Z None

NC Noncovered Procedure   LC Limited Coverage   QA Questionable OB Admit   NT New Tech Add-on   ⊞ Combination Member   ♂ Male   ♀ Female

ICD-10-PCS 2023   775

Nuclear Medicine

C   Nuclear Medicine
8   Eye
1   Planar Nuclear Medicine Imaging   Definition: Introduction of radioactive materials into the body for single plane display of images developed from the capture of radioactive emissions

Body Part Character 4	Radionuclide Character 5	Qualifier Character 6	Qualifier Character 7
9 Lacrimal Ducts, Bilateral	1 Technetium 99m (Tc-99m) Y Other Radionuclide	Z None	Z None
Y Eye	Y Other Radionuclide	Z None	Z None

C   Nuclear Medicine
9   Ear, Nose, Mouth and Throat
1   Planar Nuclear Medicine Imaging   Definition: Introduction of radioactive materials into the body for single plane display of images developed from the capture of radioactive emissions

Body Part Character 4	Radionuclide Character 5	Qualifier Character 6	Qualifier Character 7
B Salivary Glands, Bilateral	1 Technetium 99m (Tc-99m) Y Other Radionuclide	Z None	Z None
Y Ear, Nose, Mouth and Throat	Y Other Radionuclide	Z None	Z None

C   Nuclear Medicine
B   Respiratory System
1   Planar Nuclear Medicine Imaging   Definition: Introduction of radioactive materials into the body for single plane display of images developed from the capture of radioactive emissions

Body Part Character 4	Radionuclide Character 5	Qualifier Character 6	Qualifier Character 7
2 Lungs and Bronchi	1 Technetium 99m (Tc-99m) 9 Krypton (Kr-81m) T Xenon 127 (Xe-127) V Xenon 133 (Xe-133) Y Other Radionuclide	Z None	Z None
Y Respiratory System	Y Other Radionuclide	Z None	Z None

C   Nuclear Medicine
B   Respiratory System
2   Tomographic (Tomo) Nuclear Medicine Imaging   Definition: Introduction of radioactive materials into the body for three dimensional display of images developed from the capture of radioactive emissions

Body Part Character 4	Radionuclide Character 5	Qualifier Character 6	Qualifier Character 7
2 Lungs and Bronchi	1 Technetium 99m (Tc-99m) 9 Krypton (Kr-81m) Y Other Radionuclide	Z None	Z None
Y Respiratory System	Y Other Radionuclide	Z None	Z None

C   Nuclear Medicine
B   Respiratory System
3   Positron Emission Tomographic (PET) Imaging   Definition: Introduction of radioactive materials into the body for three dimensional display of images developed from the simultaneous capture, 180 degrees apart, of radioactive emissions

Body Part Character 4	Radionuclide Character 5	Qualifier Character 6	Qualifier Character 7
2 Lungs and Bronchi	K Fluorine 18 (F-18) Y Other Radionuclide	Z None	Z None
Y Respiratory System	Y Other Radionuclide	Z None	Z None

C   Nuclear Medicine
D   Gastrointestinal System
1   Planar Nuclear Medicine Imaging   Definition: Introduction of radioactive materials into the body for single plane display of images developed from the capture of radioactive emissions

Body Part Character 4	Radionuclide Character 5	Qualifier Character 6	Qualifier Character 7
5 Upper Gastrointestinal Tract 7 Gastrointestinal Tract	1 Technetium 99m (Tc-99m) D Indium 111 (In-111) Y Other Radionuclide	Z None	Z None
Y Digestive System	Y Other Radionuclide	Z None	Z None

Non-OR Procedure   DRG Non-OR Procedure   Valid OR Procedure   HAC Associated Procedure   Combination Only   New/Revised April   New/Revised October

776   ICD-10-PCS 2023

C   **Nuclear Medicine**
D   **Gastrointestinal System**
2   **Tomographic (Tomo) Nuclear Medicine Imaging**   Definition: Introduction of radioactive materials into the body for three dimensional display of images developed from the capture of radioactive emissions

Body Part Character 4	Radionuclide Character 5	Qualifier Character 6	Qualifier Character 7
7 Gastrointestinal Tract	**1** Technetium 99m (Tc-99m) **D** Indium 111 (In-111) **Y** Other Radionuclide	**Z** None	**Z** None
Y Digestive System	**Y** Other Radionuclide	**Z** None	**Z** None

C   **Nuclear Medicine**
F   **Hepatobiliary System and Pancreas**
1   **Planar Nuclear Medicine Imaging**   Definition: Introduction of radioactive materials into the body for single plane display of images developed from the capture of radioactive emissions

Body Part Character 4	Radionuclide Character 5	Qualifier Character 6	Qualifier Character 7
4 Gallbladder **5** Liver **6** Liver and Spleen **C** Hepatobiliary System, All	**1** Technetium 99m (Tc-99m) **Y** Other Radionuclide	**Z** None	**Z** None
Y Hepatobiliary System and Pancreas	**Y** Other Radionuclide	**Z** None	**Z** None

C   **Nuclear Medicine**
F   **Hepatobiliary System and Pancreas**
2   **Tomographic (Tomo) Nuclear Medicine Imaging**   Definition: Introduction of radioactive materials into the body for three dimensional display of images developed from the capture of radioactive emissions

Body Part Character 4	Radionuclide Character 5	Qualifier Character 6	Qualifier Character 7
4 Gallbladder **5** Liver **6** Liver and Spleen	**1** Technetium 99m (Tc-99m) **Y** Other Radionuclide	**Z** None	**Z** None
Y Hepatobiliary System and Pancreas	**Y** Other Radionuclide	**Z** None	**Z** None

C   **Nuclear Medicine**
G   **Endocrine System**
1   **Planar Nuclear Medicine Imaging**   Definition: Introduction of radioactive materials into the body for single plane display of images developed from the capture of radioactive emissions

Body Part Character 4	Radionuclide Character 5	Qualifier Character 6	Qualifier Character 7
1 Parathyroid Glands	**1** Technetium 99m (Tc-99m) **S** Thallium 201 (Tl-201) **Y** Other Radionuclide	**Z** None	**Z** None
2 Thyroid Gland	**1** Technetium 99m (Tc-99m) **F** Iodine 123 (I-123) **G** Iodine 131 (I-131) **Y** Other Radionuclide	**Z** None	**Z** None
4 Adrenal Glands, Bilateral	**G** Iodine 131 (I-131) **Y** Other Radionuclide	**Z** None	**Z** None
Y Endocrine System	**Y** Other Radionuclide	**Z** None	**Z** None

C   **Nuclear Medicine**
G   **Endocrine System**
2   **Tomographic (Tomo) Nuclear Medicine Imaging**   Definition: Introduction of radioactive materials into the body for three dimensional display of images developed from the capture of radioactive emissions

Body Part Character 4	Radionuclide Character 5	Qualifier Character 6	Qualifier Character 7
1 Parathyroid Glands	**1** Technetium 99m (Tc-99m) **S** Thallium 201 (Tl-201) **Y** Other Radionuclide	**Z** None	**Z** None
Y Endocrine System	**Y** Other Radionuclide	**Z** None	**Z** None

NC Noncovered Procedure   **LC** Limited Coverage   **QA** Questionable OB Admit   **NT** New Tech Add-on   ⊞ Combination Member   ♂ Male   ♀ Female

ICD-10-PCS 2023   777

C   **Nuclear Medicine**
G   **Endocrine System**
4   **Nonimaging Nuclear Medicine Uptake**   Definition: Introduction of radioactive materials into the body for measurements of organ function, from the detection of radioactive emissions

Body Part Character 4	Radionuclide Character 5	Qualifier Character 6	Qualifier Character 7
2 Thyroid Gland	1 Technetium 99m (Tc-99m) F Iodine 123 (I-123) G Iodine 131 (I-131) Y Other Radionuclide	Z None	Z None
Y Endocrine System	Y Other Radionuclide	Z None	Z None

C   **Nuclear Medicine**
H   **Skin, Subcutaneous Tissue and Breast**
1   **Planar Nuclear Medicine Imaging**   Definition: Introduction of radioactive materials into the body for single plane display of images developed from the capture of radioactive emissions

Body Part Character 4	Radionuclide Character 5	Qualifier Character 6	Qualifier Character 7
Ø Breast, Right 1 Breast, Left 2 Breasts, Bilateral	1 Technetium 99m (Tc-99m) S Thallium 201 (Tl-201) Y Other Radionuclide	Z None	Z None
Y Skin, Subcutaneous Tissue and Breast	Y Other Radionuclide	Z None	Z None

C   **Nuclear Medicine**
H   **Skin, Subcutaneous Tissue and Breast**
2   **Tomographic (Tomo) Nuclear Medicine Imaging**   Definition: Introduction of radioactive materials into the body for three dimensional display of images developed from the capture of radioactive emissions

Body Part Character 4	Radionuclide Character 5	Qualifier Character 6	Qualifier Character 7
Ø Breast, Right 1 Breast, Left 2 Breasts, Bilateral	1 Technetium 99m (Tc-99m) S Thallium 201 (Tl-201) Y Other Radionuclide	Z None	Z None
Y Skin, Subcutaneous Tissue and Breast	Y Other Radionuclide	Z None	Z None

C   **Nuclear Medicine**
P   **Musculoskeletal System**
1   **Planar Nuclear Medicine Imaging**   Definition: Introduction of radioactive materials into the body for single plane display of images developed from the capture of radioactive emissions

Body Part Character 4	Radionuclide Character 5	Qualifier Character 6	Qualifier Character 7
1 Skull 4 Thorax 5 Spine 6 Pelvis 7 Spine and Pelvis 8 Upper Extremity, Right 9 Upper Extremity, Left B Upper Extremities, Bilateral C Lower Extremity, Right D Lower Extremity, Left F Lower Extremities, Bilateral Z Musculoskeletal System, All	1 Technetium 99m (Tc-99m) Y Other Radionuclide	Z None	Z None
Y Musculoskeletal System, Other	Y Other Radionuclide	Z None	Z None

C Nuclear Medicine
P Musculoskeletal System
2 Tomographic (Tomo) Nuclear Medicine Imaging Definition: Introduction of radioactive materials into the body for three dimensional display of images developed from the capture of radioactive emissions

Body Part Character 4	Radionuclide Character 5	Qualifier Character 6	Qualifier Character 7
1 Skull 2 Cervical Spine 3 Skull and Cervical Spine 4 Thorax 6 Pelvis 7 Spine and Pelvis 8 Upper Extremity, Right 9 Upper Extremity, Left B Upper Extremities, Bilateral C Lower Extremity, Right D Lower Extremity, Left F Lower Extremities, Bilateral G Thoracic Spine H Lumbar Spine J Thoracolumbar Spine	1 Technetium 99m (Tc-99m) Y Other Radionuclide	Z None	Z None
Y Musculoskeletal System, Other	Y Other Radionuclide	Z None	Z None

C Nuclear Medicine
P Musculoskeletal System
5 Nonimaging Nuclear Medicine Probe Definition: Introduction of radioactive materials into the body for the study of distribution and fate of certain substances by the detection of radioactive emissions; or, alternatively, measurement of absorption of radioactive emissions from an external source

Body Part Character 4	Radionuclide Character 5	Qualifier Character 6	Qualifier Character 7
5 Spine N Upper Extremities P Lower Extremities	Z None	Z None	Z None
Y Musculoskeletal System, Other	Y Other Radionuclide	Z None	Z None

C Nuclear Medicine
T Urinary System
1 Planar Nuclear Medicine Imaging Definition: Introduction of radioactive materials into the body for single plane display of images developed from the capture of radioactive emissions

Body Part Character 4	Radionuclide Character 5	Qualifier Character 6	Qualifier Character 7
3 Kidneys, Ureters and Bladder	1 Technetium 99m (Tc-99m) F Iodine 123 (I-123) G Iodine 131 (I-131) Y Other Radionuclide	Z None	Z None
H Bladder and Ureters	1 Technetium 99m (Tc-99m) Y Other Radionuclide	Z None	Z None
Y Urinary System	Y Other Radionuclide	Z None	Z None

C Nuclear Medicine
T Urinary System
2 Tomographic (Tomo) Nuclear Medicine Imaging Definition: Introduction of radioactive materials into the body for three dimensional display of images developed from the capture of radioactive emissions

Body Part Character 4	Radionuclide Character 5	Qualifier Character 6	Qualifier Character 7
3 Kidneys, Ureters and Bladder	1 Technetium 99m (Tc-99m) Y Other Radionuclide	Z None	Z None
Y Urinary System	Y Other Radionuclide	Z None	Z None

C Nuclear Medicine
T Urinary System
6 Nonimaging Nuclear Medicine Assay Definition: Introduction of radioactive materials into the body for the study of body fluids and blood elements, by the detection of radioactive emissions

Body Part Character 4	Radionuclide Character 5	Qualifier Character 6	Qualifier Character 7
3 Kidneys, Ureters and Bladder	1 Technetium 99m (Tc-99m) F Iodine 123 (I-123) G Iodine 131 (I-131) H Iodine 125 (I-125) Y Other Radionuclide	Z None	Z None
Y Urinary System	Y Other Radionuclide	Z None	Z None

C   Nuclear Medicine
V   Male Reproductive System
1   Planar Nuclear Medicine Imaging   Definition: Introduction of radioactive materials into the body for single plane display of images developed from the capture of radioactive emissions

Body Part Character 4	Radionuclide Character 5	Qualifier Character 6	Qualifier Character 7
9 Testicles, Bilateral ♂	1 Technetium 99m (Tc-99m) Y Other Radionuclide	Z None	Z None
Y Male Reproductive System ♂	Y Other Radionuclide	Z None	Z None

♂   All body part, radionuclide, and qualifier values

C   Nuclear Medicine
W   Anatomical Regions
1   Planar Nuclear Medicine Imaging   Definition: Introduction of radioactive materials into the body for single plane display of images developed from the capture of radioactive emissions

Body Part Character 4	Radionuclide Character 5	Qualifier Character 6	Qualifier Character 7
Ø Abdomen 1 Abdomen and Pelvis 4 Chest and Abdomen 6 Chest and Neck B Head and Neck D Lower Extremity J Pelvic Region M Upper Extremity N Whole Body	1 Technetium 99m (Tc-99m) D Indium 111 (In-111) F Iodine 123 (I-123) G Iodine 131 (I-131) L Gallium 67 (Ga-67) S Thallium 201 (Tl-201) Y Other Radionuclide	Z None	Z None
3 Chest	1 Technetium 99m (Tc-99m) D Indium 111 (In-111) F Iodine 123 (I-123) G Iodine 131 (I-131) K Fluorine 18 (F-18) L Gallium 67 (Ga-67) S Thallium 201 (Tl-201) Y Other Radionuclide	Z None	Z None
Y Anatomical Regions, Multiple	Y Other Radionuclide	Z None	Z None
Z Anatomical Region, Other	Z None	Z None	Z None

C   Nuclear Medicine
W   Anatomical Regions
2   Tomographic (Tomo) Nuclear Medicine Imaging   Definition: Introduction of radioactive materials into the body for three dimensional display of images developed from the capture of radioactive emissions

Body Part Character 4	Radionuclide Character 5	Qualifier Character 6	Qualifier Character 7
Ø Abdomen 1 Abdomen and Pelvis 3 Chest 4 Chest and Abdomen 6 Chest and Neck B Head and Neck D Lower Extremity J Pelvic Region M Upper Extremity	1 Technetium 99m (Tc-99m) D Indium 111 (In-111) F Iodine 123 (I-123) G Iodine 131 (I-131) K Fluorine 18 (F-18) L Gallium 67 (Ga-67) S Thallium 201 (Tl-201) Y Other Radionuclide	Z None	Z None
Y Anatomical Regions, Multiple	Y Other Radionuclide	Z None	Z None

C   Nuclear Medicine
W   Anatomical Regions
3   Positron Emission Tomographic (PET) Imaging   Definition: Introduction of radioactive materials into the body for three dimensional display of images developed from the simultaneous capture, 180 degrees apart, of radioactive emissions

Body Part Character 4	Radionuclide Character 5	Qualifier Character 6	Qualifier Character 7
N Whole Body	Y Other Radionuclide	Z None	Z None

C   **Nuclear Medicine**
W   **Anatomical Regions**
5   **Nonimaging Nuclear Medicine Probe**   Definition: Introduction of radioactive materials into the body for the study of distribution and fate of certain substances by the detection of radioactive emissions; or, alternatively, measurement of absorption of radioactive emissions from an external source

Body Part Character 4	Radionuclide Character 5	Qualifier Character 6	Qualifier Character 7
Ø Abdomen 1 Abdomen and Pelvis 3 Chest 4 Chest and Abdomen 6 Chest and Neck B Head and Neck D Lower Extremity J Pelvic Region M Upper Extremity	1 Technetium 99m (Tc-99m) D Indium 111 (In-111) Y Other Radionuclide	Z None	Z None

C   **Nuclear Medicine**
W   **Anatomical Regions**
7   **Systemic Nuclear Medicine Therapy**   Definition: Introduction of unsealed radioactive materials into the body for treatment

Body Part Character 4	Radionuclide Character 5	Qualifier Character 6	Qualifier Character 7
Ø Abdomen 3 Chest	N Phosphorus 32 (P-32) Y Other Radionuclide	Z None	Z None
G Thyroid	G Iodine 131 (I-131) Y Other Radionuclide	Z None	Z None
N Whole Body	8 Samarium 153 (Sm-153) G Iodine 131 (I-131) N Phosphorus 32 (P-32) P Strontium 89 (Sr-89) Y Other Radionuclide	Z None	Z None
Y Anatomical Regions, Multiple	Y Other Radionuclide	Z None	Z None

NC Noncovered Procedure   **LC** Limited Coverage   **QA** Questionable OB Admit   **NT** New Tech Add-on   ⊞ Combination Member   ♂ Male   ♀ Female

ICD-10-PCS 2023   **781**

Radiation Therapy D00–DWY

AHA Coding Clinic for table D01

2020, 4Q, 43-44	Insertion of radioactive element
2020, 4Q, 69-70	Cesium 131 brachytherapy
2019, 4Q, 42-44	Unidirectional source brachytherapy

AHA Coding Clinic for table D0Y

2020, 4Q, 70	Intraoperative radiation therapy

AHA Coding Clinic for table D71

2020, 4Q, 43-44	Insertion of radioactive element
2020, 4Q, 69-70	Cesium 131 brachytherapy
2019, 4Q, 42-44	Unidirectional source brachytherapy

AHA Coding Clinic for table D81

2020, 4Q, 43-44	Insertion of radioactive element
2020, 4Q, 69-70	Cesium 131 brachytherapy
2019, 4Q, 42-44	Unidirectional source brachytherapy

AHA Coding Clinic for table D91

2020, 4Q, 43-44	Insertion of radioactive element
2020, 4Q, 69-70	Cesium 131 brachytherapy
2019, 4Q, 42-44	Unidirectional source brachytherapy

AHA Coding Clinic for table DB1

2020, 4Q, 43-44	Insertion of radioactive element
2020, 4Q, 69-70	Cesium 131 brachytherapy
2019, 4Q, 42-44	Unidirectional source brachytherapy

AHA Coding Clinic for table DD1

2020, 4Q, 43-44	Insertion of radioactive element
2020, 4Q, 69-70	Cesium 131 brachytherapy
2019, 4Q, 42-44	Unidirectional source brachytherapy

AHA Coding Clinic for table DF1

2022, 2Q, 26	Radioembolization of right hepatic lobe
2020, 4Q, 43-44	Insertion of radioactive element
2020, 4Q, 69-70	Cesium 131 brachytherapy
2019, 4Q, 42-44	Unidirectional source brachytherapy

AHA Coding Clinic for table DG1

2020, 4Q, 43-44	Insertion of radioactive element
2020, 4Q, 69-70	Cesium 131 brachytherapy
2019, 4Q, 42-44	Unidirectional source brachytherapy

AHA Coding Clinic for table DM1

2020, 4Q, 43-44	Insertion of radioactive element
2020, 4Q, 69-70	Cesium 131 brachytherapy
2019, 4Q, 42-44	Unidirectional source brachytherapy

AHA Coding Clinic for table DT1

2020, 4Q, 43-44	Insertion of radioactive element
2020, 4Q, 69-70	Cesium 131 brachytherapy
2019, 4Q, 42-44	Unidirectional source brachytherapy

AHA Coding Clinic for table DU1

2020, 4Q, 43-44	Insertion of radioactive element
2020, 4Q, 69-70	Cesium 131 brachytherapy
2019, 4Q, 42-44	Unidirectional source brachytherapy
2017, 4Q, 104	Intrauterine brachytherapy & placement of tandems & ovoids

AHA Coding Clinic for table DV1

2020, 4Q, 43-44	Insertion of radioactive element
2020, 4Q, 69-70	Cesium 131 brachytherapy
2019, 4Q, 42-44	Unidirectional source brachytherapy

AHA Coding Clinic for table DW1

2020, 4Q, 43-44	Insertion of radioactive element
2020, 4Q, 69-70	Cesium 131 brachytherapy
2019, 4Q, 42-44	Unidirectional source brachytherapy

AHA Coding Clinic for table DWY

2019, 4Q, 37	Hyperthermic antineoplastic chemotherapy

D   **Radiation Therapy**
0   **Central and Peripheral Nervous System**
0   **Beam Radiation**

Treatment Site Character 4	Modality Qualifier Character 5	Isotope Character 6	Qualifier Character 7
0 Brain 1 Brain Stem 6 Spinal Cord 7 Peripheral Nerve	0 Photons <1 MeV 1 Photons 1- 10 MeV 2 Photons >10 MeV 4 Heavy Particles (Protons, Ions) 5 Neutrons 6 Neutron Capture	Z None	Z None
0 Brain 1 Brain Stem 6 Spinal Cord 7 Peripheral Nerve	3 Electrons	Z None	0 Intraoperative Z None

D   **Radiation Therapy**
0   **Central and Peripheral Nervous System**
1   **Brachytherapy**

Treatment Site Character 4	Modality Qualifier Character 5	Isotope Character 6	Qualifier Character 7
0 Brain 1 Brain Stem 6 Spinal Cord 7 Peripheral Nerve	9 High Dose Rate (HDR)	7 Cesium 137 (Cs-137) 8 Iridium 192 (Ir-192) 9 Iodine 125 (I-125) B Palladium 103 (Pd-103) C Californium 252 (Cf-252) Y Other Isotope	Z None
0 Brain 1 Brain Stem 6 Spinal Cord 7 Peripheral Nerve	B Low Dose Rate (LDR)	6 Cesium 131 (Cs-131) 7 Cesium 137 (Cs-137) 8 Iridium 192 (Ir-192) 9 Iodine 125 (I-125) C Californium 252 (Cf-252) Y Other Isotope	Z None
0 Brain 1 Brain Stem 6 Spinal Cord 7 Peripheral Nerve	B Low Dose Rate (LDR)	B Palladium 103 (Pd-103)	1 Unidirectional Source Z None

NC Noncovered Procedure   LC Limited Coverage   QA Questionable OB Admit   NT New Tech Add-on   ⊞ Combination Member   ♂ Male   ♀ Female

ICD-10-PCS 2023   783

Radiation Therapy

D   Radiation Therapy
Ø   Central and Peripheral Nervous System
2   Stereotactic Radiosurgery

Treatment Site Character 4	Modality Qualifier Character 5	Isotope Character 6	Qualifier Character 7

Ø   Brain
1   Brain Stem
6   Spinal Cord
7   Peripheral Nerve
	D Stereotactic Other Photon
	     Radiosurgery
	H Stereotactic Particulate
	     Radiosurgery
	J Stereotactic Gamma Beam
	     Radiosurgery
		Z None	Z None

DRG Non-OR   All treatment site, modality, isotope, and qualifier values

D   Radiation Therapy
Ø   Central and Peripheral Nervous System
Y   Other Radiation

Treatment Site Character 4	Modality Qualifier Character 5	Isotope Character 6	Qualifier Character 7
Ø Brain 1 Brain Stem 6 Spinal Cord 7 Peripheral Nerve	7 Contact Radiation 8 Hyperthermia C Intraoperative Radiation Therapy (IORT) F Plaque Radiation	Z None	Z None

D   Radiation Therapy
7   Lymphatic and Hematologic System
Ø   Beam Radiation

Treatment Site Character 4	Modality Qualifier Character 5	Isotope Character 6	Qualifier Character 7
Ø Bone Marrow 1 Thymus 2 Spleen 3 Lymphatics, Neck 4 Lymphatics, Axillary 5 Lymphatics, Thorax 6 Lymphatics, Abdomen 7 Lymphatics, Pelvis 8 Lymphatics, Inguinal	Ø Photons <1 MeV 1 Photons 1- 10 MeV 2 Photons >10 MeV 4 Heavy Particles (Protons, Ions) 5 Neutrons 6 Neutron Capture	Z None	Z None
Ø Bone Marrow 1 Thymus 2 Spleen 3 Lymphatics, Neck 4 Lymphatics, Axillary 5 Lymphatics, Thorax 6 Lymphatics, Abdomen 7 Lymphatics, Pelvis 8 Lymphatics, Inguinal	3 Electrons	Z None	Ø Intraoperative Z None

D   **Radiation Therapy**
7   **Lymphatic and Hematologic System**
1   **Brachytherapy**

Treatment Site Character 4	Modality Qualifier Character 5	Isotope Character 6	Qualifier Character 7
Ø Bone Marrow 1 Thymus 2 Spleen 3 Lymphatics, Neck 4 Lymphatics, Axillary 5 Lymphatics, Thorax 6 Lymphatics, Abdomen 7 Lymphatics, Pelvis 8 Lymphatics, Inguinal	9 High Dose Rate (HDR)	7 Cesium 137 (Cs-137) 8 Iridium 192 (Ir-192) 9 Iodine 125 (I-125) B Palladium 103 (Pd-103) C Californium 252 (Cf-252) Y Other Isotope	Z None
Ø Bone Marrow 1 Thymus 2 Spleen 3 Lymphatics, Neck 4 Lymphatics, Axillary 5 Lymphatics, Thorax 6 Lymphatics, Abdomen 7 Lymphatics, Pelvis 8 Lymphatics, Inguinal	B Low Dose Rate (LDR)	6 Cesium 131 (Cs-131) 7 Cesium 137 (Cs-137) 8 Iridium 192 (Ir-192) 9 Iodine 125 (I-125) C Californium 252 (Cf-252) Y Other Isotope	Z None
Ø Bone Marrow 1 Thymus 2 Spleen 3 Lymphatics, Neck 4 Lymphatics, Axillary 5 Lymphatics, Thorax 6 Lymphatics, Abdomen 7 Lymphatics, Pelvis 8 Lymphatics, Inguinal	B Low Dose Rate (LDR)	B Palladium 103 (Pd-103)	1 Unidirectional Source Z None

D   **Radiation Therapy**
7   **Lymphatic and Hematologic System**
2   **Stereotactic Radiosurgery**

Treatment Site Character 4	Modality Qualifier Character 5	Isotope Character 6	Qualifier Character 7
Ø Bone Marrow 1 Thymus 2 Spleen 3 Lymphatics, Neck 4 Lymphatics, Axillary 5 Lymphatics, Thorax 6 Lymphatics, Abdomen 7 Lymphatics, Pelvis 8 Lymphatics, Inguinal	D Stereotactic Other Photon Radiosurgery H Stereotactic Particulate Radiosurgery J Stereotactic Gamma Beam Radiosurgery	Z None	Z None

DRG Non-OR   All treatment site, modality, isotope, and qualifier values

D   **Radiation Therapy**
7   **Lymphatic and Hematologic System**
Y   **Other Radiation**

Treatment Site Character 4	Modality Qualifier Character 5	Isotope Character 6	Qualifier Character 7
Ø Bone Marrow 1 Thymus 2 Spleen 3 Lymphatics, Neck 4 Lymphatics, Axillary 5 Lymphatics, Thorax 6 Lymphatics, Abdomen 7 Lymphatics, Pelvis 8 Lymphatics, Inguinal	8 Hyperthermia F Plaque Radiation	Z None	Z None

Radiation Therapy

D   Radiation Therapy
8   Eye
Ø   Beam Radiation

Treatment Site Character 4	Modality Qualifier Character 5	Isotope Character 6	Qualifier Character 7
Ø Eye	Ø Photons <1 MeV 1 Photons 1- 10 MeV 2 Photons >10 MeV 4 Heavy Particles (Protons, Ions) 5 Neutrons 6 Neutron Capture	Z None	Z None
Ø Eye	3 Electrons	Z None	Ø Intraoperative Z None

D   Radiation Therapy
8   Eye
1   Brachytherapy

Treatment Site Character 4	Modality Qualifier Character 5	Isotope Character 6	Qualifier Character 7
Ø Eye	9 High Dose Rate (HDR)	7 Cesium 137 (Cs-137) 8 Iridium 192 (Ir-192) 9 Iodine 125 (I-125) B Palladium 103 (Pd-103) C Californium 252 (Cf-252) Y Other Isotope	Z None
Ø Eye	B Low Dose Rate (LDR)	6 Cesium 131 (Cs-131) 7 Cesium 137 (Cs-137) 8 Iridium 192 (Ir-192) 9 Iodine 125 (I-125) C Californium 252 (Cf-252) Y Other Isotope	Z None
Ø Eye	B Low Dose Rate (LDR)	B Palladium 103 (Pd-103)	1 Unidirectional Source Z None

D   Radiation Therapy
8   Eye
2   Stereotactic Radiosurgery

Treatment Site Character 4	Modality Qualifier Character 5	Isotope Character 6	Qualifier Character 7

Ø Eye	D Stereotactic Other Photon
	     Radiosurgery
	H Stereotactic Particulate
	     Radiosurgery
	J Stereotactic Gamma Beam
	     Radiosurgery
		Z None	Z None

DRG Non-OR   All treatment site, modality, isotope, and qualifier values

D   Radiation Therapy
8   Eye
Y   Other Radiation

Treatment Site Character 4	Modality Qualifier Character 5	Isotope Character 6	Qualifier Character 7
Ø Eye	7 Contact Radiation 8 Hyperthermia F Plaque Radiation	Z None	Z None

Non-OR Procedure   DRG Non-OR Procedure   Valid OR Procedure   HAC Associated Procedure   Combination Only   New/Revised April   New/Revised October

786   ICD-10-PCS 2023

D   Radiation Therapy
9   Ear, Nose, Mouth and Throat
Ø   Beam Radiation

Treatment Site Character 4	Modality Qualifier Character 5	Isotope Character 6	Qualifier Character 7
Ø Ear 1 Nose 3 Hypopharynx 4 Mouth 5 Tongue 6 Salivary Glands 7 Sinuses 8 Hard Palate 9 Soft Palate B Larynx D Nasopharynx F Oropharynx	Ø Photons <1 MeV 1 Photons 1- 10 MeV 2 Photons >10 MeV 4 Heavy Particles (Protons, Ions) 5 Neutrons 6 Neutron Capture	Z None	Z None
Ø Ear 1 Nose 3 Hypopharynx 4 Mouth 5 Tongue 6 Salivary Glands 7 Sinuses 8 Hard Palate 9 Soft Palate B Larynx D Nasopharynx F Oropharynx	3 Electrons	Z None	Ø Intraoperative Z None

D   Radiation Therapy
9   Ear, Nose, Mouth and Throat
1   Brachytherapy

Treatment Site Character 4	Modality Qualifier Character 5	Isotope Character 6	Qualifier Character 7
Ø Ear 1 Nose 3 Hypopharynx 4 Mouth 5 Tongue 6 Salivary Glands 7 Sinuses 8 Hard Palate 9 Soft Palate B Larynx D Nasopharynx F Oropharynx	9 High Dose Rate (HDR)	7 Cesium 137 (Cs-137) 8 Iridium 192 (Ir-192) 9 Iodine 125 (I-125) B Palladium 103 (Pd-103) C Californium 252 (Cf-252) Y Other Isotope	Z None
Ø Ear 1 Nose 3 Hypopharynx 4 Mouth 5 Tongue 6 Salivary Glands 7 Sinuses 8 Hard Palate 9 Soft Palate B Larynx D Nasopharynx F Oropharynx	B Low Dose Rate (LDR)	6 Cesium 131 (Cs-131) 7 Cesium 137 (Cs-137) 8 Iridium 192 (Ir-192) 9 Iodine 125 (I-125) C Californium 252 (Cf-252) Y Other Isotope	Z None
Ø Ear 1 Nose 3 Hypopharynx 4 Mouth 5 Tongue 6 Salivary Glands 7 Sinuses 8 Hard Palate 9 Soft Palate B Larynx D Nasopharynx F Oropharynx	B Low Dose Rate (LDR)	B Palladium 103 (Pd-103)	1 Unidirectional Source Z None

NC Noncovered Procedure   **LC** Limited Coverage   **QA** Questionable OB Admit   **NT** New Tech Add-on   ⊞ Combination Member   ♂ Male   ♀ Female

ICD-10-PCS 2023   787

Radiation Therapy

D Radiation Therapy
9 Ear, Nose, Mouth and Throat
2 Stereotactic Radiosurgery

Treatment Site Character 4	Modality Qualifier Character 5	Isotope Character 6	Qualifier Character 7
Ø Ear 1 Nose 4 Mouth 5 Tongue 6 Salivary Glands 7 Sinuses 8 Hard Palate 9 Soft Palate B Larynx C Pharynx D Nasopharynx	D Stereotactic Other Photon Radiosurgery H Stereotactic Particulate Radiosurgery J Stereotactic Gamma Beam Radiosurgery	Z None	Z None

DRG Non-OR All treatment site, modality, isotope, and qualifier values

D Radiation Therapy
9 Ear, Nose, Mouth and Throat
Y Other Radiation

Treatment Site Character 4	Modality Qualifier Character 5	Isotope Character 6	Qualifier Character 7
Ø Ear 1 Nose 5 Tongue 6 Salivary Glands 7 Sinuses 8 Hard Palate 9 Soft Palate	7 Contact Radiation 8 Hyperthermia F Plaque Radiation	Z None	Z None
3 Hypopharynx F Oropharynx	7 Contact Radiation 8 Hyperthermia	Z None	Z None
4 Mouth B Larynx D Nasopharynx	7 Contact Radiation 8 Hyperthermia C Intraoperative Radiation Therapy (IORT) F Plaque Radiation	Z None	Z None
C Pharynx	C Intraoperative Radiation Therapy (IORT) F Plaque Radiation	Z None	Z None

D Radiation Therapy
B Respiratory System
Ø Beam Radiation

Treatment Site Character 4	Modality Qualifier Character 5	Isotope Character 6	Qualifier Character 7
Ø Trachea 1 Bronchus 2 Lung 5 Pleura 6 Mediastinum 7 Chest Wall 8 Diaphragm	Ø Photons <1 MeV 1 Photons 1- 10 MeV 2 Photons >10 MeV 4 Heavy Particles (Protons, Ions) 5 Neutrons 6 Neutron Capture	Z None	Z None
Ø Trachea 1 Bronchus 2 Lung 5 Pleura 6 Mediastinum 7 Chest Wall 8 Diaphragm	3 Electrons	Z None	Ø Intraoperative Z None

Non-OR Procedure DRG Non-OR Procedure Valid OR Procedure HAC Associated Procedure Combination Only New/Revised April New/Revised October

788

ICD-10-PCS 2023

D   **Radiation Therapy**
B   **Respiratory System**
1   **Brachytherapy**

Treatment Site Character 4	Modality Qualifier Character 5	Isotope Character 6	Qualifier Character 7
Ø Trachea 1 Bronchus 2 Lung 5 Pleura 6 Mediastinum 7 Chest Wall 8 Diaphragm	9 High Dose Rate (HDR)	7 Cesium 137 (Cs-137) 8 Iridium 192 (Ir-192) 9 Iodine 125 (I-125) B Palladium 103 (Pd-103) C Californium 252 (Cf-252) Y Other Isotope	Z None
Ø Trachea 1 Bronchus 2 Lung 5 Pleura 6 Mediastinum 7 Chest Wall 8 Diaphragm	B Low Dose Rate (LDR)	6 Cesium 131 (Cs-131) 7 Cesium 137 (Cs-137) 8 Iridium 192 (Ir-192) 9 Iodine 125 (I-125) C Californium 252 (Cf-252) Y Other Isotope	Z None
Ø Trachea 1 Bronchus 2 Lung 5 Pleura 6 Mediastinum 7 Chest Wall 8 Diaphragm	B Low Dose Rate (LDR)	B Palladium 103 (Pd-103)	1 Unidirectional Source Z None

D   **Radiation Therapy**
B   **Respiratory System**
2   **Stereotactic Radiosurgery**

Treatment Site Character 4	Modality Qualifier Character 5	Isotope Character 6	Qualifier Character 7

Ø   Trachea
1   Bronchus
2   Lung
5   Pleura
6   Mediastinum
7   Chest Wall
8   Diaphragm
	D Stereotactic Other Photon
	     Radiosurgery
	H Stereotactic Particulate
	     Radiosurgery
	J Stereotactic Gamma Beam
	     Radiosurgery
		Z None	Z None

DRG Non-OR   All treatment site, modality, isotope, and qualifier values

D   **Radiation Therapy**
B   **Respiratory System**
Y   **Other Radiation**

Treatment Site Character 4	Modality Qualifier Character 5	Isotope Character 6	Qualifier Character 7
Ø Trachea 1 Bronchus 2 Lung 5 Pleura 6 Mediastinum 7 Chest Wall 8 Diaphragm	7 Contact Radiation 8 Hyperthermia F Plaque Radiation	Z None	Z None

NC Noncovered Procedure   **LC** Limited Coverage   **QA** Questionable OB Admit   **NT** New Tech Add-on   ⊞ Combination Member   ♂ Male   ♀ Female

ICD-10-PCS 2023   **789**

Radiation Therapy

D   **Radiation Therapy**
D   **Gastrointestinal System**
Ø   **Beam Radiation**

Treatment Site Character 4	Modality Qualifier Character 5	Isotope Character 6	Qualifier Character 7
Ø Esophagus 1 Stomach 2 Duodenum 3 Jejunum 4 Ileum 5 Colon 7 Rectum	Ø Photons <1 MeV 1 Photons 1- 10 MeV 2 Photons >10 MeV 4 Heavy Particles (Protons, Ions) 5 Neutrons 6 Neutron Capture	Z None	Z None
Ø Esophagus 1 Stomach 2 Duodenum 3 Jejunum 4 Ileum 5 Colon 7 Rectum	3 Electrons	Z None	Ø Intraoperative Z None

D   **Radiation Therapy**
D   **Gastrointestinal System**
1   **Brachytherapy**

Treatment Site Character 4	Modality Qualifier Character 5	Isotope Character 6	Qualifier Character 7
Ø Esophagus 1 Stomach 2 Duodenum 3 Jejunum 4 Ileum 5 Colon 7 Rectum	9 High Dose Rate (HDR)	7 Cesium 137 (Cs-137) 8 Iridium 192 (Ir-192) 9 Iodine 125 (I-125) B Palladium 103 (Pd-103) C Californium 252 (Cf-252) Y Other Isotope	Z None
Ø Esophagus 1 Stomach 2 Duodenum 3 Jejunum 4 Ileum 5 Colon 7 Rectum	B Low Dose Rate (LDR)	6 Cesium 131 (Cs-131) 7 Cesium 137 (Cs-137) 8 Iridium 192 (Ir-192) 9 Iodine 125 (I-125) C Californium 252 (Cf-252) Y Other Isotope	Z None
Ø Esophagus 1 Stomach 2 Duodenum 3 Jejunum 4 Ileum 5 Colon 7 Rectum	B Low Dose Rate (LDR)	B Palladium 103 (Pd-103)	1 Unidirectional Source Z None

D   **Radiation Therapy**
D   **Gastrointestinal System**
2   **Stereotactic Radiosurgery**

Treatment Site Character 4	Modality Qualifier Character 5	Isotope Character 6	Qualifier Character 7
Ø Esophagus 1 Stomach 2 Duodenum 3 Jejunum 4 Ileum 5 Colon 7 Rectum	D Stereotactic Other Photon Radiosurgery H Stereotactic Particulate Radiosurgery J Stereotactic Gamma Beam Radiosurgery	Z None	Z None

DRG Non-OR   All treatment site, modality, isotope, and qualifier values

Non-OR Procedure   DRG Non-OR Procedure   Valid OR Procedure   HAC Associated Procedure   Combination Only   New/Revised April   New/Revised October

790   ICD-10-PCS 2023

D   **Radiation therapy**
D   **Gastrointestinal System**
Y   **Other Radiation**

Treatment Site Character 4	Modality Qualifier Character 5	Isotope Character 6	Qualifier Character 7
Ø Esophagus	7 Contact Radiation 8 Hyperthermia F Plaque Radiation	Z None	Z None
1 Stomach 2 Duodenum 3 Jejunum 4 Ileum 5 Colon 7 Rectum	7 Contact Radiation 8 Hyperthermia C Intraoperative Radiation Therapy (IORT) F Plaque Radiation	Z None	Z None
8 Anus	C Intraoperative Radiation Therapy (IORT) F Plaque Radiation	Z None	Z None

D   **Radiation Therapy**
F   **Hepatobiliary System and Pancreas**
Ø   **Beam Radiation**

Treatment Site Character 4	Modality Qualifier Character 5	Isotope Character 6	Qualifier Character 7
Ø Liver 1 Gallbladder 2 Bile Ducts 3 Pancreas	Ø Photons <1 MeV 1 Photons 1- 10 MeV 2 Photons >10 MeV 4 Heavy Particles (Protons, Ions) 5 Neutrons 6 Neutron Capture	Z None	Z None
Ø Liver 1 Gallbladder 2 Bile Ducts 3 Pancreas	3 Electrons	Z None	Ø Intraoperative Z None

D   **Radiation Therapy**
F   **Hepatobiliary System and Pancreas**
1   **Brachytherapy**

Treatment Site Character 4	Modality Qualifier Character 5	Isotope Character 6	Qualifier Character 7
Ø Liver 1 Gallbladder 2 Bile Ducts 3 Pancreas	9 High Dose Rate (HDR)	7 Cesium 137 (Cs-137) 8 Iridium 192 (Ir-192) 9 Iodine 125 (I-125) B Palladium 103 (Pd-103) C Californium 252 (Cf-252) Y Other Isotope	Z None
Ø Liver 1 Gallbladder 2 Bile Ducts 3 Pancreas	B Low Dose Rate (LDR)	6 Cesium 131 (Cs-131) 7 Cesium 137 (Cs-137) 8 Iridium 192 (Ir-192) 9 Iodine 125 (I-125) C Californium 252 (Cf-252) Y Other Isotope	Z None
Ø Liver 1 Gallbladder 2 Bile Ducts 3 Pancreas	B Low Dose Rate (LDR)	B Palladium 103 (Pd-103)	1 Unidirectional Source Z None

D   **Radiation Therapy**
F   **Hepatobiliary System and Pancreas**
2   **Stereotactic Radiosurgery**

Treatment Site Character 4	Modality Qualifier Character 5	Isotope Character 6	Qualifier Character 7
Ø Liver 1 Gallbladder 2 Bile Ducts 3 Pancreas	D Stereotactic Other Photon Radiosurgery H Stereotactic Particulate Radiosurgery J Stereotactic Gamma Beam Radiosurgery	Z None	Z None

DRG Non-OR   All treatment site, modality, isotope, and qualifier values

---

NC Noncovered Procedure   **LC** Limited Coverage   **QA** Questionable OB Admit   **NT** New Tech Add-on   ⊞ Combination Member   ♂ Male   ♀ Female

ICD-10-PCS 2023   **791**

D Radiation Therapy
F Hepatobiliary System and Pancreas
Y Other Radiation

Treatment Site Character 4	Modality Qualifier Character 5	Isotope Character 6	Qualifier Character 7
Ø Liver 1 Gallbladder 2 Bile Ducts 3 Pancreas	7 Contact Radiation 8 Hyperthermia C Intraoperative Radiation Therapy (IORT) F Plaque Radiation	Z None	Z None

D Radiation Therapy
G Endocrine System
Ø Beam Radiation

Treatment Site Character 4	Modality Qualifier Character 5	Isotope Character 6	Qualifier Character 7
Ø Pituitary Gland 1 Pineal Body 2 Adrenal Glands 4 Parathyroid Glands 5 Thyroid	Ø Photons <1 MeV 1 Photons 1- 10 MeV 2 Photons >10 MeV 5 Neutrons 6 Neutron Capture	Z None	Z None
Ø Pituitary Gland 1 Pineal Body 2 Adrenal Glands 4 Parathyroid Glands 5 Thyroid	3 Electrons	Z None	Ø Intraoperative Z None

D Radiation Therapy
G Endocrine System
1 Brachytherapy

Treatment Site Character 4	Modality Qualifier Character 5	Isotope Character 6	Qualifier Character 7
Ø Pituitary Gland 1 Pineal Body 2 Adrenal Glands 4 Parathyroid Glands 5 Thyroid	9 High Dose Rate (HDR)	7 Cesium 137 (Cs-137) 8 Iridium 192 (Ir-192) 9 Iodine 125 (I-125) B Palladium 103 (Pd-103) C Californium 252 (Cf-252) Y Other Isotope	Z None
Ø Pituitary Gland 1 Pineal Body 2 Adrenal Glands 4 Parathyroid Glands 5 Thyroid	B Low Dose Rate (LDR)	6 Cesium 131 (Cs-131) 7 Cesium 137 (Cs-137) 8 Iridium 192 (Ir-192) 9 Iodine 125 (I-125) C Californium 252 (Cf-252) Y Other Isotope	Z None
Ø Pituitary Gland 1 Pineal Body 2 Adrenal Glands 4 Parathyroid Glands 5 Thyroid	B Low Dose Rate (LDR)	B Palladium 103 (Pd-103)	1 Unidirectional Source Z None

D Radiation Therapy
G Endocrine System
2 Stereotactic Radiosurgery

Treatment Site Character 4	Modality Qualifier Character 5	Isotope Character 6	Qualifier Character 7
Ø Pituitary Gland 1 Pineal Body 2 Adrenal Glands 4 Parathyroid Glands 5 Thyroid	D Stereotactic Other Photon Radiosurgery H Stereotactic Particulate Radiosurgery J Stereotactic Gamma Beam Radiosurgery	Z None	Z None

DRG Non-OR All treatment site, modality, isotope, and qualifier values

D   **Radiation therapy**
G   **Endocrine System**
Y   **Other Radiation**

Treatment Site Character 4	Modality Qualifier Character 5	Isotope Character 6	Qualifier Character 7
0 Pituitary Gland	7 Contact Radiation	Z None	Z None
1 Pineal Body	8 Hyperthermia		
2 Adrenal Glands	F Plaque Radiation		
4 Parathyroid Glands			
5 Thyroid			

D   **Radiation Therapy**
H   **Skin**
0   **Beam Radiation**

Treatment Site Character 4	Modality Qualifier Character 5	Isotope Character 6	Qualifier Character 7
2 Skin, Face	0 Photons <1 MeV	Z None	Z None
3 Skin, Neck	1 Photons 1- 10 MeV		
4 Skin, Arm	2 Photons >10 MeV		
6 Skin, Chest	4 Heavy Particles (Protons, Ions)		
7 Skin, Back	5 Neutrons		
8 Skin, Abdomen	6 Neutron Capture		
9 Skin, Buttock			
B Skin, Leg			
2 Skin, Face	3 Electrons	Z None	0 Intraoperative
3 Skin, Neck			Z None
4 Skin, Arm			
6 Skin, Chest			
7 Skin, Back			
8 Skin, Abdomen			
9 Skin, Buttock			
B Skin, Leg			

D   **Radiation Therapy**
H   **Skin**
Y   **Other Radiation**

Treatment Site Character 4	Modality Qualifier Character 5	Isotope Character 6	Qualifier Character 7
2 Skin, Face	7 Contact Radiation	Z None	Z None
3 Skin, Neck	8 Hyperthermia		
4 Skin, Arm	F Plaque Radiation		
6 Skin, Chest			
7 Skin, Back			
8 Skin, Abdomen			
9 Skin, Buttock			
B Skin, Leg			
5 Skin, Hand	F Plaque Radiation	Z None	Z None
C Skin, Foot			

D   **Radiation Therapy**
M   **Breast**
0   **Beam Radiation**

Treatment Site Character 4	Modality Qualifier Character 5	Isotope Character 6	Qualifier Character 7
0 Breast, Left	0 Photons <1 MeV	Z None	Z None
1 Breast, Right	1 Photons 1- 10 MeV		
	2 Photons >10 MeV		
	4 Heavy Particles (Protons, Ions)		
	5 Neutrons		
	6 Neutron Capture		
0 Breast, Left	3 Electrons	Z None	0 Intraoperative
1 Breast, Right			Z None

NC Noncovered Procedure   **LC** Limited Coverage   **QA** Questionable OB Admit   **NT** New Tech Add-on   ⊞ Combination Member   ♂ Male   ♀ Female

ICD-10-PCS 2023   793

Radiation Therapy (sidebar)

D Radiation Therapy
M Breast
1 Brachytherapy

Treatment Site Character 4	Modality Qualifier Character 5	Isotope Character 6	Qualifier Character 7
Ø Breast, Left 1 Breast, Right	9 High Dose Rate (HDR)	7 Cesium 137 (Cs-137) 8 Iridium 192 (Ir-192) 9 Iodine 125 (I-125) B Palladium 103 (Pd-103) C Californium 252 (Cf-252) Y Other Isotope	Z None
Ø Breast, Left 1 Breast, Right	B Low Dose Rate (LDR)	6 Cesium 131 (Cs-131) 7 Cesium 137 (Cs-137) 8 Iridium 192 (Ir-192) 9 Iodine 125 (I-125) C Californium 252 (Cf-252) Y Other Isotope	Z None
Ø Breast, Left 1 Breast, Right	B Low Dose Rate (LDR)	B Palladium 103 (Pd-103)	1 Unidirectional Source Z None

D Radiation Therapy
M Breast
2 Stereotactic Radiosurgery

Treatment Site Character 4	Modality Qualifier Character 5	Isotope Character 6	Qualifier Character 7
Ø Breast, Left 1 Breast, Right	D Stereotactic Other Photon Radiosurgery H Stereotactic Particulate Radiosurgery J Stereotactic Gamma Beam Radiosurgery	Z None	Z None

DRG Non-OR All treatment site, modality, isotope, and qualifier values

D Radiation Therapy
M Breast
Y Other Radiation

Treatment Site Character 4	Modality Qualifier Character 5	Isotope Character 6	Qualifier Character 7
Ø Breast, Left 1 Breast, Right	7 Contact Radiation 8 Hyperthermia F Plaque Radiation	Z None	Z None

D Radiation Therapy
P Musculoskeletal System
Ø Beam Radiation

Treatment Site Character 4	Modality Qualifier Character 5	Isotope Character 6	Qualifier Character 7
Ø Skull 2 Maxilla 3 Mandible 4 Sternum 5 Rib(s) 6 Humerus 7 Radius/Ulna 8 Pelvic Bones 9 Femur B Tibia/Fibula C Other Bone	Ø Photons <1 MeV 1 Photons 1- 10 MeV 2 Photons >10 MeV 4 Heavy Particles (Protons, Ions) 5 Neutrons 6 Neutron Capture	Z None	Z None
Ø Skull 2 Maxilla 3 Mandible 4 Sternum 5 Rib(s) 6 Humerus 7 Radius/Ulna 8 Pelvic Bones 9 Femur B Tibia/Fibula C Other Bone	3 Electrons	Z None	Ø Intraoperative Z None

D Radiation Therapy
P Musculoskeletal System
Y Other Radiation

Treatment Site Character 4	Modality Qualifier Character 5	Isotope Character 6	Qualifier Character 7
Ø Skull 2 Maxilla 3 Mandible 4 Sternum 5 Rib(s) 6 Humerus 7 Radius/Ulna 8 Pelvic Bones 9 Femur B Tibia/Fibula C Other Bone	7 Contact Radiation 8 Hyperthermia F Plaque Radiation	Z None	Z None

D Radiation Therapy
T Urinary System
Ø Beam Radiation

Treatment Site Character 4	Modality Qualifier Character 5	Isotope Character 6	Qualifier Character 7
Ø Kidney 1 Ureter 2 Bladder 3 Urethra	Ø Photons <1 MeV 1 Photons 1- 10 MeV 2 Photons >10 MeV 4 Heavy Particles (Protons, Ions) 5 Neutrons 6 Neutron Capture	Z None	Z None
Ø Kidney 1 Ureter 2 Bladder 3 Urethra	3 Electrons	Z None	Ø Intraoperative Z None

D Radiation Therapy
T Urinary System
1 Brachytherapy

Treatment Site Character 4	Modality Qualifier Character 5	Isotope Character 6	Qualifier Character 7
Ø Kidney 1 Ureter 2 Bladder 3 Urethra	9 High Dose Rate (HDR)	7 Cesium 137 (Cs-137) 8 Iridium 192 (Ir-192) 9 Iodine 125 (I-125) B Palladium 103 (Pd-103) C Californium 252 (Cf-252) Y Other Isotope	Z None
Ø Kidney 1 Ureter 2 Bladder 3 Urethra	B Low Dose Rate (LDR)	6 Cesium 131 (Cs-131) 7 Cesium 137 (Cs-137) 8 Iridium 192 (Ir-192) 9 Iodine 125 (I-125) C Californium 252 (Cf-252) Y Other Isotope	Z None
Ø Kidney 1 Ureter 2 Bladder 3 Urethra	B Low Dose Rate (LDR)	B Palladium 103 (Pd-103)	1 Unidirectional Source Z None

D Radiation Therapy
T Urinary System
2 Stereotactic Radiosurgery

Treatment Site Character 4	Modality Qualifier Character 5	Isotope Character 6	Qualifier Character 7

Ø Kidney
1 Ureter
2 Bladder
3 Urethra
	D Stereotactic Other Photon
	    Radiosurgery
	H Stereotactic Particulate
	    Radiosurgery
	J Stereotactic Gamma Beam
	    Radiosurgery
		Z None	Z None

DRG Non-OR All treatment site, modality, isotope, and qualifier values

NC Noncovered Procedure **LC** Limited Coverage **QA** Questionable OB Admit **NT** New Tech Add-on ⊞ Combination Member ♂ Male ♀ Female

ICD-10-PCS 2023 795

Radiation Therapy

D   Radiation Therapy
T   Urinary System
Y   Other Radiation

Treatment Site Character 4	Modality Qualifier Character 5	Isotope Character 6	Qualifier Character 7
Ø Kidney 1 Ureter 2 Bladder 3 Urethra	7 Contact Radiation 8 Hyperthermia C Intraoperative Radiation Therapy (IORT) F Plaque Radiation	Z None	Z None

D   Radiation Therapy
U   Female Reproductive System
Ø   Beam Radiation

Treatment Site Character 4	Modality Qualifier Character 5	Isotope Character 6	Qualifier Character 7
Ø Ovary ♀ 1 Cervix ♀ 2 Uterus ♀	Ø Photons <1 MeV 1 Photons 1- 10 MeV 2 Photons >10 MeV 4 Heavy Particles (Protons, Ions) 5 Neutrons 6 Neutron Capture	Z None	Z None
Ø Ovary ♀ 1 Cervix ♀ 2 Uterus ♀	3 Electrons	Z None	Ø Intraoperative Z None

♀   All treatment site, modality, isotope, and qualifier values

D   Radiation Therapy
U   Female Reproductive System
1   Brachytherapy

Treatment Site Character 4	Modality Qualifier Character 5	Isotope Character 6	Qualifier Character 7
Ø Ovary ♀ 1 Cervix ♀ 2 Uterus ♀	9 High Dose Rate (HDR)	7 Cesium 137 (Cs-137) 8 Iridium 192 (Ir-192) 9 Iodine 125 (I-125) B Palladium 103 (Pd-103) C Californium 252 (Cf-252) Y Other Isotope	Z None
Ø Ovary ♀ 1 Cervix ♀ 2 Uterus ♀	B Low Dose Rate (LDR)	6 Cesium 131 (Cs-131) 7 Cesium 137 (Cs-137) 8 Iridium 192 (Ir-192) 9 Iodine 125 (I-125) C Californium 252 (Cf-252) Y Other Isotope	Z None
Ø Ovary ♀ 1 Cervix ♀ 2 Uterus ♀	B Low Dose Rate (LDR)	B Palladium 103 (Pd-103)	1 Unidirectional Source Z None

♀   All treatment site, modality, isotope, and qualifier values

D   Radiation Therapy
U   Female Reproductive System
2   Stereotactic Radiosurgery

Treatment Site Character 4	Modality Qualifier Character 5	Isotope Character 6	Qualifier Character 7
Ø Ovary ♀ 1 Cervix ♀ 2 Uterus ♀	D Stereotactic Other Photon Radiosurgery H Stereotactic Particulate Radiosurgery J Stereotactic Gamma Beam Radiosurgery	Z None	Z None

DRG Non-OR   All treatment site, modality, isotope, and qualifier values
♀   All treatment site, modality, isotope, and qualifier values

---

Non-OR Procedure   DRG Non-OR Procedure   Valid OR Procedure   HAC Associated Procedure   Combination Only   New/Revised April   New/Revised October

D Radiation Therapy
U Female Reproductive System
Y Other Radiation

Treatment Site Character 4		Modality Qualifier Character 5	Isotope Character 6	Qualifier Character 7
Ø Ovary	♀	7 Contact Radiation	Z None	Z None
1 Cervix	♀	8 Hyperthermia		
2 Uterus	♀	C Intraoperative Radiation Therapy (IORT)		
		F Plaque Radiation		

♀	All treatment site, modality, isotope, and qualifier values

D Radiation Therapy
V Male Reproductive System
Ø Beam Radiation

Treatment Site Character 4		Modality Qualifier Character 5	Isotope Character 6	Qualifier Character 7
Ø Prostate	♂	Ø Photons <1 MeV	Z None	Z None
1 Testis	♂	1 Photons 1- 10 MeV		
		2 Photons >10 MeV		
		4 Heavy Particles (Protons, Ions)		
		5 Neutrons		
		6 Neutron Capture		
Ø Prostate	♂	3 Electrons	Z None	Ø Intraoperative
1 Testis	♂			Z None

♂	All treatment site, modality, isotope, and qualifier values

D Radiation Therapy
V Male Reproductive System
1 Brachytherapy

Treatment Site Character 4		Modality Qualifier Character 5	Isotope Character 6	Qualifier Character 7
Ø Prostate	♂	9 High Dose Rate (HDR)	7 Cesium 137 (Cs-137)	Z None
1 Testis	♂		8 Iridium 192 (Ir-192)	
			9 Iodine 125 (I-125)	
			B Palladium 103 (Pd-103)	
			C Californium 252 (Cf-252)	
			Y Other Isotope	
Ø Prostate	♂	B Low Dose Rate (LDR)	6 Cesium 131 (Cs-131)	Z None
1 Testis	♂		7 Cesium 137 (Cs-137)	
			8 Iridium 192 (Ir-192)	
			9 Iodine 125 (I-125)	
			C Californium 252 (Cf-252)	
			Y Other Isotope	
Ø Prostate	♂	B Low Dose Rate (LDR)	B Palladium 103 (Pd-103)	1 Unidirectional Source
1 Testis	♂			Z None

♂	All treatment site, modality, isotope, and qualifier values

D Radiation Therapy
V Male Reproductive System
2 Stereotactic Radiosurgery

Treatment Site Character 4		Modality Qualifier Character 5	Isotope Character 6	Qualifier Character 7
Ø Prostate	♂	D Stereotactic Other Photon Radiosurgery	Z None	Z None
1 Testis	♂	H Stereotactic Particulate Radiosurgery		
		J Stereotactic Gamma Beam Radiosurgery		

DRG Non-OR	All treatment site, modality, isotope, and qualifier values
♂	All treatment site, modality, isotope, and qualifier values

NC Noncovered Procedure   **LC** Limited Coverage   **QA** Questionable OB Admit   **NT** New Tech Add-on   ✚ Combination Member   ♂ Male   ♀ Female

ICD-10-PCS 2023   **797**

Radiation Therapy

D Radiation Therapy
V Male Reproductive System
Y Other Radiation

Treatment Site Character 4		Modality Qualifier Character 5	Isotope Character 6	Qualifier Character 7
Ø Prostate	♂	7 Contact Radiation 8 Hyperthermia C Intraoperative Radiation Therapy (IORT) F Plaque Radiation	Z None	Z None
1 Testis	♂	7 Contact Radiation 8 Hyperthermia F Plaque Radiation	Z None	Z None
♂	All treatment site, modality, isotope, and qualifier values			

D Radiation Therapy
W Anatomical Regions
Ø Beam Radiation

Treatment Site Character 4	Modality Qualifier Character 5	Isotope Character 6	Qualifier Character 7
1 Head and Neck 2 Chest 3 Abdomen 4 Hemibody 5 Whole Body 6 Pelvic Region	Ø Photons <1 MeV 1 Photons 1- 10 MeV 2 Photons >10 MeV 4 Heavy Particles (Protons, Ions) 5 Neutrons 6 Neutron Capture	Z None	Z None
1 Head and Neck 2 Chest 3 Abdomen 4 Hemibody 5 Whole Body 6 Pelvic Region	3 Electrons	Z None	Ø Intraoperative Z None

D Radiation Therapy
W Anatomical Regions
1 Brachytherapy

Treatment Site Character 4	Modality Qualifier Character 5	Isotope Character 6	Qualifier Character 7
Ø Cranial Cavity K Upper Back L Lower Back P Gastrointestinal Tract Q Respiratory Tract R Genitourinary Tract X Upper Extremity Y Lower Extremity	B Low Dose Rate (LDR)	B Palladium 103 (Pd-103)	1 Unidirectional Source Z None
1 Head and Neck 2 Chest 3 Abdomen 6 Pelvic Region	9 High Dose Rate (HDR)	7 Cesium 137 (Cs-137) 8 Iridium 192 (Ir-192) 9 Iodine 125 (I-125) B Palladium 103 (Pd-103) C Californium 252 (Cf-252) Y Other Isotope	Z None
1 Head and Neck 2 Chest 3 Abdomen 6 Pelvic Region	B Low Dose Rate (LDR)	6 Cesium 131 (Cs-131) 7 Cesium 137 (Cs-137) 8 Iridium 192 (Ir-192) 9 Iodine 125 (I-125) C Californium 252 (Cf-252) Y Other Isotope	Z None
1 Head and Neck 2 Chest 3 Abdomen 6 Pelvic Region	B Low Dose Rate (LDR)	B Palladium 103 (Pd-103)	1 Unidirectional Source Z None

Non-OR Procedure   DRG Non-OR Procedure   Valid OR Procedure   HAC Associated Procedure   Combination Only   New/Revised April   New/Revised October

798   ICD-10-PCS 2023

D   **Radiation Therapy**
W   **Anatomical Regions**
2   **Stereotactic Radiosurgery**

Treatment Site Character 4	Modality Qualifier Character 5	Isotope Character 6	Qualifier Character 7

1   Head and Neck
2   Chest
3   Abdomen
6   Pelvic Region
	D Stereotactic Other Photon
	     Radiosurgery
	H Stereotactic Particulate
	     Radiosurgery
	J Stereotactic Gamma Beam
	     Radiosurgery
		Z None	Z None

DRG Non-OR   All treatment site, modality, isotope, and qualifier values

D   **Radiation Therapy**
W   **Anatomical Regions**
Y   **Other Radiation**

Treatment Site Character 4	Modality Qualifier Character 5	Isotope Character 6	Qualifier Character 7
1 Head and Neck 2 Chest 3 Abdomen 4 Hemibody 6 Pelvic Region	7 Contact Radiation 8 Hyperthermia F Plaque Radiation	Z None	Z None
5 Whole Body	7 Contact Radiation 8 Hyperthermia F Plaque Radiation	Z None	Z None
5 Whole Body	G Isotope Administration	D Iodine 131 (I-131) F Phosphorus 32 (P-32) G Strontium 89 (Sr-89) H Strontium 90 (Sr-90) Y Other Isotope	Z None

NC Noncovered Procedure   **LC** Limited Coverage   **QA** Questionable OB Admit   **NT** New Tech Add-on   ⊞ Combination Member   ♂ Male   ♀ Female

ICD-10-PCS 2023   **799**

Physical Rehabilitation and Diagnostic Audiology F00–F15

F   **Physical Rehabilitation and Diagnostic Audiology**
0   **Rehabilitation**
0   **Speech Assessment**   Definition: Measurement of speech and related functions

Body System/Region Character 4	Type Qualifier Character 5	Equipment Character 6	Qualifier Character 7

3 Neurological System - Whole Body	G Communicative/Cognitive
	     Integration Skills
		K Audiovisual
		M Augmentative / Alternative
		     Communication
		P Computer
		Y Other Equipment
		Z None
			Z None

Z None	0 Filtered Speech 3 Staggered Spondaic Word Q Performance Intensity Phonetically Balanced Speech Discrimination R Brief Tone Stimuli S Distorted Speech T Dichotic Stimuli V Temporal Ordering of Stimuli W Masking Patterns	1 Audiometer 2 Sound Field / Booth K Audiovisual Z None	Z None
Z None	1 Speech Threshold 2 Speech/Word Recognition	1 Audiometer 2 Sound Field / Booth 9 Cochlear Implant K Audiovisual Z None	Z None
Z None	4 Sensorineural Acuity Level	1 Audiometer 2 Sound Field / Booth Z None	Z None
Z None	5 Synthetic Sentence Identification	1 Audiometer 2 Sound Field / Booth 9 Cochlear Implant K Audiovisual	Z None

Z None	6 Speech and/or Language Screening
	7 Nonspoken Language
	8 Receptive/Expressive Language
	C Aphasia
	G Communicative/Cognitive
	     Integration Skills
	L Augmentative/Alternative
	     Communication System
		K Audiovisual
		M Augmentative / Alternative
		     Communication
		P Computer
		Y Other Equipment
		Z None
			Z None

Z None	9 Articulation/Phonology	K Audiovisual P Computer Q Speech Analysis Y Other Equipment Z None	Z None
Z None	B Motor Speech	K Audiovisual N Biosensory Feedback P Computer Q Speech Analysis T Aerodynamic Function Y Other Equipment Z None	Z None
Z None	D Fluency	K Audiovisual N Biosensory Feedback P Computer Q Speech Analysis S Voice Analysis T Aerodynamic Function Y Other Equipment Z None	Z None
Z None	F Voice	K Audiovisual N Biosensory Feedback P Computer S Voice Analysis T Aerodynamic Function Y Other Equipment Z None	Z None

DRG Non-OR   All body system/region, type qualifier, equipment, and qualifier values

F00 Continued on next page

NC Noncovered Procedure   **LC** Limited Coverage   **QA** Questionable OB Admit   **NT** New Tech Add-on   ⊞ Combination Member   ♂ Male   ♀ Female

Physical Rehabilitation and Diagnostic Audiology *(side tab)*

F00 Continued

F   **Physical Rehabilitation and Diagnostic Audiology**
0   **Rehabilitation**
0   **Speech Assessment**   Definition: Measurement of speech and related functions

Body System/Region Character 4	Type Qualifier Character 5	Equipment Character 6	Qualifier Character 7
Z None	H Bedside Swallowing and Oral Function P Oral Peripheral Mechanism	Y Other Equipment Z None	Z None
Z None	J Instrumental Swallowing and Oral Function	T Aerodynamic Function W Swallowing Y Other Equipment	Z None
Z None	K Orofacial Myofunctional	K Audiovisual P Computer Y Other Equipment Z None	Z None
Z None	M Voice Prosthetic	K Audiovisual P Computer S Voice Analysis V Speech Prosthesis Y Other Equipment Z None	Z None
Z None	N Non-invasive Instrumental Status	N Biosensory Feedback P Computer Q Speech Analysis S Voice Analysis T Aerodynamic Function Y Other Equipment	Z None
Z None	X Other Specified Central Auditory Processing	Z None	Z None

DRG Non-OR   All body system/region, type qualifier, equipment, and qualifier values

F   **Physical Rehabilitation and Diagnostic Audiology**
0   **Rehabilitation**
1   **Motor and/or Nerve Function Assessment**   Definition: Measurement of motor, nerve, and related functions

Body System/Region Character 4	Type Qualifier Character 5	Equipment Character 6	Qualifier Character 7
0 Neurological System - Head and Neck 1 Neurological System - Upper Back/ Upper Extremity 2 Neurological System - Lower Back/ Lower Extremity 3 Neurological System - Whole Body	0 Muscle Performance	E Orthosis F Assistive, Adaptive, Supportive or Protective U Prosthesis Y Other Equipment Z None	Z None
0 Neurological System - Head and Neck 1 Neurological System - Upper Back/ Upper Extremity 2 Neurological System - Lower Back/ Lower Extremity 3 Neurological System - Whole Body	1 Integumentary Integrity 3 Coordination/Dexterity 4 Motor Function G Reflex Integrity	Z None	Z None
0 Neurological System - Head and Neck 1 Neurological System - Upper Back/ Upper Extremity 2 Neurological System - Lower Back/ Lower Extremity 3 Neurological System - Whole Body	5 Range of Motion and Joint Integrity 6 Sensory Awareness/Processing/ Integrity	Y Other Equipment Z None	Z None
D Integumentary System - Head and Neck F Integumentary System - Upper Back/ Upper Extremity G Integumentary System - Lower Back/ Lower Extremity H Integumentary System - Whole Body J Musculoskeletal System - Head and Neck K Musculoskeletal System - Upper Back/ Upper Extremity L Musculoskeletal System - Lower Back/ Lower Extremity M Musculoskeletal System - Whole Body	0 Muscle Performance	E Orthosis F Assistive, Adaptive, Supportive or Protective U Prosthesis Y Other Equipment Z None	Z None

DRG Non-OR   All body system/region, type qualifier, equipment, and qualifier values

F01 Continued on next page

Non-OR Procedure   DRG Non-OR Procedure   Valid OR Procedure   HAC Associated Procedure   Combination Only   New/Revised April   New/Revised October

F   **Physical Rehabilitation and Diagnostic Audiology**   *F01 Continued*
Ø   **Rehabilitation**
1   **Motor and/or Nerve Function Assessment**   Definition: Measurement of motor, nerve, and related functions

Body System/Region Character 4	Type Qualifier Character 5	Equipment Character 6	Qualifier Character 7
D Integumentary System - Head and Neck **F** Integumentary System - Upper Back/ Upper Extremity **G** Integumentary System - Lower Back/ Lower Extremity **H** Integumentary System - Whole Body **J** Musculoskeletal System - Head and Neck **K** Musculoskeletal System - Upper Back/ Upper Extremity **L** Musculoskeletal System - Lower Back/ Lower Extremity **M** Musculoskeletal System - Whole Body	**1** Integumentary Integrity	**Z** None	**Z** None
D Integumentary System - Head and Neck **F** Integumentary System - Upper Back/ Upper Extremity **G** Integumentary System - Lower Back/ Lower Extremity **H** Integumentary System - Whole Body **J** Musculoskeletal System - Head and Neck **K** Musculoskeletal System - Upper Back/ Upper Extremity **L** Musculoskeletal System - Lower Back/ Lower Extremity **M** Musculoskeletal System - Whole Body	**5** Range of Motion and Joint Integrity **6** Sensory Awareness/Processing/ Integrity	**Y** Other Equipment **Z** None	**Z** None
N Genitourinary System	**Ø** Muscle Performance	**E** Orthosis **F** Assistive, Adaptive, Supportive or Protective **U** Prosthesis **Y** Other Equipment **Z** None	**Z** None
Z None	**2** Visual Motor Integration	**K** Audiovisual **M** Augmentative / Alternative Communication **N** Biosensory Feedback **P** Computer **Q** Speech Analysis **S** Voice Analysis **Y** Other Equipment **Z** None	**Z** None
Z None	**7** Facial Nerve Function	**7** Electrophysiologic	**Z** None
Z None	**9** Somatosensory Evoked Potentials	**J** Somatosensory	**Z** None
Z None	**B** Bed Mobility **C** Transfer **F** Wheelchair Mobility	**E** Orthosis **F** Assistive, Adaptive, Supportive or Protective **U** Prosthesis **Z** None	**Z** None
Z None	**D** Gait and/or Balance	**E** Orthosis **F** Assistive, Adaptive, Supportive or Protective **U** Prosthesis **Y** Other Equipment **Z** None	**Z** None

DRG Non-OR   All body system/region, type qualifier, equipment, and qualifier values

Physical Rehabilitation and Diagnostic Audiology

F   Physical Rehabilitation and Diagnostic Audiology
Ø   Rehabilitation
2   Activities of Daily Living Assessment   Definition: Measurement of functional level for activities of daily living

Body System/Region Character 4	Type Qualifier Character 5	Equipment Character 6	Qualifier Character 7
Ø Neurological System - Head and Neck	9 Cranial Nerve Integrity D Neuromotor Development	Y Other Equipment Z None	Z None
1 Neurological System - Upper Back/Upper Extremity 2 Neurological System - Lower Back/Lower Extremity 3 Neurological System - Whole Body	D Neuromotor Development	Y Other Equipment Z None	Z None
4 Circulatory System - Head and Neck 5 Circulatory System - Upper Back/Upper Extremity 6 Circulatory System - Lower Back/Lower Extremity 8 Respiratory System - Head and Neck 9 Respiratory System - Upper Back/Upper Extremity B Respiratory System - Lower Back/Lower Extremity	G Ventilation, Respiration and Circulation	C Mechanical G Aerobic Endurance and Conditioning Y Other Equipment Z None	Z None
7 Circulatory System - Whole Body C Respiratory System - Whole Body	7 Aerobic Capacity and Endurance	E Orthosis G Aerobic Endurance and Conditioning U Prosthesis Y Other Equipment Z None	Z None
7 Circulatory System - Whole Body C Respiratory System - Whole Body	G Ventilation, Respiration and Circulation	C Mechanical G Aerobic Endurance and Conditioning Y Other Equipment Z None	Z None
Z None	Ø Bathing/Showering 1 Dressing 3 Grooming/Personal Hygiene 4 Home Management	E Orthosis F Assistive, Adaptive, Supportive or Protective U Prosthesis Z None	Z None
Z None	2 Feeding/Eating 8 Anthropometric Characteristics F Pain	Y Other Equipment Z None	Z None
Z None	5 Perceptual Processing	K Audiovisual M Augmentative / Alternative Communication N Biosensory Feedback P Computer Q Speech Analysis S Voice Analysis Y Other Equipment Z None	Z None
Z None	6 Psychosocial Skills	Z None	Z None
Z None	B Environmental, Home and Work Barriers C Ergonomics and Body Mechanics	E Orthosis F Assistive, Adaptive, Supportive or Protective U Prosthesis Y Other Equipment Z None	Z None
Z None	H Vocational Activities and Functional Community or Work Reintegration Skills	E Orthosis F Assistive, Adaptive, Supportive or Protective G Aerobic Endurance and Conditioning U Prosthesis Y Other Equipment Z None	Z None

DRG Non-OR   All body system/region, type qualifier, equipment, and qualifier values

Non-OR Procedure   DRG Non-OR Procedure   Valid OR Procedure   HAC Associated Procedure   Combination Only   New/Revised April   New/Revised October

F   **Physical Rehabilitation and Diagnostic Audiology**
Ø   **Rehabilitation**
6   **Speech Treatment**   Definition: Application of techniques to improve, augment, or compensate for speech and related functional impairment

Body System/Region Character 4	Type Qualifier Character 5	Equipment Character 6	Qualifier Character 7

3 Neurological System - Whole Body	6 Communicative/Cognitive
	     Integration Skills
		K Audiovisual
		M Augmentative / Alternative
		     Communication
		P Computer
		Y Other Equipment
		Z None
			Z None

Z None	Ø Nonspoken Language
	3 Aphasia
	6 Communicative/Cognitive
	     Integration Skills
		K Audiovisual
		M Augmentative / Alternative
		     Communication
		P Computer
		Y Other Equipment
		Z None
			Z None

Z None	1 Speech-Language Pathology and
	     Related Disorders Counseling
	2 Speech-Language Pathology and
	     Related Disorders Prevention
		K Audiovisual
		Z None
			Z None

Z None	4 Articulation/Phonology	K Audiovisual P Computer Q Speech Analysis T Aerodynamic Function Y Other Equipment Z None	Z None
Z None	5 Aural Rehabilitation	K Audiovisual L Assistive Listening M Augmentative / Alternative Communication N Biosensory Feedback P Computer Q Speech Analysis S Voice Analysis Y Other Equipment Z None	Z None
Z None	7 Fluency	4 Electroacoustic Immitance / Acoustic Reflex K Audiovisual N Biosensory Feedback Q Speech Analysis S Voice Analysis T Aerodynamic Function Y Other Equipment Z None	Z None
Z None	8 Motor Speech	K Audiovisual N Biosensory Feedback P Computer Q Speech Analysis S Voice Analysis T Aerodynamic Function Y Other Equipment Z None	Z None
Z None	9 Orofacial Myofunctional	K Audiovisual P Computer Y Other Equipment Z None	Z None
Z None	B Receptive/Expressive Language	K Audiovisual L Assistive Listening M Augmentative / Alternative Communication P Computer Y Other Equipment Z None	Z None

DRG Non-OR   All body system/region, type qualifier, equipment, and qualifier values

F06 Continued on next page

F   Physical Rehabilitation and Diagnostic Audiology
0   Rehabilitation
6   Speech Treatment   Definition: Application of techniques to improve, augment, or compensate for speech and related functional impairment

Body System/Region Character 4	Type Qualifier Character 5	Equipment Character 6	Qualifier Character 7
Z None	C Voice	K Audiovisual N Biosensory Feedback P Computer S Voice Analysis T Aerodynamic Function V Speech Prosthesis Y Other Equipment Z None	Z None
Z None	D Swallowing Dysfunction	M Augmentative / Alternative Communication T Aerodynamic Function V Speech Prosthesis Y Other Equipment Z None	Z None

DRG Non-OR   All body system/region, type qualifier, equipment, and qualifier values

F   Physical Rehabilitation and Diagnostic Audiology
0   Rehabilitation
7   Motor Treatment   Definition: Exercise or activities to increase or facilitate motor function

Body System/Region Character 4	Type Qualifier Character 5	Equipment Character 6	Qualifier Character 7

0   Neurological System - Head and Neck
1   Neurological System - Upper Back/
     Upper Extremity
2   Neurological System - Lower Back/
     Lower Extremity
3   Neurological System - Whole Body
D   Integumentary System - Head and
     Neck
F   Integumentary System - Upper Back/
     Upper Extremity
G   Integumentary System - Lower Back/
     Lower Extremity
H   Integumentary System - Whole Body
J   Musculoskeletal System - Head and
     Neck
K   Musculoskeletal System - Upper Back/
     Upper Extremity
L   Musculoskeletal System - Lower Back/
     Lower Extremity
M   Musculoskeletal System - Whole Body
	0 Range of Motion and Joint
	     Mobility
	1 Muscle Performance
	2 Coordination/Dexterity
	3 Motor Function
		E Orthosis
		F Assistive, Adaptive, Supportive or
		     Protective
		U Prosthesis
		Y Other Equipment
		Z None
			Z None

0   Neurological System - Head and Neck
1   Neurological System - Upper Back/
     Upper Extremity
2   Neurological System - Lower Back/
     Lower Extremity
3   Neurological System - Whole Body
D   Integumentary System - Head and
     Neck
F   Integumentary System - Upper Back/
     Upper Extremity
G   Integumentary System - Lower Back/
     Lower Extremity
H   Integumentary System - Whole Body
J   Musculoskeletal System - Head and
     Neck
K   Musculoskeletal System - Upper Back/
     Upper Extremity
L   Musculoskeletal System - Lower Back/
     Lower Extremity
M   Musculoskeletal System - Whole Body
	6 Therapeutic Exercise	B Physical Agents
		C Mechanical
		D Electrotherapeutic
		E Orthosis
		F Assistive, Adaptive, Supportive or
		     Protective
		G Aerobic Endurance and
		     Conditioning
		H Mechanical or Electromechanical
		U Prosthesis
		Y Other Equipment
		Z None
			Z None

DRG Non-OR   All body system/region, type qualifier, equipment, and qualifier values

F07 Continued on next page

Non-OR Procedure   DRG Non-OR Procedure   Valid OR Procedure   HAC Associated Procedure   Combination Only   New/Revised April   New/Revised October

806   ICD-10-PCS 2023

F   **Physical Rehabilitation and Diagnostic Audiology**
Ø   **Rehabilitation**
7   **Motor Treatment**   Definition: Exercise or activities to increase or facilitate motor function

Body System/Region Character 4	Type Qualifier Character 5	Equipment Character 6	Qualifier Character 7
Ø Neurological System - Head and Neck **1** Neurological System - Upper Back/ Upper Extremity **2** Neurological System - Lower Back/ Lower Extremity **3** Neurological System - Whole Body **D** Integumentary System - Head and Neck **F** Integumentary System - Upper Back/ Upper Extremity **G** Integumentary System - Lower Back/ Lower Extremity **H** Integumentary System - Whole Body **J** Musculoskeletal System - Head and Neck **K** Musculoskeletal System - Upper Back/ Upper Extremity **L** Musculoskeletal System - Lower Back/ Lower Extremity **M** Musculoskeletal System - Whole Body	**7** Manual Therapy Techniques	**Z** None	**Z** None
4 Circulatory System - Head and Neck **5** Circulatory System - Upper Back / Upper Extremity **6** Circulatory System - Lower Back / Lower Extremity **7** Circulatory System - Whole Body **8** Respiratory System - Head and Neck **9** Respiratory System - Upper Back / Upper Extremity **B** Respiratory System - Lower Back / Lower Extremity **C** Respiratory System - Whole Body	**6** Therapeutic Exercise	**B** Physical Agents **C** Mechanical **D** Electrotherapeutic **E** Orthosis **F** Assistive, Adaptive, Supportive or Protective **G** Aerobic Endurance and Conditioning **H** Mechanical or Electromechanical **U** Prosthesis **Y** Other Equipment **Z** None	**Z** None
N Genitourinary System	**1** Muscle Performance	**E** Orthosis **F** Assistive, Adaptive, Supportive or Protective **U** Prosthesis **Y** Other Equipment **Z** None	**Z** None
N Genitourinary System	**6** Therapeutic Exercise	**B** Physical Agents **C** Mechanical **D** Electrotherapeutic **E** Orthosis **F** Assistive, Adaptive, Supportive or Protective **G** Aerobic Endurance and Conditioning **H** Mechanical or Electromechanical **U** Prosthesis **Y** Other Equipment **Z** None	**Z** None
Z None	**4** Wheelchair Mobility	**D** Electrotherapeutic **E** Orthosis **F** Assistive, Adaptive, Supportive or Protective **U** Prosthesis **Y** Other Equipment **Z** None	**Z** None
Z None	**5** Bed Mobility	**C** Mechanical **E** Orthosis **F** Assistive, Adaptive, Supportive or Protective **U** Prosthesis **Y** Other Equipment **Z** None	**Z** None
Z None	**8** Transfer Training	**C** Mechanical **D** Electrotherapeutic **E** Orthosis **F** Assistive, Adaptive, Supportive or Protective **U** Prosthesis **Y** Other Equipment **Z** None	**Z** None

DRG Non-OR   All body system/region, type qualifier, equipment, and qualifier values

F07 Continued on next page

NC Noncovered Procedure   **LC** Limited Coverage   **QA** Questionable OB Admit   **NT** New Tech Add-on   ⊞ Combination Member   ♂ Male   ♀ Female

F   **Physical Rehabilitation and Diagnostic Audiology**
Ø   **Rehabilitation**
7   **Motor Treatment**   Definition: Exercise or activities to increase or facilitate motor function

F07 Continued

Body System/Region Character 4	Type Qualifier Character 5	Equipment Character 6	Qualifier Character 7

Z None	9 Gait Training/Functional
	     Ambulation
		C Mechanical
		D Electrotherapeutic
		E Orthosis
		F Assistive, Adaptive, Supportive or
		     Protective
		G Aerobic Endurance and
		     Conditioning
		U Prosthesis
		Y Other Equipment
		Z None
			Z None

DRG Non-OR   All body system/region, type qualifier, equipment, and qualifier values

F   **Physical Rehabilitation and Diagnostic Audiology**
Ø   **Rehabilitation**
8   **Activities of Daily Living Treatment**   Definition: Exercise or activities to facilitate functional competence for activities of daily living

Body System/Region Character 4	Type Qualifier Character 5	Equipment Character 6	Qualifier Character 7

D   Integumentary System - Head and
     Neck
F   Integumentary System - Upper Back/
     Upper Extremity
G   Integumentary System - Lower Back/
     Lower Extremity
H   Integumentary System - Whole Body
J   Musculoskeletal System - Head and
     Neck
K   Musculoskeletal System - Upper Back/
     Upper Extremity
L   Musculoskeletal System - Lower Back/
     Lower Extremity
M   Musculoskeletal System - Whole Body
	5 Wound Management	B Physical Agents
		C Mechanical
		D Electrotherapeutic
		E Orthosis
		F Assistive, Adaptive, Supportive or
		     Protective
		U Prosthesis
		Y Other Equipment
		Z None
			Z None

Z None	Ø Bathing/Showering Techniques 1 Dressing Techniques 2 Grooming/Personal Hygiene	E Orthosis F Assistive, Adaptive, Supportive or Protective U Prosthesis Y Other Equipment Z None	Z None
Z None	3 Feeding/Eating	C Mechanical D Electrotherapeutic E Orthosis F Assistive, Adaptive, Supportive or Protective U Prosthesis Y Other Equipment Z None	Z None
Z None	4 Home Management	D Electrotherapeutic E Orthosis F Assistive, Adaptive, Supportive or Protective U Prosthesis Y Other Equipment Z None	Z None
Z None	6 Psychosocial Skills	Z None	Z None

Z None	7 Vocational Activities and
	     Functional Community or Work
	     Reintegration Skills
		B Physical Agents
		C Mechanical
		D Electrotherapeutic
		E Orthosis
		F Assistive, Adaptive, Supportive or
		     Protective
		G Aerobic Endurance and
		     Conditioning
		U Prosthesis
		Y Other Equipment
		Z None
			Z None

DRG Non-OR   All body system/region, type qualifier, equipment, and qualifier values

Non-OR Procedure   DRG Non-OR Procedure   Valid OR Procedure   HAC Associated Procedure   Combination Only   New/Revised April   New/Revised October

F   **Physical Rehabilitation and Diagnostic Audiology**
0   **Rehabilitation**
9   **Hearing Treatment**   Definition: Application of techniques to improve, augment, or compensate for hearing and related functional impairment

Body System/Region Character 4	Type Qualifier Character 5	Equipment Character 6	Qualifier Character 7

Z None	0 Hearing and Related Disorders
	     Counseling
	1 Hearing and Related Disorders
	     Prevention
		K Audiovisual
		Z None
			Z None

Z None	2 Auditory Processing	K Audiovisual L Assistive Listening P Computer Y Other Equipment Z None	Z None
Z None	3 Cerumen Management	X Cerumen Management Z None	Z None

DRG Non-OR   All body system/region, type qualifier, equipment, and qualifier values

F   **Physical Rehabilitation and Diagnostic Audiology**
0   **Rehabilitation**
B   **Cochlear Implant Treatment**   Definition: Application of techniques to improve the communication abilities of individuals with cochlear implant

Body System/Region Character 4	Type Qualifier Character 5	Equipment Character 6	Qualifier Character 7
Z None	0 Cochlear Implant Rehabilitation	1 Audiometer 2 Sound Field / Booth 9 Cochlear Implant K Audiovisual P Computer Y Other Equipment	Z None

DRG Non-OR   All body system/region, type qualifier, equipment, and qualifier values

F   **Physical Rehabilitation and Diagnostic Audiology**
0   **Rehabilitation**
C   **Vestibular Treatment**   Definition: Application of techniques to improve, augment, or compensate for vestibular and related functional impairment

Body System/Region Character 4	Type Qualifier Character 5	Equipment Character 6	Qualifier Character 7

3   Neurological System - Whole Body
H   Integumentary System - Whole
     Body
M   Musculoskeletal System - Whole
     Body
	3 Postural Control	E Orthosis
		F Assistive, Adaptive, Supportive or
		     Protective
		U Prosthesis
		Y Other Equipment
		Z None
			Z None

Z None	0 Vestibular	8 Vestibular / Balance Z None	Z None
Z None	1 Perceptual Processing 2 Visual Motor Integration	K Audiovisual L Assistive Listening N Biosensory Feedback P Computer Q Speech Analysis S Voice Analysis T Aerodynamic Function Y Other Equipment Z None	Z None

DRG Non-OR   All body system/region, type qualifier, equipment, and qualifier values

F **Physical Rehabilitation and Diagnostic Audiology**
Ø **Rehabilitation**
D **Device Fitting**   Definition: Fitting of a device designed to facilitate or support achievement of a higher level of function

Body System/Region Character 4	Type Qualifier Character 5	Equipment Character 6	Qualifier Character 7
Z None	Ø Tinnitus Masker	5 Hearing Aid Selection / Fitting / Test Z None	Z None
Z None	1 Monaural Hearing Aid 2 Binaural Hearing Aid 5 Assistive Listening Device	1 Audiometer 2 Sound Field / Booth 5 Hearing Aid Selection / Fitting / Test K Audiovisual L Assistive Listening Z None	Z None
Z None	3 Augmentative/Alternative Communication System	M Augmentative / Alternative Communication	Z None
Z None	4 Voice Prosthetic	S Voice Analysis V Speech Prosthesis	Z None
Z None	6 Dynamic Orthosis 7 Static Orthosis 8 Prosthesis 9 Assistive, Adaptive, Supportive or Protective Devices	E Orthosis F Assistive, Adaptive, Supportive or Protective U Prosthesis Z None	Z None

DRG Non-OR	FØDZØ[5,Z]Z
DRG Non-OR	FØDZ[1, 2,5][1,2,5, K,L,Z]Z
DRG Non-OR	FØDZ3MZ
DRG Non-OR	FØDZ4[S,V]Z
DRG Non-OR	FØDZ[6,7][E,F,U,Z]Z
DRG Non-OR	FØDZ8[E,F,U]Z

F **Physical Rehabilitation and Diagnostic Audiology**
Ø **Rehabilitation**
F **Caregiver Training**   Definition: Training in activities to support patient's optimal level of function

Body System/Region Character 4	Type Qualifier Character 5	Equipment Character 6	Qualifier Character 7
Z None	Ø Bathing/Showering Technique 1 Dressing 2 Feeding and Eating 3 Grooming/Personal Hygiene 4 Bed Mobility 5 Transfer 6 Wheelchair Mobility 7 Therapeutic Exercise 8 Airway Clearance Techniques 9 Wound Management B Vocational Activities and Functional Community or Work Reintegration Skills C Gait Training/Functional Ambulation D Application, Proper Use and Care of Devices F Application, Proper Use and Care of Orthoses G Application, Proper Use and Care of Prosthesis H Home Management	E Orthosis F Assistive, Adaptive, Supportive or Protective U Prosthesis Z None	Z None
Z None	J Communication Skills	K Audiovisual L Assistive Listening M Augmentative / Alternative Communication P Computer Z None	Z None

DRG Non-OR	All body system/region, type qualifier, equipment, and qualifier values

Physical Rehabilitation and Diagnostic Audiology

Non-OR Procedure   DRG Non-OR Procedure   Valid OR Procedure   HAC Associated Procedure   Combination Only   New/Revised April   New/Revised October
810   ICD-10-PCS 2023

F   Physical Rehabilitation and Diagnostic Audiology
1   Diagnostic Audiology
3   Hearing Assessment   Definition: Measurement of hearing and related functions

Body System/Region Character 4	Type Qualifier Character 5	Equipment Character 6	Qualifier Character 7
Z None	0 Hearing Screening	0 Occupational Hearing 1 Audiometer 2 Sound Field / Booth 3 Tympanometer 8 Vestibular / Balance 9 Cochlear Implant Z None	Z None
Z None	1 Pure Tone Audiometry, Air 2 Pure Tone Audiometry, Air and Bone	0 Occupational Hearing 1 Audiometer 2 Sound Field / Booth Z None	Z None
Z None	3 Bekesy Audiometry 6 Visual Reinforcement Audiometry 9 Short Increment Sensitivity Index B Stenger C Pure Tone Stenger	1 Audiometer 2 Sound Field / Booth Z None	Z None
Z None	4 Conditioned Play Audiometry 5 Select Picture Audiometry	1 Audiometer 2 Sound Field / Booth K Audiovisual Z None	Z None
Z None	7 Alternate Binaural or Monaural Loudness Balance	1 Audiometer K Audiovisual Z None	Z None
Z None	8 Tone Decay D Tympanometry F Eustachian Tube Function G Acoustic Reflex Patterns H Acoustic Reflex Threshold J Acoustic Reflex Decay	3 Tympanometer 4 Electroacoustic Immitance / Acoustic Reflex Z None	Z None
Z None	K Electrocochleography L Auditory Evoked Potentials	7 Electrophysiologic Z None	Z None

Z None	M Evoked Otoacoustic Emissions,
	     Screening
	N Evoked Otoacoustic Emissions,
	     Diagnostic
		6 Otoacoustic Emission (OAE)
		Z None
			Z None

Z None	P Aural Rehabilitation Status	1 Audiometer 2 Sound Field / Booth 4 Electroacoustic Immitance / Acoustic Reflex 9 Cochlear Implant K Audiovisual L Assistive Listening P Computer Z None	Z None
Z None	Q Auditory Processing	K Audiovisual P Computer Y Other Equipment Z None	Z None

NC Noncovered Procedure   LC Limited Coverage   QA Questionable OB Admit   NT New Tech Add-on   ⊞ Combination Member   ♂ Male   ♀ Female

ICD-10-PCS 2023   811

Physical Rehabilitation and Diagnostic Audiology

F   **Physical Rehabilitation and Diagnostic Audiology**
1   **Diagnostic Audiology**
4   **Hearing Aid Assessment**   Definition: Measurement of the appropriateness and/or effectiveness of a hearing device

Body System/Region Character 4	Type Qualifier Character 5	Equipment Character 6	Qualifier Character 7
Z None	**Ø** Cochlear Implant	**1** Audiometer **2** Sound Field / Booth **3** Tympanometer **4** Electroacoustic Immitance / Acoustic Reflex **5** Hearing Aid Selection / Fitting / Test **7** Electrophysiologic **9** Cochlear Implant **K** Audiovisual **L** Assistive Listening **P** Computer **Y** Other Equipment **Z** None	**Z** None

Z None	**1** Ear Canal Probe Microphone
	6 Binaural Electroacoustic Hearing
	    Aid Check
	8 Monaural Electroacoustic Hearing
	    Aid Check
		5 Hearing Aid Selection / Fitting / Test
		Z None
			Z None

Z None	**2** Monaural Hearing Aid **3** Binaural Hearing Aid	**1** Audiometer **2** Sound Field / Booth **3** Tympanometer **4** Electroacoustic Immitance / Acoustic Reflex **5** Hearing Aid Selection / Fitting / Test **K** Audiovisual **L** Assistive Listening **P** Computer **Z** None	**Z** None

Z None	**4** Assistive Listening System/Device
	    Selection
		1 Audiometer
		2 Sound Field / Booth
		3 Tympanometer
		4 Electroacoustic Immitance /
		    Acoustic Reflex
		K Audiovisual
		L Assistive Listening
		Z None
			Z None

Z None	**5** Sensory Aids	**1** Audiometer **2** Sound Field / Booth **3** Tympanometer **4** Electroacoustic Immitance / Acoustic Reflex **5** Hearing Aid Selection / Fitting / Test **K** Audiovisual **L** Assistive Listening **Z** None	**Z** None
Z None	**7** Ear Protector Attentuation	**Ø** Occupational Hearing **Z** None	**Z** None

F   **Physical Rehabilitation and Diagnostic Audiology**
1   **Diagnostic Audiology**
5   **Vestibular Assessment**   Definition: Measurement of the vestibular system and related functions

Body System/Region Character 4	Type Qualifier Character 5	Equipment Character 6	Qualifier Character 7

Z None	**Ø** Bithermal, Binaural Caloric
	    Irrigation
	1 Bithermal, Monaural Caloric
	    Irrigation
	2 Unithermal Binaural Screen
	3 Oscillating Tracking
	4 Sinusoidal Vertical Axis Rotational
	5 Dix-Hallpike Dynamic
	6 Computerized Dynamic
	    Posturography
		8 Vestibular / Balance
		Z None
			Z None

Z None	**7** Tinnitus Masker	**5** Hearing Aid Selection / Fitting / Test **Z** None	**Z** None

Non-OR Procedure   DRG Non-OR Procedure   Valid OR Procedure   HAC Associated Procedure   Combination Only   New/Revised April   New/Revised October

812   ICD-10-PCS 2023

Mental Health GZ1–GZJ

G   **Mental Health**
Z   **None**
1   **Psychological Tests**   Definition: The administration and interpretation of standardized psychological tests and measurement instruments for the assessment of psychological function

Qualifier Character 4	Qualifier Character 5	Qualifier Character 6	Qualifier Character 7
Ø Developmental 1 Personality and Behavioral 2 Intellectual and Psychoeducational 3 Neuropsychological 4 Neurobehavioral and Cognitive Status	Z None	Z None	Z None

G   **Mental Health**
Z   **None**
2   **Crisis Intervention**   Definition: Treatment of a traumatized, acutely disturbed or distressed individual for the purpose of short-term stabilization

Qualifier Character 4	Qualifier Character 5	Qualifier Character 6	Qualifier Character 7
Z None	Z None	Z None	Z None

G   **Mental Health**
Z   **None**
3   **Medication Management**   Definition: Monitoring and adjusting the use of medications for the treatment of a mental health disorder

Qualifier Character 4	Qualifier Character 5	Qualifier Character 6	Qualifier Character 7
Z None	Z None	Z None	Z None

G   **Mental Health**
Z   **None**
5   **Individual Psychotherapy**   Definition: Treatment of an individual with a mental health disorder by behavioral, cognitive, psychoanalytic, psychodynamic or psychophysiological means to improve functioning or well-being

Qualifier Character 4	Qualifier Character 5	Qualifier Character 6	Qualifier Character 7
Ø Interactive 1 Behavioral 2 Cognitive 3 Interpersonal 4 Psychoanalysis 5 Psychodynamic 6 Supportive 8 Cognitive-Behavioral 9 Psychophysiological	Z None	Z None	Z None

G   **Mental Health**
Z   **None**
6   **Counseling**   Definition: The application of psychological methods to treat an individual with normal developmental issues and psychological problems in order to increase function, improve well-being, alleviate distress, maladjustment or resolve crises

Qualifier Character 4	Qualifier Character 5	Qualifier Character 6	Qualifier Character 7
Ø Educational 1 Vocational 3 Other Counseling	Z None	Z None	Z None

G   **Mental Health**
Z   **None**
7   **Family Psychotherapy**   Definition: Treatment that includes one or more family members of an individual with a mental health disorder by behavioral, cognitive, psychoanalytic, psychodynamic or psychophysiological means to improve functioning or well-being

Explanation: Remediation of emotional or behavioral problems presented by one or more family members in cases where psychotherapy with more than one family member is indicated

Qualifier Character 4	Qualifier Character 5	Qualifier Character 6	Qualifier Character 7
2 Other Family Psychotherapy	Z None	Z None	Z None

NC Noncovered Procedure   **LC** Limited Coverage   **QA** Questionable OB Admit   **NT** New Tech Add-on   ⊞ Combination Member   ♂ Male   ♀ Female

Mental Health

G   **Mental Health**
Z   **None**
B   **Electroconvulsive Therapy**   Definition: The application of controlled electrical voltages to treat a mental health disorder

Qualifier Character 4	Qualifier Character 5	Qualifier Character 6	Qualifier Character 7
Ø Unilateral-Single Seizure	Z None	Z None	Z None
1 Unilateral-Multiple Seizure			
2 Bilateral-Single Seizure			
3 Bilateral-Multiple Seizure			
4 Other Electroconvulsive Therapy			

G   **Mental Health**
Z   **None**
C   **Biofeedback**   Definition: Provision of information from the monitoring and regulating of physiological processes in conjunction with cognitive-behavioral techniques to improve patient functioning or well-being

Qualifier Character 4	Qualifier Character 5	Qualifier Character 6	Qualifier Character 7
9 Other Biofeedback	Z None	Z None	Z None

G   **Mental Health**
Z   **None**
F   **Hypnosis**   Definition: Induction of a state of heightened suggestibility by auditory, visual and tactile techniques to elicit an emotional or behavioral response

Qualifier Character 4	Qualifier Character 5	Qualifier Character 6	Qualifier Character 7
Z None	Z None	Z None	Z None

G   **Mental Health**
Z   **None**
G   **Narcosynthesis**   Definition: Administration of intravenous barbiturates in order to release suppressed or repressed thoughts

Qualifier Character 4	Qualifier Character 5	Qualifier Character 6	Qualifier Character 7
Z None	Z None	Z None	Z None

G   **Mental Health**
Z   **None**
H   **Group Psychotherapy**   Definition: Treatment of two or more individuals with a mental health disorder by behavioral, cognitive, psychoanalytic, psychodynamic or psychophysiological means to improve functioning or well-being

Qualifier Character 4	Qualifier Character 5	Qualifier Character 6	Qualifier Character 7
Z None	Z None	Z None	Z None

G   **Mental Health**
Z   **None**
J   **Light Therapy**   Definition: Application of specialized light treatments to improve functioning or well-being

Qualifier Character 4	Qualifier Character 5	Qualifier Character 6	Qualifier Character 7
Z None	Z None	Z None	Z None

Non-OR Procedure   DRG Non-OR Procedure   Valid OR Procedure   HAC Associated Procedure   Combination Only   New/Revised April   New/Revised October

814   ICD-10-PCS 2023

Substance Abuse Treatment HZ2–HZ9

AHA Coding Clinic for table HZ2
2020, 1Q, 21   Inpatient detoxification services

AHA Coding Clinic for table HZ9
2020, 1Q, 21   Inpatient detoxification services

H   Substance Abuse Treatment
Z   None
2   Detoxification Services   Definition: Detoxification from alcohol and/or drugs

Explanation: Not a treatment modality, but helps the patient stabilize physically and psychologically until the body becomes free of drugs and the effects of alcohol

Qualifier Character 4	Qualifier Character 5	Qualifier Character 6	Qualifier Character 7
Z None	Z None	Z None	Z None

H   Substance Abuse Treatment
Z   None
3   Individual Counseling   Definition: The application of psychological methods to treat an individual with addictive behavior

Explanation: Comprised of several different techniques, which apply various strategies to address drug addiction

Qualifier Character 4	Qualifier Character 5	Qualifier Character 6	Qualifier Character 7
Ø Cognitive 1 Behavioral 2 Cognitive-Behavioral 3 12-Step 4 Interpersonal 5 Vocational 6 Psychoeducation 7 Motivational Enhancement 8 Confrontational 9 Continuing Care B Spiritual C Pre/Post-Test Infectious Disease	Z None	Z None	Z None

DRG Non-OR   HZ3[Ø,1,2,3,4,5,6,7,8,9,B]ZZZ

H   Substance Abuse Treatment
Z   None
4   Group Counseling   Definition: The application of psychological methods to treat two or more individuals with addictive behavior

Explanation: Provides structured group counseling sessions and healing power through the connection with others

Qualifier Character 4	Qualifier Character 5	Qualifier Character 6	Qualifier Character 7
Ø Cognitive 1 Behavioral 2 Cognitive-Behavioral 3 12-Step 4 Interpersonal 5 Vocational 6 Psychoeducation 7 Motivational Enhancement 8 Confrontational 9 Continuing Care B Spiritual C Pre/Post-Test Infectious Disease	Z None	Z None	Z None

DRG Non-OR   HZ4[Ø,1,2,3,4,5,6,7,8,9,B]ZZZ

NC Noncovered Procedure   LC Limited Coverage   ØA Questionable OB Admit   NT New Tech Add-on   ⊞ Combination Member   ♂ Male   ♀ Female

ICD-10-PCS 2023   815

H   **Substance Abuse Treatment**
Z   **None**
5   **Individual Psychotherapy**   Definition: Treatment of an individual with addictive behavior by behavioral, cognitive, psychoanalytic, psychodynamic or psychophysiological means

Qualifier Character 4	Qualifier Character 5	Qualifier Character 6	Qualifier Character 7
Ø Cognitive	Z None	Z None	Z None
1 Behavioral			
2 Cognitive-Behavioral			
3 12-Step			
4 Interpersonal			
5 Interactive			
6 Psychoeducation			
7 Motivational Enhancement			
8 Confrontational			
9 Supportive			
B Psychoanalysis			
C Psychodynamic			
D Psychophysiological			

DRG Non-OR   For all qualifier values

H   **Substance Abuse Treatment**
Z   **None**
6   **Family Counseling**   Definition: The application of psychological methods that includes one or more family members to treat an individual with addictive behavior

Explanation: Provides support and education for family members of addicted individuals. Family member participation is seen as a critical area of substance abuse treatment

Qualifier Character 4	Qualifier Character 5	Qualifier Character 6	Qualifier Character 7
3 Other Family Counseling	Z None	Z None	Z None

H   **Substance Abuse Treatment**
Z   **None**
8   **Medication Management**   Definition: Monitoring or adjusting the use of replacement medications for the treatment of addiction

Qualifier Character 4	Qualifier Character 5	Qualifier Character 6	Qualifier Character 7
Ø Nicotine Replacement	Z None	Z None	Z None
1 Methadone Maintenance			
2 Levo-alpha-acetyl-methadol (LAAM)			
3 Antabuse			
4 Naltrexone			
5 Naloxone			
6 Clonidine			
7 Bupropion			
8 Psychiatric Medication			
9 Other Replacement Medication			

H   **Substance Abuse Treatment**
Z   **None**
9   **Pharmacotherapy**   Definition: The use of replacement medications for the treatment of addiction

Qualifier Character 4	Qualifier Character 5	Qualifier Character 6	Qualifier Character 7
Ø Nicotine Replacement	Z None	Z None	Z None
1 Methadone Maintenance			
2 Levo-alpha-acetyl-methadol (LAAM)			
3 Antabuse			
4 Naltrexone			
5 Naloxone			
6 Clonidine			
7 Bupropion			
8 Psychiatric Medication			
9 Other Replacement Medication			

New Technology X27–XY0

AHA Coding Clinic for all tables in the New Technology Section
2015, 4Q, 8-11   New Section X codes - New Technology procedures

AHA Coding Clinic for table X27
2019, 4Q, 45-46   Sustained released drug-eluting stent

AHA Coding Clinic for table X2A
2021, 1Q, 16   Placement of Sentinel™ embolic protection device with deployment of single filter
2020, 4Q, 70-71   Cerebral embolic filtration extracorporeal flow reversal circuit
2019, 4Q, 46   Cerebral embolic filtration
2016, 4Q, 115-116 Cerebral embolic filtration

AHA Coding Clinic for table X2C
2021, 4Q, 58-59   Computer-aided mechanical aspiration thrombectomy
2016, 4Q, 82-83   Coronary artery, number of arteries
2015, 4Q, 8-14   New Section X codes—New Technology procedures

AHA Coding Clinic for table X2J
2021, 4Q, 59   Transthoracic echocardiography with computer-aided image acquisition

AHA Coding Clinic for table X2K
2021, 4Q, 60   Percutaneous creation of arteriovenous fistula using thermal resistance energy

AHA Coding Clinic for table X2R
2021, 4Q, 61-62   Replacement combined with restriction of descending thoracic aorta
2016, 4Q, 116   Aortic valve rapid deployment
2015, 4Q, 8-12   New Section X codes—New Technology procedures

AHA Coding Clinic for table X2V
2021, 4Q, 61-62   Replacement combined with restriction of descending thoracic aorta
2021, 4Q, 63   Restriction of coronary sinus

AHA Coding Clinic for table XD2
2021, 4Q, 63-64   Monitoring of tissue oxygen saturation in gastrointestinal tract

AHA Coding Clinic for table XDP
2021, 4Q, 64-65   Colonic irrigation for colonoscopy

AHA Coding Clinic for table XFJ
2021, 4Q, 65-66   Single-use duodenoscope during endoscopic retrograde cholangiopancreatography

AHA Coding Clinic for table XHR
2021, 4Q, 66   Application of bioengineered allogeneic construct
2016, 4Q, 116   Application of wound matrix

AHA Coding Clinic for table XK0
2017, 4Q, 74   Intramuscular autologous bone marrow cell therapy

AHA Coding Clinic for table XNS
2021, 4Q, 67   Posterior dynamic distraction
2017, 4Q, 74-75   Magnetic growth rods
2016, 4Q, 117   Placement of magnetic growth rods

AHA Coding Clinic for table XNU
2020, 4Q, 72   Implantation of vertebral mechanically expandable device

AHA Coding Clinic for table XRG
2021, 4Q, 68   Customizable interbody fusion
2017, 4Q, 76   Radiolucent porous interbody fusion device

AHA Coding Clinic for table XT2
2019, 4Q, 46-47   Renal function monitoring

AHA Coding Clinic for table XV5
2018, 4Q, 55   Robotic waterjet ablation

AHA Coding Clinic for table XW0
2022, 1Q, 5-6   COVID-19 vaccine administration
2022, 1Q, 7   Fostamatinib
2022, 1Q, 7-8   Tixagevimab and cilgavimab
2022, 1Q, 8   Other monoclonal antibody
2021, 4Q, 69-71   Introduction of new therapeutic substances
2021, 4Q, 71-74   Chimeric antigen receptor T-cell immunotherapy
2021, 4Q, 74-75   Antibiotic-eluting bone void filler
2021, 4Q, 110   New/revised frequently asked questions regarding ICD-10-CM/PCS coding for COVID-19
2021, 1Q, 49   Frequently asked questions regarding ICD-10-CM and ICD-10-PCS coding for COVID-19
2020, 4Q, 72-76   Introduction of new therapeutic substances
2020, 4Q, 95   Frequently asked questions regarding ICD-10-PCS coding for COVID-19
2020, 3Q, 17-21   New procedure codes for introduction or infusion of therapeutics
2019, 4Q, 47-50   New therapeutic substances
2018, 4Q, 56   New therapeutic substances
2015, 4Q, 8-15   New Section X codes—New Technology procedures

AHA Coding Clinic for table XW1
2021, 4Q, 76   Transfusion of hyperimmune globulin and high-dose immune globulin
2020, 3Q, 17-21   New procedure codes for introduction or infusion of therapeutics

AHA Coding Clinic for table XWH
2021, 4Q, 76-77   Pharyngeal electrical stimulation

AHA Coding Clinic for table XXE
2021, 4Q, 77   Computer-aided assessment of intracranial vascular activity
2021, 4Q, 77-78   Computer-aided triage and notification of pulmonary artery flow
2021, 4Q, 78-79   Mechanical initial specimen diversion of whole blood using active negative pressure
2021, 4Q, 79-80   Concurrent measurement of mRNA, PCR test and detection of antibodies
2020, 4Q, 78-79   Measurement of infection
2020, 4Q, 78-79   Positive blood culture fluorescence hybridization
2020, 4Q, 79   Nucleic acid-base microbial detection
2019, 4Q, 50-51   Whole blood nucleic acid-base microbial detection

AHA Coding Clinic for table XY0
2021, 4Q, 80   Regional anticoagulation for renal replacement therapy
2017, 4Q, 78   Intraoperative treatment of vascular grafts

X   **New Technology**
0   **Nervous System**
H   **Insertion**   Definition: Putting in a nonbiological appliance that monitors, assists, performs, or prevents a physiological function but does not physically take the place of a body part
     Explanation: None

Body Part Character 4	Approach Character 5	Device/Substance/Technology Character 6	Qualifier Character 7
K Sphenopalatine Ganglion	3 Percutaneous	Q Neurostimulator Lead	8 New Technology Group 8
Q Vagus Nerve	3 Percutaneous	R Neurostimulator Lead with Paired Stimulation System	8 New Technology Group 8

X   **New Technology**
0   **Nervous System**
Z   **Other Procedures**   Definition: Methodologies which attempt to remediate or cure a disorder or disease
     Explanation: None

Body Part Character 4	Approach Character 5	Device/Substance/Technology Character 6	Qualifier Character 7
0 Prefrontal Cortex	X External	1 Computer-assisted Transcranial Magnetic Stimulation	8 New Technology Group 8

NC Noncovered Procedure   **LC** Limited Coverage   **QA** Questionable OB Admit   **NT** New Tech Add-on   ✚ Combination Member   ♂ Male   ♀ Female

ICD-10-PCS 2023   **817**

X **New Technology**
2 **Cardiovascular System**
7 **Dilation**   Definition: Expanding an orifice or the lumen of a tubular body part

                     Explanation: The orifice can be a natural orifice or an artificially created orifice. Accomplished by stretching a tubular body part using intraluminal pressure or by cutting part of the orifice or wall of the tubular body part.

Body Part Character 4	Approach Character 5	Device/Substance/Technology Character 6	Qualifier Character 7
H Femoral Artery, Right **J** Femoral Artery, Left **K** Popliteal Artery, Proximal Right **L** Popliteal Artery, Proximal Left **M** Popliteal Artery, Distal Right **N** Popliteal Artery, Distal Left **P** Anterior Tibial Artery, Right **Q** Anterior Tibial Artery, Left **R** Posterior Tibial Artery, Right **S** Posterior Tibial Artery, Left **T** Peroneal Artery, Right **U** Peroneal Artery, Left	**3** Percutaneous	**8** Intraluminal Device, Sustained Release Drug-eluting **9** Intraluminal Device, Sustained Release Drug-eluting, Two **B** Intraluminal Device, Sustained Release Drug-eluting, Three **C** Intraluminal Device, Sustained Release Drug-eluting, Four or More	**5** New Technology Group 5

Valid OR   All body part, approach, device/substance/technology, and qualifier values

---

X **New Technology**
2 **Cardiovascular System**
A **Assistance**   Definition: Taking over a portion of a physiological function by extracorporeal means

                     Explanation: None

Body Part Character 4	Approach Character 5	Device/Substance/Technology Character 6	Qualifier Character 7
5 Innominate Artery and Left Common Carotid Artery	**3** Percutaneous	**1** Cerebral Embolic Filtration, Dual Filter	**2** New Technology Group 2
6 Aortic Arch	**3** Percutaneous	**2** Cerebral Embolic Filtration, Single Deflection Filter	**5** New Technology Group 5
7 Coronary Sinus	**3** Percutaneous	**5** Intermittent Coronary Sinus Occlusion	**8** New Technology Group 8
H Common Carotid Artery, Right **J** Common Carotid Artery, Left	**3** Percutaneous	**3** Cerebral Embolic Filtration, Extracorporeal Flow Reversal Circuit	**6** New Technology Group 6

DRG Non-OR   X2A7358

X **New Technology**
2 **Cardiovascular System**
C **Extirpation**   Definition: Taking or cutting out solid matter from a body part

                     Explanation: The solid matter may be an abnormal byproduct of a biological function or a foreign body; it may be imbedded in a body part or in the lumen of a tubular body part. The solid matter may or may not have been previously broken into pieces.

Body Part Character 4	Approach Character 5	Device/Substance/Technology Character 6	Qualifier Character 7
P Abdominal Aorta **Q** Upper Extremity Vein, Right **R** Upper Extremity Vein, Left **S** Lower Extremity Artery, Right **T** Lower Extremity Artery, Left **U** Lower Extremity Vein, Right **V** Lower Extremity Vein, Left **Y** Great Vessel	**3** Percutaneous	**T** Computer-aided Mechanical Aspiration	**7** New Technology Group 7

Valid OR   All body part, approach, device/substance/technology, and qualifier values

---

X **New Technology**
2 **Cardiovascular System**
J **Inspection**   Definition: Visually and/or manually exploring a body part

                     Explanation: None

Body Part Character 4	Approach Character 5	Device/Substance/Technology Character 6	Qualifier Character 7
A Heart	**X** External	**4** Transthoracic Echocardiography, Computer-aided Guidance **NT**	**7** New Technology Group 7

NT   X2JAX47 for Caption Guidance™

X **New Technology**
2 **Cardiovascular System**
K **Bypass**   Definition: Altering the route of passage of the contents of a tubular body part

                     Explanation: None

Body Part Character 4	Approach Character 5	Device/Substance/Technology Character 6	Qualifier Character 7
B Radial Artery, Right **C** Radial Artery, Left	**3** Percutaneous	**1** Thermal Resistance Energy	**7** New Technology Group 7

Valid OR   All body part, approach, device/substance/technology, and qualifier values

---

Non-OR Procedure   DRG Non-OR Procedure   Valid OR Procedure   HAC Associated Procedure   Combination Only   New/Revised April   New/Revised October

818   ICD-10-PCS 2023

X   **New Technology**
2   **Cardiovascular System**
R   **Replacement**   Definition: Putting in or on biological or synthetic material that physically takes the place and/or function of all or a portion of a body part
                        Explanation: None

Body Part Character 4	Approach Character 5	Device/Substance/Technology Character 6	Qualifier Character 7
X Thoracic Aorta, Arch	Ø Open	N Branched Synthetic Substitute with Intraluminal Device	7 New Technology Group 7

   Valid OR   All body part, approach, device/substance/technology, and qualifier values

X   **New Technology**
2   **Cardiovascular System**
V   **Restriction**   Definition: Partially closing an orifice or the lumen of a tubular body part
                        Explanation: None

Body Part Character 4	Approach Character 5	Device/Substance/Technology Character 6	Qualifier Character 7
7 Coronary Sinus	3 Percutaneous	Q Reduction Device	7 New Technology Group 7
W Thoracic Aorta, Descending	Ø Open	N Branched Synthetic Substitute with Intraluminal Device	7 New Technology Group 7

   Valid OR   All body part, approach, device/substance/technology, and qualifier values

X   **New Technology**
D   **Gastrointestinal System**
2   **Monitoring**   Definition: Determining the level of a physiological or physical function repetitively over a period of time
                        Explanation: None

Body Part Character 4	Approach Character 5	Device/Substance/Technology Character 6	Qualifier Character 7
G Upper GI H Lower GI	4 Percutaneous Endoscopic 8 Via Natural or Artificial Opening Endoscopic	V Oxygen Saturation	7 New Technology Group 7

X   **New Technology**
D   **Gastrointestinal System**
P   **Irrigation**   Definition: Putting in or on a cleansing substance
                        Explanation: None

Body Part Character 4	Approach Character 5	Device/Substance/Technology Character 6	Qualifier Character 7
H Lower GI	8 Via Natural or Artificial Opening Endoscopic	K Intraoperative Single-use Oversleeve	7 New Technology Group 7

X   **New Technology**
F   **Hepatobiliary System and Pancreas**
5   **Destruction**   Definition: Physical eradication of all or a portion of a body part by the direct use of energy, force, or a destructive agent
                        Explanation: None of the body part is physically taken out

Body Part Character 4	Approach Character 5	Device/Substance/Technology Character 6	Qualifier Character 7
Ø Liver 1 Liver, Right Lobe 2 Liver, Left Lobe	X External	Ø Ultrasound-guided Cavitation	8 New Technology Group 8

   DRG Non-OR   All body part, approach, device/substance/technology, and qualifier values

X   **New Technology**
F   **Hepatobiliary System and Pancreas**
J   **Inspection**   Definition: Visually and/or manually exploring a body part
                        Explanation: None

Body Part Character 4	Approach Character 5	Device/Substance/Technology Character 6	Qualifier Character 7
B Hepatobiliary Duct D Pancreatic Duct	8 Via Natural or Artificial Opening Endoscopic	A Single-use Duodenoscope **NT**	7 New Technology Group 7

   NT   XFJ[B,D]8A7 for aScope® Duodeno

NC Noncovered Procedure   **LC** Limited Coverage   **QA** Questionable OB Admit   **NT** New Tech Add-on   **⊞** Combination Member   ♂ Male   ♀ Female

ICD-10-PCS 2023   819

X New Technology
H Skin, Subcutaneous Tissue, Fascia and Breast
R Replacement   Definition: Putting in or on biological or synthetic material that physically takes the place and/or function of all or a portion of a body part
                    Explanation: None

Body Part Character 4	Approach Character 5	Device/Substance/Technology Character 6	Qualifier Character 7
P Skin	**X** External	**F** Bioengineered Allogeneic **NT** Construct	**7** New Technology Group 7

Valid OR	XHRPXF7
NT	XHRPXF7 for StrataGraft®

X New Technology
K Muscles, Tendons, Bursae and Ligaments
U Supplement   Definition: Putting in or on biological or synthetic material that physically reinforces and/or augments the function of a portion of a body part
                    Explanation: None

Body Part Character 4	Approach Character 5	Device/Substance/Technology Character 6	Qualifier Character 7
C Upper Spine Bursa and Ligament **D** Lower Spine Bursa and Ligament	**Ø** Open	**6** Posterior Vertebral Tether	**8** New Technology Group 8

X New Technology
N Bones
H Insertion   Definition: Putting in a nonbiological appliance that monitors, assists, performs, or prevents a physiological function but does not physically take the place of a body part
                  Explanation: None

Body Part Character 4	Approach Character 5	Device/Substance/Technology Character 6	Qualifier Character 7
6 Pelvic Bone, Right **7** Pelvic Bone, Left	**Ø** Open **3** Percutaneous	**5** Internal Fixation Device with Tulip Connector	**8** New Technology Group 8

X New Technology
N Bones
S Reposition   Definition: Moving to its normal location, or other suitable location, all or a portion of a body part
                   Explanation: The body part is moved to a new location from an abnormal location, or from a normal location where it is not functioning correctly. The body part may or may not be cut out or off to be moved to the new location.

Body Part Character 4	Approach Character 5	Device/Substance/Technology Character 6	Qualifier Character 7
Ø Lumbar Vertebra	**Ø** Open	**3** Magnetically Controlled Growth Rod(s)	**2** New Technology Group 2
Ø Lumbar Vertebra	**Ø** Open	**C** Posterior (Dynamic) Distraction Device	**7** New Technology Group 7
Ø Lumbar Vertebra	**3** Percutaneous	**3** Magnetically Controlled Growth Rod(s)	**2** New Technology Group 2
Ø Lumbar Vertebra	**3** Percutaneous	**C** Posterior (Dynamic) Distraction Device	**7** New Technology Group 7
3 Cervical Vertebra	**Ø** Open **3** Percutaneous	**3** Magnetically Controlled Growth Rod(s)	**2** New Technology Group 2
4 Thoracic Vertebra	**Ø** Open	**3** Magnetically Controlled Growth Rod(s)	**2** New Technology Group 2
4 Thoracic Vertebra	**Ø** Open	**C** Posterior (Dynamic) Distraction Device	**7** New Technology Group 7
4 Thoracic Vertebra	**3** Percutaneous	**3** Magnetically Controlled Growth Rod(s)	**2** New Technology Group 2
4 Thoracic Vertebra	**3** Percutaneous	**C** Posterior (Dynamic) Distraction Device	**7** New Technology Group 7

Valid OR	All body part, approach, device/substance/technology, and qualifier values

X New Technology
N Bones
U Supplement   Definition: Putting in or on biological or synthetic material that physically reinforces and/or augments the function of a portion of a body part
                    Explanation: None

Body Part Character 4	Approach Character 5	Device/Substance/Technology Character 6	Qualifier Character 7
Ø Lumbar Vertebra **4** Thoracic Vertebra	**3** Percutaneous	**5** Synthetic Substitute, Mechanically Expandable (Paired)	**6** New Technology Group 6

Valid OR	XNU[Ø,4]356

X New Technology
R Joints
G Fusion Definition: Joining together portions of an articular body part rendering the articular body part immobile
Explanation: None

Body Part Character 4	Approach Character 5	Device/Substance/Technology Character 6	Qualifier Character 7
A Thoracolumbar Vertebral Joint	Ø Open	R Interbody Fusion Device, NT Customizable	7 New Technology Group 7
B Lumbar Vertebral Joint	3 Percutaneous		
C Lumbar Vertebral Joints, 2 or more ⊞	4 Percutaneous Endoscopic		
D Lumbosacral Joint			
E Sacroiliac Joint, Right	Ø Open	5 Internal Fixation Device with Tulip	8 New Technology Group 8
F Sacroiliac Joint, Left	3 Percutaneous	Connector	

Valid OR XRG[A,B,C,D][Ø,3,4]R7
HAC XRG[A,B,C,D][Ø,3,4]R7 when reported with SDx K68.11 or T81.4Ø-T81.49,
T84.6Ø-T84.619, T84.63-T84.7 with 7th character A
NT XRG[A,B,C,D][Ø,3,4]R7 for aprevo® Intervertebral Body Fusion Device

See Appendix L for Procedure Combinations
⊞ XRGC[Ø,3,4]R7

X New Technology
R Joints
H Insertion Definition: Putting in a nonbiological appliance that monitors, assists, performs, or prevents a physiological function but does not physically take the place of a body part
Explanation: None

Body Part Character 4	Approach Character 5	Device/Substance/Technology Character 6	Qualifier Character 7
B Lumbar Vertebral Joint	Ø Open	1 Posterior Spinal Motion Preservation Device	8 New Technology Group 8
D Lumbosacral Joint			

X New Technology
R Joints
R Replacement Definition: Putting in or on biological or synthetic material that physically takes the place and/or function of all or a portion of a body part
Explanation: None

Body Part Character 4	Approach Character 5	Device/Substance/Technology Character 6	Qualifier Character 7
G Knee Joint, Right ⊞	Ø Open	L Synthetic Substitute, Lateral Meniscus	8 New Technology Group 8
H Knee Joint, Left ⊞		M Synthetic Substitute, Medial Meniscus	

Valid OR All body part, approach, device/substance/technology, and qualifier values
HAC XRR[G,H]Ø[L,M]8 when reported with SDx of I26.Ø2-I26.Ø9, I26.92-I26.99, or I82.4Ø1-I82.4Z9

See Appendix L for Procedure Combinations
⊞ XRR[G,H]Ø[L,M]8

X New Technology
T Urinary System
2 Monitoring Definition: Determining the level of a physiological or physical function repetitively over a period of time
Explanation: None

Body Part Character 4	Approach Character 5	Device/Substance/Technology Character 6	Qualifier Character 7
5 Kidney	X External	E Fluorescent Pyrazine	5 New Technology Group 5

X New Technology
V Male Reproductive System
5 Destruction Definition: Physical eradication of all or a portion of a body part by the direct use of energy, force, or a destructive agent
Explanation: None of the body part is physically taken out

Body Part Character 4	Approach Character 5	Device/Substance/Technology Character 6	Qualifier Character 7
Ø Prostate	8 Via Natural or Artificial Opening Endoscopic	A Robotic Waterjet Ablation	4 New Technology Group 4

Valid OR All body part, approach, device/substance/technology, and qualifier values

X **New Technology**
W **Anatomical Regions**
0 **Introduction** Definition: Putting in or on a therapeutic, diagnostic, nutritional, physiological, or prophylactic substance except blood or blood products
　　　　　　　　　Explanation: None

Body Part Character 4	Approach Character 5	Device/Substance/Technology Character 6	Qualifier Character 7
0 Skin	**X** External	**2** Bromelain-enriched Proteolytic Enzyme	**7** New Technology Group 7
1 Subcutaneous Tissue	3 Percutaneous	1 Daratumumab and Hyaluronidase-fihj 4 Teclistamab Antineoplastic	8 New Technology Group 8
1 Subcutaneous Tissue	**3** Percutaneous	**9** Satralizumab-mwge	**7** New Technology Group 7
1 Subcutaneous Tissue	**3** Percutaneous	**F** Other New Technology Therapeutic Substance	**5** New Technology Group 5
1 Subcutaneous Tissue	**3** Percutaneous	**H** Other New Technology Monoclonal Antibody **K** Leronlimab Monoclonal Antibody **S** COVID-19 Vaccine Dose 1 **T** COVID-19 Vaccine Dose 2 **U** COVID-19 Vaccine	**6** New Technology Group 6
1 Subcutaneous Tissue	**3** Percutaneous	**V** COVID-19 Vaccine Dose 3	**7** New Technology Group 7
1 Subcutaneous Tissue	**3** Percutaneous	**W** Caplacizumab	**5** New Technology Group 5
1 Subcutaneous Tissue	**3** Percutaneous	**W** COVID-19 Vaccine Booster	**7** New Technology Group 7
1 Subcutaneous Tissue	**X** External	**2** Bromelain-enriched Proteolytic Enzyme	**7** New Technology Group 7
2 Muscle	0 Open	D Engineered Allogeneic Thymus Tissue	8 New Technology Group 8
2 Muscle	**3** Percutaneous	**S** COVID-19 Vaccine Dose 1 **T** COVID-19 Vaccine Dose 2 **U** COVID-19 Vaccine	**6** New Technology Group 6
2 Muscle	**3** Percutaneous	**V** COVID-19 Vaccine Dose 3 **W** COVID-19 Vaccine Booster **X** Tixagevimab and Cilgavimab Monoclonal 　 Antibody **Y** Other New Technology Monoclonal Antibody	**7** New Technology Group 7
3 Peripheral Vein	**3** Percutaneous	**0** Brexanolone	**6** New Technology Group 6
3 Peripheral Vein	3 Percutaneous	0 Spesolimab Monoclonal Antibody	8 New Technology Group 8
3 Peripheral Vein	**3** Percutaneous	**2** Nerinitide **3** Durvalumab Antineoplastic	**6** New Technology Group 6
3 Peripheral Vein	**3** Percutaneous	**5** Narsoplimab Monoclonal Antibody	**7** New Technology Group 7
3 Peripheral Vein	3 Percutaneous	5 Mosunetuzumab Antineoplastic	8 New Technology Group 8
3 Peripheral Vein	**3** Percutaneous	**6** Lefamulin Anti-infective	**6** New Technology Group 6
3 Peripheral Vein	**3** Percutaneous	**6** Terlipressin	**7** New Technology Group 7
3 Peripheral Vein	3 Percutaneous	6 Afamitresgene Autoleucel Immunotherapy	8 New Technology Group 8
3 Peripheral Vein	**3** Percutaneous	**7** Coagulation Factor Xa, Inactivated	**2** New Technology Group 2
3 Peripheral Vein	**3** Percutaneous	**7** Trilaciclib　　　　　　　NT	**7** New Technology Group 7
3 Peripheral Vein	3 Percutaneous	7 Tabelecleucel Immunotherapy	8 New Technology Group 8
3 Peripheral Vein	**3** Percutaneous	**8** Lurbinectedin　　　　　NT	**7** New Technology Group 7
3 Peripheral Vein	3 Percutaneous	8 Treosulfan	8 New Technology Group 8
3 Peripheral Vein	**3** Percutaneous	**9** Ceftolozane/Tazobactam Anti-infective	**6** New Technology Group 6
3 Peripheral Vein	3 Percutaneous	9 Inebilizumab-cdon	8 New Technology Group 8
3 Peripheral Vein	**3** Percutaneous	**A** Cefiderocol Anti-infective　　NT	**6** New Technology Group 6
3 Peripheral Vein	**3** Percutaneous	**A** Ciltacabtagene Autoleucel	**7** New Technology Group 7
3 Peripheral Vein	**3** Percutaneous	**B** Cytarabine and Daunorubicin Liposome Antineoplastic	**3** New Technology Group 3
3 Peripheral Vein	**3** Percutaneous	**B** Omadacycline Anti-infective	**6** New Technology Group 6
3 Peripheral Vein	**3** Percutaneous	**B** Amivantamab Monoclonal Antibody　NT	**7** New Technology Group 7
3 Peripheral Vein	**3** Percutaneous	**C** Eculizumab	**6** New Technology Group 6
3 Peripheral Vein	**3** Percutaneous	**C** Engineered Chimeric Antigen Receptor T-cell Immunotherapy, Autologous	**7** New Technology Group 7
3 Peripheral Vein	**3** Percutaneous	**D** Atezolizumab Antineoplastic	**6** New Technology Group 6
3 Peripheral Vein	**3** Percutaneous	**E** Remdesivir Anti-infective　　NT	**5** New Technology Group 5
3 Peripheral Vein	**3** Percutaneous	**E** Etesevimab Monoclonal Antibody	**6** New Technology Group 6
3 Peripheral Vein	**3** Percutaneous	**F** Other New Technology Therapeutic Substance	**3** New Technology Group 3
3 Peripheral Vein	**3** Percutaneous	**F** Other New Technology Therapeutic Substance	**5** New Technology Group 5

DRG Non-OR　XW033A7
DRG Non-OR　XW033C7
　　　　　NT　XW03377
　　　　　NT　XW03387
　　　　　NT　XW033A6 in combination with dx code Y95 and one of the following: J14, J15.0, J15.1, J15.5, J15.6, J15.8, OR dx code J95.851
　　　　　　　　and one of the following: B96.1, B96.20, B96.21, B96.22, B96.23, B96.29, B96.3, B96.5, or B96.89
　　　　　NT　XW033B7
　　　　　NT　XW033E5

* For all codes with NT icon *see* Appendix I for registered or trade name of substance

XW0 Continued on next page

X New Technology
W Anatomical Regions
Ø Introduction   Definition: Putting in or on a therapeutic, diagnostic, nutritional, physiological, or prophylactic substance except blood or blood products

XWØ Continued

Explanation: None

Body Part Character 4	Approach Character 5	Device/Substance/Technology Character 6	Qualifier Character 7
3 Peripheral Vein	3 Percutaneous	F Bamlanivimab Monoclonal Antibody	6 New Technology Group 6
3 Peripheral Vein	3 Percutaneous	G Plazomicin Anti-infective	4 New Technology Group 4
3 Peripheral Vein	3 Percutaneous	G Sarilumab	5 New Technology Group 5
3 Peripheral Vein	3 Percutaneous	G REGN-COV2 Monoclonal Antibody	6 New Technology Group 6
3 Peripheral Vein	3 Percutaneous	G Engineered Chimeric Antigen Receptor T-cell Immunotherapy, Allogeneic	7 New Technology Group 7
3 Peripheral Vein	3 Percutaneous	H Synthetic Human Angiotensin II	4 New Technology Group 4
3 Peripheral Vein	3 Percutaneous	H Tocilizumab	5 New Technology Group 5
3 Peripheral Vein	3 Percutaneous	H Other New Technology Monoclonal Antibody	6 New Technology Group 6
3 Peripheral Vein	3 Percutaneous	H Axicabtagene Ciloleucel Immunotherapy J Tisagenlecleucel Immunotherapy	7 New Technology Group 7
3 Peripheral Vein	3 Percutaneous	K Fosfomycin Anti-infective	5 New Technology Group 5
3 Peripheral Vein	3 Percutaneous	K Idecabtagene Vicleucel Immunotherapy NT	7 New Technology Group 7
3 Peripheral Vein	3 Percutaneous	L CD24Fc Immunomodulator	6 New Technology Group 6
3 Peripheral Vein	3 Percutaneous	L Lifileucel Immunotherapy M Brexucabtagene Autoleucel Immunotherapy NT	7 New Technology Group 7
3 Peripheral Vein	3 Percutaneous	N Meropenem-vaborbactam Anti-infective	5 New Technology Group 5
3 Peripheral Vein	3 Percutaneous	N Lisocabtagene Maraleucel Immunotherapy	7 New Technology Group 7
3 Peripheral Vein	3 Percutaneous	Q Tagraxofusp-erzs Antineoplastic S Iobenguane I-131 Antineoplastic U Imipenem-cilastatin-relebactam Anti-infective NT W Caplacizumab	5 New Technology Group 5
4 Central Vein	3 Percutaneous	Ø Brexanolone	6 New Technology Group 6
4 Central Vein	3 Percutaneous	Ø Spesolimab Monoclonal Antibody	8 New Technology Group 8
4 Central Vein	3 Percutaneous	2 Nerinitide 3 Durvalumab Antineoplastic	6 New Technology Group 6
4 Central Vein	3 Percutaneous	5 Narsoplimab Monoclonal Antibody	7 New Technology Group 7
4 Central Vein	3 Percutaneous	5 Mosunetuzumab Antineoplastic	8 New Technology Group 8
4 Central Vein	3 Percutaneous	6 Lefamulin Anti-infective	6 New Technology Group 6
4 Central Vein	3 Percutaneous	6 Terlipressin	7 New Technology Group 7
4 Central Vein	3 Percutaneous	6 Afamitresgene Autoleucel Immunotherapy	8 New Technology Group 8
4 Central Vein	3 Percutaneous	7 Coagulation Factor Xa, Inactivated	2 New Technology Group 2
4 Central Vein	3 Percutaneous	7 Trilaciclib NT	7 New Technology Group 7
4 Central Vein	3 Percutaneous	7 Tabelecleucel Immunotherapy	8 New Technology Group 8
4 Central Vein	3 Percutaneous	8 Lurbinectedin NT	7 New Technology Group 7
4 Central Vein	3 Percutaneous	8 Treosulfan	8 New Technology Group 8
4 Central Vein	3 Percutaneous	9 Ceftolozane/Tazobactam Anti-infective	6 New Technology Group 6
4 Central Vein	3 Percutaneous	9 Inebilizumab-cdon	8 New Technology Group 8
4 Central Vein	3 Percutaneous	A Cefiderocol Anti-infective NT	6 New Technology Group 6
4 Central Vein	3 Percutaneous	A Ciltacabtagene Autoleucel	7 New Technology Group 7
4 Central Vein	3 Percutaneous	B Cytarabine and Daunorubicin Liposome Antineoplastic	3 New Technology Group 3
4 Central Vein	3 Percutaneous	B Omadacycline Anti-infective	6 New Technology Group 6
4 Central Vein	3 Percutaneous	B Amivantamab Monoclonal Antibody NT	7 New Technology Group 7
4 Central Vein	3 Percutaneous	C Eculizumab	6 New Technology Group 6
4 Central Vein	3 Percutaneous	C Engineered Chimeric Antigen Receptor T-cell Immunotherapy, Autologous	7 New Technology Group 7
4 Central Vein	3 Percutaneous	D Atezolizumab Antineoplastic	6 New Technology Group 6
4 Central Vein	3 Percutaneous	E Remdesivir Anti-infective NT	5 New Technology Group 5
4 Central Vein	3 Percutaneous	E Etesevimab Monoclonal Antibody	6 New Technology Group 6

DRG Non-OR	XWØ33G7	NT	XWØ33K7
DRG Non-OR	XWØ33[H,J]7	NT	XWØ33M7
DRG Non-OR	XWØ33K7	NT	XWØ33U5 in combination with dx code Y95 and one of the following: J14, J15.Ø, J15.1, J15.5, J15.6, J15.8, OR dx code J95.851 and one of the following: B96.1, B96.2Ø, B96.21, B96.22, B96.23, B96.29, B96.3, B96.5, or B96.89
DRG Non-OR	XWØ33[L,M]7	NT	XWØ4377
DRG Non-OR	XWØ33N7	NT	XWØ4387
DRG Non-OR	XWØ43A7		XWØ43A6 in combination with dx code Y95 and one of the following: J14, J15.Ø, J15.1, J15.5, J15.6, J15.8 OR dx code J95.851 and one of the following: B96.1, B96.2Ø, B96.21, B96.22, B96.23, B96.29, B96.3, B96.5, or B96.89
DRG Non-OR	XWØ43C7	NT	XWØ43B7
		NT	XWØ43E5

* For all codes with NT icon *see* Appendix I for registered or trade name of substance

XWØ Continued on next page

NC Noncovered Procedure   LC Limited Coverage   OA Questionable OB Admit   NT New Tech Add-on   ⊞ Combination Member   ♂ Male   ♀ Female

ICD-10-PCS 2023   823

X   New Technology
W   Anatomical Regions
Ø   Introduction   Definition: Putting in or on a therapeutic, diagnostic, nutritional, physiological, or prophylactic substance except blood or blood products
                          Explanation: None

XWØ Continued

Body Part Character 4	Approach Character 5	Device/Substance/Technology Character 6	Qualifier Character 7
4 Central Vein	3 Percutaneous	F Other New Technology Therapeutic Substance	3 New Technology Group 3
4 Central Vein	3 Percutaneous	F Other New Technology Therapeutic Substance	5 New Technology Group 5
4 Central Vein	3 Percutaneous	F Bamlanivimab Monoclonal Antibody	6 New Technology Group 6
4 Central Vein	3 Percutaneous	G Plazomicin Anti-infective	4 New Technology Group 4
4 Central Vein	3 Percutaneous	G Sarilumab	5 New Technology Group 5
4 Central Vein	3 Percutaneous	G REGN-COV2 Monoclonal Antibody	6 New Technology Group 6
4 Central Vein	3 Percutaneous	G Engineered Chimeric Antigen Receptor T-cell Immunotherapy, Allogeneic	7 New Technology Group 7
4 Central Vein	3 Percutaneous	H Synthetic Human Angiotensin II	4 New Technology Group 4
4 Central Vein	3 Percutaneous	H Tocilizumab	5 New Technology Group 5
4 Central Vein	3 Percutaneous	H Other New Technology Monoclonal Antibody	6 New Technology Group 6
4 Central Vein	3 Percutaneous	H Axicabtagene Ciloleucel Immunotherapy J Tisagenlecleucel Immunotherapy	7 New Technology Group 7
4 Central Vein	3 Percutaneous	K Fosfomycin Anti-infective	5 New Technology Group 5
4 Central Vein	3 Percutaneous	K Idecabtagene Vicleucel Immunotherapy **NT**	7 New Technology Group 7
4 Central Vein	3 Percutaneous	L CD24Fc Immunomodulator	6 New Technology Group 6
4 Central Vein	3 Percutaneous	L Lifileucel Immunotherapy M Brexucabtagene Autoleucel Immunotherapy **NT**	7 New Technology Group 7
4 Central Vein	3 Percutaneous	N Meropenem-vaborbactam Anti-infective	5 New Technology Group 5
4 Central Vein	3 Percutaneous	N Lisocabtagene Maraleucel Immunotherapy	7 New Technology Group 7
4 Central Vein	3 Percutaneous	Q Tagraxofusp-erzs Antineoplastic S Iobenguane I-131 Antineoplastic U Imipenem-cilastatin-relebactam Anti-infective **NT** W Caplacizumab	5 New Technology Group 5
9 Nose	7 Via Natural or Artificial Opening	M Esketamine Hydrochloride	5 New Technology Group 5
D Mouth and Pharynx	X External	3 Maribavir Anti-infective	8 New Technology Group 8
D Mouth and Pharynx	X External	6 Lefamulin Anti-infective	6 New Technology Group 6
D Mouth and Pharynx	X External	8 Uridine Triacetate	2 New Technology Group 2
D Mouth and Pharynx	X External	F Other New Technology Therapeutic Substance J Apalutamide Antineoplastic L Erdafitinib Antineoplastic	5 New Technology Group 5
D Mouth and Pharynx	X External	M Baricitinib **NT**	6 New Technology Group 6
D Mouth and Pharynx	X External	R Venetoclax Antineoplastic	5 New Technology Group 5
D Mouth and Pharynx	X External	R Fostamatinib	7 New Technology Group 7
D Mouth and Pharynx	X External	T Ruxolitinib V Gilteritinib Antineoplastic	5 New Technology Group 5
G Upper GI	7 Via Natural or Artificial Opening	3 Maribavir Anti-infective	8 New Technology Group 8
G Upper GI	7 Via Natural or Artificial Opening	M Baricitinib **NT**	6 New Technology Group 6
G Upper GI	7 Via Natural or Artificial Opening	R Fostamatinib	7 New Technology Group 7
G Upper GI	8 Via Natural or Artificial Opening Endoscopic	8 Mineral-based Topical Hemostatic Agent	6 New Technology Group 6
H Lower GI	7 Via Natural or Artificial Opening	3 Maribavir Anti-infective	8 New Technology Group 8
H Lower GI	7 Via Natural or Artificial Opening	M Baricitinib **NT**	6 New Technology Group 6
H Lower GI	7 Via Natural or Artificial Opening	R Fostamatinib	7 New Technology Group 7
H Lower GI	7 Via Natural or Artificial Opening	X Broad Consortium Microbiota-based Live Biotherapeutic Suspension	8 New Technology Group 8
H Lower GI	8 Via Natural or Artificial Opening Endoscopic	8 Mineral-based Topical HemostaticAgent	6 New Technology Group 6
Q Cranial Cavity and Brain	3 Percutaneous	1 Eladocagene exuparvovec	6 New Technology Group 6
V Bones	Ø Open	P Antibiotic-eluting Bone Void Filler	7 New Technology Group 7

Valid OR   XWØQ316   **NT**   XWØ43K7
DRG Non-OR   XWØ43G7   **NT**   XWØ43M7
DRG Non-OR   XWØ43[H,J]7   **NT**   XWØ43U5 in combination with dx code Y95 and one of the following: J14, J15.Ø, J15.1, J15.5, J15.6, J15.8, OR dx code
DRG Non-OR   XWØ43K7   J95.851 and one of the following: B96.1, B96.2Ø, B96.21, B96.22, B96.23, B96.29, B96.3, B96.5, or B96.89
DRG Non-OR   XWØ43[L,M]7   **NT**   XWØDXM6
DRG Non-OR   XWØ43N7   **NT**   XWØG7M6
                                    NT   XWØH7M6

* For all codes with NT icon *see* Appendix I for registered or trade name of substance

X   New Technology
W   Anatomical Regions
1   Transfusion   Definition: Putting in blood or blood products
               Explanation: None

Body Part Character 4	Approach Character 5	Device/Substance/Technology Character 6	Qualifier Character 7
3 Peripheral Vein	3 Percutaneous	2 Plasma, Convalescent **NT** (Nonautologous)	5 New Technology Group 5
3 Peripheral Vein	3 Percutaneous	B Betibeglogene Autotemcel C Omidubicel	8 New Technology Group 8
3 Peripheral Vein	3 Percutaneous	D High-Dose Intravenous Immune Globulin E Hyperimmune Globulin	7 New Technology Group 7
3 Peripheral Vein	3 Percutaneous	F OTL-103 G OTL-200	8 New Technology Group 8
4 Central Vein	3 Percutaneous	2 Plasma, Convalescent **NT** (Nonautologous)	5 New Technology Group 5
4 Central Vein	3 Percutaneous	B Betibeglogene Autotemcel C Omidubicel	8 New Technology Group 8
4 Central Vein	3 Percutaneous	D High-Dose Intravenous Immune Globulin E Hyperimmune Globulin	7 New Technology Group 7
4 Central Vein	3 Percutaneous	F OTL-103 G OTL-200	8 New Technology Group 8

NT   XW13325
NT   XW14325

X   New Technology
W   Anatomical Regions
H   Insertion   Definition: Putting in a nonbiological appliance that monitors, assists, performs, or prevents a physiological function but does not physically take the place of a body part
               Explanation: None

Body Part Character 4	Approach Character 5	Device/Substance/Technology Character 6	Qualifier Character 7
D Mouth and Pharynx	7 Via Natural or Artificial Opening	Q Neurostimulator Lead	7 New Technology Group 7

X   New Technology
X   Physiological Systems
E   Measurement   Definition: Determining the level of a physiological or physical function at a point in time
                        Explanation: None

Body Part Character 4	Approach Character 5	Device/Substance/Technology Character 6	Qualifier Character 7
Ø Central Nervous	X External	Ø Intracranial Vascular Activity, Computer-aided Assessment	7 New Technology Group 7
Ø Central Nervous	X External	4 Brain Electrical Activity, Computer-aided Semiologic Analysis	8 New Technology Group 8
3 Arterial	X External	2 Pulmonary Artery Flow, Computer-aided Triage and Notification	7 New Technology Group 7
3 Arterial	X External	5 Coronary Artery Flow, Quantitative Flow Ratio Analysis 6 Coronary Artery Flow, Computer-aided Valve Modeling and Notification	8 New Technology Group 8
5 Circulatory	X External	3 Infection, Whole Blood Reverse Transcription and Quantitative Real-time Polymerase Chain Reaction	8 New Technology Group 8
5 Circulatory	X External	M Infection, Whole Blood Nucleic Acid-base Microbial Detection	5 New Technology Group 5
5 Circulatory	X External	N Infection, Positive Blood Culture Fluorescence Hybridization for Organism Identification, Concentration and Susceptibility	6 New Technology Group 6
5 Circulatory	X External	R Infection, Mechanical Initial Specimen Diversion Technique Using Active Negative Pressure T Intracranial Arterial Flow, Whole Blood mRNA V Infection, Serum/Plasma Nanoparticle Fluorescence SARS-CoV-2 Antibody Detection	7 New Technology Group 7
9 Nose	7 Via Natural or Artificial Opening	U Infection, Nasopharyngeal Fluid SARS-CoV-2 Polymerase Chain Reaction	7 New Technology Group 7
B Respiratory	X External	Q Infection, Lower Respiratory Fluid Nucleic Acid-base Microbial Detection	6 New Technology Group 6

X   New Technology
Y   Extracorporeal
Ø   Introduction   Definition: Putting in or on a therapeutic, diagnostic, nutritional, physiological, or prophylactic substance except blood or blood products
                        Explanation: None

Body Part Character 4	Approach Character 5	Device/Substance/Technology Character 6	Qualifier Character 7
V Vein Graft	X External	8 Endothelial Damage Inhibitor	3 New Technology Group 3
Y Extracorporeal	X External	2 Taurolidine Anti-infective and Heparin Anticoagulant	8 New Technology Group 8
Y Extracorporeal	X External	3 Nafamostat Anticoagulant	7 New Technology Group 7

Appendixes

Appendix A: Components of the Medical and Surgical Approach Definitions

ICD-10-PCS Value	Definition	Access Location	Method	Type of Instrumentation	Example
Open (Ø)	Cutting through the skin or mucous membrane and any other body layers necessary to expose the site of the procedure	Skin or mucous membrane, any other body layers	Cutting	None	Abdominal hysterectomy
Percutaneous (3)	Entry, by puncture or minor incision, of instrumentation through the skin or mucous membrane and any other body layers necessary to reach the site of the procedure	Skin or mucous membrane, any other body layers	Puncture or minor incision	Without visualization	Needle biopsy of liver, Liposuction
Percutaneous endoscopic (4)	Entry, by puncture or minor incision, of instrumentation through the skin or mucous membrane and any other body layers necessary to reach and visualize the site of the procedure	Skin or mucous membrane, any other body layers	Puncture or minor incision	With visualization	Arthroscopy, Laparoscopic cholecystectomy
Via natural or artificial opening (7)	Entry of instrumentation through a natural or artificial external opening to reach the site of the procedure	Natural or artificial external opening	Direct entry	Without visualization	Endotracheal tube insertion, Foley catheter placement
Via natural or artificial opening endoscopic (8)	Entry of instrumentation through a natural or artificial external opening to reach and visualize the site of the procedure	Natural or artificial external opening	Direct entry	With visualization	Sigmoidoscopy, EGD, ERCP
Via natural or artificial opening with percutaneous endoscopic assistance (F)	Entry of instrumentation through a natural or artificial external opening and entry, by puncture or minor incision, of instrumentation through the skin or mucous membrane and any other body layers necessary to aid in the performance of the procedure	Skin or mucous membrane, any other body layers	Direct entry with puncture or minor incision for instrumentation only	With visualization	Laparoscopic-assisted vaginal hysterectomy
External (X)	Procedures performed directly on the skin or mucous membrane and procedures performed indirectly by the application of external force through the skin or mucous membrane	Skin or mucous membrane	Direct or indirect application	None	Closed fracture reduction, Resection of tonsils

The approach comprises three components: the access location, method, and type of instrumentation.

Access location: For procedures performed on an internal body part, the access location specifies the external site through which the site of the procedure is reached. There are two general types of access locations: skin or mucous membranes, and external orifices. Every approach value except external includes one of these two access locations. The skin or mucous membrane can be cut or punctured to reach the procedure site. All open and percutaneous approach values use this access location. The site of a procedure can also be reached through an external opening. External openings can be natural (e.g., mouth) or artificial (e.g., colostomy stoma).

Method: For procedures performed on an internal body part, the method specifies how the external access location is entered. An open method specifies cutting through the skin or mucous membrane and any other intervening body layers necessary to expose the site of the procedure. An instrumentation method specifies the entry of instrumentation through the access location to the internal procedure site. Instrumentation can be introduced by puncture or minor incision, or through an external opening. The puncture or minor incision does not constitute an open approach because it does not expose the site of the procedure. An approach can define multiple methods. For example, Via Natural or Artificial Opening with Percutaneous Endoscopic Assistance includes both the initial entry of instrumentation to reach the site of the procedure, and the placement of additional percutaneous instrumentation into the body part to visualize and assist in the performance of the procedure.

Type of instrumentation: For procedures performed on an internal body part, instrumentation means that specialized equipment is used to perform the procedure. Instrumentation is used in all internal approaches other than the basic open approach. Instrumentation may or may not include the capacity to visualize the procedure site. For example, the instrumentation used to perform a sigmoidoscopy permits the internal site of the procedure to be visualized, while the instrumentation used to perform a needle biopsy of the liver does not. The term "endoscopic" as used in approach values refers to instrumentation that permits a site to be visualized.

Procedures performed directly on the skin or mucous membrane are identified by the external approach (e.g., skin excision). Procedures performed indirectly by the application of external force are also identified by the external approach (e.g., closed reduction of fracture).

Open (Ø)

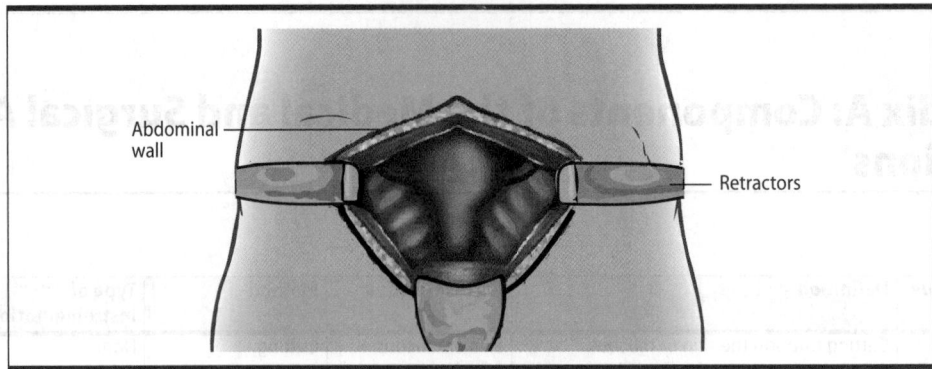

Percutaneous (3)

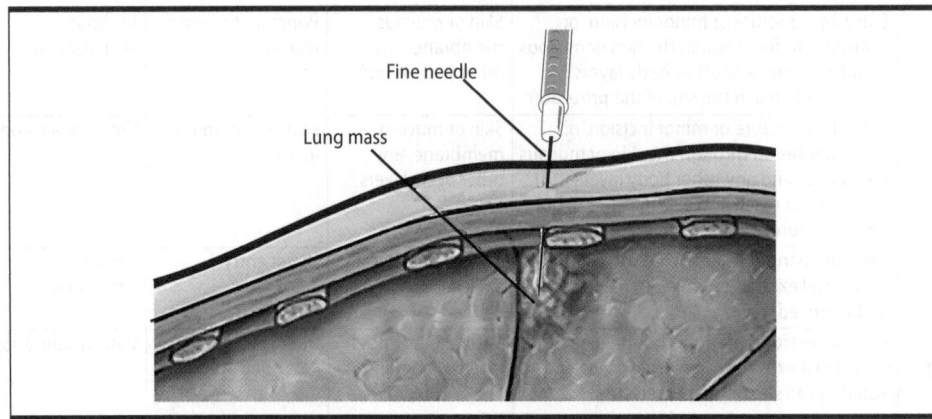

Percutaneous Endoscopic (4)

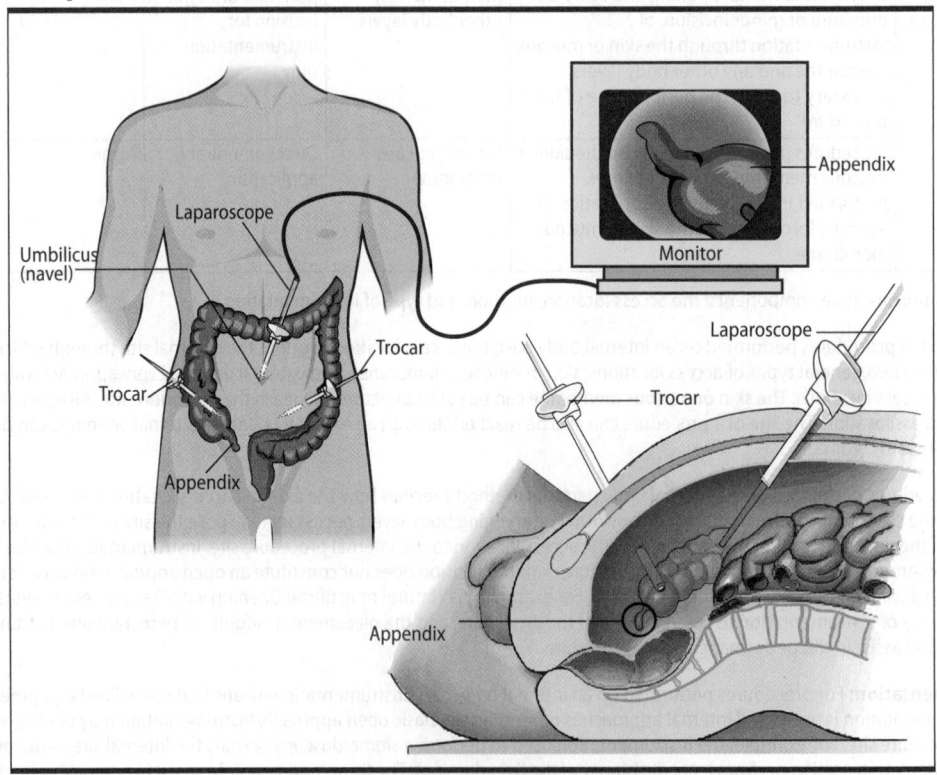

Via Natural or Artificial Opening (7)

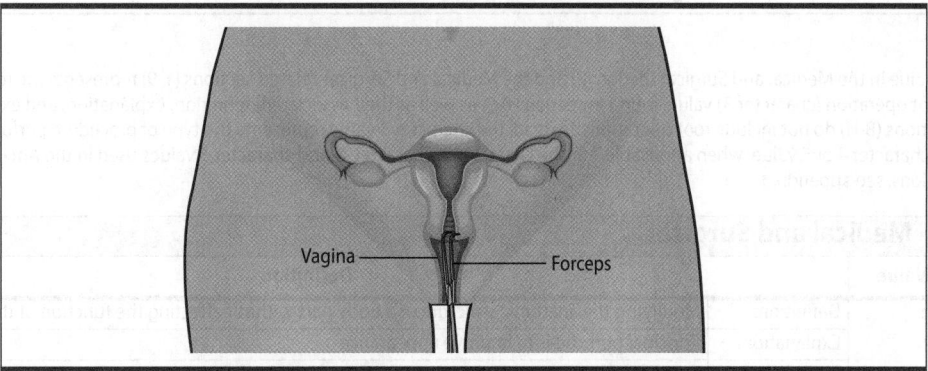

Via Natural or Artificial Opening, Endoscopic (8)

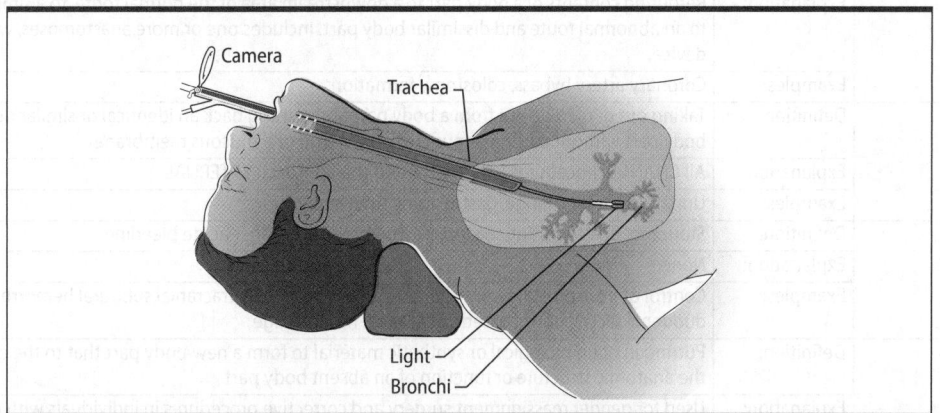

Via Natural or Artificial Opening with Percutaneous Endoscopic Assistance (F)

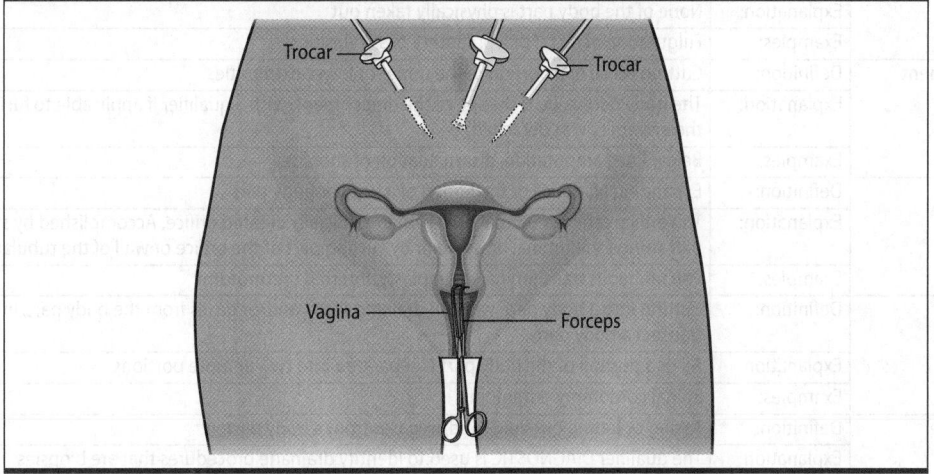

External (X)

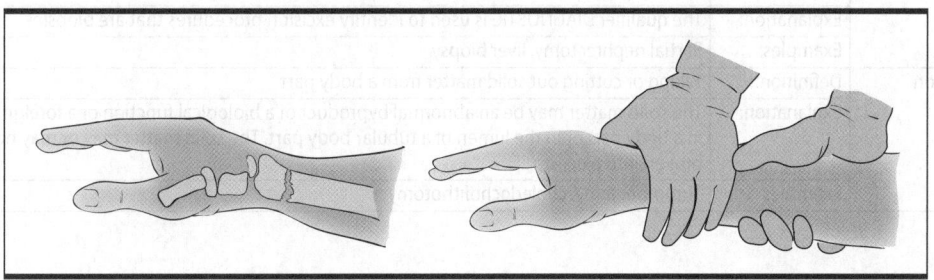

Appendix B: Root Operation Definitions

The character 3 value in the Medical and Surgical section (Ø) and the Medical and Surgical-related sections (1-9) represents the root operation. This resource provides each root operation (character 3) value, found in sections Ø-9, as well as their associated definition, explanation, and examples, where applicable. The Ancillary sections (B-H) do not include root operations; instead, the character 3 value represents the type of procedure performed with additional detail provided by the character 4 or 5 value, when applicable. For the character 3, character 4, and character 5 values used in the Ancillary sections of B-H, along with their definitions, see appendix J.

Ø	Medical and Surgical		
ICD-1Ø-PCS Value			**Definition**
Ø	Alteration	Definition:	Modifying the anatomic structure of a body part without affecting the function of the body part
		Explanation:	Principal purpose is to improve appearance
		Examples:	Face lift, breast augmentation
1	Bypass	Definition:	Altering the route of passage of the contents of a tubular body part
		Explanation:	Rerouting contents of a body part to a downstream area of the normal route, to a similar route and body part, or to an abnormal route and dissimilar body part. Includes one or more anastomoses, with or without the use of a device.
		Examples:	Coronary artery bypass, colostomy formation
2	Change	Definition:	Taking out or off a device from a body part and putting back an identical or similar device in or on the same body part without cutting or puncturing the skin or a mucous membrane
		Explanation:	All CHANGE procedures are coded using the approach EXTERNAL
		Examples:	Urinary catheter change, gastrostomy tube change
3	Control	Definition:	Stopping, or attempting to stop, postprocedural or other acute bleeding
		Explanation:	None
		Examples:	Control of post-prostatectomy hemorrhage, control of intracranial subdural hemorrhage, control of bleeding duodenal ulcer, control of retroperitoneal hemorrhage
4	Creation	Definition:	Putting in or on biological or synthetic material to form a new body part that to the extent possible replicates the anatomic structure or function of an absent body part
		Explanation:	Used for gender reassignment surgery and corrective procedures in individuals with congenital anomalies
		Examples:	Creation of vagina in a male, creation of right and left atrioventricular valve from common atrioventricular valve
5	Destruction	Definition:	Physical eradication of all or a portion of a body part by the direct use of energy, force, or a destructive agent
		Explanation:	None of the body part is physically taken out
		Examples:	Fulguration of rectal polyp, cautery of skin lesion
6	Detachment	Definition:	Cutting off all or a portion of the upper or lower extremities
		Explanation:	The body part value is the site of the detachment, with a qualifier if applicable to further specify the level where the extremity was detached
		Examples:	Below knee amputation, disarticulation of shoulder
7	Dilation	Definition:	Expanding an orifice or the lumen of a tubular body part
		Explanation:	The orifice can be a natural orifice or an artificially created orifice. Accomplished by stretching a tubular body part using intraluminal pressure or by cutting part of the orifice or wall of the tubular body part.
		Examples:	Percutaneous transluminal angioplasty, internal urethrotomy
8	Division	Definition:	Cutting into a body part, without draining fluids and/or gases from the body part, in order to separate or transect a body part
		Explanation:	All or a portion of the body part is separated into two or more portions
		Examples:	Spinal cordotomy, osteotomy
9	Drainage	Definition:	Taking or letting out fluids and/or gases from a body part
		Explanation:	The qualifier DIAGNOSTIC is used to identify drainage procedures that are biopsies
		Examples:	Thoracentesis, incision and drainage
B	Excision	Definition:	Cutting out or off, without replacement, a portion of a body part
		Explanation:	The qualifier DIAGNOSTIC is used to identify excision procedures that are biopsies
		Examples:	Partial nephrectomy, liver biopsy
C	Extirpation	Definition:	Taking or cutting out solid matter from a body part
		Explanation:	The solid matter may be an abnormal byproduct of a biological function or a foreign body; it may be imbedded in a body part or in the lumen of a tubular body part. The solid matter may or may not have been previously broken into pieces.
		Examples:	Thrombectomy, choledocholithotomy

Continued on next page

Ø		**Medical and Surgical**		*Continued from previous page*
ICD-10-PCS Value			**Definition**	
D	Extraction	Definition:	Pulling or stripping out or off all or a portion of a body part by the use of force	
		Explanation:	The qualifier DIAGNOSTIC is used to identify extractions that are biopsies	
		Examples:	Dilation and curettage, vein stripping	
F	Fragmentation	Definition:	Breaking solid matter in a body part into pieces	
		Explanation:	Physical force (e.g., manual, ultrasonic) applied directly or indirectly is used to break the solid matter into pieces. The solid matter may be an abnormal byproduct of a biological function or a foreign body. The pieces of solid matter are not taken out.	
		Examples:	Extracorporeal shockwave lithotripsy, transurethral lithotripsy	
G	Fusion	Definition:	Joining together portions of an articular body part rendering the articular body part immobile	
		Explanation:	The body part is joined together by fixation device, bone graft, or other means	
		Examples:	Spinal fusion, ankle arthrodesis	
H	Insertion	Definition:	Putting in a nonbiological appliance that monitors, assists, performs, or prevents a physiological function but does not physically take the place of a body part	
		Explanation:	None	
		Examples:	Insertion of radioactive implant, insertion of central venous catheter	
J	Inspection	Definition:	Visually and/or manually exploring a body part	
		Explanation:	Visual exploration may be performed with or without optical instrumentation. Manual exploration may be performed directly or through intervening body layers.	
		Examples:	Diagnostic arthroscopy, exploratory laparotomy	
K	Map	Definition:	Locating the route of passage of electrical impulses and/or locating functional areas in a body part	
		Explanation:	Applicable only to the cardiac conduction mechanism and the central nervous system	
		Examples:	Cardiac mapping, cortical mapping	
L	Occlusion	Definition:	Completely closing an orifice or lumen of a tubular body part	
		Explanation:	The orifice can be a natural orifice or an artificially created orifice	
		Examples:	Fallopian tube ligation, ligation of inferior vena cava	
M	Reattachment	Definition:	Putting back in or on all or a portion of a separated body part to its normal location or other suitable location	
		Explanation:	Vascular circulation and nervous pathways may or may not be reestablished	
		Examples:	Reattachment of hand, reattachment of avulsed kidney	
N	Release	Definition:	Freeing a body part from an abnormal physical constraint by cutting or by use of force	
		Explanation:	Some of the restraining tissue may be taken out but none of the body part is taken out	
		Examples:	Adhesiolysis, carpal tunnel release	
P	Removal	Definition:	Taking out or off a device from a body part	
		Explanation:	If a device is taken out and a similar device put in without cutting or puncturing the skin or mucous membrane, the procedure is coded to the root operation CHANGE. Otherwise, the procedure for taking out a device is coded to the root operation REMOVAL.	
		Examples:	Drainage tube removal, cardiac pacemaker removal	
Q	Repair	Definition:	Restoring, to the extent possible, a body part to its normal anatomic structure and function	
		Explanation:	Used only when the method to accomplish the repair is not one of the other root operations	
		Examples:	Colostomy takedown, suture of laceration	
R	Replacement	Definition:	Putting in or on biological or synthetic material that physically takes the place and/or function of all or a portion of a body part	
		Explanation:	The body part may have been taken out or replaced, or may be taken out, physically eradicated, or rendered nonfunctional during the REPLACEMENT procedure. A REMOVAL procedure is coded for taking out the device used in a previous replacement procedure.	
		Examples:	Total hip replacement, bone graft, free skin graft	
S	Reposition	Definition:	Moving to its normal location, or other suitable location, all or a portion of a body part	
		Explanation:	The body part is moved to a new location from an abnormal location, or from a normal location where it is not functioning correctly. The body part may or may not be cut out or off to be moved to the new location.	
		Examples:	Reposition of undescended testicle, fracture reduction	
T	Resection	Definition:	Cutting out or off, without replacement, all of a body part	
		Explanation:	None	
		Examples:	Total nephrectomy, total lobectomy of lung	
V	Restriction	Definition:	Partially closing an orifice or the lumen of a tubular body part	
		Explanation:	The orifice can be a natural orifice or an artificially created orifice	
		Examples:	Esophagogastric fundoplication, cervical cerclage	

Continued on next page

Ø   Medical and Surgical

Continued from previous page

ICD-1Ø-PCS Value			Definition
W	Revision	Definition:	Correcting, to the extent possible, a portion of a malfunctioning device or the position of a displaced device
		Explanation:	Revision can include correcting a malfunctioning or displaced device by taking out or putting in components of the device such as a screw or pin
		Examples:	Adjustment of position of pacemaker lead, recementing of hip prosthesis
U	Supplement	Definition:	Putting in or on biological or synthetic material that physically reinforces and/or augments the function of a portion of a body part
		Explanation:	The biological material is non-living, or is living and from the same individual. The body part may have been previously replaced, and the SUPPLEMENT procedure is performed to physically reinforce and/or augment the function of the replaced body part.
		Examples:	Herniorrhaphy using mesh, mitral valve ring annuloplasty, put a new acetabular liner in a previous hip replacement
X	Transfer	Definition:	Moving, without taking out, all or a portion of a body part to another location to take over the function of all or a portion of a body part
		Explanation:	The body part transferred remains connected to its vascular and nervous supply
		Examples:	Tendon transfer, skin pedicle flap transfer
Y	Transplantation	Definition:	Putting in or on all or a portion of a living body part taken from another individual or animal to physically take the place and/or function of all or a portion of a similar body part
		Explanation:	The native body part may or may not be taken out, and the transplanted body part may take over all or a portion of its function
		Examples:	Kidney transplant, heart transplant

Root Operation Definitions for Other Sections

1   Obstetrics

ICD-1Ø-PCS Value			Definition
2	Change	Definition:	Taking out or off a device from a body part and putting back an identical or similar device in or on the same body part without cutting or puncturing the skin or a mucous membrane
		Explanation:	None
		Example:	Replacement of fetal scalp electrode
9	Drainage	Definition:	Taking or letting out fluids and/or gases from a body part
		Explanation:	None
		Example:	Biopsy of amniotic fluid
A	Abortion	Definition:	Artificially terminating a pregnancy
		Explanation:	None
		Example:	Transvaginal abortion using vacuum aspiration technique
D	Extraction	Definition:	Pulling or stripping out or off all or a portion of a body part by the use of force
		Explanation:	None
		Example:	Low-transverse C-section
E	Delivery	Definition:	Assisting the passage of the products of conception from the genital canal
		Explanation:	None
		Example:	Manually-assisted delivery
H	Insertion	Definition:	Putting in a nonbiological appliance that monitors, assists, performs, or prevents a physiological function but does not physically take the place of a body part
		Explanation:	None
		Example:	Placement of fetal scalp electrode
J	Inspection	Definition:	Visually and/or manually exploring a body part
		Explanation:	Visual exploration may be performed with or without optical instrumentation. Manual exploration may be performed directly or through intervening body layers.
		Example:	Bimanual pregnancy exam
P	Removal	Definition:	Taking out or off a device from a body part, region or orifice
		Explanation:	If a device is taken out and a similar device put in without cutting or puncturing the skin or mucous membrane, the procedure is coded to the root operation CHANGE. Otherwise, the procedure for taking out a device is coded to the root operation REMOVAL.
		Example:	Removal of fetal monitoring electrode

Continued on next page

1   Obstetrics

Continued from previous page

ICD-10-PCS Value			Definition
Q	Repair	Definition:	Restoring, to the extent possible, a body part to its normal anatomic structure and function
		Explanation:	Used only when the method to accomplish the repair is not one of the other root operations
		Example:	In utero repair of congenital diaphragmatic hernia
S	Reposition	Definition:	Moving to its normal location, or other suitable location, all or a portion of a body part
		Explanation:	The body part is moved to a new location from an abnormal location, or from a normal location where it is not functioning correctly. The body part may or may not be cut out or off to be moved to the new location.
		Example:	External version of fetus
T	Resection	Definition:	Cutting out or off, without replacement, all of a body part
		Explanation:	None
		Example:	Total excision of tubal pregnancy
Y	Transplantation	Definition:	Putting in or on all or a portion of a living body part taken from another individual or animal to physically take the place and/or function of all or a portion of a similar body part
		Explanation:	The native body part may or may not be taken out, and the transplanted body part may take over all or a portion of its function
		Example:	In utero fetal kidney transplant

2   Placement

ICD-10-PCS Value			Definition
Ø	Change	Definition:	Taking out or off a device from a body part and putting back an identical or similar device in or on the same body part without cutting or puncturing the skin or a mucous membrane
		Example:	Change of vaginal packing
1	Compression	Definition:	Putting pressure on a body region
		Example:	Placement of pressure dressing on abdominal wall
2	Dressing	Definition:	Putting material on a body region for protection
		Example:	Application of sterile dressing to head wound
3	Immobilization	Definition:	Limiting or preventing motion of a body region
		Example:	Placement of splint on left finger
4	Packing	Definition:	Putting material in a body region or orifice
		Example:	Placement of nasal packing
5	Removal	Definition:	Taking out or off a device from a body part
		Example:	Removal of stereotactic head frame
6	Traction	Definition:	Exerting a pulling force on a body region in a distal direction
		Example:	Lumbar traction using motorized split-traction table

3   Administration

ICD-10-PCS Value			Definition
Ø	Introduction	Definition:	Putting in or on a therapeutic, diagnostic, nutritional, physiological, or prophylactic substance except blood or blood products
		Example:	Nerve block injection to median nerve
1	Irrigation	Definition:	Putting in or on a cleansing substance
		Example:	Flushing of eye
2	Transfusion	Definition:	Putting in blood or blood products
		Example:	Transfusion of cell saver red cells into central venous line

4   Measurement and Monitoring

ICD-10-PCS Value			Definition
Ø	Measurement	Definition:	Determining the level of a physiological or physical function at a point in time
		Example:	External electrocardiogram(EKG), single reading
1	Monitoring	Definition:	Determining the level of a physiological or physical function repetitively over a period of time
		Example:	Urinary pressure monitoring

5   Extracorporeal or Systemic Assistance and Performance

ICD-10-PCS Value			Definition
Ø	Assistance	Definition:	Taking over a portion of a physiological function by extracorporeal means
		Example:	Hyperbaric oxygenation of wound
1	Performance	Definition:	Completely taking over a physiological function by extracorporeal means
		Example:	Cardiopulmonary bypass in conjunction with CABG
2	Restoration	Definition:	Returning, or attempting to return, a physiological function to its original state by extracorporeal means
		Example:	Attempted cardiac defibrillation, unsuccessful

6   Extracorporeal or Systemic Therapies

ICD-10-PCS Value			Definition
Ø	Atmospheric Control	Definition:	Extracorporeal control of atmospheric pressure and composition
		Example:	Antigen-free air conditioning, series treatment
1	Decompression	Definition:	Extracorporeal elimination of undissolved gas from body fluids
		Example:	Hyperbaric decompression treatment, single
2	Electromagnetic Therapy	Definition:	Extracorporeal treatment by electromagnetic rays
		Example:	TMS (transcranial magnetic stimulation), series treatment
3	Hyperthermia	Definition:	Extracorporeal raising of body temperature
		Example:	None
4	Hypothermia	Definition:	Extracorporeal lowering of body temperature
		Example:	Whole body hypothermia treatment for temperature imbalances, series
5	Pheresis	Definition:	Extracorporeal separation of blood products
		Example:	Therapeutic leukopheresis, single treatment
6	Phototherapy	Definition:	Extracorporeal treatment by light rays
		Example:	Phototherapy of circulatory system, series treatment
7	Ultrasound Therapy	Definition:	Extracorporeal treatment by ultrasound
		Example:	Therapeutic ultrasound of peripheral vessels, single treatment
8	Ultraviolet Light Therapy	Definition:	Extracorporeal treatment by ultraviolet light
		Example:	Ultraviolet light phototherapy, series treatment
9	Shock Wave Therapy	Definition:	Extracorporeal treatment by shock waves
		Example:	Shockwave therapy of plantar fascia, single treatment
B	Perfusion	Definition:	Extracorporeal treatment by diffusion of therapeutic fluid
		Example:	Perfusion of donor liver while preparing transplant patient

7   Osteopathic

ICD-10-PCS Value			Definition
Ø	Treatment	Definition:	Manual treatment to eliminate or alleviate somatic dysfunction and related disorders
		Examples:	Fascial release of abdomen, osteopathic treatment

8   Other Procedures

ICD-10-PCS Value			Definition
Ø	Other Procedures	Definition:	Methodologies which attempt to remediate or cure a disorder or disease
		Examples:	Acupuncture, yoga therapy

9   Chiropractic

ICD-10-PCS Value			Definition
B	Manipulation	Definition:	Manual procedure that involves a directed thrust to move a joint past the physiological range of motion, without exceeding the anatomical limit
		Example:	Chiropractic treatment of cervical spine, short lever specific contact

Appendix C: Comparison of Medical and Surgical Root Operations

Note: The character associated with each operation appears in parentheses after its title.

Procedures That Take Out Some or All of a Body Part

Root Operation	Objective of Procedure	Site of Procedure	Example
Destruction (5)	Eradicating without taking out or replacement	Some/all of a body part	Fulguration of endometrium
Detachment (6)	Cutting out/off without replacement	Extremity only, any level	Amputation above elbow
Excision (B)	Cutting out/off without replacement	Some of a body part	Breast lumpectomy
Extraction (D)	Pulling out/off without replacement	Some/all of a body part	Suction D&C
Resection (T)	Cutting out/off without replacement	All of a body part	Total mastectomy

Procedures That Put In/Put Back or Move Some/All of a Body Part

Root Operation	Objective of Procedure	Site of Procedure	Example
Reattachment (M)	Putting back a detached body part	Some/all of a body part	Reattach finger
Reposition (S)	Moving a body part to normal or other suitable location	Some/all of a body part	Move undescended testicle
Transfer (X)	Moving a body part to function for a similar body part	Some/all of a body part	Skin pedicle transfer flap
Transplantation (Y)	Putting in a living body part from a person/animal	Some/all of a body part	Kidney transplant

Procedures That Take Out or Eliminate Solid Matter, Fluids, or Gases From a Body Part

Root Operation	Objective of Procedure	Site of Procedure	Example
Drainage (9)	Taking or letting out	Fluids and/or gases from a body part	Incision and drainage
Extirpation (C)	Taking or cutting out	Solid matter in a body part	Thrombectomy
Fragmentation (F)	Breaking into pieces	Solid matter within a body part	Lithotripsy

Procedures That Involve Only Examination of Body Parts and Regions

Root Operation	Objective of Procedure	Site of Procedure	Example
Inspection (J)	Visual/manual exploration	Some/all of a body part	Diagnostic cystoscopy Exploratory laparoscopy
Map (K)	Locating electrical impulse route/functional areas	Brain/cardiac conduction mechanism	Cardiac mapping

Procedures That Alter the Diameter/Route of a Tubular Body Part

Root Operation	Objective of Procedure	Site of Procedure	Example
Bypass (1)	Altering route of passage of contents	Tubular body part	Coronary artery bypass graft (CABG)
Dilation (7)	Expanding natural or artificially created orifice/lumen	Tubular body part	Percutaneous transluminal coronary angioplasty (PTCA)
Occlusion (L)	Completely closing natural or artificially created orifice/lumen	Tubular body part	Fallopian tube ligation
Restriction (V)	Partially closing natural or artificially created orifice/lumen	Tubular body part	Gastroesophageal fundoplication

Procedures That Always Involve Devices

Root Operation		Objective of Procedure	Site of Procedure	Example
Change (2)	DVC	Exchanging device w/out cutting/puncturing	In/on a body part	Gastrostomy tube change
Insertion (H)	DVC	Putting in nonbiological device	In/on a body part	Central line insertion
Removal (P)	DVC	Taking out device	In/on a body part	Central line removal
Replacement (R)	DVC	Putting in device that replaces a body part	Some/all of a body part	Total hip replacement
Revision (W)	DVC	Correcting a malfunctioning/displaced device	In/on a body part	Revision of pacemaker
Supplement (U)	DVC	Putting in device that reinforces or augments a body part	In/on a body part	Abdominal wall herniorrhaphy using mesh

DVC = Device involved in root operation

Procedures Involving Cutting or Separation Only

Root Operation	Objective of Procedure	Site of Procedure	Example
Division (8)	Cutting into/separating	A body part	Neurotomy
Release (N)	Freeing a body part from constraint	Around a body part	Adhesiolysis

Procedures That Define Other Repairs

Root Operation	Objective of Procedure	Site of Procedure	Example
Control (3)	Stopping/attempting to stop postprocedural or other acute bleeding	Anatomical region or nasal mucosa/soft tissue	Post-prostatectomy bleeding control, control subdural hemorrhage, bleeding ulcer, retroperitoneal hemorrhage
Repair (Q)	Restoring body part to its normal structure/function	Some/all of a body part	Suture laceration

Procedures That Define Other Objectives

Root Operation	Objective of Procedure	Site of Procedure	Example
Alteration (Ø)	Modifying body part for cosmetic purposes without affecting function	Some/all of a body part	Face lift
Creation (4)	Using biological or synthetic material to form a new body part that replicates the anatomic structure or function of a missing body part	Perineum, valve	Sex change/artificial vagina/penis, atrioventricular valve creation
Fusion (G)	Unification or immobilization	Joint or articular body part	Spinal fusion

Appendix D: Body Part Key

Term	ICD-10-PCS Value
Abdominal aortic plexus	Abdominal Sympathetic Nerve
Abdominal cavity	Peritoneal Cavity
Abdominal esophagus	Esophagus, Lower
Abductor hallucis muscle	Foot Muscle, Right
	Foot Muscle, Left
Accessory cephalic vein	Cephalic Vein, Right
	Cephalic Vein, Left
Accessory obturator nerve	Lumbar Plexus
Accessory phrenic nerve	Phrenic nerve
Accessory spleen	Spleen
Acetabulofemoral joint	Hip Joint, Right
	Hip Joint, Left
Achilles tendon	Lower Leg Tendon, Right
	Lower Leg Tendon, Left
Acromioclavicular ligament	Shoulder Bursa and Ligament, Right
	Shoulder Bursa and Ligament, Left
Acromion (process)	Scapula, Right
	Scapula, Left
Adductor brevis muscle	Upper Leg Muscle, Right
	Upper Leg Muscle, Left
Adductor hallucis muscle	Foot Muscle, Right
	Foot Muscle, Left
Adductor longus muscle	Upper Leg Muscle, Right
	Upper Leg Muscle, Left
Adductor magnus muscle	Upper Leg Muscle, Right
	Upper Leg Muscle, Left
Adenohypophysis	Pituitary Gland
Alar ligament of axis	Head and Neck Bursa and Ligament
Alveolar process of mandible	Mandible, Right
	Mandible, Left
Alveolar process of maxilla	Maxilla
Anal orifice	Anus
Anatomical snuffbox	Lower Arm and Wrist Muscle, Right
	Lower Arm and Wrist Muscle, Left
Angular artery	Face Artery
Angular vein	Face Vein, Right
	Face Vein, Left
Annular ligament	Elbow Bursa and Ligament, Right
	Elbow Bursa and Ligament, Left
Anorectal junction	Rectum
Ansa cervicalis	Cervical Plexus
Antebrachial fascia	Subcutaneous Tissue and Fascia, Right Lower Arm
	Subcutaneous Tissue and Fascia, Left Lower Arm
Anterior (pectoral) lymph node	Lymphatic, Right Axillary
	Lymphatic, Left Axillary
Anterior cerebral artery	Intracranial Artery
Anterior cerebral vein	Intracranial Vein
Anterior choroidal artery	Intracranial Artery
Anterior circumflex humeral artery	Axillary Artery, Right
	Axillary Artery, Left
Anterior communicating artery	Intracranial Artery

Term	ICD-10-PCS Value
Anterior cruciate ligament (ACL)	Knee Bursa and Ligament, Right
	Knee Bursa and Ligament, Left
Anterior crural nerve	Femoral Nerve
Anterior facial vein	Face Vein, Right
	Face Vein, Left
Anterior intercostal artery	Internal Mammary Artery, Right
	Internal Mammary Artery, Left
Anterior interosseous nerve	Median Nerve
Anterior lateral malleolar artery	Anterior Tibial Artery, Right
	Anterior Tibial Artery, Left
Anterior lingual gland	Minor Salivary Gland
Anterior medial malleolar artery	Anterior Tibial Artery, Right
	Anterior Tibial Artery, Left
Anterior spinal artery	Vertebral Artery, Right
	Vertebral Artery, Left
Anterior tibial recurrent artery	Anterior Tibial Artery, Right
	Anterior Tibial Artery, Left
Anterior ulnar recurrent artery	Ulnar Artery, Right
	Ulnar Artery, Left
Anterior vagal trunk	Vagus Nerve
Anterior vertebral muscle	Neck Muscle, Right
	Neck Muscle, Left
Antihelix	External Ear, Right
	External Ear, Left
	External Ear, Bilateral
Antitragus	External Ear, Right
	External Ear, Left
	External Ear, Bilateral
Antrum of Highmore	Maxillary Sinus, Right
	Maxillary Sinus, Left
Aortic annulus	Aortic Valve
Aortic arch	Thoracic Aorta, Ascending/Arch
Aortic intercostal artery	Upper Artery
Apical (subclavicular) lymph node	Lymphatic, Right Axillary
	Lymphatic, Left Axillary
Apneustic center	Pons
Aqueduct of Sylvius	Cerebral Ventricle
Aqueous humour	Anterior Chamber, Right
	Anterior Chamber, Left
Arachnoid mater, intracranial	Cerebral Meninges
Arachnoid mater, spinal	Spinal Meninges
Arcuate artery	Foot Artery, Right
	Foot Artery, Left
Areola	Nipple, Right
	Nipple, Left
Arterial canal (duct)	Pulmonary Artery, Left
Aryepiglottic fold	Larynx
Arytenoid cartilage	Larynx
Arytenoid muscle	Neck Muscle, Right
	Neck Muscle, Left
Ascending aorta	Thoracic Aorta, Ascending/Arch
Ascending palatine artery	Face Artery
Ascending pharyngeal artery	External Carotid Artery, Right
	External Carotid Artery, Left

Term	ICD-10-PCS Value
Atlantoaxial joint	Cervical Vertebral Joint
Atrioventricular node	Conduction Mechanism
Atrium dextrum cordis	Atrium, Right
Atrium pulmonale	Atrium, Left
Auditory tube	Eustachian Tube, Right
	Eustachian Tube, Left
Auerbach's (myenteric) plexus	Abdominal Sympathetic Nerve
Auricle	External Ear, Right
	External Ear, Left
	External Ear, Bilateral
Auricularis muscle	Head Muscle
Axillary fascia	Subcutaneous Tissue and Fascia, Right Upper Arm
	Subcutaneous Tissue and Fascia, Left Upper Arm
Axillary nerve	Brachial Plexus
Bartholin's (greater vestibular) gland	Vestibular Gland
Basal (internal) cerebral vein	Intracranial Vein
Basal nuclei	Basal Ganglia
Base of tongue	Pharynx
Basilar artery	Intracranial Artery
Basis pontis	Pons
Biceps brachii muscle	Upper Arm Muscle, Right
	Upper Arm Muscle, Left
Biceps femoris muscle	Upper Leg Muscle, Right
	Upper Leg Muscle, Left
Bicipital aponeurosis	Subcutaneous Tissue and Fascia, Right Lower Arm
	Subcutaneous Tissue and Fascia, Left Lower Arm
Bicuspid valve	Mitral Valve
Body of femur	Femoral Shaft, Right
	Femoral Shaft, Left
Body of fibula	Fibula, Right
	Fibula, Left
Bony labyrinth	Inner Ear, Right
	Inner Ear, Left
Bony orbit	Orbit, Right
	Orbit, Left
Bony vestibule	Inner Ear, Right
	Inner Ear, Left
Botallo's duct	Pulmonary Artery, Left
Brachial (lateral) lymph node	Lymphatic, Right Axillary
	Lymphatic, Left Axillary
Brachialis muscle	Upper Arm Muscle, Right
	Upper Arm Muscle, Left
Brachiocephalic artery	Innominate Artery
Brachiocephalic trunk	Innominate Artery
Brachiocephalic vein	Innominate Vein, Right
	Innominate Vein, Left
Brachioradialis muscle	Lower Arm and Wrist Muscle, Right
	Lower Arm and Wrist Muscle, Left
Breast procedures, skin only	Skin, Chest
Broad ligament	Uterine Supporting Structure
Bronchial artery	Upper Artery
Bronchus intermedius	Main Bronchus, Right

Term	ICD-10-PCS Value
Buccal gland	Buccal Mucosa
Buccinator lymph node	Lymphatic, Head
Buccinator muscle	Facial Muscle
Bulbospongiosus muscle	Perineum Muscle
Bulbourethral (Cowper's) gland	Urethra
Bundle of His	Conduction Mechanism
Bundle of Kent	Conduction Mechanism
Calcaneocuboid joint	Tarsal Joint, Right
	Tarsal Joint, Left
Calcaneocuboid ligament	Foot Bursa and Ligament, Right
	Foot Bursa and Ligament, Left
Calcaneofibular ligament	Ankle Bursa and Ligament, Right
	Ankle Bursa and Ligament, Left
Calcaneus	Tarsal, Right
	Tarsal, Left
Capitate bone	Carpal, Right
	Carpal, Left
Cardia	Esophagogastric Junction
Cardiac plexus	Thoracic Sympathetic Nerve
Cardioesophageal junction	Esophagogastric Junction
Caroticotympanic artery	Internal Carotid Artery, Right
	Internal Carotid Artery, Left
Carotid glomus	Carotid Body, Right
	Carotid Body, Left
	Carotid Bodies, Bilateral
Carotid sinus	Internal Carotid Artery, Right
	Internal Carotid Artery, Left
Carotid sinus nerve	Glossopharyngeal Nerve
Carpometacarpal ligament	Hand Bursa and Ligament, Right
	Hand Bursa and Ligament, Left
Cauda equina	Lumbar Spinal Cord
Cavernous plexus	Head and Neck Sympathetic Nerve
Cavoatrial junction	Superior Vena Cava
Celiac ganglion	Abdominal Sympathetic Nerve
Celiac (solar) plexus	Abdominal Sympathetic Nerve
Celiac lymph node	Lymphatic, Aortic
Celiac trunk	Celiac Artery
Central axillary lymph node	Lymphatic, Right Axillary
	Lymphatic, Left Axillary
Cerebral aqueduct (Sylvius)	Cerebral Ventricle
Cerebrum	Brain
Cervical esophagus	Esophagus, Upper
Cervical facet joint	Cervical Vertebral Joint
	Cervical Vertebral Joints, 2 or more
Cervical ganglion	Head and Neck Sympathetic Nerve
Cervical interspinous ligament	Head and Neck Bursa and Ligament
Cervical intertransverse ligament	Head and Neck Bursa and Ligament
Cervical ligamentum flavum	Head and Neck Bursa and Ligament
Cervical lymph node	Lymphatic, Right Neck
	Lymphatic, Left Neck
Cervicothoracic facet joint	Cervicothoracic Vertebral Joint
Choana	Nasopharynx
Chondroglossus muscle	Tongue, Palate, Pharynx Muscle
Chorda tympani	Facial Nerve
Choroid plexus	Cerebral Ventricle

Term	ICD-10-PCS Value
Ciliary body	Eye, Right
	Eye, Left
Ciliary ganglion	Head and Neck Sympathetic Nerve
Circle of Willis	Intracranial Artery
Circumflex iliac artery	Femoral Artery, Right
	Femoral Artery, Left
Claustrum	Basal Ganglia
Coccygeal body	Coccygeal Glomus
Coccygeus muscle	Trunk Muscle, Right
	Trunk Muscle, Left
Cochlea	Inner Ear, Right
	Inner Ear, Left
Cochlear nerve	Acoustic Nerve
Columella	Nasal Mucosa and Soft Tissue
Common digital vein	Foot Vein, Right
	Foot Vein, Left
Common facial vein	Face Vein, Right
	Face Vein, Left
Common fibular nerve	Peroneal Nerve
Common hepatic artery	Hepatic Artery
Common iliac (subaortic) lymph node	Lymphatic, Pelvis
Common interosseous artery	Ulnar Artery, Right
	Ulnar Artery, Left
Common peroneal nerve	Peroneal Nerve
Condyloid process	Mandible, Right
	Mandible, Left
Conus arteriosus	Ventricle, Right
Conus medullaris	Lumbar Spinal Cord
Coracoacromial ligament	Shoulder Bursa and Ligament, Right
	Shoulder Bursa and Ligament, Left
Coracobrachialis muscle	Upper Arm Muscle, Right
	Upper Arm Muscle, Left
Coracoclavicular ligament	Shoulder Bursa and Ligament, Right
	Shoulder Bursa and Ligament, Left
Coracohumeral ligament	Shoulder Bursa and Ligament, Right
	Shoulder Bursa and Ligament, Left
Coracoid process	Scapula, Right
	Scapula, Left
Corniculate cartilage	Larynx
Corpus callosum	Brain
Corpus cavernosum	Penis
Corpus spongiosum	Penis
Corpus striatum	Basal Ganglia
Corrugator supercilii muscle	Facial Muscle
Costocervical trunk	Subclavian Artery, Right
	Subclavian Artery, Left
Costoclavicular ligament	Shoulder Bursa and Ligament, Right
	Shoulder Bursa and Ligament, Left
Costotransverse joint	Thoracic Vertebral Joint
Costotransverse ligament	Rib(s) Bursa and Ligament
Costovertebral joint	Thoracic Vertebral Joint
Costoxiphoid ligament	Sternum Bursa and Ligament
Cowper's (bulbourethral) gland	Urethra
Cremaster muscle	Perineum Muscle
Cribriform plate	Ethmoid Bone, Right
	Ethmoid Bone, Left

Term	ICD-10-PCS Value
Cricoid cartilage	Trachea
Cricothyroid artery	Thyroid Artery, Right
	Thyroid Artery, Left
Cricothyroid muscle	Neck Muscle, Right
	Neck Muscle, Left
Crural fascia	Subcutaneous Tissue and Fascia, Right Upper Leg
	Subcutaneous Tissue and Fascia, Left Upper Leg
Cubital lymph node	Lymphatic, Right Upper Extremity
	Lymphatic, Left Upper Extremity
Cubital nerve	Ulnar Nerve
Cuboid bone	Tarsal, Right
	Tarsal, Left
Cuboideonavicular joint	Tarsal Joint, Right
	Tarsal Joint, Left
Culmen	Cerebellum
Cuneiform cartilage	Larynx
Cuneonavicular joint	Tarsal Joint, Right
	Tarsal Joint, Left
Cuneonavicular ligament	Foot Bursa and Ligament, Right
	Foot Bursa and Ligament, Left
Cutaneous (transverse) cervical nerve	Cervical Plexus
Deep cervical fascia	Subcutaneous Tissue and Fascia, Right Neck
	Subcutaneous Tissue and Fascia, Left Neck
Deep cervical vein	Vertebral Vein, Right
	Vertebral Vein, Left
Deep circumflex iliac artery	External Iliac Artery, Right
	External Iliac Artery, Left
Deep facial vein	Face Vein, Right
	Face Vein, Left
Deep femoral artery	Femoral Artery, Right
	Femoral Artery, Left
Deep femoral (profunda femoris) vein	Femoral Vein, Right
	Femoral Vein, Left
Deep palmar arch	Hand Artery, Right
	Hand Artery, Left
Deep transverse perineal muscle	Perineum Muscle
Deferential artery	Internal Iliac Artery, Right
	Internal Iliac Artery, Left
Deltoid fascia	Subcutaneous Tissue and Fascia, Right Upper Arm
	Subcutaneous Tissue and Fascia, Left Upper Arm
Deltoid ligament	Ankle Bursa and Ligament, Right
	Ankle Bursa and Ligament, Left
Deltoid muscle	Shoulder Muscle, Right
	Shoulder Muscle, Left
Deltopectoral (infraclavicular) lymph node	Lymphatic, Right Upper Extremity
	Lymphatic, Left Upper Extremity
Dens	Cervical Vertebra
Denticulate (dentate) ligament	Spinal Meninges
Depressor anguli oris muscle	Facial Muscle
Depressor labii inferioris muscle	Facial Muscle

Appendix D: Body Part Key

Term	ICD-10-PCS Value
Depressor septi nasi muscle	Facial Muscle
Depressor supercilii muscle	Facial Muscle
Dermis	Skin
Descending genicular artery	Femoral Artery, Right
	Femoral Artery, Left
Diaphragma sellae	Dura Mater
Distal humerus	Humeral Shaft, Right
	Humeral Shaft, Left
Distal humerus, involving joint	Elbow Joint, Right
	Elbow Joint, Left
Distal radioulnar joint	Wrist Joint, Right
	Wrist Joint, Left
Dorsal digital nerve	Radial Nerve
Dorsal metacarpal vein	Hand Vein, Right
	Hand Vein, Left
Dorsal metatarsal artery	Foot Artery, Right
	Foot Artery, Left
Dorsal metatarsal vein	Foot Vein, Right
	Foot Vein, Left
Dorsal root ganglion	Cervical Spinal Cord
	Lumbar Spinal Cord
	Spinal Cord
	Thoracic Spinal Cord
Dorsal scapular artery	Subclavian Artery, Right
	Subclavian Artery, Left
Dorsal scapular nerve	Brachial Plexus
Dorsal venous arch	Foot Vein, Right
	Foot Vein, Left
Dorsalis pedis artery	Anterior Tibial Artery, Right
	Anterior Tibial Artery, Left
Duct of Santorini	Pancreatic Duct, Accessory
Duct of Wirsung	Pancreatic Duct
Ductus deferens	Vas Deferens, Right
	Vas Deferens, Left
	Vas Deferens, Bilateral
	Vas Deferens
Duodenal ampulla	Ampulla of Vater
Duodenojejunal flexure	Jejunum
Dura mater, intracranial	Dura Mater
Dura mater, spinal	Spinal Meninges
Dural venous sinus	Intracranial Vein
Earlobe	External Ear, Right
	External Ear, Left
	External Ear, Bilateral
Eighth cranial nerve	Acoustic Nerve
Ejaculatory duct	Vas Deferens, Right
	Vas Deferens, Left
	Vas Deferens, Bilateral
	Vas Deferens
Eleventh cranial nerve	Accessory Nerve
Encephalon	Brain
Ependyma	Cerebral Ventricle
Epidermis	Skin
Epidural space, spinal	Spinal Canal
Epiploic foramen	Peritoneum
Epithalamus	Thalamus
Epitrochlear lymph node	Lymphatic, Right Upper Extremity
	Lymphatic, Left Upper Extremity

Term	ICD-10-PCS Value
Erector spinae muscle	Trunk Muscle, Right
	Trunk Muscle, Left
Esophageal artery	Upper Artery
Esophageal plexus	Thoracic Sympathetic Nerve
Ethmoidal air cell	Ethmoid Sinus, Right
	Ethmoid Sinus, Left
Extensor carpi radialis muscle	Lower Arm and Wrist Muscle, Right
	Lower Arm and Wrist Muscle, Left
Extensor carpi ulnaris muscle	Lower Arm and Wrist Muscle, Right
	Lower Arm and Wrist Muscle, Left
Extensor digitorum brevis muscle	Foot Muscle, Right
	Foot Muscle, Left
Extensor digitorum longus muscle	Lower Leg Muscle, Right
	Lower Leg Muscle, Left
Extensor hallucis brevis muscle	Foot Muscle, Right
	Foot Muscle, Left
Extensor hallucis longus muscle	Lower Leg Muscle, Right
	Lower Leg Muscle, Left
External anal sphincter	Anal Sphincter
External auditory meatus	External Auditory Canal, Right
	External Auditory Canal, Left
External maxillary artery	Face Artery
External naris	Nasal Mucosa and Soft Tissue
External oblique aponeurosis	Subcutaneous Tissue and Fascia, Trunk
External oblique muscle	Abdomen Muscle, Right
	Abdomen Muscle, Left
External popliteal nerve	Peroneal Nerve
External pudendal artery	Femoral Artery, Right
	Femoral Artery, Left
External pudendal vein	Saphenous Vein, Right
	Saphenous Vein, Left
External urethral sphincter	Urethra
Extradural space, intracranial	Epidural Space, Intracranial
Extradural space, spinal	Spinal Canal
Facial artery	Face Artery
False vocal cord	Larynx
Falx cerebri	Dura Mater
Fascia lata	Subcutaneous Tissue and Fascia, Right Upper Leg
	Subcutaneous Tissue and Fascia, Left Upper Leg
Femoral head	Upper Femur, Right
	Upper Femur, Left
Femoral lymph node	Lymphatic, Right Lower Extremity
	Lymphatic, Left Lower Extremity
Femoropatellar joint	Knee Joint, Right
	Knee Joint, Left
	Knee Joint, Femoral Surface, Right
	Knee Joint, Femoral Surface, Left
Femorotibial joint	Knee Joint, Right
	Knee Joint, Left
	Knee Joint, Tibial Surface, Right
	Knee Joint, Tibial Surface, Left
Fibular artery	Peroneal Artery, Right
	Peroneal Artery, Left
Fibular sesamoid	Metatarsal, Right
	Metatarsal, Left

Term	ICD-10-PCS Value
Fibularis brevis muscle	Lower Leg Muscle, Right
	Lower Leg Muscle, Left
Fibularis longus muscle	Lower Leg Muscle, Right
	Lower Leg Muscle, Left
Fifth cranial nerve	Trigeminal Nerve
Filum terminale	Spinal Meninges
First cranial nerve	Olfactory Nerve
First intercostal nerve	Brachial Plexus
Flexor carpi radialis muscle	Lower Arm and Wrist Muscle, Right
	Lower Arm and Wrist Muscle, Left
Flexor carpi ulnaris muscle	Lower Arm and Wrist Muscle, Right
	Lower Arm and Wrist Muscle, Left
Flexor digitorum brevis muscle	Foot Muscle, Right
	Foot Muscle, Left
Flexor digitorum longus muscle	Lower Leg Muscle, Right
	Lower Leg Muscle, Left
Flexor hallucis brevis muscle	Foot Muscle, Right
	Foot Muscle, Left
Flexor hallucis longus muscle	Lower Leg Muscle, Right
	Lower Leg Muscle, Left
Flexor pollicis longus muscle	Lower Arm and Wrist Muscle, Right
	Lower Arm and Wrist Muscle, Left
Foramen magnum	Occipital Bone
Foramen of Monro (intraventricular)	Cerebral Ventricle
Foreskin	Prepuce
Fossa of Rosenmuller	Nasopharynx
Fourth cranial nerve	Trochlear Nerve
Fourth ventricle	Cerebral Ventricle
Fovea	Retina, Right
	Retina, Left
Frenulum labii inferioris	Lower Lip
Frenulum labii superioris	Upper Lip
Frenulum linguae	Tongue
Frontal lobe	Cerebral Hemisphere
Frontal vein	Face Vein, Right
	Face Vein, Left
Fundus uteri	Uterus
Galea aponeurotica	Subcutaneous Tissue and Fascia, Scalp
Ganglion impar (ganglion of Walther)	Sacral Sympathetic Nerve
Gasserian ganglion	Trigeminal Nerve
Gastric lymph node	Lymphatic, Aortic
Gastric plexus	Abdominal Sympathetic Nerve
Gastrocnemius muscle	Lower Leg Muscle, Right
	Lower Leg Muscle, Left
Gastrocolic ligament	Omentum
Gastrocolic omentum	Omentum
Gastroduodenal artery	Hepatic Artery
Gastroesophageal (GE) junction	Esophagogastric Junction
Gastrohepatic omentum	Omentum
Gastrophrenic ligament	Omentum
Gastrosplenic ligament	Omentum
Gemellus muscle	Hip Muscle, Right
	Hip Muscle, Left
Geniculate ganglion	Facial Nerve
Geniculate nucleus	Thalamus
Genioglossus muscle	Tongue, Palate, Pharynx Muscle

Term	ICD-10-PCS Value
Genitofemoral nerve	Lumbar Plexus
Glans penis	Prepuce
Glenohumeral joint	Shoulder Joint, Right
	Shoulder Joint, Left
Glenohumeral ligament	Shoulder Bursa and Ligament, Right
	Shoulder Bursa and Ligament, Left
Glenoid fossa (of scapula)	Glenoid Cavity, Right
	Glenoid Cavity, Left
Glenoid ligament (labrum)	Shoulder Joint, Right
	Shoulder Joint, Left
Globus pallidus	Basal Ganglia
Glossoepiglottic fold	Epiglottis
Glottis	Larynx
Gluteal lymph node	Lymphatic, Pelvis
Gluteal vein	Hypogastric Vein, Right
	Hypogastric Vein, Left
Gluteus maximus muscle	Hip Muscle, Right
	Hip Muscle, Left
Gluteus medius muscle	Hip Muscle, Right
	Hip Muscle, Left
Gluteus minimus muscle	Hip Muscle, Right
	Hip Muscle, Left
Gracilis muscle	Upper Leg Muscle, Right
	Upper Leg Muscle, Left
Great auricular nerve	Cervical Plexus
Great cerebral vein	Intracranial Vein
Great(er) saphenous vein	Saphenous Vein, Right
	Saphenous Vein, Left
Greater alar cartilage	Nasal Mucosa and Soft Tissue
Greater occipital nerve	Cervical Nerve
Greater omentum	Omentum
Greater splanchnic nerve	Thoracic Sympathetic Nerve
Greater superficial petrosal nerve	Facial Nerve
Greater trochanter	Upper Femur, Right
	Upper Femur, Left
Greater tuberosity	Humeral Head, Right
	Humeral Head, Left
Greater vestibular (Bartholin's) gland	Vestibular Gland
Greater wing	Sphenoid Bone
Hallux	1st Toe, Right
	1st Toe, Left
Hamate bone	Carpal, Right
	Carpal, Left
Head of fibula	Fibula, Right
	Fibula, Left
Helix	External Ear, Right
	External Ear, Left
	External Ear, Bilateral
Hepatic artery proper	Hepatic Artery
Hepatic flexure	Transverse Colon
Hepatic lymph node	Lymphatic, Aortic
Hepatic plexus	Abdominal Sympathetic Nerve
Hepatic portal vein	Portal Vein
Hepatogastric ligament	Omentum
Hepatopancreatic ampulla	Ampulla of Vater

Term	ICD-10-PCS Value
Humeroradial joint	Elbow Joint, Right
	Elbow Joint, Left
Humeroulnar joint	Elbow Joint, Right
	Elbow Joint, Left
Humerus, distal	Humeral Shaft, Right
	Humeral Shaft, Left
Hyoglossus muscle	Tongue, Palate, Pharynx Muscle
Hyoid artery	Thyroid Artery, Right
	Thyroid Artery, Left
Hypogastric artery	Internal Iliac Artery, Right
	Internal Iliac Artery, Left
Hypopharynx	Pharynx
Hypophysis	Pituitary Gland
Hypothenar muscle	Hand Muscle, Right
	Hand Muscle, Left
Ileal artery	Superior Mesenteric Artery
Ileocolic artery	Superior Mesenteric Artery
Ileocolic vein	Colic Vein
Iliac crest	Pelvic Bone, Right
	Pelvic Bone, Left
Iliac fascia	Subcutaneous Tissue and Fascia, Right Upper Leg
	Subcutaneous Tissue and Fascia, Left Upper Leg
Iliac lymph node	Lymphatic, Pelvis
Iliacus muscle	Hip Muscle, Right
	Hip Muscle, Left
Iliofemoral ligament	Hip Bursa and Ligament, Right
	Hip Bursa and Ligament, Left
Iliohypogastric nerve	Lumbar Plexus
Ilioinguinal nerve	Lumbar Plexus
Iliolumbar artery	Internal Iliac Artery, Right
	Internal Iliac Artery, Left
Iliolumbar ligament	Lower Spine Bursa and Ligament
Iliotibial tract (band)	Subcutaneous Tissue and Fascia, Right Upper Leg
	Subcutaneous Tissue and Fascia, Left Upper Leg
Ilium	Pelvic Bone, Right
	Pelvic Bone, Left
Incus	Auditory Ossicle, Right
	Auditory Ossicle, Left
Inferior cardiac nerve	Thoracic Sympathetic Nerve
Inferior cerebellar vein	Intracranial Vein
Inferior cerebral vein	Intracranial Vein
Inferior epigastric artery	External Iliac Artery, Right
	External Iliac Artery, Left
Inferior epigastric lymph node	Lymphatic, Pelvis
Inferior genicular artery	Popliteal Artery, Right
	Popliteal Artery, Left
Inferior gluteal artery	Internal Iliac Artery, Right
	Internal Iliac Artery, Left
Inferior gluteal nerve	Sacral Plexus
Inferior hypogastric plexus	Abdominal Sympathetic Nerve
Inferior labial artery	Face Artery
Inferior longitudinal muscle	Tongue, Palate, Pharynx Muscle
Inferior mesenteric ganglion	Abdominal Sympathetic Nerve

Term	ICD-10-PCS Value
Inferior mesenteric lymph node	Lymphatic, Mesenteric
Inferior mesenteric plexus	Abdominal Sympathetic Nerve
Inferior oblique muscle	Extraocular Muscle, Right
	Extraocular Muscle, Left
Inferior pancreaticoduodenal artery	Superior Mesenteric Artery
Inferior phrenic artery	Abdominal Aorta
Inferior rectus muscle	Extraocular Muscle, Right
	Extraocular Muscle, Left
Inferior suprarenal artery	Renal Artery, Right
	Renal Artery, Left
Inferior tarsal plate	Lower Eyelid, Right
	Lower Eyelid, Left
Inferior thyroid vein	Innominate Vein, Right
	Innominate Vein, Left
Inferior tibiofibular joint	Ankle Joint, Right
	Ankle Joint, Left
Inferior turbinate	Nasal Turbinate
Inferior ulnar collateral artery	Brachial Artery, Right
	Brachial Artery, Left
Inferior vesical artery	Internal Iliac Artery, Right
	Internal Iliac Artery, Left
Infraauricular lymph node	Lymphatic, Head
Infraclavicular (deltopectoral) lymph node	Lymphatic, Right Upper Extremity
	Lymphatic, Left Upper Extremity
Infrahyoid muscle	Neck Muscle, Right
	Neck Muscle, Left
Infraparotid lymph node	Lymphatic, Head
Infraspinatus fascia	Subcutaneous Tissue and Fascia, Right Upper Arm
	Subcutaneous Tissue and Fascia, Left Upper Arm
Infraspinatus muscle	Shoulder Muscle, Right
	Shoulder Muscle, Left
Infundibulopelvic ligament	Uterine Supporting Structure
Inguinal canal	Inguinal Region, Right
	Inguinal Region, Left
	Inguinal Region, Bilateral
Inguinal triangle	Inguinal Region, Right
	Inguinal Region, Left
	Inguinal Region, Bilateral
Interatrial septum	Atrial Septum
Intercarpal joint	Carpal Joint, Right
	Carpal Joint, Left
Intercarpal ligament	Hand Bursa and Ligament, Right
	Hand Bursa and Ligament, Left
Interclavicular ligament	Shoulder Bursa and Ligament, Right
	Shoulder Bursa and Ligament, Left
Intercostal lymph node	Lymphatic, Thorax
Intercostal muscle	Thorax Muscle, Right
	Thorax Muscle, Left
Intercostal nerve	Thoracic Nerve
Intercostobrachial nerve	Thoracic Nerve
Intercuneiform joint	Tarsal Joint, Right
	Tarsal Joint, Left
Intercuneiform ligament	Foot Bursa and Ligament, Right
	Foot Bursa and Ligament, Left
Intermediate bronchus	Main Bronchus, Right

Term	ICD-10-PCS Value
Intermediate cuneiform bone	Tarsal, Right
	Tarsal, Left
Internal anal sphincter	Anal Sphincter
Internal (basal) cerebral vein	Intracranial Vein
Internal carotid artery, intracranial portion	Intracranial Artery
Internal carotid plexus	Head and Neck Sympathetic Nerve
Internal iliac vein	Hypogastric Vein, Right
	Hypogastric Vein, Left
Internal maxillary artery	External Carotid Artery, Right
	External Carotid Artery, Left
Internal naris	Nasal Mucosa and Soft Tissue
Internal oblique muscle	Abdomen Muscle, Right
	Abdomen Muscle, Left
Internal pudendal artery	Internal Iliac Artery, Right
	Internal Iliac Artery, Left
Internal pudendal vein	Hypogastric Vein, Right
	Hypogastric Vein, Left
Internal thoracic artery	Internal Mammary Artery, Right
	Internal Mammary Artery, Left
	Subclavian Artery, Right
	Subclavian Artery, Left
Internal urethral sphincter	Urethra
Interphalangeal (IP) joint	Finger Phalangeal Joint, Right
	Finger Phalangeal Joint, Left
	Toe Phalangeal Joint, Right
	Toe Phalangeal Joint, Left
Interphalangeal ligament	Foot Bursa and Ligament, Right
	Foot Bursa and Ligament, Left
	Hand Bursa and Ligament, Right
	Hand Bursa and Ligament, Left
Interspinalis muscle	Trunk Muscle, Right
	Trunk Muscle, Left
Interspinous ligament, cervical	Head and Neck Bursa and Ligament
Interspinous ligament, lumbar	Lower Spine Bursa and Ligament
Interspinous ligament, thoracic	Upper Spine Bursa and Ligament
Intertransversarius muscle	Trunk Muscle, Right
	Trunk Muscle, Left
Intertransverse ligament, cervical	Head and Neck Bursa and Ligament
Intertransverse ligament, lumbar	Lower Spine Bursa and Ligament
Intertransverse ligament, thoracic	Upper Spine Bursa and Ligament
Interventricular foramen (Monro)	Cerebral Ventricle
Interventricular septum	Ventricular Septum
Intestinal lymphatic trunk	Cisterna Chyli
Ischiatic nerve	Sciatic Nerve
Ischiocavernosus muscle	Perineum Muscle
Ischiofemoral ligament	Hip Bursa and Ligament, Right
	Hip Bursa and Ligament, Left
Ischium	Pelvic Bone, Right
	Pelvic Bone, Left
Jejunal artery	Superior Mesenteric Artery
Jugular body	Glomus Jugulare

Term	ICD-10-PCS Value
Jugular lymph node	Lymphatic, Right Neck
	Lymphatic, Left Neck
Labia majora	Vulva
Labia minora	Vulva
Labial gland	Upper Lip
	Lower Lip
Lacrimal canaliculus	Lacrimal Duct, Right
	Lacrimal Duct, Left
Lacrimal punctum	Lacrimal Duct, Right
	Lacrimal Duct, Left
Lacrimal sac	Lacrimal Duct, Right
	Lacrimal Duct, Left
Laryngopharynx	Pharynx
Lateral (brachial) lymph node	Lymphatic, Right Axillary
	Lymphatic, Left Axillary
Lateral canthus	Upper Eyelid, Right
	Upper Eyelid, Left
Lateral collateral ligament (LCL)	Knee Bursa and Ligament, Right
	Knee Bursa and Ligament, Left
Lateral condyle of femur	Lower Femur, Right
	Lower Femur, Left
Lateral condyle of tibia	Tibia, Right
	Tibia, Left
Lateral cuneiform bone	Tarsal, Right
	Tarsal, Left
Lateral epicondyle of femur	Lower Femur, Right
	Lower Femur, Left
Lateral epicondyle of humerus	Humeral Shaft, Right
	Humeral Shaft, Left
Lateral femoral cutaneous nerve	Lumbar Plexus
Lateral malleolus	Fibula, Right
	Fibula, Left
Lateral meniscus	Knee Joint, Right
	Knee Joint, Left
Lateral nasal cartilage	Nasal Mucosa and Soft Tissue
Lateral plantar artery	Foot Artery, Right
	Foot Artery, Left
Lateral plantar nerve	Tibial Nerve
Lateral rectus muscle	Extraocular Muscle, Right
	Extraocular Muscle, Left
Lateral sacral artery	Internal Iliac Artery, Right
	Internal Iliac Artery, Left
Lateral sacral vein	Hypogastric Vein, Right
	Hypogastric Vein, Left
Lateral sural cutaneous nerve	Peroneal Nerve
Lateral tarsal artery	Foot Artery, Right
	Foot Artery, Left
Lateral temporo-mandibular ligament	Head and Neck Bursa and Ligament
Lateral thoracic artery	Axillary Artery, Right
	Axillary Artery, Left
Latissimus dorsi muscle	Trunk Muscle, Right
	Trunk Muscle, Left
Least splanchnic nerve	Thoracic Sympathetic Nerve
Left ascending lumbar vein	Hemiazygos Vein
Left atrioventricular valve	Mitral Valve
Left auricular appendix	Atrium, Left

Term	ICD-10-PCS Value
Left colic vein	Colic Vein
Left coronary sulcus	Heart, Left
Left gastric artery	Gastric Artery
Left gastroepiploic artery	Splenic Artery
Left gastroepiploic vein	Splenic Vein
Left inferior phrenic vein	Renal Vein, Left
Left inferior pulmonary vein	Pulmonary Vein, Left
Left jugular trunk	Thoracic Duct
Left lateral ventricle	Cerebral Ventricle
Left ovarian vein	Renal Vein, Left
Left second lumbar vein	Renal Vein, Left
Left subclavian trunk	Thoracic Duct
Left subcostal vein	Hemiazygos Vein
Left superior pulmonary vein	Pulmonary Vein, Left
Left suprarenal vein	Renal Vein, Left
Left testicular vein	Renal Vein, Left
Leptomeninges, intracranial	Cerebral Meninges
Leptomeninges, spinal	Spinal Meninges
Lesser alar cartilage	Nasal Mucosa and Soft Tissue
Lesser occipital nerve	Cervical Plexus
Lesser omentum	Omentum
Lesser saphenous vein	Saphenous Vein, Right
	Saphenous Vein, Left
Lesser splanchnic nerve	Thoracic Sympathetic Nerve
Lesser trochanter	Upper Femur, Right
	Upper Femur, Left
Lesser tuberosity	Humeral Head, Right
	Humeral Head, Left
Lesser wing	Sphenoid Bone
Levator anguli oris muscle	Facial Muscle
Levator ani muscle	Perineum Muscle
Levator labii superioris alaeque nasi muscle	Facial Muscle
Levator labii superioris muscle	Facial Muscle
Levator palpebrae superioris muscle	Upper Eyelid, Right
	Upper Eyelid, Left
Levator scapulae muscle	Neck Muscle, Right
	Neck Muscle, Left
Levator veli palatini muscle	Tongue, Palate, Pharynx Muscle
Levatores costarum muscle	Thorax Muscle, Right
	Thorax Muscle, Left
Ligament of head of fibula	Knee Bursa and Ligament, Right
	Knee Bursa and Ligament, Left
Ligament of the lateral malleolus	Ankle Bursa and Ligament, Right
	Ankle Bursa and Ligament, Left
Ligamentum flavum, cervical	Head and Neck Bursa and Ligament
Ligamentum flavum, lumbar	Lower Spine Bursa and Ligament
Ligamentum flavum, thoracic	Upper Spine Bursa and Ligament
Lingual artery	External Carotid Artery, Right
	External Carotid Artery, Left
Lingual tonsil	Pharynx
Locus ceruleus	Pons
Long thoracic nerve	Brachial Plexus

Term	ICD-10-PCS Value
Lumbar artery	Abdominal Aorta
Lumbar facet joint	Lumbar Vertebral Joint
Lumbar ganglion	Lumbar Sympathetic Nerve
Lumbar lymph node	Lymphatic, Aortic
Lumbar lymphatic trunk	Cisterna Chyli
Lumbar splanchnic nerve	Lumbar Sympathetic Nerve
Lumbosacral facet joint	Lumbosacral Joint
Lumbosacral trunk	Lumbar Nerve
Lunate bone	Carpal, Right
	Carpal, Left
Lunotriquetral ligament	Hand Bursa and Ligament, Right
	Hand Bursa and Ligament, Left
Macula	Retina, Right
	Retina, Left
Malleus	Auditory Ossicle, Right
	Auditory Ossicle, Left
Mammary duct	Breast, Right
	Breast, Left
	Breast, Bilateral
Mammary gland	Breast, Right
	Breast, Left
	Breast, Bilateral
Mammillary body	Hypothalamus
Mandibular nerve	Trigeminal Nerve
Mandibular notch	Mandible, Right
	Mandible, Left
Manubrium	Sternum
Masseter muscle	Head Muscle
Masseteric fascia	Subcutaneous Tissue and Fascia, Face
Mastoid (postauricular) lymph node	Lymphatic, Right Neck
	Lymphatic, Left Neck
Mastoid air cells	Mastoid Sinus, Right
	Mastoid Sinus, Left
Mastoid process	Temporal Bone, Right
	Temporal Bone, Left
Maxillary artery	External Carotid Artery, Right
	External Carotid Artery, Left
Maxillary nerve	Trigeminal Nerve
Medial canthus	Lower Eyelid, Right
	Lower Eyelid, Left
Medial collateral ligament (MCL)	Knee Bursa and Ligament, Right
	Knee Bursa and Ligament, Left
Medial condyle of femur	Lower Femur, Right
	Lower Femur, Left
Medial condyle of tibia	Tibia, Right
	Tibia, Left
Medial cuneiform bone	Tarsal, Right
	Tarsal, Left
Medial epicondyle of femur	Lower Femur, Right
	Lower Femur, Left
Medial epicondyle of humerus	Humeral Shaft, Right
	Humeral Shaft, Left
Medial malleolus	Tibia, Right
	Tibia, Left
Medial meniscus	Knee Joint, Right
	Knee Joint, Left
Medial plantar artery	Foot Artery, Right
	Foot Artery, Left

Term	ICD-10-PCS Value
Medial plantar nerve	Tibial Nerve
Medial popliteal nerve	Tibial Nerve
Medial rectus muscle	Extraocular Muscle, Right
	Extraocular Muscle, Left
Medial sural cutaneous nerve	Tibial Nerve
Median antebrachial vein	Basilic Vein, Right
	Basilic Vein, Left
Median cubital vein	Basilic Vein, Right
	Basilic Vein, Left
Median sacral artery	Abdominal Aorta
Mediastinal cavity	Mediastinum
Mediastinal lymph node	Lymphatic, Thorax
Mediastinal space	Mediastinum
Meissner's (submucous) plexus	Abdominal Sympathetic Nerve
Membranous urethra	Urethra
Mental foramen	Mandible, Right
	Mandible, Left
Mentalis muscle	Facial Muscle
Mesoappendix	Mesentery
Mesocolon	Mesentery
Metacarpal ligament	Hand Bursa and Ligament, Right
	Hand Bursa and Ligament, Left
Metacarpophalangeal ligament	Hand Bursa and Ligament, Right
	Hand Bursa and Ligament, Left
Metatarsal ligament	Foot Bursa and Ligament, Right
	Foot Bursa and Ligament, Left
Metatarsophalangeal ligament	Foot Bursa and Ligament, Right
	Foot Bursa and Ligament, Left
Metatarsophalangeal (MTP) joint	Metatarsal-Phalangeal Joint, Right
	Metatarsal-Phalangeal Joint, Left
Metathalamus	Thalamus
Midcarpal joint	Carpal Joint, Right
	Carpal Joint, Left
Middle cardiac nerve	Thoracic Sympathetic Nerve
Middle cerebral artery	Intracranial Artery
Middle cerebral vein	Intracranial Vein
Middle colic vein	Colic Vein
Middle genicular artery	Popliteal Artery, Right
	Popliteal Artery, Left
Middle hemorrhoidal vein	Hypogastric Vein, Right
	Hypogastric Vein, Left
Middle rectal artery	Internal Iliac Artery, Right
	Internal Iliac Artery, Left
Middle suprarenal artery	Abdominal Aorta
Middle temporal artery	Temporal Artery, Right
	Temporal Artery, Left
Middle turbinate	Nasal Turbinate
Mitral annulus	Mitral Valve
Molar gland	Buccal Mucosa
Musculocutaneous nerve	Brachial Plexus
Musculophrenic artery	Internal Mammary Artery, Right
	Internal Mammary Artery, Left
Musculospiral nerve	Radial Nerve
Myelencephalon	Medulla Oblongata
Myenteric (Auerbach's) plexus	Abdominal Sympathetic Nerve
Myometrium	Uterus

Term	ICD-10-PCS Value
Nail bed	Finger Nail
	Toe Nail
Nail plate	Finger Nail
	Toe Nail
Nasal cavity	Nasal Mucosa and Soft Tissue
Nasal concha	Nasal Turbinate
Nasalis muscle	Facial Muscle
Nasolacrimal duct	Lacrimal Duct, Right
	Lacrimal Duct, Left
Navicular bone	Tarsal, Right
	Tarsal, Left
Neck of femur	Upper Femur, Right
	Upper Femur, Left
Neck of humerus (anatomical) (surgical)	Humeral Head, Right
	Humeral Head, Left
Nerve to the stapedius	Facial Nerve
Neurohypophysis	Pituitary Gland
Ninth cranial nerve	Glossopharyngeal Nerve
Nostril	Nasal Mucosa and Soft Tissue
Obturator artery	Internal Iliac Artery, Right
	Internal Iliac Artery, Left
Obturator lymph node	Lymphatic, Pelvis
Obturator muscle	Hip Muscle, Right
	Hip Muscle, Left
Obturator nerve	Lumbar Plexus
Obturator vein	Hypogastric Vein, Right
	Hypogastric Vein, Left
Obtuse margin	Heart, Left
Occipital artery	External Carotid Artery, Right
	External Carotid Artery, Left
Occipital lobe	Cerebral Hemisphere
Occipital lymph node	Lymphatic, Right Neck
	Lymphatic, Left Neck
Occipitofrontalis muscle	Facial Muscle
Odontoid process	Cervical Vertebra
Olecranon bursa	Elbow Bursa and Ligament, Right
	Elbow Bursa and Ligament, Left
Olecranon process	Ulna, Right
	Ulna, Left
Olfactory bulb	Olfactory Nerve
Ophthalmic artery	Intracranial Artery
Ophthalmic nerve	Trigeminal Nerve
Ophthalmic vein	Intracranial Vein
Optic chiasma	Optic Nerve
Optic disc	Retina, Right
	Retina, Left
Optic foramen	Sphenoid Bone
Orbicularis oculi muscle	Upper Eyelid, Right
	Upper Eyelid, Left
Orbicularis oris muscle	Facial Muscle
Orbital fascia	Subcutaneous Tissue and Fascia, Face
Orbital portion of ethmoid bone	Orbit, Right
	Orbit, Left
Orbital portion of frontal bone	Orbit, Right
	Orbit, Left
Orbital portion of lacrimal bone	Orbit, Right
	Orbit, Left

Appendix D: Body Part Key

Term	ICD-10-PCS Value
Orbital portion of maxilla	Orbit, Right
	Orbit, Left
Orbital portion of palatine bone	Orbit, Right
	Orbit, Left
Orbital portion of sphenoid bone	Orbit, Right
	Orbit, Left
Orbital portion of zygomatic bone	Orbit, Right
	Orbit, Left
Oropharynx	Pharynx
Otic ganglion	Head and Neck Sympathetic Nerve
Oval window	Middle Ear, Right
	Middle Ear, Left
Ovarian artery	Abdominal Aorta
Ovarian ligament	Uterine Supporting Structure
Oviduct	Fallopian Tube, Right
	Fallopian Tube, Left
Palatine gland	Buccal Mucosa
Palatine tonsil	Tonsils
Palatine uvula	Uvula
Palatoglossal muscle	Tongue, Palate, Pharynx Muscle
Palatopharyngeal muscle	Tongue, Palate, Pharynx Muscle
Palmar (volar) digital vein	Hand Vein, Right
	Hand Vein, Left
Palmar (volar) metacarpal vein	Hand Vein, Right
	Hand Vein, Left
Palmar cutaneous nerve	Median Nerve
	Radial Nerve
Palmar fascia (aponeurosis)	Subcutaneous Tissue and Fascia, Right Hand
	Subcutaneous Tissue and Fascia, Left Hand
Palmar interosseous muscle	Hand Muscle, Right
	Hand Muscle, Left
Palmar ulnocarpal ligament	Wrist Bursa and Ligament, Right
	Wrist Bursa and Ligament, Left
Palmaris longus muscle	Lower Arm and Wrist Muscle, Right
	Lower Arm and Wrist Muscle, Left
Pancreatic artery	Splenic Artery
Pancreatic plexus	Abdominal Sympathetic Nerve
Pancreatic vein	Splenic Vein
Pancreaticosplenic lymph node	Lymphatic, Aortic
Paraaortic lymph node	Lymphatic, Aortic
Parapharyngeal space	Neck
Pararectal lymph node	Lymphatic, Mesenteric
Parasternal lymph node	Lymphatic, Thorax
Paratracheal lymph node	Lymphatic, Thorax
Paraurethral (Skene's) gland	Vestibular Gland
Parietal lobe	Cerebral Hemisphere
Parotid lymph node	Lymphatic, Head
Parotid plexus	Facial Nerve
Pars flaccida	Tympanic Membrane, Right
	Tympanic Membrane, Left
Patellar ligament	Knee Bursa and Ligament, Right
	Knee Bursa and Ligament, Left
Patellar tendon	Knee Tendon, Right
	Knee Tendon, Left

Term	ICD-10-PCS Value
Patellofemoral joint	Knee Joint, Right
	Knee Joint, Left
	Knee Joint, Femoral Surface, Right
	Knee Joint, Femoral Surface, Left
Pectineus muscle	Upper Leg Muscle, Right
	Upper Leg Muscle, Left
Pectoral (anterior) lymph node	Lymphatic, Right Axillary
	Lymphatic, Left Axillary
Pectoral fascia	Subcutaneous Tissue and Fascia, Chest
Pectoralis major muscle	Thorax Muscle, Right
	Thorax Muscle, Left
Pectoralis minor muscle	Thorax Muscle, Right
	Thorax Muscle, Left
Pelvic splanchnic nerve	Abdominal Sympathetic Nerve
	Sacral Sympathetic Nerve
Penile urethra	Urethra
Perianal skin	Skin, Perineum
Pericardiophrenic artery	Internal Mammary Artery, Right
	Internal Mammary Artery, Left
Perimetrium	Uterus
Peroneus brevis muscle	Lower Leg Muscle, Right
	Lower Leg Muscle, Left
Peroneus longus muscle	Lower Leg Muscle, Right
	Lower Leg Muscle, Left
Petrous part of temoporal bone	Temporal Bone, Right
	Temporal Bone, Left
Pharyngeal constrictor muscle	Tongue, Palate, Pharynx Muscle
Pharyngeal plexus	Vagus Nerve
Pharyngeal recess	Nasopharynx
Pharyngeal tonsil	Adenoids
Pharyngotympanic tube	Eustachian Tube, Right
	Eustachian Tube, Left
Pia mater, intracranial	Cerebral Meninges
Pia mater, spinal	Spinal Meninges
Pinna	External Ear, Right
	External Ear, Left
	External Ear, Bilateral
Piriform recess (sinus)	Pharynx
Piriformis muscle	Hip Muscle, Right
	Hip Muscle, Left
Pisiform bone	Carpal, Right
	Carpal, Left
Pisohamate ligament	Hand Bursa and Ligament, Right
	Hand Bursa and Ligament, Left
Pisometacarpal ligament	Hand Bursa and Ligament, Right
	Hand Bursa and Ligament, Left
Plantar digital vein	Foot Vein, Right
	Foot Vein, Left
Plantar fascia (aponeurosis)	Subcutaneous Tissue and Fascia, Right Foot
	Subcutaneous Tissue and Fascia, Left Foot
Plantar metatarsal vein	Foot Vein, Right
	Foot Vein, Left
Plantar venous arch	Foot Vein, Right
	Foot Vein, Left
Platysma muscle	Neck Muscle, Right
	Neck Muscle, Left

Term	ICD-10-PCS Value
Plica semilunaris	Conjunctiva, Right
	Conjunctiva, Left
Pneumogastric nerve	Vagus Nerve
Pneumotaxic center	Pons
Pontine tegmentum	Pons
Popliteal ligament	Knee Bursa and Ligament, Right
	Knee Bursa and Ligament, Left
Popliteal lymph node	Lymphatic, Left Lower Extremity
	Lymphatic, Right Lower Extremity
Popliteal vein	Femoral Vein, Right
	Femoral Vein, Left
Popliteus muscle	Lower Leg Muscle, Right
	Lower Leg Muscle, Left
Postauricular (mastoid) lymph node	Lymphatic, Right Neck
	Lymphatic, Left Neck
Postcava	Inferior Vena Cava
Posterior (subscapular) lymph node	Lymphatic, Right Axillary
	Lymphatic, Left Axillary
Posterior auricular artery	External Carotid Artery, Right
	External Carotid Artery, Left
Posterior auricular nerve	Facial Nerve
Posterior auricular vein	External Jugular Vein, Right
	External Jugular Vein, Left
Posterior cerebral artery	Intracranial Artery
Posterior chamber	Eye, Right
	Eye, Left
Posterior circumflex humeral artery	Axillary Artery, Right
	Axillary Artery, Left
Posterior communicating artery	Intracranial Artery
Posterior cruciate ligament (PCL)	Knee Bursa and Ligament, Right
	Knee Bursa and Ligament, Left
Posterior facial (retromandibular) vein	Face Vein, Right
	Face Vein, Left
Posterior femoral cutaneous nerve	Sacral Plexus
Posterior inferior cerebellar artery (PICA)	Intracranial Artery
Posterior interosseous nerve	Radial Nerve
Posterior labial nerve	Pudendal Nerve
Posterior scrotal nerve	Pudendal Nerve
Posterior spinal artery	Vertebral Artery, Right
	Vertebral Artery, Left
Posterior tibial recurrent artery	Anterior Tibial Artery, Right
	Anterior Tibial Artery, Left
Posterior ulnar recurrent artery	Ulnar Artery, Right
	Ulnar Artery, Left
Posterior vagal trunk	Vagus Nerve
Preauricular lymph node	Lymphatic, Head
Precava	Superior Vena Cava
Prepatellar bursa	Knee Bursa and Ligament, Right
	Knee Bursa and Ligament, Left
Pretracheal fascia	Subcutaneous Tissue and Fascia, Right Neck
	Subcutaneous Tissue and Fascia, Left Neck
Prevertebral fascia	Subcutaneous Tissue and Fascia, Right Neck
	Subcutaneous Tissue and Fascia, Left Neck

Term	ICD-10-PCS Value
Princeps pollicis artery	Hand Artery, Right
	Hand Artery, Left
Procerus muscle	Facial Muscle
Profunda brachii	Brachial Artery, Right
	Brachial Artery, Left
Profunda femoris (deep femoral) vein	Femoral Vein, Right
	Femoral Vein, Left
Pronator quadratus muscle	Lower Arm and Wrist Muscle, Right
	Lower Arm and Wrist Muscle, Left
Pronator teres muscle	Lower Arm and Wrist Muscle, Right
	Lower Arm and Wrist Muscle, Left
Prostatic artery	Internal Iliac Artery, Right
	Internal Iliac Artery, Left
Prostatic urethra	Urethra
Proximal radioulnar joint	Elbow Joint, Right
	Elbow Joint, Left
Psoas muscle	Hip Muscle, Right
	Hip Muscle, Left
Pterygoid muscle	Head Muscle
Pterygoid process	Sphenoid Bone
Pterygopalatine (sphenopalatine) ganglion	Head and Neck Sympathetic Nerve
Pubis	Pelvic Bone, Right
	Pelvic Bone, Left
Pubofemoral ligament	Hip Bursa and Ligament, Right
	Hip Bursa and Ligament, Left
Pudendal nerve	Sacral Plexus
Pulmoaortic canal	Pulmonary Artery, Left
Pulmonary annulus	Pulmonary Valve
Pulmonary plexus	Thoracic Sympathetic Nerve
	Vagus Nerve
Pulmonic valve	Pulmonary Valve
Pulvinar	Thalamus
Pyloric antrum	Stomach, Pylorus
Pyloric canal	Stomach, Pylorus
Pyloric sphincter	Stomach, Pylorus
Pyramidalis muscle	Abdomen Muscle, Right
	Abdomen Muscle, Left
Quadrangular cartilage	Nasal Septum
Quadrate lobe	Liver
Quadratus femoris muscle	Hip Muscle, Right
	Hip Muscle, Left
Quadratus lumborum muscle	Trunk Muscle, Right
	Trunk Muscle, Left
Quadratus plantae muscle	Foot Muscle, Right
	Foot Muscle, Left
Quadriceps (femoris)	Upper Leg Muscle, Right
	Upper Leg Muscle, Left
Radial collateral carpal ligament	Wrist Bursa and Ligament, Right
	Wrist Bursa and Ligament, Left
Radial collateral ligament	Elbow Bursa and Ligament, Right
	Elbow Bursa and Ligament, Left
Radial notch	Ulna, Right
	Ulna, Left
Radial recurrent artery	Radial Artery, Right
	Radial Artery, Left
Radial vein	Brachial Vein, Right
	Brachial Vein, Left

Term	ICD-10-PCS Value
Radialis indicis	Hand Artery, Right
	Hand Artery, Left
Radiocarpal joint	Wrist Joint, Right
	Wrist Joint, Left
Radiocarpal ligament	Wrist Bursa and Ligament, Right
	Wrist Bursa and Ligament, Left
Radioulnar ligament	Wrist Bursa and Ligament, Right
	Wrist Bursa and Ligament, Left
Rectosigmoid junction	Sigmoid Colon
Rectus abdominis muscle	Abdomen Muscle, Right
	Abdomen Muscle, Left
Rectus femoris muscle	Upper Leg Muscle, Right
	Upper Leg Muscle, Left
Recurrent laryngeal nerve	Vagus Nerve
Renal calyx	Kidney, Right
	Kidney, Left
	Kidneys, Bilateral
	Kidney
Renal capsule	Kidney, Right
	Kidney, Left
	Kidneys, Bilateral
	Kidney
Renal cortex	Kidney, Right
	Kidney, Left
	Kidneys, Bilateral
	Kidney
Renal nerve	Abdominal sympathetic Nerve
Renal plexus	Abdominal Sympathetic Nerve
Renal segment	Kidney, Right
	Kidney, Left
	Kidneys, Bilateral
	Kidney
Renal segmental artery	Renal Artery, Right
	Renal Artery, Left
Retroperitoneal cavity	Retroperitoneum
Retroperitoneal lymph node	Lymphatic, Aortic
Retroperitoneal space	Retroperitoneum
Retropharyngeal lymph node	Lymphatic, Right Neck
	Lymphatic, Left Neck
Retropharyngeal space	Neck
Retropubic space	Pelvic Cavity
Rhinopharynx	Nasopharynx
Rhomboid major muscle	Trunk Muscle, Right
	Trunk Muscle, Left
Rhomboid minor muscle	Trunk Muscle, Right
	Trunk Muscle, Left
Right ascending lumbar vein	Azygos Vein
Right atrioventricular valve	Tricuspid Valve
Right auricular appendix	Atrium, Right
Right colic vein	Colic Vein
Right coronary sulcus	Heart, Right
Right gastric artery	Gastric Artery
Right gastroepiploic vein	Superior Mesenteric Vein
Right inferior phrenic vein	Inferior Vena Cava
Right inferior pulmonary vein	Pulmonary Vein, Right
Right jugular trunk	Lymphatic, Right Neck

Term	ICD-10-PCS Value
Right lateral ventricle	Cerebral Ventricle
Right lymphatic duct	Lymphatic, Right Neck
Right ovarian vein	Inferior Vena Cava
Right second lumbar vein	Inferior Vena Cava
Right subclavian trunk	Lymphatic, Right Neck
Right subcostal vein	Azygos Vein
Right superior pulmonary vein	Pulmonary Vein, Right
Right suprarenal vein	Inferior Vena Cava
Right testicular vein	Inferior Vena Cava
Rima glottidis	Larynx
Risorius muscle	Facial Muscle
Round ligament of uterus	Uterine Supporting Structure
Round window	Inner Ear, Right
	Inner Ear, Left
Sacral ganglion	Sacral Sympathetic Nerve
Sacral lymph node	Lymphatic, Pelvis
Sacral splanchnic nerve	Sacral Sympathetic Nerve
Sacrococcygeal ligament	Lower Spine Bursa and Ligament
Sacrococcygeal symphysis	Sacrococcygeal Joint
Sacroiliac ligament	Lower Spine Bursa and Ligament
Sacrospinous ligament	Lower Spine Bursa and Ligament
Sacrotuberous ligament	Lower Spine Bursa and Ligament
Salpingopharyngeus muscle	Tongue, Palate, Pharynx Muscle
Salpinx	Fallopian Tube, Right
	Fallopian Tube, Left
Saphenous nerve	Femoral Nerve
Sartorius muscle	Upper Leg Muscle, Right
	Upper Leg Muscle, Left
Scalene muscle	Neck Muscle, Right
	Neck Muscle, Left
Scaphoid bone	Carpal, Right
	Carpal, Left
Scapholunate ligament	Wrist Bursa and Ligament, Right
	Wrist Bursa and Ligament, Left
Scaphotrapezium ligament	Hand Bursa and Ligament, Right
	Hand Bursa and Ligament, Left
Scarpa's (vestibular) ganglion	Acoustic Nerve
Sebaceous gland	Skin
Second cranial nerve	Optic Nerve
Sella turcica	Sphenoid Bone
Semicircular canal	Inner Ear, Right
	Inner Ear, Left
Semimembranosus muscle	Upper Leg Muscle, Right
	Upper Leg Muscle, Left
Semitendinosus muscle	Upper Leg Muscle, Right
	Upper Leg Muscle, Left
Septal cartilage	Nasal Septum
Serratus anterior muscle	Thorax Muscle, Right
	Thorax Muscle, Left
Serratus posterior muscle	Trunk Muscle, Right
	Trunk Muscle, Left
Seventh cranial nerve	Facial Nerve
Short gastric artery	Splenic Artery
Sigmoid artery	Inferior Mesenteric Artery
Sigmoid flexure	Sigmoid Colon
Sigmoid vein	Inferior Mesenteric Vein

Term	ICD-10-PCS Value
Sinoatrial node	Conduction Mechanism
Sinus venosus	Atrium, Right
Sixth cranial nerve	Abducens Nerve
Skene's (paraurethral) gland	Vestibular Gland
Small saphenous vein	Saphenous Vein, Right
	Saphenous Vein, Left
Solar (celiac) plexus	Abdominal Sympathetic Nerve
Soleus muscle	Lower Leg Muscle, Right
	Lower Leg Muscle, Left
Sphenomandibular ligament	Head and Neck Bursa and Ligament
Sphenopalatine (pterygopalatine) ganglion	Head and Neck Sympathetic Nerve
Spinal nerve, cervical	Cervical Nerve
Spinal nerve, lumbar	Lumbar Nerve
Spinal nerve, sacral	Sacral Nerve
Spinal nerve, thoracic	Thoracic Nerve
Spinous process	Cervical Vertebra
	Lumbar Vertebra
	Thoracic Vertebra
Spiral ganglion	Acoustic Nerve
Splenic flexure	Transverse Colon
Splenic plexus	Abdominal Sympathetic Nerve
Splenius capitis muscle	Head Muscle
Splenius cervicis muscle	Neck Muscle, Right
	Neck Muscle, Left
Stapes	Auditory Ossicle, Right
	Auditory Ossicle, Left
Stellate ganglion	Head and Neck Sympathetic Nerve
Stensen's duct	Parotid Duct, Right
	Parotid Duct, Left
Sternoclavicular ligament	Shoulder Bursa and Ligament, Right
	Shoulder Bursa and Ligament, Left
Sternocleidomastoid artery	Thyroid Artery, Right
	Thyroid Artery, Left
Sternocleidomastoid muscle	Neck Muscle, Right
	Neck Muscle, Left
Sternocostal ligament	Sternum Bursa and Ligament
Styloglossus muscle	Tongue, Palate, Pharynx Muscle
Stylomandibular ligament	Head and Neck Bursa and Ligament
Stylopharyngeus muscle	Tongue, Palate, Pharynx Muscle
Subacromial bursa	Shoulder Bursa and Ligament, Right
	Shoulder Bursa and Ligament, Left
Subaortic (common iliac) lymph node	Lymphatic, Pelvis
Subarachnoid space, spinal	Spinal Canal
Subclavicular (apical) lymph node	Lymphatic, Right Axillary
	Lymphatic, Left Axillary
Subclavius muscle	Thorax Muscle, Right
	Thorax Muscle, Left
Subclavius nerve	Brachial Plexus
Subcostal artery	Upper Artery
Subcostal muscle	Thorax Muscle, Right
	Thorax Muscle, Left
Subcostal nerve	Thoracic Nerve
Subdural space, spinal	Spinal Canal
Submandibular ganglion	Facial Nerve
	Head and Neck Sympathetic Nerve

Term	ICD-10-PCS Value
Submandibular gland	Submaxillary Gland, Right
	Submaxillary Gland, Left
Submandibular lymph node	Lymphatic, Head
Submandibular space	Subcutaneous Tissue and Fascia, Face
Submaxillary ganglion	Head and Neck Sympathetic Nerve
Submaxillary lymph node	Lymphatic, Head
Submental artery	Face Artery
Submental lymph node	Lymphatic, Head
Submucous (Meissner's) plexus	Abdominal Sympathetic Nerve
Suboccipital nerve	Cervical Nerve
Suboccipital venous plexus	Vertebral Vein, Right
	Vertebral Vein, Left
Subparotid lymph node	Lymphatic, Head
Subscapular aponeurosis	Subcutaneous Tissue and Fascia, Right Upper Arm
	Subcutaneous Tissue and Fascia, Left Upper Arm
Subscapular artery	Axillary Artery, Right
	Axillary Artery, Left
Subscapular (posterior) lymph node	Lymphatic, Right Axillary
	Lymphatic, Left Axillary
Subscapularis muscle	Shoulder Muscle, Right
	Shoulder Muscle, Left
Substantia nigra	Basal Ganglia
Subtalar (talocalcaneal) joint	Tarsal Joint, Right
	Tarsal Joint, Left
Subtalar ligament	Foot Bursa and Ligament, Right
	Foot Bursa and Ligament, Left
Subthalamic nucleus	Basal Ganglia
Superficial circumflex iliac vein	Saphenous Vein, Right
	Saphenous Vein, Left
Superficial epigastric artery	Femoral Artery, Right
	Femoral Artery, Left
Superficial epigastric vein	Saphenous Vein, Right
	Saphenous Vein, Left
Superficial palmar arch	Hand Artery, Right
	Hand Artery, Left
Superficial palmar venous arch	Hand Vein, Right
	Hand Vein, Left
Superficial temporal artery	Temporal Artery, Right
	Temporal Artery, Left
Superficial transverse perineal muscle	Perineum Muscle
Superior cardiac nerve	Thoracic Sympathetic Nerve
Superior cerebellar vein	Intracranial Vein
Superior cerebral vein	Intracranial Vein
Superior clunic (cluneal) nerve	Lumbar Nerve
Superior epigastric artery	Internal Mammary Artery, Right
	Internal Mammary Artery, Left
Superior genicular artery	Popliteal Artery, Right
	Popliteal Artery, Left
Superior gluteal artery	Internal Iliac Artery, Right
	Internal Iliac Artery, Left
Superior gluteal nerve	Lumbar Plexus
Superior hypogastric plexus	Abdominal Sympathetic Nerve
Superior labial artery	Face Artery

Term	ICD-10-PCS Value
Superior laryngeal artery	Thyroid Artery, Right
	Thyroid Artery, Left
Superior laryngeal nerve	Vagus Nerve
Superior longitudinal muscle	Tongue, Palate, Pharynx Muscle
Superior mesenteric ganglion	Abdominal Sympathetic Nerve
Superior mesenteric lymph node	Lymphatic, Mesenteric
Superior mesenteric plexus	Abdominal Sympathetic Nerve
Superior oblique muscle	Extraocular Muscle, Right
	Extraocular Muscle, Left
Superior olivary nucleus	Pons
Superior rectal artery	Inferior Mesenteric Artery
Superior rectal vein	Inferior Mesenteric Vein
Superior rectus muscle	Extraocular Muscle, Right
	Extraocular Muscle, Left
Superior tarsal plate	Upper Eyelid, Right
	Upper Eyelid, Left
Superior thoracic artery	Axillary Artery, Right
	Axillary Artery, Left
Superior thyroid artery	External Carotid Artery, Right
	External Carotid Artery, Left
	Thyroid Artery, Right
	Thyroid Artery, Left
Superior turbinate	Nasal Turbinate
Superior ulnar collateral artery	Brachial Artery, Right
	Brachial Artery, Left
Superior vesical artery	Internal Iliac Artery, Right
	Internal Iliac Artery, Left
Supraclavicular nerve	Cervical Plexus
Supraclavicular (Virchow's) lymph node	Lymphatic, Right Neck
	Lymphatic, Left Neck
Suprahyoid lymph node	Lymphatic, Head
Suprahyoid muscle	Neck Muscle, Right
	Neck Muscle, Left
Suprainguinal lymph node	Lymphatic, Pelvis
Supraorbital vein	Face Vein, Right
	Face Vein, Left
Suprarenal gland	Adrenal Gland, Right
	Adrenal Gland, Left
	Adrenal Glands, Bilateral
	Adrenal Gland
Suprarenal plexus	Abdominal Sympathetic Nerve
Suprascapular nerve	Brachial Plexus
Supraspinatus fascia	Subcutaneous Tissue and Fascia, Right Upper Arm
	Subcutaneous Tissue and Fascia, Left Upper Arm
Supraspinatus muscle	Shoulder Muscle, Right
	Shoulder Muscle, Left
Supraspinous ligament	Upper Spine Bursa and Ligament
	Lower Spine Bursa and Ligament
Suprasternal notch	Sternum
Supratrochlear lymph node	Lymphatic, Right Upper Extremity
	Lymphatic, Left Upper Extremity
Sural artery	Popliteal Artery, Right
	Popliteal Artery, Left
Sweat gland	Skin

Term	ICD-10-PCS Value
Talocalcaneal ligament	Foot Bursa and Ligament, Right
	Foot Bursa and Ligament, Left
Talocalcaneal (subtalar) joint	Tarsal Joint, Right
	Tarsal Joint, Left
Talocalcaneonavicular joint	Tarsal Joint, Right
	Tarsal Joint, Left
Talocalcaneonavicular ligament	Foot Bursa and Ligament, Right
	Foot Bursa and Ligament, Left
Talocrural joint	Ankle Joint, Right
	Ankle Joint, Left
Talofibular ligament	Ankle Bursa and Ligament, Right
	Ankle Bursa and Ligament, Left
Talus bone	Tarsal, Right
	Tarsal, Left
Tarsometatarsal ligament	Foot Bursa and Ligament, Right
	Foot Bursa and Ligament, Left
Temporal lobe	Cerebral Hemisphere
Temporalis muscle	Head Muscle
Temporoparietalis muscle	Head Muscle
Tensor fasciae latae muscle	Hip Muscle, Right
	Hip Muscle, Left
Tensor veli palatini muscle	Tongue, Palate, Pharynx Muscle
Tenth cranial nerve	Vagus Nerve
Tentorium cerebelli	Dura Mater
Teres major muscle	Shoulder Muscle, Right
	Shoulder Muscle, Left
Teres minor muscle	Shoulder Muscle, Right
	Shoulder Muscle, Left
Testicular artery	Abdominal Aorta
Thenar muscle	Hand Muscle, Right
	Hand Muscle, Left
Third cranial nerve	Oculomotor Nerve
Third occipital nerve	Cervical Nerve
Third ventricle	Cerebral Ventricle
Thoracic aortic plexus	Thoracic Sympathetic Nerve
Thoracic esophagus	Esophagus, Middle
Thoracic facet joint	Thoracic Vertebral Joint
Thoracic ganglion	Thoracic Sympathetic Nerve
Thoracoacromial artery	Axillary Artery, Right
	Axillary Artery, Left
Thoracolumbar facet joint	Thoracolumbar Vertebral Joint
Thymus gland	Thymus
Thyroarytenoid muscle	Neck Muscle, Right
	Neck Muscle, Left
Thyrocervical trunk	Thyroid Artery, Right
	Thyroid Artery, Left
Thyroid cartilage	Larynx
Tibial sesamoid	Metatarsal, Right
	Metatarsal, Left
Tibialis anterior muscle	Lower Leg Muscle, Right
	Lower Leg Muscle, Left
Tibialis posterior muscle	Lower Leg Muscle, Right
	Lower Leg Muscle, Left
Tibiofemoral joint	Knee Joint, Right
	Knee Joint, Left
	Knee Joint, Tibial Surface, Right
	Knee Joint, Tibial Surface, Left

Term	ICD-10-PCS Value
Tibioperoneal trunk	Popliteal Artery, Right
	Popliteal Artery, Left
Tongue, base of	Pharynx
Tracheobronchial lymph node	Lymphatic, Thorax
Tragus	External Ear, Right
	External Ear, Left
	External Ear, Bilateral
Transversalis fascia	Subcutaneous Tissue and Fascia, Trunk
Transverse acetabular ligament	Hip Bursa and Ligament, Right
	Hip Bursa and Ligament, Left
Transverse (cutaneous) cervical nerve	Cervical Plexus
Transverse facial artery	Temporal Artery, Right
	Temporal Artery, Left
Transverse foramen	Cervical Vertebra
Transverse humeral ligament	Shoulder Bursa and Ligament, Right
	Shoulder Bursa and Ligament, Left
Transverse ligament of atlas	Head and Neck Bursa and Ligament
Transverse process	Cervical Vertebra
	Thoracic Vertebra
	Lumbar Vertebra
Transverse scapular ligament	Shoulder Bursa and Ligament, Right
	Shoulder Bursa and Ligament, Left
Transverse thoracis muscle	Thorax Muscle, Right
	Thorax Muscle, Left
Transversospinalis muscle	Trunk Muscle, Right
	Trunk Muscle, Left
Transversus abdominis muscle	Abdomen Muscle, Right
	Abdomen Muscle, Left
Trapezium bone	Carpal, Right
	Carpal, Left
Trapezius muscle	Trunk Muscle, Right
	Trunk Muscle, Left
Trapezoid bone	Carpal, Right
	Carpal, Left
Triceps brachii muscle	Upper Arm Muscle, Right
	Upper Arm Muscle, Left
Tricuspid annulus	Tricuspid Valve
Trifacial nerve	Trigeminal Nerve
Trigone of bladder	Bladder
Triquetral bone	Carpal, Right
	Carpal, Left
Trochanteric bursa	Hip Bursa and Ligament, Right
	Hip Bursa and Ligament, Left
Twelfth cranial nerve	Hypoglossal Nerve
Tympanic cavity	Middle Ear, Right
	Middle Ear, Left
Tympanic nerve	Glossopharyngeal Nerve
Tympanic part of temoporal bone	Temporal Bone, Right
	Temporal Bone, Left
Ulnar collateral carpal ligament	Wrist Bursa and Ligament, Right
	Wrist Bursa and Ligament, Left
Ulnar collateral ligament	Elbow Bursa and Ligament, Right
	Elbow Bursa and Ligament, Left
Ulnar notch	Radius, Right
	Radius, Left

Term	ICD-10-PCS Value
Ulnar vein	Brachial Vein, Right
	Brachial Vein, Left
Umbilical artery	Internal Iliac Artery, Right
	Internal Iliac Artery, Left
	Lower Artery
Ureteral orifice	Ureter, Right
	Ureter, Left
	Ureters, Bilateral
	Ureter
Ureteropelvic junction (UPJ)	Kidney Pelvis, Right
	Kidney Pelvis, Left
Ureterovesical orifice	Ureter, Right
	Ureter, Left
	Ureters, Bilateral
	Ureter
Uterine artery	Internal Iliac Artery, Right
	Internal Iliac Artery, Left
Uterine cornu	Uterus
Uterine tube	Fallopian Tube, Right
	Fallopian Tube, Left
Uterine vein	Hypogastric Vein, Right
	Hypogastric Vein, Left
Vaginal artery	Internal Iliac Artery, Right
	Internal Iliac Artery, Left
Vaginal vein	Hypogastric Vein, Right
	Hypogastric Vein, Left
Vastus intermedius muscle	Upper Leg Muscle, Right
	Upper Leg Muscle, Left
Vastus lateralis muscle	Upper Leg Muscle, Right
	Upper Leg Muscle, Left
Vastus medialis muscle	Upper Leg Muscle, Right
	Upper Leg Muscle, Left
Ventricular fold	Larynx
Vermiform appendix	Appendix
Vermilion border	Upper Lip
	Lower Lip
Vertebral arch	Cervical Vertebra
	Lumbar Vertebra
	Thoracic Vertebra
Vertebral body	Cervical Vertebra
	Lumbar Vertebra
	Thoracic Vertebra
Vertebral canal	Spinal Canal
Vertebral foramen	Cervical Vertebra
	Lumbar Vertebra
	Thoracic Vertebra
Vertebral lamina	Cervical Vertebra
	Lumbar Vertebra
	Thoracic Vertebra
Vertebral pedicle	Cervical Vertebra
	Lumbar Vertebra
	Thoracic Vertebra
Vesical vein	Hypogastric Vein, Right
	Hypogastric Vein, Left
Vestibular (Scarpa's) ganglion	Acoustic Nerve
Vestibular nerve	Acoustic Nerve
Vestibulocochlear nerve	Acoustic Nerve

Term	ICD-10-PCS Value
Virchow's (supraclavicular) lymph node	Lymphatic, Right Neck
	Lymphatic, Left Neck
Vitreous body	Vitreous, Right
	Vitreous, Left
Vocal fold	Vocal Cord, Right
	Vocal Cord, Left
Volar (palmar) digital vein	Hand Vein, Right
	Hand Vein, Left
Volar (palmar) metacarpal vein	Hand Vein, Right
	Hand Vein, Left
Vomer bone	Nasal Septum
Vomer of nasal septum	Nasal Bone
Xiphoid process	Sternum
Zonule of Zinn	Lens, Right
	Lens, Left
Zygomatic process of frontal bone	Frontal Bone
Zygomatic process of temporal bone	Temporal Bone, Right
	Temporal Bone, Left
Zygomaticus muscle	Facial Muscle

Appendix E: Body Part Definitions

ICD-10-PCS Value	Definition
1st Toe, Left 1st Toe, Right	**Includes:** Hallux
Abdomen Muscle, Left Abdomen Muscle, Right	**Includes:** External oblique muscle Internal oblique muscle Pyramidalis muscle Rectus abdominis muscle Transversus abdominis muscle
Abdominal Aorta	**Includes:** Inferior phrenic artery Lumbar artery Median sacral artery Middle suprarenal artery Ovarian artery Testicular artery
Abdominal Sympathetic Nerve	**Includes:** Abdominal aortic plexus Auerbach's (myenteric) plexus Celiac (solar) plexus Celiac ganglion Gastric plexus Hepatic plexus Inferior hypogastric plexus Inferior mesenteric ganglion Inferior mesenteric plexus Meissner's (submucous) plexus Myenteric (Auerbach's) plexus Pancreatic plexus Pelvic splanchnic nerve Renal nerve Renal plexus Solar (celiac) plexus Splenic plexus Submucous (Meissner's) plexus Superior hypogastric plexus Superior mesenteric ganglion Superior mesenteric plexus Suprarenal plexus
Abducens Nerve	**Includes:** Sixth cranial nerve
Accessory Nerve	**Includes:** Eleventh cranial nerve
Acoustic Nerve	**Includes:** Cochlear nerve Eighth cranial nerve Scarpa's (vestibular) ganglion Spiral ganglion Vestibular (Scarpa's) ganglion Vestibular nerve Vestibulocochlear nerve
Adenoids	**Includes:** Pharyngeal tonsil
Adrenal Gland Adrenal Gland, Left Adrenal Gland, Right Adrenal Glands, Bilateral	**Includes:** Suprarenal gland
Ampulla of Vater	**Includes:** Duodenal ampulla Hepatopancreatic ampulla
Anal Sphincter	**Includes:** External anal sphincter Internal anal sphincter

ICD-10-PCS Value	Definition
Ankle Bursa and Ligament, Left Ankle Bursa and Ligament, Right	**Includes:** Calcaneofibular ligament Deltoid ligament Ligament of the lateral malleolus Talofibular ligament
Ankle Joint, Left Ankle Joint, Right	**Includes:** Inferior tibiofibular joint Talocrural joint
Anterior Chamber, Left Anterior Chamber, Right	**Includes:** Aqueous humour
Anterior Tibial Artery, Left Anterior Tibial Artery, Right	**Includes:** Anterior lateral malleolar artery Anterior medial malleolar artery Anterior tibial recurrent artery Dorsalis pedis artery Posterior tibial recurrent artery
Anus	**Includes:** Anal orifice
Aortic Valve	**Includes:** Aortic annulus
Appendix	**Includes:** Vermiform appendix
Atrial Septum	**Includes:** Interatrial septum
Atrium, Left	**Includes:** Atrium pulmonale Left auricular appendix
Atrium, Right	**Includes:** Atrium dextrum cordis Right auricular appendix Sinus venosus
Auditory Ossicle, Left Auditory Ossicle, Right	**Includes:** Incus Malleus Stapes
Axillary Artery, Left Axillary Artery, Right	**Includes:** Anterior circumflex humeral artery Lateral thoracic artery Posterior circumflex humeral artery Subscapular artery Superior thoracic artery Thoracoacromial artery
Azygos Vein	**Includes:** Right ascending lumbar vein Right subcostal vein
Basal Ganglia	**Includes:** Basal nuclei Claustrum Corpus striatum Globus pallidus Substantia nigra Subthalamic nucleus
Basilic Vein, Left Basilic Vein, Right	**Includes:** Median antebrachial vein Median cubital vein
Bladder	**Includes:** Trigone of bladder
Brachial Artery, Left Brachial Artery, Right	**Includes:** Inferior ulnar collateral artery Profunda brachii Superior ulnar collateral artery

ICD-10-PCS Value	Definition
Brachial Plexus	**Includes:** Axillary nerve Dorsal scapular nerve First intercostal nerve Long thoracic nerve Musculocutaneous nerve Subclavius nerve Suprascapular nerve
Brachial Vein, Left Brachial Vein, Right	**Includes:** Radial vein Ulnar vein
Brain	**Includes:** Cerebrum Corpus callosum Encephalon
Breast, Bilateral Breast, Left Breast, Right	**Includes:** Mammary duct Mammary gland
Buccal Mucosa	**Includes:** Buccal gland Molar gland Palatine gland
Carotid Bodies, Bilateral Carotid Body, Left Carotid Body, Right	**Includes:** Carotid glomus
Carpal Joint, Left Carpal Joint, Right	**Includes:** Intercarpal joint Midcarpal joint
Carpal, Left Carpal, Right	**Includes:** Capitate bone Hamate bone Lunate bone Pisiform bone Scaphoid bone Trapezium bone Trapezoid bone Triquetral bone
Celiac Artery	**Includes:** Celiac trunk
Cephalic Vein, Left Cephalic Vein, Right	**Includes:** Accessory cephalic vein
Cerebellum	**Includes:** Culmen
Cerebral Hemisphere	**Includes:** Frontal lobe Occipital lobe Parietal lobe Temporal lobe
Cerebral Meninges	**Includes:** Arachnoid mater, intracranial Leptomeninges, intracranial Pia mater, intracranial
Cerebral Ventricle	**Includes:** Aqueduct of Sylvius Cerebral aqueduct (Sylvius) Choroid plexus Ependyma Foramen of Monro (intraventricular) Fourth ventricle Interventricular foramen (Monro) Left lateral ventricle Right lateral ventricle Third ventricle
Cervical Nerve	**Includes:** Greater occipital nerve Spinal nerve, cervical Suboccipital nerve Third occipital nerve

ICD-10-PCS Value	Definition
Cervical Plexus	**Includes:** Ansa cervicalis Cutaneous (transverse) cervical nerve Great auricular nerve Lesser occipital nerve Supraclavicular nerve Transverse (cutaneous) cervical nerve
Cervical Spinal Cord	**Includes:** Dorsal root ganglion
Cervical Vertebra	**Includes:** Dens Odontoid process Spinous process Transverse foramen Transverse process Vertebral arch Vertebral body Vertebral foramen Vertebral lamina Vertebral pedicle
Cervical Vertebral Joint	**Includes:** Atlantoaxial joint Cervical facet joint
Cervical Vertebral Joints, 2 or more	**Includes:** Cervical facet joint
Cervicothoracic Vertebral Joint	**Includes:** Cervicothoracic facet joint
Cisterna Chyli	**Includes:** Intestinal lymphatic trunk Lumbar lymphatic trunk
Coccygeal Glomus	**Includes:** Coccygeal body
Colic Vein	**Includes:** Ileocolic vein Left colic vein Middle colic vein Right colic vein
Conduction Mechanism	**Includes:** Atrioventricular node Bundle of His Bundle of Kent Sinoatrial node
Conjunctiva, Left Conjunctiva, Right	**Includes:** Plica semilunaris
Dura Mater	**Includes:** Diaphragma sellae Dura mater, intracranial Falx cerebri Tentorium cerebelli
Elbow Bursa and Ligament, Left Elbow Bursa and Ligament, Right	**Includes:** Annular ligament Olecranon bursa Radial collateral ligament Ulnar collateral ligament
Elbow Joint, Left Elbow Joint, Right	**Includes:** Distal humerus, involving joint Humeroradial joint Humeroulnar joint Proximal radioulnar joint
Epidural Space, Intracranial	**Includes:** Extradural space, intracranial
Epiglottis	**Includes:** Glossoepiglottic fold
Esophagogastric Junction	**Includes:** Cardia Cardioesophageal junction Gastroesophageal (GE) junction

ICD-10-PCS Value	Definition
Esophagus, Lower	**Includes:** Abdominal esophagus
Esophagus, Middle	**Includes:** Thoracic esophagus
Esophagus, Upper	**Includes:** Cervical esophagus
Ethmoid Bone, Left Ethmoid Bone, Right	**Includes:** Cribriform plate
Ethmoid Sinus, Left Ethmoid Sinus, Right	**Includes:** Ethmoidal air cell
Eustachian Tube, Left Eustachian Tube, Right	**Includes:** Auditory tube Pharyngotympanic tube
External Auditory Canal, Left External Auditory Canal, Right	**Includes:** External auditory meatus
External Carotid Artery, Left External Carotid Artery, Right	**Includes:** Ascending pharyngeal artery Internal maxillary artery Lingual artery Maxillary artery Occipital artery Posterior auricular artery Superior thyroid artery
External Ear, Bilateral External Ear, Left External Ear, Right	**Includes:** Antihelix Antitragus Auricle Earlobe Helix Pinna Tragus
External Iliac Artery, Left External Iliac Artery, Right	**Includes:** Deep circumflex iliac artery Inferior epigastric artery
External Jugular Vein, Left External Jugular Vein, Right	**Includes:** Posterior auricular vein
Extraocular Muscle, Left Extraocular Muscle, Right	**Includes:** Inferior oblique muscle Inferior rectus muscle Lateral rectus muscle Medial rectus muscle Superior oblique muscle Superior rectus muscle
Eye, Left Eye, Right	**Includes:** Ciliary body Posterior chamber
Face Artery	**Includes:** Angular artery Ascending palatine artery External maxillary artery Facial artery Inferior labial artery Submental artery Superior labial artery
Face Vein, Left Face Vein, Right	**Includes:** Angular vein Anterior facial vein Common facial vein Deep facial vein Frontal vein Posterior facial (retromandibular) vein Supraorbital vein

ICD-10-PCS Value	Definition
Facial Muscle	**Includes:** Buccinator muscle Corrugator supercilii muscle Depressor anguli oris muscle Depressor labii inferioris muscle Depressor septi nasi muscle Depressor supercilii muscle Levator anguli oris muscle Levator labii superioris alaeque nasi muscle Levator labii superioris muscle Mentalis muscle Nasalis muscle Occipitofrontalis muscle Orbicularis oris muscle Procerus muscle Risorius muscle Zygomaticus muscle
Facial Nerve	**Includes:** Chorda tympani Geniculate ganglion Greater superficial petrosal nerve Nerve to the stapedius Parotid plexus Posterior auricular nerve Seventh cranial nerve Submandibular ganglion
Fallopian Tube, Left Fallopian Tube, Right	**Includes:** Oviduct Salpinx Uterine tube
Femoral Artery, Left Femoral Artery, Right	**Includes:** Circumflex iliac artery Deep femoral artery Descending genicular artery External pudendal artery Superficial epigastric artery
Femoral Nerve	**Includes:** Anterior crural nerve Saphenous nerve
Femoral Shaft, Left Femoral Shaft, Right	**Includes:** Body of femur
Femoral Vein, Left Femoral Vein, Right	**Includes:** Deep femoral (profunda femoris) vein Popliteal vein Profunda femoris (deep femoral) vein
Fibula, Left Fibula, Right	**Includes:** Body of fibula Head of fibula Lateral malleolus
Finger Nail	**Includes:** Nail bed Nail plate
Finger Phalangeal Joint, Left Finger Phalangeal Joint, Right	**Includes:** Interphalangeal (IP) joint
Foot Artery, Left Foot Artery, Right	**Includes:** Arcuate artery Dorsal metatarsal artery Lateral plantar artery Lateral tarsal artery Medial plantar artery

ICD-10-PCS Value	Definition
Foot Bursa and Ligament, Left Foot Bursa and Ligament, Right	**Includes:** Calcaneocuboid ligament Cuneonavicular ligament Intercuneiform ligament Interphalangeal ligament Metatarsal ligament Metatarsophalangeal ligament Subtalar ligament Talocalcaneal ligament Talocalcaneonavicular ligament Tarsometatarsal ligament
Foot Muscle, Left Foot Muscle, Right	**Includes:** Abductor hallucis muscle Adductor hallucis muscle Extensor digitorum brevis muscle Extensor hallucis brevis muscle Flexor digitorum brevis muscle Flexor hallucis brevis muscle Quadratus plantae muscle
Foot Vein, Left Foot Vein, Right	**Includes:** Common digital vein Dorsal metatarsal vein Dorsal venous arch Plantar digital vein Plantar metatarsal vein Plantar venous arch
Frontal Bone	**Includes:** Zygomatic process of frontal bone
Gastric Artery	**Includes:** Left gastric artery Right gastric artery
Glenoid Cavity, Left Glenoid Cavity, Right	**Includes:** Glenoid fossa (of scapula)
Glomus Jugulare	**Includes:** Jugular body
Glossopharyngeal Nerve	**Includes:** Carotid sinus nerve Ninth cranial nerve Tympanic nerve
Hand Artery, Left Hand Artery, Right	**Includes:** Deep palmar arch Princeps pollicis artery Radialis indicis Superficial palmar arch
Hand Bursa and Ligament, Left Hand Bursa and Ligament, Right	**Includes:** Carpometacarpal ligament Intercarpal ligament Interphalangeal ligament Lunotriquetral ligament Metacarpal ligament Metacarpophalangeal ligament Pisohamate ligament Pisometacarpal ligament Scaphotrapezium ligament
Hand Muscle, Left Hand Muscle, Right	**Includes:** Hypothenar muscle Palmar interosseous muscle Thenar muscle
Hand Vein, Left Hand Vein, Right	**Includes:** Dorsal metacarpal vein Palmar (volar) digital vein Palmar (volar) metacarpal vein Superficial palmar venous arch Volar (palmar) digital vein Volar (palmar) metacarpal vein

ICD-10-PCS Value	Definition
Head and Neck Bursa and Ligament	**Includes:** Alar ligament of axis Cervical interspinous ligament Cervical intertransverse ligament Cervical ligamentum flavum Interspinous ligament, cervical Intertransverse ligament, cervical Lateral temporomandibular ligament Ligamentum flavum, cervical Sphenomandibular ligament Stylomandibular ligament Transverse ligament of atlas
Head and Neck Sympathetic Nerve	**Includes:** Cavernous plexus Cervical ganglion Ciliary ganglion Internal carotid plexus Otic ganglion Pterygopalatine (sphenopalatine) ganglion Sphenopalatine (pterygopalatine) ganglion Stellate ganglion Submandibular ganglion Submaxillary ganglion
Head Muscle	**Includes:** Auricularis muscle Masseter muscle Pterygoid muscle Splenius capitis muscle Temporalis muscle Temporoparietalis muscle
Heart, Left	**Includes:** Left coronary sulcus Obtuse margin
Heart, Right	**Includes:** Right coronary sulcus
Hemiazygos Vein	**Includes:** Left ascending lumbar vein Left subcostal vein
Hepatic Artery	**Includes:** Common hepatic artery Gastroduodenal artery Hepatic artery proper
Hip Bursa and Ligament, Left Hip Bursa and Ligament, Right	**Includes:** Iliofemoral ligament Ischiofemoral ligament Pubofemoral ligament Transverse acetabular ligament Trochanteric bursa
Hip Joint, Left Hip Joint, Right	**Includes:** Acetabulofemoral joint
Hip Muscle, Left Hip Muscle, Right	**Includes:** Gemellus muscle Gluteus maximus muscle Gluteus medius muscle Gluteus minimus muscle Iliacus muscle Obturator muscle Piriformis muscle Psoas muscle Quadratus femoris muscle Tensor fasciae latae muscle
Humeral Head, Left Humeral Head, Right	**Includes:** Greater tuberosity Lesser tuberosity Neck of humerus (anatomical)(surgical)

ICD-10-PCS Value	Definition
Humeral Shaft, Left Humeral Shaft, Right	**Includes:** Distal humerus Humerus, distal Lateral epicondyle of humerus Medial epicondyle of humerus
Hypogastric Vein, Left Hypogastric Vein, Right	**Includes:** Gluteal vein Internal iliac vein Internal pudendal vein Lateral sacral vein Middle hemorrhoidal vein Obturator vein Uterine vein Vaginal vein Vesical vein
Hypoglossal Nerve	**Includes:** Twelfth cranial nerve
Hypothalamus	**Includes:** Mammillary body
Inferior Mesenteric Artery	**Includes:** Sigmoid artery Superior rectal artery
Inferior Mesenteric Vein	**Includes:** Sigmoid vein Superior rectal vein
Inferior Vena Cava	**Includes:** Postcava Right inferior phrenic vein Right ovarian vein Right second lumbar vein Right suprarenal vein Right testicular vein
Inguinal Region, Bilateral Inguinal Region, Left Inguinal Region, Right	**Includes:** Inguinal canal Inguinal triangle
Inner Ear, Left Inner Ear, Right	**Includes:** Bony labyrinth Bony vestibule Cochlea Round window Semicircular canal
Innominate Artery	**Includes:** Brachiocephalic artery Brachiocephalic trunk
Innominate Vein, Left Innominate Vein, Right	**Includes:** Brachiocephalic vein Inferior thyroid vein
Internal Carotid Artery, Left Internal Carotid Artery, Right	**Includes:** Caroticotympanic artery Carotid sinus
Internal Iliac Artery, Left Internal Iliac Artery, Right	**Includes:** Deferential artery Hypogastric artery Iliolumbar artery Inferior gluteal artery Inferior vesical artery Internal pudendal artery Lateral sacral artery Middle rectal artery Obturator artery Prostatic artery Superior gluteal artery Superior vesical artery Umbilical artery Uterine artery Vaginal artery

ICD-10-PCS Value	Definition
Internal Mammary Artery, Left Internal Mammary Artery, Right	**Includes:** Anterior intercostal artery Internal thoracic artery Musculophrenic artery Pericardiophrenic artery Superior epigastric artery
Intracranial Artery	**Includes:** Anterior cerebral artery Anterior choroidal artery Anterior communicating artery Basilar artery Circle of Willis Internal carotid artery, intracranial portion Middle cerebral artery Ophthalmic artery Posterior cerebral artery Posterior communicating artery Posterior inferior cerebellar artery (PICA)
Intracranial Vein	**Includes:** Anterior cerebral vein Basal (internal) cerebral vein Dural venous sinus Great cerebral vein Inferior cerebellar vein Inferior cerebral vein Internal (basal) cerebral vein Middle cerebral vein Ophthalmic vein Superior cerebellar vein Superior cerebral vein
Jejunum	**Includes:** Duodenojejunal flexure
Kidney	**Includes:** Renal calyx Renal capsule Renal cortex Renal segment
Kidney Pelvis, Left Kidney Pelvis, Right	**Includes:** Ureteropelvic junction (UPJ)
Kidney, Left Kidney, Right Kidneys, Bilateral	**Includes:** Renal calyx Renal capsule Renal cortex Renal segment
Knee Bursa and Ligament, Left Knee Bursa and Ligament, Right	**Includes:** Anterior cruciate ligament (ACL) Lateral collateral ligament (LCL) Ligament of head of fibula Medial collateral ligament (MCL) Patellar ligament Popliteal ligament Posterior cruciate ligament (PCL) Prepatellar bursa
Knee Joint, Femoral Surface, Left Knee Joint, Femoral Surface, Right	**Includes:** Femoropatellar joint Patellofemoral joint
Knee Joint, Left Knee Joint, Right	**Includes:** Femoropatellar joint Femorotibial joint Lateral meniscus Medial meniscus Patellofemoral joint Tibiofemoral joint
Knee Joint, Tibial Surface, Left Knee Joint, Tibial Surface, Right	**Includes:** Femorotibial joint Tibiofemoral joint
Knee Tendon, Left Knee Tendon, Right	**Includes:** Patellar tendon

ICD-10-PCS Value	Definition
Lacrimal Duct, Left Lacrimal Duct, Right	**Includes:** Lacrimal canaliculus Lacrimal punctum Lacrimal sac Nasolacrimal duct
Larynx	**Includes:** Aryepiglottic fold Arytenoid cartilage Corniculate cartilage Cuneiform cartilage False vocal cord Glottis Rima glottidis Thyroid cartilage Ventricular fold
Lens, Left Lens, Right	**Includes:** Zonule of Zinn
Liver	**Includes:** Quadrate lobe
Lower Arm and Wrist Muscle, Left Lower Arm and Wrist Muscle, Right	**Includes:** Anatomical snuffbox Brachioradialis muscle Extensor carpi radialis muscle Extensor carpi ulnaris muscle Flexor carpi radialis muscle Flexor carpi ulnaris muscle Flexor pollicis longus muscle Palmaris longus muscle Pronator quadratus muscle Pronator teres muscle
Lower Artery	**Includes:** Umbilical artery
Lower Eyelid, Left Lower Eyelid, Right	**Includes:** Inferior tarsal plate Medial canthus
Lower Femur, Left Lower Femur, Right	**Includes:** Lateral condyle of femur Lateral epicondyle of femur Medial condyle of femur Medial epicondyle of femur
Lower Leg Muscle, Left Lower Leg Muscle, Right	**Includes:** Extensor digitorum longus muscle Extensor hallucis longus muscle Fibularis brevis muscle Fibularis longus muscle Flexor digitorum longus muscle Flexor hallucis longus muscle Gastrocnemius muscle Peroneus brevis muscle Peroneus longus muscle Popliteus muscle Soleus muscle Tibialis anterior muscle Tibialis posterior muscle
Lower Leg Tendon, Left Lower Leg Tendon, Right	**Includes:** Achilles tendon
Lower Lip	**Includes:** Frenulum labii inferioris Labial gland Vermilion border

ICD-10-PCS Value	Definition
Lower Spine Bursa and Ligament	**Includes:** Iliolumbar ligament Interspinous ligament, lumbar Intertransverse ligament, lumbar Ligamentum flavum, lumbar Sacrococcygeal ligament Sacroiliac ligament Sacrospinous ligament Sacrotuberous ligament Supraspinous ligament
Lumbar Nerve	**Includes:** Lumbosacral trunk Spinal nerve, lumbar Superior clunic (cluneal) nerve
Lumbar Plexus	**Includes:** Accessory obturator nerve Genitofemoral nerve Iliohypogastric nerve Ilioinguinal nerve Lateral femoral cutaneous nerve Obturator nerve Superior gluteal nerve
Lumbar Spinal Cord	**Includes:** Cauda equina Conus medullaris Dorsal root ganglion
Lumbar Sympathetic Nerve	**Includes:** Lumbar ganglion Lumbar splanchnic nerve
Lumbar Vertebra	**Includes:** Spinous process Transverse process Vertebral arch Vertebral body Vertebral foramen Vertebral lamina Vertebral pedicle
Lumbar Vertebral Joint	**Includes:** Lumbar facet joint
Lumbosacral Joint	**Includes:** Lumbosacral facet joint
Lymphatic, Aortic	**Includes:** Celiac lymph node Gastric lymph node Hepatic lymph node Lumbar lymph node Pancreaticosplenic lymph node Paraaortic lymph node Retroperitoneal lymph node
Lymphatic, Head	**Includes:** Buccinator lymph node Infraauricular lymph node Infraparotid lymph node Parotid lymph node Preauricular lymph node Submandibular lymph node Submaxillary lymph node Submental lymph node Subparotid lymph node Suprahyoid lymph node
Lymphatic, Left Axillary	**Includes:** Anterior (pectoral) lymph node Apical (subclavicular) lymph node Brachial (lateral) lymph node Central axillary lymph node Lateral (brachial) lymph node Pectoral (anterior) lymph node Posterior (subscapular) lymph node Subclavicular (apical) lymph node Subscapular (posterior) lymph node

ICD-10-PCS Value	Definition
Lymphatic, Left Lower Extremity	**Includes:** Femoral lymph node Popliteal lymph node
Lymphatic, Left Neck	**Includes:** Cervical lymph node Jugular lymph node Mastoid (postauricular) lymph node Occipital lymph node Postauricular (mastoid) lymph node Retropharyngeal lymph node Supraclavicular (Virchow's) lymph node Virchow's (supraclavicular) lymph node
Lymphatic, Left Upper Extremity	**Includes:** Cubital lymph node Deltopectoral (infraclavicular) lymph node Epitrochlear lymph node Infraclavicular (deltopectoral) lymph node Supratrochlear lymph node
Lymphatic, Mesenteric	**Includes:** Inferior mesenteric lymph node Pararectal lymph node Superior mesenteric lymph node
Lymphatic, Pelvis	**Includes:** Common iliac (subaortic) lymph node Gluteal lymph node Iliac lymph node Inferior epigastric lymph node Obturator lymph node Sacral lymph node Subaortic (common iliac) lymph node Suprainguinal lymph node
Lymphatic, Right Axillary	**Includes:** Anterior (pectoral) lymph node Apical (subclavicular) lymph node Brachial (lateral) lymph node Central axillary lymph node Lateral (brachial) lymph node Pectoral (anterior) lymph node Posterior (subscapular) lymph node Subclavicular (apical) lymph node Subscapular (posterior) lymph node
Lymphatic, Right Lower Extremity	**Includes:** Femoral lymph node Popliteal lymph node
Lymphatic, Right Neck	**Includes:** Cervical lymph node Jugular lymph node Mastoid (postauricular) lymph node Occipital lymph node Postauricular (mastoid) lymph node Retropharyngeal lymph node Right jugular trunk Right lymphatic duct Right subclavian trunk Supraclavicular (Virchow's) lymph node Virchow's (supraclavicular) lymph node
Lymphatic, Right Upper Extremity	**Includes:** Cubital lymph node Deltopectoral (infraclavicular) lymph node Epitrochlear lymph node Infraclavicular (deltopectoral) lymph node Supratrochlear lymph node
Lymphatic, Thorax	**Includes:** Intercostal lymph node Mediastinal lymph node Parasternal lymph node Paratracheal lymph node Tracheobronchial lymph node

ICD-10-PCS Value	Definition
Main Bronchus, Right	**Includes:** Bronchus intermedius Intermediate bronchus
Mandible, Left Mandible, Right	**Includes:** Alveolar process of mandible Condyloid process Mandibular notch Mental foramen
Mastoid Sinus, Left Mastoid Sinus, Right	**Includes:** Mastoid air cells
Metatarsal, Left Metatarsal, Right	**Includes:** Fibular sesamoid Tibial sesamoid
Maxilla	**Includes:** Alveolar process of maxilla
Maxillary Sinus, Left Maxillary Sinus, Right	**Includes:** Antrum of Highmore
Median Nerve	**Includes:** Anterior interosseous nerve Palmar cutaneous nerve
Mediastinum	**Includes:** Mediastinal cavity Mediastinal space
Medulla Oblongata	**Includes:** Myelencephalon
Mesentery	**Includes:** Mesoappendix Mesocolon
Metatarsal, Right Metatarsal, Left	**Includes:** Fibular sesamoid Tibial sesamoid
Metatarsal-Phalangeal Joint, Left Metatarsal-Phalangeal Joint, Right	**Includes:** Metatarsophalangeal (MTP) joint
Middle Ear, Left Middle Ear, Right	**Includes:** Oval window Tympanic cavity
Minor Salivary Gland	**Includes:** Anterior lingual gland
Mitral Valve	**Includes:** Bicuspid valve Left atrioventricular valve Mitral annulus
Nasal Bone	**Includes:** Vomer of nasal septum
Nasal Mucosa and Soft Tissue	**Includes:** Columella External naris Greater alar cartilage Internal naris Lateral nasal cartilage Lesser alar cartilage Nasal cavity Nostril
Nasal Septum	**Includes:** Quadrangular cartilage Septal cartilage Vomer bone
Nasal Turbinate	**Includes:** Inferior turbinate Middle turbinate Nasal concha Superior turbinate

ICD-10-PCS Value	Definition
Nasopharynx	**Includes:** Choana Fossa of Rosenmuller Pharyngeal recess Rhinopharynx
Neck	**Includes:** Parapharyngeal space Retropharyngeal space
Neck Muscle, Left Neck Muscle, Right	**Includes:** Anterior vertebral muscle Arytenoid muscle Cricothyroid muscle Infrahyoid muscle Levator scapulae muscle Platysma muscle Scalene muscle Splenius cervicis muscle Sternocleidomastoid muscle Suprahyoid muscle Thyroarytenoid muscle
Nipple, Left Nipple, Right	**Includes:** Areola
Occipital Bone	**Includes:** Foramen magnum
Oculomotor Nerve	**Includes:** Third cranial nerve
Olfactory Nerve	**Includes:** First cranial nerve Olfactory bulb
Omentum	**Includes:** Gastrocolic ligament Gastrocolic omentum Gastrohepatic omentum Gastrophrenic ligament Gastrosplenic ligament Greater Omentum Hepatogastric ligament Lesser Omentum
Optic Nerve	**Includes:** Optic chiasma Second cranial nerve
Orbit, Left Orbit, Right	**Includes:** Bony orbit Orbital portion of ethmoid bone Orbital portion of frontal bone Orbital portion of lacrimal bone Orbital portion of maxilla Orbital portion of palatine bone Orbital portion of sphenoid bone Orbital portion of zygomatic bone
Pancreatic Duct	**Includes:** Duct of Wirsung
Pancreatic Duct, Accessory	**Includes:** Duct of Santorini
Parotid Duct, Left Parotid Duct, Right	**Includes:** Stensen's duct
Pelvic Bone, Left Pelvic Bone, Right	**Includes:** Iliac crest Ilium Ischium Pubis
Pelvic Cavity	**Includes:** Retropubic space
Penis	**Includes:** Corpus cavernosum Corpus spongiosum

ICD-10-PCS Value	Definition
Perineum Muscle	**Includes:** Bulbospongiosus muscle Cremaster muscle Deep transverse perineal muscle Ischiocavernosus muscle Levator ani muscle Superficial transverse perineal muscle
Peritoneal Cavity	**Includes:** Abdominal cavity
Peritoneum	**Includes:** Epiploic foramen
Peroneal Artery, Left Peroneal Artery, Right	**Includes:** Fibular artery
Peroneal Nerve	**Includes:** Common fibular nerve Common peroneal nerve External popliteal nerve Lateral sural cutaneous nerve
Pharynx	**Includes:** Base of Tongue Hypopharynx Laryngopharynx Lingual tonsil Oropharynx Piriform recess (sinus) Tongue, base of
Phrenic Nerve	**Includes:** Accessory phrenic nerve
Pituitary Gland	**Includes:** Adenohypophysis Hypophysis Neurohypophysis
Pons	**Includes:** Apneustic center Basis pontis Locus ceruleus Pneumotaxic center Pontine tegmentum Superior olivary nucleus
Popliteal Artery, Left Popliteal Artery, Right	**Includes:** Inferior genicular artery Middle genicular artery Superior genicular artery Sural artery Tibioperoneal trunk
Portal Vein	**Includes:** Hepatic portal vein
Prepuce	**Includes:** Foreskin Glans penis
Pudendal Nerve	**Includes:** Posterior labial nerve Posterior scrotal nerve
Pulmonary Artery, Left	**Includes:** Arterial canal (duct) Botallo's duct Pulmoaortic canal
Pulmonary Valve	**Includes:** Pulmonary annulus Pulmonic valve
Pulmonary Vein, Left	**Includes:** Left inferior pulmonary vein Left superior pulmonary vein
Pulmonary Vein, Right	**Includes:** Right inferior pulmonary vein Right superior pulmonary vein
Radial Artery, Left Radial Artery, Right	**Includes:** Radial recurrent artery

ICD-10-PCS Value	Definition
Radial Nerve	**Includes:** Dorsal digital nerve Musculospiral nerve Palmar cutaneous nerve Posterior interosseous nerve
Radius, Left Radius, Right	**Includes:** Ulnar notch
Rectum	**Includes:** Anorectal junction
Renal Artery, Left Renal Artery, Right	**Includes:** Inferior suprarenal artery Renal segmental artery
Renal Vein, Left	**Includes:** Left inferior phrenic vein Left ovarian vein Left second lumbar vein Left suprarenal vein Left testicular vein
Retina, Left Retina, Right	**Includes:** Fovea Macula Optic disc
Retroperitoneum	**Includes:** Retroperitoneal cavity Retroperitoneal space
Rib(s) Bursa and Ligament	**Includes:** Costotransverse ligament
Sacral Nerve	**Includes:** Spinal nerve, sacral
Sacral Plexus	**Includes:** Inferior gluteal nerve Posterior femoral cutaneous nerve Pudendal nerve
Sacral Sympathetic Nerve	**Includes:** Ganglion impar (ganglion of Walther) Pelvic splanchnic nerve Sacral ganglion Sacral splanchnic nerve
Sacrococcygeal Joint	**Includes:** Sacrococcygeal symphysis
Saphenous Vein, Left Saphenous Vein, Right	**Includes:** External pudendal vein Great(er) saphenous vein Lesser saphenous vein Small saphenous vein Superficial circumflex iliac vein Superficial epigastric vein
Scapula, Left Scapula, Right	**Includes:** Acromion (process) Coracoid process
Sciatic Nerve	**Includes:** Ischiatic nerve
Shoulder Bursa and Ligament, Left Shoulder Bursa and Ligament, Right	**Includes:** Acromioclavicular ligament Coracoacromial ligament Coracoclavicular ligament Coracohumeral ligament Costoclavicular ligament Glenohumeral ligament Interclavicular ligament Sternoclavicular ligament Subacromial bursa Transverse humeral ligament Transverse scapular ligament
Shoulder Joint, Left Shoulder Joint, Right	**Includes:** Glenohumeral joint Glenoid ligament (labrum)

ICD-10-PCS Value	Definition
Shoulder Muscle, Left Shoulder Muscle, Right	**Includes:** Deltoid muscle Infraspinatus muscle Subscapularis muscle Supraspinatus muscle Teres major muscle Teres minor muscle
Sigmoid Colon	**Includes:** Rectosigmoid junction Sigmoid flexure
Skin	**Includes:** Dermis Epidermis Sebaceous gland Sweat gland
Skin, Chest	**Includes:** Breast procedures, skin only
Skin, Perineum	**Includes:** Perianal skin
Sphenoid Bone	**Includes:** Greater wing Lesser wing Optic foramen Pterygoid process Sella turcica
Spinal Canal	**Includes:** Epidural space, spinal Extradural space, spinal Subarachnoid space, spinal Subdural space, spinal Vertebral canal
Spinal Cord	**Includes:** Dorsal root ganglion
Spinal Meninges	**Includes:** Arachnoid mater, spinal Denticulate (dentate) ligament Dura mater, spinal Filum terminale Leptomeninges, spinal Pia mater, spinal
Spleen	**Includes:** Accessory spleen
Splenic Artery	**Includes:** Left gastroepiploic artery Pancreatic artery Short gastric artery
Splenic Vein	**Includes:** Left gastroepiploic vein Pancreatic vein
Sternum	**Includes:** Manubrium Suprasternal notch Xiphoid process
Sternum Bursa and Ligament	**Includes:** Costoxiphoid ligament Sternocostal ligament
Stomach, Pylorus	**Includes:** Pyloric antrum Pyloric canal Pyloric sphincter
Subclavian Artery, Left Subclavian Artery, Right	**Includes:** Costocervical trunk Dorsal scapular artery Internal thoracic artery
Subcutaneous Tissue and Fascia, Chest	**Includes:** Pectoral fascia

ICD-10-PCS Value	Definition
Subcutaneous Tissue and Fascia, Face	**Includes:** Masseteric fascia Orbital fascia Submandibular space
Subcutaneous Tissue and Fascia, Left Foot	**Includes:** Plantar fascia (aponeurosis)
Subcutaneous Tissue and Fascia, Left Hand	**Includes:** Palmar fascia (aponeurosis)
Subcutaneous Tissue and Fascia, Left Lower Arm	**Includes:** Antebrachial fascia Bicipital aponeurosis
Subcutaneous Tissue and Fascia, Left Neck	**Includes:** Deep cervical fascia Pretracheal fascia Prevertebral fascia
Subcutaneous Tissue and Fascia, Left Upper Arm	**Includes:** Axillary fascia Deltoid fascia Infraspinatus fascia Subscapular aponeurosis Supraspinatus fascia
Subcutaneous Tissue and Fascia, Left Upper Leg	**Includes:** Crural fascia Fascia lata Iliac fascia Iliotibial tract (band)
Subcutaneous Tissue and Fascia, Right Foot	**Includes:** Plantar fascia (aponeurosis)
Subcutaneous Tissue and Fascia, Right Hand	**Includes:** Palmar fascia (aponeurosis)
Subcutaneous Tissue and Fascia, Right Lower Arm	**Includes:** Antebrachial fascia Bicipital aponeurosis
Subcutaneous Tissue and Fascia, Right Neck	**Includes:** Deep cervical fascia Pretracheal fascia Prevertebral fascia
Subcutaneous Tissue and Fascia, Right Upper Arm	**Includes:** Axillary fascia Deltoid fascia Infraspinatus fascia Subscapular aponeurosis Supraspinatus fascia
Subcutaneous Tissue and Fascia, Right Upper Leg	**Includes:** Crural fascia Fascia lata Iliac fascia Iliotibial tract (band)
Subcutaneous Tissue and Fascia, Scalp	**Includes:** Galea aponeurotica
Subcutaneous Tissue and Fascia, Trunk	**Includes:** External oblique aponeurosis Transversalis fascia
Submaxillary Gland, Left Submaxillary Gland, Right	**Includes:** Submandibular gland
Superior Mesenteric Artery	**Includes:** Ileal artery Ileocolic artery Inferior pancreaticoduodenal artery Jejunal artery
Superior Mesenteric Vein	**Includes:** Right gastroepiploic vein
Superior Vena Cava	**Includes:** Cavoatrial junction Precava

ICD-10-PCS Value	Definition
Tarsal Joint, Left Tarsal Joint, Right	**Includes:** Calcaneocuboid joint Cuboideonavicular joint Cuneonavicular joint Intercuneiform joint Subtalar (talocalcaneal) joint Talocalcaneal (subtalar) joint Talocalcaneonavicular joint
Tarsal, Left Tarsal, Right	**Includes:** Calcaneus Cuboid bone Intermediate cuneiform bone Lateral cuneiform bone Medial cuneiform bone Navicular bone Talus bone
Temporal Artery, Left Temporal Artery, Right	**Includes:** Middle temporal artery Superficial temporal artery Transverse facial artery
Temporal Bone, Left Temporal Bone, Right	**Includes:** Mastoid process Petrous part of temoporal bone Tympanic part of temoporal bone Zygomatic process of temporal bone
Thalamus	**Includes:** Epithalamus Geniculate nucleus Metathalamus Pulvinar
Thoracic Aorta, Ascending/Arch	**Includes:** Aortic arch Ascending aorta
Thoracic Duct	**Includes:** Left jugular trunk Left subclavian trunk
Thoracic Nerve	**Includes:** Intercostal nerve Intercostobrachial nerve Spinal nerve, thoracic Subcostal nerve
Thoracic Spinal Cord	**Includes:** Dorsal root ganglion
Thoracic Sympathetic Nerve	**Includes:** Cardiac plexus Esophageal plexus Greater splanchnic nerve Inferior cardiac nerve Least splanchnic nerve Lesser splanchnic nerve Middle cardiac nerve Pulmonary plexus Superior cardiac nerve Thoracic aortic plexus Thoracic ganglion
Thoracic Vertebra	**Includes:** Spinous process Transverse process Vertebral arch Vertebral body Vertebral foramen Vertebral lamina Vertebral pedicle
Thoracic Vertebral Joint	**Includes:** Costotransverse joint Costovertebral joint Thoracic facet joint
Thoracolumbar Vertebral Joint	**Includes:** Thoracolumbar facet joint

ICD-10-PCS Value	Definition
Thorax Muscle, Left **Thorax Muscle, Right**	**Includes:** Intercostal muscle Levatores costarum muscle Pectoralis major muscle Pectoralis minor muscle Serratus anterior muscle Subclavius muscle Subcostal muscle Transverse thoracis muscle
Thymus	**Includes:** Thymus gland
Thyroid Artery, Left **Thyroid Artery, Right**	**Includes:** Cricothyroid artery Hyoid artery Sternocleidomastoid artery Superior laryngeal artery Superior thyroid artery Thyrocervical trunk
Tibia, Left **Tibia, Right**	**Includes:** Lateral condyle of tibia Medial condyle of tibia Medial malleolus
Tibial Nerve	**Includes:** Lateral plantar nerve Medial plantar nerve Medial popliteal nerve Medial sural cutaneous nerve
Toe Nail	**Includes:** Nail bed Nail plate
Toe Phalangeal Joint, Left **Toe Phalangeal Joint, Right**	**Includes:** Interphalangeal (IP) joint
Tongue	**Includes:** Frenulum linguae
Tongue, Palate, Pharynx Muscle	**Includes:** Chondroglossus muscle Genioglossus muscle Hyoglossus muscle Inferior longitudinal muscle Levator veli palatini muscle Palatoglossal muscle Palatopharyngeal muscle Pharyngeal constrictor muscle Salpingopharyngeus muscle Styloglossus muscle Stylopharyngeus muscle Superior longitudinal muscle Tensor veli palatini muscle
Tonsils	**Includes:** Palatine tonsil
Trachea	**Includes:** Cricoid cartilage
Transverse Colon	**Includes:** Hepatic flexure Splenic flexure
Tricuspid Valve	**Includes:** Right atrioventricular valve Tricuspid annulus
Trigeminal Nerve	**Includes:** Fifth cranial nerve Gasserian ganglion Mandibular nerve Maxillary nerve Ophthalmic nerve Trifacial nerve
Trochlear Nerve	**Includes:** Fourth cranial nerve

ICD-10-PCS Value	Definition
Trunk Muscle, Left **Trunk Muscle, Right**	**Includes:** Coccygeus muscle Erector spinae muscle Interspinalis muscle Intertransversarius muscle Latissimus dorsi muscle Quadratus lumborum muscle Rhomboid major muscle Rhomboid minor muscle Serratus posterior muscle Transversospinalis muscle Trapezius muscle
Tympanic Membrane, Left **Tympanic Membrane, Right**	**Includes:** Pars flaccida
Ulna, Left **Ulna, Right**	**Includes:** Olecranon process Radial notch
Ulnar Artery, Left **Ulnar Artery, Right**	**Includes:** Anterior ulnar recurrent artery Common interosseous artery Posterior ulnar recurrent artery
Ulnar Nerve	**Includes:** Cubital nerve
Upper Arm Muscle, Left **Upper Arm Muscle, Right**	**Includes:** Biceps brachii muscle Brachialis muscle Coracobrachialis muscle Triceps brachii muscle
Upper Artery	**Includes:** Aortic intercostal artery Bronchial artery Esophageal artery Subcostal artery
Upper Eyelid, Left **Upper Eyelid, Right**	**Includes:** Lateral canthus Levator palpebrae superioris muscle Orbicularis oculi muscle Superior tarsal plate
Upper Femur, Left **Upper Femur, Right**	**Includes:** Femoral head Greater trochanter Lesser trochanter Neck of femur
Upper Leg Muscle, Left **Upper Leg Muscle, Right**	**Includes:** Adductor brevis muscle Adductor longus muscle Adductor magnus muscle Biceps femoris muscle Gracilis muscle Pectineus muscle Quadriceps (femoris) Rectus femoris muscle Sartorius muscle Semimembranosus muscle Semitendinosus muscle Vastus intermedius muscle Vastus lateralis muscle Vastus medialis muscle
Upper Lip	**Includes:** Frenulum labii superioris Labial gland Vermilion border
Upper Spine Bursa and Ligament	**Includes:** Interspinous ligament, thoracic Intertransverse ligament, thoracic Ligamentum flavum, thoracic Supraspinous ligament

ICD-10-PCS Value	Definition
Ureter Ureter, Left Ureter, Right Ureters, Bilateral	**Includes:** Ureteral orifice Ureterovesical orifice
Urethra	**Includes:** Bulbourethral (Cowper's) gland Cowper's (bulbourethral) gland External urethral sphincter Internal urethral sphincter Membranous urethra Penile urethra Prostatic urethra
Uterine Supporting Structure	**Includes:** Broad ligament Infundibulopelvic ligament Ovarian ligament Round ligament of uterus
Uterus	**Includes:** Fundus uteri Myometrium Perimetrium Uterine cornu
Uvula	**Includes:** Palatine uvula
Vagus Nerve	**Includes:** Anterior vagal trunk Pharyngeal plexus Pneumogastric nerve Posterior vagal trunk Pulmonary plexus Recurrent laryngeal nerve Superior laryngeal nerve Tenth cranial nerve
Vas Deferens Vas Deferens, Bilateral Vas Deferens, Left Vas Deferens, Right	**Includes:** Ductus deferens Ejaculatory duct
Ventricle, Right	**Includes:** Conus arteriosus
Ventricular Septum	**Includes:** Interventricular septum
Vertebral Artery, Left Vertebral Artery, Right	**Includes:** Anterior spinal artery Posterior spinal artery
Vertebral Vein, Left Vertebral Vein, Right	**Includes:** Deep cervical vein Suboccipital venous plexus
Vestibular Gland	**Includes:** Bartholin's (greater vestibular) gland Greater vestibular (Bartholin's) gland Paraurethral (Skene's) gland Skene's (paraurethral) gland
Vitreous, Left Vitreous, Right	**Includes:** Vitreous body
Vocal Cord, Left Vocal Cord, Right	**Includes:** Vocal fold
Vulva	**Includes:** Labia majora Labia minora
Wrist Bursa and Ligament, Left Wrist Bursa and Ligament, Right	**Includes:** Palmar ulnocarpal ligament Radial collateral carpal ligament Radiocarpal ligament Radioulnar ligament Scapholunate ligament Ulnar collateral carpal ligament
Wrist Joint, Left Wrist Joint, Right	**Includes:** Distal radioulnar joint Radiocarpal joint

Appendix F: Device Classification

In most PCS codes, the sixth character of the code classifies the device. The sixth character device value "defines the material or appliance used to accomplish the objective of the procedure that remains in or on the procedure site at the end of the procedure." If the device is the means by which the procedural objective is accomplished, then a specific device value is coded in the sixth character. If no device is used to accomplish the objective of the procedure, the device value *No Device* is coded in the sixth character. In limited root operations, the classification provides the qualifier values *Temporary* and *Intraoperative*, for specific procedures involving clinically significant devices whose purpose is brief use during the procedure or current inpatient stay.

Material that is classified as a PCS device is distinguished from material classified as a PCS substance by its having a specific location. A device is intended to maintain a fixed location at the procedure site where it was put, whereas a substance is intended to disperse or be absorbed in the body. There are circumstances in which a device does not stay where it was put and may need to be "revised" in a subsequent procedure to move the device back to its intended location.

Material classified as a PCS device is also distinguishable by the fact that it is removable. Although it may not be practical to remove some types of devices, once they become established at the site, it is physically possible to remove a device for some time after the procedure. A skin graft, for example, once it "takes," may be nearly indistinguishable from the surrounding skin and so is no longer clearly identifiable as a device. Nevertheless, procedures that involve material coded as a device can for the most part be "reversed" by removing the device from the procedure site.

General Device Types

Device Type	Definition	Examples
Grafts	Biological or synthetic material that **takes the place of all or a portion of a body part.**	Full- or partial-thickness skin grafts: • Autologous • Nonautologous • Synthetic • Zooplastic Other tissue grafts: • Bone • Tendon • Vascular
Prosthesis	Biological or synthetic material that **takes the place of all or a portion of a body part.**	Joint prosthesis: • Autologous • Nonautologous • Synthetic
Implants	**Therapeutic** material that is not absorbed by, eliminated by, or incorporated into a body part.	External fixation device Internal fixation device: • Orthopaedic pins • Intramedullary rods Radioactive element implant Mesh
Simple or mechanical appliances	Biological or synthetic material that **assists or prevents a physiological function.**	Drainage device Extraluminal device Endobrachial device Fusion device Intraluminal device (can be temporary) Tracheostomy device IUD
Electronic appliances	Electronic appliances used to **assist, monitor, take the pace of, or prevent a physiological function.**	Cardiac leads Diaphragmatic pacemaker External heart assist system Short-term external heart assist system (Intraoperative) Fetal monitoring Hearing device Monitoring device Neurostimulator
External appliances	Performed without making an incision or a puncture, external appliances are used for the purpose of **protection, immobilization, stretching, compression, or packing.**	Bandage Cast Packing material Pressure dressing Traction apparatus

Transplant/Grafting Tissue Type Terminology

Tissue Type	Terminology
Tissue or organ transferred into a new position in **the body of the same individual**	Autograft Autologous Autoplastic
Having to do with individuals or tissues that have **identical genes**, such as identical twins	Isograft Isologous Syngeneic Syngraft
Tissue or organ taken from **different individuals** of the same species	Allogeneic Allograft Homologous Homograft
Tissue or organ from a **cadaver**	Nonautologous
Tissue or organ from individuals of **different species**	Heterogeneic Heterologous Xenogeneic Xenograft Zooplastic

Appendix G: Device Key and Aggregation Table

This 🔳 symbol next to a device in the Term column identifies that the device has been approved for NTAP (new technology add-on payment). CMS provides incremental payment, in addition to the DRG payment, for technologies that have received an NTAP designation.

Device Key

Term	ICD-10-PCS Value
3f (Aortic) Bioprosthesis valve	Zooplastic Tissue in Heart and Great Vessels
AbioCor® Total Replacement Heart	Synthetic Substitute
Absolute Pro Vascular (OTW) Self-Expanding Stent System	Intraluminal Device
Acculink (RX) Carotid Stent System	Intraluminal Device
Acellular Hydrated Dermis	Nonautologous Tissue Substitute
Acetabular cup	Liner in Lower Joints
Activa PC neurostimulator	Stimulator Generator, Multiple Array for Insertion in Subcutaneous Tissue and Fascia
Activa RC neurostimulator	Stimulator Generator, Multiple Array Rechargeable for Insertion in Subcutaneous Tissue and Fascia
Activa SC neurostimulator	Stimulator Generator, Single Array for Insertion in Subcutaneous Tissue and Fascia
ACUITY™ Steerable Lead	Cardiac Lead, Pacemaker for Insertion in Heart and Great Vessels Cardiac Lead, Defibrillator for Insertion in Heart and Great Vessels
Advisa (MRI)	Pacemaker, Dual Chamber for Insertion in Subcutaneous Tissue and Fascia
AFX® Endovascular AAA System	Intraluminal Device
Alfapump® system	Other Device
AMPLATZER® Muscular VSD Occluder	Synthetic Substitute
AMS 800® Urinary Control System	Artificial Sphincter in Urinary System
AneuRx® AAA Advantage®	Intraluminal Device
Annuloplasty ring	Synthetic Substitute
ApiFix® Minimally Invasive Deformity Correction (MID-C) System (C)	Posterior (Dynamic) Distraction Device in New Technology
aprevo™	Interbody Fusion Device, Customizable in New Technology
Articulating Spacer (Antibiotic)	Articulating Spacer in Lower Joints
Artificial anal sphincter (AAS)	Artificial Sphincter in Gastrointestinal System
Artificial bowel sphincter (neosphincter)	Artificial Sphincter in Gastrointestinal System
Artificial urinary sphincter (AUS)	Artificial Sphincter in Urinary System
Ascenda Intrathecal Catheter	Infusion Device
Assurant (Cobalt) stent	Intraluminal Device
AtriClip LAA Exclusion System	Extraluminal Device
Attain Ability® Lead	Cardiac Lead, Pacemaker for Insertion in Heart and Great Vessels Cardiac Lead, Defibrillator for Insertion in Heart and Great Vessels

Term	ICD-10-PCS Value
Attain StarFix® (OTW) Lead	Cardiac Lead, Pacemaker for Insertion in Heart and Great Vessels Cardiac Lead, Defibrillator for Insertion in Heart and Great Vessels
Autograft	Autologous Tissue Substitute
Autologous artery graft	Autologous Arterial Tissue in Heart and Great Vessels Autologous Arterial Tissue in Upper Arteries Autologous Arterial Tissue in Lower Arteries Autologous Arterial Tissue in Upper Veins Autologous Arterial Tissue in Lower Veins
Autologous vein graft	Autologous Venous Tissue in Heart and Great Vessels Autologous Venous Tissue in Upper Arteries Autologous Venous Tissue in Lower Arteries Autologous Venous Tissue in Upper Veins Autologous Venous Tissue in Lower Veins
Axial Lumbar Interbody Fusion System	Interbody Fusion Device in Lower Joints
AxiaLIF® System	Interbody Fusion Device in Lower Joints
BAK/C® Interbody Cervical Fusion System	Interbody Fusion Device in Upper Joints
Bard® Composix® (E/X)(LP) mesh	Synthetic Substitute
Bard® Composix® Kugel® patch	Synthetic Substitute
Bard® Dulex™ mesh	Synthetic Substitute
Bard® Ventralex™ hernia patch	Synthetic Substitute
Baroreflex Activation Therapy® (BAT®)	Stimulator Lead in Upper Arteries Stimulator Generator in Subcutaneous Tissue and Fascia
Barricaid® Annular Closure Device (ACD)	Synthetic Substitute
Berlin Heart Ventricular Assist Device	Implantable Heart Assist System in Heart and Great Vessels
Bioactive embolization coil(s)	Intraluminal Device, Bioactive in Upper Arteries
Biventricular external heart assist system	Short-term External Heart Assist System in Heart and Great Vessels
Blood glucose monitoring system	Monitoring Device
Bone anchored hearing device	Hearing Device, Bone Conduction for Insertion in Ear, Nose, Sinus Hearing Device, in Head and Facial Bones
Bone bank bone graft	Nonautologous Tissue Substitute
Bone screw (interlocking)(lag)(pedicle)(recessed)	Internal Fixation Device in Head and Facial Bones Internal Fixation Device in Upper Bones Internal Fixation Device in Lower Bones
Bovine pericardial valve	Zooplastic Tissue in Heart and Great Vessels
Bovine pericardium graft	Zooplastic Tissue in Heart and Great Vessels
Brachytherapy seeds	Radioactive Element
BRYAN® Cervical Disc System	Synthetic Substitute
BVS 5000 Ventricular Assist Device	Short-term External Heart Assist System in Heart and Great Vessels

Term	ICD-10-PCS Value
Cardiac contractility modulation lead	Cardiac Lead in Heart and Great Vessels
Cardiac event recorder	Monitoring Device
Cardiac resynchronization therapy (CRT) lead	Cardiac Lead, Pacemaker for Insertion in Heart and Great Vessels Cardiac Lead, Defibrillator for Insertion in Heart and Great Vessels
CardioMEMS® pressure sensor	Monitoring Device, Pressure Sensor for Insertion in Heart and Great Vessels
Carmat total artificial heart (TAH)	Biologic with Synthetic Substitute, Autoregulated Electrohydraulic for Replacement in Heart and Great Vessels
Carotid (artery) sinus (baroreceptor) lead	Stimulator Lead in Upper Arteries
Carotid WALLSTENT® Monorail® Endoprosthesis	Intraluminal Device
Centrimag® Blood Pump	Short-term External Heart Assist System in Heart and Great Vessels
Ceramic on ceramic bearing surface	Synthetic Substitute, Ceramic for Replacement in Lower Joints
Cesium-131 Collagen Implant	Radioactive Element, Cesium-131 Collagen Implant for Insertion in Central Nervous System and Cranial Nerves
CivaSheet®	Radioactive Element
Clamp and rod internal fixation system (CRIF)	Internal Fixation Device in Upper Bones Internal Fixation Device in Lower Bones
COALESCE® radiolucent interbody fusion device	Interbody Fusion Device in Upper Joints Interbody Fusion Device in Lower Joints
CoAxia NeuroFlo catheter	Intraluminal Device
Cobalt/chromium head and polyethylene socket	Synthetic Substitute, Metal on Polyethylene for Replacement in Lower Joints
Cobalt/chromium head and socket	Synthetic Substitute, Metal for Replacement in Lower Joints
Cochlear implant (CI), multiple channel (electrode)	Hearing Device, Multiple Channel Cochlear Prosthesis for Insertion in Ear, Nose, Sinus
Cochlear implant (CI), single channel (electrode)	Hearing Device, Single Channel Cochlear Prosthesis for Insertion in Ear, Nose, Sinus
COGNIS® CRT-D	Cardiac Resynchronization Defibrillator Pulse Generator for Insertion in Subcutaneous Tissue and Fascia
COHERE® radiolucent interbody fusion device	Interbody Fusion Device in Upper Joints Interbody Fusion Device in Lower Joints
Colonic Z-Stent®	Intraluminal Device
Complete (SE) stent	Intraluminal Device
Concerto II CRT-D	Cardiac Resynchronization Defibrillator Pulse Generator for Insertion in Subcutaneous Tissue and Fascia
CONSERVE® PLUS Total Resurfacing Hip System	Resurfacing Device in Lower Joints
Consulta CRT-D	Cardiac Resynchronization Defibrillator Pulse Generator for Insertion in Subcutaneous Tissue and Fascia
Consulta CRT-P	Cardiac Resynchronization Pacemaker Pulse Generator for Insertion in Subcutaneous Tissue and Fascia
CONTAK RENEWAL® 3 RF (HE) CRT-D	Cardiac Resynchronization Defibrillator Pulse Generator for Insertion in Subcutaneous Tissue and Fascia
Contegra Pulmonary Valved Conduit	Zooplastic Tissue in Heart and Great Vessels

Term	ICD-10-PCS Value
Continuous Glucose Monitoring (CGM) device	Monitoring Device
Cook Biodesign® Fistula Plug(s)	Nonautologous Tissue Substitute
Cook Biodesign® Hernia Graft(s)	Nonautologous Tissue Substitute
Cook Biodesign® Layered Graft(s)	Nonautologous Tissue Substitute
Cook Zenapro™ Layered Graft(s)	Nonautologous Tissue Substitute
Cook Zenith AAA Endovascular Graft	Intraluminal Device
Cook Zenith® Fenestrated AAA Endovascular Graft	Intraluminal Device, Branched or Fenestrated, One or Two Arteries for Restriction in Lower Arteries Intraluminal Device, Branched or Fenestrated, Three or More Arteries for Restriction in Lower Arteries
CoreValve transcatheter aortic valve	Zooplastic Tissue in Heart and Great Vessels
Cormet Hip Resurfacing System	Resurfacing Device in Lower Joints
CoRoent® XL	Interbody Fusion Device in Lower Joints
Corox (OTW) Bipolar Lead	Cardiac Lead, Pacemaker for Insertion in Heart and Great Vessels Cardiac Lead, Defibrillator for Insertion in Heart and Great Vessels
Cortical strip neurostimulator lead	Neurostimulator Lead in Central Nervous System and Cranial Nerves
Corvia IASD®	Synthetic Substitute
Cultured epidermal cell autograft	Autologous Tissue Substitute
CYPHER® Stent	Intraluminal Device, Drug-eluting in Heart and Great Vessels
Cystostomy tube	Drainage Device
DBS lead	Neurostimulator Lead in Central Nervous System and Cranial Nerves
DeBakey Left Ventricular Assist Device	Implantable Heart Assist System in Heart and Great Vessels
Deep brain neurostimulator lead	Neurostimulator Lead in Central Nervous System and Cranial Nerves
Delta frame external fixator	External Fixation Device, Hybrid for Insertion in Upper Bones External Fixation Device, Hybrid for Reposition in Upper Bones External Fixation Device, Hybrid for Insertion in Lower Bones External Fixation Device, Hybrid for Reposition in Lower Bones
Delta III Reverse shoulder prosthesis	Synthetic Substitute, Reverse Ball and Socket for Replacement in Upper Joints
Diaphragmatic pacemaker generator	Stimulator Generator in Subcutaneous Tissue and Fascia
Direct Lateral Interbody Fusion (DLIF) device	Interbody Fusion Device in Lower Joints
Driver stent (RX) (OTW)	Intraluminal Device
DuraHeart Left Ventricular Assist System	Implantable Heart Assist System in Heart and Great Vessels
Durata® Defibrillation Lead	Cardiac Lead, Defibrillator for Insertion in Heart and Great Vessels
DynaClip® (Forte)	Internal Fixation Device, Sustained Compression for Fusion in Upper Joints Internal Fixation Device, Sustained Compression for Fusion in Lower Joints

Term	ICD-10-PCS Value
DynaNail® (Hybrid) (Mini)	Internal Fixation Device, Sustained Compression for Fusion in Upper Joints Internal Fixation Device, Sustained Compression for Fusion in Lower Joints
Dynesys® Dynamic Stabilization System	Spinal Stabilization Device, Pedicle-Based for Insertion in Upper Joints Spinal Stabilization Device, Pedicle-Based for Insertion in Lower Joints
E-Luminexx™ (Biliary)(Vascular) Stent	Intraluminal Device
Electrical bone growth stimulator (EBGS)	Bone Growth Stimulator in Head and Facial Bones Bone Growth Stimulator in Upper Bones Bone Growth Stimulator in Lower Bones
Electrical muscle stimulation (EMS) lead	Stimulator Lead in Muscles
Electronic muscle stimulator lead	Stimulator Lead in Muscles
Eluvia™ Drug-eluting Vascular Stent System	Intraluminal Device, Sustained Release Drug-eluting in New Technology Intraluminal Device, Sustained Release Drug-eluting, Two in New Technology Intraluminal Device, Sustained Release Drug-eluting, Three in New Technology Intraluminal Device, Sustained Release Drug-eluting, Four or More in New Technology
Embolization coil(s)	Intraluminal Device
Endeavor® (III)(IV) (Sprint) Zotarolimus-eluting Coronary Stent System	Intraluminal Device, Drug-eluting in Heart and Great Vessels
Endologix AFX® Endovascular AAA System	Intraluminal Device
EndoSure® sensor	Monitoring Device, Pressure Sensor for Insertion in Heart and Great Vessels
ENDOTAK RELIANCE® (G) Defibrillation Lead	Cardiac Lead, Defibrillator for Insertion in Heart and Great Vessels
Endotracheal tube (cuffed)(double-lumen)	Intraluminal Device, Endotracheal Airway in Respiratory System
Endurant® Endovascular Stent Graft	Intraluminal Device
Endurant® II AAA stent graft system	Intraluminal Device
EnRhythm	Pacemaker, Dual Chamber for Insertion in Subcutaneous Tissue and Fascia
Enterra gastric neurostimulator	Stimulator Generator, Multiple Array for Insertion in Subcutaneous Tissue and Fascia
Epic™ Stented Tissue Valve (aortic)	Zooplastic Tissue in Heart and Great Vessels
Epicel® cultured epidermal autograft	Autologous Tissue Substitute
Esophageal obturator airway (EOA)	Intraluminal Device, Airway in Gastrointestinal System
Esteem® implantable hearing system	Hearing Device in Ear, Nose, Sinus
Evera (XT)(S)(DR/VR)	Defibrillator Generator for Insertion in Subcutaneous Tissue and Fascia
Everolimus-eluting coronary stent	Intraluminal Device, Drug-eluting in Heart and Great Vessels
Ex-PRESS™ mini glaucoma shunt	Synthetic Substitute

Term	ICD-10-PCS Value
EXCLUDER® AAA Endoprosthesis	Intraluminal Device Intraluminal Device, Branched or Fenestrated, One or Two Arteries for Restriction in Lower Arteries Intraluminal Device, Branched or Fenestrated, Three or More Arteries for Restriction in Lower Arteries
EXCLUDER® IBE Endoprosthesis	Intraluminal Device, Branched or Fenestrated, One or Two Arteries for Restriction in Lower Arteries
Express® (LD) Premounted Stent System	Intraluminal Device
Express® Biliary SD Monorail® Premounted Stent System	Intraluminal Device
Express® SD Renal Monorail® Premounted Stent System	Intraluminal Device
External fixator	External Fixation Device in Head and Facial Bones External Fixation Device in Upper Bones External Fixation Device in Lower Bones External Fixation Device in Upper Joints External Fixation Device in Lower Joints
EXtreme Lateral Interbody Fusion (XLIF) device	Interbody Fusion Device in Lower Joints
Facet replacement spinal stabilization device	Spinal Stabilization Device, Facet Replacement for Insertion in Upper Joints Spinal Stabilization Device, Facet Replacement for Insertion in Lower Joints
FLAIR® Endovascular Stent Graft	Intraluminal Device
Flexible Composite Mesh	Synthetic Substitute
Flow Diverter embolization device	Intraluminal Device, Flow Diverter for Restriction in Upper Arteries
Foley catheter	Drainage Device
Formula™ Balloon-Expandable Renal Stent System	Intraluminal Device
Freestyle (Stentless) Aortic Root Bioprosthesis	Zooplastic Tissue in Heart and Great Vessels
Fusion screw (compression)(lag)(locking)	Internal Fixation Device in Upper Joints Internal Fixation Device in Lower Joints
GammaTile™	Radioactive Element, Cesium-131 Collagen Implant for Insertion in Central Nervous System and Cranial Nerves
Gastric electrical stimulation (GES) lead	Stimulator Lead in Gastrointestinal System
Gastric pacemaker lead	Stimulator Lead in Gastrointestinal System
GORE EXCLUDER® AAA Endoprosthesis	Intraluminal Device Intraluminal Device, Branched or Fenestrated, One or Two Arteries for Restriction in Lower Arteries Intraluminal Device, Branched or Fenestrated, Three or More Arteries for Restriction in Lower Arteries
GORE EXCLUDER® IBE Endoprosthesis	Intraluminal Device, Branched or Fenestrated, One or Two Arteries for Restriction in Lower Arteries
GORE TAG® Thoracic Endoprosthesis	Intraluminal Device
GORE® DUALMESH®	Synthetic Substitute
Guedel airway	Intraluminal Device, Airway in Mouth and Throat

Term	ICD-10-PCS Value
Hancock Bioprosthesis (aortic)(mitral) valve	Zooplastic Tissue in Heart and Great Vessels
Hancock Bioprosthetic Valved Conduit	Zooplastic Tissue in Heart and Great Vessels
HeartMate 3™ LVAS	Implantable Heart Assist System in Heart and Great Vessels
HeartMate II® Left Ventricular Assist Device (LVAD)	Implantable Heart Assist System in Heart and Great Vessels
HeartMate XVE® Left Ventricular Assist Device (LVAD)	Implantable Heart Assist System in Heart and Great Vessels
Herculink (RX) Elite Renal Stent System	Intraluminal Device
Hip (joint) liner	Liner in Lower Joints
Holter valve ventricular shunt	Synthetic Substitute
IASD® (InterAtrial Shunt Device), Corvia	Synthetic Substitute
iFuse Bedrock™ Granite Implant System	Internal Fixation Device with Tulip Connector in New Technology
Ilizarov external fixator	External Fixation Device, Ring for Insertion in Upper Bones External Fixation Device, Ring for Reposition in Upper Bones External Fixation Device, Ring for Insertion in Lower Bones External Fixation Device, Ring for Reposition in Lower Bones
Ilizarov-Vecklich device	External Fixation Device, Limb Lengthening for Insertion in Upper Bones External Fixation Device, Limb Lengthening for Insertion in Lower Bones
Impella® heart pump	Short-term External Heart Assist System in Heart and Great Vessels
Implantable cardioverter-defibrillator (ICD)	Defibrillator Generator for Insertion in Subcutaneous Tissue and Fascia
Implantable drug infusion pump (anti-spasmodic) (chemotherapy)(pain)	Infusion Device, Pump in Subcutaneous Tissue and Fascia
Implantable glucose monitoring device	Monitoring Device
Implantable hemodynamic monitor (IHM)	Monitoring Device, Hemodynamic for Insertion in Subcutaneous Tissue and Fascia
Implantable hemodynamic monitoring system (IHMS)	Monitoring Device, Hemodynamic for Insertion in Subcutaneous Tissue and Fascia
Implantable Miniature Telescope™ (IMT)	Synthetic Substitute, Intraocular Telescope for Replacement in Eye
Implanted (venous)(access) port	Vascular Access Device, Totally Implantable in Subcutaneous Tissue and Fascia
InDura, intrathecal catheter (1P) (spinal)	Infusion Device
Injection reservoir, port	Vascular Access Device, Totally Implantable in Subcutaneous Tissue and Fascia
Injection reservoir, pump	Infusion Device, Pump in Subcutaneous Tissue and Fascia
InterAtrial Shunt Device IASD®, Corvia	Synthetic Substitute
Interbody fusion (spine) cage	Interbody Fusion Device in Upper Joints Interbody Fusion Device in Lower Joints

Term	ICD-10-PCS Value
Interspinous process spinal stabilization device	Spinal Stabilization Device, Interspinous Process for Insertion in Upper Joints Spinal Stabilization Device, Interspinous Process for Insertion in Lower Joints
InterStim™ Micro Therapy neurostimulator	Stimulator Generator, Single Array Rechargeable for Insertion in Subcutaneous Tissue and Fascia
InterStim® Therapy lead	Neurostimulator Lead in Peripheral Nervous System
InterStim™ II Therapy neurostimulator	Stimulator Generator, Single Array for Insertion in Subcutaneous Tissue and Fascia
Intramedullary (IM) rod (nail)	Internal Fixation Device, Intramedullary in Upper Bones Internal Fixation Device, Intramedullary in Lower Bones
Intramedullary skeletal kinetic distractor (ISKD)	Internal Fixation Device, Intramedullary in Upper Bones Internal Fixation Device, Intramedullary in Lower Bones
Intrauterine Device (IUD)	Contraceptive Device in Female Reproductive System
Ischemic Stroke System (ISS500)	Neurostimulator Lead in New Technology
ISS500 (Ischemic Stroke System)	Neurostimulator Lead in New Technology
Itrel (3)(4) neurostimulator	Stimulator Generator, Single Array for Insertion in Subcutaneous Tissue and Fascia
Joint fixation plate	Internal Fixation Device in Upper Joints Internal Fixation Device in Lower Joints
Joint liner (insert)	Liner in Lower Joints
Joint spacer (antibiotic)	Spacer in Upper Joints Spacer in Lower Joints
Kappa	Pacemaker, Dual Chamber for Insertion in Subcutaneous Tissue and Fascia
Kirschner wire (K-wire)	Internal Fixation Device in Head and Facial Bones Internal Fixation Device in Upper Bones Internal Fixation Device in Lower Bones Internal Fixation Device in Upper Joints Internal Fixation Device in Lower Joints
Knee (implant) insert	Liner in Lower Joints
Kuntscher nail	Internal Fixation Device, Intramedullary in Upper Bones Internal Fixation Device, Intramedullary in Lower Bones
LAP-BAND® adjustable gastric banding system	Extraluminal Device
LifeStent® (Flexstar)(XL) Vascular Stent System	Intraluminal Device
LigaPASS 2.0™ PJK Prevention System	Posterior Vertebral Tether in New Technology
LIVIAN™ CRT-D	Cardiac Resynchronization Defibrillator Pulse Generator for Insertion in Subcutaneous Tissue and Fascia
Loop recorder, implantable	Monitoring Device
MAGEC® Spinal Bracing and Distraction System	Magnetically Controlled Growth Rod(s) in New Technology
Mark IV Breathing Pacemaker System	Stimulator Generator in Subcutaneous Tissue and Fascia
Maximo II DR (VR)	Defibrillator Generator for Insertion in Subcutaneous Tissue and Fascia

Term	ICD-10-PCS Value
Maximo II DR CRT-D	Cardiac Resynchronization Defibrillator Pulse Generator for Insertion in Subcutaneous Tissue and Fascia
Medtronic Endurant® II AAA stent graft system	Intraluminal Device
Melody® transcatheter pulmonary valve	Zooplastic Tissue in Heart and Great Vessels
Metal on metal bearing surface	Synthetic Substitute, Metal for Replacement in Lower Joints
Micro-Driver stent (RX) (OTW)	Intraluminal Device
MicroMed HeartAssist	Implantable Heart Assist System in Heart and Great Vessels
Micrus CERECYTE microcoil	Intraluminal Device, Bioactive in Upper Arteries
MIRODERM™ Biologic Wound Matrix	Nonautologous Tissue Substitute
MitraClip valve repair system	Synthetic Substitute
Mitroflow® Aortic Pericardial Heart Valve	Zooplastic Tissue in Heart and Great Vessels
Mosaic Bioprosthesis (aortic) (mitral) valve	Zooplastic Tissue in Heart and Great Vessels
MULTI-LINK (VISION)(MINI-VISION)(ULTRA) Coronary Stent System	Intraluminal Device
nanoLOCK™ interbody fusion device	Interbody Fusion Device in Upper Joints Interbody Fusion Device in Lower Joints
Nasopharyngeal airway (NPA)	Intraluminal Device, Airway in Ear, Nose, Sinus
Neovasc Reducer™	Reduction Device in New Technology
Neuromuscular electrical stimulation (NEMS) lead	Stimulator Lead in Muscles
Neurostimulator generator, multiple channel	Stimulator Generator, Multiple Array for Insertion in Subcutaneous Tissue and Fascia
Neurostimulator generator, multiple channel rechargeable	Stimulator Generator, Multiple Array Rechargeable for Insertion in Subcutaneous Tissue and Fascia
Neurostimulator generator, single channel	Stimulator Generator, Single Array for Insertion in Subcutaneous Tissue and Fascia
Neurostimulator generator, single channel rechargeable	Stimulator Generator, Single Array Rechargeable for Insertion in Subcutaneous Tissue and Fascia
Neutralization plate	Internal Fixation Device in Head and Facial Bones Internal Fixation Device in Upper Bones Internal Fixation Device in Lower Bones
Nitinol framed polymer mesh	Synthetic Substitute
Non-tunneled central venous catheter	Infusion Device
Novacor Left Ventricular Assist Device	Implantable Heart Assist System in Heart and Great Vessels
Novation® Ceramic AHS® (Articulation Hip System)	Synthetic Substitute, Ceramic for Replacement in Lower Joints
NUsurface® Meniscus Implant	Synthetic Substitute, Lateral Meniscus in New Technology Synthetic Substitute, Medial Meniscus in New Technology
Omnilink Elite Vascular Balloon Expandable Stent System	Intraluminal Device

Term	ICD-10-PCS Value
Open Pivot Aortic Valve Graft (AVG)	Synthetic Substitute
Open Pivot (mechanical) Valve	Synthetic Substitute
Optimizer™ III implantable pulse generator	Contractility Modulation Device for Insertion in Subcutaneous Tissue and Fascia
Oropharyngeal airway (OPA)	Intraluminal Device, Airway in Mouth and Throat
Ovatio™ CRT-D	Cardiac Resynchronization Defibrillator Pulse Generator for Insertion in Subcutaneous Tissue and Fascia
OXINIUM	Synthetic Substitute, Oxidized Zirconium on Polyethylene for Replacement in Lower Joints
Paclitaxel-eluting coronary stent	Intraluminal Device, Drug-eluting in Heart and Great Vessels
Paclitaxel-eluting peripheral stent	Intraluminal Device, Drug-eluting in Upper Arteries Intraluminal Device, Drug-eluting in Lower Arteries
Partially absorbable mesh	Synthetic Substitute
Pedicle-based dynamic stabilization device	Spinal Stabilization Device, Pedicle-Based for Insertion in Upper Joints Spinal Stabilization Device, Pedicle-Based for Insertion in Lower Joints
PERCEPT™ PC neurostimulator	Stimulator Generator, Multiple Array for Insertion in Subcutaneous Tissue and Fascia
Percutaneous endoscopic gastrojejunostomy (PEG/J) tube	Feeding Device in Gastrointestinal System
Percutaneous endoscopic gastrostomy (PEG) tube	Feeding Device in Gastrointestinal System
Percutaneous nephrostomy catheter	Drainage Device
Peripherally inserted central catheter (PICC)	Infusion Device
Pessary ring	Intraluminal Device, Pessary in Female Reproductive System
Phrenic nerve stimulator generator	Stimulator Generator in Subcutaneous Tissue and Fascia
Phrenic nerve stimulator lead	Diaphragmatic Pacemaker Lead in Respiratory System
PHYSIOMESH™ Flexible Composite Mesh	Synthetic Substitute
Pipeline™ (Flex) embolization device	Intraluminal Device, Flow Diverter for Restriction in Upper Arteries
Polyethylene socket	Synthetic Substitute, Polyethylene for Replacement in Lower Joints
Polymethylmethacrylate (PMMA)	Synthetic Substitute
Polypropylene mesh	Synthetic Substitute
Porcine (bioprosthetic) valve	Zooplastic Tissue in Heart and Great Vessels
PRECICE intramedullary limb lengthening system	Internal Fixation Device, Intramedullary Limb Lengthening for Insertion in Upper Bones Internal Fixation Device, Intramedullary Limb Lengthening for Insertion in Lower Bones
PRESTIGE® Cervical Disc	Synthetic Substitute
PrimeAdvanced neurostimulator (SureScan)(MRI Safe)	Stimulator Generator, Multiple Array for Insertion in Subcutaneous Tissue and Fascia

Term	ICD-10-PCS Value
PROCEED™ Ventral Patch	Synthetic Substitute
Prodisc-C	Synthetic Substitute
Prodisc-L	Synthetic Substitute
PROLENE Polypropylene Hernia System (PHS)	Synthetic Substitute
Protecta XT CRT-D	Cardiac Resynchronization Defibrillator Pulse Generator for Insertion in Subcutaneous Tissue and Fascia
Protecta XT DR (XT VR)	Defibrillator Generator for Insertion in Subcutaneous Tissue and Fascia
Protégé® RX Carotid Stent System	Intraluminal Device
Pump reservoir	Infusion Device, Pump in Subcutaneous Tissue and Fascia
REALIZE® Adjustable Gastric Band	Extraluminal Device
Rebound HRD® (Hernia Repair Device)	Synthetic Substitute
Reducer™ System	Reduction Device in New Technology
RestoreAdvanced neurostimulator (SureScan)(MRI Safe)	Stimulator Generator, Multiple Array Rechargeable for Insertion in Subcutaneous Tissue and Fascia
RestoreSensor neurostimulator (SureScan)(MRI Safe)	Stimulator Generator, Multiple Array Rechargeable for Insertion in Subcutaneous Tissue and Fascia
RestoreUltra neurostimulator (SureScan)(MRI Safe)	Stimulator Generator, Multiple Array Rechargeable for Insertion in Subcutaneous Tissue and Fascia
Reveal (LINQ)(DX)(XT)	Monitoring Device
Reverse® Shoulder Prosthesis	Synthetic Substitute, Reverse Ball and Socket for Replacement in Upper Joints
Revo MRI™ SureScan® pacemaker	Pacemaker, Dual Chamber for Insertion in Subcutaneous Tissue and Fascia
Rheos® System device	Stimulator Generator in Subcutaneous Tissue and Fascia
Rheos® System lead	Stimulator Lead in Upper Arteries
RNS System lead	Neurostimulator Lead in Central Nervous System and Cranial Nerves
RNS system neurostimulator generator	Neurostimulator Generator in Head and Facial Bones
S-ICD™ lead	Subcutaneous Defibrillator Lead in Subcutaneous Tissue and Fascia
Sacral nerve modulation (SNM) lead	Stimulator Lead in Urinary System
Sacral neuromodulation lead	Stimulator Lead in Urinary System
SAPIEN transcatheter aortic valve	Zooplastic Tissue in Heart and Great Vessels
SAVAL below-the-knee (BTK) drug-eluting stent system	Intraluminal Device, Sustained Release Drug-eluting in New Technology Intraluminal Device, Sustained Release Drug-eluting, Two in New Technology Intraluminal Device, Sustained Release Drug-eluting, Three in New Technology Intraluminal Device, Sustained Release Drug-eluting, Four or More in New Technology
Secura (DR) (VR)	Defibrillator Generator for Insertion in Subcutaneous Tissue and Fascia

Term	ICD-10-PCS Value
Sheffield hybrid external fixator	External Fixation Device, Hybrid for Insertion in Upper Bones External Fixation Device, Hybrid for Reposition in Upper Bones External Fixation Device, Hybrid for Insertion in Lower Bones External Fixation Device, Hybrid for Reposition in Lower Bones
Sheffield ring external fixator	External Fixation Device, Ring for Insertion in Upper Bones External Fixation Device, Ring for Reposition in Upper Bones External Fixation Device, Ring for Insertion in Lower Bones External Fixation Device, Ring for Reposition in Lower Bones
Single lead pacemaker (atrium)(ventricle)	Pacemaker, Single Chamber for Insertion in Subcutaneous Tissue and Fascia
Single lead rate responsive pacemaker (atrium)(ventricle)	Pacemaker, Single Chamber Rate Responsive for Insertion in Subcutaneous Tissue and Fascia
Sirolimus-eluting coronary stent	Intraluminal Device, Drug-eluting in Heart and Great Vessels
SJM Biocor® Stented Valve System	Zooplastic Tissue in Heart and Great Vessels
Spacer, Articulating (Antibiotic)	Articulating Spacer in Lower Joints
Spacer, Static (Antibiotic)	Spacer in Lower Joints
Spinal cord neurostimulator lead	Neurostimulator Lead in Central Nervous System and Cranial Nerves
Spinal growth rods, magnetically controlled	Magnetically Controlled Growth Rod(s) in New Technology
SpineJack® system	Synthetic Substitute, Mechanically Expandable (Paired) in New Technology
Spiration IBV™ Valve System	Intraluminal Device, Endobronchial Valve in Respiratory System
Static Spacer (Antibiotic)	Spacer in Lower Joints
Stent, intraluminal (cardiovascular) (gastrointestinal) (hepatobiliary)(urinary)	Intraluminal Device
Stented tissue valve	Zooplastic Tissue in Heart and Great Vessels
Stratos LV	Cardiac Resynchronization Pacemaker Pulse Generator for Insertion in Subcutaneous Tissue and Fascia
Subcutaneous injection reservoir, port	Vascular Access Device, Totally Implantable in Subcutaneous Tissue and Fascia
Subcutaneous injection reservoir, pump	Infusion Device, Pump in Subcutaneous Tissue and Fascia
Subdermal progesterone implant	Contraceptive Device in Subcutaneous Tissue and Fascia
Surpass Streamline™ Flow Diverter	Intraluminal Device, Flow Diverter for Restriction in Upper Arteries
SynCardia (temporary) Total Artificial Heart (TAH)	Synthetic Substitute, Pneumatic for Replacement in Heart and Great Vessels
SynCardia Total Artificial Heart	Synthetic Substitute
Synchra CRT-P	Cardiac Resynchronization Pacemaker Pulse Generator for Insertion in Subcutaneous Tissue and Fascia
SynchroMed Pump	Infusion Device, Pump in Subcutaneous Tissue and Fascia
Talent® Converter	Intraluminal Device

Term	ICD-10-PCS Value
Talent® Occluder	Intraluminal Device
Talent® Stent Graft (abdominal)(thoracic)	Intraluminal Device
TandemHeart® System	Short-term External Heart Assist System in Heart and Great Vessels
TAXUS® Liberté® Paclitaxel-eluting Coronary Stent System	Intraluminal Device, Drug-eluting in Heart and Great Vessels
Therapeutic occlusion coil(s)	Intraluminal Device
Thoracostomy tube	Drainage Device
Thoraflex™ Hybrid device	Branched Synthetic Substitute with Intraluminal Device in New Technology
Thoratec IVAD (Implantable Ventricular Assist Device)	Implantable Heart Assist System in Heart and Great Vessels
Thoratec Paracorporeal Ventricular Assist Device	Short-term External Heart Assist System in Heart and Great Vessels
Tibial insert	Liner in Lower Joints
Tissue bank graft	Nonautologous Tissue Substitute
Tissue expander (inflatable)(injectable)	Tissue Expander in Skin and Breast Tissue Expander in Subcutaneous Tissue and Fascia
Titan Endoskeleton™	Interbody Fusion Device in Upper Joints Interbody Fusion Device in Lower Joints
Titanium Sternal Fixation System (TSFS)	Internal Fixation Device, Rigid Plate for Insertion in Upper Bones Internal Fixation Device, Rigid Plate for Reposition in Upper Bones
TOPS™ System	Posterior Spinal Motion Preservation Device in New Technology
Total artificial (replacement) heart	Synthetic Substitute
Tracheostomy tube	Tracheostomy Device in Respiratory System
Trifecta™ Valve (aortic)	Zooplastic Tissue in Heart and Great Vessels
Tunneled central venous catheter	Vascular Access Device, Tunneled in Subcutaneous Tissue and Fascia
Tunneled spinal (intrathecal) catheter	Infusion Device
Two lead pacemaker	Pacemaker, Dual Chamber for Insertion in Subcutaneous Tissue and Fascia
Ultraflex™ Precision Colonic Stent System	Intraluminal Device
ULTRAPRO Hernia System (UHS)	Synthetic Substitute
ULTRAPRO Partially Absorbable Lightweight Mesh	Synthetic Substitute
ULTRAPRO Plug	Synthetic Substitute
Ultrasonic osteogenic stimulator	Bone Growth Stimulator in Head and Facial Bones Bone Growth Stimulator in Upper Bones Bone Growth Stimulator in Lower Bones
Ultrasound bone healing system	Bone Growth Stimulator in Head and Facial Bones Bone Growth Stimulator in Upper Bones Bone Growth Stimulator in Lower Bones
Uniplanar external fixator	External Fixation Device, Monoplanar for Insertion in Upper Bones External Fixation Device, Monoplanar for Reposition in Upper Bones External Fixation Device, Monoplanar for Insertion in Lower Bones External Fixation Device, Monoplanar for Reposition in Lower Bones

Term	ICD-10-PCS Value
Urinary incontinence stimulator lead	Stimulator Lead in Urinary System
V-Wave Interatrial Shunt System	Synthetic Substitute
Vaginal pessary	Intraluminal Device, Pessary in Female Reproductive System
Valiant Thoracic Stent Graft	Intraluminal Device
Vectra® Vascular Access Graft	Vascular Access Device, Tunneled in Subcutaneous Tissue and Fascia
Ventrio™ Hernia Patch	Synthetic Substitute
Versa	Pacemaker, Dual Chamber for Insertion in Subcutaneous Tissue and Fascia
Virtuoso (II) (DR) (VR)	Defibrillator Generator for Insertion in Subcutaneous Tissue and Fascia
Viva(XT)(S)	Cardiac Resynchronization Defibrillator Pulse Generator for Insertion in Subcutaneous Tissue and Fascia
Vivistim® Paired VNS System Lead	Neurostimulator Lead with Paired Stimulation System in New Technology
WALLSTENT® Endoprosthesis	Intraluminal Device
X-Spine Axle Cage	Spinal Stabilization Device, Interspinous Process for Insertion in Upper Joints Spinal Stabilization Device, Interspinous Process for Insertion in Lower Joints
X-STOP® Spacer	Spinal Stabilization Device, Interspinous Process for Insertion in Upper Joints Spinal Stabilization Device, Interspinous Process for Insertion in Lower Joints
Xact Carotid Stent System	Intraluminal Device
Xenograft	Zooplastic Tissue in Heart and Great Vessels
XIENCE Everolimus Eluting Coronary Stent System	Intraluminal Device, Drug-eluting in Heart and Great Vessels
XLIF® System	Interbody Fusion Device in Lower Joints
Zenith AAA Endovascular Graft	Intraluminal Device
Zenith® Fenestrated AAA Endovascular Graft	Intraluminal Device, Branched or Fenestrated, One or Two Arteries for Restriction in Lower Arteries Intraluminal Device, Branched or Fenestrated, Three or More Arteries for Restriction in Lower Arteries
Zenith Flex® AAA Endovascular Graft	Intraluminal Device
Zenith® Renu™ AAA Ancillary Graft	Intraluminal Device
Zenith TX2® TAA Endovascular Graft	Intraluminal Device
Zilver® PTX® (paclitaxel) Drug-Eluting Peripheral Stent	Intraluminal Device, Drug-eluting in Upper Arteries Intraluminal Device, Drug-eluting in Lower Arteries
Zimmer® NexGen® LPS Mobile Bearing Knee	Synthetic Substitute
Zimmer® NexGen® LPS-Flex Mobile Knee	Synthetic Substitute
Zotarolimus-eluting coronary stent	Intraluminal Device, Drug-eluting in Heart and Great Vessels

Device Aggregation Table

This table crosswalks specific device character value definitions for specific root operations in a specific body system to the more general device character value to be used when the root operation covers a wide range of body parts and the device character represents an entire family of devices.

Specific Device	for Operation	in Body System	General Device	
Autologous Arterial Tissue (A)	All applicable	Heart and Great Vessels Lower Arteries Lower Veins Upper Arteries Upper Veins	7	Autologous Tissue Substitute
Autologous Venous Tissue (9)	All applicable	Heart and Great Vessels Lower Arteries Lower Veins Upper Arteries Upper Veins	7	Autologous Tissue Substitute
Cardiac Lead, Defibrillator (K)	Insertion	Heart and Great Vessels	M	Cardiac Lead
Cardiac Lead, Pacemaker (J)	Insertion	Heart and Great Vessels	M	Cardiac Lead
Cardiac Resynchronization Defibrillator Pulse Generator (9)	Insertion	Subcutaneous Tissue and Fascia	P	Cardiac Rhythm Related Device
Cardiac Resynchronization Pacemaker Pulse Generator (7)	Insertion	Subcutaneous Tissue and Fascia	P	Cardiac Rhythm Related Device
Contractility Modulation Device (A)	Insertion	Subcutaneous Tissue and Fascia	P	Cardiac Rhythm Related Device
Defibrillator Generator (8)	Insertion	Subcutaneous Tissue and Fascia	P	Cardiac Rhythm Related Device
Epiretinal Visual Prosthesis (5)	All applicable	Eye	J	Synthetic Substitute
External Fixation Device, Hybrid (D)	Insertion	Lower Bones Upper Bones	5	External Fixation Device
External Fixation Device, Hybrid (D)	Reposition	Lower Bones Upper Bones	5	External Fixation Device
External Fixation Device, Limb Lengthening (8)	Insertion	Lower Bones Upper Bones	5	External Fixation Device
External Fixation Device, Monoplanar (B)	Insertion	Lower Bones Upper Bones	5	External Fixation Device
External Fixation Device, Monoplanar (B)	Reposition	Lower Bones Upper Bones	5	External Fixation Device
External Fixation Device, Ring (C)	Insertion	Lower Bones Upper Bones	5	External Fixation Device
External Fixation Device, Ring (C)	Reposition	Lower Bones Upper Bones	5	External Fixation Device
Hearing Device, Bone Conduction (4)	Insertion	Ear, Nose, Sinus	S	Hearing Device
Hearing Device, Multiple Channel Cochlear Prosthesis (6)	Insertion	Ear, Nose, Sinus	S	Hearing Device
Hearing Device, Single Channel Cochlear Prosthesis (5)	Insertion	Ear, Nose, Sinus	S	Hearing Device
Internal Fixation Device, Intramedullary (6)	All applicable	Lower Bones Upper Bones	4	Internal Fixation Device
Internal Fixation Device, Intramedullary Limb Lengthening (7)	Insertion	Lower Bones Upper Bones	6	Internal Fixation Device, Intramedullary
Internal Fixation Device, Rigid Plate (Ø)	Insertion	Upper Bones	4	Internal Fixation Device
Internal Fixation Device, Rigid Plate (Ø)	Reposition	Upper Bones	4	Internal Fixation Device
Intraluminal Device, Airway (B)	All applicable	Ear, Nose, Sinus Gastrointestinal System Mouth and Throat	D	Intraluminal Device
Intraluminal Device, Bioactive (B)	All applicable	Upper Arteries	D	Intraluminal Device
Intraluminal Device, Branched or Fenestrated, One or Two Arteries (E)	Restriction	Heart and Great Vessels Lower Arteries	D	Intraluminal Device
Intraluminal Device, Branched or Fenestrated, Three or More Arteries (F)	Restriction	Heart and Great Vessels Lower Arteries	D	Intraluminal Device
Intraluminal Device, Drug-eluting (4)	All applicable	Heart and Great Vessels Lower Arteries Upper Arteries	D	Intraluminal Device
Intraluminal Device, Drug-eluting, Four or More (7)	All applicable	Heart and Great Vessels Lower Arteries Upper Arteries	D	Intraluminal Device

Specific Device	for Operation	in Body System	General Device	
Intraluminal Device, Drug-eluting, Three (6)	All applicable	Heart and Great Vessels Lower Arteries Upper Arteries	D	Intraluminal Device
Intraluminal Device, Drug-eluting, Two (5)	All applicable	Heart and Great Vessels Lower Arteries Upper Arteries	D	Intraluminal Device
Intraluminal Device, Endobronchial Valve (G)	All applicable	Respiratory System	D	Intraluminal Device
Intraluminal Device, Endotracheal Airway (E)	All applicable	Respiratory System	D	Intraluminal Device
Intraluminal Device, Flow Diverter (H)	Restriction	Upper Arteries	D	Intraluminal Device
Intraluminal Device, Four or More (G)	All applicable	Heart and Great Vessels Lower Arteries Upper Arteries	D	Intraluminal Device
Intraluminal Device, Pessary (G)	All applicable	Female Reproductive System	D	Intraluminal Device
Intraluminal Device, Radioactive (T)	All applicable	Heart and Great Vessels	D	Intraluminal Device
Intraluminal Device, Three (F)	All applicable	Heart and Great Vessels Lower Arteries Upper Arteries	D	Intraluminal Device
Intraluminal Device, Two (E)	All applicable	Heart and Great Vessels Lower Arteries Upper Arteries	D	Intraluminal Device
Monitoring Device, Hemodynamic (Ø)	Insertion	Subcutaneous Tissue and Fascia	2	Monitoring Device
Monitoring Device, Pressure Sensor (Ø)	Insertion	Heart and Great Vessels	2	Monitoring Device
Pacemaker, Dual Chamber (6)	Insertion	Subcutaneous Tissue and Fascia	P	Cardiac Rhythm Related Device
Pacemaker, Single Chamber (4)	Insertion	Subcutaneous Tissue and Fascia	P	Cardiac Rhythm Related Device
Pacemaker, Single Chamber Rate Responsive (5)	Insertion	Subcutaneous Tissue and Fascia	P	Cardiac Rhythm Related Device
Spinal Stabilization Device, Facet Replacement (D)	Insertion	Lower Joints Upper Joints	4	Internal Fixation Device
Spinal Stabilization Device, Interspinous Process (B)	Insertion	Lower Joints Upper Joints	4	Internal Fixation Device
Spinal Stabilization Device, Pedicle-Based (C)	Insertion	Lower Joints Upper Joints	4	Internal Fixation Device
Spinal Stabilization Device, Vertebral Body Tether (3)	Reposition	Lower Bones Upper Bones	4	Internal Fixation Device
Stimulator Generator, Multiple Array (D)	Insertion	Subcutaneous Tissue and Fascia	M	Stimulator Generator
Stimulator Generator, Multiple Array Rechargeable (E)	Insertion	Subcutaneous Tissue and Fascia	M	Stimulator Generator
Stimulator Generator, Single Array (B)	Insertion	Subcutaneous Tissue and Fascia	M	Stimulator Generator
Stimulator Generator, Single Array Rechargeable (C)	Insertion	Subcutaneous Tissue and Fascia	M	Stimulator Generator
Synthetic Substitute, Ceramic (3)	Replacement	Lower Joints	J	Synthetic Substitute
Synthetic Substitute, Ceramic on Polyethylene (4)	Replacement	Lower Joints	J	Synthetic Substitute
Synthetic Substitute, Intraocular Telescope (Ø)	Replacement	Eye	J	Synthetic Substitute
Synthetic Substitute, Metal (1)	Replacement	Lower Joints	J	Synthetic Substitute
Synthetic Substitute, Metal on Polyethylene (2)	Replacement	Lower Joints	J	Synthetic Substitute
Synthetic Substitute, Oxidized Zirconium on Polyethylene (6)	Replacement	Lower Joints	J	Synthetic Substitute
Synthetic Substitute, Polyethylene (Ø)	Replacement	Lower Joints	J	Synthetic Substitute
Synthetic Substitute, Reverse Ball and Socket (Ø)	Replacement	Upper Joints	J	Synthetic Substitute

Appendix H: Device Definitions

This **NT** symbol next to a device in the Definition column identifies that the device has been approved for NTAP (new technology add-on payment). CMS provides incremental payment, in addition to the DRG payment, for technologies that have received an NTAP designation.

ICD-10-PCS Value	Definition
Articulating Spacer in Lower Joints	**Includes:** Articulating Spacer (Antibiotic) Spacer, Articulating (Antibiotic)
Artificial Sphincter in Gastrointestinal System	**Includes:** Artificial anal sphincter (AAS) Artificial bowel sphincter (neosphincter)
Artificial Sphincter in Urinary System	**Includes:** AMS 800® Urinary Control System Artificial urinary sphincter (AUS)
Autologous Arterial Tissue in Heart and Great Vessels	**Includes:** Autologous artery graft
Autologous Arterial Tissue in Lower Arteries	**Includes:** Autologous artery graft
Autologous Arterial Tissue in Lower Veins	**Includes:** Autologous artery graft
Autologous Arterial Tissue in Upper Arteries	**Includes:** Autologous artery graft
Autologous Arterial Tissue in Upper Veins	**Includes:** Autologous artery graft
Autologous Tissue Substitute	**Includes:** Autograft Cultured epidermal cell autograft Epicel® cultured epidermal autograft
Autologous Venous Tissue in Heart and Great Vessels	**Includes:** Autologous vein graft
Autologous Venous Tissue in Lower Arteries	**Includes:** Autologous vein graft
Autologous Venous Tissue in Lower Veins	**Includes:** Autologous vein graft
Autologous Venous Tissue in Upper Arteries	**Includes:** Autologous vein graft
Autologous Venous Tissue in Upper Veins	**Includes:** Autologous vein graft
Biologic with Synthetic Substitute, Autoregulated Electrohydraulic for Replacement in Heart and Great Vessels	**Includes:** Carmat total artificial heart (TAH)
Bone Growth Stimulator in Head and Facial Bones	**Includes:** Electrical bone growth stimulator (EBGS) Ultrasonic osteogenic stimulator Ultrasound bone healing system
Bone Growth Stimulator in Lower Bones	**Includes:** Electrical bone growth stimulator (EBGS) Ultrasonic osteogenic stimulator Ultrasound bone healing system
Bone Growth Stimulator in Upper Bones	**Includes:** Electrical bone growth stimulator (EBGS) Ultrasonic osteogenic stimulator Ultrasound bone healing system
Branched Synthetic Substitute with Intraluminal Device in New Technology	**Includes:** Thoraflex™ Hybrid device
Cardiac Lead in Heart and Great Vessels	**Includes:** Cardiac contractility modulation lead

ICD-10-PCS Value	Definition
Cardiac Lead, Defibrillator for Insertion in Heart and Great Vessels	**Includes:** ACUITY™ Steerable Lead Attain Ability® lead Attain StarFix® (OTW) lead Cardiac resynchronization therapy (CRT) lead Corox (OTW) Bipolar Lead Durata® Defibrillation Lead ENDOTAK RELIANCE® (G) Defibrillation Lead
Cardiac Lead, Pacemaker for Insertion in Heart and Great Vessels	**Includes:** ACUITY™ Steerable Lead Attain Ability® lead Attain StarFix® (OTW) lead Cardiac resynchronization therapy (CRT) lead Corox (OTW) Bipolar Lead
Cardiac Resynchronization Defibrillator Pulse Generator for Insertion in Subcutaneous Tissue and Fascia	**Includes:** COGNIS® CRT-D Concerto II CRT-D Consulta CRT-D CONTAK RENEWA® 3 RF (HE) CRT-D LIVIAN™ CRT-D Maximo II DR CRT-D Ovatio™ CRT-D Protecta XT CRT-D Viva (XT)(S)
Cardiac Resynchronization Pacemaker Pulse Generator for Insertion in Subcutaneous Tissue and Fascia	**Includes:** Consulta CRT-P Stratos LV Synchra CRT-P
Contraceptive Device in Female Reproductive System	**Includes:** Intrauterine device (IUD)
Contraceptive Device in Subcutaneous Tissue and Fascia	**Includes:** Subdermal progesterone implant
Contractility Modulation Device for Insertion in Subcutaneous Tissue and Fascia	**Includes:** Optimizer™ III implantable pulse generator
Defibrillator Generator for Insertion in Subcutaneous Tissue and Fascia	**Includes:** Evera (XT)(S)(DR/VR) Implantable cardioverter-defibrillator (ICD) Maximo II DR (VR) Protecta XT DR (XT VR) Secura (DR) (VR) Virtuoso (II) (DR) (VR)
Diaphragmatic Pacemaker Lead in Respiratory System	**Includes:** Phrenic nerve stimulator lead
Drainage Device	**Includes:** Cystostomy tube Foley catheter Percutaneous nephrostomy catheter Thoracostomy tube
External Fixation Device in Head and Facial Bones	**Includes:** External fixator

ICD-10-PCS Value	Definition
External Fixation Device in Lower Bones	**Includes:** External fixator
External Fixation Device in Lower Joints	**Includes:** External fixator
External Fixation Device in Upper Bones	**Includes:** External fixator
External Fixation Device in Upper Joints	**Includes:** External fixator
External Fixation Device, Hybrid for Insertion in Lower Bones	**Includes:** Delta frame external fixator Sheffield hybrid external fixator
External Fixation Device, Hybrid for Insertion in Upper Bones	**Includes:** Delta frame external fixator Sheffield hybrid external fixator
External Fixation Device, Hybrid for Reposition in Lower Bones	**Includes:** Delta frame external fixator Sheffield hybrid external fixator
External Fixation Device, Hybrid for Reposition in Upper Bones	**Includes:** Delta frame external fixator Sheffield hybrid external fixator
External Fixation Device, Limb Lengthening for Insertion in Lower Bones	**Includes:** Ilizarov-Vecklich device
External Fixation Device, Limb Lengthening for Insertion in Upper Bones	**Includes:** Ilizarov-Vecklich device
External Fixation Device, Monoplanar for Insertion in Lower Bones	**Includes:** Uniplanar external fixator
External Fixation Device, Monoplanar for Insertion in Upper Bones	**Includes:** Uniplanar external fixator
External Fixation Device, Monoplanar for Reposition in Lower Bones	**Includes:** Uniplanar external fixator
External Fixation Device, Monoplanar for Reposition in Upper Bones	**Includes:** Uniplanar external fixator
External Fixation Device, Ring for Insertion in Lower Bones	**Includes:** Ilizarov external fixator Sheffield ring external fixator
External Fixation Device, Ring for Insertion in Upper Bones	**Includes:** Ilizarov external fixator Sheffield ring external fixator
External Fixation Device, Ring for Reposition in Lower Bones	**Includes:** Ilizarov external fixator Sheffield ring external fixator
External Fixation Device, Ring for Reposition in Upper Bones	**Includes:** Ilizarov external fixator Sheffield ring external fixator
Extraluminal Device	**Includes:** AtriClip LAA Exclusion System LAP-BAND® adjustable gastric banding system REALIZE® Adjustable Gastric Band
Feeding Device in Gastrointestinal System	**Includes:** Percutaneous endoscopic gastrojejunostomy (PEG/J) tube Percutaneous endoscopic gastrostomy (PEG) tube
Hearing Device in Ear, Nose, Sinus	**Includes:** Esteem® implantable hearing system
Hearing Device in Head and Facial Bones	**Includes:** Bone anchored hearing device

ICD-10-PCS Value	Definition
Hearing Device, Bone Conduction for Insertion in Ear, Nose, Sinus	**Includes:** Bone anchored hearing device
Hearing Device, Multiple Channel Cochlear Prosthesis for Insertion in Ear, Nose, Sinus	**Includes:** Cochlear implant (CI), multiple channel (electrode)
Hearing Device, Single Channel Cochlear Prosthesis for Insertion in Ear, Nose, Sinus	**Includes:** Cochlear implant (CI), single channel (electrode)
Implantable Heart Assist System in Heart and Great Vessels	**Includes:** Berlin Heart Ventricular Assist Device DeBakey Left Ventricular Assist Device DuraHeart Left Ventricular Assist System HeartMate 3™ LVAS HeartMate II® Left Ventricular Assist Device (LVAD) HeartMate XVE® Left Ventricular Assist Device (LVAD) MicroMed HeartAssist Novacor Left Ventricular Assist Device Thoratec IVAD (Implantable Ventricular Assist Device)
Infusion Device	**Includes:** Ascenda Intrathecal Catheter InDura, intrathecal catheter (1P) (spinal) Non-tunneled central venous catheter Peripherally inserted central catheter (PICC) Tunneled spinal (intrathecal) catheter
Infusion Device, Pump in Subcutaneous Tissue and Fascia	**Includes:** Implantable drug infusion pump (anti-spasmodic)(chemotherapy) (pain) Injection reservoir, pump Pump reservoir Subcutaneous injection reservoir, pump SynchroMed pump
Interbody Fusion Device, Customizable in New Technology	**Includes:** aprevo™
Interbody Fusion Device in Lower Joints	**Includes:** Axial Lumbar Interbody Fusion System AxiaLIF® System COALESCE® radiolucent interbody fusion device COHERE® radiolucent interbody fusion device CoRoent® XL Direct Lateral Interbody Fusion (DLIF) device EXtreme Lateral Interbody Fusion (XLIF) device Interbody fusion (spine) cage nanoLOCK™ interbody fusion device Titan Endoskeleton™ XLIF® System
Interbody Fusion Device in Upper Joints	**Includes:** BAK/C® Interbody Cervical Fusion System COALESCE® radiolucent interbody fusion device COHERE® radiolucent interbody fusion device Interbody fusion (spine) cage nanoLOCK™ interbody fusion device Titan Endoskeleton™

ICD-10-PCS Value	Definition
Internal Fixation Device in Head and Facial Bones	**Includes:** Bone screw (interlocking)(lag)(pedicle) (recessed) Kirschner wire (K-wire) Neutralization plate
Internal Fixation Device in Lower Bones	**Includes:** Bone screw (interlocking)(lag)(pedicle) (recessed) Clamp and rod internal fixation system (CRIF) Kirschner wire (K-wire) Neutralization plate
Internal Fixation Device in Lower Joints	**Includes:** Fusion screw (compression)(lag)(locking) Joint fixation plate Kirschner wire (K-wire)
Internal Fixation Device in Upper Bones	**Includes:** Bone screw (interlocking)(lag)(pedicle) (recessed) Clamp and rod internal fixation system (CRIF) Kirschner wire (K-wire) Neutralization plate
Internal Fixation Device in Upper Joints	**Includes:** Fusion screw (compression)(lag)(locking) Joint fixation plate Kirschner wire (K-wire)
Internal Fixation Device, Intramedullary in Lower Bones	**Includes:** Intramedullary (IM) rod (nail) Intramedullary skeletal kinetic distractor (ISKD) Kuntscher nail
Internal Fixation Device, Intramedullary in Upper Bones	**Includes:** Intramedullary (IM) rod (nail) Intramedullary skeletal kinetic distractor (ISKD) Kuntscher nail
Internal Fixation Device Intramedullary Limb Lengthening for Insertion in Lower Bones	**Includes:** PRECICE intramedullary limb lengthening system
Internal Fixation Device Intramedullary Limb Lengthening for Insertion in Upper Bones	**Includes:** PRECICE intramedullary limb lengthening system
Internal Fixation Device, Rigid Plate for Insertion in Upper Bones	**Includes:** Titanium Sternal Fixation System (TSFS)
Internal Fixation Device, Rigid Plate for Reposition in Upper Bones	**Includes:** Titanium Sternal Fixation System (TSFS)
Internal Fixation Device, Sustained Compression for Fusion in Lower Joints	**Includes:** DynaClip® (Forte) DynaNail® (Hybrid) (Mini)
Internal Fixation Device, Sustained Compression for Fusion in Upper Joints	**Includes:** DynaClip® (Forte) DynaNail® (Hybrid) (Mini)
Internal Fixation Device with Tulip Connector in New Technology	**Includes:** iFuse Bedrock™ Granite Implant System

ICD-10-PCS Value	Definition
Intraluminal Device	**Includes:** Absolute Pro Vascular (OTW) Self-Expanding Stent System Acculink (RX) Carotid Stent System AFX® Endovascular AAA System AneuRx® AAA Advantage® Assurant (Cobalt) stent Carotid WALLSTENT® Monorail® Endoprosthesis CoAxia NeuroFlo catheter Colonic Z-Stent® Complete (SE) stent Cook Zenith AAA Endovascular Graft Driver stent (RX) (OTW) E-Luminexx™ (Biliary)(Vascular) Stent Embolization coil(s) Endologix AFX® Endovascular AAA System Endurant® Endovascular Stent Graft Endurant® II AAA stent graft system EXCLUDER® AAA Endoprosthesis Express® (LD) Premounted Stent System Express® Biliary SD Monorail® Premounted Stent System Express® SD Renal Monorail® Premounted Stent System FLAIR® Endovascular Stent Graft Formula™ Balloon-Expandable Renal Stent System GORE EXCLUDER® AAA Endoprosthesis GORE TAG® Thoracic Endoprosthesis Herculink (RX) Elite Renal Stent System LifeStent® (Flexstar)(XL) Vascular Stent System Medtronic Endurant® II AAA stent graft system Micro-Driver stent (RX) (OTW) MULTI-LINK (VISION)(MINI-VISION)(ULTRA) Coronary Stent System Omnilink Elite Vascular Balloon Expandable Stent System Protege® RX Carotid Stent System Stent, intraluminal (cardiovascular) (gastrointestinal)(hepatobiliary) (urinary) Talent® Converter Talent® Occluder Talent® Stent Graft (abdominal)(thoracic) Therapeutic occlusion coil(s) Ultraflex™ Precision Colonic Stent System Valiant Thoracic Stent Graft WALLSTENT® Endoprosthesis Xact Carotid Stent System Zenith AAA Endovascular Graft Zenith Flex® AAA Endovascular Graft Zenith TX2® TAA Endovascular Graft Zenith® Renu™ AAA Ancillary Graft
Intraluminal Device, Airway in Ear, Nose, Sinus	**Includes:** Nasopharyngeal airway (NPA)
Intraluminal Device, Airway in Gastrointestinal System	**Includes:** Esophageal obturator airway (EOA)
Intraluminal Device, Airway in Mouth and Throat	**Includes:** Guedel airway Oropharyngeal airway (OPA)
Intraluminal Device, Bioactive in Upper Arteries	**Includes:** Bioactive embolization coil(s) Micrus CERECYTE microcoil

ICD-10-PCS Value	Definition
Intraluminal Device, Branched or Fenestrated, One or Two Arteries for Restriction in Lower Arteries	**Includes:** Cook Zenith® Fenestrated AAA Endovascular Graft EXCLUDER® AAA Endoprosthesis EXCLUDER® IBE Endoprosthesis GORE EXCLUDER® AAA Endoprosthesis GORE EXCLUDER®IBE Endoprosthesis Zenith® Fenestrated AAA Endovascular Graft
Intraluminal Device, Branched or Fenestrated, Three or More Arteries for Restriction in Lower Arteries	**Includes:** Cook Zenith® Fenestrated AAA Endovascular Graft EXCLUDER® AAA Endoprosthesis GORE EXCLUDER® AAA Endoprosthesis Zenith® Fenestrated AAA Endovascular Graft
Intraluminal Device, Drug-eluting in Heart and Great Vessels	**Includes:** CYPHER® Stent Endeavor® (III)(IV) (Sprint) Zotarolimus-eluting Coronary Stent System Everolimus-eluting coronary stent Paclitaxel-eluting coronary stent Sirolimus-eluting coronary stent TAXUS® Liberte® Paclitaxel-eluting Coronary Stent System XIENCE Everolimus Eluting Coronary Stent System Zotarolimus-eluting coronary stent
Intraluminal Device, Drug-eluting in Lower Arteries	**Includes:** Paclitaxel-eluting peripheral stent Zilver® PTX® (paclitaxel) Drug-Eluting Peripheral Stent
Intraluminal Device, Drug-eluting in Upper Arteries	**Includes:** Paclitaxel-eluting peripheral stent Zilver® PTX® (paclitaxel) Drug-Eluting Peripheral Stent
Intraluminal Device, Endobronchial Valve in Respiratory System	**Includes:** Spiration IBV™ Valve System
Intraluminal Device, Endotracheal Airway in Respiratory System	**Includes:** Endotracheal tube (cuffed)(double-lumen)
Intraluminal Device, Flow Diverter for Restriction in Upper Arteries	**Includes:** Flow Diverter embolization device Pipeline™ (Flex) embolization device Surpass Streamline™ Flow Diverter
Intraluminal Device, Pessary in Female Reproductive System	**Includes:** Pessary ring Vaginal pessary
Intraluminal Device, Sustained Release Drug-eluting in New Technology	**Includes:** Eluvia™ Drug-eluting Vascular Stent System SAVAL below-the-knee (BTK) drug-eluting stent system
Intraluminal Device, Sustained Release Drug-eluting, Four or More in New Technology	**Includes:** Eluvia™ Drug-eluting Vascular Stent System SAVAL below-the-knee (BTK) drug-eluting stent system
Intraluminal Device, Sustained Release Drug-eluting, Three in New Technology	**Includes:** Eluvia™ Drug-eluting Vascular Stent System SAVAL below-the-knee (BTK) drug-eluting stent system

ICD-10-PCS Value	Definition
Intraluminal Device, Sustained Release Drug-eluting, Two in New Technology	**Includes:** Eluvia™ Drug-eluting Vascular Stent System SAVAL below-the-knee (BTK) drug-eluting stent system
Liner in Lower Joints	**Includes:** Acetabular cup Hip (joint) liner Joint liner (insert) Knee (implant) insert Tibial insert
Magnetically Controlled Growth Rod(s) in New Technology	**Includes:** MAGEC® Spinal Bracing and Distraction System Spinal growth rods, magnetically controlled
Monitoring Device	**Includes:** Blood glucose monitoring system Cardiac event recorder Continuous Glucose Monitoring (CGM) device Implantable glucose monitoring device Loop recorder, implantable Reveal (LINQ)(DX)(XT)
Monitoring Device, Hemodynamic for Insertion in Subcutaneous Tissue and Fascia	**Includes:** Implantable hemodynamic monitor (IHM) Implantable hemodynamic monitoring system (IHMS)
Monitoring Device, Pressure Sensor for Insertion in Heart and Great Vessels	**Includes:** CardioMEMS® pressure sensor EndoSure® sensor
Neurostimulator Generator in Head and Facial Bones	**Includes:** RNS system neurostimulator generator
Neurostimulator Lead in Central Nervous System and Cranial Nerves	**Includes:** Cortical strip neurostimulator lead DBS lead Deep brain neurostimulator lead RNS System lead Spinal cord neurostimulator lead
Neurostimulator Lead in Peripheral Nervous System	**Includes:** InterStim® Therapy lead
Neurostimulator Lead in New Technology	Ischemic Stroke System (ISS500) ISS500 (Ischemic Stroke System)
Neurostimulator Lead with Paired Stimulation System in New Technology	**Includes:** Vivistim® Paired VNS System Lead
Nonautologous Tissue Substitute	**Includes:** Acellular Hydrated Dermis Bone bank bone graft Cook Biodesign® Fistula Plug(s) Cook Biodesign® Hernia Graft(s) Cook Biodesign® Layered Graft(s) Cook Zenapro™ Layered Graft(s) MIRODERM™ Biologic Wound Matrix Tissue bank graft
Other Device	**Includes:** Alfapump® system
Pacemaker, Dual Chamber for Insertion in Subcutaneous Tissue and Fascia	**Includes:** Advisa (MRI) EnRhythm Kappa Revo MRI™ SureScan® pacemaker Two lead pacemaker Versa

Appendix H: Device Definitions

ICD-10-PCS Value	Definition
Pacemaker, Single Chamber for Insertion in Subcutaneous Tissue and Fascia	Includes: Single lead pacemaker (atrium)(ventricle)
Pacemaker, Single Chamber Rate Responsive for Insertion in Subcutaneous Tissue and Fascia	Includes: Single lead rate responsive pacemaker (atrium)(ventricle)
Posterior (Dynamic) Distraction Device in New Technology	Includes: ApiFix® Minimally Invasive Deformity Correction (MID-C) System
Posterior Spinal Motion Preservation Device in New Technology	Includes: TOPS™ System
Posterior Vertebral Tether in New Technology	Includes: LigaPASS 2.0™ PJK Prevention System
Radioactive Element	Includes: Brachytherapy seeds CivaSheet®
Radioactive Element, Cesium-131 Collagen Implant for Insertion in Central Nervous System and Cranial Nerves	Includes: Cesium-131 Collagen Implant GammaTile™
Reduction Device in New Technology	Includes: Neovasc Reducer™ Reducer™ System
Resurfacing Device in Lower Joints	Includes: CONSERVE® PLUS Total Resurfacing Hip System Cormet Hip Resurfacing System
Short-term External Heart Assist System in Heart and Great Vessels	Includes: Biventricular external heart assist system BVS 5000 Ventricular Assist Device Centrimag® Blood Pump Impella® heart pump TandemHeart® System Thoratec Paracorporeal Ventricular Assist Device
Spacer in Lower Joints	Includes: Joint spacer (antibiotic) Spacer, Static (Antibiotic) Static Spacer (Antibiotic)
Spacer in Upper Joints	Includes: Joint spacer (antibiotic)
Spinal Stabilization Device, Facet Replacement for Insertion in Lower Joints	Includes: Facet replacement spinal stabilization device
Spinal Stabilization Device, Facet Replacement for Insertion in Upper Joints	Includes: Facet replacement spinal stabilization device
Spinal Stabilization Device, Interspinous Process for Insertion in Lower Joints	Includes: Interspinous process spinal stabilization device X-Spine Axle Cage X-STOP® Spacer
Spinal Stabilization Device, Interspinous Process for Insertion in Upper Joints	Includes: Interspinous process spinal stabilization device X-Spine Axle Cage X-STOP® Spacer

ICD-10-PCS Value	Definition
Spinal Stabilization Device, Pedicle- Based for Insertion in Lower Joints	Includes: Dynesys® Dynamic Stabilization System Pedicle-based dynamic stabilization device
Spinal Stabilization Device, Pedicle-Based for Insertion in Upper Joints	Includes: Dynesys® Dynamic Stabilization System Pedicle-based dynamic stabilization device
Stimulator Generator in Subcutaneous Tissue and Fascia	Includes: Baroreflex Activation Therapy® (BAT®) Diaphragmatic pacemaker generator Mark IV Breathing Pacemaker System Phrenic nerve stimulator generator Rheos® System device
Stimulator Generator, Multiple Array for Insertion in Subcutaneous Tissue and Fascia	Includes: Activa PC neurostimulator Enterra gastric neurostimulator Neurostimulator generator, multiple channel PERCEPT™ PC neurostimulator PrimeAdvanced neurostimulator (SureScan)(MRI Safe)
Stimulator Generator, Multiple Array Rechargeable for Insertion in Subcutaneous Tissue and Fascia	Includes: Activa RC neurostimulator Neurostimulator generator, multiple channel rechargeable RestoreAdvanced neurostimulator (SureScan)(MRI Safe) RestoreSensor neurostimulator (SureScan)(MRI Safe) RestoreUltra neurostimulator (SureScan)(MRI Safe)
Stimulator Generator, Single Array for Insertion in Subcutaneous Tissue and Fascia	Includes: Activa SC neurostimulator InterStim™ II Therapy neurostimulator Itrel (3)(4) neurostimulator Neurostimulator generator, single channel
Stimulator Generator, Single Array Rechargeable for Insertion in Subcutaneous Tissue and Fascia	Includes: InterStim™ Micro Therapy neurostimulator Neurostimulator generator, single channel rechargeable
Stimulator Lead in Gastrointestinal System	Includes: Gastric electrical stimulation (GES) lead Gastric pacemaker lead
Stimulator Lead in Muscles	Includes: Electrical muscle stimulation (EMS) lead Electronic muscle stimulator lead Neuromuscular electrical stimulation (NEMS) lead
Stimulator Lead in Upper Arteries	Includes: Baroreflex Activation Therapy® (BAT®) Carotid (artery) sinus (baroreceptor) lead Rheos® System lead
Stimulator Lead in Urinary System	Includes: Sacral nerve modulation (SNM) lead Sacral neuromodulation lead Urinary incontinence stimulator lead
Subcutaneous Defibrillator Lead in Subcutaneous Tissue and Fascia	Includes: S-ICD™ lead

ICD-10-PCS Value	Definition
Synthetic Substitute	**Includes:** AbioCor® Total Replacement Heart AMPLATZER® Muscular VSD Occluder Annuloplasty ring Bard® Composix® (E/X) (LP) mesh Bard® Composix® Kugel® patch Bard® Dulex™ mesh Bard® Ventralex™ hernia patch Barricaid® Annular Closure Device (ACD) BRYAN® Cervical Disc System Corvia IASD® Ex-PRESS™ mini glaucoma shunt Flexible Composite Mesh GORE® DUALMESH® Holter valve ventricular shunt IASD® (InterAtrial Shunt Device), Corvia InterAtrial Shunt Device IASD®, Corvia MitraClip valve repair system Nitinol framed polymer mesh Open Pivot (mechanical) valve Open Pivot Aortic Valve Graft (AVG) Partially absorbable mesh PHYSIOMESH™ Flexible Composite Mesh Polymethylmethacrylate (PMMA) Polypropylene mesh PRESTIGE® Cervical Disc PROCEED™ Ventral Patch Prodisc-C Prodisc-L PROLENE Polypropylene Hernia System (PHS) Rebound HRD® (Hernia Repair Device) SynCardia Total Artificial Heart Total artificial (replacement) heart ULTRAPRO Hernia System (UHS) ULTRAPRO Partially Absorbable Lightweight Mesh ULTRAPRO Plug V-Wave Interatrial Shunt System Ventrio™ Hernia Patch Zimmer® NexGen® LPS Mobile Bearing Knee Zimmer® NexGen® LPS-Flex Mobile Knee
Synthetic Substitute, Ceramic for Replacement in Lower Joints	**Includes:** Ceramic on ceramic bearing surface Novation® Ceramic AHS® (Articulation Hip System)
Synthetic Substitute, Intraocular Telescope for Replacement in Eye	**Includes:** Implantable Miniature Telescope™ (IMT)
Synthetic Substitute, Lateral Meniscus in New Technology	**Includes:** NUsurface® Meniscus Implant
Synthetic Substitute, Mechanically Expandable (Paired) in New Technology	**Includes:** SpineJack® system
Synthetic Substitute, Medial Meniscus in New Technology	**Includes:** NUsurface® Meniscus Implant
Synthetic Substitute, Metal for Replacement in Lower Joints	**Includes:** Cobalt/chromium head and socket Metal on metal bearing surface
Synthetic Substitute, Metal on Polyethylene for Replacement in Lower Joints	**Includes:** Cobalt/chromium head and polyethylene socket

ICD-10-PCS Value	Definition
Synthetic Substitute, Oxidized Zirconium on Polyethylene for Replacement in Lower Joints	**Includes:** OXINIUM
Synthetic Substitute, Pneumatic for Replacement in Heart and Great Vessels	**Includes:** SynCardia (temporary) total artificial heart (TAH)
Synthetic Substitute, Polyethylene for Replacement in Lower Joints	**Includes:** Polyethylene socket
Synthetic Substitute, Reverse Ball and Socket for Replacement in Upper Joints	**Includes:** Delta III Reverse shoulder prosthesis Reverse® Shoulder Prosthesis
Tissue Expander in Skin and Breast	**Includes:** Tissue expander (inflatable) (injectable)
Tissue Expander in Subcutaneous Tissue and Fascia	**Includes:** Tissue expander (inflatable) (injectable)
Tracheostomy Device in Respiratory System	**Includes:** Tracheostomy tube
Vascular Access Device, Totally Implantable in Subcutaneous Tissue and Fascia	**Includes:** Implanted (venous)(access) port Injection reservoir, port Subcutaneous injection reservoir, port
Vascular Access Device, Tunneled in Subcutaneous Tissue and Fascia	**Includes:** Tunneled central venous catheter Vectra® Vascular Access Graft
Zooplastic Tissue in Heart and Great Vessels	**Includes:** 3f (Aortic) Bioprosthesis valve Bovine pericardial valve Bovine pericardium graft Contegra Pulmonary Valved Conduit CoreValve transcatheter aortic valve Epic™ Stented Tissue Valve (aortic) Freestyle (Stentless) Aortic Root Bioprosthesis Hancock Bioprosthesis (aortic) (mitral) valve Hancock Bioprosthetic Valved Conduit Melody® transcatheter pulmonary valve Mitroflow® Aortic Pericardial Heart Valve Mosaic Bioprosthesis (aortic) (mitral) valve Porcine (bioprosthetic) valve SAPIEN transcatheter aortic valve SJM Biocor® Stented Valve System Stented tissue valve Trifecta™ Valve (aortic) Xenograft

Appendix I: Substance Key/Substance Definitions

Substance Key

This table crosswalks a specific substance, listed by trade name or synonym, to the PCS value that would be used to represent that substance in either the Administration or New Technology section. The ICD-10-PCS value may be located in either the 6th-character Substance column or the 7th-character Qualifier column depending on the section/table to which it is classified. The most specific character is listed in the table.

This **NT** symbol next to a substance/technology in the Trade Name or Synonym column identifies that the substance/technology has been approved for NTAP (new technology add-on payment). CMS provides incremental payment, in addition to the DRG payment, for technologies that have received an NTAP designation.

Substances denoted by an asterisk (*) in the Trade Name or Synonym column, although not included in the official ICD-10-PCS classification, were added based on information provided in the FY 2023 IPPS proposed rule.

Trade Name or Synonym	ICD-10-PCS Value	PCS Section
ABECMA® **NT**	Idecabtagene Vicleucel Immunotherapy (K)	New Technology (X)
ACTEMRA®	Tocilizumab (H)	New Technology (X)
afami-cel	Afamitresgene Autoleucel Immunotherapy (6)	New Technology (X)
AIGISRx Antibacterial Envelope	Anti-Infective Envelope (A)	Administration (3)
Andexanet Alfa, Factor Xa Inhibitor Reversal Agent	Coagulation Factor Xa, Inactivated (7)	New Technology (X)
Andexxa	Coagulation Factor Xa, Inactivated (7)	New Technology (X)
Angiotensin II	Synthetic Human Angiotensin II (H)	New Technology (X)
Antibacterial Envelope (TYRX) (AIGISRx)	Anti-Infective Envelope (A)	Administration (3)
Antimicrobial envelope	Anti-Infective Envelope (A)	Administration (3)
Anti-SARS-CoV-2 hyperimmune globulin	Hyperimmune Globulin (E)	New Technology (X)
AVYCAZ® (ceftazidime-avibactam)	Other Anti-infective (9)	Administration (3)
Axicabtagene Ciloleucel	Axicabtagene Ciloleucel Immunotherapy (H)	New Technology (X)
AZEDRA®	Iobenguane I-131 Antineoplastic (S)	New Technology (X)
*Balversa™	Erdafitinib Antineoplastic (L)	New Technology (X)
beti-cel	Betibeglogene Autotemcel (B)	New Technology (X)
Blinatumomab	Other Antineoplastic (5)	Administration (3)
BLINCYTO® (blinatumomab)	Other Antineoplastic (5)	Administration (3)
Bone morphogenetic protein 2 (BMP 2)	Recombinant Bone Morphogenetic Protein (B)	Administration (3)
Brexucabtagene Autoleucel	Brexucabtagene Autoleucel Immunotherapy (4)	New Technology (X)
Breyanzi®	Lisocabtagene Maraleucel Immunotherapy (N)	New Technology (X)
*CABLIVI®	Caplacizumab (W)	New Technology (X)
CARVYKTI™	Ciltacabtagene Autoleucel (A)	New Technology (X)
Casirivimab (REGN10933) and Imdevimab (REGN10987)	REGN-COV2 Monoclonal Antibody (G)	New Technology (X)
CBMA (Concentrated Bone Marrow Aspirate)	Other Substance (C)	Administration (3)
Ceftazidime-avibactam	Other Anti-infective (9)	Administration (3)
CERAMENT® G	Antibiotic-eluting Bone Void Filler (P)	New Technology (X)
cilta-cel	Ciltacabtagene Autoleucel (A)	New Technology (X)
Clolar	Clofarabine (P)	Administration (3)
Coagulation Factor Xa, (Recombinant) Inactivated	Coagulation Factor Xa, Inactivated (7)	New Technology (X)
CONTEPO™	Fosfomycin Anti-infective (K)	New Technology (X)
COSELA™ **NT**	Trilaciclib (7)	New Technology (X)
CRESEMBA® (isavuconazonium sulfate)	Other Anti-infective (9)	Administration (3)
Darzalex Faspro®	Daratumumab and Hyaluronidase-fihj (1)	New Technology (X)
DefenCath™	Taurolidine Anti-infective and Heparin Anticoagulant (2)	New Technology (X)
Defitelio	Other Substance (C)	Administration (3)
DuraGraft® Endothelial Damage Inhibitor	Endothelial Damage Inhibitor (8)	New Technology (X)
ELZONRIS™	Tagraxofusp-erzs Antineoplastic (Q)	New Technology (X)
ENSPRYNG™	Satralizumab-mwge (9)	New Technology (X)
ERLEADA™	Apalutamide Antineoplastic (J)	New Technology (X)
EVUSHELD™	Tixagevimab and Cilgavimab Monoclonal Antibody (X)	New Technology (X)
Factor Xa Inhibitor Reversal Agent, Andexanet Alfa	Coagulation Factor Xa, Inactivated (7)	New Technology (X)
FETROJA® **NT**	Cefiderocol Anti-infective (A)	New Technology (X)
Fosfomycin injection	Fosfomycin Anti-infective (K)	New Technology (X)
Gammaglobulin	Globulin (S)	Administration (3)

Trade Name or Synonym	ICD-10-PCS Value	PCS Section
GAMUNEX-C, for COVID-19 treatment	High-Dose Intravenous Immune Globulin (D)	New Technology (X)
GIAPREZA™	Synthetic Human Angiotensin II (H)	New Technology (X)
GS-5734	Remdesivir Anti-infective (E)	New Technology (X)
hdIVIG (high-dose intravenous immunoglobulin), for COVID-19 treatment	High-Dose Intravenous Immune Globulin (D)	New Technology (X)
Hemospray® Endoscopic Hemostat	Mineral-based Topical Hemostatic Agent (8)	New Technology (X)
HIG (hyperimmune globulin), for COVID-19 treatment	Hyperimmune Globulin (E)	New Technology (X)
High-dose intravenous immunoglobulin (hdIVIG), for COVID-19 treatment	High-Dose Intravenous Immune Globulin (D)	New Technology (X)
hIVIG (hyperimmune intravenous immunoglobulin), for COVID-19 treatment	Hyperimmune Globulin (E)	New Technology (X)
Human angiotensin II, synthetic	Synthetic Human Angiotensin II (H)	New Technology (X)
Hyperimmune globulin	Globulin (S)	Administration (3)
Hyperimmune intravenous immunoglobulin (hIVIG), for COVID-19 treatment	Hyperimmune Globulin (E)	New Technology (X)
Idarucizumab, Pradaxa® (dabigatran) reversal agent	Other Therapeutic Substance (G)	Administration (3)
Idecabtagene Vicleucel	Idecabtagene Vicleucel Immunotherapy (K)	New Technology (X)
Ide-cel	Idecabtagene Vicleucel Immunotherapy (K)	New Technology (X)
IGIV-C, for COVID-19 treatment	Hyperimmune Globulin (E)	New Technology (X)
Imdevimab (REGN10987) and Casirivimab (REGN10933)	REGN-COV2 Monoclonal Antibody (G)	New Technology (X)
IMFINZI®	Durvalumab Antineoplastic (3)	New Technology (X)
IMI/REL	Imipenem-cilastatin-relebactam Anti-infective (U)	New Technology (X)
Immunoglobulin	Globulin (S)	Administration (3)
INTERCEPT Blood System for Plasma Pathogen Reduced Cryoprecipitated Fibrinogen Complex [NT]	Pathogen Reduced Cryoprecipitated Fibrinogen Complex (D)	Administration (3)
INTERCEPT Fibrinogen Complex [NT]	Pathogen Reduced Cryoprecipitated Fibrinogen Complex (D)	Administration (3)
Iobenguane I-131, High Specific Activity (HSA)	Iobenguane I-131 Antineoplastic (S)	New Technology (X)
Isavuconazole (isavuconazonium sulfate)	Other Anti-infective (9)	Administration (3)
Jakafi®	Ruxolitinib (T)	New Technology (X)
Kcentra	4-Factor Prothrombin Complex Concentrate (B)	Administration (3)
KEVZARA®	Sarilumab (G)	New Technology (X)
KYMRIAH®	Tisagenlecleucel Immunotherapy (J)	New Technology (X)
Lifileucel	Lifileucel Immunotherapy (L)	New Technology (X)
Lisocabtagene Maraleucel	Lisocabtagene Maraleucel Immunotherapy (7)	New Technology (X)
LIVTENCITY™	Maribavir Anti-infective (3)	New Technology (X)
LTX Regional Anticoagulant	Nafamostat Anticoagulant (3)	New Technology (X)
MarrowStim™ PAD Kit for CBMA (Concentrated Bone Marrow Aspirate)	Other Substance (C)	Administration (3)
NA-1 (Nerinitide)	Nerinitide (2)	New Technology (X)
Nesiritide	Human B-type Natriuretic Peptide (H)	Administration (3)
NexoBrid™	Bromelain-enriched Proteolytic Enzyme (2)	New Technology (X)
Niyad™	Nafamostat Anticoagulant (3)	New Technology (X)
NUZYRA™	Omadacycline Anti-infective (B)	New Technology (X)
Octagam 10%, for COVID-19 treatment	High-Dose Intravenous Immune Globulin (D)	New Technology (X)
Olumiant® [NT]	Baricitinib (M)	New Technology (X)
OTL-101	Hematopoietic Stem/Progenitor Cells, Genetically Modified (C)	Administration (3)
Polyclonal hyperimmune globulin	Globulin (S)	Administration (3)
Praxbind® (idarucizumab), Pradaxa® (dabigatran) reversal agent	Other Therapeutic Substance (G)	Administration (3)
REBYOTA®	Broad Consortium Microbiota-based Live Biotherapeutic Suspension (X)	New Technology (X)
*RECARBRIO™ [NT]	Imipenem-cilastatin-relebactam Anti-infective (U)	New Technology (X)
RETHYMIC®	Engineered Allogeneic Thymus Tissue (D)	New Technology (X)
rhBMP-2	Recombinant Bone Morphogenetic Protein (B)	Administration (3)
RYBREVANT™ [NT]	Amivantamab Monoclonal Antibody (B)	New Technology (X)
Seprafilm	Adhesion Barrier (5)	Administration (3)
Soliris®	Eculizumab (C)	New Technology (X)
SPRAVATO™	Esketamine Hydrochloride (M)	New Technology (X)
STELARA®	Other New Technology Therapeutic Substance (F)	New Technology (X)

Trade Name or Synonym	ICD-10-PCS Value	PCS Section
StrataGraft® **NT**	Bioengineered Allogeneic Construct (F)	New Technology (X)
tab-cel®	Tabelecleucel Immunotherapy (7)	New Technology (X)
TECARTUS™ **NT**	Brexucabtagene Autoleucel Immunotherapy (M)	New Technology (X)
TECENTRIQ®	Atezolizumab Antineoplastic (D)	New Technology (X)
TERLIVAZ®	Terlipressin (6)	New Technology (X)
Tisagenlecleucel	Tisagenlecleucel Immunotherapy (J)	New Technology (X)
Tissue Plasminogen Activator (tPA)(r-tPA)	Other Thrombolytic (7)	Administration (3)
TYRX Antibacterial Envelope	Anti-Infective Envelope (A)	Administration (3)
UPLIZNA®	Inebilizumab-cdon (9)	New Technology (X)
Ustekinumab	Other New Technology Therapeutic Substance (F)	New Technology (X)
Vabomere™	Meropenem-vaborbactam Anti-infective (N)	New Technology (X)
Veklury **NT**	Remdesivir Anti-infective (E)	New Technology (X)
Venclexta®	Venetoclax Antineoplastic (R)	New Technology (X)
Vistogard®	Uridine Triacetate (8)	New Technology (X)
Voraxaze	Glucarpidase (Q)	Administration (3)
VYXEOS™	Cytarabine and Daunorubicin Liposome Antineoplastic (B)	New Technology (X)
XENLETA™	Lefamulin Anti-infective (6)	New Technology (X)
XOSPATA®	Gilteritinib Antineoplastic (V)	New Technology (X)
Yescarta®	Axicabtagene Ciloleucel Immunotherapy (H)	New Technology (X)
*ZEMDRI®	Plazomicin Anti-infective (6)	New Technology (X)
ZEPZELCA™ **NT**	Lurbinectedin (8)	New Technology (X)
ZERBAXA®	Ceftolozane/Tazobactam Anti-infective (9)	New Technology (X)
ZULRESSO™	Brexanolone (Ø)	New Technology (X)
Zyvox	Oxazolidinones (8)	Administration (3)

Substance Definitions

This table crosswalks a PCS value, used in the Administration or New Technology section, to a specific substance. The specific substances are listed by trade name or synonym. The ICD-10-PCS value may be located in either the 6th-character Substance column or the 7th-character Qualifier column depending on the section/table to which it is classified.

This **NT** symbol next to a substance/technology in the Trade Name or Synonym column identifies that the substance/technology has been approved for NTAP (new technology add-on payment). CMS provides incremental payment, in addition to the DRG payment, for technologies that have received an NTAP designation.

Substances denoted by an asterisk (*) in the Trade Name or Synonym column, although not included in the official ICD-10-PCS classification, were added based on information provided in the FY 2023 IPPS proposed rule.

ICD-10-PCS Value	Trade Name or Synonym		PCS Section
4-Factor Prothrombin Complex Concentrate (B)	Includes:	Kcentra	Administration (3)
Afamitresgene Autoleucel Immunotherapy (6)	Includes:	afami-cel	New Technology (X)
Adhesion Barrier (5)	Includes:	Seprafilm	Administration (3)
Amivantamab Monoclonal Antibody (B)	Includes:	RYBREVANT™ **NT**	New Technology (X)
Antibiotic-eluting Bone Void Filler (P)	Includes:	CERAMENT® G	New Technology (X)
Anti-Infective Envelope (A)	Includes:	AIGISRx Antibacterial Envelope Antibacterial Envelope (TYRX) (AIGISRx) Antimicrobial envelope TYRX Antibacterial Envelope	Administration (3)
Apalutamide Antineoplastic (J)	Includes:	ERLEADA™	New Technology (X)
Atezolizumab Antineoplastic (D)	Includes:	TECENTRIQ®	New Technology (X)
Axicabtagene Ciloleucel Immunotherapy (H)	Includes:	Axicabtagene Ciloleucel Yescarta®	New Technology (X)
Baricitinib (M)	Includes:	Olumiant® **NT**	New Technology (X)
Betibeglogene Autotemcel (B)	Includes:	beti-cel	New Technology (X)
Bioengineered Allogeneic Construct (F)	Includes:	StrataGraft® **NT**	New Technology (X)
Brexanolone (Ø)	Includes:	ZULRESSO™	New Technology (X)
Brexucabtagene Autoleucel Immunotherapy (M)	Includes:	TECARTUS™ **NT**	New Technology (X)
Broad Consortium Microbiota-based Live Biotherapeutic Suspension (X)	Includes:	REBYOTA®	New Technology (X)
Bromelain-enriched Proteolytic Enzyme (2)	Includes:	NexoBrid™	New Technology (X)
Caplacizumab (W)	Includes:	*CABLIVI®	New Technology (X)

ICD-10-PCS Value	Trade Name or Synonym		PCS Section
Cefiderocol Anti-infective (A)	Includes:	FETROJA® **NT**	New Technology (X)
Ceftolozane/Tazobactam Anti- infective (9)	Includes:	ZERBAXA®	New Technology (X)
Ciltacabtagene Autoleucel (A)	Includes:	CARVYKTI™ cilta-cel	New Technology (X)
Clofarabine (P)	Includes:	Clolar	Administration (3)
Coagulation Factor Xa, Inactivated (7)	Includes:	Andexanet Alfa, Factor Xa Inhibitor Reversal Agent Andexxa Coagulation Factor Xa, (Recombinant) Inactivated Factor Xa Inhibitor Reversal Agent, Andexanet Alfa	New Technology (X)
Cytarabine and Daunorubicin Liposome Antineoplastic (B)	Includes:	VYXEOS™	New Technology (X)
Daratumumab and Hyaluronidase-fihj (1)	Includes:	Darzalex Faspro®	New Technology (X)
Durvalumab Antineoplastic (3)	Includes:	IMFINZI®	New Technology (X)
Eculizumab (C)	Includes:	Soliris®	New Technology (X)
Endothelial Damage Inhibitor (8)	Includes:	DuraGraft® Endothelial Damage Inhibitor	New Technology (X)
Erdafitinib Antineoplastic (L)	Includes:	*Balversa™	New Technology (X)
Engineered Allogeneic Thymus Tissue (D)	Includes:	RETHYMIC®	New Technology (X)
Esketamine Hydrochloride (M)	Includes:	SPRAVATO™	New Technology (X)
Fosfomycin Anti-infective (K)	Includes:	CONTEPO™ Fosfomycin injection	New Technology (X)
Gilteritinib Antineoplastic (V)	Includes:	XOSPATA®	New Technology (X)
Globulin (S)	Includes:	Gammaglobulin Hyperimmune globulin Immunoglobulin Polyclonal hyperimmune globulin	Administration (3)
Glucarpidase (Q)	Includes:	Voraxaze	Administration (3)
Hematopoietic Stem/Progenitor Cells, Genetically Modified (C)	Includes:	OTL-101	Administration (3)
High-Dose Intravenous Immune Globulin (D)	Includes:	GAMUNEX-C, for COVID-19 treatment hdIVIG (high-dose intravenous immunoglobulin), for COVID-19 treatment High-dose intravenous immunoglobulin (hdIVIG), for COVID-19 treatment Octagam 10%, for COVID-19 treatment	New Technology (X)
Human B-type Natriuretic Peptide (H)	Includes:	Nesiritide	Administration (3)
Hyperimmune Globulin (E)	Includes:	Anti-SARS-CoV-2 hyperimmune globulin HIG (hyperimmune globulin), for COVID-19 treatment hIVIG (hyperimmune intravenous immunoglobulin), for COVID-19 treatment Hyperimmune intravenous immunoglobulin (hIVIG), for COVID-19 treatment IGIV-C, for COVID-19 treatment	New Technology (X)
Idecabtagene Vicleucel Immunotherapy (K)	Includes:	ABECMA® **NT** Idecabtagene Vicleucel Ide-cel	New Technology (X)
Imipenem-cilastatin-relebactam Anti-infective (U)	Includes:	IMI/REL *RECARBRIO™ **NT**	New Technology (X)
Inebilizumab-cdon (9)	Includes:	UPLIZNA®	New Technology (X)
Iobenguane I-131 Antineoplastic (S)	Includes:	AZEDRA® Iobenguane I-131, High Specific Activity (HSA)	New Technology (X)
Lefamulin Anti-infective (6)	Includes:	XENLETA™	New Technology (X)
Lifileucel Immunotherapy (L)	Includes:	Lifileucel	New Technology (X)
Lisocabtagene Maraleucel Immunotherapy (7)	Includes:	Breyanzi® Lisocabtagene Maraleucel	New Technology (X)
Lurbinectedin (8)	Includes:	ZEPZELCA™ **NT**	New Technology (X)
Maribavir Anti-infective (3)	Includes:	LIVTENCITY™	New Technology (X)
Meropenem-vaborbactam Anti-infective (N)	Includes:	Vabomere™	New Technology (X)
Mineral-based Topical Hemostatic Agent (8)	Includes:	Hemospray® Endoscopic Hemostat	New Technology (X)
Nafamostat Anticoagulant (3)	Includes:	LTX Regional Anticoagulant Niyad™	New Technology (X)
Nerinitide (2)	Includes:	NA-1 (Nerinitide)	New Technology (X)
Omadacycline Anti-infective (B)	Includes:	NUZYRA™	New Technology (X)

ICD-10-PCS Value	Trade Name or Synonym		PCS Section
Other Anti-infective (9)	Includes:	AVYCAZ® (ceftazidime-avibactam) Ceftazidime-avibactam CRESEMBA® (isavuconazonium sulfate) Isavuconazole (isavuconazonium sulfate)	Administration (3)
Other Antineoplastic (5)	Includes:	Blinatumomab BLINCYTO® (blinatumomab)	Administration (3)
Other New Technology Therapeutic Substance (F)	Includes:	STELARA® Ustekinumab	New Technology (X)
Other Substance (C)	Includes:	CBMA (Concentrated Bone Marrow Aspirate) Defitelio MarrowStim™ PAD Kit for CBMA (Concentrated Bone Marrow Aspirate)	Administration (3)
Other Therapeutic Substance (G)	Includes:	Idarucizumab, Pradaxa® (dabigatran) reversal agent Praxbind® (idarucizumab), Pradaxa® (dabigatran) reversal agent	Administration (3)
Other Thrombolytic (7)	Includes:	Tissue Plasminogen Activator (tPA)(r-tPA)	Administration (3)
Oxazolidinones (8)	Includes:	Zyvox	Administration (3)
Pathogen Reduced Cryoprecipitated Fibrinogen Complex (D)	Includes:	INTERCEPT Blood System for Plasma Pathogen Reduced Cryoprecipitated Fibrinogen Complex **NT** INTERCEPT Fibrinogen Complex **NT**	Administration (3)
Plazomicin Anti-infective (G)	Includes:	*ZEMDRI®	New Technology (X)
Recombinant Bone Morphogenetic Protein (B)	Includes:	Bone morphogenetic protein 2 (BMP 2) rhBMP-2	Administration (3)
REGN-COV2 Monoclonal Antibody (G)	Includes:	Casirivimab (REGN10933) and Imdevimab (REGN10987) Imdevimab (REGN10987) and Casirivimab (REGN10933)	New Technology (X)
Remdesivir Anti-infective (E)	Includes:	GS-5734 Veklury **NT**	New Technology (X)
Ruxolitinib (T)	Includes:	Jakafi®	New Technology (X)
Sarilumab (G)	Includes:	KEVZARA®	New Technology (X)
Satralizumab-mwge (9)	Includes:	ENSPRYNG™	New Technology (X)
Synthetic Human Angiotensin II (H)	Includes:	Angiotensin II GIAPREZA™ Human angiotensin II, synthetic	New Technology (X)
Tabelecleucel Immunotherapy (7)	Includes:	tab-cel®	New Technology (X)
Tagraxofusp-erzs Antineoplastic (Q)	Includes:	ELZONRIS™	New Technology (X)
Taurolidine Anti-infective and Heparin Anticoagulant (2)	Includes:	DefenCath™	New Technology (X)
Terlipressin (6)	Includes:	TERLIVAZ®	New Technology (X)
Tisagenlecleucel Immunotherapy (J)	Includes:	KYMRIAH® Tisagenlecleucel	New Technology (X)
Tixagevimab and Cilgavimab Monoclonal Antibody (X)	Includes:	EVUSHELD™	New Technology (X)
Tocilizumab (H)	Includes:	ACTEMRA®	New Technology (X)
Trilaciclib (7)	Includes:	COSELA™ **NT**	New Technology (X)
Uridine Triacetate (8)	Includes:	Vistogard®	New Technology (X)
Venetoclax Antineoplastic (R)	Includes:	Venclexta®	New Technology (X)

Appendix J: Sections B–H Character Definitions

Sections B-H (Imaging through Substance Abuse Treatment) do not include root operations. Instead, the character 3 value represents the type of procedure performed with additional details about that procedure provided by the character 4 or 5 value, when appropriate. This resource provides the specific ICD-10-PCS value and its associated definition for the character 3, character 4, and character 5 values in the ancillary sections of B-H.

Section B–Imaging

ICD-10-PCS Value (Character 3)	Definition
Computerized Tomography (CT Scan) (2)	Computer reformatted digital display of multiplanar images developed from the capture of multiple exposures of external ionizing radiation
Fluoroscopy (1)	Single plane or bi-plane real time display of an image developed from the capture of external ionizing radiation on a fluorescent screen. The image may also be stored by either digital or analog means.
Magnetic Resonance Imaging (MRI) (3)	Computer reformatted digital display of multiplanar images developed from the capture of radiofrequency signals emitted by nuclei in a body site excited within a magnetic field
Other Imaging (5)	Other specified modality for visualizing a body part
Plain Radiography (Ø)	Planar display of an image developed from the capture of external ionizing radiation on photographic or photoconductive plate
Ultrasonography (4)	Real time display of images of anatomy or flow information developed from the capture of reflected and attenuated high frequency sound waves

Section C–Nuclear Medicine

ICD-10-PCS Value (Character 3)	Definition
Nonimaging Nuclear Medicine Assay (6)	Introduction of radioactive materials into the body for the study of body fluids and blood elements, by the detection of radioactive emissions
Nonimaging Nuclear Medicine Probe (5)	Introduction of radioactive materials into the body for the study of distribution and fate of certain substances by the detection of radioactive emissions; or, alternatively, measurement of absorption of radioactive emissions from an external source
Nonimaging Nuclear Medicine Uptake (4)	Introduction of radioactive materials into the body for measurements of organ function, from the detection of radioactive emissions
Planar Nuclear Medicine Imaging (1)	Introduction of radioactive materials into the body for single plane display of images developed from the capture of radioactive emissions
Positron Emission Tomographic (PET) Imaging (3)	Introduction of radioactive materials into the body for three dimensional display of images developed from the simultaneous capture, 18Ø degrees apart, of radioactive emissions
Systemic Nuclear Medicine Therapy (7)	Introduction of unsealed radioactive materials into the body for treatment
Tomographic (Tomo) Nuclear Medicine Imaging (2)	Introduction of radioactive materials into the body for three dimensional display of images developed from the capture of radioactive emissions

Section F–Physical Rehabilitation and Diagnostic Audiology

ICD-10-PCS Value (Character 3)	Definition
Activities of Daily Living Assessment (2)	Measurement of functional level for activities of daily living
Activities of Daily Living Treatment (8)	Exercise or activities to facilitate functional competence for activities of daily living
Caregiver Training (F)	Training in activities to support patient's optimal level of function
Cochlear Implant Treatment (B)	Application of techniques to improve the communication abilities of individuals with cochlear implant
Device Fitting (D)	Fitting of a device designed to facilitate or support achievement of a higher level of function
Hearing Aid Assessment (4)	Measurement of the appropriateness and/or effectiveness of a hearing device
Hearing Assessment (3)	Measurement of hearing and related functions
Hearing Treatment (9)	Application of techniques to improve, augment, or compensate for hearing and related functional impairment
Motor and/or Nerve Function Assessment (1)	Measurement of motor, nerve, and related functions

Continued on next page

Section F–Physical Rehabilitation and Diagnostic Audiology

Continued from previous page

ICD-10-PCS Value (Character 3)	Definition
Motor Treatment (7)	Exercise or activities to increase or facilitate motor function
Speech Assessment (Ø)	Measurement of speech and related functions
Speech Treatment (6)	Application of techniques to improve, augment, or compensate for speech and related functional impairment
Vestibular Assessment (5)	Measurement of the vestibular system and related functions
Vestibular Treatment (C)	Application of techniques to improve, augment, or compensate for vestibular and related functional impairment

Section F–Physical Rehabilitation and Diagnostic Audiology

ICD-10-PCS Value Qualifier (Character 5)	Definition
Acoustic Reflex Decay (J)	Measures reduction in size/strength of acoustic reflex over time Includes/Examples: Includes site of lesion test
Acoustic Reflex Patterns (G)	Defines site of lesion based upon presence/absence of acoustic reflexes with ipsilateral vs. contralateral stimulation
Acoustic Reflex Threshold (H)	Determines minimal intensity that acoustic reflex occurs with ipsilateral and/or contralateral stimulation
Aerobic Capacity and Endurance (7)	Measures autonomic responses to positional changes; perceived exertion, dyspnea or angina during activity; performance during exercise protocols; standard vital signs; and blood gas analysis or oxygen consumption
Alternate Binaural or Monaural Loudness Balance (7)	Determines auditory stimulus parameter that yields the same objective sensation Includes/Examples: Sound intensities that yield same loudness perception
Anthropometric Characteristics (B)	Measures edema, body fat composition, height, weight, length and girth
Aphasia (Assessment) (C)	Measures expressive and receptive speech and language function including reading and writing
Aphasia (Treatment) (3)	Applying techniques to improve, augment, or compensate for receptive/ expressive language impairments
Articulation/Phonology (Assessment) (9)	Measures speech production
Articulation/Phonology (Treatment) (4)	Applying techniques to correct, improve, or compensate for speech productive impairment
Assistive Listening Device (5)	Assists in use of effective and appropriate assistive listening device/system
Assistive Listening System/Device Selection (4)	Measures the effectiveness and appropriateness of assistive listening systems/devices
Assistive, Adaptive, Supportive or Protective Devices (9)	Explanation: Devices to facilitate or support achievement of a higher level of function in wheelchair mobility; bed mobility; transfer or ambulation ability; bath and showering ability; dressing; grooming; personal hygiene; play or leisure
Auditory Evoked Potentials (L)	Measures electric responses produced by the VIIIth cranial nerve and brainstem following auditory stimulation
Auditory Processing (Assessment) (Q)	Evaluates ability to receive and process auditory information and comprehension of spoken language
Auditory Processing (Treatment) (2)	Applying techniques to improve the receiving and processing of auditory information and comprehension of spoken language
Augmentative/Alternative Communication System (Assessment) (L)	Determines the appropriateness of aids, techniques, symbols, and/or strategies to augment or replace speech and enhance communication Includes/Examples: Includes the use of telephones, writing equipment, emergency equipment, and TDD
Augmentative/Alternative Communication System (Treatment) (3)	Includes/Examples: Includes augmentative communication devices and aids
Aural Rehabilitation (5)	Applying techniques to improve the communication abilities associated with hearing loss
Aural Rehabilitation Status (P)	Measures impact of a hearing loss including evaluation of receptive and expressive communication skills
Bathing/Showering (Ø)	Includes/Examples: Includes obtaining and using supplies; soaping, rinsing, and drying body parts; maintaining bathing position; and transferring to and from bathing positions

Continued on next page

Section F–Physical Rehabilitation and Diagnostic Audiology

Continued from previous page

ICD-10-PCS Value Qualifier (Character 5)	Definition
Bathing/Showering Techniques (Ø)	Activities to facilitate obtaining and using supplies, soaping, rinsing and drying body parts, maintaining bathing position, and transferring to and from bathing positions
Bed Mobility (Assessment) (B)	Transitional movement within bed
Bed Mobility (Treatment) (5)	Exercise or activities to facilitate transitional movements within bed
Bedside Swallowing and Oral Function (H)	Includes/Examples: Bedside swallowing includes assessment of sucking, masticating, coughing, and swallowing. Oral function includes assessment of musculature for controlled movements, structures, and functions to determine coordination and phonation.
Bekesy Audiometry (3)	Uses an instrument that provides a choice of discrete or continuously varying pure tones; choice of pulsed or continuous signal
Binaural Electroacoustic Hearing Aid Check (6)	Determines mechanical and electroacoustic function of bilateral hearing aids using hearing aid test box
Binaural Hearing Aid (Assessment) (3)	Measures the candidacy, effectiveness, and appropriateness of a hearing aid Explanation: Measures bilateral fit
Binaural Hearing Aid (Treatment) (2)	Explanation: Assists in achieving maximum understanding and performance
Bithermal, Binaural Caloric Irrigation (Ø)	Measures the rhythmic eye movements stimulated by changing the temperature of the vestibular system
Bithermal, Monaural Caloric Irrigation (1)	Measures the rhythmic eye movements stimulated by changing the temperature of the vestibular system in one ear
Brief Tone Stimuli (R)	Measures specific central auditory process
Cerumen Management (3)	Includes examination of external auditory canal and tympanic membrane and removal of cerumen from external ear canal
Cochlear Implant (Ø)	Measures candidacy for cochlear implant
Cochlear Implant Rehabilitation (Ø)	Applying techniques to improve the communication abilities of individuals with cochlear implant; includes programming the device, providing patients/families with information
Communicative/Cognitive Integration Skills (Assessment) (G)	Measures ability to use higher cortical functions Includes/Examples: Includes orientation, recognition, attention span, initiation and termination of activity, memory, sequencing, categorizing, concept formation, spatial operations, judgment, problem solving, generalization and pragmatic communication
Communicative/Cognitive Integration Skills (Treatment) (6)	Activities to facilitate the use of higher cortical functions Includes/Examples: Includes level of arousal, orientation, recognition, attention span, initiation and termination of activity, memory sequencing, judgment and problem solving, learning and generalization, and pragmatic communication
Computerized Dynamic Posturography (6)	Measures the status of the peripheral and central vestibular system and the sensory/motor component of balance; evaluates the efficacy of vestibular rehabilitation
Conditioned Play Audiometry (4)	Behavioral measures using nonspeech and speech stimuli to obtain frequency-specific and ear-specific information on auditory status from the patient Explanation: Obtains speech reception threshold by having patient point to pictures of spondaic words
Coordination/Dexterity (Assessment) (3)	Measures large and small muscle groups for controlled goal-directed movements Explanation: Dexterity includes object manipulation
Coordination/Dexterity (Treatment) (2)	Exercise or activities to facilitate gross coordination and fine coordination
Cranial Nerve Integrity (9)	Measures cranial nerve sensory and motor functions, including tastes, smell and facial expression
Dichotic Stimuli (T)	Measures specific central auditory process
Distorted Speech (S)	Measures specific central auditory process
Dix-Hallpike Dynamic (5)	Measures nystagmus following Dix-Hallpike maneuver
Dressing (1)	Includes/Examples: Includes selecting clothing and accessories, obtaining clothing from storage, dressing, fastening and adjusting clothing and shoes, and applying and removing personal devices, prosthesis or orthosis
Dressing Techniques (1)	Activities to facilitate selecting clothing and accessories, dressing and undressing, adjusting clothing and shoes, applying and removing devices, prostheses or orthoses
Dynamic Orthosis (6)	Includes/Examples: Includes customized and prefabricated splints, inhibitory casts, spinal and other braces, and protective devices; allows motion through transfer of movement from other body parts or by use of outside forces

Continued on next page

Section F–Physical Rehabilitation and Diagnostic Audiology

Continued from previous page

ICD-10-PCS Value Qualifier (Character 5)	Definition
Ear Canal Probe Microphone (1)	Real ear measures
Ear Protector Attentuation (7)	Measures ear protector fit and effectiveness
Electrocochleography (K)	Measures the VIIIth cranial nerve action potential
Environmental, Home, Work Barriers (B)	Measures current and potential barriers to optimal function, including safety hazards, access problems and home or office design
Ergonomics and Body Mechanics (C)	Ergonomic measurement of job tasks, work hardening or work conditioning needs; functional capacity; and body mechanics
Eustachian Tube Function (F)	Measures eustachian tube function and patency of eustachian tube
Evoked Otoacoustic Emissions, Diagnostic (N)	Measures auditory evoked potentials in a diagnostic format
Evoked Otoacoustic Emissions, Screening (M)	Measures auditory evoked potentials in a screening format
Facial Nerve Function (7)	Measures electrical activity of the VIIth cranial nerve (facial nerve)
Feeding/Eating (Assessment) (2)	Includes/Examples: Includes setting up food, selecting and using utensils and tableware, bringing food or drink to mouth, cleaning face, hands, and clothing, and management of alternative methods of nourishment
Feeding/Eating (Treatment) (3)	Exercise or activities to facilitate setting up food, selecting and using utensils and tableware, bringing food or drink to mouth, cleaning face, hands, and clothing, and management of alternative methods of nourishment
Filtered Speech (Ø)	Uses high or low pass filtered speech stimuli to assess central auditory processing disorders, site of lesion testing
Fluency (Assessment) (D)	Measures speech fluency or stuttering
Fluency (Treatment) (7)	Applying techniques to improve and augment fluent speech
Gait and/or Balance (D)	Measures biomechanical, arthrokinematic and other spatial and temporal characteristics of gait and balance
Gait Training/Functional Ambulation (9)	Exercise or activities to facilitate ambulation on a variety of surfaces and in a variety of environments
Grooming/Personal Hygiene (Assessment) (3)	Includes/Examples: Includes ability to obtain and use supplies in a sequential fashion, general grooming, oral hygiene, toilet hygiene, personal care devices, including care for artificial airways
Grooming/Personal Hygiene (Treatment) (2)	Activities to facilitate obtaining and using supplies in a sequential fashion: general grooming, oral hygiene, toilet hygiene, cleaning body, and personal care devices, including artificial airways
Hearing and Related Disorders Counseling (Ø)	Provides patients/families/caregivers with information, support, referrals to facilitate recovery from a communication disorder Includes/Examples: Includes strategies for psychosocial adjustment to hearing loss for clients and families/caregivers
Hearing and Related Disorders Prevention (1)	Provides patients/families/caregivers with information and support to prevent communication disorders
Hearing Screening (Ø)	Pass/refer measures designed to identify need for further audiologic assessment
Home Management (Assessment) (4)	Obtaining and maintaining personal and household possessions and environment Includes/Examples: Includes clothing care, cleaning, meal preparation and cleanup, shopping, money management, household maintenance, safety procedures, and childcare/parenting
Home Management (Treatment) (4)	Activities to facilitate obtaining and maintaining personal household possessions and environment Includes/Examples: Includes clothing care, cleaning, meal preparation and clean-up, shopping, money management, household maintenance, safety procedures, childcare/parenting
Instrumental Swallowing and Oral Function (J)	Measures swallowing function using instrumental diagnostic procedures Explanation: Methods include videofluoroscopy, ultrasound, manometry, endoscopy
Integumentary Integrity (1)	Includes/Examples: Includes burns, skin conditions, ecchymosis, bleeding, blisters, scar tissue, wounds and other traumas, tissue mobility, turgor and texture
Manual Therapy Techniques (7)	Techniques in which the therapist uses his/her hands to administer skilled movements Includes/Examples: Includes connective tissue massage, joint mobilization and manipulation, manual lymph drainage, manual traction, soft tissue mobilization and manipulation
Masking Patterns (W)	Measures central auditory processing status

Continued on next page

Section F–Physical Rehabilitation and Diagnostic Audiology
Continued from previous page

ICD-10-PCS Value Qualifier (Character 5)	Definition
Monaural Electroacoustic Hearing Aid Check (8)	Determines mechanical and electroacoustic function of one hearing aid using hearing aid test box
Monaural Hearing Aid (Assessment) (2)	Measures the candidacy, effectiveness, and appropriateness of a hearing aid Explanation: Measures unilateral fit
Monaural Hearing Aid (Treatment) (1)	Explanation: Assists in achieving maximum understanding and performance
Motor Function (Assessment) (4)	Measures the body's functional and versatile movement patterns Includes/Examples: Includes motor assessment scales, analysis of head, trunk and limb movement, and assessment of motor learning
Motor Function (Treatment) (3)	Exercise or activities to facilitate crossing midline, laterality, bilateral integration, praxis, neuromuscular relaxation, inhibition, facilitation, motor function and motor learning
Motor Speech (Assessment) (B)	Measures neurological motor aspects of speech production
Motor Speech (Treatment) (8)	Applying techniques to improve and augment the impaired neurological motor aspects of speech production
Muscle Performance (Assessment) (Ø)	Measures muscle strength, power and endurance using manual testing, dynamometry or computer-assisted electromechanical muscle test; functional muscle strength, power and endurance; muscle pain, tone, or soreness; or pelvic-floor musculature Explanation: Muscle endurance refers to the ability to contract a muscle repeatedly over time
Muscle Performance (Treatment) (1)	Exercise or activities to increase the capacity of a muscle to do work in terms of strength, power, and/or endurance Explanation: Muscle strength is the force exerted to overcome resistance in one maximal effort. Muscle power is work produced per unit of time, or the product of strength and speed. Muscle endurance is the ability to contract a muscle repeatedly over time.
Neuromotor Development (D)	Measures motor development, righting and equilibrium reactions, and reflex and equilibrium reactions
Non-invasive Instrumental Status (N)	Instrumental measures of oral, nasal, vocal, and velopharyngeal functions as they pertain to speech production
Nonspoken Language (Assessment) (7)	Measures nonspoken language (print, sign, symbols) for communication
Nonspoken Language (Treatment) (Ø)	Applying techniques that improve, augment, or compensate spoken communication
Oral Peripheral Mechanism (P)	Structural measures of face, jaw, lips, tongue, teeth, hard and soft palate, pharynx as related to speech production
Orofacial Myofunctional (Assessment) (K)	Measures orofacial myofunctional patterns for speech and related functions
Orofacial Myofunctional (Treatment) (9)	Applying techniques to improve, alter, or augment impaired orofacial myofunctional patterns and related speech production errors
Oscillating Tracking (3)	Measures ability to visually track
Pain (F)	Measures muscle soreness, pain and soreness with joint movement, and pain perception Includes/Examples: Includes questionnaires, graphs, symptom magnification scales or visual analog scales
Perceptual Processing (Assessment) (5)	Measures stereognosis, kinesthesia, body schema, right-left discrimination, form constancy, position in space, visual closure, figure-ground, depth perception, spatial relations and topographical orientation
Perceptual Processing (Treatment) (1)	Exercise and activities to facilitate perceptual processing Explanation: Includes stereognosis, kinesthesia, body schema, right-left discrimination, form constancy, position in space, visual closure, figure-ground, depth perception, spatial relations, and topographical orientation Includes/Examples: Includes stereognosis, kinesthesia, body schema, right-left discrimination, form constancy, position in space, visual closure, figure-ground, depth perception, spatial relations, and topographical orientation
Performance Intensity Phonetically Balanced Speech Discrimination (Q)	Measures word recognition over varying intensity levels
Postural Control (3)	Exercise or activities to increase postural alignment and control
Prosthesis (8)	Explanation: Artificial substitutes for missing body parts that augment performance or function Includes/Examples: Limb prosthesis, ocular prosthesis

Continued on next page

Section F–Physical Rehabilitation and Diagnostic Audiology   *Continued from previous page*

ICD-10-PCS Value Qualifier (Character 5)	Definition
Psychosocial Skills (Assessment) (6)	The ability to interact in society and to process emotions Includes/Examples: Includes psychological (values, interests, self-concept); social (role performance, social conduct, interpersonal skills, self expression); self-management (coping skills, time management, self-control)
Psychosocial Skills (Treatment) (6)	The ability to interact in society and to process emotions Includes/Examples: Includes psychological (values, interests, self-concept); social (role performance, social conduct, interpersonal skills, self expression); self-management (coping skills, time management, self-control)
Pure Tone Audiometry, Air (1)	Air-conduction pure tone threshold measures with appropriate masking
Pure Tone Audiometry, Air and Bone (2)	Air-conduction and bone-conduction pure tone threshold measures with appropriate masking
Pure Tone Stenger (C)	Measures unilateral nonorganic hearing loss based on simultaneous presentation of pure tones of differing volume
Range of Motion and Joint Integrity (5)	Measures quantity, quality, grade, and classification of joint movement and/or mobility Explanation: Range of Motion is the space, distance or angle through which movement occurs at a joint or series of joints. Joint integrity is the conformance of joints to expected anatomic, biomechanical and kinematic norms.
Range of Motion and Joint Mobility (Ø)	Exercise or activities to increase muscle length and joint mobility
Receptive/Expressive Language (Assessment) (8)	Measures receptive and expressive language
Receptive/Expressive Language (Treatment) (B)	Applying techniques to improve and augment receptive/expressive language
Reflex Integrity (G)	Measures the presence, absence, or exaggeration of developmentally appropriate, pathologic or normal reflexes
Select Picture Audiometry (5)	Establishes hearing threshold levels for speech using pictures
Sensorineural Acuity Level (4)	Measures sensorineural acuity masking presented via bone conduction
Sensory Aids (5)	Determines the appropriateness of a sensory prosthetic device, other than a hearing aid or assistive listening system/device
Sensory Awareness/ Processing/ Integrity (6)	Includes/Examples: Includes light touch, pressure, temperature, pain, sharp/dull, proprioception, vestibular, visual, auditory, gustatory, and olfactory
Short Increment Sensitivity Index (9)	Measures the ear's ability to detect small intensity changes; site of lesion test requiring a behavioral response
Sinusoidal Vertical Axis Rotational (4)	Measures nystagmus following rotation
Somatosensory Evoked Potentials (9)	Measures neural activity from sites throughout the body
Speech/Language Screening (6)	Identifies need for further speech and/or language evaluation
Speech Threshold (1)	Measures minimal intensity needed to repeat spondaic words
Speech-Language Pathology and Related Disorders Counseling (1)	Provides patients/families with information, support, referrals to facilitate recovery from a communication disorder
Speech-Language Pathology and Related Disorders Prevention (2)	Applying techniques to avoid or minimize onset and/or development of a communication disorder
Speech/Word Recognition (2)	Measures ability to repeat/identify single syllable words; scores given as a percentage; includes word recognition/speech discrimination
Staggered Spondaic Word (3)	Measures central auditory processing site of lesion based upon dichotic presentation of spondaic words
Static Orthosis (7)	Includes/Examples: Includes customized and prefabricated splints, inhibitory casts, spinal and other braces, and protective devices; has no moving parts, maintains joint(s) in desired position
Stenger (B)	Measures unilateral nonorganic hearing loss based on simultaneous presentation of signals of differing volume
Swallowing Dysfunction (D)	Activities to improve swallowing function in coordination with respiratory function Includes/Examples: Includes function and coordination of sucking, mastication, coughing, swallowing
Synthetic Sentence Identification (5)	Measures central auditory dysfunction using identification of third order approximations of sentences and competing messages

Continued on next page

Section F–Physical Rehabilitation and Diagnostic Audiology

Continued from previous page

ICD-10-PCS Value Qualifier (Character 5)	Definition
Temporal Ordering of Stimuli (V)	Measures specific central auditory process
Therapeutic Exercise (6)	Exercise or activities to facilitate sensory awareness, sensory processing, sensory integration, balance training, conditioning, reconditioning Includes/Examples: Includes developmental activities, breathing exercises, aerobic endurance activities, aquatic exercises, stretching and ventilatory muscle training
Tinnitus Masker (Assessment) (7)	Determines candidacy for tinnitus masker
Tinnitus Masker (Treatment) (Ø)	Explanation: Used to verify physical fit, acoustic appropriateness, and benefit; assists in achieving maximum benefit
Tone Decay (8)	Measures decrease in hearing sensitivity to a tone; site of lesion test requiring a behavioral response
Transfer (C)	Transitional movement from one surface to another
Transfer Training (8)	Exercise or activities to facilitate movement from one surface to another
Tympanometry (D)	Measures the integrity of the middle ear; measures ease at which sound flows through the tympanic membrane while air pressure against the membrane is varied
Unithermal Binaural Screen (2)	Measures the rhythmic eye movements stimulated by changing the temperature of the vestibular system in both ears using warm water, screening format
Ventilation/Respiration/Circulation (G)	Measures ventilatory muscle strength, power and endurance, pulmonary function and ventilatory mechanics Includes/Examples: Includes ability to clear airway, activities that aggravate or relieve edema, pain, dyspnea or other symptoms, chest wall mobility, cardiopulmonary response to performance of ADL and IAD, cough and sputum, standard vital signs
Vestibular (Ø)	Applying techniques to compensate for balance disorders; includes habituation, exercise therapy, and balance retraining
Visual Motor Integration (Assessment) (2)	Coordinating the interaction of information from the eyes with body movement during activity
Visual Motor Integration (Treatment) (2)	Exercise or activities to facilitate coordinating the interaction of information from eyes with body movement during activity
Visual Reinforcement Audiometry (6)	Behavioral measures using nonspeech and speech stimuli to obtain frequency/ear-specific information on auditory status Includes/Examples: Includes a conditioned response of looking toward a visual reinforcer (e.g., lights, animated toy) every time auditory stimuli are heard
Vocational Activities and Functional Community or Work Reintegration Skills (Assessment) (H)	Measures environmental, home, work (job/school/play) barriers that keep patients from functioning optimally in their environment Includes/Examples: Includes assessment of vocational skills and interests, environment of work (job/school/play), injury potential and injury prevention or reduction, ergonomic stressors, transportation skills, and ability to access and use community resources
Vocational Activities and Functional Community or Work Reintegration Skills (Treatment) (7)	Activities to facilitate vocational exploration, body mechanics training, job acquisition, and environmental or work (job/school/play) task adaptation Includes/Examples: Includes injury prevention and reduction, ergonomic stressor reduction, job coaching and simulation, work hardening and conditioning, driving training, transportation skills, and use of community resources
Voice (Assessment) (F)	Measures vocal structure, function and production
Voice (Treatment) (C)	Applying techniques to improve voice and vocal function
Voice Prosthetic (Assessment) (M)	Determines the appropriateness of voice prosthetic/adaptive device to enhance or facilitate communication
Voice Prosthetic (Treatment) (4)	Includes/Examples: Includes electrolarynx, and other assistive, adaptive, supportive devices
Wheelchair Mobility (Assessment) (F)	Measures fit and functional abilities within wheelchair in a variety of environments
Wheelchair Mobility (Treatment) (4)	Management, maintenance and controlled operation of a wheelchair, scooter or other device, in and on a variety of surfaces and environments
Wound Management (5)	Includes/Examples: Includes non-selective and selective debridement (enzymes, autolysis, sharp debridement), dressings (wound coverings, hydrogel, vacuum-assisted closure), topical agents, etc.

Section G–Mental Health

ICD-10-PCS Value (Character 3)	Definition
Biofeedback (C)	Provision of information from the monitoring and regulating of physiological processes in conjunction with cognitive-behavioral techniques to improve patient functioning or well-being Includes/Examples: Includes EEG, blood pressure, skin temperature or peripheral blood flow, ECG, electrooculogram, EMG, respirometry or capnometry, GSR/EDR, perineometry to monitor/regulate bowel/bladder activity, electrogastrogram to monitor/regulate gastric motility
Counseling (6)	The application of psychological methods to treat an individual with normal developmental issues and psychological problems in order to increase function, improve well-being, alleviate distress, maladjustment or resolve crises
Crisis Intervention (2)	Treatment of a traumatized, acutely disturbed or distressed individual for the purpose of short-term stabilization Includes/Examples: Includes defusing, debriefing, counseling, psychotherapy and/or coordination of care with other providers or agencies
Electroconvulsive Therapy (B)	The application of controlled electrical voltages to treat a mental health disorder Includes/Examples: Includes appropriate sedation and other preparation of the individual
Family Psychotherapy (7)	Treatment that includes one or more family members of an individual with a mental health disorder by behavioral, cognitive, psychoanalytic, psychodynamic or psychophysiological means to improve functioning or well-being Explanation: Remediation of emotional or behavioral problems presented by one or more family members in cases where psychotherapy with more than one family member is indicated
Group Psychotherapy (H)	Treatment of two or more individuals with a mental health disorder by behavioral, cognitive, psychoanalytic, psychodynamic or psychophysiological means to improve functioning or well-being
Hypnosis (F)	Induction of a state of heightened suggestibility by auditory, visual and tactile techniques to elicit an emotional or behavioral response
Individual Psychotherapy (5)	Treatment of an individual with a mental health disorder by behavioral, cognitive, psychoanalytic, psychodynamic or psychophysiological means to improve functioning or well-being
Light Therapy (J)	Application of specialized light treatments to improve functioning or well-being
Medication Management (3)	Monitoring and adjusting the use of medications for the treatment of a mental health disorder
Narcosynthesis (G)	Administration of intravenous barbiturates in order to release suppressed or repressed thoughts
Psychological Tests (1)	The administration and interpretation of standardized psychological tests and measurement instruments for the assessment of psychological function
Behavioral (1)	Primarily to modify behavior Includes/Examples: Includes modeling and role playing, positive reinforcement of target behaviors, response cost, and training of self-management skills
Cognitive (2)	Primarily to correct cognitive distortions and errors
Cognitive-Behavioral (8)	Combining cognitive and behavioral treatment strategies to improve functioning Explanation: Maladaptive responses are examined to determine how cognitions relate to behavior patterns in response to an event. Uses learning principles and information-processing models.
Developmental (Ø)	Age-normed developmental status of cognitive, social and adaptive behavior skills
Intellectual and Psychoeducational (2)	Intellectual abilities, academic achievement and learning capabilities (including behaviors and emotional factors affecting learning)
Interactive (Ø)	Uses primarily physical aids and other forms of non-oral interaction with a patient who is physically, psychologically or developmentally unable to use ordinary language for communication Includes/Examples: Includes the use of toys in symbolic play
Interpersonal (3)	Helps an individual make changes in interpersonal behaviors to reduce psychological dysfunction Includes/Examples: Includes exploratory techniques, encouragement of affective expression, clarification of patient statements, analysis of communication patterns, use of therapy relationship and behavior change techniques
Neurobehavioral and Cognitive Status (4)	Includes neurobehavioral status exam, interview(s), and observation for the clinical assessment of thinking, reasoning and judgment, acquired knowledge, attention, memory, visual spatial abilities, language functions, and planning
Neuropsychological (3)	Thinking, reasoning and judgment, acquired knowledge, attention, memory, visual spatial abilities, language functions, planning
Personality and Behavioral (1)	Mood, emotion, behavior, social functioning, psychopathological conditions, personality traits and characteristics

Continued on next page

Section G–Mental Health   *Continued from previous page*

ICD-10-PCS Value (Character 3)	Definition
Psychoanalysis (4)	Methods of obtaining a detailed account of past and present mental and emotional experiences to determine the source and eliminate or diminish the undesirable effects of unconscious conflicts Explanation: Accomplished by making the individual aware of their existence, origin, and inappropriate expression in emotions and behavior
Psychodynamic (5)	Exploration of past and present emotional experiences to understand motives and drives using insight-oriented techniques to reduce the undesirable effects of internal conflicts on emotions and behavior Explanation: Techniques include empathetic listening, clarifying self-defeating behavior patterns, and exploring adaptive alternatives
Psychophysiological (9)	Monitoring and alteration of physiological processes to help the individual associate physiological reactions combined with cognitive and behavioral strategies to gain improved control of these processes to help the individual cope more effectively
Supportive (6)	Formation of therapeutic relationship primarily for providing emotional support to prevent further deterioration in functioning during periods of particular stress Explanation: Often used in conjunction with other therapeutic approaches
Vocational (1)	Exploration of vocational interests, aptitudes and required adaptive behavior skills to develop and carry out a plan for achieving a successful vocational placement Includes/Examples: Includes enhancing work related adjustment and/or pursuing viable options in training education or preparation

Section H–Substance Abuse Treatment

ICD-10-PCS Value (Character 3)	Definition
Detoxification Services (2)	Detoxification from alcohol and/or drugs Explanation: Not a treatment modality, but helps the patient stabilize physically and psychologically until the body becomes free of drugs and the effects of alcohol
Family Counseling (6)	The application of psychological methods that includes one or more family members to treat an individual with addictive behavior Explanation: Provides support and education for family members of addicted individuals. Family member participation is seen as a critical area of substance abuse treatment.
Group Counseling (4)	The application of psychological methods to treat two or more individuals with addictive behavior Explanation: Provides structured group counseling sessions and healing power through the connection with others
Individual Counseling (3)	The application of psychological methods to treat an individual with addictive behavior Explanation: Comprised of several different techniques, which apply various strategies to address drug addiction
Individual Psychotherapy (5)	Treatment of an individual with addictive behavior by behavioral, cognitive, psychoanalytic, psychodynamic or psychophysiological means
Medication Management (8)	Monitoring and adjusting the use of replacement medications for the treatment of addiction
Pharmacotherapy (9)	The use of replacement medications for the treatment of addiction

Appendix K: Hospital Acquired Conditions

Hospital acquired conditions (HACs) are conditions considered reasonably preventable through the application of evidence-based guidelines. Although it is the ICD-10-CM diagnosis code that drives a HAC designation, in some cases a specific ICD-10-PCS procedure code must also be present before that diagnosis code can be considered a HAC. This resource provides only those HAC categories that require both an ICD-10-PCS code and an ICD-10-CM diagnosis code. The official descriptions for each code are also provided. To see all 14 HAC categories and their corresponding codes, refer to Optum's *ICD-10-CM Expert for Hospitals*.

Note: The resource used to compile this list is the proposed, version 40, MS-DRG Grouper software and Definitions Manual files published with the fiscal 2023 IPPS proposed rule. For the most current files, refer to the following: https://www.cms.gov/Medicare/Medicare-Fee-for-Service-Payment/AcuteInpatientPPS/MS-DRG-Classifications-and-Software.

HAC 08: Surgical Site Infection of Mediastinitis After Coronary Bypass Graft (CABG) Procedures

Secondary diagnosis not POA:

J98.51	Mediastinitis
J98.59	Other diseases of mediastinum, not elsewhere classified

AND

Any of the following procedures:

0210083	Bypass Coronary Artery, One Artery from Coronary Artery with Zooplastic Tissue, Open Approach
0210088	Bypass Coronary Artery, One Artery from Right Internal Mammary with Zooplastic Tissue, Open Approach
0210089	Bypass Coronary Artery, One Artery from Left Internal Mammary with Zooplastic Tissue, Open Approach
021008C	Bypass Coronary Artery, One Artery from Thoracic Artery with Zooplastic Tissue, Open Approach
021008F	Bypass Coronary Artery, One Artery from Abdominal Artery with Zooplastic Tissue, Open Approach
021008W	Bypass Coronary Artery, One Artery from Aorta with Zooplastic Tissue, Open Approach
0210093	Bypass Coronary Artery, One Artery from Coronary Artery with Autologous Venous Tissue, Open Approach
0210098	Bypass Coronary Artery, One Artery from Right Internal Mammary with Autologous Venous Tissue, Open Approach
0210099	Bypass Coronary Artery, One Artery from Left Internal Mammary with Autologous Venous Tissue, Open Approach
021009C	Bypass Coronary Artery, One Artery from Thoracic Artery with Autologous Venous Tissue, Open Approach
021009F	Bypass Coronary Artery, One Artery from Abdominal Artery with Autologous Venous Tissue, Open Approach
021009W	Bypass Coronary Artery, One Artery from Aorta with Autologous Venous Tissue, Open Approach
02100A3	Bypass Coronary Artery, One Artery from Coronary Artery with Autologous Arterial Tissue, Open Approach
02100A8	Bypass Coronary Artery, One Artery from Right Internal Mammary with Autologous Arterial Tissue, Open Approach
02100A9	Bypass Coronary Artery, One Artery from Left Internal Mammary with Autologous Arterial Tissue, Open Approach
02100AC	Bypass Coronary Artery, One Artery from Thoracic Artery with Autologous Arterial Tissue, Open Approach
02100AF	Bypass Coronary Artery, One Artery from Abdominal Artery with Autologous Arterial Tissue, Open Approach
02100AW	Bypass Coronary Artery, One Artery from Aorta with Autologous Arterial Tissue, Open Approach

02100J3	Bypass Coronary Artery, One Artery from Coronary Artery with Synthetic Substitute, Open Approach
02100J8	Bypass Coronary Artery, One Artery from Right Internal Mammary with Synthetic Substitute, Open Approach
02100J9	Bypass Coronary Artery, One Artery from Left Internal Mammary with Synthetic Substitute, Open Approach
02100JC	Bypass Coronary Artery, One Artery from Thoracic Artery with Synthetic Substitute, Open Approach
02100JF	Bypass Coronary Artery, One Artery from Abdominal Artery with Synthetic Substitute, Open Approach
02100JW	Bypass Coronary Artery, One Artery from Aorta with Synthetic Substitute, Open Approach
02100K3	Bypass Coronary Artery, One Artery from Coronary Artery with Nonautologous Tissue Substitute, Open Approach
02100K8	Bypass Coronary Artery, One Artery from Right Internal Mammary with Nonautologous Tissue Substitute, Open Approach
02100K9	Bypass Coronary Artery, One Artery from Left Internal Mammary with Nonautologous Tissue Substitute, Open Approach
02100KC	Bypass Coronary Artery, One Artery from Thoracic Artery with Nonautologous Tissue Substitute, Open Approach
02100KF	Bypass Coronary Artery, One Artery from Abdominal Artery with Nonautologous Tissue Substitute, Open Approach
02100KW	Bypass Coronary Artery, One Artery from Aorta with Nonautologous Tissue Substitute, Open Approach
02100Z3	Bypass Coronary Artery, One Artery from Coronary Artery, Open Approach
02100Z8	Bypass Coronary Artery, One Artery from Right Internal Mammary, Open Approach
02100Z9	Bypass Coronary Artery, One Artery from Left Internal Mammary, Open Approach
02100ZC	Bypass Coronary Artery, One Artery from Thoracic Artery, Open Approach
02100ZF	Bypass Coronary Artery, One Artery from Abdominal Artery, Open Approach
0210483	Bypass Coronary Artery, One Artery from Coronary Artery with Zooplastic Tissue, Percutaneous Endoscopic Approach
0210488	Bypass Coronary Artery, One Artery from Right Internal Mammary with Zooplastic Tissue, Percutaneous Endoscopic Approach
0210489	Bypass Coronary Artery, One Artery from Left Internal Mammary with Zooplastic Tissue, Percutaneous Endoscopic Approach

021048C	Bypass Coronary Artery, One Artery from Thoracic Artery with Zooplastic Tissue, Percutaneous Endoscopic Approach
021048F	Bypass Coronary Artery, One Artery from Abdominal Artery with Zooplastic Tissue, Percutaneous Endoscopic Approach
021048W	Bypass Coronary Artery, One Artery from Aorta with Zooplastic Tissue, Percutaneous Endoscopic Approach
0210493	Bypass Coronary Artery, One Artery from Coronary Artery with Autologous Venous Tissue, Percutaneous Endoscopic Approach
0210498	Bypass Coronary Artery, One Artery from Right Internal Mammary with Autologous Venous Tissue, Percutaneous Endoscopic Approach
0210499	Bypass Coronary Artery, One Artery from Left Internal Mammary with Autologous Venous Tissue, Percutaneous Endoscopic Approach
021049C	Bypass Coronary Artery, One Artery from Thoracic Artery with Autologous Venous Tissue, Percutaneous Endoscopic Approach
021049F	Bypass Coronary Artery, One Artery from Abdominal Artery with Autologous Venous Tissue, Percutaneous Endoscopic Approach
021049W	Bypass Coronary Artery, One Artery from Aorta with Autologous Venous Tissue, Percutaneous Endoscopic Approach
02104A3	Bypass Coronary Artery, One Artery from Coronary Artery with Autologous Arterial Tissue, Percutaneous Endoscopic Approach
02104A8	Bypass Coronary Artery, One Artery from Right Internal Mammary with Autologous Arterial Tissue, Percutaneous Endoscopic Approach
02104A9	Bypass Coronary Artery, One Artery from Left Internal Mammary with Autologous Arterial Tissue, Percutaneous Endoscopic Approach
02104AC	Bypass Coronary Artery, One Artery from Thoracic Artery with Autologous Arterial Tissue, Percutaneous Endoscopic Approach
02104AF	Bypass Coronary Artery, One Artery from Abdominal Artery with Autologous Arterial Tissue, Percutaneous Endoscopic Approach
02104AW	Bypass Coronary Artery, One Artery from Aorta with Autologous Arterial Tissue, Percutaneous Endoscopic Approach
02104J3	Bypass Coronary Artery, One Artery from Coronary Artery with Synthetic Substitute, Percutaneous Endoscopic Approach

HAC 08: Surgical Site Infection of Mediastinitis After Coronary Bypass Graft (CABG) Procedures (continued)

02104J8　Bypass Coronary Artery, One Artery from Right Internal Mammary with Synthetic Substitute, Percutaneous Endoscopic Approach

02104J9　Bypass Coronary Artery, One Artery from Left Internal Mammary with Synthetic Substitute, Percutaneous Endoscopic Approach

02104JC　Bypass Coronary Artery, One Artery from Thoracic Artery with Synthetic Substitute, Percutaneous Endoscopic Approach

02104JF　Bypass Coronary Artery, One Artery from Abdominal Artery with Synthetic Substitute, Percutaneous Endoscopic Approach

02104JW　Bypass Coronary Artery, One Artery from Aorta with Synthetic Substitute, Percutaneous Endoscopic Approach

02104K3　Bypass Coronary Artery, One Artery from Coronary Artery with Nonautologous Tissue Substitute, Percutaneous Endoscopic Approach

02104K8　Bypass Coronary Artery, One Artery from Right Internal Mammary with Nonautologous Tissue Substitute, Percutaneous Endoscopic Approach

02104K9　Bypass Coronary Artery, One Artery from Left Internal Mammary with Nonautologous Tissue Substitute, Percutaneous Endoscopic Approach

02104KC　Bypass Coronary Artery, One Artery from Thoracic Artery with Nonautologous Tissue Substitute, Percutaneous Endoscopic Approach

02104KF　Bypass Coronary Artery, One Artery from Abdominal Artery with Nonautologous Tissue Substitute, Percutaneous Endoscopic Approach

02104KW　Bypass Coronary Artery, One Artery from Aorta with Nonautologous Tissue Substitute, Percutaneous Endoscopic Approach

02104Z3　Bypass Coronary Artery, One Artery from Coronary Artery, Percutaneous Endoscopic Approach

02104Z8　Bypass Coronary Artery, One Artery from Right Internal Mammary, Percutaneous Endoscopic Approach

02104Z9　Bypass Coronary Artery, One Artery from Left Internal Mammary, Percutaneous Endoscopic Approach

02104ZC　Bypass Coronary Artery, One Artery from Thoracic Artery, Percutaneous Endoscopic Approach

02104ZF　Bypass Coronary Artery, One Artery from Abdominal Artery, Percutaneous Endoscopic Approach

0211083　Bypass Coronary Artery, Two Arteries from Coronary Artery with Zooplastic Tissue, Open Approach

0211088　Bypass Coronary Artery, Two Arteries from Right Internal Mammary with Zooplastic Tissue, Open Approach

0211089　Bypass Coronary Artery, Two Arteries from Left Internal Mammary with Zooplastic Tissue, Open Approach

021108C　Bypass Coronary Artery, Two Arteries from Thoracic Artery with Zooplastic Tissue, Open Approach

021108F　Bypass Coronary Artery, Two Arteries from Abdominal Artery with Zooplastic Tissue, Open Approach

021108W　Bypass Coronary Artery, Two Arteries from Aorta with Zooplastic Tissue, Open Approach

0211093　Bypass Coronary Artery, Two Arteries from Coronary Artery with Autologous Venous Tissue, Open Approach

0211098　Bypass Coronary Artery, Two Arteries from Right Internal Mammary with Autologous Venous Tissue, Open Approach

0211099　Bypass Coronary Artery, Two Arteries from Left Internal Mammary with Autologous Venous Tissue, Open Approach

021109C　Bypass Coronary Artery, Two Arteries from Thoracic Artery with Autologous Venous Tissue, Open Approach

021109F　Bypass Coronary Artery, Two Arteries from Abdominal Artery with Autologous Venous Tissue, Open Approach

021109W　Bypass Coronary Artery, Two Arteries from Aorta with Autologous Venous Tissue, Open Approach

02110A3　Bypass Coronary Artery, Two Arteries from Coronary Artery with Autologous Arterial Tissue, Open Approach

02110A8　Bypass Coronary Artery, Two Arteries from Right Internal Mammary with Autologous Arterial Tissue, Open Approach

02110A9　Bypass Coronary Artery, Two Arteries from Left Internal Mammary with Autologous Arterial Tissue, Open Approach

02110AC　Bypass Coronary Artery, Two Arteries from Thoracic Artery with Autologous Arterial Tissue, Open Approach

02110AF　Bypass Coronary Artery, Two Arteries from Abdominal Artery with Autologous Arterial Tissue, Open Approach

02110AW　Bypass Coronary Artery, Two Arteries from Aorta with Autologous Arterial Tissue, Open Approach

02110J3　Bypass Coronary Artery, Two Arteries from Coronary Artery with Synthetic Substitute, Open Approach

02110J8　Bypass Coronary Artery, Two Arteries from Right Internal Mammary with Synthetic Substitute, Open Approach

02110J9　Bypass Coronary Artery, Two Arteries from Left Internal Mammary with Synthetic Substitute, Open Approach

02110JC　Bypass Coronary Artery, Two Arteries from Thoracic Artery with Synthetic Substitute, Open Approach

02110JF　Bypass Coronary Artery, Two Arteries from Abdominal Artery with Synthetic Substitute, Open Approach

02110JW　Bypass Coronary Artery, Two Arteries from Aorta with Synthetic Substitute, Open Approach

02110K3　Bypass Coronary Artery, Two Arteries from Coronary Artery with Nonautologous Tissue Substitute, Open Approach

02110K8　Bypass Coronary Artery, Two Arteries from Right Internal Mammary with Nonautologous Tissue Substitute, Open Approach

02110K9　Bypass Coronary Artery, Two Arteries from Left Internal Mammary with Nonautologous Tissue Substitute, Open Approach

02110KC　Bypass Coronary Artery, Two Arteries from Thoracic Artery with Nonautologous Tissue Substitute, Open Approach

02110KF　Bypass Coronary Artery, Two Arteries from Abdominal Artery with Nonautologous Tissue Substitute, Open Approach

02110KW　Bypass Coronary Artery, Two Arteries from Aorta with Nonautologous Tissue Substitute, Open Approach

02110Z3　Bypass Coronary Artery, Two Arteries from Coronary Artery, Open Approach

02110Z8　Bypass Coronary Artery, Two Arteries from Right Internal Mammary, Open Approach

02110Z9　Bypass Coronary Artery, Two Arteries from Left Internal Mammary, Open Approach

02110ZC　Bypass Coronary Artery, Two Arteries from Thoracic Artery, Open Approach

02110ZF　Bypass Coronary Artery, Two Arteries from Abdominal Artery, Open Approach

0211483　Bypass Coronary Artery, Two Arteries from Coronary Artery with Zooplastic Tissue, Percutaneous Endoscopic Approach

0211488　Bypass Coronary Artery, Two Arteries from Right Internal Mammary with Zooplastic Tissue, Percutaneous Endoscopic Approach

0211489　Bypass Coronary Artery, Two Arteries from Left Internal Mammary with Zooplastic Tissue, Percutaneous Endoscopic Approach

021148C　Bypass Coronary Artery, Two Arteries from Thoracic Artery with Zooplastic Tissue, Percutaneous Endoscopic Approach

021148F　Bypass Coronary Artery, Two Arteries from Abdominal Artery with Zooplastic Tissue, Percutaneous Endoscopic Approach

021148W　Bypass Coronary Artery, Two Arteries from Aorta with Zooplastic Tissue, Percutaneous Endoscopic Approach

0211493　Bypass Coronary Artery, Two Arteries from Coronary Artery with Autologous Venous Tissue, Percutaneous Endoscopic Approach

0211498　Bypass Coronary Artery, Two Arteries from Right Internal Mammary with Autologous Venous Tissue, Percutaneous Endoscopic Approach

0211499　Bypass Coronary Artery, Two Arteries from Left Internal Mammary with Autologous Venous Tissue, Percutaneous Endoscopic Approach

021149C　Bypass Coronary Artery, Two Arteries from Thoracic Artery with Autologous Venous Tissue, Percutaneous Endoscopic Approach

021149F　Bypass Coronary Artery, Two Arteries from Abdominal Artery with Autologous Venous Tissue, Percutaneous Endoscopic Approach

021149W　Bypass Coronary Artery, Two Arteries from Aorta with Autologous Venous Tissue, Percutaneous Endoscopic Approach

02114A3　Bypass Coronary Artery, Two Arteries from Coronary Artery with Autologous Arterial Tissue, Percutaneous Endoscopic Approach

02114A8　Bypass Coronary Artery, Two Arteries from Right Internal Mammary with Autologous Arterial Tissue, Percutaneous Endoscopic Approach

02114A9　Bypass Coronary Artery, Two Arteries from Left Internal Mammary with Autologous Arterial Tissue, Percutaneous Endoscopic Approach

02114AC　Bypass Coronary Artery, Two Arteries from Thoracic Artery with Autologous Arterial Tissue, Percutaneous Endoscopic Approach

02114AF　Bypass Coronary Artery, Two Arteries from Abdominal Artery with Autologous Arterial Tissue, Percutaneous Endoscopic Approach

HAC 08: Surgical Site Infection of Mediastinitis After Coronary Bypass Graft (CABG) Procedures (continued)

02114AW Bypass Coronary Artery, Two Arteries from Aorta with Autologous Arterial Tissue, Percutaneous Endoscopic Approach

02114J3 Bypass Coronary Artery, Two Arteries from Coronary Artery with Synthetic Substitute, Percutaneous Endoscopic Approach

02114J8 Bypass Coronary Artery, Two Arteries from Right Internal Mammary with Synthetic Substitute, Percutaneous Endoscopic Approach

02114J9 Bypass Coronary Artery, Two Arteries from Left Internal Mammary with Synthetic Substitute, Percutaneous Endoscopic Approach

02114JC Bypass Coronary Artery, Two Arteries from Thoracic Artery with Synthetic Substitute, Percutaneous Endoscopic Approach

02114JF Bypass Coronary Artery, Two Arteries from Abdominal Artery with Synthetic Substitute, Percutaneous Endoscopic Approach

02114JW Bypass Coronary Artery, Two Arteries from Aorta with Synthetic Substitute, Percutaneous Endoscopic Approach

02114K3 Bypass Coronary Artery, Two Arteries from Coronary Artery with Nonautologous Tissue Substitute, Percutaneous Endoscopic Approach

02114K8 Bypass Coronary Artery, Two Arteries from Right Internal Mammary with Nonautologous Tissue Substitute, Percutaneous Endoscopic Approach

02114K9 Bypass Coronary Artery, Two Arteries from Left Internal Mammary with Nonautologous Tissue Substitute, Percutaneous Endoscopic Approach

02114KC Bypass Coronary Artery, Two Arteries from Thoracic Artery with Nonautologous Tissue Substitute, Percutaneous Endoscopic Approach

02114KF Bypass Coronary Artery, Two Arteries from Abdominal Artery with Nonautologous Tissue Substitute, Percutaneous Endoscopic Approach

02114KW Bypass Coronary Artery, Two Arteries from Aorta with Nonautologous Tissue Substitute, Percutaneous Endoscopic Approach

02114Z3 Bypass Coronary Artery, Two Arteries from Coronary Artery, Percutaneous Endoscopic Approach

02114Z8 Bypass Coronary Artery, Two Arteries from Right Internal Mammary, Percutaneous Endoscopic Approach

02114Z9 Bypass Coronary Artery, Two Arteries from Left Internal Mammary, Percutaneous Endoscopic Approach

02114ZC Bypass Coronary Artery, Two Arteries from Thoracic Artery, Percutaneous Endoscopic Approach

02114ZF Bypass Coronary Artery, Two Arteries from Abdominal Artery, Percutaneous Endoscopic Approach

02120B3 Bypass Coronary Artery, Three Arteries from Coronary Artery with Zooplastic Tissue, Open Approach

02120B8 Bypass Coronary Artery, Three Arteries from Right Internal Mammary with Zooplastic Tissue, Open Approach

02120B9 Bypass Coronary Artery, Three Arteries from Left Internal Mammary with Zooplastic Tissue, Open Approach

02120BC Bypass Coronary Artery, Three Arteries from Thoracic Artery with Zooplastic Tissue, Open Approach

02120BF Bypass Coronary Artery, Three Arteries from Abdominal Artery with Zooplastic Tissue, Open Approach

02120BW Bypass Coronary Artery, Three Arteries from Aorta with Zooplastic Tissue, Open Approach

02120B3 Bypass Coronary Artery, Three Arteries from Coronary Artery with Autologous Venous Tissue, Open Approach

02120B8 Bypass Coronary Artery, Three Arteries from Right Internal Mammary with Autologous Venous Tissue, Open Approach

02120B9 Bypass Coronary Artery, Three Arteries from Left Internal Mammary with Autologous Venous Tissue, Open Approach

02120BC Bypass Coronary Artery, Three Arteries from Thoracic Artery with Autologous Venous Tissue, Open Approach

02120BF Bypass Coronary Artery, Three Arteries from Abdominal Artery with Autologous Venous Tissue, Open Approach

02120BW Bypass Coronary Artery, Three Arteries from Aorta with Autologous Venous Tissue, Open Approach

02120A3 Bypass Coronary Artery, Three Arteries from Coronary Artery with Autologous Arterial Tissue, Open Approach

02120A8 Bypass Coronary Artery, Three Arteries from Right Internal Mammary with Autologous Arterial Tissue, Open Approach

02120A9 Bypass Coronary Artery, Three Arteries from Left Internal Mammary with Autologous Arterial Tissue, Open Approach

02120AC Bypass Coronary Artery, Three Arteries from Thoracic Artery with Autologous Arterial Tissue, Open Approach

02120AF Bypass Coronary Artery, Three Arteries from Abdominal Artery with Autologous Arterial Tissue, Open Approach

02120AW Bypass Coronary Artery, Three Arteries from Aorta with Autologous Arterial Tissue, Open Approach

02120J3 Bypass Coronary Artery, Three Arteries from Coronary Artery with Synthetic Substitute, Open Approach

02120J8 Bypass Coronary Artery, Three Arteries from Right Internal Mammary with Synthetic Substitute, Open Approach

02120J9 Bypass Coronary Artery, Three Arteries from Left Internal Mammary with Synthetic Substitute, Open Approach

02120JC Bypass Coronary Artery, Three Arteries from Thoracic Artery with Synthetic Substitute, Open Approach

02120JF Bypass Coronary Artery, Three Arteries from Abdominal Artery with Synthetic Substitute, Open Approach

02120JW Bypass Coronary Artery, Three Arteries from Aorta with Synthetic Substitute, Open Approach

02120K3 Bypass Coronary Artery, Three Arteries from Coronary Artery with Nonautologous Tissue Substitute, Open Approach

02120K8 Bypass Coronary Artery, Three Arteries from Right Internal Mammary with Nonautologous Tissue Substitute, Open Approach

02120K9 Bypass Coronary Artery, Three Arteries from Left Internal Mammary with Nonautologous Tissue Substitute, Open Approach

02120KC Bypass Coronary Artery, Three Arteries from Thoracic Artery with Nonautologous Tissue Substitute, Open Approach

02120KF Bypass Coronary Artery, Three Arteries from Abdominal Artery with Nonautologous Tissue Substitute, Open Approach

02120KW Bypass Coronary Artery, Three Arteries from Aorta with Nonautologous Tissue Substitute, Open Approach

02120Z3 Bypass Coronary Artery, Three Arteries from Coronary Artery, Open Approach

02120Z8 Bypass Coronary Artery, Three Arteries from Right Internal Mammary, Open Approach

02120Z9 Bypass Coronary Artery, Three Arteries from Left Internal Mammary, Open Approach

02120ZC Bypass Coronary Artery, Three Arteries from Thoracic Artery, Open Approach

02120ZF Bypass Coronary Artery, Three Arteries from Abdominal Artery, Open Approach

02124B3 Bypass Coronary Artery, Three Arteries from Coronary Artery with Zooplastic Tissue, Percutaneous Endoscopic Approach

02124B8 Bypass Coronary Artery, Three Arteries from Right Internal Mammary with Zooplastic Tissue, Percutaneous Endoscopic Approach

02124B9 Bypass Coronary Artery, Three Arteries from Left Internal Mammary with Zooplastic Tissue, Percutaneous Endoscopic Approach

02124BC Bypass Coronary Artery, Three Arteries from Thoracic Artery with Zooplastic Tissue, Percutaneous Endoscopic Approach

02124BF Bypass Coronary Artery, Three Arteries from Abdominal Artery with Zooplastic Tissue, Percutaneous Endoscopic Approach

02124BW Bypass Coronary Artery, Three Arteries from Aorta with Zooplastic Tissue, Percutaneous Endoscopic Approach

02124B3 Bypass Coronary Artery, Three Arteries from Coronary Artery with Autologous Venous Tissue, Percutaneous Endoscopic Approach

02124B8 Bypass Coronary Artery, Three Arteries from Right Internal Mammary with Autologous Venous Tissue, Percutaneous Endoscopic Approach

02124B9 Bypass Coronary Artery, Three Arteries from Left Internal Mammary with Autologous Venous Tissue, Percutaneous Endoscopic Approach

02124BC Bypass Coronary Artery, Three Arteries from Thoracic Artery with Autologous Venous Tissue, Percutaneous Endoscopic Approach

02124BF Bypass Coronary Artery, Three Arteries from Abdominal Artery with Autologous Venous Tissue, Percutaneous Endoscopic Approach

02124BW Bypass Coronary Artery, Three Arteries from Aorta with Autologous Venous Tissue, Percutaneous Endoscopic Approach

02124A3 Bypass Coronary Artery, Three Arteries from Coronary Artery with Autologous Arterial Tissue, Percutaneous Endoscopic Approach

HAC 08: Surgical Site Infection of Mediastinitis After Coronary Bypass Graft (CABG) Procedures (continued)

Ø2124A8 Bypass Coronary Artery, Three Arteries from Right Internal Mammary with Autologous Arterial Tissue, Percutaneous Endoscopic Approach

Ø2124A9 Bypass Coronary Artery, Three Arteries from Left Internal Mammary with Autologous Arterial Tissue, Percutaneous Endoscopic Approach

Ø2124AC Bypass Coronary Artery, Three Arteries from Thoracic Artery with Autologous Arterial Tissue, Percutaneous Endoscopic Approach

Ø2124AF Bypass Coronary Artery, Three Arteries from Abdominal Artery with Autologous Arterial Tissue, Percutaneous Endoscopic Approach

Ø2124AW Bypass Coronary Artery, Three Arteries from Aorta with Autologous Arterial Tissue, Percutaneous Endoscopic Approach

Ø2124J3 Bypass Coronary Artery, Three Arteries from Coronary Artery with Synthetic Substitute, Percutaneous Endoscopic Approach

Ø2124J8 Bypass Coronary Artery, Three Arteries from Right Internal Mammary with Synthetic Substitute, Percutaneous Endoscopic Approach

Ø2124J9 Bypass Coronary Artery, Three Arteries from Left Internal Mammary with Synthetic Substitute, Percutaneous Endoscopic Approach

Ø2124JC Bypass Coronary Artery, Three Arteries from Thoracic Artery with Synthetic Substitute, Percutaneous Endoscopic Approach

Ø2124JF Bypass Coronary Artery, Three Arteries from Abdominal Artery with Synthetic Substitute, Percutaneous Endoscopic Approach

Ø2124JW Bypass Coronary Artery, Three Arteries from Aorta with Synthetic Substitute, Percutaneous Endoscopic Approach

Ø2124K3 Bypass Coronary Artery, Three Arteries from Coronary Artery with Nonautologous Tissue Substitute, Percutaneous Endoscopic Approach

Ø2124K8 Bypass Coronary Artery, Three Arteries from Right Internal Mammary with Nonautologous Tissue Substitute, Percutaneous Endoscopic Approach

Ø2124K9 Bypass Coronary Artery, Three Arteries from Left Internal Mammary with Nonautologous Tissue Substitute, Percutaneous Endoscopic Approach

Ø2124KC Bypass Coronary Artery, Three Arteries from Thoracic Artery with Nonautologous Tissue Substitute, Percutaneous Endoscopic Approach

Ø2124KF Bypass Coronary Artery, Three Arteries from Abdominal Artery with Nonautologous Tissue Substitute, Percutaneous Endoscopic Approach

Ø2124KW Bypass Coronary Artery, Three Arteries from Aorta with Nonautologous Tissue Substitute, Percutaneous Endoscopic Approach

Ø2124Z3 Bypass Coronary Artery, Three Arteries from Coronary Artery, Percutaneous Endoscopic Approach

Ø2124Z8 Bypass Coronary Artery, Three Arteries from Right Internal Mammary, Percutaneous Endoscopic Approach

Ø2124Z9 Bypass Coronary Artery, Three Arteries from Left Internal Mammary, Percutaneous Endoscopic Approach

Ø2124ZC Bypass Coronary Artery, Three Arteries from Thoracic Artery, Percutaneous Endoscopic Approach

Ø2124ZF Bypass Coronary Artery, Three Arteries from Abdominal Artery, Percutaneous Endoscopic Approach

Ø213Ø83 Bypass Coronary Artery, Four or More Arteries from Coronary Artery with Zooplastic Tissue, Open Approach

Ø213Ø88 Bypass Coronary Artery, Four or More Arteries from Right Internal Mammary with Zooplastic Tissue, Open Approach

Ø213Ø89 Bypass Coronary Artery, Four or More Arteries from Left Internal Mammary with Zooplastic Tissue, Open Approach

Ø213Ø8C Bypass Coronary Artery, Four or More Arteries from Thoracic Artery with Zooplastic Tissue, Open Approach

Ø213Ø8F Bypass Coronary Artery, Four or More Arteries from Abdominal Artery with Zooplastic Tissue, Open Approach

Ø213Ø8W Bypass Coronary Artery, Four or More Arteries from Aorta with Zooplastic Tissue, Open Approach

Ø213Ø93 Bypass Coronary Artery, Four or More Arteries from Coronary Artery with Autologous Venous Tissue, Open Approach

Ø213Ø98 Bypass Coronary Artery, Four or More Arteries from Right Internal Mammary with Autologous Venous Tissue, Open Approach

Ø213Ø99 Bypass Coronary Artery, Four or More Arteries from Left Internal Mammary with Autologous Venous Tissue, Open Approach

Ø213Ø9C Bypass Coronary Artery, Four or More Arteries from Thoracic Artery with Autologous Venous Tissue, Open Approach

Ø213Ø9F Bypass Coronary Artery, Four or More Arteries from Abdominal Artery with Autologous Venous Tissue, Open Approach

Ø213Ø9W Bypass Coronary Artery, Four or More Arteries from Aorta with Autologous Venous Tissue, Open Approach

Ø213ØA3 Bypass Coronary Artery, Four or More Arteries from Coronary Artery with Autologous Arterial Tissue, Open Approach

Ø213ØA8 Bypass Coronary Artery, Four or More Arteries from Right Internal Mammary with Autologous Arterial Tissue, Open Approach

Ø213ØA9 Bypass Coronary Artery, Four or More Arteries from Left Internal Mammary with Autologous Arterial Tissue, Open Approach

Ø213ØAC Bypass Coronary Artery, Four or More Arteries from Thoracic Artery with Autologous Arterial Tissue, Open Approach

Ø213ØAF Bypass Coronary Artery, Four or More Arteries from Abdominal Artery with Autologous Arterial Tissue, Open Approach

Ø213ØAW Bypass Coronary Artery, Four or More Arteries from Aorta with Autologous Arterial Tissue, Open Approach

Ø213ØJ3 Bypass Coronary Artery, Four or More Arteries from Coronary Artery with Synthetic Substitute, Open Approach

Ø213ØJ8 Bypass Coronary Artery, Four or More Arteries from Right Internal Mammary with Synthetic Substitute, Open Approach

Ø213ØJ9 Bypass Coronary Artery, Four or More Arteries from Left Internal Mammary with Synthetic Substitute, Open Approach

Ø213ØJC Bypass Coronary Artery, Four or More Arteries from Thoracic Artery with Synthetic Substitute, Open Approach

Ø213ØJF Bypass Coronary Artery, Four or More Arteries from Abdominal Artery with Synthetic Substitute, Open Approach

Ø213ØJW Bypass Coronary Artery, Four or More Arteries from Aorta with Synthetic Substitute, Open Approach

Ø213ØK3 Bypass Coronary Artery, Four or More Arteries from Coronary Artery with Nonautologous Tissue Substitute, Open Approach

Ø213ØK8 Bypass Coronary Artery, Four or More Arteries from Right Internal Mammary with Nonautologous Tissue Substitute, Open Approach

Ø213ØK9 Bypass Coronary Artery, Four or More Arteries from Left Internal Mammary with Nonautologous Tissue Substitute, Open Approach

Ø213ØKC Bypass Coronary Artery, Four or More Arteries from Thoracic Artery with Nonautologous Tissue Substitute, Open Approach

Ø213ØKF Bypass Coronary Artery, Four or More Arteries from Abdominal Artery with Nonautologous Tissue Substitute, Open Approach

Ø213ØKW Bypass Coronary Artery, Four or More Arteries from Aorta with Nonautologous Tissue Substitute, Open Approach

Ø213ØZ3 Bypass Coronary Artery, Four or More Arteries from Coronary Artery, Open Approach

Ø213ØZ8 Bypass Coronary Artery, Four or More Arteries from Right Internal Mammary, Open Approach

Ø213ØZ9 Bypass Coronary Artery, Four or More Arteries from Left Internal Mammary, Open Approach

Ø213ØZC Bypass Coronary Artery, Four or More Arteries from Thoracic Artery, Open Approach

Ø213ØZF Bypass Coronary Artery, Four or More Arteries from Abdominal Artery, Open Approach

Ø213483 Bypass Coronary Artery, Four or More Arteries from Coronary Artery with Zooplastic Tissue, Percutaneous Endoscopic Approach

Ø213488 Bypass Coronary Artery, Four or More Arteries from Right Internal Mammary with Zooplastic Tissue, Percutaneous Endoscopic Approach

Ø213489 Bypass Coronary Artery, Four or More Arteries from Left Internal Mammary with Zooplastic Tissue, Percutaneous Endoscopic Approach

Ø21348C Bypass Coronary Artery, Four or More Arteries from Thoracic Artery with Zooplastic Tissue, Percutaneous Endoscopic Approach

Ø21348F Bypass Coronary Artery, Four or More Arteries from Abdominal Artery with Zooplastic Tissue, Percutaneous Endoscopic Approach

Ø21348W Bypass Coronary Artery, Four or More Arteries from Aorta with Zooplastic Tissue, Percutaneous Endoscopic Approach

HAC 08: Surgical Site Infection of Mediastinitis After Coronary Bypass Graft (CABG) Procedures (continued)

Ø213493   Bypass Coronary Artery, Four or More Arteries from Coronary Artery with Autologous Venous Tissue, Percutaneous Endoscopic Approach

Ø213498   Bypass Coronary Artery, Four or More Arteries from Right Internal Mammary with Autologous Venous Tissue, Percutaneous Endoscopic Approach

Ø213499   Bypass Coronary Artery, Four or More Arteries from Left Internal Mammary with Autologous Venous Tissue, Percutaneous Endoscopic Approach

Ø21349C   Bypass Coronary Artery, Four or More Arteries from Thoracic Artery with Autologous Venous Tissue, Percutaneous Endoscopic Approach

Ø21349F   Bypass Coronary Artery, Four or More Arteries from Abdominal Artery with Autologous Venous Tissue, Percutaneous Endoscopic Approach

Ø21349W   Bypass Coronary Artery, Four or More Arteries from Aorta with Autologous Venous Tissue, Percutaneous Endoscopic Approach

Ø2134A3   Bypass Coronary Artery, Four or More Arteries from Coronary Artery with Autologous Arterial Tissue, Percutaneous Endoscopic Approach

Ø2134A8   Bypass Coronary Artery, Four or More Arteries from Right Internal Mammary with Autologous Arterial Tissue, Percutaneous Endoscopic Approach

Ø2134A9   Bypass Coronary Artery, Four or More Arteries from Left Internal Mammary with Autologous Arterial Tissue, Percutaneous Endoscopic Approach

Ø2134AC   Bypass Coronary Artery, Four or More Arteries from Thoracic Artery with Autologous Arterial Tissue, Percutaneous Endoscopic Approach

Ø2134AF   Bypass Coronary Artery, Four or More Arteries from Abdominal Artery with Autologous Arterial Tissue, Percutaneous Endoscopic Approach

Ø2134AW   Bypass Coronary Artery, Four or More Arteries from Aorta with Autologous Arterial Tissue, Percutaneous Endoscopic Approach

Ø2134J3   Bypass Coronary Artery, Four or More Arteries from Coronary Artery with Synthetic Substitute, Percutaneous Endoscopic Approach

Ø2134J8   Bypass Coronary Artery, Four or More Arteries from Right Internal Mammary with Synthetic Substitute, Percutaneous Endoscopic Approach

Ø2134J9   Bypass Coronary Artery, Four or More Arteries from Left Internal Mammary with Synthetic Substitute, Percutaneous Endoscopic Approach

Ø2134JC   Bypass Coronary Artery, Four or More Arteries from Thoracic Artery with Synthetic Substitute, Percutaneous Endoscopic Approach

Ø2134JF   Bypass Coronary Artery, Four or More Arteries from Abdominal Artery with Synthetic Substitute, Percutaneous Endoscopic Approach

Ø2134JW   Bypass Coronary Artery, Four or More Arteries from Aorta with Synthetic Substitute, Percutaneous Endoscopic Approach

Ø2134K3   Bypass Coronary Artery, Four or More Arteries from Coronary Artery with Nonautologous Tissue Substitute, Percutaneous Endoscopic Approach

Ø2134K8   Bypass Coronary Artery, Four or More Arteries from Right Internal Mammary with Nonautologous Tissue Substitute, Percutaneous Endoscopic Approach

Ø2134K9   Bypass Coronary Artery, Four or More Arteries from Left Internal Mammary with Nonautologous Tissue Substitute, Percutaneous Endoscopic Approach

Ø2134KC   Bypass Coronary Artery, Four or More Arteries from Thoracic Artery with Nonautologous Tissue Substitute, Percutaneous Endoscopic Approach

Ø2134KF   Bypass Coronary Artery, Four or More Arteries from Abdominal Artery with Nonautologous Tissue Substitute, Percutaneous Endoscopic Approach

Ø2134KW   Bypass Coronary Artery, Four or More Arteries from Aorta with Nonautologous Tissue Substitute, Percutaneous Endoscopic Approach

Ø2134Z3   Bypass Coronary Artery, Four or More Arteries from Coronary Artery, Percutaneous Endoscopic Approach

Ø2134Z8   Bypass Coronary Artery, Four or More Arteries from Right Internal Mammary, Percutaneous Endoscopic Approach

Ø2134Z9   Bypass Coronary Artery, Four or More Arteries from Left Internal Mammary, Percutaneous Endoscopic Approach

Ø2134ZC   Bypass Coronary Artery, Four or More Arteries from Thoracic Artery, Percutaneous Endoscopic Approach

Ø2134ZF   Bypass Coronary Artery, Four or More Arteries from Abdominal Artery, Percutaneous Endoscopic Approach

HAC 10: Deep Vein Thrombosis (DVT) or Pulmonary Embolism (PE) with Total Knee or Hip Replacement

Secondary diagnosis not POA:

I26.Ø2   Saddle embolus of pulmonary artery with acute cor pulmonale

I26.Ø9   Other pulmonary embolism with acute cor pulmonale

I26.92   Saddle embolus of pulmonary artery without acute cor pulmonale

I26.93   Single subsegmental pulmonary embolism without acute cor pulmonale

I26.94   Multiple subsegmental pulmonary emboli without acute cor pulmonale

I26.99   Other pulmonary embolism without acute cor pulmonale

I82.4Ø1   Acute embolism and thrombosis of unspecified deep veins of right lower extremity

I82.4Ø2   Acute embolism and thrombosis of unspecified deep veins of left lower extremity

I82.4Ø3   Acute embolism and thrombosis of unspecified deep veins of lower extremity, bilateral

I82.4Ø9   Acute embolism and thrombosis of unspecified deep veins of unspecified lower extremity

I82.411   Acute embolism and thrombosis of right femoral vein

I82.412   Acute embolism and thrombosis of left femoral vein

I82.413   Acute embolism and thrombosis of femoral vein, bilateral

I82.419   Acute embolism and thrombosis of unspecified femoral vein

I82.421   Acute embolism and thrombosis of right iliac vein

I82.422   Acute embolism and thrombosis of left iliac vein

I82.423   Acute embolism and thrombosis of iliac vein, bilateral

I82.429   Acute embolism and thrombosis of unspecified iliac vein

I82.431   Acute embolism and thrombosis of right popliteal vein

I82.432   Acute embolism and thrombosis of left popliteal vein

I82.433   Acute embolism and thrombosis of popliteal vein, bilateral

I82.439   Acute embolism and thrombosis of unspecified popliteal vein

I82.441   Acute embolism and thrombosis of right tibial vein

I82.442   Acute embolism and thrombosis of left tibial vein

I82.443   Acute embolism and thrombosis of tibial vein, bilateral

I82.449   Acute embolism and thrombosis of unspecified tibial vein

I82.451   Acute embolism and thrombosis of right peroneal vein

I82.452   Acute embolism and thrombosis of left peroneal vein

I82.453   Acute embolism and thrombosis of peroneal vein, bilateral

I82.459   Acute embolism and thrombosis of unspecified peroneal vein

I82.491   Acute embolism and thrombosis of other specified deep vein of right lower extremity

I82.492   Acute embolism and thrombosis of other specified deep vein of left lower extremity

I82.493   Acute embolism and thrombosis of other specified deep vein of lower extremity, bilateral

I82.499   Acute embolism and thrombosis of other specified deep vein of unspecified lower extremity

I82.4Y1   Acute embolism and thrombosis of unspecified deep veins of right proximal lower extremity

I82.4Y2   Acute embolism and thrombosis of unspecified deep veins of left proximal lower extremity

I82.4Y3   Acute embolism and thrombosis of unspecified deep veins of proximal lower extremity, bilateral

I82.4Y9   Acute embolism and thrombosis of unspecified deep veins of unspecified proximal lower extremity

I82.4Z1   Acute embolism and thrombosis of unspecified deep veins of right distal lower extremity

I82.4Z2   Acute embolism and thrombosis of unspecified deep veins of left distal lower extremity

I82.4Z3   Acute embolism and thrombosis of unspecified deep veins of distal lower extremity, bilateral

I82.4Z9   Acute embolism and thrombosis of unspecified deep veins of unspecified distal lower extremity

AND

Any of the following procedures:

ØSR9Ø19   Replacement of Right Hip Joint with Metal Synthetic Substitute, Cemented, Open Approach

ØSR9Ø1A   Replacement of Right Hip Joint with Metal Synthetic Substitute, Uncemented, Open Approach

HAC 10: Deep Vein Thrombosis (DVT) or Pulmonary Embolism (PE) with Total Knee or Hip Replacement (continued)

ØSR901Z   Replacement of Right Hip Joint with Metal Synthetic Substitute, Open Approach

ØSR9029   Replacement of Right Hip Joint with Metal on Polyethylene Synthetic Substitute, Cemented, Open Approach

ØSR902A   Replacement of Right Hip Joint with Metal on Polyethylene Synthetic Substitute, Uncemented, Open Approach

ØSR902Z   Replacement of Right Hip Joint with Metal on Polyethylene Synthetic Substitute, Open Approach

ØSR9039   Replacement of Right Hip Joint with Ceramic Synthetic Substitute, Cemented, Open Approach

ØSR903A   Replacement of Right Hip Joint with Ceramic Synthetic Substitute, Uncemented, Open Approach

ØSR903Z   Replacement of Right Hip Joint with Ceramic Synthetic Substitute, Open Approach

ØSR9049   Replacement of Right Hip Joint with Ceramic on Polyethylene Synthetic Substitute, Cemented, Open Approach

ØSR904A   Replacement of Right Hip Joint with Ceramic on Polyethylene Synthetic Substitute, Uncemented, Open Approach

ØSR904Z   Replacement of Right Hip Joint with Ceramic on Polyethylene Synthetic Substitute, Open Approach

ØSR9069   Replacement of Right Hip Joint with Oxidized Zirconium on Polyethylene Synthetic Substitute, Cemented, Open Approach

ØSR906A   Replacement of Right Hip Joint with Oxidized Zirconium on Polyethylene Synthetic Substitute, Uncemented, Open Approach

ØSR906Z   Replacement of Right Hip Joint with Oxidized Zirconium on Polyethylene Synthetic Substitute, Open Approach

ØSR907Z   Replacement of Right Hip Joint with Autologous Tissue Substitute, Open Approach

ØSR90EZ   Replacement of Right Hip Joint with Articulating Spacer, Open Approach

ØSR90J9   Replacement of Right Hip Joint with Synthetic Substitute, Cemented, Open Approach

ØSR90JA   Replacement of Right Hip Joint with Synthetic Substitute, Uncemented, Open Approach

ØSR90JZ   Replacement of Right Hip Joint with Synthetic Substitute, Open Approach

ØSR90KZ   Replacement of Right Hip Joint with Nonautologous Tissue Substitute, Open Approach

ØSRA009   Replacement of Right Hip Joint, Acetabular Surface with Polyethylene Synthetic Substitute, Cemented, Open Approach

ØSRA00A   Replacement of Right Hip Joint, Acetabular Surface with Polyethylene Synthetic Substitute, Uncemented, Open Approach

ØSRA00Z   Replacement of Right Hip Joint, Acetabular Surface with Polyethylene Synthetic Substitute, Open Approach

ØSRA019   Replacement of Right Hip Joint, Acetabular Surface with Metal Synthetic Substitute, Cemented, Open Approach

ØSRA01A   Replacement of Right Hip Joint, Acetabular Surface with Metal Synthetic Substitute, Uncemented, Open Approach

ØSRA01Z   Replacement of Right Hip Joint, Acetabular Surface with Metal Synthetic Substitute, Open Approach

ØSRA039   Replacement of Right Hip Joint, Acetabular Surface with Ceramic Synthetic Substitute, Cemented, Open Approach

ØSRA03A   Replacement of Right Hip Joint, Acetabular Surface with Ceramic Synthetic Substitute, Uncemented, Open Approach

ØSRA03Z   Replacement of Right Hip Joint, Acetabular Surface with Ceramic Synthetic Substitute, Open Approach

ØSRA07Z   Replacement of Right Hip Joint, Acetabular Surface with Autologous Tissue Substitute, Open Approach

ØSRA0J9   Replacement of Right Hip Joint, Acetabular Surface with Synthetic Substitute, Cemented, Open Approach

ØSRA0JA   Replacement of Right Hip Joint, Acetabular Surface with Synthetic Substitute, Uncemented, Open Approach

ØSRA0JZ   Replacement of Right Hip Joint, Acetabular Surface with Synthetic Substitute, Open Approach

ØSRA0KZ   Replacement of Right Hip Joint, Acetabular Surface with Nonautologous Tissue Substitute, Open Approach

ØSRB019   Replacement of Left Hip Joint with Metal Synthetic Substitute, Cemented, Open Approach

ØSRB01A   Replacement of Left Hip Joint with Metal Synthetic Substitute, Uncemented, Open Approach

ØSRB01Z   Replacement of Left Hip Joint with Metal Synthetic Substitute, Open Approach

ØSRB029   Replacement of Left Hip Joint with Metal on Polyethylene Synthetic Substitute, Cemented, Open Approach

ØSRB02A   Replacement of Left Hip Joint with Metal on Polyethylene Synthetic Substitute, Uncemented, Open Approach

ØSRB02Z   Replacement of Left Hip Joint with Metal on Polyethylene Synthetic Substitute, Open Approach

ØSRB039   Replacement of Left Hip Joint with Ceramic Synthetic Substitute, Cemented, Open Approach

ØSRB03A   Replacement of Left Hip Joint with Ceramic Synthetic Substitute, Uncemented, Open Approach

ØSRB03Z   Replacement of Left Hip Joint with Ceramic Synthetic Substitute, Open Approach

ØSRB049   Replacement of Left Hip Joint with Ceramic on Polyethylene Synthetic Substitute, Cemented, Open Approach

ØSRB04A   Replacement of Left Hip Joint with Ceramic on Polyethylene Synthetic Substitute, Uncemented, Open Approach

ØSRB04Z   Replacement of Left Hip Joint with Ceramic on Polyethylene Synthetic Substitute, Open Approach

ØSRB069   Replacement of Left Hip Joint with Oxidized Zirconium on Polyethylene Synthetic Substitute, Cemented, Open Approach

ØSRB06A   Replacement of Left Hip Joint with Oxidized Zirconium on Polyethylene Synthetic Substitute, Uncemented, Open Approach

ØSRB06Z   Replacement of Left Hip Joint with Oxidized Zirconium on Polyethylene Synthetic Substitute, Open Approach

ØSRB07Z   Replacement of Left Hip Joint with Autologous Tissue Substitute, Open Approach

ØSRB0EZ   Replacement of Left Hip Joint with Articulating Spacer, Open Approach

ØSRB0J9   Replacement of Left Hip Joint with Synthetic Substitute, Cemented, Open Approach

ØSRB0JA   Replacement of Left Hip Joint with Synthetic Substitute, Uncemented, Open Approach

ØSRB0JZ   Replacement of Left Hip Joint with Synthetic Substitute, Open Approach

ØSRB0KZ   Replacement of Left Hip Joint with Nonautologous Tissue Substitute, Open Approach

ØSRC069   Replacement of Right Knee Joint with Oxidized Zirconium on Polyethylene Synthetic Substitute, Cemented, Open Approach

ØSRC06A   Replacement of Right Knee Joint with Oxidized Zirconium on Polyethylene Synthetic Substitute, Uncemented, Open Approach

ØSRC06Z   Replacement of Right Knee Joint with Oxidized Zirconium on Polyethylene Synthetic Substitute, Open Approach

ØSRC07Z   Replacement of Right Knee Joint with Autologous Tissue Substitute, Open Approach

ØSRC0EZ   Replacement of Right Knee Joint with Articulating Spacer, Open Approach

ØSRC0J9   Replacement of Right Knee Joint with Synthetic Substitute, Cemented, Open Approach

ØSRC0JA   Replacement of Right Knee Joint with Synthetic Substitute, Uncemented, Open Approach

ØSRC0JZ   Replacement of Right Knee Joint with Synthetic Substitute, Open Approach

ØSRC0KZ   Replacement of Right Knee Joint with Nonautologous Tissue Substitute, Open Approach

ØSRC0L9   Replacement of Right Knee Joint with Medial Unicondylar Synthetic Substitute, Cemented, Open Approach

ØSRC0LA   Replacement of Right Knee Joint with Medial Unicondylar Synthetic Substitute, Uncemented, Open Approach

ØSRC0LZ   Replacement of Right Knee Joint with Medial Unicondylar Synthetic Substitute, Open Approach

ØSRC0M9   Replacement of Right Knee Joint with Lateral Unicondylar Synthetic Substitute, Cemented, Open Approach

ØSRC0MA   Replacement of Right Knee Joint with Lateral Unicondylar Synthetic Substitute, Uncemented, Open Approach

ØSRC0MZ   Replacement of Right Knee Joint with Lateral Unicondylar Synthetic Substitute, Open Approach

ØSRC0N9   Replacement of Right Knee Joint with Patellofemoral Synthetic Substitute, Cemented, Open Approach

ØSRC0NA   Replacement of Right Knee Joint with Patellofemoral Synthetic Substitute, Uncemented, Open Approach

ØSRC0NZ   Replacement of Right Knee Joint with Patellofemoral Synthetic Substitute, Open Approach

ØSRD069   Replacement of Left Knee Joint with Oxidized Zirconium on Polyethylene Synthetic Substitute, Cemented, Open Approach

ØSRD06A   Replacement of Left Knee Joint with Oxidized Zirconium on Polyethylene Synthetic Substitute, Uncemented, Open Approach

HAC 10: Deep Vein Thrombosis (DVT) or Pulmonary Embolism (PE) with Total Knee or Hip Replacement (continued)

ØSRDØ6Z Replacement of Left Knee Joint with Oxidized Zirconium on Polyethylene Synthetic Substitute, Open Approach

ØSRDØ7Z Replacement of Left Knee Joint with Autologous Tissue Substitute, Open Approach

ØSRDØEZ Replacement of Left Knee Joint with Articulating Spacer, Open Approach

ØSRDØJ9 Replacement of Left Knee Joint with Synthetic Substitute, Cemented, Open Approach

ØSRDØJA Replacement of Left Knee Joint with Synthetic Substitute, Uncemented, Open Approach

ØSRDØJZ Replacement of Left Knee Joint with Synthetic Substitute, Open Approach

ØSRDØKZ Replacement of Left Knee Joint with Nonautologous Tissue Substitute, Open Approach

ØSRDØL9 Replacement of Left Knee Joint with Medial Unicondylar Synthetic Substitute, Cemented, Open Approach

ØSRDØLA Replacement of Left Knee Joint with Medial Unicondylar Synthetic Substitute, Uncemented, Open Approach

ØSRDØLZ Replacement of Left Knee Joint with Medial Unicondylar Synthetic Substitute, Open Approach

ØSRDØM9 Replacement of Left Knee Joint with Lateral Unicondylar Synthetic Substitute, Cemented, Open Approach

ØSRDØMA Replacement of Left Knee Joint with Lateral Unicondylar Synthetic Substitute, Uncemented, Open Approach

ØSRDØMZ Replacement of Left Knee Joint with Lateral Unicondylar Synthetic Substitute, Open Approach

ØSRDØN9 Replacement of Left Knee Joint with Patellofemoral Synthetic Substitute, Cemented, Open Approach

ØSRDØNA Replacement of Left Knee Joint with Patellofemoral Synthetic Substitute, Uncemented, Open Approach

ØSRDØNZ Replacement of Left Knee Joint with Patellofemoral Synthetic Substitute, Open Approach

ØSRE009 Replacement of Left Hip Joint, Acetabular Surface with Polyethylene Synthetic Substitute, Cemented, Open Approach

ØSRE00A Replacement of Left Hip Joint, Acetabular Surface with Polyethylene Synthetic Substitute, Uncemented, Open Approach

ØSRE00Z Replacement of Left Hip Joint, Acetabular Surface with Polyethylene Synthetic Substitute, Open Approach

ØSRE019 Replacement of Left Hip Joint, Acetabular Surface with Metal Synthetic Substitute, Cemented, Open Approach

ØSRE01A Replacement of Left Hip Joint, Acetabular Surface with Metal Synthetic Substitute, Uncemented, Open Approach

ØSRE01Z Replacement of Left Hip Joint, Acetabular Surface with Metal Synthetic Substitute, Open Approach

ØSRE039 Replacement of Left Hip Joint, Acetabular Surface with Ceramic Synthetic Substitute, Cemented, Open Approach

ØSRE03A Replacement of Left Hip Joint, Acetabular Surface with Ceramic Synthetic Substitute, Uncemented, Open Approach

ØSRE03Z Replacement of Left Hip Joint, Acetabular Surface with Ceramic Synthetic Substitute, Open Approach

ØSRE07Z Replacement of Left Hip Joint, Acetabular Surface with Autologous Tissue Substitute, Open Approach

ØSRE0J9 Replacement of Left Hip Joint, Acetabular Surface with Synthetic Substitute, Cemented, Open Approach

ØSRE0JA Replacement of Left Hip Joint, Acetabular Surface with Synthetic Substitute, Uncemented, Open Approach

ØSRE0JZ Replacement of Left Hip Joint, Acetabular Surface with Synthetic Substitute, Open Approach

ØSRE0KZ Replacement of Left Hip Joint, Acetabular Surface with Nonautologous Tissue Substitute, Open Approach

ØSRR019 Replacement of Right Hip Joint, Femoral Surface with Metal Synthetic Substitute, Cemented, Open Approach

ØSRR01A Replacement of Right Hip Joint, Femoral Surface with Metal Synthetic Substitute, Uncemented, Open Approach

ØSRR01Z Replacement of Right Hip Joint, Femoral Surface with Metal Synthetic Substitute, Open Approach

ØSRR039 Replacement of Right Hip Joint, Femoral Surface with Ceramic Synthetic Substitute, Cemented, Open Approach

ØSRR03A Replacement of Right Hip Joint, Femoral Surface with Ceramic Synthetic Substitute, Uncemented, Open Approach

ØSRR03Z Replacement of Right Hip Joint, Femoral Surface with Ceramic Synthetic Substitute, Open Approach

ØSRR07Z Replacement of Right Hip Joint, Femoral Surface with Autologous Tissue Substitute, Open Approach

ØSRR0J9 Replacement of Right Hip Joint, Femoral Surface with Synthetic Substitute, Cemented, Open Approach

ØSRR0JA Replacement of Right Hip Joint, Femoral Surface with Synthetic Substitute, Uncemented, Open Approach

ØSRR0JZ Replacement of Right Hip Joint, Femoral Surface with Synthetic Substitute, Open Approach

ØSRR0KZ Replacement of Right Hip Joint, Femoral Surface with Nonautologous Tissue Substitute, Open Approach

ØSRS019 Replacement of Left Hip Joint, Femoral Surface with Metal Synthetic Substitute, Cemented, Open Approach

ØSRS01A Replacement of Left Hip Joint, Femoral Surface with Metal Synthetic Substitute, Uncemented, Open Approach

ØSRS01Z Replacement of Left Hip Joint, Femoral Surface with Metal Synthetic Substitute, Open Approach

ØSRS039 Replacement of Left Hip Joint, Femoral Surface with Ceramic Synthetic Substitute, Cemented, Open Approach

ØSRS03A Replacement of Left Hip Joint, Femoral Surface with Ceramic Synthetic Substitute, Uncemented, Open Approach

ØSRS03Z Replacement of Left Hip Joint, Femoral Surface with Ceramic Synthetic Substitute, Open Approach

ØSRS07Z Replacement of Left Hip Joint, Femoral Surface with Autologous Tissue Substitute, Open Approach

ØSRS0J9 Replacement of Left Hip Joint, Femoral Surface with Synthetic Substitute, Cemented, Open Approach

ØSRS0JA Replacement of Left Hip Joint, Femoral Surface with Synthetic Substitute, Uncemented, Open Approach

ØSRS0JZ Replacement of Left Hip Joint, Femoral Surface with Synthetic Substitute, Open Approach

ØSRS0KZ Replacement of Left Hip Joint, Femoral Surface with Nonautologous Tissue Substitute, Open Approach

ØSRT07Z Replacement of Right Knee Joint, Femoral Surface with Autologous Tissue Substitute, Open Approach

ØSRT0J9 Replacement of Right Knee Joint, Femoral Surface with Synthetic Substitute, Cemented, Open Approach

ØSRT0JA Replacement of Right Knee Joint, Femoral Surface with Synthetic Substitute, Uncemented, Open Approach

ØSRT0JZ Replacement of Right Knee Joint, Femoral Surface with Synthetic Substitute, Open Approach

ØSRT0KZ Replacement of Right Knee Joint, Femoral Surface with Nonautologous Tissue Substitute, Open Approach

ØSRU07Z Replacement of Left Knee Joint, Femoral Surface with Autologous Tissue Substitute, Open Approach

ØSRU0J9 Replacement of Left Knee Joint, Femoral Surface with Synthetic Substitute, Cemented, Open Approach

ØSRU0JA Replacement of Left Knee Joint, Femoral Surface with Synthetic Substitute, Uncemented, Open Approach

ØSRU0JZ Replacement of Left Knee Joint, Femoral Surface with Synthetic Substitute, Open Approach

ØSRU0KZ Replacement of Left Knee Joint, Femoral Surface with Nonautologous Tissue Substitute, Open Approach

ØSRV07Z Replacement of Right Knee Joint, Tibial Surface with Autologous Tissue Substitute, Open Approach

ØSRV0J9 Replacement of Right Knee Joint, Tibial Surface with Synthetic Substitute, Cemented, Open Approach

ØSRV0JA Replacement of Right Knee Joint, Tibial Surface with Synthetic Substitute, Uncemented, Open Approach

ØSRV0JZ Replacement of Right Knee Joint, Tibial Surface with Synthetic Substitute, Open Approach

ØSRV0KZ Replacement of Right Knee Joint, Tibial Surface with Nonautologous Tissue Substitute, Open Approach

ØSRW07Z Replacement of Left Knee Joint, Tibial Surface with Autologous Tissue Substitute, Open Approach

ØSRW0J9 Replacement of Left Knee Joint, Tibial Surface with Synthetic Substitute, Cemented, Open Approach

ØSRW0JA Replacement of Left Knee Joint, Tibial Surface with Synthetic Substitute, Uncemented, Open Approach

ØSRW0JZ Replacement of Left Knee Joint, Tibial Surface with Synthetic Substitute, Open Approach

ØSRW0KZ Replacement of Left Knee Joint, Tibial Surface with Nonautologous Tissue Substitute, Open Approach

ØSU90BZ Supplement Right Hip Joint with Resurfacing Device, Open Approach

ØSUA0BZ Supplement Right Hip Joint, Acetabular Surface with Resurfacing Device, Open Approach

ØSUB0BZ Supplement Left Hip Joint with Resurfacing Device, Open Approach

ØSUE0BZ Supplement Left Hip Joint, Acetabular Surface with Resurfacing Device, Open Approach

HAC 10: Deep Vein Thrombosis (DVT) or Pulmonary Embolism (PE) with Total Knee or Hip Replacement (continued)

ØSURØBZ Supplement Right Hip Joint, Femoral Surface with Resurfacing Device, Open Approach

ØSUSØBZ Supplement Left Hip Joint, Femoral Surface with Resurfacing Device, Open Approach

XRRGØL8 Replacement of Right Knee Joint with Synthetic Substitute, Lateral Meniscus, Open Approach, New Technology Group 8

XRRGØM8 Replacement of Right Knee Joint with Synthetic Substitute, Medial Meniscus, Open Approach, New Technology Group 8

XRRHØL8 Replacement of Left Knee Joint with Synthetic Substitute, Lateral Meniscus, Open Approach, New Technology Group 8

XRRHØM8 Replacement of Left Knee Joint with Synthetic Substitute, Medial Meniscus, Open Approach, New Technology Group 8

HAC 11: Surgical Site Infection-Bariatric Surgery

Principal diagnosis of:

E66.Ø1 Morbid (severe) obesity due to excess calories

AND

Secondary diagnosis not POA:

K68.11 Postprocedural retroperitoneal abscess
K95.Ø1 Infection due to gastric band procedure
K95.81 Infection due to other bariatric procedure
T81.4ØXA Infection following a procedure, unspecified, initial encounter
T81.41XA Infection following a procedure, superficial incisional surgical site, initial encounter
T81.42XA Infection following a procedure, deep incisional surgical site, initial encounter
T81.43XA Infection following a procedure, organ and space surgical site, initial encounter
T81.44XA Sepsis following a procedure, initial encounter
T81.49XA Infection following a procedure, other surgical site, initial encounter

AND

Any of the following procedures:

ØD16Ø79 Bypass Stomach to Duodenum with Autologous Tissue Substitute, Open Approach

ØD16Ø7A Bypass Stomach to Jejunum with Autologous Tissue Substitute, Open Approach

ØD16Ø7B Bypass Stomach to Ileum with Autologous Tissue Substitute, Open Approach

ØD16Ø7L Bypass Stomach to Transverse Colon with Autologous Tissue Substitute, Open Approach

ØD16ØJ9 Bypass Stomach to Duodenum with Synthetic Substitute, Open Approach

ØD16ØJA Bypass Stomach to Jejunum with Synthetic Substitute, Open Approach

ØD16ØJB Bypass Stomach to Ileum with Synthetic Substitute, Open Approach

ØD16ØJL Bypass Stomach to Transverse Colon with Synthetic Substitute, Open Approach

ØD16ØK9 Bypass Stomach to Duodenum with Nonautologous Tissue Substitute, Open Approach

ØD16ØKA Bypass Stomach to Jejunum with Nonautologous Tissue Substitute, Open Approach

ØD16ØKB Bypass Stomach to Ileum with Nonautologous Tissue Substitute, Open Approach

ØD16ØKL Bypass Stomach to Transverse Colon with Nonautologous Tissue Substitute, Open Approach

ØD16ØZ9 Bypass Stomach to Duodenum, Open Approach

ØD16ØZA Bypass Stomach to Jejunum, Open Approach

ØD16ØZB Bypass Stomach to Ileum, Open Approach

ØD16ØZL Bypass Stomach to Transverse Colon, Open Approach

ØD16479 Bypass Stomach to Duodenum with Autologous Tissue Substitute, Percutaneous Endoscopic Approach

ØD1647A Bypass Stomach to Jejunum with Autologous Tissue Substitute, Percutaneous Endoscopic Approach

ØD1647B Bypass Stomach to Ileum with Autologous Tissue Substitute, Percutaneous Endoscopic Approach

ØD1647L Bypass Stomach to Transverse Colon with Autologous Tissue Substitute, Percutaneous Endoscopic Approach

ØD164J9 Bypass Stomach to Duodenum with Synthetic Substitute, Percutaneous Endoscopic Approach

ØD164JA Bypass Stomach to Jejunum with Synthetic Substitute, Percutaneous Endoscopic Approach

ØD164JB Bypass Stomach to Ileum with Synthetic Substitute, Percutaneous Endoscopic Approach

ØD164JL Bypass Stomach to Transverse Colon with Synthetic Substitute, Percutaneous Endoscopic Approach

ØD164K9 Bypass Stomach to Duodenum with Nonautologous Tissue Substitute, Percutaneous Endoscopic Approach

ØD164KA Bypass Stomach to Jejunum with Nonautologous Tissue Substitute, Percutaneous Endoscopic Approach

ØD164KB Bypass Stomach to Ileum with Nonautologous Tissue Substitute, Percutaneous Endoscopic Approach

ØD164KL Bypass Stomach to Transverse Colon with Nonautologous Tissue Substitute, Percutaneous Endoscopic Approach

ØD164Z9 Bypass Stomach to Duodenum, Percutaneous Endoscopic Approach

ØD164ZA Bypass Stomach to Jejunum, Percutaneous Endoscopic Approach

ØD164ZB Bypass Stomach to Ileum, Percutaneous Endoscopic Approach

ØD164ZL Bypass Stomach to Transverse Colon, Percutaneous Endoscopic Approach

ØD16879 Bypass Stomach to Duodenum with Autologous Tissue Substitute, Via Natural or Artificial Opening Endoscopic

ØD1687A Bypass Stomach to Jejunum with Autologous Tissue Substitute, Via Natural or Artificial Opening Endoscopic

ØD1687B Bypass Stomach to Ileum with Autologous Tissue Substitute, Via Natural or Artificial Opening Endoscopic

ØD1687L Bypass Stomach to Transverse Colon with Autologous Tissue Substitute, Via Natural or Artificial Opening Endoscopic

ØD168J9 Bypass Stomach to Duodenum with Synthetic Substitute, Via Natural or Artificial Opening Endoscopic

ØD168JA Bypass Stomach to Jejunum with Synthetic Substitute, Via Natural or Artificial Opening Endoscopic

ØD168JB Bypass Stomach to Ileum with Synthetic Substitute, Via Natural or Artificial Opening Endoscopic

ØD168JL Bypass Stomach to Transverse Colon with Synthetic Substitute, Via Natural or Artificial Opening Endoscopic

ØD168K9 Bypass Stomach to Duodenum with Nonautologous Tissue Substitute, Via Natural or Artificial Opening Endoscopic

ØD168KA Bypass Stomach to Jejunum with Nonautologous Tissue Substitute, Via Natural or Artificial Opening Endoscopic

ØD168KB Bypass Stomach to Ileum with Nonautologous Tissue Substitute, Via Natural or Artificial Opening Endoscopic

ØD168KL Bypass Stomach to Transverse Colon with Nonautologous Tissue Substitute, Via Natural or Artificial Opening Endoscopic

ØD168Z9 Bypass Stomach to Duodenum, Via Natural or Artificial Opening Endoscopic

ØD168ZA Bypass Stomach to Jejunum, Via Natural or Artificial Opening Endoscopic

ØD168ZB Bypass Stomach to Ileum, Via Natural or Artificial Opening Endoscopic

ØD168ZL Bypass Stomach to Transverse Colon, Via Natural or Artificial Opening Endoscopic

ØDV64CZ Restriction of Stomach with Extraluminal Device, Percutaneous Endoscopic Approach

HAC 12: Surgical Site Infection-Certain Orthopedic Procedures of the Spine, Shoulder, and Elbow

Secondary diagnosis not POA:

K68.11 Postprocedural retroperitoneal abscess
T81.4ØXA Infection following a procedure, unspecified, initial encounter
T81.41XA Infection following a procedure, superficial incisional surgical site, initial encounter
T81.42XA Infection following a procedure, deep incisional surgical site, initial encounter
T81.43XA Infection following a procedure, organ and space surgical site, initial encounter
T81.44XA Sepsis following a procedure, initial encounter
T81.49XA Infection following a procedure, other surgical site, initial encounter
T84.6ØXA Infection and inflammatory reaction due to internal fixation device of unspecified site, initial encounter
T84.61ØA Infection and inflammatory reaction due to internal fixation device of right humerus, initial encounter
T84.611A Infection and inflammatory reaction due to internal fixation device of left humerus, initial encounter
T84.612A Infection and inflammatory reaction due to internal fixation device of right radius, initial encounter
T84.613A Infection and inflammatory reaction due to internal fixation device of left radius, initial encounter
T84.614A Infection and inflammatory reaction due to internal fixation device of right ulna, initial encounter
T84.615A Infection and inflammatory reaction due to internal fixation device of left ulna, initial encounter
T84.619A Infection and inflammatory reaction due to internal fixation device of unspecified bone of arm, initial encounter
T84.63XA Infection and inflammatory reaction due to internal fixation device of spine, initial encounter
T84.69XA Infection and inflammatory reaction due to internal fixation device of other site, initial encounter
T84.7XXA Infection and inflammatory reaction due to other internal orthopedic prosthetic devices, implants and grafts, initial encounter

AND

Any of the following procedures:

ØRGØØ7Ø Fusion of Occipital-cervical Joint with Autologous Tissue Substitute, Anterior Approach, Anterior Column, Open Approach

HAC 12: Surgical Site Infection-Certain Orthopedic Procedures of the Spine, Shoulder, and Elbow (continued)

ØRG0071   Fusion of Occipital-cervical Joint with Autologous Tissue Substitute, Posterior Approach, Posterior Column, Open Approach

ØRG007J   Fusion of Occipital-cervical Joint with Autologous Tissue Substitute, Posterior Approach, Anterior Column, Open Approach

ØRG00A0   Fusion of Occipital-cervical Joint with Interbody Fusion Device, Anterior Approach, Anterior Column, Open Approach

ØRG00AJ   Fusion of Occipital-cervical Joint with Interbody Fusion Device, Posterior Approach, Anterior Column, Open Approach

ØRG00J0   Fusion of Occipital-cervical Joint with Synthetic Substitute, Anterior Approach, Anterior Column, Open Approach

ØRG00J1   Fusion of Occipital-cervical Joint with Synthetic Substitute, Posterior Approach, Posterior Column, Open Approach

ØRG00JJ   Fusion of Occipital-cervical Joint with Synthetic Substitute, Posterior Approach, Anterior Column, Open Approach

ØRG00K0   Fusion of Occipital-cervical Joint with Nonautologous Tissue Substitute, Anterior Approach, Anterior Column, Open Approach

ØRG00K1   Fusion of Occipital-cervical Joint with Nonautologous Tissue Substitute, Posterior Approach, Posterior Column, Open Approach

ØRG00KJ   Fusion of Occipital-cervical Joint with Nonautologous Tissue Substitute, Posterior Approach, Anterior Column, Open Approach

ØRG0370   Fusion of Occipital-cervical Joint with Autologous Tissue Substitute, Anterior Approach, Anterior Column, Percutaneous Approach

ØRG0371   Fusion of Occipital-cervical Joint with Autologous Tissue Substitute, Posterior Approach, Posterior Column, Percutaneous Approach

ØRG037J   Fusion of Occipital-cervical Joint with Autologous Tissue Substitute, Posterior Approach, Anterior Column, Percutaneous Approach

ØRG03A0   Fusion of Occipital-cervical Joint with Interbody Fusion Device, Anterior Approach, Anterior Column, Percutaneous Approach

ØRG03AJ   Fusion of Occipital-cervical Joint with Interbody Fusion Device, Posterior Approach, Anterior Column, Percutaneous Approach

ØRG03J0   Fusion of Occipital-cervical Joint with Synthetic Substitute, Anterior Approach, Anterior Column, Percutaneous Approach

ØRG03J1   Fusion of Occipital-cervical Joint with Synthetic Substitute, Posterior Approach, Posterior Column, Percutaneous Approach

ØRG03JJ   Fusion of Occipital-cervical Joint with Synthetic Substitute, Posterior Approach, Anterior Column, Percutaneous Approach

ØRG03K0   Fusion of Occipital-cervical Joint with Nonautologous Tissue Substitute, Anterior Approach, Anterior Column, Percutaneous Approach

ØRG03K1   Fusion of Occipital-cervical Joint with Nonautologous Tissue Substitute, Posterior Approach, Posterior Column, Percutaneous Approach

ØRG03KJ   Fusion of Occipital-cervical Joint with Nonautologous Tissue Substitute, Posterior Approach, Anterior Column, Percutaneous Approach

ØRG0470   Fusion of Occipital-cervical Joint with Autologous Tissue Substitute, Anterior Approach, Anterior Column, Percutaneous Endoscopic Approach

ØRG0471   Fusion of Occipital-cervical Joint with Autologous Tissue Substitute, Posterior Approach, Posterior Column, Percutaneous Endoscopic Approach

ØRG047J   Fusion of Occipital-cervical Joint with Autologous Tissue Substitute, Posterior Approach, Anterior Column, Percutaneous Endoscopic Approach

ØRG04A0   Fusion of Occipital-cervical Joint with Interbody Fusion Device, Anterior Approach, Anterior Column, Percutaneous Endoscopic Approach

ØRG04AJ   Fusion of Occipital-cervical Joint with Interbody Fusion Device, Posterior Approach, Anterior Column, Percutaneous Endoscopic Approach

ØRG04J0   Fusion of Occipital-cervical Joint with Synthetic Substitute, Anterior Approach, Anterior Column, Percutaneous Endoscopic Approach

ØRG04J1   Fusion of Occipital-cervical Joint with Synthetic Substitute, Posterior Approach, Posterior Column, Percutaneous Endoscopic Approach

ØRG04JJ   Fusion of Occipital-cervical Joint with Synthetic Substitute, Posterior Approach, Anterior Column, Percutaneous Endoscopic Approach

ØRG04K0   Fusion of Occipital-cervical Joint with Nonautologous Tissue Substitute, Anterior Approach, Anterior Column, Percutaneous Endoscopic Approach

ØRG04K1   Fusion of Occipital-cervical Joint with Nonautologous Tissue Substitute, Posterior Approach, Posterior Column, Percutaneous Endoscopic Approach

ØRG04KJ   Fusion of Occipital-cervical Joint with Nonautologous Tissue Substitute, Posterior Approach, Anterior Column, Percutaneous Endoscopic Approach

ØRG1070   Fusion of Cervical Vertebral Joint with Autologous Tissue Substitute, Anterior Approach, Anterior Column, Open Approach

ØRG1071   Fusion of Cervical Vertebral Joint with Autologous Tissue Substitute, Posterior Approach, Posterior Column, Open Approach

ØRG107J   Fusion of Cervical Vertebral Joint with Autologous Tissue Substitute, Posterior Approach, Anterior Column, Open Approach

ØRG10A0   Fusion of Cervical Vertebral Joint with Interbody Fusion Device, Anterior Approach, Anterior Column, Open Approach

ØRG10AJ   Fusion of Cervical Vertebral Joint with Interbody Fusion Device, Posterior Approach, Anterior Column, Open Approach

ØRG10J0   Fusion of Cervical Vertebral Joint with Synthetic Substitute, Anterior Approach, Anterior Column, Open Approach

ØRG10J1   Fusion of Cervical Vertebral Joint with Synthetic Substitute, Posterior Approach, Posterior Column, Open Approach

ØRG10JJ   Fusion of Cervical Vertebral Joint with Synthetic Substitute, Posterior Approach, Anterior Column, Open Approach

ØRG10K0   Fusion of Cervical Vertebral Joint with Nonautologous Tissue Substitute, Anterior Approach, Anterior Column, Open Approach

ØRG10K1   Fusion of Cervical Vertebral Joint with Nonautologous Tissue Substitute, Posterior Approach, Posterior Column, Open Approach

ØRG10KJ   Fusion of Cervical Vertebral Joint with Nonautologous Tissue Substitute, Posterior Approach, Anterior Column, Open Approach

ØRG1370   Fusion of Cervical Vertebral Joint with Autologous Tissue Substitute, Anterior Approach, Anterior Column, Percutaneous Approach

ØRG1371   Fusion of Cervical Vertebral Joint with Autologous Tissue Substitute, Posterior Approach, Posterior Column, Percutaneous Approach

ØRG137J   Fusion of Cervical Vertebral Joint with Autologous Tissue Substitute, Posterior Approach, Anterior Column, Percutaneous Approach

ØRG13A0   Fusion of Cervical Vertebral Joint with Interbody Fusion Device, Anterior Approach, Anterior Column, Percutaneous Approach

ØRG13AJ   Fusion of Cervical Vertebral Joint with Interbody Fusion Device, Posterior Approach, Anterior Column, Percutaneous Approach

ØRG13J0   Fusion of Cervical Vertebral Joint with Synthetic Substitute, Anterior Approach, Anterior Column, Percutaneous Approach

ØRG13J1   Fusion of Cervical Vertebral Joint with Synthetic Substitute, Posterior Approach, Posterior Column, Percutaneous Approach

ØRG13JJ   Fusion of Cervical Vertebral Joint with Synthetic Substitute, Posterior Approach, Anterior Column, Percutaneous Approach

ØRG13K0   Fusion of Cervical Vertebral Joint with Nonautologous Tissue Substitute, Anterior Approach, Anterior Column, Percutaneous Approach

ØRG13K1   Fusion of Cervical Vertebral Joint with Nonautologous Tissue Substitute, Posterior Approach, Posterior Column, Percutaneous Approach

ØRG13KJ   Fusion of Cervical Vertebral Joint with Nonautologous Tissue Substitute, Posterior Approach, Anterior Column, Percutaneous Approach

ØRG1470   Fusion of Cervical Vertebral Joint with Autologous Tissue Substitute, Anterior Approach, Anterior Column, Percutaneous Endoscopic Approach

ØRG1471   Fusion of Cervical Vertebral Joint with Autologous Tissue Substitute, Posterior Approach, Posterior Column, Percutaneous Endoscopic Approach

ØRG147J   Fusion of Cervical Vertebral Joint with Autologous Tissue Substitute, Posterior Approach, Anterior Column, Percutaneous Endoscopic Approach

ØRG14A0   Fusion of Cervical Vertebral Joint with Interbody Fusion Device, Anterior Approach, Anterior Column, Percutaneous Endoscopic Approach

HAC 12: Surgical Site Infection-Certain Orthopedic Procedures of the Spine, Shoulder, and Elbow (continued)

ØRG14AJ Fusion of Cervical Vertebral Joint with Interbody Fusion Device, Posterior Approach, Anterior Column, Percutaneous Endoscopic Approach

ØRG14JØ Fusion of Cervical Vertebral Joint with Synthetic Substitute, Anterior Approach, Anterior Column, Percutaneous Endoscopic Approach

ØRG14J1 Fusion of Cervical Vertebral Joint with Synthetic Substitute, Posterior Approach, Posterior Column, Percutaneous Endoscopic Approach

ØRG14JJ Fusion of Cervical Vertebral Joint with Synthetic Substitute, Posterior Approach, Anterior Column, Percutaneous Endoscopic Approach

ØRG14KØ Fusion of Cervical Vertebral Joint with Nonautologous Tissue Substitute, Anterior Approach, Anterior Column, Percutaneous Endoscopic Approach

ØRG14K1 Fusion of Cervical Vertebral Joint with Nonautologous Tissue Substitute, Posterior Approach, Posterior Column, Percutaneous Endoscopic Approach

ØRG14KJ Fusion of Cervical Vertebral Joint with Nonautologous Tissue Substitute, Posterior Approach, Anterior Column, Percutaneous Endoscopic Approach

ØRG2Ø7Ø Fusion of 2 or more Cervical Vertebral Joints with Autologous Tissue Substitute, Anterior Approach, Anterior Column, Open Approach

ØRG2Ø71 Fusion of 2 or more Cervical Vertebral Joints with Autologous Tissue Substitute, Posterior Approach, Posterior Column, Open Approach

ØRG2Ø7J Fusion of 2 or more Cervical Vertebral Joints with Autologous Tissue Substitute, Posterior Approach, Anterior Column, Open Approach

ØRG2ØAØ Fusion of 2 or more Cervical Vertebral Joints with Interbody Fusion Device, Anterior Approach, Anterior Column, Open Approach

ØRG2ØAJ Fusion of 2 or more Cervical Vertebral Joints with Interbody Fusion Device, Posterior Approach, Anterior Column, Open Approach

ØRG2ØJØ Fusion of 2 or more Cervical Vertebral Joints with Synthetic Substitute, Anterior Approach, Anterior Column, Open Approach

ØRG2ØJ1 Fusion of 2 or more Cervical Vertebral Joints with Synthetic Substitute, Posterior Approach, Posterior Column, Open Approach

ØRG2ØJJ Fusion of 2 or more Cervical Vertebral Joints with Synthetic Substitute, Posterior Approach, Anterior Column, Open Approach

ØRG2ØKØ Fusion of 2 or more Cervical Vertebral Joints with Nonautologous Tissue Substitute, Anterior Approach, Anterior Column, Open Approach

ØRG2ØK1 Fusion of 2 or more Cervical Vertebral Joints with Nonautologous Tissue Substitute, Posterior Approach, Posterior Column, Open Approach

ØRG2ØKJ Fusion of 2 or more Cervical Vertebral Joints with Nonautologous Tissue Substitute, Posterior Approach, Anterior Column, Open Approach

ØRG237Ø Fusion of 2 or more Cervical Vertebral Joints with Autologous Tissue Substitute, Anterior Approach, Anterior Column, Percutaneous Approach

ØRG2371 Fusion of 2 or more Cervical Vertebral Joints with Autologous Tissue Substitute, Posterior Approach, Posterior Column, Percutaneous Approach

ØRG237J Fusion of 2 or more Cervical Vertebral Joints with Autologous Tissue Substitute, Posterior Approach, Anterior Column, Percutaneous Approach

ØRG23AØ Fusion of 2 or more Cervical Vertebral Joints with Interbody Fusion Device, Anterior Approach, Anterior Column, Percutaneous Approach

ØRG23AJ Fusion of 2 or more Cervical Vertebral Joints with Interbody Fusion Device, Posterior Approach, Anterior Column, Percutaneous Approach

ØRG23JØ Fusion of 2 or more Cervical Vertebral Joints with Synthetic Substitute, Anterior Approach, Anterior Column, Percutaneous Approach

ØRG23J1 Fusion of 2 or more Cervical Vertebral Joints with Synthetic Substitute, Posterior Approach, Posterior Column, Percutaneous Approach

ØRG23JJ Fusion of 2 or more Cervical Vertebral Joints with Synthetic Substitute, Posterior Approach, Anterior Column, Percutaneous Approach

ØRG23KØ Fusion of 2 or more Cervical Vertebral Joints with Nonautologous Tissue Substitute, Anterior Approach, Anterior Column, Percutaneous Approach

ØRG23K1 Fusion of 2 or more Cervical Vertebral Joints with Nonautologous Tissue Substitute, Posterior Approach, Posterior Column, Percutaneous Approach

ØRG23KJ Fusion of 2 or more Cervical Vertebral Joints with Nonautologous Tissue Substitute, Posterior Approach, Anterior Column, Percutaneous Approach

ØRG247Ø Fusion of 2 or more Cervical Vertebral Joints with Autologous Tissue Substitute, Anterior Approach, Anterior Column, Percutaneous Endoscopic Approach

ØRG2471 Fusion of 2 or more Cervical Vertebral Joints with Autologous Tissue Substitute, Posterior Approach, Posterior Column, Percutaneous Endoscopic Approach

ØRG247J Fusion of 2 or more Cervical Vertebral Joints with Autologous Tissue Substitute, Posterior Approach, Anterior Column, Percutaneous Endoscopic Approach

ØRG24AØ Fusion of 2 or more Cervical Vertebral Joints with Interbody Fusion Device, Anterior Approach, Anterior Column, Percutaneous Endoscopic Approach

ØRG24AJ Fusion of 2 or more Cervical Vertebral Joints with Interbody Fusion Device, Posterior Approach, Anterior Column, Percutaneous Endoscopic Approach

ØRG24JØ Fusion of 2 or more Cervical Vertebral Joints with Synthetic Substitute, Anterior Approach, Anterior Column, Percutaneous Endoscopic Approach

ØRG24J1 Fusion of 2 or more Cervical Vertebral Joints with Synthetic Substitute, Posterior Approach, Posterior Column, Percutaneous Endoscopic Approach

ØRG24JJ Fusion of 2 or more Cervical Vertebral Joints with Synthetic Substitute, Posterior Approach, Anterior Column, Percutaneous Endoscopic Approach

ØRG24KØ Fusion of 2 or more Cervical Vertebral Joints with Nonautologous Tissue Substitute, Anterior Approach, Anterior Column, Percutaneous Endoscopic Approach

ØRG24K1 Fusion of 2 or more Cervical Vertebral Joints with Nonautologous Tissue Substitute, Posterior Approach, Posterior Column, Percutaneous Endoscopic Approach

ØRG24KJ Fusion of 2 or more Cervical Vertebral Joints with Nonautologous Tissue Substitute, Posterior Approach, Anterior Column, Percutaneous Endoscopic Approach

ØRG4Ø7Ø Fusion of Cervicothoracic Vertebral Joint with Autologous Tissue Substitute, Anterior Approach, Anterior Column, Open Approach

ØRG4Ø71 Fusion of Cervicothoracic Vertebral Joint with Autologous Tissue Substitute, Posterior Approach, Posterior Column, Open Approach

ØRG4Ø7J Fusion of Cervicothoracic Vertebral Joint with Autologous Tissue Substitute, Posterior Approach, Anterior Column, Open Approach

ØRG4ØAØ Fusion of Cervicothoracic Vertebral Joint with Interbody Fusion Device, Anterior Approach, Anterior Column, Open Approach

ØRG4ØAJ Fusion of Cervicothoracic Vertebral Joint with Interbody Fusion Device, Posterior Approach, Anterior Column, Open Approach

ØRG4ØJØ Fusion of Cervicothoracic Vertebral Joint with Synthetic Substitute, Anterior Approach, Anterior Column, Open Approach

ØRG4ØJ1 Fusion of Cervicothoracic Vertebral Joint with Synthetic Substitute, Posterior Approach, Posterior Column, Open Approach

ØRG4ØJJ Fusion of Cervicothoracic Vertebral Joint with Synthetic Substitute, Posterior Approach, Anterior Column, Open Approach

ØRG4ØKØ Fusion of Cervicothoracic Vertebral Joint with Nonautologous Tissue Substitute, Anterior Approach, Anterior Column, Open Approach

ØRG4ØK1 Fusion of Cervicothoracic Vertebral Joint with Nonautologous Tissue Substitute, Posterior Approach, Posterior Column, Open Approach

ØRG4ØKJ Fusion of Cervicothoracic Vertebral Joint with Nonautologous Tissue Substitute, Posterior Approach, Anterior Column, Open Approach

ØRG437Ø Fusion of Cervicothoracic Vertebral Joint with Autologous Tissue Substitute, Anterior Approach, Anterior Column, Percutaneous Approach

ØRG4371 Fusion of Cervicothoracic Vertebral Joint with Autologous Tissue Substitute, Posterior Approach, Posterior Column, Percutaneous Approach

ØRG437J Fusion of Cervicothoracic Vertebral Joint with Autologous Tissue Substitute, Posterior Approach, Anterior Column, Percutaneous Approach

ØRG43AØ Fusion of Cervicothoracic Vertebral Joint with Interbody Fusion Device, Anterior Approach, Anterior Column, Percutaneous Approach

HAC 12: Surgical Site Infection-Certain Orthopedic Procedures of the Spine, Shoulder, and Elbow (continued)

ØRG43AJ Fusion of Cervicothoracic Vertebral Joint with Interbody Fusion Device, Posterior Approach, Anterior Column, Percutaneous Approach

ØRG43J0 Fusion of Cervicothoracic Vertebral Joint with Synthetic Substitute, Anterior Approach, Anterior Column, Percutaneous Approach

ØRG43J1 Fusion of Cervicothoracic Vertebral Joint with Synthetic Substitute, Posterior Approach, Posterior Column, Percutaneous Approach

ØRG43JJ Fusion of Cervicothoracic Vertebral Joint with Synthetic Substitute, Posterior Approach, Anterior Column, Percutaneous Approach

ØRG43K0 Fusion of Cervicothoracic Vertebral Joint with Nonautologous Tissue Substitute, Anterior Approach, Anterior Column, Percutaneous Approach

ØRG43K1 Fusion of Cervicothoracic Vertebral Joint with Nonautologous Tissue Substitute, Posterior Approach, Posterior Column, Percutaneous Approach

ØRG43KJ Fusion of Cervicothoracic Vertebral Joint with Nonautologous Tissue Substitute, Posterior Approach, Anterior Column, Percutaneous Approach

ØRG4470 Fusion of Cervicothoracic Vertebral Joint with Autologous Tissue Substitute, Anterior Approach, Anterior Column, Percutaneous Endoscopic Approach

ØRG4471 Fusion of Cervicothoracic Vertebral Joint with Autologous Tissue Substitute, Posterior Approach, Posterior Column, Percutaneous Endoscopic Approach

ØRG447J Fusion of Cervicothoracic Vertebral Joint with Autologous Tissue Substitute, Posterior Approach, Anterior Column, Percutaneous Endoscopic Approach

ØRG44A0 Fusion of Cervicothoracic Vertebral Joint with Interbody Fusion Device, Anterior Approach, Anterior Column, Percutaneous Endoscopic Approach

ØRG44AJ Fusion of Cervicothoracic Vertebral Joint with Interbody Fusion Device, Posterior Approach, Anterior Column, Percutaneous Endoscopic Approach

ØRG44J0 Fusion of Cervicothoracic Vertebral Joint with Synthetic Substitute, Anterior Approach, Anterior Column, Percutaneous Endoscopic Approach

ØRG44J1 Fusion of Cervicothoracic Vertebral Joint with Synthetic Substitute, Posterior Approach, Posterior Column, Percutaneous Endoscopic Approach

ØRG44JJ Fusion of Cervicothoracic Vertebral Joint with Synthetic Substitute, Posterior Approach, Anterior Column, Percutaneous Endoscopic Approach

ØRG44K0 Fusion of Cervicothoracic Vertebral Joint with Nonautologous Tissue Substitute, Anterior Approach, Anterior Column, Percutaneous Endoscopic Approach

ØRG44K1 Fusion of Cervicothoracic Vertebral Joint with Nonautologous Tissue Substitute, Posterior Approach, Posterior Column, Percutaneous Endoscopic Approach

ØRG44KJ Fusion of Cervicothoracic Vertebral Joint with Nonautologous Tissue Substitute, Posterior Approach, Anterior Column, Percutaneous Endoscopic Approach

ØRG6070 Fusion of Thoracic Vertebral Joint with Autologous Tissue Substitute, Anterior Approach, Anterior Column, Open Approach

ØRG6071 Fusion of Thoracic Vertebral Joint with Autologous Tissue Substitute, Posterior Approach, Posterior Column, Open Approach

ØRG607J Fusion of Thoracic Vertebral Joint with Autologous Tissue Substitute, Posterior Approach, Anterior Column, Open Approach

ØRG60A0 Fusion of Thoracic Vertebral Joint with Interbody Fusion Device, Anterior Approach, Anterior Column, Open Approach

ØRG60AJ Fusion of Thoracic Vertebral Joint with Interbody Fusion Device, Posterior Approach, Anterior Column, Open Approach

ØRG60J0 Fusion of Thoracic Vertebral Joint with Synthetic Substitute, Anterior Approach, Anterior Column, Open Approach

ØRG60J1 Fusion of Thoracic Vertebral Joint with Synthetic Substitute, Posterior Approach, Posterior Column, Open Approach

ØRG60JJ Fusion of Thoracic Vertebral Joint with Synthetic Substitute, Posterior Approach, Anterior Column, Open Approach

ØRG60K0 Fusion of Thoracic Vertebral Joint with Nonautologous Tissue Substitute, Anterior Approach, Anterior Column, Open Approach

ØRG60K1 Fusion of Thoracic Vertebral Joint with Nonautologous Tissue Substitute, Posterior Approach, Posterior Column, Open Approach

ØRG60KJ Fusion of Thoracic Vertebral Joint with Nonautologous Tissue Substitute, Posterior Approach, Anterior Column, Open Approach

ØRG6370 Fusion of Thoracic Vertebral Joint with Autologous Tissue Substitute, Anterior Approach, Anterior Column, Percutaneous Approach

ØRG6371 Fusion of Thoracic Vertebral Joint with Autologous Tissue Substitute, Posterior Approach, Posterior Column, Percutaneous Approach

ØRG637J Fusion of Thoracic Vertebral Joint with Autologous Tissue Substitute, Posterior Approach, Anterior Column, Percutaneous Approach

ØRG63A0 Fusion of Thoracic Vertebral Joint with Interbody Fusion Device, Anterior Approach, Anterior Column, Percutaneous Approach

ØRG63AJ Fusion of Thoracic Vertebral Joint with Interbody Fusion Device, Posterior Approach, Anterior Column, Percutaneous Approach

ØRG63J0 Fusion of Thoracic Vertebral Joint with Synthetic Substitute, Anterior Approach, Anterior Column, Percutaneous Approach

ØRG63J1 Fusion of Thoracic Vertebral Joint with Synthetic Substitute, Posterior Approach, Posterior Column, Percutaneous Approach

ØRG63JJ Fusion of Thoracic Vertebral Joint with Synthetic Substitute, Posterior Approach, Anterior Column, Percutaneous Approach

ØRG63K0 Fusion of Thoracic Vertebral Joint with Nonautologous Tissue Substitute, Anterior Approach, Anterior Column, Percutaneous Approach

ØRG63K1 Fusion of Thoracic Vertebral Joint with Nonautologous Tissue Substitute, Posterior Approach, Posterior Column, Percutaneous Approach

ØRG63KJ Fusion of Thoracic Vertebral Joint with Nonautologous Tissue Substitute, Posterior Approach, Anterior Column, Percutaneous Approach

ØRG6470 Fusion of Thoracic Vertebral Joint with Autologous Tissue Substitute, Anterior Approach, Anterior Column, Percutaneous Endoscopic Approach

ØRG6471 Fusion of Thoracic Vertebral Joint with Autologous Tissue Substitute, Posterior Approach, Posterior Column, Percutaneous Endoscopic Approach

ØRG647J Fusion of Thoracic Vertebral Joint with Autologous Tissue Substitute, Posterior Approach, Anterior Column, Percutaneous Endoscopic Approach

ØRG64A0 Fusion of Thoracic Vertebral Joint with Interbody Fusion Device, Anterior Approach, Anterior Column, Percutaneous Endoscopic Approach

ØRG64AJ Fusion of Thoracic Vertebral Joint with Interbody Fusion Device, Posterior Approach, Anterior Column, Percutaneous Endoscopic Approach

ØRG64J0 Fusion of Thoracic Vertebral Joint with Synthetic Substitute, Anterior Approach, Anterior Column, Percutaneous Endoscopic Approach

ØRG64J1 Fusion of Thoracic Vertebral Joint with Synthetic Substitute, Posterior Approach, Posterior Column, Percutaneous Endoscopic Approach

ØRG64JJ Fusion of Thoracic Vertebral Joint with Synthetic Substitute, Posterior Approach, Anterior Column, Percutaneous Endoscopic Approach

ØRG64K0 Fusion of Thoracic Vertebral Joint with Nonautologous Tissue Substitute, Anterior Approach, Anterior Column, Percutaneous Endoscopic Approach

ØRG64K1 Fusion of Thoracic Vertebral Joint with Nonautologous Tissue Substitute, Posterior Approach, Posterior Column, Percutaneous Endoscopic Approach

ØRG64KJ Fusion of Thoracic Vertebral Joint with Nonautologous Tissue Substitute, Posterior Approach, Anterior Column, Percutaneous Endoscopic Approach

ØRG7070 Fusion of 2 to 7 Thoracic Vertebral Joints with Autologous Tissue Substitute, Anterior Approach, Anterior Column, Open Approach

ØRG7071 Fusion of 2 to 7 Thoracic Vertebral Joints with Autologous Tissue Substitute, Posterior Approach, Posterior Column, Open Approach

ØRG707J Fusion of 2 to 7 Thoracic Vertebral Joints with Autologous Tissue Substitute, Posterior Approach, Anterior Column, Open Approach

ØRG70A0 Fusion of 2 to 7 Thoracic Vertebral Joints with Interbody Fusion Device, Anterior Approach, Anterior Column, Open Approach

ØRG70AJ Fusion of 2 to 7 Thoracic Vertebral Joints with Interbody Fusion Device, Posterior Approach, Anterior Column, Open Approach

ØRG70J0 Fusion of 2 to 7 Thoracic Vertebral Joints with Synthetic Substitute, Anterior Approach, Anterior Column, Open Approach

HAC 12: Surgical Site Infection-Certain Orthopedic Procedures of the Spine, Shoulder, and Elbow (continued)

ØRG70J1 Fusion of 2 to 7 Thoracic Vertebral Joints with Synthetic Substitute, Posterior Approach, Posterior Column, Open Approach

ØRG70JJ Fusion of 2 to 7 Thoracic Vertebral Joints with Synthetic Substitute, Posterior Approach, Anterior Column, Open Approach

ØRG70KØ Fusion of 2 to 7 Thoracic Vertebral Joints with Nonautologous Tissue Substitute, Anterior Approach, Anterior Column, Open Approach

ØRG70K1 Fusion of 2 to 7 Thoracic Vertebral Joints with Nonautologous Tissue Substitute, Posterior Approach, Posterior Column, Open Approach

ØRG70KJ Fusion of 2 to 7 Thoracic Vertebral Joints with Nonautologous Tissue Substitute, Posterior Approach, Anterior Column, Open Approach

ØRG737Ø Fusion of 2 to 7 Thoracic Vertebral Joints with Autologous Tissue Substitute, Anterior Approach, Anterior Column, Percutaneous Approach

ØRG7371 Fusion of 2 to 7 Thoracic Vertebral Joints with Autologous Tissue Substitute, Posterior Approach, Posterior Column, Percutaneous Approach

ØRG737J Fusion of 2 to 7 Thoracic Vertebral Joints with Autologous Tissue Substitute, Posterior Approach, Anterior Column, Percutaneous Approach

ØRG73AØ Fusion of 2 to 7 Thoracic Vertebral Joints with Interbody Fusion Device, Anterior Approach, Anterior Column, Percutaneous Approach

ØRG73AJ Fusion of 2 to 7 Thoracic Vertebral Joints with Interbody Fusion Device, Posterior Approach, Anterior Column, Percutaneous Approach

ØRG73JØ Fusion of 2 to 7 Thoracic Vertebral Joints with Synthetic Substitute, Anterior Approach, Anterior Column, Percutaneous Approach

ØRG73J1 Fusion of 2 to 7 Thoracic Vertebral Joints with Synthetic Substitute, Posterior Approach, Posterior Column, Percutaneous Approach

ØRG73JJ Fusion of 2 to 7 Thoracic Vertebral Joints with Synthetic Substitute, Posterior Approach, Anterior Column, Percutaneous Approach

ØRG73KØ Fusion of 2 to 7 Thoracic Vertebral Joints with Nonautologous Tissue Substitute, Anterior Approach, Anterior Column, Percutaneous Approach

ØRG73K1 Fusion of 2 to 7 Thoracic Vertebral Joints with Nonautologous Tissue Substitute, Posterior Approach, Posterior Column, Percutaneous Approach

ØRG73KJ Fusion of 2 to 7 Thoracic Vertebral Joints with Nonautologous Tissue Substitute, Posterior Approach, Anterior Column, Percutaneous Approach

ØRG747Ø Fusion of 2 to 7 Thoracic Vertebral Joints with Autologous Tissue Substitute, Anterior Approach, Anterior Column, Percutaneous Endoscopic Approach

ØRG7471 Fusion of 2 to 7 Thoracic Vertebral Joints with Autologous Tissue Substitute, Posterior Approach, Posterior Column, Percutaneous Endoscopic Approach

ØRG747J Fusion of 2 to 7 Thoracic Vertebral Joints with Autologous Tissue Substitute, Posterior Approach, Anterior Column, Percutaneous Endoscopic Approach

ØRG74AØ Fusion of 2 to 7 Thoracic Vertebral Joints with Interbody Fusion Device, Anterior Approach, Anterior Column, Percutaneous Endoscopic Approach

ØRG74AJ Fusion of 2 to 7 Thoracic Vertebral Joints with Interbody Fusion Device, Posterior Approach, Anterior Column, Percutaneous Endoscopic Approach

ØRG74JØ Fusion of 2 to 7 Thoracic Vertebral Joints with Synthetic Substitute, Anterior Approach, Anterior Column, Percutaneous Endoscopic Approach

ØRG74J1 Fusion of 2 to 7 Thoracic Vertebral Joints with Synthetic Substitute, Posterior Approach, Posterior Column, Percutaneous Endoscopic Approach

ØRG74JJ Fusion of 2 to 7 Thoracic Vertebral Joints with Synthetic Substitute, Posterior Approach, Anterior Column, Percutaneous Endoscopic Approach

ØRG74KØ Fusion of 2 to 7 Thoracic Vertebral Joints with Nonautologous Tissue Substitute, Anterior Approach, Anterior Column, Percutaneous Endoscopic Approach

ØRG74K1 Fusion of 2 to 7 Thoracic Vertebral Joints with Nonautologous Tissue Substitute, Posterior Approach, Posterior Column, Percutaneous Endoscopic Approach

ØRG74KJ Fusion of 2 to 7 Thoracic Vertebral Joints with Nonautologous Tissue Substitute, Posterior Approach, Anterior Column, Percutaneous Endoscopic Approach

ØRG80 7Ø Fusion of 8 or More Thoracic Vertebral Joints with Autologous Tissue Substitute, Anterior Approach, Anterior Column, Open Approach

ØRG80 71 Fusion of 8 or More Thoracic Vertebral Joints with Autologous Tissue Substitute, Posterior Approach, Posterior Column, Open Approach

ØRG807J Fusion of 8 or More Thoracic Vertebral Joints with Autologous Tissue Substitute, Posterior Approach, Anterior Column, Open Approach

ØRG80AØ Fusion of 8 or More Thoracic Vertebral Joints with Interbody Fusion Device, Anterior Approach, Anterior Column, Open Approach

ØRG80AJ Fusion of 8 or More Thoracic Vertebral Joints with Interbody Fusion Device, Posterior Approach, Anterior Column, Open Approach

ØRG80JØ Fusion of 8 or More Thoracic Vertebral Joints with Synthetic Substitute, Anterior Approach, Anterior Column, Open Approach

ØRG80J1 Fusion of 8 or More Thoracic Vertebral Joints with Synthetic Substitute, Posterior Approach, Posterior Column, Open Approach

ØRG80JJ Fusion of 8 or More Thoracic Vertebral Joints with Synthetic Substitute, Posterior Approach, Anterior Column, Open Approach

ØRG80KØ Fusion of 8 or More Thoracic Vertebral Joints with Nonautologous Tissue Substitute, Anterior Approach, Anterior Column, Open Approach

ØRG80K1 Fusion of 8 or More Thoracic Vertebral Joints with Nonautologous Tissue Substitute, Posterior Approach, Posterior Column, Open Approach

ØRG80KJ Fusion of 8 or More Thoracic Vertebral Joints with Nonautologous Tissue Substitute, Posterior Approach, Anterior Column, Open Approach

ØRG8370 Fusion of 8 or More Thoracic Vertebral Joints with Autologous Tissue Substitute, Anterior Approach, Anterior Column, Percutaneous Approach

ØRG8371 Fusion of 8 or More Thoracic Vertebral Joints with Autologous Tissue Substitute, Posterior Approach, Posterior Column, Percutaneous Approach

ØRG837J Fusion of 8 or More Thoracic Vertebral Joints with Autologous Tissue Substitute, Posterior Approach, Anterior Column, Percutaneous Approach

ØRG83AØ Fusion of 8 or More Thoracic Vertebral Joints with Interbody Fusion Device, Anterior Approach, Anterior Column, Percutaneous Approach

ØRG83AJ Fusion of 8 or More Thoracic Vertebral Joints with Interbody Fusion Device, Posterior Approach, Anterior Column, Percutaneous Approach

ØRG83JØ Fusion of 8 or More Thoracic Vertebral Joints with Synthetic Substitute, Anterior Approach, Anterior Column, Percutaneous Approach

ØRG83J1 Fusion of 8 or More Thoracic Vertebral Joints with Synthetic Substitute, Posterior Approach, Posterior Column, Percutaneous Approach

ØRG83JJ Fusion of 8 or More Thoracic Vertebral Joints with Synthetic Substitute, Posterior Approach, Anterior Column, Percutaneous Approach

ØRG83KØ Fusion of 8 or More Thoracic Vertebral Joints with Nonautologous Tissue Substitute, Anterior Approach, Anterior Column, Percutaneous Approach

ØRG83K1 Fusion of 8 or More Thoracic Vertebral Joints with Nonautologous Tissue Substitute, Posterior Approach, Posterior Column, Percutaneous Approach

ØRG83KJ Fusion of 8 or More Thoracic Vertebral Joints with Nonautologous Tissue Substitute, Posterior Approach, Anterior Column, Percutaneous Approach

ØRG8470 Fusion of 8 or More Thoracic Vertebral Joints with Autologous Tissue Substitute, Anterior Approach, Anterior Column, Percutaneous Endoscopic Approach

ØRG8471 Fusion of 8 or More Thoracic Vertebral Joints with Autologous Tissue Substitute, Posterior Approach, Posterior Column, Percutaneous Endoscopic Approach

ØRG847J Fusion of 8 or More Thoracic Vertebral Joints with Autologous Tissue Substitute, Posterior Approach, Anterior Column, Percutaneous Endoscopic Approach

ØRG84AØ Fusion of 8 or More Thoracic Vertebral Joints with Interbody Fusion Device, Anterior Approach, Anterior Column, Percutaneous Endoscopic Approach

ØRG84AJ Fusion of 8 or More Thoracic Vertebral Joints with Interbody Fusion Device, Posterior Approach, Anterior Column, Percutaneous Endoscopic Approach

ØRG84JØ Fusion of 8 or More Thoracic Vertebral Joints with Synthetic Substitute, Anterior Approach, Anterior Column, Percutaneous Endoscopic Approach

ØRG84J1 Fusion of 8 or More Thoracic Vertebral Joints with Synthetic Substitute, Posterior Approach, Posterior Column, Percutaneous Endoscopic Approach

HAC 12: Surgical Site Infection-Certain Orthopedic Procedures of the Spine, Shoulder, and Elbow (continued)

ØRG84JJ Fusion of 8 or More Thoracic Vertebral Joints with Synthetic Substitute, Posterior Approach, Anterior Column, Percutaneous Endoscopic Approach

ØRG84KØ Fusion of 8 or More Thoracic Vertebral Joints with Nonautologous Tissue Substitute, Anterior Approach, Anterior Column, Percutaneous Endoscopic Approach

ØRG84K1 Fusion of 8 or More Thoracic Vertebral Joints with Nonautologous Tissue Substitute, Posterior Approach, Posterior Column, Percutaneous Endoscopic Approach

ØRG84KJ Fusion of 8 or More Thoracic Vertebral Joints with Nonautologous Tissue Substitute, Posterior Approach, Anterior Column, Percutaneous Endoscopic Approach

ØRGA07Ø Fusion of Thoracolumbar Vertebral Joint with Autologous Tissue Substitute, Anterior Approach, Anterior Column, Open Approach

ØRGA071 Fusion of Thoracolumbar Vertebral Joint with Autologous Tissue Substitute, Posterior Approach, Posterior Column, Open Approach

ØRGA07J Fusion of Thoracolumbar Vertebral Joint with Autologous Tissue Substitute, Posterior Approach, Anterior Column, Open Approach

ØRGAØAØ Fusion of Thoracolumbar Vertebral Joint with Interbody Fusion Device, Anterior Approach, Anterior Column, Open Approach

ØRGAØAJ Fusion of Thoracolumbar Vertebral Joint with Interbody Fusion Device, Posterior Approach, Anterior Column, Open Approach

ØRGAØJØ Fusion of Thoracolumbar Vertebral Joint with Synthetic Substitute, Anterior Approach, Anterior Column, Open Approach

ØRGAØJ1 Fusion of Thoracolumbar Vertebral Joint with Synthetic Substitute, Posterior Approach, Posterior Column, Open Approach

ØRGAØJJ Fusion of Thoracolumbar Vertebral Joint with Synthetic Substitute, Posterior Approach, Anterior Column, Open Approach

ØRGAØKØ Fusion of Thoracolumbar Vertebral Joint with Nonautologous Tissue Substitute, Anterior Approach, Anterior Column, Open Approach

ØRGAØK1 Fusion of Thoracolumbar Vertebral Joint with Nonautologous Tissue Substitute, Posterior Approach, Posterior Column, Open Approach

ØRGAØKJ Fusion of Thoracolumbar Vertebral Joint with Nonautologous Tissue Substitute, Posterior Approach, Anterior Column, Open Approach

ØRGA37Ø Fusion of Thoracolumbar Vertebral Joint with Autologous Tissue Substitute, Anterior Approach, Anterior Column, Percutaneous Approach

ØRGA371 Fusion of Thoracolumbar Vertebral Joint with Autologous Tissue Substitute, Posterior Approach, Posterior Column, Percutaneous Approach

ØRGA37J Fusion of Thoracolumbar Vertebral Joint with Autologous Tissue Substitute, Posterior Approach, Anterior Column, Percutaneous Approach

ØRGA3AØ Fusion of Thoracolumbar Vertebral Joint with Interbody Fusion Device, Anterior Approach, Anterior Column, Percutaneous Approach

ØRGA3AJ Fusion of Thoracolumbar Vertebral Joint with Interbody Fusion Device, Posterior Approach, Anterior Column, Percutaneous Approach

ØRGA3JØ Fusion of Thoracolumbar Vertebral Joint with Synthetic Substitute, Anterior Approach, Anterior Column, Percutaneous Approach

ØRGA3J1 Fusion of Thoracolumbar Vertebral Joint with Synthetic Substitute, Posterior Approach, Posterior Column, Percutaneous Approach

ØRGA3JJ Fusion of Thoracolumbar Vertebral Joint with Synthetic Substitute, Posterior Approach, Anterior Column, Percutaneous Approach

ØRGA3KØ Fusion of Thoracolumbar Vertebral Joint with Nonautologous Tissue Substitute, Anterior Approach, Anterior Column, Percutaneous Approach

ØRGA3K1 Fusion of Thoracolumbar Vertebral Joint with Nonautologous Tissue Substitute, Posterior Approach, Posterior Column, Percutaneous Approach

ØRGA3KJ Fusion of Thoracolumbar Vertebral Joint with Nonautologous Tissue Substitute, Posterior Approach, Anterior Column, Percutaneous Approach

ØRGA47Ø Fusion of Thoracolumbar Vertebral Joint with Autologous Tissue Substitute, Anterior Approach, Anterior Column, Percutaneous Endoscopic Approach

ØRGA471 Fusion of Thoracolumbar Vertebral Joint with Autologous Tissue Substitute, Posterior Approach, Posterior Column, Percutaneous Endoscopic Approach

ØRGA47J Fusion of Thoracolumbar Vertebral Joint with Autologous Tissue Substitute, Posterior Approach, Anterior Column, Percutaneous Endoscopic Approach

ØRGA4AØ Fusion of Thoracolumbar Vertebral Joint with Interbody Fusion Device, Anterior Approach, Anterior Column, Percutaneous Endoscopic Approach

ØRGA4AJ Fusion of Thoracolumbar Vertebral Joint with Interbody Fusion Device, Posterior Approach, Anterior Column, Percutaneous Endoscopic Approach

ØRGA4JØ Fusion of Thoracolumbar Vertebral Joint with Synthetic Substitute, Anterior Approach, Anterior Column, Percutaneous Endoscopic Approach

ØRGA4J1 Fusion of Thoracolumbar Vertebral Joint with Synthetic Substitute, Posterior Approach, Posterior Column, Percutaneous Endoscopic Approach

ØRGA4JJ Fusion of Thoracolumbar Vertebral Joint with Synthetic Substitute, Posterior Approach, Anterior Column, Percutaneous Endoscopic Approach

ØRGA4KØ Fusion of Thoracolumbar Vertebral Joint with Nonautologous Tissue Substitute, Anterior Approach, Anterior Column, Percutaneous Endoscopic Approach

ØRGA4K1 Fusion of Thoracolumbar Vertebral Joint with Nonautologous Tissue Substitute, Posterior Approach, Posterior Column, Percutaneous Endoscopic Approach

ØRGA4KJ Fusion of Thoracolumbar Vertebral Joint with Nonautologous Tissue Substitute, Posterior Approach, Anterior Column, Percutaneous Endoscopic Approach

ØRGE04Z Fusion of Right Sternoclavicular Joint with Internal Fixation Device, Open Approach

ØRGE07Z Fusion of Right Sternoclavicular Joint with Autologous Tissue Substitute, Open Approach

ØRGEØJZ Fusion of Right Sternoclavicular Joint with Synthetic Substitute, Open Approach

ØRGEØKZ Fusion of Right Sternoclavicular Joint with Nonautologous Tissue Substitute, Open Approach

ØRGE34Z Fusion of Right Sternoclavicular Joint with Internal Fixation Device, Percutaneous Approach

ØRGE37Z Fusion of Right Sternoclavicular Joint with Autologous Tissue Substitute, Percutaneous Approach

ØRGE3JZ Fusion of Right Sternoclavicular Joint with Synthetic Substitute, Percutaneous Approach

ØRGE3KZ Fusion of Right Sternoclavicular Joint with Nonautologous Tissue Substitute, Percutaneous Approach

ØRGE44Z Fusion of Right Sternoclavicular Joint with Internal Fixation Device, Percutaneous Endoscopic Approach

ØRGE47Z Fusion of Right Sternoclavicular Joint with Autologous Tissue Substitute, Percutaneous Endoscopic Approach

ØRGE4JZ Fusion of Right Sternoclavicular Joint with Synthetic Substitute, Percutaneous Endoscopic Approach

ØRGE4KZ Fusion of Right Sternoclavicular Joint with Nonautologous Tissue Substitute, Percutaneous Endoscopic Approach

ØRGF04Z Fusion of Left Sternoclavicular Joint with Internal Fixation Device, Open Approach

ØRGF07Z Fusion of Left Sternoclavicular Joint with Autologous Tissue Substitute, Open Approach

ØRGFØJZ Fusion of Left Sternoclavicular Joint with Synthetic Substitute, Open Approach

ØRGFØKZ Fusion of Left Sternoclavicular Joint with Nonautologous Tissue Substitute, Open Approach

ØRGF34Z Fusion of Left Sternoclavicular Joint with Internal Fixation Device, Percutaneous Approach

ØRGF37Z Fusion of Left Sternoclavicular Joint with Autologous Tissue Substitute, Percutaneous Approach

ØRGF3JZ Fusion of Left Sternoclavicular Joint with Synthetic Substitute, Percutaneous Approach

ØRGF3KZ Fusion of Left Sternoclavicular Joint with Nonautologous Tissue Substitute, Percutaneous Approach

ØRGF44Z Fusion of Left Sternoclavicular Joint with Internal Fixation Device, Percutaneous Endoscopic Approach

ØRGF47Z Fusion of Left Sternoclavicular Joint with Autologous Tissue Substitute, Percutaneous Endoscopic Approach

ØRGF4JZ Fusion of Left Sternoclavicular Joint with Synthetic Substitute, Percutaneous Endoscopic Approach

ØRGF4KZ Fusion of Left Sternoclavicular Joint with Nonautologous Tissue Substitute, Percutaneous Endoscopic Approach

ØRGG04Z Fusion of Right Acromioclavicular Joint with Internal Fixation Device, Open Approach

HAC 12: Surgical Site Infection-Certain Orthopedic Procedures of the Spine, Shoulder, and Elbow (continued)

ØRGGØ7Z Fusion of Right Acromioclavicular Joint with Autologous Tissue Substitute, Open Approach

ØRGGØJZ Fusion of Right Acromioclavicular Joint with Synthetic Substitute, Open Approach

ØRGGØKZ Fusion of Right Acromioclavicular Joint with Nonautologous Tissue Substitute, Open Approach

ØRGG34Z Fusion of Right Acromioclavicular Joint with Internal Fixation Device, Percutaneous Approach

ØRGG37Z Fusion of Right Acromioclavicular Joint with Autologous Tissue Substitute, Percutaneous Approach

ØRGG3JZ Fusion of Right Acromioclavicular Joint with Synthetic Substitute, Percutaneous Approach

ØRGG3KZ Fusion of Right Acromioclavicular Joint with Nonautologous Tissue Substitute, Percutaneous Approach

ØRGG44Z Fusion of Right Acromioclavicular Joint with Internal Fixation Device, Percutaneous Endoscopic Approach

ØRGG47Z Fusion of Right Acromioclavicular Joint with Autologous Tissue Substitute, Percutaneous Endoscopic Approach

ØRGG4JZ Fusion of Right Acromioclavicular Joint with Synthetic Substitute, Percutaneous Endoscopic Approach

ØRGG4KZ Fusion of Right Acromioclavicular Joint with Nonautologous Tissue Substitute, Percutaneous Endoscopic Approach

ØRGHØ4Z Fusion of Left Acromioclavicular Joint with Internal Fixation Device, Open Approach

ØRGHØ7Z Fusion of Left Acromioclavicular Joint with Autologous Tissue Substitute, Open Approach

ØRGHØJZ Fusion of Left Acromioclavicular Joint with Synthetic Substitute, Open Approach

ØRGHØKZ Fusion of Left Acromioclavicular Joint with Nonautologous Tissue Substitute, Open Approach

ØRGH34Z Fusion of Left Acromioclavicular Joint with Internal Fixation Device, Percutaneous Approach

ØRGH37Z Fusion of Left Acromioclavicular Joint with Autologous Tissue Substitute, Percutaneous Approach

ØRGH3JZ Fusion of Left Acromioclavicular Joint with Synthetic Substitute, Percutaneous Approach

ØRGH3KZ Fusion of Left Acromioclavicular Joint with Nonautologous Tissue Substitute, Percutaneous Approach

ØRGH44Z Fusion of Left Acromioclavicular Joint with Internal Fixation Device, Percutaneous Endoscopic Approach

ØRGH47Z Fusion of Left Acromioclavicular Joint with Autologous Tissue Substitute, Percutaneous Endoscopic Approach

ØRGH4JZ Fusion of Left Acromioclavicular Joint with Synthetic Substitute, Percutaneous Endoscopic Approach

ØRGH4KZ Fusion of Left Acromioclavicular Joint with Nonautologous Tissue Substitute, Percutaneous Endoscopic Approach

ØRGJØ4Z Fusion of Right Shoulder Joint with Internal Fixation Device, Open Approach

ØRGJØ7Z Fusion of Right Shoulder Joint with Autologous Tissue Substitute, Open Approach

ØRGJØJZ Fusion of Right Shoulder Joint with Synthetic Substitute, Open Approach

ØRGJØKZ Fusion of Right Shoulder Joint with Nonautologous Tissue Substitute, Open Approach

ØRGJ34Z Fusion of Right Shoulder Joint with Internal Fixation Device, Percutaneous Approach

ØRGJ37Z Fusion of Right Shoulder Joint with Autologous Tissue Substitute, Percutaneous Approach

ØRGJ3JZ Fusion of Right Shoulder Joint with Synthetic Substitute, Percutaneous Approach

ØRGJ3KZ Fusion of Right Shoulder Joint with Nonautologous Tissue Substitute, Percutaneous Approach

ØRGJ44Z Fusion of Right Shoulder Joint with Internal Fixation Device, Percutaneous Endoscopic Approach

ØRGJ47Z Fusion of Right Shoulder Joint with Autologous Tissue Substitute, Percutaneous Endoscopic Approach

ØRGJ4JZ Fusion of Right Shoulder Joint with Synthetic Substitute, Percutaneous Endoscopic Approach

ØRGJ4KZ Fusion of Right Shoulder Joint with Nonautologous Tissue Substitute, Percutaneous Endoscopic Approach

ØRGKØ4Z Fusion of Left Shoulder Joint with Internal Fixation Device, Open Approach

ØRGKØ7Z Fusion of Left Shoulder Joint with Autologous Tissue Substitute, Open Approach

ØRGKØJZ Fusion of Left Shoulder Joint with Synthetic Substitute, Open Approach

ØRGKØKZ Fusion of Left Shoulder Joint with Nonautologous Tissue Substitute, Open Approach

ØRGK34Z Fusion of Left Shoulder Joint with Internal Fixation Device, Percutaneous Approach

ØRGK37Z Fusion of Left Shoulder Joint with Autologous Tissue Substitute, Percutaneous Approach

ØRGK3JZ Fusion of Left Shoulder Joint with Synthetic Substitute, Percutaneous Approach

ØRGK3KZ Fusion of Left Shoulder Joint with Nonautologous Tissue Substitute, Percutaneous Approach

ØRGK44Z Fusion of Left Shoulder Joint with Internal Fixation Device, Percutaneous Endoscopic Approach

ØRGK47Z Fusion of Left Shoulder Joint with Autologous Tissue Substitute, Percutaneous Endoscopic Approach

ØRGK4JZ Fusion of Left Shoulder Joint with Synthetic Substitute, Percutaneous Endoscopic Approach

ØRGK4KZ Fusion of Left Shoulder Joint with Nonautologous Tissue Substitute, Percutaneous Endoscopic Approach

ØRGLØ3Z Fusion of Right Elbow Joint with Sustained Compression Internal Fixation Device, Open Approach

ØRGLØ4Z Fusion of Right Elbow Joint with Internal Fixation Device, Open Approach

ØRGLØ5Z Fusion of Right Elbow Joint with External Fixation Device, Open Approach

ØRGLØ7Z Fusion of Right Elbow Joint with Autologous Tissue Substitute, Open Approach

ØRGLØJZ Fusion of Right Elbow Joint with Synthetic Substitute, Open Approach

ØRGLØKZ Fusion of Right Elbow Joint with Nonautologous Tissue Substitute, Open Approach

ØRGL33Z Fusion of Right Elbow Joint with Sustained Compression Internal Fixation Device, Percutaneous Approach

ØRGL34Z Fusion of Right Elbow Joint with Internal Fixation Device, Percutaneous Approach

ØRGL35Z Fusion of Right Elbow Joint with External Fixation Device, Percutaneous Approach

ØRGL37Z Fusion of Right Elbow Joint with Autologous Tissue Substitute, Percutaneous Approach

ØRGL3JZ Fusion of Right Elbow Joint with Synthetic Substitute, Percutaneous Approach

ØRGL3KZ Fusion of Right Elbow Joint with Nonautologous Tissue Substitute, Percutaneous Approach

ØRGL43Z Fusion of Right Elbow Joint with Sustained Compression Internal Fixation Device, Percutaneous Endoscopic Approach

ØRGL44Z Fusion of Right Elbow Joint with Internal Fixation Device, Percutaneous Endoscopic Approach

ØRGL45Z Fusion of Right Elbow Joint with External Fixation Device, Percutaneous Endoscopic Approach

ØRGL47Z Fusion of Right Elbow Joint with Autologous Tissue Substitute, Percutaneous Endoscopic Approach

ØRGL4JZ Fusion of Right Elbow Joint with Synthetic Substitute, Percutaneous Endoscopic Approach

ØRGL4KZ Fusion of Right Elbow Joint with Nonautologous Tissue Substitute, Percutaneous Endoscopic Approach

ØRGMØ3Z Fusion of Left Elbow Joint with Sustained Compression Internal Fixation Device, Open Approach

ØRGMØ4Z Fusion of Left Elbow Joint with Internal Fixation Device, Open Approach

ØRGMØ5Z Fusion of Left Elbow Joint with External Fixation Device, Open Approach

ØRGMØ7Z Fusion of Left Elbow Joint with Autologous Tissue Substitute, Open Approach

ØRGMØJZ Fusion of Left Elbow Joint with Synthetic Substitute, Open Approach

ØRGMØKZ Fusion of Left Elbow Joint with Nonautologous Tissue Substitute, Open Approach

ØRGM33Z Fusion of Left Elbow Joint with Sustained Compression Internal Fixation Device, Percutaneous Approach

ØRGM34Z Fusion of Left Elbow Joint with Internal Fixation Device, Percutaneous Approach

ØRGM35Z Fusion of Left Elbow Joint with External Fixation Device, Percutaneous Approach

ØRGM37Z Fusion of Left Elbow Joint with Autologous Tissue Substitute, Percutaneous Approach

ØRGM3JZ Fusion of Left Elbow Joint with Synthetic Substitute, Percutaneous Approach

ØRGM3KZ Fusion of Left Elbow Joint with Nonautologous Tissue Substitute, Percutaneous Approach

ØRGM43Z Fusion of Left Elbow Joint with Sustained Compression Internal Fixation Device, Percutaneous Endoscopic Approach

ØRGM44Z Fusion of Left Elbow Joint with Internal Fixation Device, Percutaneous Endoscopic Approach

ØRGM45Z Fusion of Left Elbow Joint with External Fixation Device, Percutaneous Endoscopic Approach

ØRGM47Z Fusion of Left Elbow Joint with Autologous Tissue Substitute, Percutaneous Endoscopic Approach

ØRGM4JZ Fusion of Left Elbow Joint with Synthetic Substitute, Percutaneous Endoscopic Approach

HAC 12: Surgical Site Infection-Certain Orthopedic Procedures of the Spine, Shoulder, and Elbow (continued)

ØRGM4KZ Fusion of Left Elbow Joint with Nonautologous Tissue Substitute, Percutaneous Endoscopic Approach

ØRQEØZZ Repair Right Sternoclavicular Joint, Open Approach

ØRQE3ZZ Repair Right Sternoclavicular Joint, Percutaneous Approach

ØRQE4ZZ Repair Right Sternoclavicular Joint, Percutaneous Endoscopic Approach

ØRQEXZZ Repair Right Sternoclavicular Joint, External Approach

ØRQFØZZ Repair Left Sternoclavicular Joint, Open Approach

ØRQF3ZZ Repair Left Sternoclavicular Joint, Percutaneous Approach

ØRQF4ZZ Repair Left Sternoclavicular Joint, Percutaneous Endoscopic Approach

ØRQFXZZ Repair Left Sternoclavicular Joint, External Approach

ØRQGØZZ Repair Right Acromioclavicular Joint, Open Approach

ØRQG3ZZ Repair Right Acromioclavicular Joint, Percutaneous Approach

ØRQG4ZZ Repair Right Acromioclavicular Joint, Percutaneous Endoscopic Approach

ØRQGXZZ Repair Right Acromioclavicular Joint, External Approach

ØRQHØZZ Repair Left Acromioclavicular Joint, Open Approach

ØRQH3ZZ Repair Left Acromioclavicular Joint, Percutaneous Approach

ØRQH4ZZ Repair Left Acromioclavicular Joint, Percutaneous Endoscopic Approach

ØRQHXZZ Repair Left Acromioclavicular Joint, External Approach

ØRQJØZZ Repair Right Shoulder Joint, Open Approach

ØRQJ3ZZ Repair Right Shoulder Joint, Percutaneous Approach

ØRQJ4ZZ Repair Right Shoulder Joint, Percutaneous Endoscopic Approach

ØRQJXZZ Repair Right Shoulder Joint, External Approach

ØRQKØZZ Repair Left Shoulder Joint, Open Approach

ØRQK3ZZ Repair Left Shoulder Joint, Percutaneous Approach

ØRQK4ZZ Repair Left Shoulder Joint, Percutaneous Endoscopic Approach

ØRQKXZZ Repair Left Shoulder Joint, External Approach

ØRQLØZZ Repair Right Elbow Joint, Open Approach

ØRQL3ZZ Repair Right Elbow Joint, Percutaneous Approach

ØRQL4ZZ Repair Right Elbow Joint, Percutaneous Endoscopic Approach

ØRQLXZZ Repair Right Elbow Joint, External Approach

ØRQMØZZ Repair Left Elbow Joint, Open Approach

ØRQM3ZZ Repair Left Elbow Joint, Percutaneous Approach

ØRQM4ZZ Repair Left Elbow Joint, Percutaneous Endoscopic Approach

ØRQMXZZ Repair Left Elbow Joint, External Approach

ØRUEØ7Z Supplement Right Sternoclavicular Joint with Autologous Tissue Substitute, Open Approach

ØRUEØJZ Supplement Right Sternoclavicular Joint with Synthetic Substitute, Open Approach

ØRUEØKZ Supplement Right Sternoclavicular Joint with Nonautologous Tissue Substitute, Open Approach

ØRUE37Z Supplement Right Sternoclavicular Joint with Autologous Tissue Substitute, Percutaneous Approach

ØRUE3JZ Supplement Right Sternoclavicular Joint with Synthetic Substitute, Percutaneous Approach

ØRUE3KZ Supplement Right Sternoclavicular Joint with Nonautologous Tissue Substitute, Percutaneous Approach

ØRUE47Z Supplement Right Sternoclavicular Joint with Autologous Tissue Substitute, Percutaneous Endoscopic Approach

ØRUE4JZ Supplement Right Sternoclavicular Joint with Synthetic Substitute, Percutaneous Endoscopic Approach

ØRUE4KZ Supplement Right Sternoclavicular Joint with Nonautologous Tissue Substitute, Percutaneous Endoscopic Approach

ØRUFØ7Z Supplement Left Sternoclavicular Joint with Autologous Tissue Substitute, Open Approach

ØRUFØJZ Supplement Left Sternoclavicular Joint with Synthetic Substitute, Open Approach

ØRUFØKZ Supplement Left Sternoclavicular Joint with Nonautologous Tissue Substitute, Open Approach

ØRUF37Z Supplement Left Sternoclavicular Joint with Autologous Tissue Substitute, Percutaneous Approach

ØRUF3JZ Supplement Left Sternoclavicular Joint with Synthetic Substitute, Percutaneous Approach

ØRUF3KZ Supplement Left Sternoclavicular Joint with Nonautologous Tissue Substitute, Percutaneous Approach

ØRUF47Z Supplement Left Sternoclavicular Joint with Autologous Tissue Substitute, Percutaneous Endoscopic Approach

ØRUF4JZ Supplement Left Sternoclavicular Joint with Synthetic Substitute, Percutaneous Endoscopic Approach

ØRUF4KZ Supplement Left Sternoclavicular Joint with Nonautologous Tissue Substitute, Percutaneous Endoscopic Approach

ØRUGØ7Z Supplement Right Acromioclavicular Joint with Autologous Tissue Substitute, Open Approach

ØRUGØJZ Supplement Right Acromioclavicular Joint with Synthetic Substitute, Open Approach

ØRUGØKZ Supplement Right Acromioclavicular Joint with Nonautologous Tissue Substitute, Open Approach

ØRUG37Z Supplement Right Acromioclavicular Joint with Autologous Tissue Substitute, Percutaneous Approach

ØRUG3JZ Supplement Right Acromioclavicular Joint with Synthetic Substitute, Percutaneous Approach

ØRUG3KZ Supplement Right Acromioclavicular Joint with Nonautologous Tissue Substitute, Percutaneous Approach

ØRUG47Z Supplement Right Acromioclavicular Joint with Autologous Tissue Substitute, Percutaneous Endoscopic Approach

ØRUG4JZ Supplement Right Acromioclavicular Joint with Synthetic Substitute, Percutaneous Endoscopic Approach

ØRUG4KZ Supplement Right Acromioclavicular Joint with Nonautologous Tissue Substitute, Percutaneous Endoscopic Approach

ØRUHØ7Z Supplement Left Acromioclavicular Joint with Autologous Tissue Substitute, Open Approach

ØRUHØJZ Supplement Left Acromioclavicular Joint with Synthetic Substitute, Open Approach

ØRUHØKZ Supplement Left Acromioclavicular Joint with Nonautologous Tissue Substitute, Open Approach

ØRUH37Z Supplement Left Acromioclavicular Joint with Autologous Tissue Substitute, Percutaneous Approach

ØRUH3JZ Supplement Left Acromioclavicular Joint with Synthetic Substitute, Percutaneous Approach

ØRUH3KZ Supplement Left Acromioclavicular Joint with Nonautologous Tissue Substitute, Percutaneous Approach

ØRUH47Z Supplement Left Acromioclavicular Joint with Autologous Tissue Substitute, Percutaneous Endoscopic Approach

ØRUH4JZ Supplement Left Acromioclavicular Joint with Synthetic Substitute, Percutaneous Endoscopic Approach

ØRUH4KZ Supplement Left Acromioclavicular Joint with Nonautologous Tissue Substitute, Percutaneous Endoscopic Approach

ØRUJØ7Z Supplement Right Shoulder Joint with Autologous Tissue Substitute, Open Approach

ØRUJØJZ Supplement Right Shoulder Joint with Synthetic Substitute, Open Approach

ØRUJØKZ Supplement Right Shoulder Joint with Nonautologous Tissue Substitute, Open Approach

ØRUJ37Z Supplement Right Shoulder Joint with Autologous Tissue Substitute, Percutaneous Approach

ØRUJ3JZ Supplement Right Shoulder Joint with Synthetic Substitute, Percutaneous Approach

ØRUJ3KZ Supplement Right Shoulder Joint with Nonautologous Tissue Substitute, Percutaneous Approach

ØRUJ47Z Supplement Right Shoulder Joint with Autologous Tissue Substitute, Percutaneous Endoscopic Approach

ØRUJ4JZ Supplement Right Shoulder Joint with Synthetic Substitute, Percutaneous Endoscopic Approach

ØRUJ4KZ Supplement Right Shoulder Joint with Nonautologous Tissue Substitute, Percutaneous Endoscopic Approach

ØRUKØ7Z Supplement Left Shoulder Joint with Autologous Tissue Substitute, Open Approach

ØRUKØJZ Supplement Left Shoulder Joint with Synthetic Substitute, Open Approach

ØRUKØKZ Supplement Left Shoulder Joint with Nonautologous Tissue Substitute, Open Approach

ØRUK37Z Supplement Left Shoulder Joint with Autologous Tissue Substitute, Percutaneous Approach

ØRUK3JZ Supplement Left Shoulder Joint with Synthetic Substitute, Percutaneous Approach

ØRUK3KZ Supplement Left Shoulder Joint with Nonautologous Tissue Substitute, Percutaneous Approach

ØRUK47Z Supplement Left Shoulder Joint with Autologous Tissue Substitute, Percutaneous Endoscopic Approach

ØRUK4JZ Supplement Left Shoulder Joint with Synthetic Substitute, Percutaneous Endoscopic Approach

ØRUK4KZ Supplement Left Shoulder Joint with Nonautologous Tissue Substitute, Percutaneous Endoscopic Approach

ØRULØ7Z Supplement Right Elbow Joint with Autologous Tissue Substitute, Open Approach

HAC 12: Surgical Site Infection-Certain Orthopedic Procedures of the Spine, Shoulder, and Elbow (continued)

ØRULØJZ   Supplement Right Elbow Joint with Synthetic Substitute, Open Approach

ØRULØKZ   Supplement Right Elbow Joint with Nonautologous Tissue Substitute, Open Approach

ØRUL37Z   Supplement Right Elbow Joint with Autologous Tissue Substitute, Percutaneous Approach

ØRUL3JZ   Supplement Right Elbow Joint with Synthetic Substitute, Percutaneous Approach

ØRUL3KZ   Supplement Right Elbow Joint with Nonautologous Tissue Substitute, Percutaneous Approach

ØRUL47Z   Supplement Right Elbow Joint with Autologous Tissue Substitute, Percutaneous Endoscopic Approach

ØRUL4JZ   Supplement Right Elbow Joint with Synthetic Substitute, Percutaneous Endoscopic Approach

ØRUL4KZ   Supplement Right Elbow Joint with Nonautologous Tissue Substitute, Percutaneous Endoscopic Approach

ØRUM07Z   Supplement Left Elbow Joint with Autologous Tissue Substitute, Open Approach

ØRUMØJZ   Supplement Left Elbow Joint with Synthetic Substitute, Open Approach

ØRUMØKZ   Supplement Left Elbow Joint with Nonautologous Tissue Substitute, Open Approach

ØRUM37Z   Supplement Left Elbow Joint with Autologous Tissue Substitute, Percutaneous Approach

ØRUM3JZ   Supplement Left Elbow Joint with Synthetic Substitute, Percutaneous Approach

ØRUM3KZ   Supplement Left Elbow Joint with Nonautologous Tissue Substitute, Percutaneous Approach

ØRUM47Z   Supplement Left Elbow Joint with Autologous Tissue Substitute, Percutaneous Endoscopic Approach

ØRUM4JZ   Supplement Left Elbow Joint with Synthetic Substitute, Percutaneous Endoscopic Approach

ØRUM4KZ   Supplement Left Elbow Joint with Nonautologous Tissue Substitute, Percutaneous Endoscopic Approach

ØSG0070   Fusion of Lumbar Vertebral Joint with Autologous Tissue Substitute, Anterior Approach, Anterior Column, Open Approach

ØSG0071   Fusion of Lumbar Vertebral Joint with Autologous Tissue Substitute, Posterior Approach, Posterior Column, Open Approach

ØSG007J   Fusion of Lumbar Vertebral Joint with Autologous Tissue Substitute, Posterior Approach, Anterior Column, Open Approach

ØSG00A0   Fusion of Lumbar Vertebral Joint with Interbody Fusion Device, Anterior Approach, Anterior Column, Open Approach

ØSG00AJ   Fusion of Lumbar Vertebral Joint with Interbody Fusion Device, Posterior Approach, Anterior Column, Open Approach

ØSG00J0   Fusion of Lumbar Vertebral Joint with Synthetic Substitute, Anterior Approach, Anterior Column, Open Approach

ØSG00J1   Fusion of Lumbar Vertebral Joint with Synthetic Substitute, Posterior Approach, Posterior Column, Open Approach

ØSG00JJ   Fusion of Lumbar Vertebral Joint with Synthetic Substitute, Posterior Approach, Anterior Column, Open Approach

ØSG00K0   Fusion of Lumbar Vertebral Joint with Nonautologous Tissue Substitute, Anterior Approach, Anterior Column, Open Approach

ØSG00K1   Fusion of Lumbar Vertebral Joint with Nonautologous Tissue Substitute, Posterior Approach, Posterior Column, Open Approach

ØSG00KJ   Fusion of Lumbar Vertebral Joint with Nonautologous Tissue Substitute, Posterior Approach, Anterior Column, Open Approach

ØSG0370   Fusion of Lumbar Vertebral Joint with Autologous Tissue Substitute, Anterior Approach, Anterior Column, Percutaneous Approach

ØSG0371   Fusion of Lumbar Vertebral Joint with Autologous Tissue Substitute, Posterior Approach, Posterior Column, Percutaneous Approach

ØSG037J   Fusion of Lumbar Vertebral Joint with Autologous Tissue Substitute, Posterior Approach, Anterior Column, Percutaneous Approach

ØSG03A0   Fusion of Lumbar Vertebral Joint with Interbody Fusion Device, Anterior Approach, Anterior Column, Percutaneous Approach

ØSG03AJ   Fusion of Lumbar Vertebral Joint with Interbody Fusion Device, Posterior Approach, Anterior Column, Percutaneous Approach

ØSG03J0   Fusion of Lumbar Vertebral Joint with Synthetic Substitute, Anterior Approach, Anterior Column, Percutaneous Approach

ØSG03J1   Fusion of Lumbar Vertebral Joint with Synthetic Substitute, Posterior Approach, Posterior Column, Percutaneous Approach

ØSG03JJ   Fusion of Lumbar Vertebral Joint with Synthetic Substitute, Posterior Approach, Anterior Column, Percutaneous Approach

ØSG03K0   Fusion of Lumbar Vertebral Joint with Nonautologous Tissue Substitute, Anterior Approach, Anterior Column, Percutaneous Approach

ØSG03K1   Fusion of Lumbar Vertebral Joint with Nonautologous Tissue Substitute, Posterior Approach, Posterior Column, Percutaneous Approach

ØSG03KJ   Fusion of Lumbar Vertebral Joint with Nonautologous Tissue Substitute, Posterior Approach, Anterior Column, Percutaneous Approach

ØSG0470   Fusion of Lumbar Vertebral Joint with Autologous Tissue Substitute, Anterior Approach, Anterior Column, Percutaneous Endoscopic Approach

ØSG0471   Fusion of Lumbar Vertebral Joint with Autologous Tissue Substitute, Posterior Approach, Posterior Column, Percutaneous Endoscopic Approach

ØSG047J   Fusion of Lumbar Vertebral Joint with Autologous Tissue Substitute, Posterior Approach, Anterior Column, Percutaneous Endoscopic Approach

ØSG04A0   Fusion of Lumbar Vertebral Joint with Interbody Fusion Device, Anterior Approach, Anterior Column, Percutaneous Endoscopic Approach

ØSG04AJ   Fusion of Lumbar Vertebral Joint with Interbody Fusion Device, Posterior Approach, Anterior Column, Percutaneous Endoscopic Approach

ØSG04J0   Fusion of Lumbar Vertebral Joint with Synthetic Substitute, Anterior Approach, Anterior Column, Percutaneous Endoscopic Approach

ØSG04J1   Fusion of Lumbar Vertebral Joint with Synthetic Substitute, Posterior Approach, Posterior Column, Percutaneous Endoscopic Approach

ØSG04JJ   Fusion of Lumbar Vertebral Joint with Synthetic Substitute, Posterior Approach, Anterior Column, Percutaneous Endoscopic Approach

ØSG04K0   Fusion of Lumbar Vertebral Joint with Nonautologous Tissue Substitute, Anterior Approach, Anterior Column, Percutaneous Endoscopic Approach

ØSG04K1   Fusion of Lumbar Vertebral Joint with Nonautologous Tissue Substitute, Posterior Approach, Posterior Column, Percutaneous Endoscopic Approach

ØSG04KJ   Fusion of Lumbar Vertebral Joint with Nonautologous Tissue Substitute, Posterior Approach, Anterior Column, Percutaneous Endoscopic Approach

ØSG1070   Fusion of 2 or More Lumbar Vertebral Joints with Autologous Tissue Substitute, Anterior Approach, Anterior Column, Open Approach

ØSG1071   Fusion of 2 or More Lumbar Vertebral Joints with Autologous Tissue Substitute, Posterior Approach, Posterior Column, Open Approach

ØSG107J   Fusion of 2 or More Lumbar Vertebral Joints with Autologous Tissue Substitute, Posterior Approach, Anterior Column, Open Approach

ØSG10A0   Fusion of 2 or More Lumbar Vertebral Joints with Interbody Fusion Device, Anterior Approach, Anterior Column, Open Approach

ØSG10AJ   Fusion of 2 or More Lumbar Vertebral Joints with Interbody Fusion Device, Posterior Approach, Anterior Column, Open Approach

ØSG10J0   Fusion of 2 or More Lumbar Vertebral Joints with Synthetic Substitute, Anterior Approach, Anterior Column, Open Approach

ØSG10J1   Fusion of 2 or More Lumbar Vertebral Joints with Synthetic Substitute, Posterior Approach, Posterior Column, Open Approach

ØSG10JJ   Fusion of 2 or More Lumbar Vertebral Joints with Synthetic Substitute, Posterior Approach, Anterior Column, Open Approach

ØSG10K0   Fusion of 2 or More Lumbar Vertebral Joints with Nonautologous Tissue Substitute, Anterior Approach, Anterior Column, Open Approach

ØSG10K1   Fusion of 2 or More Lumbar Vertebral Joints with Nonautologous Tissue Substitute, Posterior Approach, Posterior Column, Open Approach

ØSG10KJ   Fusion of 2 or More Lumbar Vertebral Joints with Nonautologous Tissue Substitute, Posterior Approach, Anterior Column, Open Approach

ØSG1370   Fusion of 2 or More Lumbar Vertebral Joints with Autologous Tissue Substitute, Anterior Approach, Anterior Column, Percutaneous Approach

HAC 12: Surgical Site Infection-Certain Orthopedic Procedures of the Spine, Shoulder, and Elbow (continued)

ØSG1371 Fusion of 2 or More Lumbar Vertebral Joints with Autologous Tissue Substitute, Posterior Approach, Posterior Column, Percutaneous Approach

ØSG137J Fusion of 2 or More Lumbar Vertebral Joints with Autologous Tissue Substitute, Posterior Approach, Anterior Column, Percutaneous Approach

ØSG13A0 Fusion of 2 or More Lumbar Vertebral Joints with Interbody Fusion Device, Anterior Approach, Anterior Column, Percutaneous Approach

ØSG13AJ Fusion of 2 or More Lumbar Vertebral Joints with Interbody Fusion Device, Posterior Approach, Anterior Column, Percutaneous Approach

ØSG13J0 Fusion of 2 or More Lumbar Vertebral Joints with Synthetic Substitute, Anterior Approach, Anterior Column, Percutaneous Approach

ØSG13J1 Fusion of 2 or More Lumbar Vertebral Joints with Synthetic Substitute, Posterior Approach, Posterior Column, Percutaneous Approach

ØSG13JJ Fusion of 2 or More Lumbar Vertebral Joints with Synthetic Substitute, Posterior Approach, Anterior Column, Percutaneous Approach

ØSG13K0 Fusion of 2 or More Lumbar Vertebral Joints with Nonautologous Tissue Substitute, Anterior Approach, Anterior Column, Percutaneous Approach

ØSG13K1 Fusion of 2 or More Lumbar Vertebral Joints with Nonautologous Tissue Substitute, Posterior Approach, Posterior Column, Percutaneous Approach

ØSG13KJ Fusion of 2 or More Lumbar Vertebral Joints with Nonautologous Tissue Substitute, Posterior Approach, Anterior Column, Percutaneous Approach

ØSG1470 Fusion of 2 or More Lumbar Vertebral Joints with Autologous Tissue Substitute, Anterior Approach, Anterior Column, Percutaneous Endoscopic Approach

ØSG1471 Fusion of 2 or More Lumbar Vertebral Joints with Autologous Tissue Substitute, Posterior Approach, Posterior Column, Percutaneous Endoscopic Approach

ØSG147J Fusion of 2 or More Lumbar Vertebral Joints with Autologous Tissue Substitute, Posterior Approach, Anterior Column, Percutaneous Endoscopic Approach

ØSG14A0 Fusion of 2 or More Lumbar Vertebral Joints with Interbody Fusion Device, Anterior Approach, Anterior Column, Percutaneous Endoscopic Approach

ØSG14AJ Fusion of 2 or More Lumbar Vertebral Joints with Interbody Fusion Device, Posterior Approach, Anterior Column, Percutaneous Endoscopic Approach

ØSG14J0 Fusion of 2 or More Lumbar Vertebral Joints with Synthetic Substitute, Anterior Approach, Anterior Column, Percutaneous Endoscopic Approach

ØSG14J1 Fusion of 2 or More Lumbar Vertebral Joints with Synthetic Substitute, Posterior Approach, Posterior Column, Percutaneous Endoscopic Approach

ØSG14JJ Fusion of 2 or More Lumbar Vertebral Joints with Synthetic Substitute, Posterior Approach, Anterior Column, Percutaneous Endoscopic Approach

ØSG14K0 Fusion of 2 or More Lumbar Vertebral Joints with Nonautologous Tissue Substitute, Anterior Approach, Anterior Column, Percutaneous Endoscopic Approach

ØSG14K1 Fusion of 2 or More Lumbar Vertebral Joints with Nonautologous Tissue Substitute, Posterior Approach, Posterior Column, Percutaneous Endoscopic Approach

ØSG14KJ Fusion of 2 or More Lumbar Vertebral Joints with Nonautologous Tissue Substitute, Posterior Approach, Anterior Column, Percutaneous Endoscopic Approach

ØSG3070 Fusion of Lumbosacral Joint with Autologous Tissue Substitute, Anterior Approach, Anterior Column, Open Approach

ØSG3071 Fusion of Lumbosacral Joint with Autologous Tissue Substitute, Posterior Approach, Posterior Column, Open Approach

ØSG307J Fusion of Lumbosacral Joint with Autologous Tissue Substitute, Posterior Approach, Anterior Column, Open Approach

ØSG30A0 Fusion of Lumbosacral Joint with Interbody Fusion Device, Anterior Approach, Anterior Column, Open Approach

ØSG30AJ Fusion of Lumbosacral Joint with Interbody Fusion Device, Posterior Approach, Anterior Column, Open Approach

ØSG30J0 Fusion of Lumbosacral Joint with Synthetic Substitute, Anterior Approach, Anterior Column, Open Approach

ØSG30J1 Fusion of Lumbosacral Joint with Synthetic Substitute, Posterior Approach, Posterior Column, Open Approach

ØSG30JJ Fusion of Lumbosacral Joint with Synthetic Substitute, Posterior Approach, Anterior Column, Open Approach

ØSG30K0 Fusion of Lumbosacral Joint with Nonautologous Tissue Substitute, Anterior Approach, Anterior Column, Open Approach

ØSG30K1 Fusion of Lumbosacral Joint with Nonautologous Tissue Substitute, Posterior Approach, Posterior Column, Open Approach

ØSG30KJ Fusion of Lumbosacral Joint with Nonautologous Tissue Substitute, Posterior Approach, Anterior Column, Open Approach

ØSG3370 Fusion of Lumbosacral Joint with Autologous Tissue Substitute, Anterior Approach, Anterior Column, Percutaneous Approach

ØSG3371 Fusion of Lumbosacral Joint with Autologous Tissue Substitute, Posterior Approach, Posterior Column, Percutaneous Approach

ØSG337J Fusion of Lumbosacral Joint with Autologous Tissue Substitute, Posterior Approach, Anterior Column, Percutaneous Approach

ØSG33A0 Fusion of Lumbosacral Joint with Interbody Fusion Device, Anterior Approach, Anterior Column, Percutaneous Approach

ØSG33AJ Fusion of Lumbosacral Joint with Interbody Fusion Device, Posterior Approach, Anterior Column, Percutaneous Approach

ØSG33J0 Fusion of Lumbosacral Joint with Synthetic Substitute, Anterior Approach, Anterior Column, Percutaneous Approach

ØSG33J1 Fusion of Lumbosacral Joint with Synthetic Substitute, Posterior Approach, Posterior Column, Percutaneous Approach

ØSG33JJ Fusion of Lumbosacral Joint with Synthetic Substitute, Posterior Approach, Anterior Column, Percutaneous Approach

ØSG33K0 Fusion of Lumbosacral Joint with Nonautologous Tissue Substitute, Anterior Approach, Anterior Column, Percutaneous Approach

ØSG33K1 Fusion of Lumbosacral Joint with Nonautologous Tissue Substitute, Posterior Approach, Posterior Column, Percutaneous Approach

ØSG33KJ Fusion of Lumbosacral Joint with Nonautologous Tissue Substitute, Posterior Approach, Anterior Column, Percutaneous Approach

ØSG3470 Fusion of Lumbosacral Joint with Autologous Tissue Substitute, Anterior Approach, Anterior Column, Percutaneous Endoscopic Approach

ØSG3471 Fusion of Lumbosacral Joint with Autologous Tissue Substitute, Posterior Approach, Posterior Column, Percutaneous Endoscopic Approach

ØSG347J Fusion of Lumbosacral Joint with Autologous Tissue Substitute, Posterior Approach, Anterior Column, Percutaneous Endoscopic Approach

ØSG34A0 Fusion of Lumbosacral Joint with Interbody Fusion Device, Anterior Approach, Anterior Column, Percutaneous Endoscopic Approach

ØSG34AJ Fusion of Lumbosacral Joint with Interbody Fusion Device, Posterior Approach, Anterior Column, Percutaneous Endoscopic Approach

ØSG34J0 Fusion of Lumbosacral Joint with Synthetic Substitute, Anterior Approach, Anterior Column, Percutaneous Endoscopic Approach

ØSG34J1 Fusion of Lumbosacral Joint with Synthetic Substitute, Posterior Approach, Posterior Column, Percutaneous Endoscopic Approach

ØSG34JJ Fusion of Lumbosacral Joint with Synthetic Substitute, Posterior Approach, Anterior Column, Percutaneous Endoscopic Approach

ØSG34K0 Fusion of Lumbosacral Joint with Nonautologous Tissue Substitute, Anterior Approach, Anterior Column, Percutaneous Endoscopic Approach

ØSG34K1 Fusion of Lumbosacral Joint with Nonautologous Tissue Substitute, Posterior Approach, Posterior Column, Percutaneous Endoscopic Approach

ØSG34KJ Fusion of Lumbosacral Joint with Nonautologous Tissue Substitute, Posterior Approach, Anterior Column, Percutaneous Endoscopic Approach

ØSG704Z Fusion of Right Sacroiliac Joint with Internal Fixation Device, Open Approach

ØSG707Z Fusion of Right Sacroiliac Joint with Autologous Tissue Substitute, Open Approach

ØSG70JZ Fusion of Right Sacroiliac Joint with Synthetic Substitute, Open Approach

ØSG70KZ Fusion of Right Sacroiliac Joint with Nonautologous Tissue Substitute, Open Approach

HAC 12: Surgical Site Infection-Certain Orthopedic Procedures of the Spine, Shoulder, and Elbow (continued)

ØSG734Z Fusion of Right Sacroiliac Joint with Internal Fixation Device, Percutaneous Approach

ØSG737Z Fusion of Right Sacroiliac Joint with Autologous Tissue Substitute, Percutaneous Approach

ØSG73JZ Fusion of Right Sacroiliac Joint with Synthetic Substitute, Percutaneous Approach

ØSG73KZ Fusion of Right Sacroiliac Joint with Nonautologous Tissue Substitute, Percutaneous Approach

ØSG744Z Fusion of Right Sacroiliac Joint with Internal Fixation Device, Percutaneous Endoscopic Approach

ØSG747Z Fusion of Right Sacroiliac Joint with Autologous Tissue Substitute, Percutaneous Endoscopic Approach

ØSG74JZ Fusion of Right Sacroiliac Joint with Synthetic Substitute, Percutaneous Endoscopic Approach

ØSG74KZ Fusion of Right Sacroiliac Joint with Nonautologous Tissue Substitute, Percutaneous Endoscopic Approach

ØSG804Z Fusion of Left Sacroiliac Joint with Internal Fixation Device, Open Approach

ØSG807Z Fusion of Left Sacroiliac Joint with Autologous Tissue Substitute, Open Approach

ØSG80JZ Fusion of Left Sacroiliac Joint with Synthetic Substitute, Open Approach

ØSG80KZ Fusion of Left Sacroiliac Joint with Nonautologous Tissue Substitute, Open Approach

ØSG834Z Fusion of Left Sacroiliac Joint with Internal Fixation Device, Percutaneous Approach

ØSG837Z Fusion of Left Sacroiliac Joint with Autologous Tissue Substitute, Percutaneous Approach

ØSG83JZ Fusion of Left Sacroiliac Joint with Synthetic Substitute, Percutaneous Approach

ØSG83KZ Fusion of Left Sacroiliac Joint with Nonautologous Tissue Substitute, Percutaneous Approach

ØSG844Z Fusion of Left Sacroiliac Joint with Internal Fixation Device, Percutaneous Endoscopic Approach

ØSG847Z Fusion of Left Sacroiliac Joint with Autologous Tissue Substitute, Percutaneous Endoscopic Approach

ØSG84JZ Fusion of Left Sacroiliac Joint with Synthetic Substitute, Percutaneous Endoscopic Approach

ØSG84KZ Fusion of Left Sacroiliac Joint with Nonautologous Tissue Substitute, Percutaneous Endoscopic Approach

XRGAØR7 Fusion of Thoracolumbar Vertebral Joint using Customizable Interbody Fusion Device, Open Approach, New Technology Group 7

XRGA3R7 Fusion of Thoracolumbar Vertebral Joint using Customizable Interbody Fusion Device, Percutaneous Approach, New Technology Group 7

XRGA4R7 Fusion of Thoracolumbar Vertebral Joint using Customizable Interbody Fusion Device, Percutaneous Endoscopic Approach, New Technology Group 7

XRGBØR7 Fusion of Lumbar Vertebral Joint using Customizable Interbody Fusion Device, Open Approach, New Technology Group 7

XRGB3R7 Fusion of Lumbar Vertebral Joint using Customizable Interbody Fusion Device, Percutaneous Approach, New Technology Group 7

XRGB4R7 Fusion of Lumbar Vertebral Joint using Customizable Interbody Fusion Device, Percutaneous Endoscopic Approach, New Technology Group 7

XRGCØR7 Fusion of 2 or more Lumbar Vertebral Joints using Customizable Interbody Fusion Device, Open Approach, New Technology Group 7

XRGC3R7 Fusion of 2 or more Lumbar Vertebral Joints using Customizable Interbody Fusion Device, Percutaneous Approach, New Technology Group 7

XRGC4R7 Fusion of 2 or more Lumbar Vertebral Joints using Customizable Interbody Fusion Device, Percutaneous Endoscopic Approach, New Technology Group 7

XRGDØR7 Fusion of Lumbosacral Joint using Customizable Interbody Fusion Device, Open Approach, New Technology Group 7

XRGD3R7 Fusion of Lumbosacral Joint using Customizable Interbody Fusion Device, Percutaneous Approach, New Technology Group 7

XRGD4R7 Fusion of Lumbosacral Joint using Customizable Interbody Fusion Device, Percutaneous Endoscopic Approach, New Technology Group 7

HAC 13: Surgical Site Infection (SSI) Following Cardiac Implantable Electronic Device (CIED) Procedures

Secondary diagnosis not POA:

K68.11 Postprocedural retroperitoneal abscess

T81.40XA Infection following a procedure, unspecified, initial encounter

T81.41XA Infection following a procedure, superficial incisional surgical site, initial encounter

T81.42XA Infection following a procedure, deep incisional surgical site, initial encounter

T81.43XA Infection following a procedure, organ and space surgical site, initial encounter

T81.44XA Sepsis following a procedure, initial encounter

T81.49XA Infection following a procedure, other surgical site, initial encounter

T82.7XXA Infection and inflammatory reaction due to other internal orthopedic prosthetic devices, implants and grafts, initial encounter

AND

Any of the following procedures:

02H43JZ Insertion of Pacemaker Lead into Coronary Vein, Percutaneous Approach

02H43KZ Insertion of Defibrillator Lead into Coronary Vein, Percutaneous Approach

02H43MZ Insertion of Cardiac Lead into Coronary Vein, Percutaneous Approach

02H63JZ Insertion of Pacemaker Lead into Right Atrium, Percutaneous Approach

02H63MZ Insertion of Cardiac Lead into Right Atrium, Percutaneous Approach

02H73JZ Insertion of Pacemaker Lead into Left Atrium, Percutaneous Approach

02H73MZ Insertion of Cardiac Lead into Left Atrium, Percutaneous Approach

02HK3JZ Insertion of Pacemaker Lead into Right Ventricle, Percutaneous Approach

02HL3JZ Insertion of Pacemaker Lead into Left Ventricle, Percutaneous Approach

02HNØJZ Insertion of Pacemaker Lead into Pericardium, Open Approach

02HNØMZ Insertion of Cardiac Lead into Pericardium, Open Approach

02HN3JZ Insertion of Pacemaker Lead into Pericardium, Percutaneous Approach

02HN3MZ Insertion of Cardiac Lead into Pericardium, Percutaneous Approach

02HN4JZ Insertion of Pacemaker Lead into Pericardium, Percutaneous Endoscopic Approach

02HN4MZ Insertion of Cardiac Lead into Pericardium, Percutaneous Endoscopic Approach

02PAØMZ Removal of Cardiac Lead from Heart, Open Approach

02PA3MZ Removal of Cardiac Lead from Heart, Percutaneous Approach

02PA4MZ Removal of Cardiac Lead from Heart, Percutaneous Endoscopic Approach

02PAXMZ Removal of Cardiac Lead from Heart, External Approach

02WAØMZ Revision of Cardiac Lead in Heart, Open Approach

02WA3MZ Revision of Cardiac Lead in Heart, Percutaneous Approach

02WA4MZ Revision of Cardiac Lead in Heart, Percutaneous Endoscopic Approach

0JH604Z Insertion of Pacemaker, Single Chamber into Chest Subcutaneous Tissue and Fascia, Open Approach

0JH605Z Insertion of Pacemaker, Single Chamber Rate Responsive into Chest Subcutaneous Tissue and Fascia, Open Approach

0JH606Z Insertion of Pacemaker, Dual Chamber into Chest Subcutaneous Tissue and Fascia, Open Approach

0JH607Z Insertion of Cardiac Resynchronization Pacemaker Pulse Generator into Chest Subcutaneous Tissue and Fascia, Open Approach

0JH608Z Insertion of Defibrillator Generator into Chest Subcutaneous Tissue and Fascia, Open Approach

0JH609Z Insertion of Cardiac Resynchronization Defibrillator Pulse Generator into Chest Subcutaneous Tissue and Fascia, Open Approach

0JH60PZ Insertion of Cardiac Rhythm Related Device into Chest Subcutaneous Tissue and Fascia, Open Approach

0JH634Z Insertion of Pacemaker, Single Chamber into Chest Subcutaneous Tissue and Fascia, Percutaneous Approach

0JH635Z Insertion of Pacemaker, Single Chamber Rate Responsive into Chest Subcutaneous Tissue and Fascia, Percutaneous Approach

0JH636Z Insertion of Pacemaker, Dual Chamber into Chest Subcutaneous Tissue and Fascia, Percutaneous Approach

0JH637Z Insertion of Cardiac Resynchronization Pacemaker Pulse Generator into Chest Subcutaneous Tissue and Fascia, Percutaneous Approach

0JH638Z Insertion of Defibrillator Generator into Chest Subcutaneous Tissue and Fascia, Percutaneous Approach

0JH639Z Insertion of Cardiac Resynchronization Defibrillator Pulse Generator into Chest Subcutaneous Tissue and Fascia, Percutaneous Approach

0JH63PZ Insertion of Cardiac Rhythm Related Device into Chest Subcutaneous Tissue and Fascia, Percutaneous Approach

0JH804Z Insertion of Pacemaker, Single Chamber into Abdomen Subcutaneous Tissue and Fascia, Open Approach

HAC 13: Surgical Site Infection (SSI) Following Cardiac Implantable Electronic Device (CIED) Procedures (continued)

ØJH805Z   Insertion of Pacemaker, Single Chamber Rate Responsive into Abdomen Subcutaneous Tissue and Fascia, Open Approach

ØJH806Z   Insertion of Pacemaker, Dual Chamber into Abdomen Subcutaneous Tissue and Fascia, Open Approach

ØJH807Z   Insertion of Cardiac Resynchronization Pacemaker Pulse Generator into Abdomen Subcutaneous Tissue and Fascia, Open Approach

ØJH808Z   Insertion of Defibrillator Generator into Abdomen Subcutaneous Tissue and Fascia, Open Approach

ØJH809Z   Insertion of Cardiac Resynchronization Defibrillator Pulse Generator into Abdomen Subcutaneous Tissue and Fascia, Open Approach

ØJH80PZ   Insertion of Cardiac Rhythm Related Device into Abdomen Subcutaneous Tissue and Fascia, Open Approach

ØJH834Z   Insertion of Pacemaker, Single Chamber into Abdomen Subcutaneous Tissue and Fascia, Percutaneous Approach

ØJH835Z   Insertion of Pacemaker, Single Chamber Rate Responsive into Abdomen Subcutaneous Tissue and Fascia, Percutaneous Approach

ØJH836Z   Insertion of Pacemaker, Dual Chamber into Abdomen Subcutaneous Tissue and Fascia, Percutaneous Approach

ØJH837Z   Insertion of Cardiac Resynchronization Pacemaker Pulse Generator into Abdomen Subcutaneous Tissue and Fascia, Percutaneous Approach

ØJH838Z   Insertion of Defibrillator Generator into Abdomen Subcutaneous Tissue and Fascia, Percutaneous Approach

ØJH839Z   Insertion of Cardiac Resynchronization Defibrillator Pulse Generator into Abdomen Subcutaneous Tissue and Fascia, Percutaneous Approach

ØJH83PZ   Insertion of Cardiac Rhythm Related Device into Abdomen Subcutaneous Tissue and Fascia, Percutaneous Approach

ØJPTØFZ   Removal of Subcutaneous Defibrillator Lead from Trunk Subcutaneous Tissue and Fascia, Open Approach

ØJPTØPZ   Removal of Cardiac Rhythm Related Device from Trunk Subcutaneous Tissue and Fascia, Open Approach

ØJPT3FZ   Removal of Subcutaneous Defibrillator Lead from Trunk Subcutaneous Tissue and Fascia, Percutaneous Approach

ØJPT3PZ   Removal of Cardiac Rhythm Related Device from Trunk Subcutaneous Tissue and Fascia, Percutaneous Approach

ØJWTØFZ   Revision of Subcutaneous Defibrillator Lead in Trunk Subcutaneous Tissue and Fascia, Open Approach

ØJWTØPZ   Revision of Cardiac Rhythm Related Device in Trunk Subcutaneous Tissue and Fascia, Open Approach

ØJWT3FZ   Revision of Subcutaneous Defibrillator Lead in Trunk Subcutaneous Tissue and Fascia, Percutaneous Approach

ØJWT3PZ   Revision of Cardiac Rhythm Related Device in Trunk Subcutaneous Tissue and Fascia, Percutaneous Approach

HAC 14: Iatrogenic Pneumothorax with Venous Catheterization

Secondary diagnosis not POA:

J95.811   Postprocedural pneumothorax

AND

Any of the following procedures:

02H633Z   Insertion of Infusion Device into Right Atrium, Percutaneous Approach

02HK33Z   Insertion of Infusion Device into Right Ventricle, Percutaneous Approach

02HS33Z   Insertion of Infusion Device into Right Pulmonary Vein, Percutaneous Approach

02HS43Z   Insertion of Infusion Device into Right Pulmonary Vein, Percutaneous Endoscopic Approach

02HT33Z   Insertion of Infusion Device into Left Pulmonary Vein, Percutaneous Approach

02HT43Z   Insertion of Infusion Device into Left Pulmonary Vein, Percutaneous Endoscopic Approach

02HV33Z   Insertion of Infusion Device into Superior Vena Cava, Percutaneous Approach

02HV43Z   Insertion of Infusion Device into Superior Vena Cava, Percutaneous Endoscopic Approach

05H033Z   Insertion of Infusion Device into Azygos Vein, Percutaneous Approach

05H043Z   Insertion of Infusion Device into Azygos Vein, Percutaneous Endoscopic Approach

05H133Z   Insertion of Infusion Device into Hemiazygos Vein, Percutaneous Approach

05H143Z   Insertion of Infusion Device into Hemiazygos Vein, Percutaneous Endoscopic Approach

05H333Z   Insertion of Infusion Device into Right Innominate Vein, Percutaneous Approach

05H343Z   Insertion of Infusion Device into Right Innominate Vein, Percutaneous Endoscopic Approach

05H433Z   Insertion of Infusion Device into Left Innominate Vein, Percutaneous Approach

05H443Z   Insertion of Infusion Device into Left Innominate Vein, Percutaneous Endoscopic Approach

05H533Z   Insertion of Infusion Device into Right Subclavian Vein, Percutaneous Approach

05H543Z   Insertion of Infusion Device into Right Subclavian Vein, Percutaneous Endoscopic Approach

05H633Z   Insertion of Infusion Device into Left Subclavian Vein, Percutaneous Approach

05H643Z   Insertion of Infusion Device into Left Subclavian Vein, Percutaneous Endoscopic Approach

05HM33Z   Insertion of Infusion Device into Right Internal Jugular Vein, Percutaneous Approach

05HN33Z   Insertion of Infusion Device into Left Internal Jugular Vein, Percutaneous Approach

05HP33Z   Insertion of Infusion Device into Right External Jugular Vein, Percutaneous Approach

05HQ33Z   Insertion of Infusion Device into Left External Jugular Vein, Percutaneous Approach

ØJH63XZ   Insertion of Vascular Access Device into Chest Subcutaneous Tissue and Fascia, Percutaneous Approach

Appendix L: Procedure Combination Tables

The tables below were developed to help simplify the relationship between ICD-10-PCS coding and MS-DRG assignment. The Centers for Medicare & Medicaid Services (CMS) has identified in the MS-DRG Definitions Manual certain procedure combinations that must occur in order to assign a specific MS-DRG. There are many factors influencing MS-DRG assignment, including principal and secondary diagnoses, MCC or CC use, sex of the patient, and discharge status. These tables should be used only as a guide. These tables were created based on the proposed, version 40, MS-DRG Grouper software and Definitions Manual files published with the fiscal 2023 IPPS proposed rule. To view the most current files, refer to the following:
https://www.cms.gov/Medicare/Medicare-Fee-for-Service-Payment/AcuteInpatientPPS/MS-DRG-Classifications-and-Software.

DRG 001-002 Heart Transplant or Implant of Heart Assist System

Heart Transplant
Replacement of Right and Left Ventricle 02RK0JZ and 02RL0JZ

Insertion With Removal of Heart Assist System

Type of Heart Assist System	Code as appropriate Insertion by approach	Code also as appropriate Removal of Heart Assist System by approach
Biventricular External	02HA[0,3,4]RS	02PA[0,3,4]RZ
External	02HA[0,4]RZ	02PA[0,3,4]RZ

Revision With Removal of Heart Assist System

Type of Heart Assist System	Code as appropriate Revision by approach	Code also as appropriate Removal of Heart Assist System by approach
Implantable	02WA[0,3,4]QZ	02PA[0,3,4]RZ
External	02WA[0,3,4]RZ	02PA[0,3,4]RZ

DRG 008 Simultaneous Pancreas/Kidney Transplant

Transplanted Body Part	Code Transplant as appropriate by tissue type			Code also Pancreas Transplant as appropriate by tissue type		
	Allogeneic	Syngeneic	Zooplastic	Allogeneic	Syngeneic	Zooplastic
Kidney, Right	0TY00Z0	0TY00Z1	0TY00Z2	0FYG0Z0	0FYG0Z1	0FYG0Z2
Kidney, Left	0TY10Z0	0TY10Z1	0TY10Z2			

DRG 019 Simultaneous Pancreas/Kidney Transplant with Hemodialysis

Transplanted Body Part	Code Transplant as appropriate by tissue type			Code also Pancreas Transplant as appropriate by tissue type			Code also Hemodialysis		
	Allogeneic	Syngeneic	Zooplastic	Allogeneic	Syngeneic	Zooplastic	< 6 Hours	6-18 Hours	> 18 Hours
Kidney, Right	0TY00Z0	0TY00Z1	0TY00Z2	0FYG0Z0	0FYG0Z1	0FYG0Z2	5A1D07Z	5A1D80Z	5A1D90Z
Kidney, Left	0TY10Z0	0TY10Z1	0TY10Z2						

DRG 023-027 Craniotomy

Site of Neurostimulator Lead	Code as appropriate Insertion of Lead by approach	Code also as appropriate Insertion of Device by type and subcutaneous site						
		Neuro-stimulator Generator	Stimulator Multiple Array Code as appropriate by approach			Stimulator Multiple Array, Rechargeable Code as appropriate by approach		
		Skull	Chest	Back	Abdomen	Chest	Back	Abdomen
Brain	00H0[0,3,4]MZ	0NH00NZ	0JH6[0,3]DZ	0JH7[0,3]DZ	0JH8[0,3]DZ	0JH6[0,3]EZ	0JH7[0,3]EZ	0JH8[0,3]EZ
Cerebral Ventricle	00H6[0,3,4]MZ	0NH00NZ	0JH6[0,3]DZ	0JH7[0,3]DZ	0JH8[0,3]DZ	0JH6[0,3]EZ	0JH7[0,3]EZ	0JH8[0,3]EZ

DRG 028-030 Spinal Procedures

Generator Type	Insertion of Generator by Site			Code also as appropriate Insertion of Neurostimulator Lead by approach	
	Chest	Abdomen	Back	Spinal Canal	Spinal Cord
Single Array	0JH6[0,3]BZ	0JH8[0,3]BZ	0JH7[0,3]BZ	00HU[0,3,4]MZ	00HV[0,3,4]MZ
Single Array, Rechargeable	0JH6[0,3]CZ	0JH8[0,3]CZ	0JH7[0,3]CZ	00HU[0,3,4]MZ	00HV[0,3,4]MZ
Multiple Array	0JH6[0,3]DZ	0JH8[0,3]DZ	0JH7[0,3]DZ	00HU[0,3,4]MZ	00HV[0,3,4]MZ
Multiple Array, Rechargeable	0JH6[0,3]EZ	—	0JH7[0,3]EZ	00HU[0,3,4]MZ	00HV[0,3,4]MZ
Multiple Array, Rechargeable	—	0JH8[0,3]EZ	—	00HU[0,3,4]MZ	00HV[0,3,4]MZ

DRG 040-042 Peripheral and Cranial Nerve and Other Nervous System Procedures

Insertion of Neurostimulator Generator and Lead

Insertion Single Array Generator, by Site		Code also Lead Insertion, by Site					
		Cranial Nerve	Peripheral Nerve	Azygos Vein	Innominate Vein, RT	Innominate Vein, LT	Stomach
Chest	0JH6[0,3]BZ						
Back	0JH7[0,3]BZ	00HE[0,3,4]MZ	01HY[0,3,4]MZ	05H0[0,3,4]MZ	05H3[0,3,4]MZ	05H4[0,3,4]MZ	0DH6[0,3,4]MZ
Abdomen	0JH8[0,3]BZ						

Insertion Single Array, Rechargeable Generator, by Site		Code also Lead Insertion, by Site					
		Cranial Nerve	Peripheral Nerve	Azygos Vein	Innominate Vein, RT	Innominate Vein, LT	Stomach
Chest	0JH6[0,3]CZ						
Back	0JH7[0,3]CZ	00HE[0,3,4]MZ	01HY[0,3,4]MZ	05H0[0,3,4]MZ	05H3[0,3,4]MZ	05H4[0,3,4]MZ	0DH6[0,3,4]MZ
Abdomen	0JH8[0,3]CZ						

Insertion Multiple Array Generator, by Site		Code also Lead Insertion, by Site					
		Cranial Nerve	Peripheral Nerve	Azygos Vein	Innominate Vein, RT	Innominate Vein, LT	Stomach
Chest	0JH6[0,3]DZ						
Back	0JH7[0,3]DZ	00HE[0,3,4]MZ	01HY[0,3,4]MZ	05H0[0,3,4]MZ	05H3[0,3,4]MZ	05H4[0,3,4]MZ	0DH6[0,3,4]MZ
Abdomen	0JH8[0,3]DZ						

Insertion Multiple Array, Rechargeable Generator, by Site		Code also Lead Insertion, by Site					
		Cranial Nerve	Peripheral Nerve	Azygos Vein	Innominate Vein, RT	Innominate Vein, LT	Stomach
Chest	0JH6[0,3]EZ						
Back	0JH7[0,3]EZ	00HE[0,3,4]MZ	01HY[0,3,4]MZ	05H0[0,3,4]MZ	05H3[0,3,4]MZ	05H4[0,3,4]MZ	0DH6[0,3,4]MZ
Abdomen	0JH8[0,3]EZ						

Insertion Stimulator Generator, by Site		Code also Lead Insertion, by Site					
		Cranial Nerve	Peripheral Nerve	Azygos Vein	Innominate Vein, RT	Innominate Vein, LT	Stomach
Chest	0JH6[0,3]MZ						
Back	0JH7[0,3]MZ	00HE[0,3,4]MZ	01HY[0,3,4]MZ	05H0[0,3,4]MZ	05H3[0,3,4]MZ	05H4[0,3,4]MZ	0DH6[0,3,4]MZ
Abdomen	0JH8[0,3]MZ						

DRG 222-227 Cardiac Defibrillator Implant

Insertion of Generator With Insertion of Lead(s) into Coronary Vein, Atrium or Ventricle

Generator Type	Insertion of Generator by Site		Code also as appropriate Insertion of Leads by site					
	Chest	Abdomen	Coronary Vein	Atrium		Ventricle		
				Right	Left	Right	Left	
Defibrillator	ØJH6[Ø,3]8Z	ØJH8[Ø,3]8Z	02H4[Ø,4]KZ	02H6[Ø,3,4]KZ	02H7[Ø,3,4]KZ	02HK[Ø,3,4]KZ	02HL[Ø,3,4]KZ	
Cardiac Resynch Defibrillator Pulse Generator	ØJH6[Ø,3]9Z	ØJH8[Ø,3]9Z	02H4[Ø,3,4]KZ or 02H43[J,M]Z	02H6[Ø,3,4]KZ	02H7[Ø,3,4]KZ	02HK[Ø,3,4]KZ	02HL[Ø,3,4]KZ	
Contractility Modulation Device	ØJH6[Ø,3]AZ	ØJH8[Ø,3]AZ	—	02H6[Ø,3,4]MZ	—	02HK[Ø,3,4]MZ	—	

Insertion of Generator with Insertion of Lead(s) into Pericardium or Chest

Generator Type	Insertion of Generator by Site		Code also as appropriate Insertion of Leads by Site and Type			
	Chest	Abdomen	Pericardium			Chest
			Pacemaker	Defibrillator	Cardiac	Subcutaneous
Defibrillator	ØJH6[Ø,3]8Z	ØJH8[Ø,3]8Z	02HN[Ø,3,4]JZ	02HN[Ø,3,4]KZ	02HN[Ø,3,4]MZ	ØJH6[Ø,3]FZ
Cardiac Resynch Defibrillator Pulse Generator	ØJH6[Ø,3]9Z	ØJH8[Ø,3]9Z	02HN[Ø,3,4]JZ	02HN[Ø,3,4]KZ	02HN[Ø,3,4]MZ	ØJH6[Ø,3]FZ

DRG 242-244 Permanent Cardiac Pacemaker Implant

Insertion of Generator and Lead(s) Only

Generator Type	Insertion of Generator by Site		Code also Insertion of Lead, by Site			
	Chest	Abdomen	Coronary Vein	Right Atrium (6)/Left Atrium (7)	Right Ventricle (K)/ Left Ventricle (L)	Pericardium
Single Chamber	ØJH6[Ø,3]4Z	ØJH8[Ø,3]4Z	02H4[Ø,3,4][J,M]Z	02H[6,7][Ø,3,4][J,M]Z	02H[K,L][Ø,3,4][J,M]Z	02HN[Ø,3,4][J,M]Z
Single Chamber RR	ØJH6[Ø,3]5Z	ØJH8[Ø,3]5Z	02H4[Ø,3,4][J,M]Z	02H[6,7][Ø,3,4][J,M]Z	02H[K,L][Ø,3,4][J,M]Z	02HN[Ø,3,4][J,M]Z
Dual Chamber	ØJH6[Ø,3]6Z	ØJH8[Ø,3]6Z	02H4[Ø,3,4][J,M]Z	02H[6,7][Ø,3,4][J,M]Z	02H[K,L][Ø,3,4][J,M]Z	02HN[Ø,3,4][J,M]Z
Cardiac Resynch	ØJH6[Ø,3]7Z	ØJH8[Ø,3]7Z	02H4[Ø,3,4][J,M]Z	02H[6,7][Ø,3,4][J,M]Z	02H[K,L][Ø,3,4][J,M]Z	02HN[Ø,3,4][J,M]Z
Cardiac Rhythm Related	ØJH6[Ø,3]PZ	ØJH8[Ø,3]PZ	02H4[Ø,3,4][J,M]Z	02H[6,7][Ø,3,4][J,M]Z	02H[K,L][Ø,3,4][J,M]Z	02HN[Ø,3,4][J,M]Z

DRG 326-328 Stomach, Esophageal and Duodenal Procedures

Site	Resection by Open Approach	Code also as appropriate Resection of Pancreas by Open Approach
Duodenum	ØDT90ZZ	ØFTGØZZ

DRG 344-346 Minor Small and Large Bowel Procedures

Site	Repair by Open Approach	Code also as appropriate Repair by external approach of Abdominal Wall Stoma
Small Intestine	ØDQ80ZZ	ØWQFXZ2
Duodenum	ØDQ90ZZ	ØWQFXZ2
Jejunum	ØDQAØZZ	ØWQFXZ2
Ileum	ØDQBØZZ	ØWQFXZ2
Large Intestine	ØDQEØZZ	ØWQFXZ2
Large Intestine, Right	ØDQFØZZ	ØWQFXZ2
Large Intestine, Left	ØDQGØZZ	ØWQFXZ2
Cecum	ØDQHØZZ	ØWQFXZ2
Ascending Colon	ØDQKØZZ	ØWQFXZ2
Transverse Colon	ØDQLØZZ	ØWQFXZ2
Descending Colon	ØDQMØZZ	ØWQFXZ2
Sigmoid Colon	ØDQNØZZ	ØWQFXZ2

DRG 456-458 Spinal Fusion Except Cervical with Spinal Curvature/Malignancy/Infection or Extensive Fusions

Fusion of Thoracic and Lumbar Vertebra, Anterior Column

2 to 7 Thoracic Vertebra		Code also 2 or more Lumbar Vertebra	
ØRG[Ø,3,4][7,A,J,K]Ø	XRG70F3	ØSG1[Ø,3,4][7,A,J,K]Ø	XRGCØF3

Fusion of Thoracic and Lumbar Vertebra, Posterior Column

2 to 7 Thoracic Vertebra			Code also 2 or more Lumbar Vertebra		
Posterior Approach	Anterior Approach	New Technology	Posterior Approach	Anterior Approach	New Technology
ØRG7[Ø,3,4][7,J,K]1	ØRG7[Ø,3,4][7,A,J,K]J	XRG7092 XRG70F3	ØSG1[Ø,3,4][7,J,K]1	ØSG1[Ø,3,4][7,A,J,K]J	XRGC092 XRGCØF3

DRG 461-462 Bilateral or Multiple Major Joint Procedures of Lower Extremity

For procedures to qualify as bilateral or multiple joint procedures, at least one replacement code or combination removal and replacement code from two different lower extremity sites from the following table(s) must be reported.

Examples: Left hip and right hip codes (bilateral); left hip and left knee codes (multiple); left hip and right ankle codes (multiple); left knee and right knee codes (bilateral); right hip removal and replacement, with right knee replacement

Hip, RT	Hip, LT	Knee, RT	Knee, LT	Ankle, RT	Ankle, LT
ØSR9019	ØSRBØ19	ØSRCØ69	ØSRDØ69	ØSRFØ7Z	ØSRGØ7Z
ØSR901A	ØSRB01A	ØSRCØ6A	ØSRDØ6A	ØSRFØJ9	ØSRGØJ9
ØSR901Z	ØSRB01Z	ØSRCØ6Z	ØSRDØ6Z	ØSRFØJA	ØSRGØJA
ØSR9029	ØSRBØ29	ØSRCØ7Z	ØSRDØ7Z	ØSRFØJZ	ØSRGØJZ
ØSR902A	ØSRBØ2A	ØSRCØJ9	ØSRDØJ9	ØSRFØKZ	ØSRGØKZ
ØSR902Z	ØSRBØ2Z	ØSRCØJA	ØSRDØJA		
ØSR9039	ØSRBØ39	ØSRCØJZ	ØSRDØJZ		
ØSR903A	ØSRBØ3A	ØSRCØKZ	ØSRDØKZ		
ØSR903Z	ØSRBØ3Z	ØSRCØL9	ØSRDØL9		
ØSR9049	ØSRBØ49	ØSRCØLA	ØSRDØLA		
ØSR904A	ØSRBØ4A	ØSRCØLZ	ØSRDØLZ		
ØSR904Z	ØSRBØ4Z	ØSRCØM9	ØSRDØM9		
ØSR9069	ØSRBØ69	ØSRCØMA	ØSRDØMA		
ØSR906A	ØSRBØ6A	ØSRCØMZ	ØSRDØMZ		
ØSR906Z	ØSRBØ6Z	ØSRCØN9	ØSRDØN9		
ØSR907Z	ØSRBØ7Z	ØSRCØNA	ØSRDØNA		
ØSR90J9	ØSRBØJ9	ØSRCØNZ	ØSRDØNZ		
ØSR90JA	ØSRBØJA	ØSRTØ7Z	ØSRUØ7Z		
ØSR90JZ	ØSRBØJZ	ØSRTØJ9	ØSRUØJ9		
ØSR90KZ	ØSRBØKZ	ØSRTØJA	ØSRUØJA		
ØSRA009	ØSRE009	ØSRTØJZ	ØSRUØJZ		
ØSRA00A	ØSRE00A	ØSRTØKZ	ØSRUØKZ		
ØSRA00Z	ØSRE00Z	ØSRVØ7Z	ØSRWØ7Z		
ØSRA019	ØSRE019	ØSRVØJ9	ØSRWØJ9		
ØSRA01A	ØSRE01A	ØSRVØJA	ØSRWØJA		

Hip, RT	Hip, LT	Knee, RT	Knee, LT	Ankle, RT	Ankle, LT
ØSRA01Z	ØSRE01Z	ØSRVØJZ	ØSRWØJZ		
ØSRA039	ØSRE039	ØSRVØKZ	ØSRWØKZ		
ØSRA03A	ØSRE03A	ØSPCØJZ	ØSPDØJZ		
ØSRA03Z	ØSRE03Z				
ØSRA07Z	ØSRE07Z				
ØSRAØJ9	ØSREØJ9				
ØSRAØJA	ØSREØJA				
ØSRAØJZ	ØSREØJZ				
ØSRAØKZ	ØSREØKZ				
ØSRR019	ØSRS019				
ØSRR01A	ØSRS01A				
ØSRR01Z	ØSRS01Z				
ØSRR039	ØSRS039				
ØSRR03A	ØSRS03A				
ØSRR03Z	ØSRS03Z				
ØSRR07Z	ØSRS07Z				
ØSRRØJ9	ØSRSØJ9				
ØSRRØJA	ØSRSØJA				
ØSRRØJZ	ØSRSØJZ				
ØSRRØKZ	ØSRSØKZ				
ØSU90BZ	ØSUBØBZ				
ØSUAØBZ	ØSUEØBZ				
ØSURØBZ	ØSUSØBZ				
ØSP90JZ	ØSPBØJZ				

Hip Procedure Combinations

Open Removal of Hip Spacer with Replacement

Removal of Spacer		Code also as appropriate Replacement by Device Type					
		Metal	Metal on Poly	Ceramic	Ceramic on Poly	Oxidized Zirc on Poly	Synth Subst
Hip, RT	ØSP908Z	ØSR901[9,A,Z]	ØSR902[9,A,Z]	ØSR903[9,A,Z]	ØSR904[9,A,Z]	ØSR906[9,A,Z]	ØSR90J[9,A,Z]
Hip, LT	ØSPBØ8Z	ØSRBØ1[9,A,Z]	ØSRBØ2[9,A,Z]	ØSRBØ3[9,A,Z]	ØSRBØ4[9,A,Z]	ØSRBØ6[9,A,Z]	ØSRBØJ[9,A,Z]

Open Removal of Hip Spacer with Replacement

Removal of Spacer		Code also as appropriate Replacement by Device Type						
		Acetabular Surface				Femoral Surface		
		Poly	Metal	Ceramic	Synthetic	Metal	Ceramic	Synth
Hip, RT	ØSP9Ø8Z	ØSRAØØ[9,A,Z]	ØSRAØ1[9,A,Z]	ØSRAØ3[9,A,Z]	ØSRAØJ[9,A,Z]	ØSRRØ1[9,A,Z]	ØSRRØ3[9,A,Z]	ØSRRØJ[9,A,Z]
Hip, LT	ØSPBØ8Z	ØSREØØ[9,A,Z]	ØSREØ1[9,A,Z]	ØSREØ3[9,A,Z]	ØSREØJ[9,A,Z]	ØSRSØ1[9,A,Z]	ØSRSØ3[9,A,Z]	ØSRSØJ[9,A,Z]

Open Removal of Hip Liner with Replacement

Removal of Liner		Code also as appropriate Replacement by Device Type					
		Metal	Metal on Poly	Ceramic	Ceramic on Poly	Oxidized Zirc on Poly	Synth Subst
Hip, RT	ØSP9Ø9Z	ØSR9Ø1[9,A,Z]	ØSR9Ø2[9,A,Z]	ØSR9Ø3[9,A,Z]	ØSR9Ø4[9,A,Z]	ØSR9Ø6[9,A,Z]	ØSR9ØJ[9,A,Z]
Hip, LT	ØSPBØ9Z	ØSRBØ1[9,A,Z]	ØSRBØ2[9,A,Z]	ØSRBØ3[9,A,Z]	ØSRBØ4[9,A,Z]	ØSRBØ6[9,A,Z]	ØSRBØJ[9,A,Z]

Open Removal of Hip Liner with Replacement

Removal of Liner		Code also as appropriate Replacement by Device Type						
		Acetabular Surface				Femoral Surface		
		Poly	Metal	Ceramic	Synthetic	Metal	Ceramic	Synth
Hip, RT	ØSP9Ø9Z	ØSRAØØ[9,A,Z]	ØSRAØ1[9,A,Z]	ØSRAØ3[9,A,Z]	ØSRAØJ[9,A,Z]	ØSRRØ1[9,A,Z]	ØSRRØ3[9,A,Z]	ØSRRØJ[9,A,Z]
Hip, LT	ØSPBØ9Z	ØSREØØ[9,A,Z]	ØSREØ1[9,A,Z]	ØSREØ3[9,A,Z]	ØSREØJ[9,A,Z]	ØSRSØ1[9,A,Z]	ØSRSØ3[9,A,Z]	ØSRSØJ[9,A,Z]

Open Removal of Hip Resurfacing Device with Replacement

Removal of Resurfacing Device		Code also as appropriate Replacement by Device Type					
		Metal	Metal on Poly	Ceramic	Ceramic on Poly	Oxidized Zirc on Poly	Synth Subst
Hip, RT	ØSP9ØBZ	ØSR9Ø1[9,A,Z]	ØSR9Ø2[9,A,Z]	ØSR9Ø3[9,A,Z]	ØSR9Ø4[9,A,Z]	ØSR9Ø6[9,A,Z]	ØSR9ØJ[9,A,Z]
Hip, LT	ØSPBØBZ	ØSRBØ1[9,A,Z]	ØSRBØ2[9,A,Z]	ØSRBØ3[9,A,Z]	ØSRBØ4[9,A,Z]	ØSRBØ6[9,A,Z]	ØSRBØJ[9,A,Z]

Open Removal of Hip Resurfacing Device with Replacement

Removal of Resurfacing Device		Code also as appropriate Replacement by Device Type						
		Acetabular Surface				Femoral Surface		
		Poly	Metal	Ceramic	Synthetic	Metal	Ceramic	Synth
Hip, RT	ØSP9ØBZ	ØSRAØØ[9,A,Z]	ØSRAØ1[9,A,Z]	ØSRAØ3[9,A,Z]	ØSRAØJ[9,A,Z]	ØSRRØ1[9,A,Z]	ØSRRØ3[9,A,Z]	ØSRRØJ[9,A,Z]
Hip, LT	ØSPBØBZ	ØSREØØ[9,A,Z]	ØSREØ1[9,A,Z]	ØSREØ3[9,A,Z]	ØSREØJ[9,A,Z]	ØSRSØ1[9,A,Z]	ØSRSØ3[9,A,Z]	ØSRSØJ[9,A,Z]

Open Removal of Hip Articulating Spacer with Replacement

Removal of Articulating Spacer		Code also as appropriate Replacement by Device Type					
		Metal	Metal on Poly	Ceramic	Ceramic on Poly	Oxidized Zirc on Poly	Synth Subst
Hip, RT	ØSP9ØEZ	ØSR9Ø1[9,A,Z]	ØSR9Ø2[9,A,Z]	ØSR9Ø3[9,A,Z]	ØSR9Ø4[9,A,Z]	ØSR9Ø6[9,A,Z]	ØSR9ØJ[9,A,Z]
Hip, LT	ØSPBØEZ	ØSRBØ1[9,A,Z]	ØSRBØ2[9,A,Z]	ØSRBØ3[9,A,Z]	ØSRBØ4[9,A,Z]	ØSRBØ6[9,A,Z]	ØSRBØJ[9,A,Z]

Open Removal of Hip Articulating Spacer with Replacement

Removal of Articulating Spacer		Code also as appropriate Replacement by Device Type						
		Acetabular Surface				Femoral Surface		
		Poly	Metal	Ceramic	Synthetic	Metal	Ceramic	Synth
Hip, RT	ØSP9ØEZ	ØSRAØØ[9,A,Z]	ØSRAØ1[9,A,Z]	ØSRAØ3[9,A,Z]	ØSRAØJ[9,A,Z]	ØSRRØ1[9,A,Z]	ØSRRØ3[9,A,Z]	ØSRRØJ[9,A,Z]
Hip, LT	ØSPBØEZ	ØSREØØ[9,A,Z]	ØSREØ1[9,A,Z]	ØSREØ3[9,A,Z]	ØSREØJ[9,A,Z]	ØSRSØ1[9,A,Z]	ØSRSØ3[9,A,Z]	ØSRSØJ[9,A,Z]

Open Removal of Hip Synthetic Substitute with Replacement

Removal of Synthetic Substitute		Code also as appropriate Replacement by Device Type					
		Metal	Metal on Poly	Ceramic	Ceramic on Poly	Oxidized Zirc on Poly	Synth Subst
Hip, RT	ØSP[9,A,R]ØJZ	ØSR9Ø1[9,A,Z]	ØSR9Ø2[9,A,Z]	ØSR9Ø3[9,A,Z]	ØSR9Ø4[9,A,Z]	ØSR9Ø6[9,A,Z]	ØSR9ØJ[9,A,Z]
Hip, LT	ØSP[B,E,S]ØJZ	ØSRBØ1[9,A,Z]	ØSRBØ2[9,A,Z]	ØSRBØ3[9,A,Z]	ØSRBØ4[9,A,Z]	ØSRBØ6[9,A,Z]	ØSRBØJ[9,A,Z]

Open Removal of Hip Synthetic Substitute with Replacement

Removal of Synthetic Substitute		Code also as appropriate Replacement by Device Type						
		Acetabular Surface				Femoral Surface		
		Poly	Metal	Ceramic	Synthetic	Metal	Ceramic	Synth
Hip, RT	ØSP[9,A,R]ØJZ	ØSRAØØ[9,A,Z]	ØSRAØ1[9,A,Z]	ØSRAØ3[9,A,Z]	ØSRAØJ[9,A,Z]	ØSRRØ1[9,A,Z]	ØSRRØ3[9,A,Z]	ØSRRØJ[9,A,Z]
Hip, LT	ØSP[B,E,S]ØJZ	ØSREØØ[9,A,Z]	ØSREØ1[9,A,Z]	ØSREØ3[9,A,Z]	ØSREØJ[9,A,Z]	ØSRSØ1[9,A,Z]	ØSRSØ3[9,A,Z]	ØSRSØJ[9,A,Z]

Percutaneous Endoscopic Removal of Hip Spacer with Open Replacement

Removal of Spacer		Code also as appropriate Replacement by Device Type					
		Metal	Metal on Poly	Ceramic	Ceramic on Poly	Oxidized Zirc on Poly	Synth Subst
Hip, RT	ØSP948Z	ØSR9Ø1[9,A,Z]	ØSR9Ø2[9,A,Z]	ØSR9Ø3[9,A,Z]	ØSR9Ø4[9,A,Z]	ØSR9Ø6[9,A,Z]	ØSR9ØJ[9,A,Z]
Hip, LT	ØSPB48Z	ØSRBØ1[9,A,Z]	ØSRBØ2[9,A,Z]	ØSRBØ3[9,A,Z]	ØSRBØ4[9,A,Z]	ØSRBØ6[9,A,Z]	ØSRBØJ[9,A,Z]

Percutaneous Endoscopic Removal of Hip Spacer with Open Replacement

Removal of Spacer		Code also as appropriate Replacement by Device Type						
		Acetabular Surface				Femoral Surface		
		Poly	Metal	Ceramic	Synthetic	Metal	Ceramic	Synth
Hip, RT	ØSP948Z	ØSRAØØ[9,A,Z]	ØSRAØ1[9,A,Z]	ØSRAØ3[9,A,Z]	ØSRAØJ[9,A,Z]	ØSRRØ1[9,A,Z]	ØSRRØ3[9,A,Z]	ØSRRØJ[9,A,Z]
Hip, LT	ØSPB48Z	ØSREØØ[9,A,Z]	ØSREØ1[9,A,Z]	ØSREØ3[9,A,Z]	ØSREØJ[9,A,Z]	ØSRSØ1[9,A,Z]	ØSRSØ3[9,A,Z]	ØSRSØJ[9,A,Z]

Percutaneous Endoscopic Removal of Hip Synthetic Substitute with Open Replacement

Removal of Synthetic Substitute		Code also as appropriate Replacement by Device Type					
		Metal	Metal on Poly	Ceramic	Ceramic on Poly	Oxidized Zirc on Poly	Synth Subst
Hip, RT	ØSP[9,A,R]4JZ	ØSR9Ø1[9,A,Z]	ØSR9Ø2[9,A,Z]	ØSR9Ø3[9,A,Z]	ØSR9Ø4[9,A,Z]	ØSR9Ø6[9,A,Z]	ØSR9ØJ[9,A,Z]
Hip, LT	ØSP[B,E,S]4JZ	ØSRBØ1[9,A,Z]	ØSRBØ2[9,A,Z]	ØSRBØ3[9,A,Z]	ØSRBØ4[9,A,Z]	ØSRBØ6[9,A,Z]	ØSRBØJ[9,A,Z]

Percutaneous Endoscopic Removal of Hip Synthetic Substitute with Open Replacement

Removal of Synthetic Substitute		Code also as appropriate Replacement by Device Type						
		Acetabular Surface				Femoral Surface		
		Poly	Metal	Ceramic	Synthetic	Metal	Ceramic	Synth
Hip, RT	ØSP[9,A,R]4JZ	ØSRAØØ[9,A,Z]	ØSRAØ1[9,A,Z]	ØSRAØ3[9,A,Z]	ØSRAØJ[9,A,Z]	ØSRRØ1[9,A,Z]	ØSRRØ3[9,A,Z]	ØSRRØJ[9,A,Z]
Hip, LT	ØSP[B,E,S]4JZ	ØSREØØ[9,A,Z]	ØSREØ1[9,A,Z]	ØSREØ3[9,A,Z]	ØSREØJ[9,A,Z]	ØSRSØ1[9,A,Z]	ØSRSØ3[9,A,Z]	ØSRSØJ[9,A,Z]

Knee Procedure Combinations

Removal of Knee Spacer with Replacement

Removal of Spacer		Code also Replacement by Type of Synthetic Substitute					
		Oxidized Zirc on Poly	Synthetic Substitute	Patello-femoral	Femoral Surface	Tibial Surface	Medial (L)/Lateral (M) Meniscus
Knee, RT	ØSPC[Ø,3,4]8Z	ØSRCØ6[9,A,Z]	ØSRCØJ[9,A,Z]	ØSRCØN[9,A,Z]	ØSRTØJ[9,A,Z]	ØSRVØJ[9,A,Z]	XRRGØ[L,M]8
Knee, LT	ØSPD[Ø,3,4]8Z	ØSRDØ6[9,A,Z]	ØSRDØJ[9,A,Z]	ØSRDØN[9,A,Z]	ØSRUØJ[9,A,Z]	ØSRWØJ[9,A,Z]	XRRHØ[L,M]8

Removal of Knee Liner with Replacement

Removal of Liner		Code also Replacement by Type of Synthetic Substitute						
		Oxidized Zirc on Poly	Synthetic Substitute	Medial (L)/Lateral (M) Unicondylar	Patello-femoral	Femoral Surface	Tibial Surface	Medial (L)/Lateral (M) Meniscus
Knee, RT	ØSPCØ9Z	ØSRCØ6[9,A,Z]	ØSRCØJ[9,A,Z]	ØSRCØ[L,M][9,A,Z]	ØSRCØN[9,A,Z]	ØSRTØJ[9,A,Z]	ØSRVØJ[9,A,Z]	XRRGØ[L,M]8
Knee, LT	ØSPDØ9Z	ØSRDØ6[9,A,Z]	ØSRDØJ[9,A,Z]	ØSRDØ[L,M][9,A,Z]	ØSRDØN[9,A,Z]	ØSRUØJ[9,A,Z]	ØSRWØJ[9,A,Z]	XRRHØ[L,M]8

Removal of Knee Articulating Spacer with Replacement

Removal of Articulating Spacer		Code also Replacement by Type of Synthetic Substitute				
		Oxidized Zirc on Poly	Synthetic Substitute	Femoral Surface	Tibial Surface	Medial (L)/Lateral (M) Meniscus
Knee, RT	ØSPCØEZ	ØSRCØ6[9,A,Z]	ØSRCØJ[9,A,Z]	ØSRTØJ[9,A,Z]	ØSRVØJ[9,A,Z]	XRRGØ[L,M]8
Knee, LT	ØSPDØEZ	ØSRDØ6[9,A,Z]	ØSRDØJ[9,A,Z]	ØSRUØJ[9,A,Z]	ØSRWØJ[9,A,Z]	XRRHØ[L,M]8

Removal of Knee Patellar Surface with Replacement

Removal of Patellar Surface		Code also Replacement by Type of Synthetic Substitute					
		Oxidized Zirc on Poly	Synthetic Substitute	Patello-femoral	Femoral Surface	Tibial Surface	Medial (L)/Lateral (M) Meniscus
Knee, RT	ØSPC[Ø,4]JC	ØSRCØ6[9,A,Z]	ØSRCØJ[9,A,Z]	ØSRCØN[9,A,Z]	ØSRTØJ[9,A,Z]	ØSRVØJ[9,A,Z]	XRRGØ[L,M]8
Knee, LT	ØSPD[Ø,4]JC	ØSRDØ6[9,A,Z]	ØSRDØJ[9,A,Z]	ØSRDØN[9,A,Z]	ØSRUØJ[9,A,Z]	ØSRWØJ[9,A,Z]	XRRHØ[L,M]8

Removal of Knee Synthetic Substitute with Replacement

Removal of Synthetic Substitute		Code also Replacement by Type of Synthetic Substitute						
		Oxidized Zirc on Poly	Synthetic Substitute	Medial (L)/Lateral (M) Unicondylar	Patello-femoral	Femoral Surface	Tibial Surface	Medial (L)/Lateral (M) Meniscus
Knee, RT	ØSPC[Ø,4]JZ	ØSRCØ6[9,A,Z]	ØSRCØJ[9,A,Z]	ØSRCØ[L,M][9,A,Z]	ØSRCØN[9,A,Z]	ØSRTØJ[9,A,Z]	ØSRVØJ[9,A,Z]	XRRGØ[L,M]8
Knee, LT	ØSPD[Ø,4]JZ	ØSRDØ6[9,A,Z]	ØSRDØJ[9,A,Z]	ØSRDØ[L,M][9,A,Z]	ØSRDØN[9,A,Z]	ØSRUØJ[9,A,Z]	ØSRWØJ[9,A,Z]	XRRHØ[L,M]8

Removal of Knee Unicondylar Device with Replacement

Removal of Medial (L)/Lateral (M) Unicondylar Device		Code also Replacement by Type of Synthetic Substitute					
		Oxidized Zirc on Poly	Synthetic Substitute	Medial Unicondylar	Femoral Surface	Tibial Surface	Medial (L)/Lateral (M) Meniscus
Knee, RT	ØSPC[Ø,4][L,M]Z	ØSRCØ6[9,A,Z]	ØSRCØJ[9,A,Z]	ØSRCØL[9,A,Z]	ØSRTØJ[9,A,Z]	ØSRVØJ[9,A,Z]	XRRGØ[L,M]8
Knee, LT	ØSPD[Ø,4][L,M]Z	ØSRDØ6[9,A,Z]	ØSRDØJ[9,A,Z]	ØSRDØL[9,A,Z]	ØSRUØJ[9,A,Z]	ØSRWØJ[9,A,Z]	XRRHØ[L,M]8

Removal of Knee Patellofemoral Device with Replacement

Removal of Patellofemoral Device		Code also Replacement by Type of Synthetic Substitute					
		Oxidized Zirc on Poly	Synthetic Substitute	Medial Unicondylar	Femoral Surface	Tibial Surface	Medial (L)/Lateral (M) Meniscus
Knee, RT	ØSPC[Ø,4]NZ	ØSRCØ6[9,A,Z]	ØSRCØJ[9,A,Z]	ØSRCØL[9,A,Z]	ØSRTØJ[9,A,Z]	ØSRVØJ[9,A,Z]	XRRGØ[L,M]8
Knee, LT	ØSPD[Ø,4]NZ	ØSRDØ6[9,A,Z]	ØSRDØJ[9,A,Z]	ØSRDØL[9,A,Z]	ØSRUØJ[9,A,Z]	ØSRWØJ[9,A,Z]	XRRHØ[L,M]8

Removal of Knee Femoral/Tibial Surface Device with Replacement

Removal of Femoral (T,U)/Tibial (V,W) Surface		Code also Replacement by Type of Synthetic Substitute						
		Oxidized Zirc on Poly	Synthetic Substitute	Articulating Spacer	Patello-femoral	Femoral Surface	Tibial Surface	Medial (L)/Lateral (M) Meniscus
Knee, RT	ØSP[T,V][Ø,4]JZ	ØSRCØ6[9,A,Z]	ØSRCØJ[9,A,Z]	ØSRCØEZ	ØSRCØN[9,A,Z]	ØSRTØJ[9,A,Z]	ØSRVØJ[9,A,Z]	XRRGØ[L,M]8
Knee, LT	ØSP[U,W][Ø,4]JZ	ØSRDØ6[9,A,Z]	ØSRDØJ[9,A,Z]	ØSRDØEZ	ØSRDØN[9,A,Z]	ØSRUØJ[9,A,Z]	ØSRWØJ[9,A,Z]	XRRHØ[L,M]8

466-468 Revision of Hip or Knee Replacement

Hip Procedure Combinations

Open Removal of Hip Spacer with Replacement

Removal of Spacer		Code also as appropriate Replacement by Device Type						
		Metal	Metal on Poly	Ceramic	Ceramic on Poly	Oxidized Zirc on Poly	Articulating Spacer	Synth Subst
Hip, RT	0SP908Z	0SR901[9,A,Z]	0SR902[9,A,Z]	0SR903[9,A,Z]	0SR904[9,A,Z]	0SR906[9,A,Z]	0SR90EZ	0SR90J[9,A,Z]
Hip, LT	0SPB08Z	0SRB01[9,A,Z]	0SRB02[9,A,Z]	0SRB03[9,A,Z]	0SRB04[9,A,Z]	0SRB06[9,A,Z]	0SRB0EZ	0SRB0J[9,A,Z]

Open Removal of Hip Spacer with Replacement

Removal of Spacer		Code also as appropriate Replacement by Device Type						
		Acetabular Surface				Femoral Surface		
		Poly	Metal	Ceramic	Synthetic	Metal	Ceramic	Synth
Hip, RT	0SP908Z	0SRA00[9,A,Z]	0SRA01[9,A,Z]	0SRA03[9,A,Z]	0SRA0J[9,A,Z]	0SRR01[9,A,Z]	0SRR03[9,A,Z]	0SRR0J[9,A,Z]
Hip, LT	0SPB08Z	0SRE00[9,A,Z]	0SRE01[9,A,Z]	0SRE03[9,A,Z]	0SRE0J[9,A,Z]	0SRS01[9,A,Z]	0SRS03[9,A,Z]	0SRS0J[9,A,Z]

Open Removal of Hip Spacer with Liner Insertion (supplement)

Removal of Spacer		Code also as appropriate Supplement of Body Part by Site		
		Joint	Acetabular Surface	Femoral Surface
Hip, RT	0SP908Z	0SU909Z	0SUA09Z	0SUR09Z
Hip, LT	0SPB08Z	0SUB09Z	0SUE09Z	0SUS09Z

Open Removal of Hip Liner with Replacement

Removal of Liner		Code also as appropriate Replacement by Device Type						
		Metal	Metal on Poly	Ceramic	Ceramic on Poly	Oxidized Zirc on Poly	Articulating Spacer	Synth Subst
Hip, RT	0SP909Z	0SR901[9,A,Z]	0SR902[9,A,Z]	0SR903[9,A,Z]	0SR904[9,A,Z]	0SR906[9,A,Z]	0SR90EZ	0SR90J[9,A,Z]
Hip, LT	0SPB09Z	0SRB01[9,A,Z]	0SRB02[9,A,Z]	0SRB03[9,A,Z]	0SRB04[9,A,Z]	0SRB06[9,A,Z]	0SRB0EZ	0SRB0J[9,A,Z]

Open Removal of Hip Liner with Replacement

Removal of Liner		Code also as appropriate Replacement by Device Type						
		Acetabular Surface				Femoral Surface		
		Poly	Metal	Ceramic	Synthetic	Metal	Ceramic	Synth
Hip, RT	0SP909Z	0SRA00[9,A,Z]	0SRA01[9,A,Z]	0SRA03[9,A,Z]	0SRA0J[9,A,Z]	0SRR01[9,A,Z]	0SRR03[9,A,Z]	0SRR0J[9,A,Z]
Hip, LT	0SPB09Z	0SRE00[9,A,Z]	0SRE01[9,A,Z]	0SRE03[9,A,Z]	0SRE0J[9,A,Z]	0SRS01[9,A,Z]	0SRS03[9,A,Z]	0SRS0J[9,A,Z]

Open Removal of Hip Liner with Liner Insertion (supplement)

Removal of Liner		Code also as appropriate Supplement of Body Part by Site		
		Joint	Acetabular Surface	Femoral Surface
Hip, RT	0SP909Z	0SU909Z	0SUA09Z	0SUR09Z
Hip, LT	0SPB09Z	0SUB09Z	0SUE09Z	0SUS09Z

Open Removal of Hip Resurfacing Device with Replacement

Removal of Resurfacing Device		Code also as appropriate Replacement by Device Type						
		Metal	Metal on Poly	Ceramic	Ceramic on Poly	Oxidized Zirc on Poly	Articulating Spacer	Synth Subst
Hip, RT	0SP90BZ	0SR901[9,A,Z]	0SR902[9,A,Z]	0SR903[9,A,Z]	0SR904[9,A,Z]	0SR906[9,A,Z]	0SR90EZ	0SR90J[9,A,Z]
Hip, LT	0SPB0BZ	0SRB01[9,A,Z]	0SRB02[9,A,Z]	0SRB03[9,A,Z]	0SRB04[9,A,Z]	0SRB06[9,A,Z]	0SRB0EZ	0SRB0J[9,A,Z]

Open Removal of Hip Resurfacing Device with Replacement

Removal of Resurfacing Device		Code also as appropriate Replacement by Device Type						
		Acetabular Surface				Femoral Surface		
		Poly	Metal	Ceramic	Synthetic	Metal	Ceramic	Synth
Hip, RT	ØSP9ØBZ	ØSRAØØ[9,A,Z]	ØSRAØ1[9,A,Z]	ØSRAØ3[9,A,Z]	ØSRAØJ[9,A,Z]	ØSRRØ1[9,A,Z]	ØSRRØ3[9,A,Z]	ØSRRØJ[9,A,Z]
Hip, LT	ØSPBØBZ	ØSREØØ[9,A,Z]	ØSREØ1[9,A,Z]	ØSREØ3[9,A,Z]	ØSREØJ[9,A,Z]	ØSRSØ1[9,A,Z]	ØSRSØ3[9,A,Z]	ØSRSØJ[9,A,Z]

Open Removal of Hip Resurfacing Device with Liner Insertion (supplement)

Removal of Resurfacing Device		Code also as appropriate Supplement of Body Part by Site		
		Joint	Acetabular Surface	Femoral Surface
Hip, RT	ØSP9ØBZ	ØSU9Ø9Z	ØSUAØ9Z	ØSURØ9Z
Hip, LT	ØSPBØBZ	ØSUBØ9Z	ØSUEØ9Z	ØSUSØ9Z

Open Removal of Hip Articulating Spacer with Replacement

Removal of Articulating Spacer		Code also as appropriate Replacement by Device Type					
		Metal	Metal on Poly	Ceramic	Ceramic on Poly	Oxidized Zirc on Poly	Synth Subst
Hip, RT	ØSP9ØEZ	ØSR9Ø1[9,A,Z]	ØSR9Ø2[9,A,Z]	ØSR9Ø3[9,A,Z]	ØSR9Ø4[9,A,Z]	ØSR9Ø6[9,A,Z]	ØSR9ØJ[9,A,Z]
Hip, LT	ØSPBØEZ	ØSRBØ1[9,A,Z]	ØSRBØ2[9,A,Z]	ØSRBØ3[9,A,Z]	ØSRBØ4[9,A,Z]	ØSRBØ6[9,A,Z]	ØSRBØJ[9,A,Z]

Open Removal of Hip Articulating Spacer with Replacement

Removal of Articulating Spacer		Code also as appropriate Replacement by Device Type						
		Acetabular Surface				Femoral Surface		
		Poly	Metal	Ceramic	Synthetic	Metal	Ceramic	Synth
Hip, RT	ØSP9ØEZ	ØSRAØØ[9,A,Z]	ØSRAØ1[9,A,Z]	ØSRAØ3[9,A,Z]	ØSRAØJ[9,A,Z]	ØSRRØ1[9,A,Z]	ØSRRØ3[9,A,Z]	ØSRRØJ[9,A,Z]
Hip, LT	ØSPBØEZ	ØSREØØ[9,A,Z]	ØSREØ1[9,A,Z]	ØSREØ3[9,A,Z]	ØSREØJ[9,A,Z]	ØSRSØ1[9,A,Z]	ØSRSØ3[9,A,Z]	ØSRSØJ[9,A,Z]

Open Removal of Hip Articulating Spacer with Liner Insertion (supplement)

Removal of Articulating Spacer		Code also as appropriate Supplement of Body Part by Site		
		Joint	Acetabular Surface	Femoral Surface
Hip, RT	ØSP9ØEZ	ØSU9Ø9Z	ØSUAØ9Z	ØSURØ9Z
Hip, LT	ØSPBØEZ	ØSUBØ9Z	ØSUEØ9Z	ØSUSØ9Z

Open Removal of Hip Synthetic Substitute with Replacement

Removal of Synthetic Substitute		Code also as appropriate Replacement by Device Type						
		Metal	Metal on Poly	Ceramic	Ceramic on Poly	Oxidized Zirc on Poly	Articulating Spacer	Synth Subst
Hip, RT	ØSP[9,A,R]ØJZ	ØSR9Ø1[9,A,Z]	ØSR9Ø2[9,A,Z]	ØSR9Ø3[9,A,Z]	ØSR9Ø4[9,A,Z]	ØSR9Ø6[9,A,Z]	ØSR9ØEZ	ØSR9ØJ[9,A,Z]
Hip, LT	ØSP[B,E,S]ØJZ	ØSRBØ1[9,A,Z]	ØSRBØ2[9,A,Z]	ØSRBØ3[9,A,Z]	ØSRBØ4[9,A,Z]	ØSRBØ6[9,A,Z]	ØSRBØEZ	ØSRBØJ[9,A,Z]

Open Removal of Hip Synthetic Substitute with Replacement

Removal of Synthetic Substitute		Code also as appropriate Replacement by Device Type						
		Acetabular Surface				Femoral Surface		
		Poly	Metal	Ceramic	Synthetic	Metal	Ceramic	Synth
Hip, RT	ØSP[9,A,R]ØJZ	ØSRAØØ[9,A,Z]	ØSRAØ1[9,A,Z]	ØSRAØ3[9,A,Z]	ØSRAØJ[9,A,Z]	ØSRRØ1[9,A,Z]	ØSRRØ3[9,A,Z]	ØSRRØJ[9,A,Z]
Hip, LT	ØSP[B,E,S]ØJZ	ØSREØØ[9,A,Z]	ØSREØ1[9,A,Z]	ØSREØ3[9,A,Z]	ØSREØJ[9,A,Z]	ØSRSØ1[9,A,Z]	ØSRSØ3[9,A,Z]	ØSRSØJ[9,A,Z]

Percutaneous Endoscopic Removal of Hip Spacer with Open Replacement

Removal of Spacer		Code also as appropriate Replacement by Device Type						
		Metal	Metal on Poly	Ceramic	Ceramic on Poly	Oxidized Zirc on Poly	Articulating Spacer	Synth Subst
Hip, RT	ØSP948Z	ØSR9Ø1[9,A,Z]	ØSR9Ø2[9,A,Z]	ØSR9Ø3[9,A,Z]	ØSR9Ø4[9,A,Z]	ØSR9Ø6[9,A,Z]	ØSR9ØEZ	ØSR9ØJ[9,A,Z]
Hip, LT	ØSPB48Z	ØSRBØ1[9,A,Z]	ØSRBØ2[9,A,Z]	ØSRBØ3[9,A,Z]	ØSRBØ4[9,A,Z]	ØSRBØ6[9,A,Z]	ØSRBØEZ	ØSRBØJ[9,A,Z]

Percutaneous Endoscopic Removal of Hip Spacer with Open Replacement

Removal of Spacer		Code also as appropriate Replacement by Device Type						
		Acetabular Surface				Femoral Surface		
		Poly	Metal	Ceramic	Synthetic	Metal	Ceramic	Synth
Hip, RT	ØSP948Z	ØSRAØØ[9,A,Z]	ØSRAØ1[9,A,Z]	ØSRAØ3[9,A,Z]	ØSRAØJ[9,A,Z]	ØSRRØ1[9,A,Z]	ØSRRØ3[9,A,Z]	ØSRRØJ[9,A,Z]
Hip, LT	ØSPB48Z	ØSREØØ[9,A,Z]	ØSREØ1[9,A,Z]	ØSREØ3[9,A,Z]	ØSREØJ[9,A,Z]	ØSRSØ1[9,A,Z]	ØSRSØ3[9,A,Z]	ØSRSØJ[9,A,Z]

Percutaneous Endoscopic Removal of Hip Spacer with Open Liner Insertion (supplement)

Removal of Spacer		Code also as appropriate Supplement of Body Part by Site		
		Joint	Acetabular Surface	Femoral Surface
Hip, RT	ØSP948Z	ØSU9Ø9Z	ØSUAØ9Z	ØSURØ9Z
Hip, LT	ØSPB48Z	ØSUBØ9Z	ØSUEØ9Z	ØSUSØ9Z

Percutaneous Endoscopic Removal of Hip Synthetic Substitute with Open Replacement

Removal of Synthetic Substitute		Code also as appropriate Replacement by Device Type						
		Metal	Metal on Poly	Ceramic	Ceramic on Poly	Oxidized Zirc on Poly	Articulating Spacer	Synth Subst
Hip, RT	ØSP[9,A,R]4JZ	ØSR9Ø1[9,A,Z]	ØSR9Ø2[9,A,Z]	ØSR9Ø3[9,A,Z]	ØSR9Ø4[9,A,Z]	ØSR9Ø6[9,A,Z]	ØSR9ØEZ	ØSR9ØJ[9,A,Z]
Hip, LT	ØSP[B,E,S]4JZ	ØSRBØ1[9,A,Z]	ØSRBØ2[9,A,Z]	ØSRBØ3[9,A,Z]	ØSRBØ4[9,A,Z]	ØSRBØ6[9,A,Z]	ØSRBØEZ	ØSRBØJ[9,A,Z]

Percutaneous Endoscopic Removal of Hip Synthetic Substitute with Open Replacement

Removal of Synthetic Substitute		Code also as appropriate Replacement by Device Type						
		Acetabular Surface				Femoral Surface		
		Poly	Metal	Ceramic	Synthetic	Metal	Ceramic	Synth
Hip, RT	ØSP[9,A,R]4JZ	ØSRAØØ[9,A,Z]	ØSRAØ1[9,A,Z]	ØSRAØ3[9,A,Z]	ØSRAØJ[9,A,Z]	ØSRRØ1[9,A,Z]	ØSRRØ3[9,A,Z]	ØSRRØJ[9,A,Z]
Hip, LT	ØSP[B,E,S]4JZ	ØSREØØ[9,A,Z]	ØSREØ1[9,A,Z]	ØSREØ3[9,A,Z]	ØSREØJ[9,A,Z]	ØSRSØ1[9,A,Z]	ØSRSØ3[9,A,Z]	ØSRSØJ[9,A,Z]

Percutaneous Endoscopic Removal of Hip Synthetic Substitute with Open Liner Insertion (supplement)

Removal of Synthetic Substitute		Code also as appropriate Supplement of Body Part by Site		
		Joint	Acetabular Surface	Femoral Surface
Hip, RT	ØSP[9,A,R]4JZ	ØSU9Ø9Z	ØSUAØ9Z	ØSURØ9Z
Hip, LT	ØSP[B,E,S]4JZ	ØSUBØ9Z	ØSUEØ9Z	ØSUSØ9Z

Knee Procedure Combinations

Removal of Knee Spacer with Replacement

Removal of Spacer		Code also Replacement by Type of Synthetic Substitute						
		Oxidized Zirc on Poly	Synthetic Substitute	Articulating Spacer	Patello-femoral	Femoral Surface	Tibial Surface	Medial (L)/ Lateral (M) Meniscus
Knee, RT	ØSPC[Ø,3,4]8Z	ØSRCØ6[9,A,Z]	ØSRCØJ[9,A,Z]	ØSRCØEZ	ØSRCØN[9,A,Z]	ØSRTØJ[9,A,Z]	ØSRVØJ[9,A,Z]	XRRGØ[L,M]8
Knee, LT	ØSPD[Ø,3,4]8Z	ØSRDØ6[9,A,Z]	ØSRDØJ[9,A,Z]	ØSRDØEZ	ØSRDØN[9,A,Z]	ØSRUØJ[9,A,Z]	ØSRWØJ[9,A,Z]	XRRHØ[L,M]8

Removal of Knee Liner with Replacement

Removal of Liner		Code also Replacement by Type of Synthetic Substitute							
		Oxidized Zirc on Poly	Synthetic Substitute	Articulating Spacer	Medial (L)/ Lateral (M) Unicondylar	Patello-femoral	Femoral Surface	Tibial Surface	Medial (L)/Lateral (M) Meniscus
Knee, RT	ØSPCØ9Z	ØSRCØ6[9,A,Z]	ØSRCØJ[9,A,Z]	ØSRCØEZ	ØSRCØ[L,M][9,A,Z]	ØSRCØN[9,A,Z]	ØSRTØJ[9,A,Z]	ØSRVØJ[9,A,Z]	XRRGØ[L,M]8
Knee, LT	ØSPDØ9Z	ØSRDØ6[9,A,Z]	ØSRDØJ[9,A,Z]	ØSRDØEZ	ØSRDØ[L,M][9,A,Z]	ØSRDØN[9,A,Z]	ØSRUØJ[9,A,Z]	ØSRWØJ[9,A,Z]	XRRHØ[L,M]8

Removal of Knee Articulating Spacer with Replacement

Removal of Articulating Spacer		Code also Replacement by Type of Synthetic Substitute				
		Oxidized Zirc on Poly	Synthetic Substitute	Femoral Surface	Tibial Surface	Medial (L)/Lateral (M) Meniscus
Knee, RT	ØSPCØEZ	ØSRCØ6[9,A,Z]	ØSRCØJ[9,A,Z]	ØSRTØJ[9,A,Z]	ØSRVØJ[9,A,Z]	XRRGØ[L,M]8
Knee, LT	ØSPDØEZ	ØSRDØ6[9,A,Z]	ØSRDØJ[9,A,Z]	ØSRUØJ[9,A,Z]	ØSRWØJ[9,A,Z]	XRRHØ[L,M]8

Removal of Knee Patellar Surface with Replacement

Removal of Patellar Surface		Code also Replacement by Type of Synthetic Substitute						
		Oxidized Zirc on Poly	Synthetic Substitute	Articulating Spacer	Patello-femoral	Femoral Surface	Tibial Surface	Medial (L)/Lateral (M) Meniscus
Knee, RT	ØSPC[Ø,4]JC	ØSRCØ6[9,A,Z]	ØSRCØJ[9,A,Z]	ØSRCØEZ	ØSRCØN[9,A,Z]	ØSRTØJ[9,A,Z]	ØSRVØJ[9,A,Z]	XRRGØ[L,M]8
Knee, LT	ØSPD[Ø,4]JC	ØSRDØ6[9,A,Z]	ØSRDØJ[9,A,Z]	ØSRDØEZ	ØSRDØN[9,A,Z]	ØSRUØJ[9,A,Z]	ØSRWØJ[9,A,Z]	XRRHØ[L,M]8

Removal of Knee Synthetic Substitute with Replacement

Removal of Synthetic Substitute		Code also Replacement by Type of Synthetic Substitute							
		Oxidized Zirc on Poly	Synthetic Substitute	Articulating Spacer	Medial (L)/Lateral (M) Unicondylar	Patello-femoral	Femoral Surface	Tibial Surface	Medial (L)/Lateral (M) Meniscus
Knee, RT	ØSPC[Ø,4]JZ	ØSRCØ6[9,A,Z]	ØSRCØJ[9,A,Z]	ØSRCØEZ	ØSRCØ[L,M][9,A,Z]	ØSRCØN[9,A,Z]	ØSRTØJ[9,A,Z]	ØSRVØJ[9,A,Z]	XRRGØ[L,M]8
Knee, LT	ØSPD[Ø,4]JZ	ØSRDØ6[9,A,Z]	ØSRDØJ[9,A,Z]	ØSRDØEZ	ØSRDØ[L,M][9,A,Z]	ØSRDØN[9,A,Z]	ØSRUØJ[9,A,Z]	ØSRWØJ[9,A,Z]	XRRHØ[L,M]8

Removal of Knee Unicondylar Device with Replacement

Removal of Medial (L)/Lateral (M) Unicondylar Device		Code also Replacement by Type of Synthetic Substitute					
		Oxidized Zirc on Poly	Synthetic Substitute	Medial Unicondylar	Femoral Surface	Tibial Surface	Medial (L)/Lateral (M) Meniscus
Knee, RT	ØSPC[Ø,4][L,M]Z	ØSRCØ6[9,A,Z]	ØSRCØJ[9,A,Z]	ØSRCØL[9,A,Z]	ØSRTØJ[9,A,Z]	ØSRVØJ[9,A,Z]	XRRGØ[L,M]8
Knee, LT	ØSPD[Ø,4][L,M]Z	ØSRDØ6[9,A,Z]	ØSRDØJ[9,A,Z]	ØSRDØL[9,A,Z]	ØSRUØJ[9,A,Z]	ØSRWØJ[9,A,Z]	XRRHØ[L,M]8

Removal of Knee Patellofemoral Device with Replacement

Removal of Patellofemoral Device		Code also Replacement by Type of Synthetic Substitute					
		Oxidized Zirc on Poly	Synthetic Substitute	Medial Unicondylar	Femoral Surface	Tibial Surface	Medial (L)/Lateral (M) Meniscus
Knee, RT	ØSPC[Ø,4]NZ	ØSRCØ6[9,A,Z]	ØSRCØJ[9,A,Z]	ØSRCØL[9,A,Z]	ØSRTØJ[9,A,Z]	ØSRVØJ[9,A,Z]	XRRGØ[L,M]8
Knee, LT	ØSPD[Ø,4]NZ	ØSRDØ6[9,A,Z]	ØSRDØJ[9,A,Z]	ØSRDØL[9,A,Z]	ØSRUØJ[9,A,Z]	ØSRWØJ[9,A,Z]	XRRHØ[L,M]8

Removal of Knee Femoral/Tibial Surface Device with Replacement

Removal of Femoral (T,U)/Tibial (V,W) Surface		Code also Replacement by Type of Synthetic Substitute						
		Oxidized Zirc on Poly	Synthetic Substitute	Articulating Spacer	Patello-femoral	Femoral Surface	Tibial Surface	Medial (L)/Lateral (M) Meniscus
Knee, RT	ØSP[T,V][Ø,4]JZ	ØSRCØ6[9,A,Z]	ØSRCØJ[9,A,Z]	ØSRCØEZ	ØSRCØN[9,A,Z]	ØSRTØJ[9,A,Z]	ØSRVØJ[9,A,Z]	XRRGØ[L,M]8
Knee, LT	ØSP[U,W][Ø,4]JZ	ØSRDØ6[9,A,Z]	ØSRDØJ[9,A,Z]	ØSRDØEZ	ØSRDØN[9,A,Z]	ØSRUØJ[9,A,Z]	ØSRWØJ[9,A,Z]	XRRHØ[L,M]8

DRG 485-489 Knee Procedures

Joint	Removal of Liner by open approach	Code also as appropriate Supplement of Tibial Surface by Site
Knee, RT	ØSPCØ9Z	ØSUVØ9Z
Knee, LT	ØSPDØ9Z	ØSUWØ9Z

DRG 515-517 Other Musculoskeletal System and Connective Tissue Procedures

Site	Reposition of Vertebra by percutaneous approach	Code also as appropriate Supplement With Synthetic Substitute by Percutaneous Approach at site of Repositioned Vertebra
Cervical	0PS33ZZ	0PU33JZ
Coccyx	0QSS3ZZ	0QUS3JZ
Lumbar	0QS03ZZ	0QU03JZ
Sacrum	0QS13ZZ	0QU13JZ
Thoracic	0PS43ZZ	0PU43JZ

DRG 518-520 Back and Neck Procedures, Except Spinal Fusion, or Disc Devices/Neurostimulators

Generator Type	Insertion of Generator by Site			Code also as appropriate Insertion Neurostimulator Lead by approach and Site	
	Chest	Abdomen	Back	Spinal Canal	Spinal Cord
Single Array	0JH6[0,3]BZ	0JH8[0,3]BZ	0JH7[0,3]BZ	00HU[0,3,4]MZ	00HV[0,3,4]MZ
Single Array, Rechargeable	0JH6[0,3]CZ	0JH8[0,3]CZ	0JH7[0,3]CZ	00HU[0,3,4]MZ	00HV[0,3,4]MZ
Multiple Array	0JH6[0,3]DZ	0JH8[0,3]DZ	0JH7[0,3]DZ	00HU[0,3,4]MZ	00HV[0,3,4]MZ
Multiple Array, Rechargeable	0JH6[0,3]EZ	—	0JH7[0,3]EZ	00HU[0,3,4]MZ	00HV[0,3,4]MZ
Multiple Array, Rechargeable	—	0JH8[0,3]EZ	—	00HU[0,3,4]MZ	00HV[0,3,4]MZ

DRG 582-583 Mastectomy for Malignancy

Site	Resection by Open approach	Code also as appropriate Resection of Lymph Nodes by Open approach by site			Code also as appropriate Resection of Thorax Muscle by Open approach	
		Axillary	Internal Mammary	Thorax	Right	Left
Breast, Right	0HTT0ZZ	07T50ZZ	07T80ZZ	07T70ZZ	0KTH0ZZ	—
Breast, Left	0HTU0ZZ	07T60ZZ	07T90ZZ	07T70ZZ	—	0KTJ0ZZ
Breast, Bilateral	0HTV0ZZ	07T50ZZ and 07T60ZZ	07T80ZZ and 07T90ZZ	07T70ZZ	0KTH0ZZ	0KTJ0ZZ

DRG 584-585 Breast Biopsy, Local Excision and Other Breast Procedures

Resection of Breast With Resection of Lymph Nodes and Thorax Muscle

Site	Resection by Open approach	Code also as appropriate Resection of Lymph Nodes by Open approach by site			Code also as appropriate Resection of Thorax Muscle by Open approach	
		Axillary	Internal Mammary	Thorax	Right	Left
Breast, Right	0HTT0ZZ	07T50ZZ	07T80ZZ	07T70ZZ	0KTH0ZZ	—
Breast, Left	0HTU0ZZ	07T60ZZ	07T90ZZ	07T70ZZ	—	0KTJ0ZZ
Breast, Bilateral	0HTV0ZZ	07T50ZZ and 07T60ZZ	07T80ZZ and 07T90ZZ	07T70ZZ	0KTH0ZZ	0KTJ0ZZ

Replacement of Breast Tissue

Site	Replacement by Percutaneous approach with Autologous Tissue	Code also as appropriate Extraction of Subcutaneous Tissue by Percutaneous approach					
		Abdomen	Back	Buttock	Chest	Leg, Upper, Right	Leg, Upper, Left
Breast, Right	0HRT37Z	0JD83ZZ	0JD73ZZ	0JD93ZZ	0JD63ZZ	0JDL3ZZ	0JDM3ZZ
Breast, Left	0HRU37Z	0JD83ZZ	0JD73ZZ	0JD93ZZ	0JD63ZZ	0JDL3ZZ	0JDM3ZZ
Breast, Bilateral	0HRV37Z	0JD83ZZ	0JD73ZZ	0JD93ZZ	0JD63ZZ	0JDL3ZZ	0JDM3ZZ

DRG 628-630 Other Endocrine, Nutritional and Metabolic Procedures

Hip Procedure Combinations

Open Removal of Hip Spacer with Replacement

Removal of Spacer		Code also as appropriate Replacement by Device Type					
		Metal	Metal on Poly	Ceramic	Ceramic on Poly	Oxidized Zirc on Poly	Synthetic Substitute
Hip, RT	0SP908Z	0SR901[9,A,Z]	0SR902[9,A,Z]	0SR903[9,A,Z]	0SR904[9,A,Z]	0SR906[9,A,Z]	0SR90J[9,A,Z]
Hip, LT	0SPB08Z	0SRB01[9,A,Z]	0SRB02[9,A,Z]	0SRB03[9,A,Z]	0SRB04[9,A,Z]	0SRB06[9,A,Z]	0SRB0J[9,A,Z]

Open Removal of Hip Spacer with Replacement

Removal of Spacer		Code also as appropriate Replacement by Device Type						
		Acetabular Surface				Femoral Surface		
		Poly	Metal	Ceramic	Synthetic	Metal	Ceramic	Synthetic
Hip, RT	0SP908Z	0SRA00[9,A,Z]	0SRA01[9,A,Z]	0SRA03[9,A,Z]	0SRA0J[9,A,Z]	0SRR01[9,A,Z]	0SRR03[9,A,Z]	0SRR0J[9,A,Z]
Hip, LT	0SPB08Z	0SRE00[9,A,Z]	0SRE01[9,A,Z]	0SRE03[9,A,Z]	0SRE0J[9,A,Z]	0SRS01[9,A,Z]	0SRS03[9,A,Z]	0SRS0J[9,A,Z]

Open Removal of Hip Spacer with Liner Insertion (supplement)

Removal of Spacer		Code also as appropriate Supplement of Body Part by Site		
		Joint	Acetabular Surface	Femoral Surface
Hip, RT	0SP908Z	0SU909Z	0SUA09Z	0SUR09Z
Hip, LT	0SPB08Z	0SUB09Z	0SUE09Z	0SUS09Z

Open Removal of Hip Liner with Replacement

Removal of Liner		Code also as appropriate Replacement by Device Type					
		Metal	Metal on Poly	Ceramic	Ceramic on Poly	Oxidized Zirc on Poly	Synthetic Substitute
Hip, RT	0SP909Z	0SR901[9,A,Z]	0SR902[9,A,Z]	0SR903[9,A,Z]	0SR904[9,A,Z]	0SR906[9,A,Z]	0SR90J[9,A,Z]
Hip, LT	0SPB09Z	0SRB01[9,A,Z]	0SRB02[9,A,Z]	0SRB03[9,A,Z]	0SRB04[9,A,Z]	0SRB06[9,A,Z]	0SRB0J[9,A,Z]

Open Removal of Hip Liner with Replacement

Removal of Liner		Code also as appropriate Replacement by Device Type						
		Acetabular Surface				Femoral Surface		
		Poly	Metal	Ceramic	Synthetic	Metal	Ceramic	Synthetic
Hip, RT	0SP909Z	0SRA00[9,A,Z]	0SRA01[9,A,Z]	0SRA03[9,A,Z]	0SRA0J[9,A,Z]	0SRR01[9,A,Z]	0SRR03[9,A,Z]	0SRR0J[9,A,Z]
Hip, LT	0SPB09Z	0SRE00[9,A,Z]	0SRE01[9,A,Z]	0SRE03[9,A,Z]	0SRE0J[9,A,Z]	0SRS01[9,A,Z]	0SRS03[9,A,Z]	0SRS0J[9,A,Z]

Open Removal of Hip Liner with Liner Insertion (supplement)

Removal of Liner		Code also as appropriate Supplement of Body Part by Site		
		Joint	Acetabular Surface	Femoral Surface
Hip, RT	0SP909Z	0SU909Z	0SUA09Z	0SUR09Z
Hip, LT	0SPB09Z	0SUB09Z	0SUE09Z	0SUS09Z

Open Removal of Hip Resurfacing Device with Replacement

Removal of Resurfacing Device		Code also as appropriate Replacement by Device Type					
		Metal	Metal on Poly	Ceramic	Ceramic on Poly	Oxidized Zirc on Poly	Synthetic Substitute
Hip, RT	0SP90BZ	0SR901[9,A,Z]	0SR902[9,A,Z]	0SR903[9,A,Z]	0SR904[9,A,Z]	0SR906[9,A,Z]	0SR90J[9,A,Z]
Hip, LT	0SPB0BZ	0SRB01[9,A,Z]	0SRB02[9,A,Z]	0SRB03[9,A,Z]	0SRB04[9,A,Z]	0SRB06[9,A,Z]	0SRB0J[9,A,Z]

Open Removal of Hip Resurfacing Device with Replacement

Removal of Resurfacing Device		Code also as appropriate Replacement by Device Type						
		Acetabular Surface				Femoral Surface		
		Poly	Metal	Ceramic	Synthetic	Metal	Ceramic	Synthetic
Hip, RT	0SP90BZ	0SRA00[9,A,Z]	0SRA01[9,A,Z]	0SRA03[9,A,Z]	0SRA0J[9,A,Z]	0SRR01[9,A,Z]	0SRR03[9,A,Z]	0SRR0J[9,A,Z]
Hip, LT	0SPB0BZ	0SRE00[9,A,Z]	0SRE01[9,A,Z]	0SRE03[9,A,Z]	0SRE0J[9,A,Z]	0SRS01[9,A,Z]	0SRS03[9,A,Z]	0SRS0J[9,A,Z]

Open Removal of Hip Resurfacing Device with Liner Insertion (supplement)

Removal of Resurfacing Device		Code also as appropriate Supplement of Body Part by Site		
		Joint	Acetabular Surface	Femoral Surface
Hip, RT	0SP90BZ	0SU909Z	0SUA09Z	0SUR09Z
Hip, LT	0SPB0BZ	0SUB09Z	0SUE09Z	0SUS09Z

Open Removal of Hip Synthetic Substitute with Replacement

Removal of Synthetic Substitute		Code also as appropriate Replacement by Device Type					
		Metal	Metal on Poly	Ceramic	Ceramic on Poly	Oxidized Zirc on Poly	Synthetic Substitute
Hip, RT	ØSP9ØJZ	ØSR9Ø1[9,A,Z]	ØSR9Ø2[9,A,Z]	ØSR9Ø3[9,A,Z]	ØSR9Ø4[9,A,Z]	ØSR9Ø6[9,A,Z]	ØSR9ØJ[9,A,Z]
Hip, LT	ØSPBØJZ	ØSRBØ1[9,A,Z]	ØSRBØ2[9,A,Z]	ØSRBØ3[9,A,Z]	ØSRBØ4[9,A,Z]	ØSRBØ6[9,A,Z]	ØSRBØJ[9,A,Z]

Open Removal of Hip Synthetic Substitute with Replacement

Removal of Synthetic Substitute		Code also as appropriate Replacement by Device Type						
		Acetabular Surface				Femoral Surface		
		Poly	Metal	Ceramic	Synthetic	Metal	Ceramic	Synthetic
Hip, RT	ØSP9ØJZ	ØSRAØØ[9,A,Z]	ØSRAØ1[9,A,Z]	ØSRAØ3[9,A,Z]	ØSRAØJ[9,A,Z]	ØSRRØ1[9,A,Z]	ØSRRØ3[9,A,Z]	ØSRRØJ[9,A,Z]
Hip, LT	ØSPBØJZ	ØSREØØ[9,A,Z]	ØSREØ1[9,A,Z]	ØSREØ3[9,A,Z]	ØSREØJ[9,A,Z]	ØSRSØ1[9,A,Z]	ØSRSØ3[9,A,Z]	ØSRSØJ[9,A,Z]

Open Removal of Hip Acetabular/Femoral Surface with Replacement

Removal of Acetabular/Femoral Surface		Code also as appropriate Replacement by Device Type					
		Metal	Metal on Poly	Ceramic	Ceramic on Poly	Oxidized Zirc on Poly	Synthetic Substitute
Hip, RT	ØSP[A,R]ØJZ	ØSR9Ø1[9,A,Z]	ØSR9Ø2[9,A,Z]	ØSR9Ø3[9,A,Z]	ØSR9Ø4[9,A,Z]	ØSR9Ø6[9,A,Z]	ØSR9ØJ[9,A,Z]
Hip, LT	ØSP[E,S]ØJZ	ØSRBØ1[9,A,Z]	ØSRBØ2[9,A,Z]	ØSRBØ3[9,A,Z]	ØSRBØ4[9,A,Z]	ØSRBØ6[9,A,Z]	ØSRBØJ[9,A,Z]

Open Removal of Hip Acetabular/Femoral Surface with Replacement

Removal of Acetabular/Femoral Surface		Code also as appropriate Replacement by Device Type						
		Acetabular Surface				Femoral Surface		
		Poly	Metal	Ceramic	Synthetic	Metal	Ceramic	Synthetic
Hip, RT	ØSP[A,R]ØJZ	ØSRAØØ[9,A,Z]	ØSRAØ1[9,A,Z]	ØSRAØ3[9,A,Z]	ØSRAØJ[9,A,Z]	ØSRRØ1[9,A,Z]	ØSRRØ3[9,A,Z]	ØSRRØJ[9,A,Z]
Hip, LT	ØSP[E,S]ØJZ	ØSREØØ[9,A,Z]	ØSREØ1[9,A,Z]	ØSREØ3[9,A,Z]	ØSREØJ[9,A,Z]	ØSRSØ1[9,A,Z]	ØSRSØ3[9,A,Z]	ØSRSØJ[9,A,Z]

Percutaneous Endoscopic Removal of Hip Spacer with Replacement

Removal of Spacer		Code also as appropriate Replacement by Device Type					
		Metal	Metal on Poly	Ceramic	Ceramic on Poly	Oxidized Zirc on Poly	Synthetic Substitute
Hip, RT	ØSP948Z	ØSR9Ø1[9,A,Z]	ØSR9Ø2[9,A,Z]	ØSR9Ø3[9,A,Z]	ØSR9Ø4[9,A,Z]	ØSR9Ø6[9,A,Z]	ØSR9ØJ[9,A,Z]
Hip, LT	ØSPB48Z	ØSRBØ1[9,A,Z]	ØSRBØ2[9,A,Z]	ØSRBØ3[9,A,Z]	ØSRBØ4[9,A,Z]	ØSRBØ6[9,A,Z]	ØSRBØJ[9,A,Z]

Percutaneous Endoscopic Removal of Hip Spacer with Replacement

Removal of Spacer		Code also as appropriate Replacement by Device Type						
		Acetabular Surface				Femoral Surface		
		Poly	Metal	Ceramic	Synthetic	Metal	Ceramic	Synthetic
Hip, RT	ØSP948Z	ØSRAØØ[9,A,Z]	ØSRAØ1[9,A,Z]	ØSRAØ3[9,A,Z]	ØSRAØJ[9,A,Z]	ØSRRØ1[9,A,Z]	ØSRRØ3[9,A,Z]	ØSRRØJ[9,A,Z]
Hip, LT	ØSPB48Z	ØSREØØ[9,A,Z]	ØSREØ1[9,A,Z]	ØSREØ3[9,A,Z]	ØSREØJ[9,A,Z]	ØSRSØ1[9,A,Z]	ØSRSØ3[9,A,Z]	ØSRSØJ[9,A,Z]

Percutaneous Endoscopic Removal of Hip Spacer with Liner Insertion (supplement)

Removal of Spacer		Code also as appropriate Supplement of Body Part by Site		
		Joint	Acetabular Surface	Femoral Surface
Hip, RT	ØSP948Z	ØSU9Ø9Z	ØSUAØ9Z	ØSURØ9Z
Hip, LT	ØSPB48Z	ØSUBØ9Z	ØSUEØ9Z	ØSUSØ9Z

Percutaneous Endoscopic Removal of Hip Synthetic Substitute with Replacement

Removal of Synthetic Substitute		Code also as appropriate Replacement by Device Type					
		Metal	Metal on Poly	Ceramic	Ceramic on Poly	Oxidized Zirc on Poly	Synthetic Substitute
Hip, RT	ØSP94JZ	ØSR9Ø1[9,A,Z]	ØSR9Ø2[9,A,Z]	ØSR9Ø3[9,A,Z]	ØSR9Ø4[9,A,Z]	ØSR9Ø6[9,A,Z]	ØSR9ØJ[9,A,Z]
Hip, LT	ØSPB4JZ	ØSRBØ1[9,A,Z]	ØSRBØ2[9,A,Z]	ØSRBØ3[9,A,Z]	ØSRBØ4[9,A,Z]	ØSRBØ6[9,A,Z]	ØSRBØJ[9,A,Z]

Percutaneous Endoscopic of Hip Synthetic Substitute with Replacement

Removal of Synthetic Substitute		Code also as appropriate Replacement by Device Type						
		Acetabular Surface				Femoral Surface		
		Poly	Metal	Ceramic	Synthetic	Metal	Ceramic	Synthetic
Hip, RT	ØSP94JZ	ØSRAØØ[9,A,Z]	ØSRAØ1[9,A,Z]	ØSRAØ3[9,A,Z]	ØSRAØJ[9,A,Z]	ØSRRØ1[9,A,Z]	ØSRRØ3[9,A,Z]	ØSRRØJ[9,A,Z]
Hip, LT	ØSPB4JZ	ØSREØØ[9,A,Z]	ØSREØ1[9,A,Z]	ØSREØ3[9,A,Z]	ØSREØJ[9,A,Z]	ØSRSØ1[9,A,Z]	ØSRSØ3[9,A,Z]	ØSRSØJ[9,A,Z]

Percutaneous Endoscopic Removal of Hip Synthetic Substitute with Liner Insertion (supplement)

Removal of Synthetic Substitute		Code also as appropriate Supplement of Body Part by Site		
		Joint	Acetabular Surface	Femoral Surface
Hip, RT	ØSP94JZ	ØSU9Ø9Z	ØSUAØ9Z	ØSURØ9Z
Hip, LT	ØSPB4JZ	ØSUBØ9Z	ØSUEØ9Z	ØSUSØ9Z

Percutaneous Endoscopic Removal of Hip Acetabular/Femoral Surface with Replacement

Removal of Acetabular/Femoral Surface		Code also as appropriate Replacement by Device Type					
		Metal	Metal on Poly	Ceramic	Ceramic on Poly	Oxidized Zirc on Poly	Synthetic Substitute
Hip, RT	ØSP[A,R]4JZ	ØSR9Ø1[9,A,Z]	ØSR9Ø2[9,A,Z]	ØSR9Ø3[9,A,Z]	ØSR9Ø4[9,A,Z]	ØSR9Ø6[9,A,Z]	ØSR9ØJ[9,A,Z]
Hip, LT	ØSP[E,S]4JZ	ØSRBØ1[9,A,Z]	ØSRBØ2[9,A,Z]	ØSRBØ3[9,A,Z]	ØSRBØ4[9,A,Z]	ØSRBØ6[9,A,Z]	ØSRBØJ[9,A,Z]

Percutaneous Endoscopic of Hip Acetabular/Femoral Surface with Replacement

Removal of Acetabular/Femoral Surface		Code also as appropriate Replacement by Device Type						
		Acetabular Surface				Femoral Surface		
		Poly	Metal	Ceramic	Synthetic	Metal	Ceramic	Synthetic
Hip, RT	ØSP[A,R]4JZ	ØSRAØØ[9,A,Z]	ØSRAØ1[9,A,Z]	ØSRAØ3[9,A,Z]	ØSRAØJ[9,A,Z]	ØSRRØ1[9,A,Z]	ØSRRØ3[9,A,Z]	ØSRRØJ[9,A,Z]
Hip, LT	ØSP[E,S]4JZ	ØSREØØ[9,A,Z]	ØSREØ1[9,A,Z]	ØSREØ3[9,A,Z]	ØSREØJ[9,A,Z]	ØSRSØ1[9,A,Z]	ØSRSØ3[9,A,Z]	ØSRSØJ[9,A,Z]

Percutaneous Endoscopic Removal of Hip Acetabular/Femoral Surface with Liner Insertion (supplement)

Removal of Acetabular/Femoral Surface		Code also as appropriate Supplement of Body Part by Site		
		Joint	Acetabular Surface	Femoral Surface
Hip, RT	ØSP[A,R]4JZ	ØSU9Ø9Z	ØSUAØ9Z	ØSURØ9Z
Hip, LT	ØSP[E,S]4JZ	ØSUBØ9Z	ØSUEØ9Z	ØSUSØ9Z

Knee Procedure Combinations

Removal of Knee Liner with Replacement

Removal of Liner		Code also Replacement by Device Type						
		Oxidized Zirc on Poly	Synthetic Substitute	Medial (L)/ Lateral (M) Unicondylar	Patello-femoral	Femoral Surface	Tibial Surface	Medial (L)/ Lateral (M) Meniscus
Knee, RT	ØSPCØ9Z	ØSRCØ6[9,A,Z]	ØSRCØJ[9,A,Z]	ØSRCØ[L,M][9,A,Z]	ØSRCØN[9,A,Z]	ØSRTØJ[9,A,Z]	ØSRVØJ[9,A,Z]	XRRGØ[L,M]8
Knee, LT	ØSPDØ9Z	ØSRDØ6[9,A,Z]	ØSRDØJ[9,A,Z]	ØSRDØ[L,M][9,A,Z]	ØSRDØN[9,A,Z]	ØSRUØJ[9,A,Z]	ØSRWØJ[9,A,Z]	XRRHØ[L,M]8

Removal of Knee Patellar Surface with Replacement

Removal of Patellar Surface		Code also Replacement by Device Type	
		Femoral Surface	Tibial Surface
Knee, RT	ØSPC[Ø,4]JC	ØSRTØJ[9,A,Z]	ØSRVØJ[9,A,Z]
Knee, LT	ØSPD[Ø,4]JC	ØSRUØJ[9,A,Z]	ØSRWØJ[9,A,Z]

Removal of Knee Synthetic Substitute with Replacement

Removal of Synthetic Substitute		Code also Replacement by Device Type	
		Femoral Surface	Tibial Surface
Knee, RT	ØSPC[Ø,4]JZ	ØSRTØJ[9,A,Z]	ØSRVØJ[9,A,Z]
Knee, LT	ØSPD[Ø,4]JZ	ØSRUØJ[9,A,Z]	ØSRWØJ[9,A,Z]

Removal of Knee Unicondylar Device with Replacement

Removal of Medial (L)/ Lateral (M) Unicondylar Device		Code also Replacement by Device Type	
		Femoral Surface	Tibial Surface
Knee, RT	ØSPC[Ø,4][L,M]Z	ØSRTØJ[9,A,Z]	ØSRVØJ[9,A,Z]
Knee, LT	ØSPD[Ø,4][L,M]Z	ØSRUØJ[9,A,Z]	ØSRWØJ[9,A,Z]

Removal of Knee Patellofemoral Device with Replacement

Removal of Patellofemoral Device		Code also Replacement by Device Type	
		Femoral Surface	Tibial Surface
Knee, RT	ØSPC[Ø,4]NZ	ØSRTØJ[9,A,Z]	ØSRVØJ[9,A,Z]
Knee, LT	ØSPD[Ø,4]NZ	ØSRUØJ[9,A,Z]	ØSRWØJ[9,A,Z]

Removal of Knee Femoral/Tibial Surface Device with Replacement

Removal of Femoral (T,U)/Tibial (V,W) Surface		Code also Replacement by Device Type	
		Femoral Surface	Tibial Surface
Knee, RT	ØSP[T,V][Ø,4]JZ	ØSRTØJ[9,A,Z]	ØSRVØJ[9,A,Z]
Knee, LT	ØSP[U,W][Ø,4]JZ	ØSRUØJ[9,A,Z]	ØSRWØJ[9,A,Z]

DRG 662-664 Minor Bladder Procedure

Repair of Bladder	Code also as appropriate Repair of Abdominal Wall	
	with Stoma	without Stoma
ØTQB[Ø,3,4]ZZ	ØWQFXZ2	ØWQFXZZ

DRG 665-667 Prostatectomy

Site	Resection by approach				Code also as appropriate Resection of Seminal Vesicles, Bilateral by approach	
	Open	Percutaneous Endoscopic	Via Natural or Artificial Opening	Via Natural or Artificial Opening Endoscopic	Open	Percutaneous Endoscopic
Prostate	ØVTØØZZ	ØVTØ4ZZ	ØVTØ7ZZ	ØVTØ8ZZ	ØVT3ØZZ	ØVT34ZZ

DRG 7Ø7-7Ø8 Major Male Pelvic Procedures

Site	Resection by approach				Code also as appropriate Resection of Seminal Vesicles, Bilateral by approach	
	Open	Percutaneous Endoscopic	Via Natural or Artificial Opening	Via Natural or Artificial Opening Endoscopic	Open	Percutaneous Endoscopic
Prostate	ØVTØØZZ	ØVTØ4ZZ	ØVTØ7ZZ	ØVTØ8ZZ	ØVT3ØZZ	ØVT34ZZ

DRG 734-735 Pelvic Evisceration, Radical Hysterectomy and Radical Vulvectomy

Pelvic Evisceration

Resection by Site						
Bladder	Cervix	Fallopian Tubes, Bilateral	Ovaries, Bilateral	Urethra	Uterus	Vagina
ØTTBØZZ	ØUTCØZZ	ØUT7ØZZ	ØUT2ØZZ	ØTTDØZZ	ØUT9ØZZ	ØUTGØZZ

Radical Hysterectomy

Approach	Resection by Site		
	Cervix	Uterus	Uterine Support Structure
Vaginal	ØUTC[7,8]ZZ	ØUT9[7,8]ZZ	ØUT4[7,8]ZZ
Abdominal, Endoscopic	ØUTC4ZZ	ØUT9[4,F]ZZ	ØUT44ZZ
Abdominal, Open	ØUTCØZZ	ØUT9ØZZ	ØUT4ØZZ

Radical Vulvectomy

Resection by Site	Code also as appropriate Excision of Inguinal Lymph Nodes by Approach	
Vulva	Right	Left
ØUTM[0,X]ZZ	Ø7BH[0,4]ZZ	Ø7BJ[0,4]ZZ

Non-OR procedure combinations

Note: The following table identifies procedure combinations that are considered Non-OR even though one or more procedures of the combination are considered valid DRG OR procedures

Insertion With Removal of Intraluminal Device

Code as appropriate Insertion of Intraluminal Device into Hepatobiliary Duct	Code also as appropriate Removal of Intraluminal Device by Approach and Site			
	Via Natural or Artificial Opening		External	
	Hepatobiliary Duct	Pancreatic Duct	Hepatobiliary Duct	Pancreatic Duct
ØFHB7DZ	ØFPB[7,8]DZ	ØFPD[7,8]DZ	ØFPBXDZ	ØFPDXDZ

Appendix M: Coding Exercises and Answers

Using the ICD-10-PCS tables construct the code that accurately represents the procedure performed.

Medical Surgical Section

Procedure	Code
1. Excision of malignant melanoma from skin of right ear	
2. Laparoscopy with excision of endometrial implant from left ovary	
3. Percutaneous needle core biopsy of right kidney	
4. EGD with excisional gastric biopsy	
5. Open endarterectomy of left common carotid artery	
6. Excision of basal cell carcinoma of lower lip	
7. Open excision of tail of pancreas	
8. Percutaneous biopsy of right gastrocnemius muscle	
9. Sigmoidoscopy with sigmoid polypectomy	
10. Open excision of lesion from right Achilles tendon	
11. Open resection of cecum	
12. Total excision of pituitary gland, open	
13. Explantation of left failed kidney, open	
14. Open left axillary total lymphadenectomy	
15. Laparoscopic-assisted vaginal hysterectomy	
16. Right total mastectomy, open	
17. Open resection of papillary muscle	
18. Total retropubic prostatectomy, open	
19. Laparoscopic cholecystectomy	
20. Endoscopic bilateral total maxillary sinusectomy	
21. Amputation at right elbow level	
22. Right below-knee amputation, proximal tibia/fibula	
23. Fifth ray carpometacarpal joint amputation, left hand	
24. Right leg and hip amputation through ischium	
25. DIP joint amputation of right thumb	
26. Right wrist joint amputation	
27. Trans-metatarsal amputation of foot at left big toe	
28. Mid-shaft amputation, right humerus	
29. Left fourth toe amputation, mid-proximal phalanx	
30. Right above-knee amputation, distal femur	
31. Cryotherapy of wart on left hand	
32. Percutaneous radiofrequency ablation of right vocal cord lesion	
33. Left heart catheterization with laser destruction of arrhythmogenic focus, A-V node	
34. Cautery of nosebleed	
35. Transurethral endoscopic laser ablation of prostate	
36. Percutaneous cautery of oozing varicose vein, left calf	
37. Laparoscopy with destruction of endometriosis, bilateral ovaries	
38. Laser coagulation of right retinal vessel, percutaneous	
39. Thoracoscopic pleurodesis, left side	
40. Percutaneous insertion of Greenfield IVC filter	
41. Forceps total mouth extraction, upper and lower teeth	

Procedure	Code
42. Removal of left thumbnail	
43. Extraction of right intraocular lens without replacement, percutaneous	
44. Laparoscopy with needle aspiration of ova for in vitro fertilization	
45. Nonexcisional debridement of skin ulcer, right foot	
46. Open stripping of abdominal fascia, right side	
47. Hysteroscopy with D&C, diagnostic	
48. Liposuction for medical purposes, left upper arm	
49. Removal of tattered right ear drum fragments with tweezers	
50. Microincisional phlebectomy of spider veins, right lower leg	
51. Routine Foley catheter placement	
52. Incision and drainage of external anal abscess	
53. Percutaneous drainage of ascites	
54. Laparoscopy with left ovarian cystotomy and drainage	
55. Laparotomy and drain placement for liver abscess, right lobe	
56. Right knee arthrotomy with drain placement	
57. Thoracentesis of left pleural effusion	
58. Phlebotomy of left median cubital vein for polycythemia vera	
59. Percutaneous chest tube placement for right pneumothorax	
60. Endoscopic drainage of left ethmoid sinus	
61. External ventricular CSF drainage catheter placement via burr hole	
62. Removal of foreign body, right cornea	
63. Percutaneous mechanical thrombectomy, left brachial artery	
64. Esophagogastroscopy with removal of bezoar from stomach	
65. Foreign body removal, skin of left thumb	
66. Transurethral cystoscopy with removal of bladder stone	
67. Forceps removal of foreign body in right nostril	
68. Laparoscopy with excision of old suture from mesentery	
69. Incision and removal of right lacrimal duct stone	
70. Nonincisional removal of intraluminal foreign body from vagina	
71. Right common carotid endarterectomy, open	
72. Open excision of retained sliver, subcutaneous tissue of left foot	
73. Extracorporeal shockwave lithotripsy (ESWL), bilateral ureters	
74. Endoscopic retrograde cholangiopancreatography (ERCP) with lithotripsy of common bile duct stone	
75. Thoracotomy with crushing of pericardial calcifications	
76. Transurethral cystoscopy with fragmentation of bladder calculus	
77. Hysteroscopy with intraluminal lithotripsy of left fallopian tube calcification	
78. Division of right foot tendon, percutaneous	

Procedure	Code
79. Left heart catheterization with division of bundle of HIS	
80. Open osteotomy of capitate, left hand	
81. EGD with esophagotomy of esophagogastric junction	
82. Sacral rhizotomy for pain control, percutaneous	
83. Laparotomy with exploration and adhesiolysis of right ureter	
84. Incision of scar contracture, right elbow	
85. Frenulotomy for treatment of tongue-tie syndrome	
86. Right shoulder arthroscopy with coracoacromial ligament release	
87. Mitral valvulotomy for release of fused leaflets, open approach	
88. Percutaneous left Achilles tendon release	
89. Laparoscopy with lysis of peritoneal adhesions	
90. Manual rupture of right shoulder joint adhesions under general anesthesia	
91. Open posterior tarsal tunnel release	
92. Laparoscopy with freeing of left ovary and fallopian tube	
93. Liver transplant with donor matched liver	
94. Orthotopic heart transplant using porcine heart	
95. Right lung transplant, open, using organ donor match	
96. Transplant of large intestine, organ donor match	
97. Left kidney/pancreas organ bank transplant	
98. Replantation of avulsed scalp	
99. Reattachment of severed right ear	
100. Reattachment of traumatic left gastrocnemius avulsion, open	
101. Closed replantation of three avulsed teeth, lower jaw	
102. Reattachment of severed left hand	
103. Right open palmaris longus tendon transfer	
104. Endoscopic radial to median nerve transfer	
105. Fasciocutaneous flap closure of left thigh, open	
106. Transfer left index finger to left thumb position, open	
107. Percutaneous fascia transfer to fill defect, right neck	
108. Trigeminal to facial nerve transfer, percutaneous endoscopic	
109. Endoscopic left leg flexor hallucis longus tendon transfer	
110. Right scalp advancement flap to right temple	
111. Resection right breast with TRAM flap reconstruction, open	
112. Skin transfer flap closure of complex open wound, left lower back	
113. Open fracture reduction, right tibia	
114. Laparoscopy with gastropexy for malrotation	
115. Left knee arthroscopy with reposition of anterior cruciate ligament	
116. Open transposition of ulnar nerve	
117. Closed reduction with percutaneous internal fixation of right femoral neck fracture	
118. Trans-vaginal intraluminal cervical cerclage	
119. Cervical cerclage using Shirodkar technique	
120. Thoracotomy with banding of left pulmonary artery using extraluminal device	
121. Restriction of thoracic duct with intraluminal stent, percutaneous	

Procedure	Code
122. Craniotomy with clipping of cerebral aneurysm	
123. Nonincisional, transnasal placement of restrictive stent in right lacrimal duct	
124. Catheter-based temporary restriction of blood flow in abdominal aorta for treatment of cerebral ischemia	
125. Percutaneous ligation of esophageal vein	
126. Percutaneous embolization of left internal carotid-cavernous fistula	
127. Laparoscopy with bilateral occlusion of fallopian tubes using Hulka extraluminal clips	
128. Open suture ligation of failed AV graft, left brachial artery	
129. Percutaneous embolization of vascular supply, intracranial meningioma	
130. Percutaneous embolization of right uterine artery, using coils	
131. Open occlusion of left atrial appendage, using extraluminal pressure clips	
132. Percutaneous suture exclusion of left atrial appendage, via femoral artery access	
133. ERCP with balloon dilation of common bile duct	
134. PTCA of two coronary arteries, LAD with stent placement, RCA with no stent	
135. Cystoscopy with intraluminal dilation of bladder neck stricture	
136. Open dilation of old anastomosis, left femoral artery	
137. Dilation of upper esophageal stricture, direct visualization, with Bougie sound	
138. PTA of right brachial artery stenosis	
139. Transnasal dilation and stent placement in right lacrimal duct	
140. Hysteroscopy with balloon dilation of bilateral fallopian tubes	
141. Tracheoscopy with intraluminal dilation of tracheal stenosis	
142. Cystoscopy with dilation of left ureteral stricture, with stent placement	
143. Open gastric bypass with Roux-en-Y limb to jejunum	
144. Right temporal artery to intracranial artery bypass using Gore-Tex graft, open	
145. Tracheostomy formation with tracheostomy tube placement, percutaneous	
146. PICVA (percutaneous in situ coronary venous arterialization) of single coronary artery	
147. Open left femoral-popliteal artery bypass using cadaver vein graft	
148. Shunting of intrathecal cerebrospinal fluid to peritoneal cavity using synthetic shunt	
149. Colostomy formation, open, transverse colon to abdominal wall	
150. Open urinary diversion, left ureter, using ileal conduit to skin	
151. CABG of LAD using pedicled left internal mammary artery, open off-bypass	
152. Open pleuroperitoneal shunt, right pleural cavity, using synthetic device	
153. Percutaneous placement of ventriculoperitoneal shunt for treatment of hydrocephalus	
154. End-of-life replacement of spinal neurostimulator generator, multiple array, in lower abdomen	
155. Percutaneous insertion of spinal neurostimulator lead, lumbar spinal cord	

Appendix M: Coding Exercises and Answers

Procedure	Code
156. Percutaneous replacement of broken pacemaker lead in left atrium	
157. Open placement of dual chamber pacemaker generator in chest wall	
158. Percutaneous placement of venous central line in right internal jugular, with tip in superior vena cava	
159. Open insertion of multiple channel cochlear implant, left ear	
160. Percutaneous placement of Swan-Ganz catheter in pulmonary trunk	
161. Bronchoscopy with insertion of Low Dose, Pd-103 brachytherapy seeds, right lung	
162. Open insertion of interspinous process device into lumbar vertebral joint	
163. Open placement of bone growth stimulator, left femoral shaft	
164. Cystoscopy with placement of brachytherapy seeds in prostate gland	
165. Percutaneous insertion of Greenfield IVC filter	
166. Full-thickness skin graft to right lower arm, autograft (do not code graft harvest for this exercise)	
167. Excision of necrosed left femoral head with bone bank bone graft to fill the defect, open	
168. Penetrating keratoplasty of right cornea with donor matched cornea, percutaneous approach	
169. Excision of abdominal aorta with Gore-Tex graft replacement, open	
170. Total right knee arthroplasty with insertion of total knee prosthesis	
171. Tenonectomy with graft to right ankle using cadaver graft, open	
172. Mitral valve replacement using porcine valve, open	
173. Percutaneous phacoemulsification of right eye cataract with prosthetic lens insertion	
174. Transcatheter replacement of pulmonary valve using of bovine jugular vein valve	
175. Total left hip replacement using ceramic on ceramic prosthesis, without bone cement	
176. Aortic valve annuloplasty using ring, open	
177. Laparoscopic repair of left inguinal hernia with marlex plug	
178. Autograft nerve graft to right median nerve, percutaneous endoscopic (do not code graft harvest for this exercise)	
179. Exchange of liner in femoral component of previous left hip replacement, open approach	
180. Anterior colporrhaphy with polypropylene mesh reinforcement, open approach	
181. Implantation of CorCap cardiac support device, open approach	
182. Abdominal wall herniorrhaphy, open, using synthetic mesh	
183. Tendon graft to strengthen injured left shoulder using autograft, open (do not code graft harvest for this exercise)	
184. Onlay lamellar keratoplasty of left cornea using autograft, external approach	
185. Resurfacing procedure on right femoral head, open approach	
186. Exchange of drainage tube from right hip joint	
187. Tracheostomy tube exchange	
188. Change chest tube for left pneumothorax	
189. Exchange of cerebral ventriculostomy drainage tube	

Procedure	Code
190. Foley urinary catheter exchange	
191. Open removal of lumbar sympathetic neurostimulator lead	
192. Nonincisional removal of Swan-Ganz catheter from right pulmonary artery	
193. Laparotomy with removal of pancreatic drain	
194. Extubation, endotracheal tube	
195. Nonincisional PEG tube removal	
196. Transvaginal removal of brachytherapy seeds	
197. Transvaginal removal of extraluminal cervical cerclage	
198. Incision with removal of K-wire fixation, right first metatarsal	
199. Cystoscopy with retrieval of left ureteral stent	
200. Removal of nasogastric drainage tube for decompression	
201. Removal of external fixator, left radial fracture	
202. Trimming and reanastomosis of stenosed femorofemoral synthetic bypass graft, open	
203. Open revision of right hip replacement, with readjustment of prosthesis	
204. Adjustment of position, pacemaker lead in left ventricle, percutaneous	
205. External repositioning of Foley catheter to bladder	
206. Taking out loose screw and putting larger screw in fracture repair plate, left tibia	
207. Revision of totally implantable VAD port placement in chest wall, causing patient discomfort, open	
208. Thoracotomy with exploration of right pleural cavity	
209. Diagnostic laryngoscopy	
210. Exploratory arthrotomy of left knee	
211. Colposcopy with diagnostic hysteroscopy	
212. Digital rectal exam	
213. Diagnostic arthroscopy of right shoulder	
214. Endoscopy of maxillary sinus	
215. Laparotomy with palpation of liver	
216. Transurethral diagnostic cystoscopy	
217. Colonoscopy, discontinued at sigmoid colon	
218. Percutaneous mapping of basal ganglia	
219. Heart catheterization with cardiac mapping	
220. Intraoperative whole brain mapping via craniotomy	
221. Mapping of left cerebral hemisphere, percutaneous endoscopic	
222. Intraoperative cardiac mapping during open heart surgery	
223. Hysteroscopy with cautery of post-hysterectomy oozing and evacuation of clot	
224. Open exploration and ligation of post-op arterial bleeder, left forearm	
225. Control of post-operative retroperitoneal bleeding via laparotomy	
226. Reopening of thoracotomy site with drainage and control of post-op hemopericardium	
227. Arthroscopy with drainage of hemarthrosis at previous operative site, right knee	
228. Radiocarpal fusion of left hand with internal fixation, open	
229. Posterior approach spinal fusion at L1-L3 level with BAK cage interbody fusion device, open	
230. Intercarpal fusion of right hand with bone bank bone graft, open	